PRACTICAL GUIDE TO GERIATRIC

INE

Dedication

To James R. Lawrence AO, pioneer nephrologist and outstanding physician, exceptional and inspiring teacher who understood the need for geriatric medicine.

PRACTICAL GUIDE TO GERIATRIC MEDICINE

EDITED BY
RANJIT N RATNAIKE

The McGraw-Hill Companies, Inc.

Sydney New York San Francisco Auckland
Bangkok Bogotá Caracas Hong Kong
Kuala Lumpur Lisbon London Madrid
Mexico City Milan New Delhi San Juan
Seoul Singapore Taipei Toronto

McGraw·Hill Australia

A Division of The ***McGraw·Hill*** *Companies*

National Library of Australia Cataloguing-in-Publication data:

Practical guide to geriatric medicine.

Bibliography.
Includes index.
ISBN 0 074 40801 5.
ISBN 0 074 71033 8 (pbk.).

1. Geriatrics. I. Ratnaike, Ranjit N.

618.97

Published in Australia by
McGraw-Hill Australia Pty Limited
4 Barcoo Street, Roseville NSW 2069, Australia
Acquisitions Editor: Meiling Voon
Production Editor: Sybil Kesteven
Editors: Sarah Baker and Carolyn Pike
Proofreader: Tim Learner
Indexer: Dianne Harriman
Designer (cover and interior): Jan Schmoeger
Illustrator: Alan Laver, Shelly Communications
Typeset in 9/12 pt Slimbach by Midland Typesetters
Printed on 80 gsm matt art by Best Tri Colour Printing & Packaging Co., Hong Kong

Contents

Preface

Practical Guide to Geriatric Medicine intends to meet the needs of general practitioners (community physicians), geriatricians and nurse practitioners involved in the care of older patients. The text recognises that the focus of care is shifting from the hospital setting to the community. The acute hospital is not the centre of the older person's universe.

Practical Guide to Geriatric Medicine addresses specific medical conditions especially important to the older person, as well as a variety of other issues essential for their optimal care, including elder abuse, palliative care, euthanasia, ethical dilemmas, and sexuality.

Prevention is indeed better than cure! Separate chapters on health promotion, home and family care, falls, osteoporosis and prescription of drugs are included in the text.

A frequent criticism of texts by reviewers is of repetition. Unlike reviewers, most of us do not have the luxury of reading the text from cover to cover. Rather we refer to selected chapters or sections when the need arises. Primarily for this reason the text does not always instruct the reader to refer to other chapters for information, but provides contextually appropriate information without delay. It is hoped that any repetition of material would be regarded, not as negligent editing, but as a convenience to the reader. Cognisant of the busy lives many of us lead, the text provides rapid and convenient access to up-to-date information that is clear and concise.

Unfortunately the chapter 'Coagulation disorders' which was commissioned could not be included due to the serious illness the author suffered.

Acknowledgments

A number of colleagues at The Queen Elizabeth Hospital, Woodville, South Australia were extremely generous with their time in regard to a variety of issues: Ms. Kamaleswary Arumugam, Ms. Rebecca Black, Ms. Sue Dowsett, Ms. Doan Ngo, Dr. John Peireides, Mr. Basil Popowycz and Dr. Adam Sheridan.

I am especially grateful to Dr. Phillip Henschke (also a chapter author), Dr. Adrian Cummins, Dr. Joe Frasca, Dr. Sugit Hattotuwa, Dr. Catherine Hurworth, Dr. John Norman, Dr. Margaret Davy, Mr. David Walsh, Dr. Sunil Chandy and Dr. D.J. Christopher (also a chapter author) who reviewed chapters or sections of chapters.

Mr. Austin Milton, Senior Medical Scientist, was tireless in helping me to submit to the publishers as perfect a text as possible. His commendable vigilance and unfailing good humour made my task as editor easier and enjoyable. Despite this being the third text he has assisted me with, his enthusiasm, contrary to mine, is unabated. I am very indebted to him.

Mrs. Lina Wharton provided excellent secretarial assistance and Mrs. Ellie Giardini helped considerably during the initial stages of the project.

I am grateful for the assistance and wise counsel Ms. Meiling Voon and Ms. Sybil Kesteven from McGraw-Hill provided throughout the project.

Editors under stress can be quite cantankerous, and I am very conscious of the support and forebearance of my wife, Stephanie and our children, Alinta and Christen.

Editor

Ranjit N. Ratnaike MD, FRACP, FAFPHM
Associate Professor of Medicine
Head, Geriatric Unit
Department of Medicine
The Queen Elizabeth Hospital
The University of Adelaide
Woodville, SA 5011
Australia

Contributors

Michal Ahern MBBS(NSW), FRCP(UK), FRACP, MD
Associate Professor of Medicine
Rheumatology Unit
School of Medicine
Flinders University
GPO Box 2001
Adelaide, SA 5001
Australia

Samir Array MD
Clinical Associate Professor
Department of Community Health and
Family Medicine
College of Medicine
University of Florida
PO Box 103462
Gainesville, Florida 32610-3462
USA

Ben Barnett MD
Associate Professor of Medicine
Infectious Disease
Medical School
University of Texas-Houston Health Science Center
6431 Fannin
Houston, Texas 77030-1503
USA

Eteri Bibileishvili MD
Stroke Research Fellow
Department of Neurology
Stroke Research Centre
School of Medicine
Wake Forest University
Medical Centre Boulevard
Winston-Salem, North Carolina 27157-1068
USA

Lesley Bowker BM MRCP (UK)
Senior Lecturer in Geriatric Medicine
Royal Perth Hospital
GPO Box 2213
Perth, WA 6847
Australia

Andrew Braganza MS (Ophthalmology)
Reader
Department of Ophthalmology
Christian Medical College Hospital
Vellore, Tamil Nadu 632 004
India

Paula Brindley
Regional Palliative Care Program
Grey Nuns Community Hospital and Health Centre
1100 Youville Drive West
Edmonton, Alberta T6L 5X8
Canada

Margaret Bulling MBBS, FRACP
Senior Consultant Physician
Department of Rehabilitation and Aged Care
Repatriation General Hospital
Daws Road
Daw Park, SA 5041
Australia

Simon Burnet MBBS
Specialist Registrar in Rheumatology
Rheumatology Research Unit
Addenbrooke's Hospital
Box 194
Hills Road
Cambridge, CB2 2QQ
United Kingdom

Wade Bushman MD, PhD
Assistant Professor
Department of Medical Urology
School of Medicine
Northwestern University
303 E. Chicago Ave
Tarry Building 11.715
Chicago, Illinois 60611-3008
USA

Julie Byles BMed, PhD
Senior Lecturer in Clinical Epidemiology
Centre for Clinical Epidemiology and Biostatistics
Royal Newcastle Hospital
Level 3, Room 361
David Madison Building
Newcastle, NSW 2300
Australia

Alistair Cameron-Strange MBChB, FRCS (Ed), FRACS
Consultant Urologist
Prince of Wales Private Hospital
Barker Street
Randwick, NSW 2031
Australia

Karen E. Charlton MSc MPhil (Epidemiology) PGDipDiet SRD
Associate Professor
Head, Nutrition & Dietetics Unit
Faculty of Medicine
University of Cape Town
Observatory 7925
South Africa

Vera Chiamvimonvat MD, FRCP(C)
Cardiologist
Sunnbrook & Women's College
Health Science Centre
76 Grenville Street
Toronto, Ontario M5S 1B2
Canada

Harvey Max Chochinov MD, PhD, FRCP(C)
Department of Psychiatry
University of Manitoba
PsycHealth Centre
771 Bannatyne Avenue
Winnipeg, Manitoba R3E 3N4
Canada

Devasahayam J Christopher BSC, MBBS, DTCD, Dip NB (Resp Med), FCCP
Associate Professor and Head
Department of Pulmonary Medicine
The Christian Medical College & Hospital
Vellore, Tamil Nadu 632 004
India

Penelope Coates MBBS, FRACP
Research Fellow
Division of Clinical Biochemistry,
Institute of Medical and Veterinary Science
Frome Road
Adelaide, SA 5000
Australia

E. Terry Coyne BSc, MSc, PhD (U. Pitts)
Senior Lecturer
Nutrition Program
School of Population Health
Medical School
University of Queensland
Herston Road
Herston, Qld 4029
Australia

Ian Darnton-Hill MBBS, MPH, MSc(Med.), DipNutrDiet, FAFPHM
Vice-President for Helen Keller International Programs
Helen Keller Worldwide
90 West Street
New York, NY 10006
USA

Shelley de la Vega MD
Associate Clinical Professor in Gerontology
Department of Internal Medicine
University of the Philippines
Philippine General Hospital & Medical Centre
Manila
Philippines

Rohan S. Dhillon MBBS, FRANZCP, M.Clin. Sc
Clinical Director
West Adelaide Team
Crammond Clinic
The Queen Elizabeth Hospital
Woodville, SA 5011
Australia

Bette Emery BSW
Acute Palliative Care Unit
Grey Nuns Community Hospital and Health Centre
1100 Youville Drive West
Edmonton, Alberta T6L 5X8
Canada

Ronald L Ettinger BDS, MDS, DDSc, FACD, FICD, FASGD
Professor
Department of Prosthodontics and
Dows Institute for Dental Research
University of Iowa
418 Dental Science Building North
Iowa City, Iowa 52242-1010
USA

Paul Finucane FRCPI, FRACP
Head of Geriatric Medicine
Repatriation General Hospital
Daws Road
Daw Park, SA 5041
Australia

William M. H. Goh MBBS, FRANZCP
Consultant Psychiatrist
Crammond Clinic
The Queen Elizabeth Hospital
Woodville, SA 5011
Australia

Fiona Goldblatt MBBS (Hons), FRACP
Rheumatologist
Department of Immunology, Allergy and Arthritis
Flinders Medical Centre
Flinders Drive
Bedford Park, SA 5042
Australia

Ehud Goldhammer MD
Deputy Director
Department of Cardiology
Director
Sport Medicine and Cardiac Rehabilitation Center
Bnei-Zion Medical Center
Haifa 31048
Israel
Associate Professor
Faculty of Medicine
Technion—Israel Institute of Technology
Haifa 31048
Israel

Sarah Hatherly BAppSc (Sp. Path)
Senior Speech Pathologist
Department of Speech Pathology
The Queen Elizabeth Hospital
Woodville, SA 5011
Australia

Brian Hazleman MA, MB, FRCP
Consultant Rheumatologist
Director
Rheumatology Research Unit
Addenbrooke's Hospital
Hills Road
Cambridge, CB2 2QQ
United Kingdom

Jane Hecker MBBS FRACP
Senior Consultant Physician
Director
Memory Disorders Study Unit
Division of Medicine
Repatriation General Hospital
Daws Road
Daw Park, SA 5041
Australia

Philip Henschke MBBS(Adel), FRACP, FRCP(C), FAFRM
Senior Director
Department of Rehabilitation and Aged Care
Repatriation General Hospital
Daws Road
Daw Park, SA 5041
Australia

Keith Hill PhD
Physiotherapist
Senior Research Fellow
Falls and Balance Clinic
National Ageing Research Institute
PO Box 31
Parkville, VIC 3052
Australia

Robin Holliday FRS
12 Roma Court
West Pennant Hills, NSW 2125
Australia

Mary Ip MD, FRCP (Edin), FHKCP, FHKAM (Med)
Personal Chair Professor
Division of Respiratory and Critical Care Medicine
Department of Medicine
University of Hong Kong
Professorial Block
Queen Mary Hospital
Pok Ful Lam
Hong Kong

George T. John MD, DM, MNAMS, FRACP (Neph)
Associate Professor
Department of Nephrology
Christian Medical College and Hospital
Vellore, Tamil Nadu 632004
India

Fran Kaiser MD
Senior Regional Medical Director
Merck and Co Inc
222 W Las Colinas Blvd–Suite 1465
Irving, Texas 75039-5429
USA

Alexander Kalache MD, PhD
Chief
Aging and Health Program
World Health Organization
CH—1211
Geneva 27
Switzerland

Richard Kimber FRACP
Visiting Medical Specialist
Department of Gastroenterology
The Queen Elizabeth Hospital
Woodville, SA 5011
Australia

Susan Kurrle MBBS DipGerMed
Director and Senior Staff Specialist
Rehabilitation and Aged Care Service
Geriatric Medicine
Hornsby Ku-ring-gai Hospital
Palmerston Road
Hornsby, NSW 2077
Australia

Wah Kit Lam MD, FRCP (Lond, Edin and Glas), FRACP, FHKAM (Med), FHKCP
Chair Professor of Respiratory Medicine
Division of Respiratory and Critical Care Medicine
Department of Medicine
University of Hong Kong
Professorial Block
Queen Mary Hospital
Pok Ful Lam
Hong Kong

Per-Anders Larsson MD, PhD
Head
Department of Surgery
Ængelholm Hospital
Hindervägen 2
252 86 Helsingborg 042/92 762
Sweden

David Lowenthal MD, PhD
Professor of Medicine, Pharmacology, and Exercise Science
GRECC Director
University of Florida
VA Medical Center
GRECC—182
1601 SW Archer Road
Gainesville, Florida 32608-1197
USA

Laura Mazzenga RN, MSN, ANP
Urology Advanced Practitioner
Centre for Urology
Northwestern Memorial Hospital
251 East Huron St
Chicago, Illinois 60611
USA

John R Meuleman, MD
GRECC Clinical Director
Associate Professor of Medicine
University of Florida
VA Medical Center
GRECC—182
1601 SW Archer Road
Gainesville, Florida 32608-6142
USA

Lu J. Mykyta MBBS, MRCP (UK), FRACP, FACRM, FFRM (RACP)
Clinical Director/Executive Officer
Consultant in Geriatric Medicine
Western Domiciliary Care & Rehabilitation Services
21A Belmore Terrace
Woodville Park, SA 5011
Australia

Peter Nash MBBS (Hons), FRACP
Rheumatologist
Sunshine Coast Rheumatology Research Unit
Cotton Tree, Qld 4558
Australia

Daphne Nahmiash PhD
Professor in Social Gerontology
Chairperson
Community Committee on Elder Abuse
Montreal
Canada

Jonathan Newbury MBBS, DA, DRCOG, FRACGP
Lecturer
Department of General Practice
Royal Adelaide Hospital
North Terrace
Adelaide, SA 5000
Australia

Katina Overell MBBS
RACGP Registrar
Royal Adelaide Hospital
North Terrace
Adelaide, SA 5000
Australia

Chung Owyang MD
Division of Gastroenterology
Department of Internal Medicine
University of Michigan
3912 Taubman Centre
Ann Arbor, MI 48109
USA

Sheel M. Pandya MPH
Technical Officer
Ageing and Health Programme
World Health Organization
20 Avenue Appia,
1211 Geneva 27
Switzerland

Kelly Papanaoum MBBS, FRACP, FRCPA
Specialist Physician
Infectious Diseases Unit
Internal Medicine
Institute of Medical and Veterinary Science
Level 1
Royal Adelaide Hospital
North Terrace
Adelaide, SA 5000
Australia

A Peter Passmore BSC, MD, FRCP (Lond, Glasg)
Senior Lecturer in Geriatric Medicine
Department of Health Care for the Elderly
Belfast City Hospital
Lisburn Road
Belfast, BT9 7AB
Northern Ireland

Jose Pereira MBChB, DA(SA), CCFP
Associate Professor
Departments of Oncology/Family Medicine
Faculty of Medicine
University of Calgary
Medical Director
Palliative Care Office
Foothills Medical Centre
South Tower
1403–29 Street NW
Calgary, Alberta T2N 2T9
Canada

Kevin Pile MB, ChB, MD, FRACP
Senior Lecturer in Medicine
University of Adelaide
Director
Rheumatology Unit
The Queen Elizabeth Hospital
Woodville, SA 5011
Australia

Gurcharan Rai MD, MSc, FRCP
Consultant Physician
Care of the Elderly
Whittington Hospital
Highgate Hill, N19 5NF
United Kingdom

Ranjit N. Ratnaike MD, FRACP, FAFPHM
Associate Professor of Medicine
Head, Geriatric Unit
Department of Medicine
The Queen Elizabeth Hospital
The University of Adelaide
Woodville, SA 5011
Australia

Joel Rich MD
Fellow in Geriatric Medicine
VA Medical Center
GRECC—182
1601 SW Archer Road
Gainesville, Florida 32608-6142
USA

Ian Roberts-Thomson MD, FRACP
Senior Director
Department of Gastroenterology
The Queen Elizabeth Hospital
Woodville, SA 5011
Australia

Bernard A. Roos MD
Professor of Medicine
School of Medicine
University of Miami
VA Medical Centre
(11GRC)
1201 NW 16 ST
Miami, Florida 33125
USA

Richard E. Ruffin BSc(Hons), MD, FRACP, MBBS (Hons), PhD, FCCP
Professor of Medicine
Department of Medicine
University of Adelaide
The Queen Elizabeth Hospital
Woodville, SA 5011
Australia

Jorge Ruiz MD
Assistant Professor of Clinical Medicine
Division of Gerontology and Geriatric Medicine
School of Medicine
University of Miami
Coral Gables, Florida 33124
USA

Hussain Saba MD, PhD
Professor of Medicine
Hematologic Malignancies/Senior Adult Oncology
H Lee Moffit Cancer Center and Research Institute
Suite 3157
12092 Magnolia Drive
Tampa, Florida 33612-9497
USA

L Fernando Samos MD
Assistant Professor of Medicine
Division of Gerontology and Geriatric Medicine
Department of Medicine
University of Miami
Medical Director
Nursing Home Care Unit
VA Medical Center
(11GRC)
1201 NW 16 ST
Miami, Florida 33125
USA

Ingrid C. Schloss BScMed(Hons)Diet SRD
Lecturer, Nutrition and Dietetics Unit
Department of Medicine
Faculty of Health Sciences
University of Cape Town
Observatory 7925
South Africa

Leonard Schwartz LLB, LLM, MD
Department of Psychiatry
University of Manitoba
c/o PZ438 PsycHealth Centre
771 Bannatyne Avenue
Winnipeg, Manitoba R3E 3N4
Canada

Jennifer Schwarz FRACP
Senior Consultant Physician
Department of Geriatric Medicine
Melbourne Extended Care and Rehabilitation Service
Poplar Road
Parkville, VIC 3052
Australia

Jane Sims PhD
Senior Lecturer
Department of General Practice and Public Health
School of Medicine
University of Melbourne
200 Berkeley Street
Carlton, VIC 3053
Australia

Claire Spice MB MRCP (UK)
Specialist Registrar
Geriatric Medicine
Royal Hampshire County Hospital
Romsey Road
Winchester, Hants SO22 5DG
United Kingdom

Brian Stein MBBS, FRACP
Medical Oncologist
Ashford Cancer Centre
15 Alexander Ave
Ashford, SA 5035
Australia

Kevin Stewart BM, FRCP
Consultant Physician
Royal Hampshire County Hospital
Romsey Road
Winchester, Hants SO22 5DG
United Kingdom

Christopher R. Strakosch FRACP
Associate Professor
University Endocrine Unit
Greenslopes Private Hospital
Newdegate Street
Greenslopes, Qld 4120
Australia

Nicholas P Strong FRCS
Department of Ophthalmology
Royal Victoria Infirmary
Queen Victoria Road
Newcastle-Upon-Tyne, NE1 4LP
United Kingdom

Gabriel Sukumar MBBS, MS
Department of Surgery
Christian Medical College Hospital
Vellore, Tamil Nadu 632 004
India

Wei Ming Sun MD, PhD
Assistant Professor of Medicine
Director
Gastrointestinal Motility Laboratory
Department of Internal Medicine
University of Michigan
3912 Taubman Centre
Ann Arbor, MI 48109
USA

Ravi Thomas MD (Ophthalmology)
Head
Department of Ophthalmology
Schell Eye Hospital
Christian Medical College Hospital
Vellore, Tamil Nadu 632 004
India

James F. Toole MD
Director
Stroke Research Centre
Bowman Gray School of Medicine
Wake Forest University
Winston-Salem, North Carolina 27157—1068
USA

Mark Wahlqvist AO, MDBS, MD, FRACP, FAFPHM
Professor of Medicine
Associate Dean and Director
International Health and Development Unit
Faculty of Medicine
Monash University
Building 64
Clayton, VIC 3800
Australia

Judith A Whitworth DSc MD PhD BS (Melb) FRACP
Director
John Curtin School of Medical Research
Australian National University
PO Box 334
Canberra, ACT 2600
Australia

Nicholas Wickham MA, MRCP, FRCPath. FRCPA, FRACP
Director of Haematology
North QLD Oncology Services
Townsville General Hospital
PO Box 670
Townsville, QLD 4810
Australia

Gary Wittert MB, BCH, MD, FRACP
Associate Professor of Medicine
Senior Consultant
Royal Adelaide Hospital
North Terrace
Adelaide, SA 5000
Australia

Michael Woodward MBBS, FRACP
Director, Aged Care Services
Austin and Repatriation Medical Centre
Banksia Street
Heidelberg West, VIC 3081
Australia

Peter-John Wormald MD, FCS(SA), FRCS (Ed)
Professor and Head of Otolaryngology Head and Neck Surgery
University of Adelaide and Flinders University
The Queen Elizabeth Hospital
Woodville, SA 5011
Australia

Part 1

The ageing patient

Chapter 1

Mechanisms of ageing

ROBIN HOLLIDAY

Introduction

It is widely believed that ageing is a major unsolved problem in biology. This is no longer true, because a broad view, which encompasses a considerable proportion of the whole of biological knowledge, makes it clear why ageing exists in mammals and many other animals. There are three basic questions. Why do we age? Why do we live as long as we do? And why do different mammalian species have very different maximum lifespans? In answering these questions, a great deal is revealed about the mechanisms which underpin eventual senescence and death. Almost all the material in the following discussion will be found in my book *Understanding Ageing*,[1] which is fully referenced; other recent reviews are also available.[2]

Early evolutionary origins of ageing

The ageing of somatic cells must have occurred quite early in the evolution of multicellular animals. Initially, primitive animals probably had considerable powers of regeneration and renewal, as do the coelenterates and flatworms today. Such organisms may be potentially immortal, although in natural environments their lives would be ended by one of many environmental hazards. As more complex animals evolved, the distinction between the germ line and the soma, or body, becomes much more clear cut, and in particular organisms evolved where all the cells of the body are post-mitotic, except the germ line cells. This is the case in nematodes and many insects. When kept under good environmental conditions, such animals clearly have a finite lifespan. This can be attributed to the fact that non-dividing cells, active in metabolism, cannot be expected to survive indefinitely.

At first sight, it seems that ageing is non-adaptive, since an organism that can survive and reproduce indefinitely is fitter in Darwinian terms than one which reproduces for a given period of time and then dies. Why then did ageing evolve in the first place? The answer to this question, oddly enough, lies in Darwin's realisation that organisms normally produce far more offspring than can possibly survive and reproduce themselves. The environment is hostile, and individuals are competing for limited resources. This competition results in the natural selection of the fittest. In these circumstances the probability of an organism surviving and reproducing for a long period became very small, so potential immortality confers very little, if any, adaptive advantage. In other words, such organisms are not necessarily the fittest because resources are used to maintain the soma for a long period of time. It is a better strategy for the survival of an organism's lineage to invest resources into growth to adulthood and reproduction, rather than in long-term maintenance of the soma. Thus, the organism that evolves a soma with a limited survival time is at an advantage over one that attempts to maintain the soma indefinitely. This disposable soma theory neatly explains the early origins of ageing in animals.[3]

Subsequently, as evolution proceeded, there arose many variations in the pattern of ageing. Many adult vertebrates grow continuously, and these tend to have very long lifespans. Although the signs of senescence may be less obvious than in species that have constant adult body size, their survival for a century or so is still a minute fraction of evolutionary time. Lifespan variability is seen particularly in fish, where small species may survive for a year, and very large ones for several decades.[4]

Mammals and birds clearly evolved from cold-blooded vertebrates which have finite lifespan, so in a sense they merely inherited the lifestyle strategy that includes senescence and ageing. The next section briefly reviews some features of the mammalian body plan which make ageing inevitable.

The evolved design of mammals

A vast amount of information is available about the cells, tissues and organs of mammals. Much of this comes from the biomedical investigations of the human body encompassing many disciplines. These show that many organ systems have very limited capacity for regeneration and renewal, and it is these features of our anatomy which make senescence and ageing inevitable. The neurons of the brain are post-mitotic and very active in metabolism. Although DNA can be repaired and proteins turned over, cells that are lost cannot be replaced. There are many reasons why one individual cell cannot survive indefinitely. Some DNA lesions are not repaired, and some altered or abnormal proteins cannot be degraded by proteases and therefore accumulate. The brain is very definitely a non-renewable structure. The same applies to the retina (an extension of the brain). The rods and cones continually synthesise photoreceptors, and the oldest are removed. This process does not achieve a steady state and remnants of partially degraded photoreceptor elements accumulate in the cells themselves, or in the underlying epithelial layer. Eventually the degenerative process of retinopathy occurs. The crystallin proteins of the lens of the eye are laid down at an early stage and cannot be replaced. Lens transparency depends on their molecular homogeneity. Unfortunately, proteins are subject to many chemical changes, including the processes of oxidation, glycation, racemisation of amino acids, deamidation, and so on. Since these cannot be prevented or reversed, the molecules gradually lose their initial properties and cataracts may occur.

Collagen and elastin are also very long-lived proteins which are subject to chemical change. It is well established that collagen becomes progressively cross-linked with age, thereby losing its initial elasticity. The heart is a highly efficient pump but, like the brain, it has very limited capacity for repair or renewal. The muscle cells are post-mitotic and, unlike most skeletal muscle, they cannot be replaced by the division of myoblasts. The anatomy of the major blood vessels is also incompatible with efficient repair. The cross-linking of elastin and collagen results in hardening of arteries, and the inner wall is subject to damage, including the build-up of atherosclerotic plaques. The basic anatomical problem is that there is only one vascular system and it cannot be shut down for repair. It is in fact very difficult to repair a machine while it is operating, and the same is true of the vascular system. A potentially immortal organism would have to have two vascular systems, one of which could be shut down and repaired, while the other could be kept operating. We did not evolve in that way.

Teeth provide an instructive example of the way components of the body have evolved 'to last a lifetime'. Clearly the shape and size of adult teeth are genetically determined, but they are also subject to wear and tear, as well as decay. This is one of many examples that demonstrate the artificiality of the distinction which is often made between 'wear and tear' theories of ageing (or the stochastic accumulation of various defects) and the 'program' theories. Both, in fact, are interrelated and important. Some herbivores that continually crop plants have incisors which keep growing at the base, which is clearly a secondary adaptation to produce 'immortal' teeth, but many other herbivores do not have this ability, and it is well known that an estimate of a horse's age can be made by examination of the wear on its teeth.

Maintenance of the organism

Although the evolved design of many body components is incompatible with indefinite survival, this does not mean that maintenance mechanisms are unsuccessful. The life history of a mammalian organism comprises development and growth to the adult, a fairly long period of reproduction, followed by loss of fertility, senescence and death. Maintenance of cell, tissue and organ function is essential during development and reproduction. The total resources available to a mammalian organism are allocated to three major functions: first, ongoing metabolism; second, all aspects of reproduction; and third, a set of maintenance mechanisms. These three functions consume all available metabolic energy and, although there may be some overlap between them, it is possible to itemise their main features, as shown in Figure 1.1.

The major mechanisms of maintenance are discussed below.

Wound-healing

Damage to skin and muscle can be effectively repaired, and broken bones can rejoin. Loss of blood is prevented by clotting, and the smaller arteries and veins can be replaced. Nevertheless, mammals do not have strong regenerative capacity. Severed limbs or digits are not replaced, and when major nerves are cut, they cannot be rejoined. In this respect, some lower vertebrates

Normal functions
Biochemical synthesis
Metabolism
Respiration
Cell turnover
Movement
Feeding and digestion
Excretion

Reproduction
Gonads, gametes and sex
Development
Gestation
Suckling
Care of offspring
Growth to adult

Maintenance
Wound healing
Immunity
Protein turnover
Defence against free radicals
Proofreading
DNA repair
Detoxification
Epigenetic stability
Apoptosis
Fat storage
Homeostasis

Figure 1.1 The allocation of all available energy resources in mammals

have greater regenerative capacity, since lost limbs can be regrown.

Immunity

All organisms are subject to attack by pathogens and parasites, and a complex immune system has evolved to protect the organism. Immunology is, of course, a science in its own right, and leaving aside the 'immunologic' theory of ageing,[5] the immune response is not thought to have any relationship to the study of longevity or ageing. Nevertheless, it is a vital maintenance mechanism and without it an organism does not survive very long.

DNA repair

Although DNA is a stable molecule, it is continually subject to intrinsic and extrinsic damage. It is highly likely that oxygen free radicals are an important source of damage.[6] There is a battery of repair enzymes which continually monitor DNA for abnormalities in structure, excise or remove such damage, and then fill in any gaps by repair synthesis and rejoining. One of the most common defects in DNA is the loss of purine residues. Indeed, it has been estimated that up to 10 000 of these lesions occur in each cell per day.[7] All this damage is effectively repaired. There may be lesions which are not repaired, however, perhaps because they are less common, and the necessary enzymes have never evolved to deal with them.[8] Also, there may be adjacent lesions on both strands of a DNA molecule which are difficult to repair, and which can lead to chromosome breaks.

Accuracy in the synthesis of macromolecules

DNA repair overlaps with mechanisms to ensure that DNA is synthesised with extreme accuracy. The insertion of an incorrect base by the replicating polymerase is usually corrected by an editing excision/replacement mechanism. However, if this fails, there is a backup mismatch repair system. The removal of errors in DNA synthesis depends on many enzymes and accessory proteins. RNA and proteins are made with less accuracy; nevertheless, it would be wasteful, as well as harmful, to synthesise defective molecules, so it is not surprising that proofreading mechanisms exist to detect and remove errors. All these proofreading mechanisms consume energy. The question of the optimum accuracy of synthesis of macromolecules is an interesting one. In general, it seems to be the case that rapid synthesis results in more errors and slower synthesis allows time for more efficient editing. There must be optimum or some balance between the two which may well not be the same for all mammalian species (see below).

Protein turnover

As has been mentioned, protein molecules are subject to many post-synthetic modifications. Some modifications are, of course, a normal part of the maturation of proteins and play essential roles in their function. But there are many others which are abnormal, with potentially deleterious effects on the cell. These molecules are usually recognised and removed by proteases and the proteosome. This is a very important ongoing process, essential for the normal function of cells. Amino acids that cannot be reutilised are broken down and the nitrogen excreted in the form of urea. The removal of abnormal proteins is not completely successful, particularly if the protein is inaccessible or is part of a non-replaceable structure (such as the walls of major arteries). Also, altered proteins may form high molecular weight aggregates which are resistant to proteolytic digestion such as AGEs (advanced glycation end products) or the amyloid plaques in Alzheimer's disease. The gradual accumulation of these high molecular weight protein or peptide aggregates is an important part of the ageing process.

Detoxification

Animals have complex diets, and toxic chemicals are a common component. In particular, plants often defend themselves against animals by synthesising such compounds. In response, mammals have evolved a large set of detoxifying enzymes, collectively known as the P450 cytochromes. These comprise a very complex family of enzymes located in the liver, but also in other tissues, that can degrade a very wide range of chemicals. Nowadays, these include many artificial chemicals which would never have been encountered during evolution. Thus, the detoxification system has an inbuilt 'overkill' capacity to deal with any new chemicals which may arise in the diet or environment.

Defences against free radicals

Oxygen free radicals are continually generated by respiration, and some other metabolic processes. Although very short-lived, they are highly reactive and can damage DNA, proteins and membranes. Organisms have developed major defences against free radical attack. There are enzymes that break down free radicals, such as superoxide dismutase, catalase, glutathione peroxidase and reductase. There are also metabolites which react with free radicals, acting as free radical 'sinks', such as carotenoids or other anti-oxidants. It is likely that the evolution of the respiratory organelle, the mitochondrion, protects the chromosomal DNA in the nucleus from free radical attack. It is well known that the small mitochondria DNA genome mutates at a much higher rate than chromosomal DNA.

Epigenetic controls

Differentiated cells stably maintain their particular biochemical and morphological characteristics. This depends on the activities of genes responsible for the cells' specialised functions, together with the inactivity of all the genes needed for all other specialised cells. These controls of gene activity are generally referred to as epigenetic, and they are superimposed on the information in DNA, which is present in all cells. Many believe that epigenetic controls are entirely due to proteins which bind to specific DNA sequences, but there are now many indications that chemical modification of DNA is an essential component. The major modified base in mammals is 5-methylcytosine, and it is known that the pattern of this methylation is inherited through mitotic division, and therefore stably maintained in those specialised cells that are capable of division, as well as in post-mitotic cells. Obviously, it is extremely important to maintain epigenetic controls, because if normal regulation is lost, then a cell can adopt an abnormal phenotype, and become, for example, a neoplastic cell. This can occur through mutation, but epigenetic defects are also likely to be involved.[9]

Apoptosis

The suicide mechanism known as apoptosis is triggered in a variety of contexts. It removes unwanted cells during development, or in the immune system, but it also comes into play when damaged or abnormal cells arise. Otherwise such cells would have harmful effects on the organism. Although it has been suggested that ageing and apoptosis may be linked, the relationship is not at all simple. Apoptosis is, at least in part, a maintenance process to prevent deleterious changes. If apoptosis does not come into play, for whatever reason, then an abnormal cell will survive, and this may contribute to senescence and ageing.

Homeostatic mechanisms

These comprise a large set of physiological or regulatory processes which maintain cells, tissues and organs in a normal functional state. The most important homeostatic mechanism in mammals and birds is the control of body temperature. This produces a much more uniform internal environment, with less dependence on the external one. Therefore, mammals and birds can colonise a wider range of environments than cold-blooded vertebrates. It also allows many biochemical processes to be optimised, with the activity of many proteins adapted to body temperature. Many other homeostatic mechanisms depend on hormones or growth factors, which ensure that potential variables (such as blood-sugar levels) are controlled. Too many examples exist to review here, but it is worth mentioning that a stress response, such as the heat shock response, can be regarded as a cellular homeostatic maintenance mechanism, which protects cells from an even greater rise in temperature.

Fat storage

In natural environments it is common for the availability of food to vary considerably. Thus, periods of glut may alternate with periods of scarcity. To ensure survival in the absence of food, mammals have evolved an efficient energy storage mechanism which can tide them over periods in a harsh environment. The laying down and reutilisation of fat can therefore be regarded as a maintenance mechanism.

There are several features of these eleven maintenance mechanisms, discussed above, which should be emphasised. First, the study of all these processes comprises a major part of all biological research. Since, ultimately, ageing and death is the result of failure of maintenance, it is not unreasonable to propose that all this research is in one way or another related to the study of ageing itself. Second, it is fashionable to invoke specific 'gerontogenes' which in some way control longevity and ageing, but there are innumerable genes that specify the components of all maintenance mechanisms. All of these relate in one way or another to the efficiency and also to the eventual failure of maintenance. We know of many examples of single gene mutations which have multiple effects on the phenotype, and some of these clearly relate to ageing. Third, the various theories of ageing that have been proposed usually relate quite closely to failure of maintenance. Thus, the oxygen free radical theory of ageing is directly related to the failure to nullify their dangerous effects. This in turn overlaps with the somatic mutation theory, which is clearly related to the failure of DNA repair. The protein error theory proposes that abnormal proteins can cause escalating damage by reducing the accuracy of synthesis. Clearly this is related to the failure to remove abnormal molecules by proteolysis. This failure also results in the accumulation of abnormal protein molecules, which comprises another theory of ageing. The immunologic theory of ageing suggests that the immune system eventually loses its ability to distinguish self from non-self antigens, and therefore inflicts pathological damage on cells and tissues. The dysdifferentiation theory of ageing proposes that ectopic protein synthesis (i.e. the synthesis of a specialised protein in an inappropriate cell) is an important feature of senescence. This is related to the loss of epigenetic controls. It is very likely that there is some truth in all these theories of ageing, because ageing is multicausal.[10]

Finally, new information about the importance and complexity of maintenance is continually being obtained, and a recent example is the discovery of a peptide antibiotic in human skin.[11] Clearly this is an important defence mechanism against bacterial infection, which is rather distinct from the more familiar immune responses to infection.

Reproduction, maintenance and longevity

The 'disposable soma' theory of the evolution of ageing and longevity predicts that there should be some trade-off between resources invested in rapid growth and reproduction, and resources invested in maintenance of the soma.[12] The balance between reproduction and maintenance depends on the level of environmental hazard. In a high-risk environment, where annual mortality is very high, then it would be expected that development and reproduction would be rapid, fewer resources would be devoted to maintenance, and therefore a shorter lifespan would be seen. In a low-risk environment, the annual mortality is much less, and we would expect the evolution of slow-breeding long-lived species. In the evolution of mammals, there have been evolutionary trends which increase reproduction and reduce longevity. The carnivores provide one example, because the highly specialised stoats and weasels need a continual supply of food (i.e. they live in a high-risk environment), produce large litters which mature rapidly, and have a short lifespan in captivity. The other trend is an increase in longevity, exemplified by the primates. Small monkeys reproduce rapidly and have short lifespans; larger monkeys, small apes, the great apes and man have progressively longer lifespans. This is associated with fewer offspring and a much lower annual mortality. If lower mortality is regarded as a 'successful' adaptation to the environment, then it is also clearly associated with natural selection for longer lifespans.

The foregoing use of the terms 'lifespan' and 'longevity' refers to the documented length of life of mammalian species kept in captivity—that is, the protected environment of a zoo, or a laboratory cage. There is some relationship of this measured lifespan with the likely survival of that species in a natural environment, which is usually hard to determine. However, if it is assumed that the population size is constant, it is possible to calculate the average expectation of life at birth, provided the various reproductive parameters are known. These are the gestation period, the litter size, the time to develop to a fertile adult, and the interlitter interval. For early human hunter-gatherers, and assuming a constant population size, the expectation of life at birth is only about 16 years, and for females who reach reproductive age, it is about 28 years.[13]

The best available reproductive and lifespan-in-captivity data for 49 mammalian species demonstrates a clear inverse relationship between maximum lifespan and reproductive potential.[14] The fecundity/lifespan ratio is highest in small rodents and rabbits, then decreases through small carnivores, small primates, large carnivores, larger herbivores, pachyderms, the great apes and man. Many attempts have been made over the years to relate maximum lifespan to metabolic rate, weight and brain size, or any combination of these, in mammalian species. It is often found that bats (Chiroptera) with a high metabolic rate provide an exception to any general rule. It is striking that bats have long lifespans and low rates of reproduction, as expected from their low-risk lifestyle. The analysis of reproductive potential and maximum lifespan strongly confirm a prediction of the disposable soma theory.

Another prediction is that the efficiency of maintenance should relate to maximum longevity. A number of comparative studies have been carried out, although more are needed. In almost every case there is the expected relationship between efficiency of the maintenance parameter studied and the maximum lifespan of the species. In other cases, the relationship is inverse, but this is also in the expected direction. The studies which have been published are listed in Box 1.1.

Box 1.1 Correlation between maintenance parameters and maximum lifespan of mammalian species

Positive correlations

Longevity of fibroblasts *in vitro*
Longevity of erythrocytes *in vitro*
DNA repair
Poly-ADP ribose polymerase
γ-ray induced ADP-ribose transferase
Carotenoids in serum

Negative correlations

Cross-linking of collagen
Production of oxygen free radicals
Auto-oxidation of tissues
Metabolic rate and oxidised DNA bases
DNA methylation decline
Carcinogen binding to DNA
Mutagenicity of activated carcinogen
Incidence of cancer

Sources: R. Holliday (1995), *Understanding Ageing*, Cambridge University Press, Cambridge; R. Holliday (1996a), 'Neoplastic transformation: The contrasting stability of human and mouse cells', in T. Lindahl (ed.), *Genetic Instability in Cancer*, Cancer Surveys, 18, Cold Spring Harbor Laboratory Press, New York, pp. 103–15; and R. Holliday (1998), 'Understanding aging', *Philosophical Transactions of The Royal Society of London. Series B: Biological Sciences*, 352, pp. 1793–7.

Age-related diseases

It is sometimes maintained that 'natural ageing' is in some way distinct from the onset of age-associated disease. It is true that the changes that occur in skin, muscle or hair are not pathological. Nevertheless, when the process of degeneration we know as ageing affects an essential organ, then it is labelled a disease. More specifically, we can say that ageing is multicausal, but that the onset of deterioration in tissue and organ function is not fully synchronised, so it is inevitable that when one system fails in advance of others, it is labelled a disease. A few examples will suffice to illustrate the point (see also Table 1.1).

The brain and eye

An essential feature of the brain is the extreme localisation of function. When combined with a very limited capacity for regeneration and repair, this

Table 1.1 General relationships between cell or tissue maintenance and some major human age-associated diseases

Failure of maintenance	Major pathologies
Neurones	Dementias
Retina, lens	Blindness
Insulin metabolism	Type II diabetes
Blood vessels and heart	Cardiovascular and cerebrovascular disease
Bone structure	Osteoporosis
Immune system	Auto-immune disorders
Epigenetic controls	Cancer
Joints	Osteoarthritis
Glomeruli	Renal failure

means that the brain is a very sensitive target for pathological changes, including those that occur during ageing. The causes of brain damage can be classified as extrinsic or intrinsic. One of the most common extrinsic causes is failure of blood supply. This can be due to high blood pressure which ruptures a major blood vessel. This results in hypoxia, and in the space of a few minutes cells in brain tissue begin to die. Another cause of stroke is a blood clot, which again blocks normal blood supply. Intrinsic damage is due to changes in the neurons themselves. With increasing age, neurofibrillary tangles and neuritic or senile plaques accumulate and the latter are associated with large amounts of amyloid. In particular, a peptide fragment of amyloid protein accumulates, and this may be due to imperfect processing of the precursor protein, or to a failure to remove the peptide by proteolysis. When this occurs in relatively young individuals, say in their 50s or 60s, then Alzheimer's disease is diagnosed, the major effect being loss of memory and then premature death. Alzheimer's is a disease, because much older individuals are often free from the symptoms. Nevertheless, the pathological changes that occur in younger individuals are the same as those that can occur later in very old ones. In Down's syndrome patients, Alzheimer's disease occurs about 30 years earlier than in the general population, and there are now known familial cases where mutations have occurred in the amyloid protein.

The retina can be regarded as an extension of the brain. Photoreceptor cells reside on a layer of pigmented epithelium. They transmit signals to bipolar cells and thence to ganglion cells with axons that extend to the visual cortex of the brain. Oxygen is supplied to the retina by an extensive capillary network. Several features of the retina illustrate the inevitability of age-related changes. The photoreceptor elements are continually turned over, the rate being about 90 new receptor elements in each rod cell. Removal of these elements at the end of their useful life depends on lysosomal activity, and most protein is degraded. However, some is insoluble and this accumulates in secondary lysosomes in the underlying epithelium. Damage to the epithelium and its underlying membrane can result in detachment of the retina. The macula is the most sensitive part of the retina, and its degeneration leads to age-related blindness. The capillaries are sensitive to increased sugar levels in the blood, which occurs in diabetes, and this can lead to retinopathy.

The lens of the eye is also a sensitive target for age-associated changes. The crystallins that comprise most of the lens are laid down early in life, and are never replaced. They are subject to a number of intrinsic changes, including non-enzymic glycosylation, oxidation, cross-linking of molecules and partial denaturation. First there is loss of elasticity, with reduced ability to focus, and later the lens may lose transparency, leading to the formation of cataracts. The ear provides another notable example of a highly specialised structure with extremely limited capacity for repair of damaged components. With time, hair cells are lost and other structures may accumulate damage, with a reduced or complete loss of hearing.

The vascular system

The structure of the major arteries is not conducive to efficient maintenance and repair. The walls of arteries contain very long-lived structural proteins, such as collagen and elastin. It is well known that one of the changes associated with ageing is the cross-linking of such molecules. This in turn results in the loss of arterial elasticity which is a major cause of high blood pressure. Another cause is due to the gradual thickening of arterial walls, which is in part due to the glycation of proteins, since it is common in diabetes. High blood pressure affects other organs, such as the kidney and brain.

In the extensive research on heart disease, most attention is paid to atherosclerosis, which is due to the accumulation of atherosclerotic plaques on the inner surface of the major arteries. The origin of plaques is the subject of intense debate, but it is widely believed that they result from injury to the endothelium which lines the inner surface of arterial walls. The composition of the plaque is complex, consisting of smooth muscle cells, lipid laden foam cells, derived primarily from macrophages, and a mixture of structural proteins, including proteoglycan, elastin and collagen. It is clear from extensive studies of heart disease that arteries are unable to sustain their structure indefinitely.

The heart itself is a very efficient pump, but its muscle cells do not turn over during our lifetime and it has very limited capacity for repair. 'Heart disease' is often the result of the blockage of a coronary artery, and therefore loss of oxygen to heart muscle, but intrinsic changes occur as well, such as a loss of compliance or hardening of the muscle walls of the heart. The valves are also subject to gradual failure after prolonged use, and they may become calcified in old people. It is now well known that the incidence of heart disease—or ageing of the heart—is strongly influenced by diet and lifestyle. Smoking, a large intake of animal fat and lack of exercise are major features in promoting degeneration of the vascular system.

Late onset diabetes

Diabetes affects carbohydrate, fat and protein metabolism, primarily as a result of abnormally high glucose in blood and tissues (hyperglycaemia). Type I diabetes is of early onset, due to the loss of insulin-secreting cells, and we are concerned here with the much more common late onset type II diabetes. Although it is agreed that this is due to a failure of normal insulin metabolism, the actual cause of this is still the subject of some controversy. It could be due to a failure to produce enough insulin in response to sugar load, the existence of defective receptor or target cells, or abnormalities in the processing of the signal from the receptor, or any combination of these three. The end result is hyperglycaemia, which results in several important pathological changes. One of the most consistent features is the diffuse thickening of basement membranes in blood vessels, skin, muscle, retina and kidney. It is probable that AGEs are an important component, and the resulting complications include atherosclerosis, renal failure, cataracts, retinopathy, defects in the peripheral nerve or other components of the central nervous system. Although the causes of late onset diabetes are not altogether clear, it is well known that lifestyle, particularly a high carbohydrate diet and obesity, can induce the disease prematurely. Nevertheless, type II diabetes can be regarded as one of a whole spectrum of age-related pathological changes.

Osteoarthritis and osteoporosis

Osteoarthritis is due to endogenous changes in the joints. There is loss of chondrocytes, and proteoglycans which are essential for cartilage maintenance. There is probably an imbalance between the synthesis and removal of cartilage components. As a result, cartilage becomes pitted and fissured and this is associated with inflammation. There is release of degradative enzymes, cytokines and possibly free radicals. All these changes result in malformation of the normal contours of the ends of bones. Osteoporosis is due to a reduction in bone mass, which commonly results in fracture. Bone structure is normally maintained by a balance between formation and reabsorption, but with ageing the latter outpaces formation, the steady state is lost and bone mass declines. This decline commonly accelerates in women after the menopause, so it is clear that hormonal changes are involved, which in turn relate to calcium metabolism. Osteoporosis commonly occurs in the later decades in men and is then referred to as 'senile osteoporosis'. Both this disease and osteoarthritis are essentially due to the failure to maintain the steady state in bone and joint metabolism which is present throughout most of the lifespan.

Renal function

The kidney is far less sensitive than the brain or heart to tissue damage, since its function can be maintained even if about two-thirds of its mass is damaged. The glomeruli of the kidney are sensitive to hypertension, and the kidney itself has an active role in the control of blood pressure. This operates through the homeostatic mechanisms that normally maintain water balance and the quality of blood supply. With ageing, the number of glomeruli decline and those that remain can become abnormal through a thickening of membranes. Sclerotic and fibrotic changes occur in blood vessels. These anatomical and histological signs of deterioration are associated with a loss of physiological function. It is significant that the filtration rate of glomeruli is maintained until about the age of 40, and thereafter declines at a rate of about 1% per year, with considerable variation between individuals. Since the kidney has considerable reserve capacity, degenerative changes may have reached an advanced state before 'kidney disease' is diagnosed.

Cancer

Cancer is the result of a breakdown in the normal controls of development and tissue integrity, and the resulting cell growth may be malignant or benign. Cancers are of clonal origin and the phenotypes of the cells are heritable. Malignant cancers characteristically produce secondary tumours derived from the primary outgrowth. There is now good evidence that both the initial and subsequent events depend on changes at the DNA level. Much information is available about mutations in tumour suppressor genes and oncogenes, but it is now realised that epigenetic events (e.g., those that inactivate a gene) are also important. Some cancers occur in childhood and may develop quickly, such as leukaemias and brain tumours, but the onset of most carcinomas is age related. The epidemiological evidence indicates that several sequential events are necessary during tumour progression and the emergence of malignant cells. This has given rise to the view that cancer has nothing to do with ageing per se. In fact, ageing is clearly a temporal process, or set of processes, as are most cancers. To put it another way, both depend on 'multiple hit' events, even though the actual number of hits may be very different. It is well known that the incidence of various types of cancer are related to environmental effects, since cancers that are common in the US and Europe may be rare in Japan, and vice versa. This may be due to the existence of particular chemicals, or carcinogens, in diet. Such chemicals can be activated by the enzymes that are an essential part of the process of detoxification (see above). For example, an artificial hydrocarbon, not normally found in a natural diet, may be activated to a highly reactive epoxide that can damage DNA. Most damage to DNA is effectively repaired, but some escapes repair,[15] and thus can contribute, whether by mutation or by an 'epimutation', to tumour progression. The result is an age-related increase in the incidence of carcinoma.

It cannot be overemphasised that the research devoted to the study of all the above and many other age-associated diseases is in fact related to gerontology itself. This research has three aims:

1. better treatment of the disease in question
2. the elucidation of the cause, or causes, of the disease and
3. the development of procedures to postpone or prevent the onset of the disease.

Points 2 and 3 can certainly be regarded as being within the province of gerontology, and therefore more research on ageing itself is very likely to throw much light on the origins and development of age-related disease. Unfortunately, much persuasion is necessary to convince the present community of clinical and biomedical research scientists. Hopefully, there will be a fundamental change in the 21st century, and the significance of ageing research will be recognised by this community.[16]

Conclusions

We now have answers to the three basic questions in the 'Introduction'. We age because we evolved from organisms which also age. We age because our evolved body structure is incompatible with continual survival. We age because our various maintenance mechanisms eventually fail to preserve the normal structure and function of cells and tissues (see Table 1.1). We live as long as we do because we have evolved a lifestyle with low annual mortality.[17] This has allowed more resources to be invested in maintenance and less in reproduction. In contrast, species which live in a high-risk environment can only survive by investing much more heavily in reproduction, with correspondingly fewer resources allocated to maintenance. Thus, the adaptive radiation of mammals to many ecological niches has also resulted in the evolution of longevities over an approximately fiftyfold range. Thus, when considered at the level of the organism, ageing is no longer an unsolved problem in biology.

Nevertheless, at the level of fine detail—the actual molecular and cellular changes which produce the ageing phenotype—there is a great deal to learn. An understanding of these changes will come from further studies of maintenance mechanisms and, more importantly, the reasons why maintenance eventually fails. This new knowledge will greatly increase our understanding of the origins of age-associated disease, and will concomitantly make it possible to prevent or delay the onset of these diseases. The aim of all this research is not to increase the overall lifespan, but to significantly extend the 'health span' so that the quality of life of the elderly is greatly improved, and the costs of health care for the aged is greatly reduced.

Acknowledgment

This is an expanded version of an article which first appeared in the *New York Academy of Science*, 854, pp. 61–71 (1998). Permission to republish much of the same text has been granted by the Academy.

References

1. Holliday, R. (1995), *Understanding Ageing*, Cambridge University Press, Cambridge.
2. Finch, C. E. (1990), *Longevity, Senescence and the Genome*, University Press, Chicago; Grimley Evans, J. & Franklin Williams, T. (eds) (1992), *Oxford Textbook of Geriatric Medicine*, Oxford University Press, Oxford; and Martin, G. M., Austad, S. N. & Johnson, T. K. (1996), 'Genetic analysis of aging: Role of oxidative damage and environmental stress', *Nature Genetics*, 13, pp. 25–34.
3. Kirkwood, T. B. L. & Holliday, R. (1979), 'The evolution of ageing and longevity', *Proceedings of The Royal Society of London. Series B: Biological Sciences*, 205, pp. 531–46; and Kirkwood, T. B. L. (1985), 'Comparative and evolutionary aspects of longevity', in Finch, C. E. & Schneider, E. L., *Handbook of the Biology of Aging*, Van Nostrand Reinhold, New York, pp. 27–44.
4. Finch (1990), op. cit.; and Comfort, A. (1979), *The Biology of Senescence*, 3rd edn, Churchill Livingstone, London.
5. Walford R. L. (1969), *The Immunologic Theory of Ageing*, Munksgaard, Copenhagen.
6. Martin, Austad & Johnson (1996), op. cit.
7. Lindahl, T. (1979), 'DNA glycosylases, endonucleases for apurinic/pyrimidinic sites and base excision-repair', *Progress in Nucleic Acid Research and Molecular Biology*, 22, pp. 135–92.
8. Lindahl, T. (1993), 'Instability and decay of the primary structure of DNA', *Nature*, 362, pp. 709–15.
9. Holliday, R. (1996a), 'Neoplastic transformation: The contrasting stability of human and mouse cells', in Lindahl, T. (ed.), *Genetic Instability in Cancer*, Cancer Surveys, 18, Cold Spring Harbor Laboratory Press, New York, pp. 103–15.
10. Holliday (1995), op. cit.
11. Harder, J., Bartels, J., Christophers, E. & Schroder, J.-M. (1997), 'A peptide antibiotic from human skin', *Nature*, 387, p. 861.
12. Holliday (1995), op. cit; Kirkwood & Holliday (1979), op. cit.; and Kirkwood (1985), op. cit.
13. Holliday, R. (1996b), 'The evolution of human longevity', *Perspectives in Biology and Medicine*, 40, pp. 100–7.
14. Holliday (1995), op. cit.; and Holliday, R. (1994), 'Longevity and fecundity in eutherian mammals', in Rose, M. R. & Finch, C. E. (eds), *Genetics and Evolution of Aging*, Kluwar Academic Publishers, The Netherlands, pp. 217–25.
15. Lindahl (1993), op. cit.
16. Holliday, R. (2000), 'Ageing research in the next century', *Biogerontology*, 1, pp. 97–101.
17. Holliday (1996b), op. cit.

Chapter 2

The doctor–patient–family relationship

WILLIAM M. H. GOH and ROHAN S. DHILLON

Introduction

In geriatric practice, as in all medical practice, diagnosis and treatment begin with the interview. Gathering data about the patient's illness, evaluating it, discussing the findings with the patient, planning treatment and monitoring progress all depend on interviews. The greater the skills of the interviewer, the more accurate and pertinent will be the information obtained to formulate a diagnosis and management plan.

A skilfully conducted interview will inspire trust and confidence in the doctor. This will enhance a good doctor–patient relationship, which will in turn increase the likelihood of compliance with the doctor's recommendations.

In most instances interviewing the elderly patient does not greatly differ from interviewing younger patients, as advanced chronological age alone does not necessitate a change in the approach to medical evaluation. However, the strong association of old age with chronic disease and related impairments may increase the need for emphasis on certain aspects of evaluation.

An important consideration is that the elderly patient may not be able to give relevant or reliable information due to memory difficulty or other impairments. Consequently the doctor may need to interview family, friends, carers or other health practitioners. In many cases the doctor–patient relationship needs to be expanded to the doctor–patient–family relationship.

Evaluating the elderly patient

Older people are at the sunset of their lives and usually do not tend to look too far into the future. They may derive some pleasure and satisfaction from memories of past accomplishments and achievements, and so they tend to appreciate any attention paid to these meaningful parts of their lives. By listening and accepting them it is possible to help restore their sense of self-worth, dignity and usefulness.

Some older people may feel a sense of failure or emptiness if they consider they have failed and not achieved much in their lives. So feelings of isolation, frustration, despair and increasing dependency become prominent. The effort to see beyond immediate health problems to the strengths and accomplishments of an elderly patient can lay the foundation of a positive relationship based on acceptance, trust and mutual respect.

The elderly patient is almost invariably older than her doctor. Despite this there is a tendency for health professionals, including the doctor, to treat her as if she is a child. Doing this tends to demean the patient and can engender feelings of anger, frustration and antagonism.

Potential difficulties in geriatric assessment

In the elderly several factors make medical evaluation more challenging, complicated and time-consuming. Table 2.1 illustrates the potential difficulties encountered in interviews and assessments of the elderly.

With elderly patients their impaired hearing or vision commonly hampers history taking. Communication can be improved significantly by facing the patient in a well lit room so that the patient can lip read if necessary. Speaking at a slower pace and articulating clearly may also be helpful. Finally, when severe hearing impairment exists, the doctor may need to write in order to communicate.

Elderly patients tend to have a reduced reaction time so that their physical movements, thought processes and verbalisation are slower. They should be allowed sufficient time to answer questions and, more importantly, time to disclose information spontaneously. All this seems time consuming so patience is truly a virtue in geriatric assessment.

Older people are generally more cautious in their response to questions and tend to be reticent about disclosing their personal problems and affairs. It is not unusual for the elderly not to volunteer information about their symptoms. They have lived through many years of hardship and their bodies have experienced various aches and pains. So they may under-report potentially important symptoms because they think their symptoms are part of growing old.

Those elderly patients who suffer depression with psychomotor retardation, pessimism, feelings of futility and hopelessness may think it is not worthwhile telling the doctor of their complaints. If cognitive impairment is present, older people may not be aware of their complaints or even deny them. The elderly patients' altered physiological responses to the disease process may also result in vague and non-specific symptoms. In these cases family, friends, colleagues, carers and other health workers are important sources of information and collateral data should always be sought.

On the other hand, some elderly patients present with a myriad of symptoms which can frustrate and confuse the doctor. These multiple complaints usually indicate the presence of co-existing

Table 2.1 Potential difficulties in geriatric evaluation

Difficulty	Factors involved	Suggestions
Communication	Diminished hearing	Face patient to allow lip reading Speak more slowly Write down questions
	Impaired vision	Use well lit room
	Reduced reaction time	Allow enough time for answers
Under-reporting of symptoms	Depression	Ask specific questions to determine if depression is present
	Altered physiological responses and cognitive impairment	Interview family, friends or carers for ancillary data
Multiple symptoms	Co-existing diseases	Attend to all symptoms to elicit the treatable ones
Vague symptoms	Altered physiological responses to disease process	Rule out treatable diseases

diseases. The doctor needs to distinguish the symptoms of more recent onset and the conditions that are potentially treatable from conditions that are chronic and likely to be less amenable to treatment.

Some older people are set in their ways and are secure in their familiar environment. They have difficulty with or dislike change. This may be a normal chronological effect of ageing or its presence may be socioculturally determined. As a consequence some older people often delay consulting their doctor until late in the course of their illness.

Finally, elderly patients may resist or be non-compliant with treatment recommended by the doctor because of their fear of change, especially if major changes such as leaving home or accepting home help are recommended. Considerable time, patience and gentle persuasion are necessary to enable the patient to accept novel management initiatives.

The role of the doctor

Doctors who show an interest in geriatric practice have developed sensitivity to the concerns of elderly patients and an understanding of the multiform presentation of their medical problems. They need to be able to extend their work role to involve others associated with their patients—family members, friends, carers and other health workers.

Skills of the doctor that will enhance rapport with the patient include the following:

- The doctor needs to have a good knowledge base and appropriate clinical skills.
- The doctor needs to develop an effective means of communication.
- Certain personality characteristics such as accurate empathy, non-possessive warmth and genuineness are considered to promote rapport.

A good knowledge base

Having a good knowledge base helps the doctor to identify important symptoms and signs. When the doctor entertains different diagnostic possibilities during the interview, his line of questioning will demonstrate to the patient that he is an expert in his business and he knows what he is looking for. This will inspire confidence in the patient and promote a better relationship.

Consequently, the doctor who demonstrates a good knowledge base, effective clinical skills and sound judgment will earn the patient's acceptance, trust and respect, thereby promoting rapport for further therapeutic work. Because the person examining her is a doctor, confidence and hope will be engendered in the patient as it is assumed that the doctor has these attributes.

A good first impression is a great help in establishing rapport, as there is no second chance to create a first impression. It has been shown that patients consider doctors who wear white coats over conventional street clothes to be more competent than those who are shabbily dressed. So personal appearance can immediately inspire confidence and help establish rapport.

Maintaining good eye contact with the patient is generally interpreted positively by the patient, who feels the doctor is interested and concerned. Studies also reveal that patients are more positively disposed to doctors who smile. A good approach is to maintain an open and curious attitude with a mild healthy suspicion.

Effective communication

Sir William Osler once said, 'Listen to the patient, he will tell you the diagnosis'. This is as applicable today as it was in his time and it is as true for the elderly as for the young.

The language of medicine is characterised by medical terminology, objective descriptions of physical complaints and a classification of these within a reductionist biomedical model. The language of patients, on the other hand, is characterised by non-technical discourse about the subjective experience of illness within the context of social relationships and the patient's everyday world. When doctors and patients talk to each other they may do so in different languages, thereby causing communication difficulties.

Generally, doctors have more power than patients to structure, alter and maintain the context of the interaction between them. If doctors do not attempt to relate to the patients in their language, patients may believe that they have not been heard or understood and feel powerless to do anything about it. To improve communication, doctors and patients need to understand the process of decision making that is taking place during the consultation. Communication misunderstandings almost invariably are attributed to a lack of patient participation in the decision process, often because the patient does not understand the doctor's language.

Personality characteristics of doctors

Medical competence and skills of the highest order may only produce a sub-optimal outcome in the absence of rapport. Patients may tolerate a tactless and insensitive doctor of exceptional ability but such relationships are fraught with conflicts, anger and disloyalty, and are prone to litigation.

Studies reveal that effective therapists are able to accurately empathise with their patients' suffering. They exhibit a degree of non-possessive warmth towards their patients, and they show genuine concern for their patients' wellbeing. Although some doctors are naturally endowed with these characteristics, others can acquire them through practice and experience. Empathy will always be enhanced by identifying with the patient's suffering and showing compassion.

The doctor–patient relationship

There is a close relationship between interviewing and medical management. During interviews patients reveal personal and intimate details about themselves and in this way a relationship between doctor and patient evolves.

Clinical decision making in geriatric practice is usually not an isolated event, except in an emergency situation when it may be a single encounter and the doctor–patient relationship begins and ends there. More commonly medical management is continuous over the given course of the illness and often includes intervals of relatively good health.

Astute doctors are aware that diagnostic appraisal and therapeutic planning begin with the first interview. With subsequent interviews they build an increasing database from which to confirm, modify or refute diagnostic and therapeutic postulation.

Transference

Illnesses that cause the elderly to seek help often evoke anxiety, a feeling of helplessness, and disturbances of their relationships with others. Patients come to the doctor with an admixture of hope and fear. They hope that the doctor will be able to find the cause of their suffering and remove it. At the same time they fear that the doctor may not be able to help them or that help is not possible.

Patients also come to the doctor with feelings and expectations about consulting a healer built on their experiences of past encounters with doctors. Some of these feelings may stem from as far back as childhood interaction with their parents, who were the earliest carers for their pain and suffering. Such feelings become unconsciously displaced on to the treating doctor in a process called transference.

In geriatric practice doctors are inevitably younger than their elderly patients. Despite this, it is not unusual for the elderly patients to relate to them as if there were older and wiser. However, some elderly patients may see their doctors as inexperienced people needing to be protected from unpleasant reality.

Each interview affects subsequent interviews and the patient. Impressions, attitudes and expectations learnt by the patient in each encounter have a significant impact on the patient's response to the doctor in subsequent interviews. The first interview can have a particularly powerful influence on the development of the transference.

If the patient feels understood, accepted and valued and has confidence in the doctor, a positive transference is enhanced and a productive therapeutic relationship ensues. If, on the other hand, the patient feels disregarded, slighted or rejected, a negative transference will complicate further management.

Ideally, an effective doctor–patient relationship is characterised by trust and confidence in the doctor. The patient's initial trust in the doctor's professional skill is created by the confidence with which the doctor assesses the problems and by his qualifications. On the other hand, the establishment of personal trust and confidence in the doctor can only be built over time.

Counter-transference

In the doctor–patient relationship the doctor also harbours feelings, attitudes, expectations and beliefs about the patient. Past experiences with elderly patients, as well as previous life experiences as far back as childhood, contribute to this counter-transference. So managing an elderly patient who resembles his parent, or even grandparent, provides a unique challenge to a doctor. The counter-transference commences on a positive note if the doctor had previously enjoyed stable and meaningful relationships with elderly people, including his parents and grandparents.

In the same vein negative counter-transference frequently stems from the doctor's past experiences. Some doctors seem to think or act as if elderly people have inevitably led sheltered and protected lives, and so they avoid asking potentially important questions about usage of drugs and alcohol. Even worse, there is a tendency by some doctors to infantilise elderly patients, so that they 'talk down' to their patients, and fail to explain the interview process or provide feedback to the patients. Such an attitude implies that the doctors believe their patients lack intelligence, knowledge or comprehension. Doctors may also relate to patients' families as if they are the parents. Insight and awareness of counter-transference help doctors to objectify their management plan and be more effective in geriatric practice.

Types of doctor–patient relationships

A functional doctor–patient relationship is ideally characterised by trust and confidence in the doctor as well as allowing patients the autonomy to participate appropriately in the management process. It is recognised that there are several distinct approaches to treatment decision making that doctors can use with their patients. These include paternalistic, shared and informed (or consumerist) approaches. Each has different implications for patient management.

The paternalistic doctor–patient relationship

In the paternalistic approach, doctors use all of the authority inherent in their status and role. The process of interview is characterised by an activity–passivity interaction. The patient feels no autonomy, tries to please the doctor, and passively obeys the doctor's instructions.

Doctors using this model are not likely to be too interested in a patient's concerns and feelings, but are more likely to want brief descriptions of physical symptoms which help them formulate a diagnostic plan in the patient's best interest.

This is certainly advantageous in a medical emergency, when a patient is acutely ill and requires urgent medical attention. It is the least efficient type of relationship for diagnostic interviewing, data gathering and for most treatment.

The shared type of doctor–patient relationship

In the shared approach, doctors also exercise much authority, but create an atmosphere in which patients feel they have the power to communicate openly. This type of doctor–patient relationship emphasises a guidance–co-operation communication style. The patients have greater autonomy and participate more actively in the relationship. A guidance–co-operation relationship may not encourage spontaneous revelations of the widest possible range of information.

However, in this approach information exchange helps doctors understand their patients and ensure that patients are informed of treatment options and the potential risks and benefits of treatment. Studies reveal that patient satisfaction depends on the information patients obtain from their doctors and the degree to which they understand their illness.

The informed type of doctor–patient relationship

In the informed or consumerist approach there is mutual participation. Patients have a more active role in both defining the problem for which they seek help and in determining appropriate treatment. Here patients assume more responsibility for a successful outcome. This is created by appropriate moderation of the doctors' authority.

In such a relationship the widest range of relevant diagnostic information tends to emerge and a more successful treatment outcome is likely to occur. In the purest type of informed decision making the doctor's role is limited to providing research data about treatment options and their benefits and risks so that patients can make an informed decision.

Finally, effective doctor–patient relationships encourage patients to take appropriate responsibility for their own treatment. In geriatric practice, the unique difficulties of assessing elderly people present challenges that may require modifications to these techniques. Despite this, the models of doctor–patient relationship mentioned above should provide a useful format for a sound clinical approach to geriatric practice.

The emotional aspect of the physical examination

During a well conducted interview when the doctor–patient relationship is established, the doctor is no longer seen as a stranger but as a concerned person who is trying to help. The physical examination is the next step in the information-gathering process. Patients who gain trust and confidence in their doctors will willingly submit to such a procedure.

Undressing in front of someone is usually done in private in intimate situations. So doctors must always be aware of the issues of shame, embarrassment and feelings of vulnerability that the semi-dressed or undressed patient may experience. Doctors should allow patients their rights to preserve dignity and modesty by seeing to it that they are discreetly and appropriately covered up.

Doctors need to be alert to evidence of shame and embarrassment when examining the emotion laden parts of the body such as the breasts, genitals or rectum. Elderly patients are less likely to sexualise physical contact with doctors or see themselves as objects of sexual attention. They are also less likely to act seductively. (Such behaviour in younger patients can engender great difficulties in the doctor–patient relationship.)

Some patients may have specific anxiety about certain areas of the body. These can usually be identified during history taking. Otherwise the physical examination presents another opportunity to detect the patient's physical concerns, and invaluable data can occasionally be gathered for effective management.

Difficult doctor–patient relationships

The vast majority of geriatric patients are rewarding to deal with as they have accrued knowledge, experience, wisdom and insight from having successfully negotiated the sufferings and gratifications that are an inevitable part of longevity. However, it has been shown that 15% of consultations in general practice are deemed difficult, and some elderly patients can be difficult to deal with on a constructive basis.

It is helpful to understand that there is no such thing as a difficult patient. There are patients who present with difficult problems, and there are difficult doctor–patient relationships. When interviews get out of control, both doctor and patient experience increasing frustration and anger, which may become progressively more disturbing as each attempts to get their point across.

If adequate steps are taken to establish rapport and communication is open and meaningful, it is unlikely that such a situation would arise. Nonetheless, even experienced and skilled practitioners occasionally have a difficult doctor–patient relationship develop to a point where there is considerable frustration and anger for everyone involved.

There are a few simple steps that can help address and resolve this problem. First, do not do 'more of the same' by continuing to put your point across, as that had not worked. Doing so could further inflame the situation. Second, take a step back to evaluate the situation. Recognise your feelings about the interaction and not just your reaction towards the patient. Then verbalise your feeling and give a reason for it. For example, 'I am having difficulty with the interview at the moment because...' Finally, encourage the patient to express her feelings and then work with the patient to co-operatively resolve the impasse. Often the successful resolution of a crisis will foster a more productive doctor–patient relationship with mutual acceptance and respect.

There are more complaints against doctors that derive from a breakdown in the caring aspect of the doctor–patient relationship than there are complaints from the technical outcome of the treatment. Unresolved conflicts all too frequently lead to poor therapeutic outcome and occasionally to litigation.

The role of the family

Managing the geriatric patient can be a rewarding experience. Medical problems once thought to be hopeless or frustrating can now be seen more optimistically as treatable.

However, the geriatric patient does not exist in a social vacuum. The family usually has a stronger emotional influence on the patient than the doctor does, so comprehensive management of geriatric patients must take into consideration communication with the patient's family.

In this century, as in the previous one, the trend is towards a greater number of people surviving to their seventh, eighth and ninth decades of life. The popular belief is that family closeness in previous generations stemmed from economic necessity rather than from tender sentiments, loyalty or filial piety. Economic affluence and increased geographic mobility have resulted in a general tendency towards a more nuclear family. This has resulted in the disruption of family ties and marked changes in intergeneration relationships.

A number of social and interpersonal myths exist around the geriatric population. It is popularly held that, first, most elderly people live either alone or with their partners. Second, they are often isolated from their offspring and do not have frequent contact with them. Third, there is a 'generation gap' which strains communication and loosens family ties. Fourth, with intergeneration relationships older people are receivers rather than givers.

However, sociological and demographic studies reveal that older people neither live alone nor are isolated from their families. They have frequent contact with their families, and relations between generations appear warm and close. In fact older people are more often the givers rather than the recipients of intergenerational exchanges of assistance and support.

Unsatisfactory communication with the doctor and a misunderstanding by the doctor of family concerns for the patient are major factors leading to litigation and malpractice suits. Other reasons given by the plaintiffs for malpractice suits include the perception that the doctor devalues the patient or family views, perceptions of abandonment by the doctor, and a belief that the doctor has let the patient down by not visiting them as promised.

Family and physical illness

When elderly people become ill, family interactions and relationships may undergo some degree of upheaval. If the illness is relatively mild, minor adjustment will probably suffice. In a major illness, substantial changes in family dynamics may occur. Just as the illness has an impact on the family, the family's beliefs and reaction has an impact on the presentation of the illness (see Box 2.1).

Most patients with an acute illness accept a biomedical explanation for it. However, with a chronic illness they often seek an alternate explanation. Patients frequently share and discuss their symptoms with their families prior to seeking medical help. When the family is in agreement about the patient's illness and need for medical help, an uncomplicated medical consultation with a successful outcome is more likely to occur. The fear and uncertainty that patients entertain about their illness are greatly influenced by the family's past experience of illness. This often extends over a few generations and becomes a part of the family's 'medical myth'.

Box 2.1 The family and physical illness

- A person's definition of her illness is largely derived from consultation with family members.
- Agreement among family members about the concept of illness has been related to successful treatment outcome.
- Family attitudes are a major factor in patient compliance with treatment.
- Chronic illness in a family member adversely affects other family members.
- Maladaptive family interaction patterns can be a precipitating factor in illness onset and can affect the course of the illness.

A prolonged illness acts as a chronic stressor on the family. It initially disrupts the usual pattern of interaction in the family. Adjustment and adaptation then follow this. Successful adaptation to illness is associated with role flexibility and family rules that permit emotional expression.

Maladaptive family interaction patterns engender considerable anxiety and tension in everyone. Emotional crises are frequent, and illness onset and relapses increased. 'Medical family therapy' aims to enhance the role of the patient and family members and facilitate their relationship to reduce morbidity and relapses and to minimise the impact of the illness on family life.

Family as source of information

In general medical practice, it is usual for patients to be able to give information about their illnesses to allow accurate diagnoses. This is much less true in geriatric practice where elderly patients may only be able to give limited history because of their age related impairments. This is especially true when there is an organic brain disorder, such as dementia, when cognitive deficits would ensure that the patient could never give a reliable or comprehensive history.

Consequently, family members and, to a lesser extent friends and colleagues, can be valuable sources of important information regarding the patient's illness beyond that given by the patient. It is advantageous for communication to be established through the most responsible family member.

It is important that the patient knows of such contact so that misunderstanding is avoided. Generally, patients who seek medical help would welcome such a request, as family members can not only provide information to the doctor but also assist in management.

The family's history itself may be inaccurate because some families wish to emphasise the need for help, and exaggerate the patient's complaints. Other families may, on the other hand, underestimate the patient's symptoms when they wish to avoid outside intrusion.

Family as carer

In relation to the normal dependencies of ageing, families frequently provide direct assistance for the elderly. The family has long been considered the social institution that deals with the physical, emotional, social and economic needs of elderly people. Outside the hospital, the actual care of an elderly patient is usually provided by the patient—that is, self-care—or by family members.

Over 70% of sickness episodes are handled outside the formal health system, and self-treatment, with the family providing a substantial proportion of health care, is a common occurrence. One study found that almost 40% of offspring who care for elderly patients in their homes devote the equivalent of a full-time job plus overtime to domestic and custodial tasks. It is now appreciated that family care giving has led to increasing physical and psychological burdens on family members.

Family support of the doctor's management plan can help ensure that the patient adheres appropriately to treatment, be it taking medication, rest, diet or exercise. A hostile or antagonistic family could easily negate or severely jeopardise any treatment plan, however carefully thought out.

Family as victim

In serious illness, the family members are usually the main providers of information for the doctor.

They also need information from the doctor, as they are the principal source of support and care for the patient. As well, they can be seen as victims who have been inadvertently inflicted with a helpless and dependent sick person.

When very ill patients deny illness or refuse doctors permission to interview the family, doctors should remember that they are patients' advocates as well as being their physicians. They have to delicately balance the distress and needs of the family against resistance from patients who do not believe that any help is warranted. The responsibilities of caring for the patient's day-to-day living problems fall on the shoulders of the family.

When considering the family members as victims rather than carers, doctors need to be aware of their distress and be sensitive to their needs. Even in dire circumstances, a few friendly words of comfort from the doctor will go a long way to allay the family's anxiety and fear, and increase their trust and confidence.

Even very sick patients are aware that they may cause considerable hardship to the family. Concerns of the patient for the family can be real and moving. These also need to be understood and addressed.

Factors promoting doctor–patient–family interactions

Confidentiality is a cardinal principle of professionalism and the patient should feel secure in the knowledge that all communication with the doctor will be kept strictly confidential. The family doctor must appreciate this intimate and confidential bond and avoid any threat to its disruption. In dealing with elderly patients, communication with family members is advantageous and often essential. According to the principle of utilitarianism, the patient and family can be viewed as a unit and the doctor–patient relationship expanded to the doctor–patient–family relationship. To establish rapport with the family, two important issues need to be addressed—namely family needs and strategies for engaging the family.

Family needs

The family may be viewed as a significant resource for data gathering, for assisting with management, as a causal or precipitating factor in the illness, and as an influence on the course of the illness. A busy practitioner with a tight schedule may find it difficult to consider the family's needs, but it is important that the emotional, physical and psychosocial needs of family members not be overlooked (see Box 2.2).

Box 2.2 Family needs

- Family members' contributions need to be acknowledged.
- They need to feel that they are actively participating.
- They need information about the illness.
- They require support for the concerns and hardships in managing the patient.
- They need to be involved in post-discharge planning.

The family needs to feel acknowledged and valued for taking time out to come along with their sick relative. They would appreciate being listened to and they need to be seen as people who are attempting to contribute actively to the patient's management.

They need to be given information about the illness, its likely course, its probable consequences, the management plan and their roles. As far as possible communicate with them in simple, non-technical language that they can understand. When the family members fail to understand the doctor's explanation, it is usually because they are too preoccupied or distracted by their own distress or they do not comprehend technical terms.

It is important to recognise that family members are ordinary people trying to cope with their anxiety, fear, anger, guilt and ambivalence when someone close to them suffers an illness that they feel powerless to do anything about. Consequently, they should be given the opportunity to express and ventilate these distressing feelings. A little understanding and compassion shown by the doctor will be an immense help. When discharge is planned, family members may be the principal caregivers and need as much information as is practicable.

Engaging the family

Concepts about what caregiving is and how family members participate in providing care differ between family members and doctors and among family members themselves. Communication with concerned family members, friends or colleagues need not be time-consuming. It is usually possible to identify one family member as the communication channel to whom further reports will be given, thus avoiding frequent and repetitious calls. By initiating the calls themselves doctors can maintain effective control over the situation and derive greater satisfaction in communicating with the family. The main points in engaging the family are summarised in Box 2.3.

Whenever possible patients should be asked for permission to speak to the family. Give a brief explanation that more data is needed to complete the diagnosis and management plan. Even in severe dementia an attempt should be made to seek the patient's permission. The family often needs to be reminded that they are not legally in charge of the elderly patient even though they may feel or act *in loco parentis*. It is important that the patient know of any discussion about them.

If one or more family members are present with the patient during the interview, involve them as soon as possible. It is essential that the patient consents to their presence and involvement. If there is any doubt, this should be immediately clarified with the patient. It is helpful to clarify the reason why the family members are present. Family members should be asked for their observations and opinions of the problem. Then, if appropriate, ask the family for their assistance with patient management.

If the details provided by the patient conflict with that obtained from the family, do not take sides but remain impartial. Maintain objectivity, focus on the issues and do not become emotionally involved.

When seeing the family without the patient present, explain the purpose, structure and timing of the interview. Obtain as many details as possible of the current illness and of relevant past medical history. Ask about living arrangements and current supports. The doctor should be able to talk to the patient's family and discuss difficult issues without breaking confidentiality.

If any family member shows signs of not coping, the doctor may need to provide support and treatment for any identifiable disorders. Signs that the family is not coping include increasing tension and anger, conflicts between members of the family, emerging physical symptoms and psychological decompensation in family members.

Box 2.3 Engaging family

- When the patient is seen alone, obtain permission from the patient to speak with family members.
- If a family member is present, involve them as soon as possible.
- When there are conflicting details, remain impartial.
- When seeing family members in the absence of the patient, encourage reciprocal exchanges of information.
- If the family is not coping, provide or arrange support.

Conclusion

An ageing population, deinstitutionalisation, lack of funding and dissatisfaction with government organised health services have increasingly relegated more responsibility for the care of the elderly patient to the family. Carers are organising themselves into self-help groups, support networks and political lobby groups. Despite this the family doctor plays a crucial role in the care of the elderly patient. Consequently, comprehensive medical management of the elderly patient needs to take into consideration the interactions between the doctor, the patient and the family.

In this chapter the factors that contribute to the doctor–patient–family relationship arising in the course of managing the elderly patient are examined. There are unique issues for the doctor when dealing with an elderly patient who is invariably older and may remind the doctor of his own parents or grandparents. The potential difficulties that may arise in managing the elderly patient are described.

The skills and approach of the doctor that contribute to establishing rapport are delineated. Transference and counter-transference issues as well as treatment decision-making approaches are discussed. Issues in the family, such as how the illness affects the family, the family as a source of information, the family as carer, the family as victim, family needs and how to engage the family in management are elaborated. Finally, the doctor–patient–family relationship is described.

Acknowledgment

The authors wish to thank Dr Patrick Flynn, Director of Psycho-geriatrics, South Australian Mental Health Services, Australia, for his help in the preparation of this chapter.

Bibliography and further reading

Balint, M. (1964), *The Doctor, His Patient and the Illness*, Pitman, London.

Charles, C., Gafni, A. & Whelan, T. (1999), 'What do we mean by partnership in decisions about treatment?', *British Medical Journal*, 319, pp. 780–2.

Creed, F. & Guthrie, E. (1993), 'Techniques for interviewing the somatising patient', *British Journal of Psychiatry*, 162, pp. 467–71.

Epstein, R. M., Campbell, T. C., Cohen-Cole, S., McWhinney, I. R. & Similtstein, G. (1993), 'Perspective on patient–doctor communication', *Journal of Family Practice*, 37, pp. 377–88.

Gafni, A., Charles, C. & Whelan, T. (1998), 'The physician–patient encounter: The physician as a perfect agent for the patient versus the informed treatment decision-making model', *Social Science and Medicine*, 47, pp. 347–54.

McDaniel, S. H. & Campbell, T. L. (1998), 'Family caregiving and coping with chronic illness. Editorial', *Families, Systems & Health*, 16(3), pp. 195–6.

Newman, S. (1976), 'Housing Adjustments of Older People: A Report from the Second Phase', Institute of Social Research, University of Michigan, Ann Arbor.

Othmer, E. & Othmer, S. C. (1994), *Strategies for Rapport: The Clinical Interview Using DSM-IV*, vol. 1, American Psychiatric Press, Inc., Washington, pp. 13–24.

Simpson, M., Buckman, R., Stewart, M. et al. (1991), 'Doctor–patient communication: The Toronto consensus statement', *British Medical Journal*, 303, pp. 1385–7.

Winefield, H. R., Murrell, T. G. C., Clifford, J. V. & Farmer, E. A. (1995), 'The usefulness of distinguishing different types of general practice consultation, or are needed skills always the same?', *Family Practice*, 12, pp. 402–7.

Chapter 3

History taking and physical examination: special considerations

KATINA OVERELL and RANJIT N. RATNAIKE

Introduction

The clinical history and physical examination, the cornerstones of assessment and management, are a more difficult task in many older patients. In younger patients, the history taking and physical examination usually focus on a specific acute medical illness (or impairment) and the patient–doctor interaction not uncommonly culminates in a cure. In older persons, multiple illnesses co-exist, many of them chronic. An essential component of geriatric medical care is the need to review the disabling aspects of illness and the life impact (handicap) that may ensue from such illness. The clinician's aim is to maintain (or enhance) autonomy and to achieve an optimal quality of life.

The accuracy of information from the elderly is often presumed as being unreliable. Such attitudes may discourage obtaining a comprehensive history from the patient. Numerous studies document that the history from an older patient is accurate. A well-taken history in the oldest of patients, even those over 85, or those with some degree of cognitive impairment, can provide accurate and valuable information on current and past medical problems.

The history

The clinical setting is important. A well-lit, comfortable consulting room potentially decreases confusion and has a calming influence. For some older patients, the offer of a late morning or early afternoon clinical appointment may be appropriate to ensure attendance. Experienced clinicians project an unhurried stance in the opening remarks to optimise reporting by the patient. Recent reports suggest that autobiographical recall in patients with dementia improves significantly when background music is playing.

Typically, the history taking and physical examination should be at a slower pace than with a younger patient. A more flexible interview style is advisable. Hasty and impatient questioning will alienate older patients, who reasonably expect some deference to their seniority. The traditional methodical history taking may not be appropriate. Patients often need triggers to remember past significant events. For example, questions may be prompted during the examination when surgical scars are noted. The question, 'What is the problem that bothers you the most at the moment?', is often a useful starting point to the interview. Once this has been established, other complaints can be dealt with. Difficulties may arise in providing all the information requested with a complex past medical history—details of numerous hospitalisations, current medical issues and their treatment, including medications and dosages. Such information is best sought by contact with key clinicians or hospitals. The clinician must be alert to patient fatigue. Sometimes, more than one session may be required, especially if large amounts of information are required or many issues have to be considered.

Optimal clinical interaction occurs when the patient can hear well. Assumptions about an older patient's hearing should not be made. If there is a hearing problem, the clinician should speak loudly without shouting or with unnecessary slowness that may cause offence. Facing the patient directly helps with lip reading and provides visual clues. Shouting obliterates consonants, which often have a higher frequency, and are less well perceived by the ageing ear. Questions may need to be written. Amplification devices that can enhance communication are widely available, inexpensive, simple to use and not daunting to older patients. The patient should always be asked to use their dentures as this facilitates clarity of speech.

Elderly patients may not volunteer information about problems. Typically, these include a failing memory, abuse by a carer, or psychiatric problems such as depression. Problems of bowel or bladder dysfunction may not be raised because of embarrassment. Urinary incontinence affects 5–15% of elderly people living in the community and over 50% in institutionalised populations, and causes significant morbidity (Chapters 39 and 40). Breathlessness may be attributed to ageing and lack of physical fitness. Patients may decrease their activity to cope. Alternatively, physical incapacity may not 'expose' the problems of dyspnoea due to lung or cardiac abnormalities or angina pectoris. Thus, one problem may mask another.

A major challenge of history taking in an older patient is that the presentation of many medical and psychiatric illnesses can be associated with non-specific features. During the interview, older patients may minimise their symptoms, sometimes out of fear of the doctor's response, which in their minds may include invasive tests, hospitalisation or loss of independence. In others, such reticence may reflect acceptance of symptoms as part of normal ageing. The seriousness of a problem may be underestimated or viewed as temporary. Patients may regard some medical problems, such as constipation, not important enough to mention, thus compromising the illness profile.

Falls are a major and common problem in geriatric practice and have a significant impact on quality of life. Many older patients tend to minimise the fall and attribute it to 'just tripping'. Seventy-five per cent of falls, despite their severity, are not reported to health professionals. Recurrent falls specially require detailed questioning. It is important to determine the environment in which the fall occurred (e.g. slippery floors, multiple obstacles) and footing attire (Table 3.1). A careful review of medications is essential. Many therapeutic agents can contribute to falls due to their adverse effects or incorrect dosage (Box 3.1). The clinician must be vigilant to the possibility that an injury attributed to a fall may be due to elder abuse (Chapter 59).

Under-reporting may also occur due to other factors. A health facility must not only be available but also conveniently accessible. Formidable considerations to older persons include the ease of parking a car, the accessibility and cost of public transport, and for those without a vehicle or with physical limitations, the expense of a taxi.

Family, friends or carers can provide valuable and essential information and are often indispensable in obtaining a complete history, notably in the setting of cognitive impairment. Their presence at

Table 3.1 Falls history

Description of fall	Environment, time, circumstances, day/night
Pre-fall	Vertigo/balance, palpitations/chest pain, muscle weakness, neurological symptoms
Loss of consciousness	Length of time
Post-fall events	Oriented, alert, able to mobilise, pain, injuries sustained

Box 3.1 Medications contributing to falls

- Benzodiazepines
- Chlorpropramide
- Major tranquillisers
- Narcotics
- Alcohol
- Tricyclic antidepressants
- Antihypertensives
- Diuretics
- Digoxin
- L-dopa

the interview can be reassuring to the patient and experienced clinicians readily agree to a patient request that they attend in the clinic room. Such attendees often help the practitioner to assess current living conditions and to plan further strategies to improve the quality of life of the patient. However, it is important that the patient is not ignored in such an interaction with the family. If elder abuse and/or neglect is obvious or suspected (Chapter 59), the presence of a carer is, of course, inappropriate. In many situations, history taking in the older person is incomplete without addressing issues of sexuality, as discussed in Chapter 8.

An accurate drug history is vital. Elderly patients are more prone to adverse drug reactions and this should be considered in every acute illness. Polypharmacy due to the treatment of multiple illnesses increases the likelihood of drug–drug interactions and drug 'consumption' errors, especially if there is cognitive impairment (Chapters 15 and 16). Alcohol intake must be carefully documented. Apart from its direct toxicity, alcohol increases the hepatic metabolism of drugs such as warfarin and phenytoin. Patients or their carers should be requested to bring in all medications, including over-the-counter medications, herbal and other preparations from health food shops or prescribed by practitioners of alternative medicine. Pharmacists invariably keep a record of current and previous prescription medication, and are a useful source of information. However, patients may shop at two or more pharmacies.

Box 3.2 summarises a variety of aspects of geriatric history taking.

Box 3.2 Factors that promote good history taking in geriatric patients

- A good rapport.
- A comfortable environment.
- An appropriate level and pace of communication.
- Flexibility: frequent visits to avoid fatigue.
- Presence of family or carers.
- Accessibility of medical records.
- Sighting of all medications.
- Identifying and facilitating initiatives to maintain independence and quality of life.

Review of systems

Many older patients who are unwell fatigue easily. Instead of an exhaustive review of systems, one could concentrate on common problems in the elderly, such as decreased mobility, falls (Chapter 13), incontinence (Chapters 36, 39 and 40) and intellectual impairment (Chapters 14–16). Many medical illnesses precipitate the sudden onset or worsening of confusion (Chapters 9, 15 and 16), falls or urinary incontinence. Multisystem involvement is common in older patients. However, depression may manifest as multisystem somatic problems (Chapter 9). Sleep disorders are more prevalent than is appreciated. Sleep-disordered breathing is common in the elderly and therefore it is important to inquire about breathing disturbances, frequent awakening, restlessness during sleep and daytime sleepiness.

Physical examination

The clinical examination should not unduly tire the patient yet not be cursory. Many sick patients, especially with cognitive problems, find it difficult to co-operate with the examiner. Traditional examination procedures, such as lying flat on the bed to examine the abdomen or at 45 degrees to examine the jugular venous pressure, may be difficult to carry out. Compromises are necessary to minimise patient inconvenience.

Observation provides valuable information on grooming and gait, the ability to remove clothing unaided, and the ease of transferring from the chair to the examination couch. The patient's height and weight should be documented to assess nutritional status (Chapter 30). Recording the body temperature is important, but the elderly may not be febrile despite an infective illness and may even be hypothermic.

Determining the state of hydration of an elderly patient is essential but difficult. Reduced skin turgor and a decreased sense of thirst are features seen in normal ageing. Postural hypotension is a misleading indicator of dehydration as it is common secondary to autonomic neuropathy or medications. The sensation of thirst, a reliable indicator of dehydration in younger populations, is unreliable as thirst sensation diminishes with age. More reliable features of dehydration in older patients, reported by Gross et al. (1992), are:

- dry tongue and mucous membranes of the nose and mouth
- longitudinal tongue furrows
- upper body muscle weakness
- speech difficulty
- sunken eyes
- confusion.

The mouth should be examined to assess oral health (Chapter 29) after the dentures are removed. The gums are inspected for ulcers due to poorly fitting dentures and the dentures for denture hygiene. Other conditions to note are tooth decay, periodontal disease and oral mucosal disease, such as leucoplakia, malignancy and candidiasis.

Vision

Visual acuity should be tested routinely and fundoscopy performed to check for cataracts, senile macular degeneration and for the changes due to hypertension and diabetes mellitus (Chapter 20). Suspicion of retinal abnormality warrants referral to an ophthalmologist. Intraocular pressure testing to screen for glaucoma is recommended every 2 years unless there are symptoms and/or a family history of glaucoma (Chapter 21).

Hearing

Hearing loss increases with age. High-frequency hearing loss is common and female voices may not be heard as distinctly as (deeper) male voices. Other contributory factors are drug toxicity. Medications that are ototoxic include aminoglycosides, such as gentamicin, tobramycin and neomycin (not used frequently except in topical preparations), cytotoxic agents (e.g. cisplatin and carboplatin) and high-dose loop diuretics (e.g. frusemide and ethacrynic acid). Erythromycin can cause transient deafness with high-dose intravenous use. Many elderly persons maintain that their hearing is unimpaired despite having hearing problems. Hearing loss seriously affects the health and well being of the older patient and often leads to social isolation and depression. Otitis externa should be looked for as it commonly occurs due to allergy or infection associated with the use of a hearing aid. It is essential to remove wax to visualise the tympanic membrane (Chapter 18). Causes of conduction deafness, such as wax impaction, a foreign body and, more rarely in the elderly, otitis media are easy to identify.

Neck

The neck should be examined for lumps, including the thyroid gland (Chapter 42), and for lymphadenopathy. If a lymph gland is larger than or equal to 2 cm or is firm, feels rubbery or hard and is not painful, malignancy should be excluded. Tender nodes are more likely to be due to acute infection. An unexplainable increase in lymph node size is also suspicious of malignancy. Left supraclavicular lymphadenopathy must be looked for as it may indicate, for example, an upper gastrointestinal malignancy, a lymphoma or melanoma. Palpation of the epitrochlear, axillary and inguinal lymph nodes completes the examination of the reticulo-nodular system. Table 3.2 lists some of the more common causes of lymphadenopathy. If lymphadenopathy is present, the abdomen should be

Table 3.2 Common causes of lymphadenopathy

Infective	Viral: Epstein-Barr virus, cytomegalovirus, hepatitis, human immunodeficiency virus Bacterial: *Streptococcus*, *Staphylococcus*, tuberculosis Fungal: histoplasmosis, coccidioidomycosis
Immunological	Rheumatoid arthritis, systemic lupus erythematosus, drug hypersensitivity
Malignant	Haematological, metastatic
Other	Hyperthyroidism, sarcoidosis

palpated for hepatomegaly and/or splenomegaly. Large intra-abdominal lymph nodes or other masses may also be palpable if malignancy is present.

Breasts

In women over the age of 50 an annual clinical examination of the breasts to screen for breast cancer is essential. Clinical examination of the breasts includes inspection and palpation. Inspection is performed with the patient sitting up. The breasts are checked for asymmetry, puckering of the skin, discolouration and nipple inversion. Nipples that have inverted due to benign processes can be everted with gentle pressure on either side of the nipple. A retracted nipple due to malignancy will not easily evert. The best position to examine for lumps is with the patient lying down with the arms raised above the head. The entire breast is examined, including the axillary tail and the area behind the nipple. Using the flat of the fingers rather than the tips aids the detection of significant lumps in the otherwise nodular breast tissue. Breast examination should include axillary and supraclavicular lymph node palpation.

Cardiovascular and respiratory systems

In the cardiovascular system, the peripheral pulses, including the temporal artery, should be palpated. A pulseless temporal artery may indicate arteritis or severe atherosclerosis. Other signs of temporal arteritis are a prominent artery and tenderness on palpation. The diagnosis of hypertension is ideally established by 24-hour blood-pressure monitoring. This eliminates 'white coat hypertension', which may persist despite serial visits to the doctor. In older patients, the view that high blood pressure, especially the common finding of elevated systolic pressure, should not be treated is incorrect. Evidence of end organ damage due to hypertension, such as cardiomegaly and retinopathy, should be sought. Postural changes in blood pressure are important to document. Postural hypotension is a decrease, on standing, in systolic blood pressure of 20 mmHg and in diastolic pressure of 10 mmHg. Postural hypotension is most often due to drugs such as tricyclic antidepressants, prolonged bed rest, low cardiac output from heart failure or autonomic dysfunction due to, for example, diabetes mellitus. The blood pressure and pulse rate are ideally measured half an hour after a meal to avoid prandial blood pressure reductions, after the patient has been lying down for at least 5 minutes and then recorded on standing, both immediately and, ideally, 2 minutes later. A drop in blood pressure with no accompanying rise in pulse rate reflects baroreceptor reflex impairment.

Bruits over the carotid arteries have a variety of possible causes. They may be due to carotid artery stenosis, increased flow in a normal carotid artery, narrowing in the external carotid artery, or the transmitted murmur of aortic stenosis. As such, carotid bruits are often of little discriminatory value in the older patient. Asymptomatic carotid artery stenosis in older patients is best ignored. Effort is best directed to possible symptoms of monocular visual loss or contralateral motor or sensory symptoms (Chapter 17). These are key pointers to a possible remedial lesion in the carotid. On cardiac auscultation, the most common murmurs heard in the elderly are due to aortic stenosis, aortic sclerosis and mitral regurgitation. The murmur of aortic sclerosis is not transmitted to the carotid arteries. An ejection click may not be heard due to calcification or fibrosis of the valve. In the elderly, the common causes of mitral regurgitation are left ventricular dilatation irrespective of aetiology, myocardial ischaemia leading to ischaemic damage and dysfunction of a papillary muscle, posterior mitral valve rupture or mitral valve prolapse. In older female patients, degeneration and calcification of the mitral annulus can cause regurgitation. Chronic rheumatic heart disease is the aetiological factor in many of these patients. The echocardiogram is invaluable to confirm the diagnosis of valvular abnormalities. In many older patients, the increasingly successful outcome of valvular surgery has significantly improved quality of life.

Features of a poor arterial supply are most evident on examining the legs, which show absent pulses and reduced capillary return, loss of hair, a waxy, thin, shiny skin, coolness to the touch, and the presence of ulcers over pressure areas. Another sign is increased pallor of the soles on raising the leg and flexing the calf, and redness when the legs are dependent. Signs of venous insufficiency include deeply pigmented skin from haemosiderin deposition, and often eczema.

In the lung bases, not infrequently, basal crackles that clear during coughing occur due to atelectasis. A high index of suspicion for pneumonia in older patients with an acute onset cough is important. The classic signs and symptoms are reduced or absent. Fever and tachycardia may not be present and dyspnoea not prominent. Indeed, the presentation may centre on non-respiratory symptoms such as weakness, functional decline, falls, vague abdominal symptoms and anorexia. Older patients with pulmonary tuberculosis (Chapter 50) present with similar symptoms to younger patients, namely fever, weight loss, chronic cough and haemoptysis. In communities with a low prevalence of tuberculosis, the elderly are at risk as these symptoms are often attributed to chronic bronchitis. Compared to younger patients, anorexia and weight loss are more frequent and night sweats less common.

Abdomen

Surgical scars, if present, would assist in obtaining more information on a surgical history. Spurious hepatomegaly could be due to ptosis from lung abnormalities associated with overexpanded lungs. The spleen is palpable only when it is enlarged one and a half to two times. The examination for the spleen should include rolling the patient partially on to the right side to palpate adequately below the left costal margin for enlargement.

Severe to moderate hepatomegaly in the older patient suggests malignancy (primary or metastatic), a myeloproliferative disorder (e.g. chronic myeloid leukaemia or myelofibrosis), a lymphoproliferative disorder, alcoholic liver disease, or right heart failure. Apart from right heart failure, these conditions, and chronic anaemias with shortened erythrocyte survival, may be associated with significant splenomegaly.

Abdominal examination should include checking for the pulsatile abdominal mass of an aortic aneurysm. Note that an acute abdomen in older persons may not have the classic features of rigidity, guarding and rebound as in younger patients, particularly if they are being treated with an inflammation suppressant such as a corticosteroid. Muscle mass may be minimal and therefore rigidity may not be a prominent feature. The bladder should be percussed and palpated for urinary retention, a not uncommon finding in the elderly. Chronic urine retention in older patients will commonly not produce a palpable bladder. A history of frequent 'wetting' or dribbling warrants ultrasonographic examination of the bladder. Portable office units are commonly used.

The perianal area is inspected for skin tags, fissures and abscesses. Digital rectal examination may detect faecal impaction or a mass that is suggestive of malignancy. An empty rectum on digital examination does not rule out the possibility of faecal impaction. The presence of blood or mucus on the glove indicates large bowel abnormality. Although there is debate regarding the value of routine digital rectal examination for detecting carcinoma of the prostate, the examination may nevertheless be of extreme value. Suspicious features include nodules, hardened areas and general enlargement.

Proctosigmoidoscopy is a valuable bedside investigation to detect rectal and anal abnormalities. The proctoscope, due to its rigidity and large diameter, overcomes the firm anal tone, enabling good visualisation of the anorectal region. Sigmoidoscopy is indicated in patients with a change in bowel habit, diarrhoea with blood and mucus or rectal bleeding, but should always be followed by an adequate examination of the entire large bowel.

Musculoskeletal

The musculoskeletal examination begins by observing how a patient walks, sits and rises from the chair or examination couch. Before the examination, screening questions should focus on simple activities of daily living. Both the axial and peripheral skeleton should be examined and the 'musculo' component of the musculoskeletal system not forgotten. Findings can then be efficiently recorded under the headings of gait, arms, legs and spine (GALS; Chapter 53).

Gynaecology

When examining the female genital tract, many factors related to ageing should be considered. For example, the older patient may not be able to flex and abduct the hips due to bilateral osteoarthritis. If so, the left lateral position is more convenient. The vulva is examined for thickening, ulceration or indurated areas suspicious of malignancy. Signs of inflammation include patch erythema, increased vascularity, friability and petechiae. The patient should be asked to bear down to check for prolapse, both anterior and posterior. The odour, colour and consistency of vaginal discharge are noted. In postmenopausal patients, the examination is more comfortable using a small speculum that still provides a good view of the vaginal walls and cervix. The Australian government National Health and Medical Research Council guidelines recommend that all women up to 70 years of age should have a Pap smear biannually to screen for precursors of cervical cancer. Pap smears are recommended for women over 70 years of age if they are healthy and can undergo the examination. A woman with a previous abnormality should be advised to have regular smears indefinitely. Women with symptoms of vaginal bleeding or discharge postmenopausally should be investigated. Inspection of the cervix is mandatory, and while a Pap smear may be part of the investigation, a normal Pap smear does not exclude other serious abnormalities. A specialist gynaecological opinion is advisable.

Central and peripheral nervous systems

Examining balance and gait is an essential part of a routine examination, especially if falls have occurred. The 'get up and go and return' test, whereby the patient leaves a chair to walk 10 m and turn, is most revealing and often overlooked. Cerebellar function is assessed by the finger–nose–finger test and the heel–knee–shin test, past pointing, intention tremor and general inco-ordination. Romberg's test is not a test of cerebellar function, but tests proprioception (a modality carried by the dorsal column). The test requires the patient, with eyes open, to stand with the feet together, to observe if balance is maintained. The test is repeated with the eyes closed. If unsteadiness occurs with the eyes closed, Romberg's test is positive, indicating reduced proprioception.

Numerous tests are available to detect gait abnormalities, ranging from single to complex (Chapter 13). The more common gait abnormalities are:

- *Ataxic* (cerebellar). Wide based, patient staggers to the affected side if there is a unilateral lesion. Midline lesions result in truncal ataxia. There is loss of balance on changing position.
- *Dyspraxic*. Here the patient is typically upright and has trouble initiating gait. Once gait is entrained, it may proceed without impediment until the patient turns, which produces a 'frozen' or 'slipping clutch' effect. In later stages, such gait may be both mildly ataxic and dyspraxic. Such gait failure can produce 'lower-half parkinsonism', wherein shortened gait is unaccompanied by upper limb dysfunction.
- *Hemiparetic*. The affected leg is flexed less than the non-affected leg and is more externally rotated. The leg is swung in an arc laterally to take a step. Examination of the shoe will often reveal differential wear in the toe and outer sole due to the equinovarus deformity of mild spasticity.
- *Parkinsonian*. There is a hesitancy in starting, a forward stoop with flexion at the hips and knees, and shuffling with acceleration of the pace, known as festinating.
- *Steppage*. Foot drop requiring the patient to lift the foot higher than usual to avoid hitting it on

the floor. This is typically a feature of a lower motor neuron lesion.

- *Waddling*. Due to proximal muscle weakness, the patient uses the trunk to help lift the leg by swinging to the opposite side of the leg, and then to the other side, producing a waddling gait.

Various types of tremor may occur in the elderly. The nature of the tremor suggests the aetiology. The classic tremor present at rest, described as 'pill-rolling', is due to Parkinson's disease (Chapter 14). This tremor disappears on willed movement and is exaggerated by movement of the contralateral limb. Postural tremor occurs when the limbs are outstretched but absent when the limb is relaxed. This type of tremor occurs with anxiety, thyrotoxicosis, benign essential tremor, which is commonly familial, β-adrenergic agonists (e.g. salbutamol, salmeterol and terbutaline) and as a manifestation of the withdrawal effects of drugs such as alcohol. Benign essential tremor occurs in later years and has been inappropriately termed 'senile tremor'. Essential tremor is a preferable term as it does not differ from that seen in people of younger years. The lower limbs are not affected. This familial tremor is partially suppressed by alcohol, barbiturates or β-adrenergic agents. Each of these agents has a potential adverse effect in older people and is not recommended as therapy. A more prominent tremor when movement is initiated, the intention tremor, is invariably due to cerebellar disease. The tremor is maximal at the extreme point of the movement.

In elderly patients, signs of peripheral neuropathy should be sought. Vibration and proprioception are the first modalities affected. Neuropathy begins peripherally and extends proximally with time. Light touch and pinprick sensory loss occur in the classic 'glove and stocking' distribution. A sensory neuropathy increases the risk of a foot ulcer in a diabetic person. The risk is greater in patients with reduced pain sensation in the feet, a bony prominence and/or poorly fitting shoes.

Skin

The aged skin is less elastic and demonstrates reduced tensile strength. A number of normal variants exist. Seborrhoeic warts are tan brown to darkly pigmented plaques 1–6 cm in diameter with a 'stuck on' appearance and are usually found on the trunk or face. Lentigines are flat, brown macules on sun-exposed skin. Purpura may be a normal finding often secondary to minor trauma but may arise spontaneously. The entire skin should be examined annually to check for malignancy. Solar (actinic) keratoses with further exposure to the sun may rarely progress to squamous cell carcinoma. These scaly hyperkeratotic lesions are usually less than 1 cm in diameter, and multiple.

Pressure ulcers occur over pressure areas such as the sacrum, buttocks and heels in bed- or chair-bound patients. Factors that contribute to an increased risk of development of pressure ulcers include immobility, malnutrition, reduced cutaneous sensation and arterial insufficiency. They begin as an area of erythema and progress to widespread necrosis and ulceration.

Conclusion

In summary, the clinician must regard illness not so much in a cloistered, disease-specific context but rather explore strategies to maintain the older person's independence and improve the quality of life. The patient–doctor interaction is also a powerful platform to promote the importance of disease prevention and early detection, especially of malignancy. Recent and increasing evidence supports the dramatic and rapid benefits that occur in the health status of an individual (even after years of neglect) by weight reduction through lifestyle changes. Even small amounts of exercise are of significant benefit. As little as 225 g of fish a week decreases the risk of stroke by half. Increased consumption of fruits, vegetables and fibre alters the sensitivity to insulin within 2 weeks, thus decreasing the risk of diabetes. Cessation of cigarette smoking dramatically decreases carbon dioxide levels within 24 hours and decreases blood viscosity within a week.

In the ideal clinical interview, the medical practitioner should have addressed the patient's illness and explored strategies to maintain the older person's independence and improve quality of life.

Bibliography and further reading

Chan, E. D. & Welsh, C. H. (1998), 'Geriatric respiratory medicine', *Chest*, 114, pp. 1704–33.

Davis, P. B. & Robins, L. N. (1989), 'History-taking in the elderly with and without cognitive impairment. How useful is it?', *Journal of the American Geriatrics Society*, 37, pp. 249–55.

Espino, D., Jules-Bradley, A. C. A., Johnston, C. & Mouton, C. P. (1998), 'Diagnostic approach to the confused elderly patient', *American Family Physician*, 57, pp. 1358–66.

Folstein, M. F., Folstein, S. E. & McHugh, P. R. (1975), 'Mini mental state: a practical method for grading the cognitive state of patients for the clinician', *Journal of Psychiatric Research*, 57, pp. 189–98.

Gawkrodger, D. J. (1997), 'The skin in old age', in Gawkrodger, D. J. (ed.), *Dermatology. An Illustrated Colour Text*, Churchill Livingstone, New York, pp. 110–12.

Gross, C. R., Lindquist, R. D., Woolley A. C., Granieri, R., Allard, K. & Webster, B. (1992), 'Clinical indicators of dehydration severity in elderly patients', *Journal of Emergency Medicine*, 10, pp. 267–74.

Jarrett, P. G., Rockwood, K., Carver, D., Stolee, P. & Cosway, S. (1995), 'Illness presentation in elderly patients', *Archives of Internal Medicine*, 155, pp. 1060–4.

Kane, R. L., Ouslander, J. G. & Abrass, I. B. (eds). (1994), *Essentials of Clinical Geriatrics*, 3rd edn, McGraw-Hill, New York.

Lipsitz, L. A. (1989), 'Orthostatic hypotension in the elderly', *The New England Journal of Medicine*, 321, pp. 952–7.

Nathan, L. (1996), 'Vulvovaginal disorders in the elderly woman', *Clinical Obstetrics and Gynecology*, 39, pp. 993–95.

Pedersen, K. V., Carlsson, P., Varenhorst, E., Lofman, O. & Berglund, K. (1990), 'Screening for carcinoma of the prostate by digital rectal examination in a randomly selected population', *British Medical Journal*, 300, pp. 1041–3.

Quail, G. G. (1994), 'An approach to the assessment of falls in the elderly', *Australian Family Physician*, 23, pp. 873–82.

Swannell, A. J. (1997), 'Polymyalgia rheumatica and temporal arteritis: diagnosis and management', *British Medical Journal*, 314, pp. 1329–32.

Vestal, R. E. (1997), 'Aging and pharmacology', *Cancer*, 80, pp. 1302–9.

Chapter 4

Functional assessment: 75+ Health Assessment in Australia

JONATHAN NEWBURY and JULIE BYLES

Introduction

'Anticipatory care' of the independent elderly was proposed by Williamson et al. in 1964 following their study of the 65 and over population. They were distressed with the advanced stage of disease in which people were presenting to geriatric units. They advocated that 'timely medical and social intervention might have prevented much of the disability'. Acknowledging that consulting the general practitioner (GP) was the main way in which needs were met, they attempted to discover how many of these needs were recognised by the person's GP. Their results were a 'striking observation of the frequency of multiple disabilities', more than half of which were unknown to the GP.

Williamson et al. emphasise the importance of preventive health care in the elderly, arguing that there are few conditions where early intervention will not be of some help. Given their reported incidence of unmet needs, they proposed a system of 'periodic examination' to include all old people. This system would depend on an up-to-date practice register, nurses or allied health professionals to conduct 'screening on behalf of the GP' and would focus on functional ability, depression, social services, diet, budgeting and avoidance of accidents in the home. Thirty-five years later in Australia we are instituting a system of 75+ Health Assessments similar to that proposed by Williamson et al. in 1964.

A number of trials of functional assessment of the elderly at home have been undertaken. Mostly these studies have been in Great Britain, Europe and the US. The form of the assessment has varied but functional ability has been the common theme. Home based assessments have been demonstrated to yield the most information. Nurses or allied health professionals have performed most of the assessments. Medical practitioners, mostly GPs, have the task of integrating the information and co-ordinating service provision by local agencies.

Several publications have reviewed this system of health care (see the 'Bibliography and further reading' list at the end of this chapter). They have tried to establish if the elderly have improved outcome from this form of care.

Stuck et al. conducted a meta-analysis of Comprehensive Geriatric Assessment (CGA) trials. They included the results from 28 controlled trials of five different types of CGA, comprising 4859 intervention and 4912 control participants. One of the five types of CGA involved home based functional assessments. They found that the trials with more intensive supervision of recommendations and more ambulatory follow-up increased the proportion of participants remaining independent in their own home. However, such quantitative overviews are fraught with difficulty when the interventions compared are widely heterogeneous.

Van Haastregt et al. have recently published a qualitative systematic review. They included all trials conducted in people 65 years and over. Overall they report findings of erratic improvement in physical functioning, psychosocial functioning, falls, admission to institutions and mortality. Further analysis of their results suggest that improvement is much more likely if this system of care is provided for people 75 years and over.

A similar review published in the *Australian and New Zealand Journal of Public Health* concluded that the majority of the more rigorous and scientifically valid trials did observe improvements in health in the intervention group. However, it was difficult to determine which aspects of assessments were associated with improvement in outcome.

Protocol for home visit

Assessment involves the formal examination of a person's health and functional status. There is no standard list or structure for the conduct of 75+ Health Assessments, but they should include medical history and medications, lifestyle, hearing and vision, activities of daily living, home safety, cognition, mood and social support. There should be less emphasis on physical examination and laboratory testing and a greater emphasis on patient education and counselling for healthy lifestyle. 75+ Health Assessment must also include some expectation of and mechanism for effective treatment. Frequently, only minimal assistance or intervention is required, and the needs may be more for social and instrumental support or aids than for medical intervention. Assessments should be structured so that repeated measures can be compared and require methods that are accurate in discriminating those people who have problems and needs from those who do not. The discrimination of health and illness is much more difficult when dealing with older patients. Assessment is complicated by multiple co-morbidities, multiple aetiologies and degradation of clinical information. It is therefore important to apply assessment methods that are:

- sensitive in correctly identifying those people who have the condition of interest
- specific in correctly classifying those people who do not have the condition of interest
- reliable in providing consistent results when applied by different people, at different times, in different circumstances (the underlying condition being unchanged)
- sensitive to change in the true condition of the individual being assessed
- feasible to administer, brief and acceptable to the elderly
- easy to score or interpret.

Importantly, results of any formal instrument used in the assessment must be interpreted taking into account clinical judgment and the individual's values and circumstances: symptoms, co-morbidities, functional capacity and resources. Needs and actions should be determined in negotiation with the person and/or her carers.

In Australia the Enhanced Primary Care (EPC) package was implemented from 1 November 1999. Part of the EPC is new Medicare (Australia's universal health insurance scheme) item numbers for annual health assessments for people aged 75 years and over (75+ Health Assessments). Guidelines for these item numbers are that they are for a GP's patients only and can be performed in the GP's consulting rooms or in the patients' homes. These item numbers are not available for inpatients of hospitals or day hospital facilities or residents of nursing homes. Importantly, the information collection component can be performed 'on behalf of' a GP by nursing or allied health staff under the supervision of the GP. 75+ Health Assessments should not be in the form of screening by diagnostic imaging or pathology testing. The Medicare item number description stresses the importance of assessing the person's 'health and physical, psychological and social functioning'. Nurses or other allied health professionals conducting home visits need to be able to interpret the relatively rigid assessment instruments based on their clinical skill. Experience in Great Britain suggests that nurses or allied health professionals are more suited to performing this data collection phase than GPs. The assessment should then prompt preventive health care and education initiatives. Conceptually this means creating an integrated picture of the elderly person's functioning and the potential that exists to improve her functional abilities.

A suggested protocol for a 75+ Health Assessment that fulfils these criteria is described in the format given in Box 4.1.

Box 4.1 Components of 75+ Health Assessment

Medical history
- Self-rated health
- Past medical history
- Diabetes
- Feet and footcare
- Blood pressure
- Pulse rate and rhythm
- Body mass index
- Medication
- Hormone replacement therapy

Lifestyle
- Immunisation
- Smoking
- Alcohol
- Sleep
- Oral health
- Nutrition

Functional status
- Hearing
- Vision
- Activities of Daily Living/Barthel Index
- Continence
- Gait, balance and falls
- Home safety

Cognition and mood
- Cognitive function
- The Folstein Mini-Mental State Examination
- Abbreviated Mental Test Score
- Mood/depression

Social
- Social and community services
- Physical activities

Medical history

Self-rated health

Subjective appraisals of health are robust predictors of functional transitions and mortality even when activities of daily living are impaired. The simple 'Self-rated health' question is 'How would you rate your health?' and the choice of answers are poor, fair, good, very good and excellent. Reporting health status as excellent or very good is strongly associated with less disability over the subsequent two years and a lower probability of death or institutionalisation after adjusting for other co-variates.

Past medical history

A review of symptoms and medical problems is useful in accounting for co-morbidity and for identifying health problems that may not be presented by the patient without prompting. Physical problems need to be asked about with an emphasis on whether they have resolved or remain ongoing. A fracture sustained in a fall that has healed is no longer a problem but a tendency to fall again is a problem. A complete physical examination may be easier if left for a subsequent consultation at the surgery.

Diabetes

There are two facets of diabetes management that can be targeted in the 75+ Health Assessment: early diagnosis and monitoring. Advice on the specific management of non-insulin dependent diabetes mellitus (NIDDM) can be found in Chapter 41.

Early diagnosis

It is worth inquiring about symptoms of diabetes, particularly polydipsia and polyuria. Large numbers of people with diabetes are not diagnosed early. Even once the condition is clinically apparent, the diagnosis is often delayed. The symptoms of NIDDM may be present without the patient being aware of their significance. Alternatively, the presence of other problems may indicate the need for a diabetes test (heart disease, cataracts, overweight, leg ulcers, skin infections, etc.). This group of undiagnosed diabetics can be detected easily with a fasting sugar. The important principle in 75+ Health Assessment is clinical acumen, not merely an annual screen with a number of pathology and imaging tests.

Monitoring

For those with diabetes, the assessment provides an opportunity to check for problems with management and monitoring. Intensive management of NIDDM has a beneficial effect on outcomes by reduction in frequency and severity of complications. Advancing years and longer duration of NIDDM is also associated with increasing difficulty in maintaining control. Insulin resistance in peripheral tissues increases and medications become less effective. Medication regimens become more complex and complications, such as peripheral neuropathy and visual impairment, make insulin self-treatment harder to achieve. Good control is best achieved through co-ordinating services with allied health staff (dietitians, diabetic nurses, podiatrists, etc.) and medical specialists (ophthalmologists, physicians, endocrinologists, etc.).

Feet and footcare

Almost 80% of the population over the age of 50 will suffer at some time from at least one significant foot problem. Early detection of abnormalities allows for appropriate management for existing conditions, prompt referral for specialist care, and provides an opportunity for patient education to prevent further foot problems. A simple approach is to ask 'Do you have problems with one or both feet?', but there are also standard screening tools available (see Box 4.2).

Box 4.2 Foot care assessment

FOOT CARE ASSESSMENT

Name: **Date:**

Previous Medical History:
Arthritis
Bunions
Diabetes
Hammertoes
Pain
Peripheral vascular disease
Smoking
Spurs
Trauma
Ulcerations
Vision problems
Have you fallen in the past year?

Observe:
Gait
- Proper
- Improper
- Devices

Box continues

Box 4.2 *continued*

Ambulates
- With help
- Without help

Foot hygiene
- Proper
- Improper
- Specify

Footwear
- Proper
- Improper
- Specify

Assess (normal, abnormal)	**Problem**	**Location**	**Describe:**
Colour	Callus		
Pulses	Corn		
Structure	Cracks/ulcerations		
Temperature	Oedema		
	Long toenails		
	Thick toenails		
	Other		

Comments

Interventions: **Describe:**

Foot soak

Foot hygiene

Toenails
- Trimmed

Corns/calluses
- Buffed

Foot massage

Follow-up plan:

Return appointment: **Referral to:**

Nurse:

Source: T. Kelechi & K. Lukacs (1991), 'Nursing foot care for the aged', *Journal of Gerontological Nursing*, 17, pp. 40–3.

Blood pressure

There is a well established and strong relationship between high blood pressure (> 90 mmHg diastolic; > 140 mmHg systolic) and mortality, particularly from stroke and myocardial infarction. Blood pressure needs to be reviewed and mercury sphygmomanometry in the GP's clinic is the most appropriate screening test. Measurement is subject to error due to instrument, observer and patient related factors. It is therefore recommended that hypertension be diagnosed only after more than one elevated reading is obtained over 6 measurements, conducted on 3 separate clinic visits. Use of self-measured (home) blood pressure and ambulatory blood pressure monitoring in screening is not supported by evidence. There is better justification for measuring blood pressure in a subsequent clinic consultation rather than at the home visit.

Interpretation of the recorded blood pressure depends on the indications for treatment and current guidelines of blood pressure reduction. Considerable evidence supports the benefits of treating hypertension in the elderly. The 75+ Health Assessment provides an opportunity to enquire whether blood pressure has been measured, to check whether treatment has been initiated or maintained, and to review any problems associated with antihypertensive medications (e.g. postural hypotension, sleep disturbance).

Pulse rate and rhythm

Pulse rate and rhythm need to be checked; look paticularly for atrial fibrillation. Embolic stroke and briefer cerebral ischaemic events may be prevented by using antiplatelet agents such as aspirin. Other sources of potential emboli are damaged areas of myocardium, prosthetic valves and carotid artery atheroma. Large scale trials in patients with recent or remote myocardial infarction have shown a substantial reduction in the incidence of subsequent stroke among patients treated with aspirin. Low dose warfarin can substantially reduce stroke (by up to 86%) with minimal risk of significant haemorrhage.

Body mass index

Body mass index (BMI) is calculated to identify obesity or underweight as a surrogate measure for inappropriate nutrition (see Chapters 30 and 32). Height and weight are measured and then BMI calculated (weight/height^2, where weight is in kilograms and height in metres). A BMI of less than 20 kg/m^2 suggests undernutrition; a BMI greater than 30 suggests overweight. The relationship between BMI and health in older persons is controversial. There appears to be a 'U'-shaped relationship between BMI and mortality, and optimum BMI for health increases with age.

Medication

A multitude of problems can occur with medication use in the elderly. Inappropriate medication use in the elderly is frequently associated with adverse reactions and poor health outcomes. Common problems include the use of drugs that accumulate (due to altered drug metabolism), high doses or duplicate doses, interactions between medications, and problems with side effects and/or compliance. Polypharmacy (defined as 4 or more regular medications) is also common among the elderly and increases the risk of adverse medication effects and drug interactions (see also Chapter 5).

Periodic review of medications is an essential component of care in the elderly, but does not occur routinely. The most useful function is to visit the home and inspect the 'pharmacy'. Non-prescription medications need to be included in this assessment, whether they are over-the-counter medicines, herbal or naturopathic remedies. Record what is actually being taken. Any apparent problems in compliance and interactions arising from prescriptions from different doctors unaware of each other's prescriptions should be noted. The elderly may be inclined to hoard medication even from their departed spouse, they may not get prescriptions filled or open bottles that have been dispensed. A gentle inquiry couched in sensitive terms will usually reveal the real picture of their medication consumption. Decisions about a prepackaged medication system from pharmacy or carer are easier to make when the formal assessment of cognition has been completed.

Common interactions to be alert for include:

- warfarin with allopurinol and/or thyroxine (both potentiate the actions of warfarin)
- amiodarone and diltiazem (can have additive effects on cardiac muscle)
- digoxin with amiodorone, quinidine or verapamil (reduced clearance of digoxin)
- theophylline and allopurinol (increased plasma theophylline concentrations)
- amiloride and potassium (increased risk of hyperkalaemia)
- methotrexate and non-steroidal anti-inflammatory drugs (increased risk of methotrexate toxicity)

Hormone replacement therapy

Cross-sectional, case control and cohort studies suggest that long-term postmenopausal oestrogen therapy has important effects on a number of clinical outcomes, including prevention of osteoporotic fractures, coronary heart disease and lipids, cerebrovascular disease, vulvovaginal atrophy and relief of urogenital symptoms. However, prolonged use of unopposed oestrogen therapy is associated with increased risk of endometrial hyperplasia and endometrial cancer. The effect on breast cancer risk is uncertain.

Lifestyle

Immunisation

You should ask about the patient's immunisation status for tetanus, influenza and pneumococcus. National Health and Medical Research Council (NHMRC) advice for people above the age of 65 years is to repeat:

- tetanus vaccine once only over age 50 years, if fully vaccinated previously
- pneumococcal vaccine every 5 years
- influenza vaccine every year in the immediate pre-winter period.

Information on all three vaccinations should be entered into a general practice recall system. This would provide a prompt when the next dose is due. An effective recall system should obviate the need to inquire annually about immunisation status once all patient data are entered.

Smoking

While many have quit, a proportion of people 75 and over are current smokers. Quitting smoking will reduce the risk of heart disease and lung cancer even for those in their 70s and after a myocardial infarct. Face-to-face advice to quit is effective, is reinforced by increasing the number of people giving advice, and the number of times and ways in which the advice is given.

All adults should be asked if they smoke cigarettes, pipes or cigars. Smokers should be advised to quit and should be provided with brief motivational counselling emphasising the risks of smoking and the benefits of quitting. Assess readiness to change. For those who are ready to quit, assist by setting a quit date, identifying triggers, providing self-help materials, arranging follow-up visits and considering referral to a quit program. For smokers who are not ready to quit, reassess the readiness to quit at every opportunity.

Alcohol

Problems may be apparent as a result of current drinking or past heavy consumption. The incidence of alcohol consumption, like smoking, is less in this age group but occasionally a serious problem exists. Denial of problem drinking is common in the elderly and it may not be obvious in a surgery consultation. A home visit has the advantage of revealing visual clues such as the state of the home, presence of alcohol and general observations of self-neglect. In addition, past heavy alcohol consumption, even though the patient may no longer drink, can result in cerebellar impairment, causing unsteadiness and falls. Alcoholic cirrhosis is uncommon in the elderly as frequently it has taken its toll at a younger age.

Screening to detect problem drinking is recommended for all adults. Brief, structured questionnaires, suitable for use in clinical practice and with acceptable validity, include the CAGE (see Box 4.3) and the 10 item AUDIT (see 'Bibliography and further reading' list).

Box 4.3 The CAGE questionnaire to detect problem drinking

C: Have you ever felt you ought to **C**ut down on drinking?

A: Have people **A**nnoyed you by criticising your drinking?

G: Have you ever felt bad or **G**uilty about your drinking?

E: Have you ever had a drink first thing in the morning to steady your nerves or to get rid of a hangover (**E**ye opener)?

Source: J. Ewing (1984), 'Detecting alcoholism. The CAGE questionnaire', *Journal of the American Medical Association*, 252, pp. 1905–7. Copyright (1984) American Medical Association.

Sleep

Sleeping difficulty is common among older people, particularly women. However, the fact that older people sleep less is not a rationale for ignoring the subjective complaint of 'difficulty sleeping' and for simply writing this off to 'old age'. It has been argued that for older people it is the ability to sleep that is diminished and not the need for sleep. Sleep disturbance can be associated with clinical conditions, such as cardiovascular and respiratory disease, and people who complain of difficulty sleeping have been shown to be at increased risk of clinical depression. Other potential causes of sleeping difficulty include urinary incontinence and frequency, arthritis and joint pain, medications and sleep apnoea. The sleeping habits of the partner may also be the cause of disturbed sleep. All of these possible causes provide paths for intervention that should be considered before initiating drug therapy.

A simple question is 'Do you have trouble sleeping?', but more can be elicited using questions from the Nottingham Health Profile (see Box 4.4).

Regular benzodiazepine use is contraindicated in this age group. Benzodiazepine use incurs adverse consequences, such as drowsiness, confusion, ataxia, dizziness and impaired motor co-ordination. Increased risk of falling and fall related fractures are serious consequences. Physiological changes associated with ageing lead to changes in pharmacokinetic processes (absorption, distribution, metabolism and excretion) and may predispose older people to adverse effects. Long elimination half-lives and accumulation of commonly used sleeping tablets may lead to enhanced severity of adverse effects in older people. Negotiating an effective strategy for benzodiazepine withdrawal leads to success in a significant number of long-term users.

Box 4.4 Do you have trouble sleeping?

- Do you take tablets to help sleep?
- Do you wake early in the morning?
- Do you lie awake most of the night?
- Does it take a long time to get to sleep?
- Do you sleep badly?

Source: S. M. Hunt, S. P. McKenna, J. McEwen, J. Williams & E. Papp (1981), 'The Nottingham Health Profile: Subjective health status and medical consultations', *Social Science and Medicine [A]*, 15(3 Pt 1), pp. 221–9.

Appropriate management of sleeping difficulty obviously depends on the underlying cause, and it is important to recognise that chronic insomnia has many causes. Behavioural interventions provide a simple, safe and effective alternative to drug therapy, and appear to produce more sustained effects. Other alternatives include reassurance, sleep hygiene (such as limited use of nicotine, caffeine and alcohol), regular exercise, avoidance of daytime naps, avoidance of heavy meals before sleep, and relaxation techniques. Medication review is also a pillar in the effective management of sleep disturbance.

Oral health

The purpose of assessing oral health is to identify teeth, mouth and swallowing problems that may interfere with the older person's dietary intake and social functions. One standard method is the D-E-N-T-A-L (see Box 4.5). Compared to physical examination, D-E-N-T-A-L has a sensitivity of 82% and a specificity of 90% for detecting 'compromising oral health conditions'.

Specific questions about dentition should be included, particularly as dentures become loose with wear and resorption of bone in maxilla and mandible (see also Chapter 29).

Nutrition

Many older adults suffer from protein-kilojoule malnutrition which is often underdiagnosed, and can have serious consequences for cognitive and physical performance and overall sense of wellbeing. Older people can also have special nutritional requirements and it can be necessary to modify recommended daily intake levels of kilojoules, sodium, calcium, water, dietary fat, fibre, protein and other nutrients. Nutritional status reflects dietary intake and metabolic processes and interactions (see also Chapter 30). Nutritional status can be assessed from

Box 4.5 D-E-N-T-A-L Screening Initiative (St Louis University Health Sciences Center, Division of Geriatric Medicine)

Certain dental conditions have been known to interfere with proper nutritional intake possibly disposing a person to involuntary weight loss. Please answer the following questions regarding your dental health by placing a check in the box of those conditions which apply to you.

	Point value
☐ Dry mouth	2
☐ Eating difficulty	1
☐ No recent dental care (within 2 years)	1
☐ Tooth or mouth pain	2
☐ Alteration or change in food selection	1
☐ Lesions, sores, or lumps in the mouth	2

If you have scored more than 2 points on this survey you may have a dental problem which could be affecting your overall health and general wellbeing. We urge you to seek dental care as soon as possible for a check.

Source: L. A. Bush, N. Horenkamp, J. E. Morley & A. Spiro III (1996), 'D-E-N-T-A-L: A rapid self-administered screening instrument to promote referrals for further evaluation in older adults', *Journal of the American Geriatrics Society*, 44, pp. 979–81.

anthropomorphic measures such as height and weight (see earlier) and measures of fat distribution such as waist–hip ratio or skin-fold thickness. Dietary intake can be assessed from food records and food frequency questionnaires, but these all have obvious problems with accuracy of recall. Nutrition screening initiatives have been established in the US and Australia, but direct evidence of clinical benefit is not yet apparent.

The Australian Nutritional Screening Initiative (ANSI) is a screening tool designed to detect older people at risk of poor nutrition but is not diagnostic of a nutritional problem. The ANSI checklist has been described as more appropriately used as a basis for nutrition counselling. Questions include weight loss, alcohol intake, three or more medications, fluid intake and whether they eat alone (see Box 4.6). There is overlap among the ANSI questions with questions that may be asked in other parts of a 75+ Health Assessment. ANSI is very sensitive (but may lack specificity), as answers suggesting risk to any two of the questions places the person in the 'moderate risk' (4–5) or 'high risk' (6+) groups. In practice approximately 60% of the 75+ age group have scores suggesting moderate or high nutrition risk. Interpretation of the risk category, further assessment requirements with a dietitian and consideration of ability to bring about change in the elderly person's nutrition will influence decisions about how to proceed. Divisions of general practice in Australia have improved the availability of nutritionists.

Functional status

Hearing

Hearing declines with age in most people and is quite marked in some people. The loss can be due to a variety of mechanical and neurological processes. There is a strong tendency for people to deny hearing loss, compounding the social consequences of the hearing impairment. These consequences include isolation, depression and low self-esteem. On a day-to-day basis the functional ability of the hearing is most important. Can the elderly person hear conversation in social settings? Can she hear danger approaching when driving or walking/crossing roads? Hearing tests are of limited use in the elderly. Precise measurement of hearing levels at different pitch is useful for diagnosis but this is rarely an issue in this age group. The recommended methods for screening for hearing loss in older people include patient self-report and simple clinical techniques, such as the whisper test. The whisper test is reported to have sensitivity and specificity of 70–100% using pure-tone audiometry as the 'gold standard'. Self-assessment questionnaires to identify hearing impairment have been said to be the most rapid and least expensive way of screening for hearing loss in the adult (70–80% accurate).

Box 4.6 Australian Nutrition Screening Initiative

	YES	NO
Do you have an illness or condition that has made you change the kind and/or amount of food you eat	☐ 2	☐ 0
Do you eat at least three meals per day?	☐ 0	☐ 3
Do you eat fruit or vegetables most days?	☐ 0	☐ 2
Do you eat dairy products most days?	☐ 0	☐ 2
Do you have three or more glasses of beer, wine or spirits almost every day?	☐ 3	☐ 0
Do you have 6 to 8 cups of fluid (e.g. water, juice, tea or coffee) most days?	☐ 0	☐ 1
Do you have teeth, mouth, or swallowing problems that make it hard for you to eat?	☐ 4	☐ 0
Do you always have enough money to buy food?	☐ 0	☐ 3
Do you eat alone most of the time?	☐ 2	☐ 0
Do you take 3 or more different prescribed or over-the-counter medicines every day?	☐ 3	☐ 0
Have you lost or gained 5 kg in the last 6 months, without wanting to?	☐ 2	☐ 0
Are you always able to shop, cook and/or feed yourself?	☐ 0	☐ 2

Source: P. Lipski (1996), 'Australian Nutrition Screening Initiative', *Australian Journal on Ageing*, 15, pp. 14–17.

The traditional solution to hearing loss has been electronic amplification by hearing aids. Hearing aids can be effective but are underprescribed and underused. The amplification can distort sound and so hearing is not necessarily improved by the wearing of a hearing aid. In addition, vanity and comfort are significant contributors to not wearing aids. Size of devices has decreased with improvements in electronics, although cost is significantly greater for smaller devices. Flat batteries need replacement but this task requires nimble fingers. The elderly frequently lose sight of the fact that hearing aids do not work if they are not in the ears! Alterations in hearing over a short time frame are frequently due to changes in the hearing aid in use. Wax can clog the orifice of the aid or the external ear canal. Options for removing wax include syringing, wax-softening oils and solutions for dissolving wax (see also Chapter 18).

To maximise the hearing of the hearing impaired elderly person, it is recommended that you follow these guidelines:

- Inquire whether the hearing aid is being worn regularly.
- Check the age of the aid.
- Check and, if necessary, replace the battery.
- Accept that better quality aids are more expensive.
- Accept that more expensive aids are less intrusive to wear and more acceptable to the vain elderly.
- Clean obstructing wax out of ear canals and the orifices of hearing aids.
- Provide advice about high frequency sounds being harder to hear and the confusion of sounds when more than one person is speaking. Hearing will be facilitated by having to listen to one person only in a quiet room.
- Telephones can have amplified ringing tones to increase the likelihood of the deaf hearing them, as well as lights that flash when they 'ring'. In Australia these facilities are provided free to the hearing impaired by Telstra.

Vision

The functional problem frequently encountered is deterioration of vision that has not been noticed, reported to a professional or investigated. Visual impairment is strongly related to age, and the most common disorders are age-related lens changes, cataract, age-related macular degeneration, chronic open angle glaucoma and diabetic retinopathy. Some of the pathologies causing visual loss are amenable to prevention (diabetic retinopathy), treatment (cataract surgery) or are assisted by refraction (diminished acuity). For some, however, there are limited therapeutic options. The frequently occurring pathologies and treatments are:

- Diabetes mellitus (usually type 2): insulin resistance increases with age and treatment to achieve good sugar control becomes more difficult. Newer treatments (e.g. glitazones) are aimed at decreasing insulin resistance.
- Cataracts may have specific causes but importantly have one remedy: surgery. Cataract extraction and intra-ocular lens implantation has become progressively more refined. Day case surgery is now the norm, recovery is quicker and vision is predictably better.
- Macular degeneration is a leading cause of blindness in this age group in our society. Laser therapy is of some use but continuing deterioration is common. Occasionally this deterioration occurs as sudden change that can be helped with laser therapy as an urgent procedure.
- Field defects are most commonly due to cerebrovascular accidents affecting the occipital cortex or more proximally in the optic pathway. Secondary prevention can be achieved through antiplatelet agents (aspirin), antihypertensive agents and cessation of smoking.

Simple assessment of visual acuity can be performed by self-report, or using the distance-vision (Snellen) chart. Compared to the Snellen chart, self-report is less sensitive in detecting loss of visual acuity. However, a brief 3 item questionnaire used in the Wisconsin Epidemiologic Survey of Diabetic Retinopathy has been shown to have 86% sensitivity and 90% specificity (Fryback et al. 1993).

On a more mundane level we can usefully inquire as follows:

- What visual aids are in use (glasses, bifocals, contacts or magnifying lens)?
- How recently have glasses been prescribed?
- If not newly prescribed, has the prescription been checked in the recent past?
- Do they help with vision? Are they being worn for a problem not amenable to correction of acuity? Has a cataract developed but not been assessed because the person has assumed deterioration was occurring for some other reason?

Further discussion of visual impairment and cataracts can be found in Chapter 20.

Activities of Daily Living/Barthel Index

Measures of functional status include Activities of Daily Living (ADL) and Instrumental Activities of Daily Living (IADL). Rather than measure physical impairment, these measures assess the interaction between the individual, her impairment (if any) and her environment. The focus is on the individual's independence in performing daily activities.

A number of standard instruments, including the Barthel Index of ADL, are available. In well populations, these instruments have limited use because most people will achieve high scores. The main uses are to assess change in function over time, and to assess rehabilitation and needs for institutional care.

The Medical Outcomes Study measurement of physical functioning offers an extended ADL scale that is sensitive to variations at relatively high levels of physical function (see 'Bibliography and further reading').

Again an holistic understanding of the individual is more important than the number scored with these instruments. Frequently the elderly will be unable to climb stairs because of severe osteoarthritis, but a 75+ Health Assessment will include an inspection of the stairs, if any, in their home.

Continence

Urinary incontinence is common among older people. In the Australian Longitudinal Study on

Women's Health the prevalence of 'leaking urine' among community-dwelling women aged 70–75 years was 35%. The condition is also common among older men due to prostatic obstruction (see also Chapters 39 and 40).

A major problem in the management of incontinence is that many cases go unreported, with only around one-third of people reporting the problem to their doctor. Similarly, it is estimated that fewer than 4% of patients with faecal incontinence receive medical attention (see also Chapter 36). A first step in continence management, then, has to be raising awareness of the problem and encouraging reporting. A simple inquiry may be all that is required to give the person the opportunity to discuss her problem.

Incontinence has many causes and treatments. Prevention and treatment of stress incontinence is possible through protection and strengthening of the pelvic floor. Improvement can also be achieved through bladder retraining, medications and surgery. In intractable cases, social continence can be achieved through the use of pads and other devices, allowing the person to continue to enjoy her life.

Gait, balance and falls

A stable, safe gait is vital for independence with functional activities of daily living. Impaired gait and balance function has been shown to be an important risk factor for falls (see also Chapters 13 and 19). Being unable to stand unassisted on one leg for 5 seconds has been shown to be associated with a doubled risk of falls. Exercise has been shown to be effective in improving gait and balance. The Tinetti Gait and Balance test is the most widely used tool for measuring gait and balance. Tinetti et al. (1990) have also developed a Falls Efficacy Scale which is a 10 item self-report measure of fear of falling to the extent that this fear may impact on activity and function (see 'Bibliography and further reading').

Recent falls are an indicator of the likelihood of subsequent falls. With the annual use of 75+ Health Assessments, it seems necessary to ask about falls in the last 12 months or since last assessment. Was she able to get herself up after a fall or did she need to summon assistance? Was a satisfactory explanation of the fall found? The elderly frequently have an excuse to explain why they fell rather than an honest evaluation of their balance problem.

Currently under trial is the 'stops walking when talking' test. If the elderly stop walking in order to reply when spoken to, they are at increased risk of falls. Falls may indicate the need for mobility aids (stick, Zimmer frames, etc.) and existing aids should be reviewed for their appropriateness, including size.

Home safety

Housing assessment requires a guided tour of the home by the elderly person. Inspection of the bathroom and toilet for safety is most important. If rails are already installed, are they in the correct place and strong enough? Bedroom aids may be necessary for the patient or for the carer's benefit. Is the kitchen safe? Information can be gathered surreptitiously. Always say 'yes' to the offered cup of tea and watch it being made. Is he safe in the kitchen with balance, dexterity and memory? Standard checklists can be used to identify home hazards.

Several specific environmental risk factors thought to be implicated in falls have been identified. These include inadequate lighting, bed too high/low, slippery floors, loose electrical cords, cluttered passageways, decreased visual stimuli on walls, unstable or inadequate furniture, lack of definition of steps, kitchen storage too high/low, insufficient light on stairs, slippery shower/bath area, slippery floor surfaces, no stair rails, unstable towel rails used for support, steps too high, toilet seat too low, difficult door locks/handles, outside toilets and hazards outside the house. Many of these items are only relevant in the presence of a functional deficit, additional to the environmental problem.

Cognition and mood

Cognitive function

Dementia screening has been included in all the studies of functional assessment programs for older people. The benefits of detecting dementia before patients are severely impaired include: treatment of reversible causes, treatment to slow progression of disease, measures to reduce morbidity, and preparation and support for carers. Dementia is an area where research evidence is accumulating rapidly, and must be carefully monitored to allow appropriate policy and practice.

The Folstein Mini-Mental State Examination

One of the most commonly used screening tests is the Folstein Mini-Mental State Examination (MMSE). This 30 item test is traditionally the 'gold standard' by which others are judged (see Box 4.7). Reproducibility of the test requires careful, consistent administration. Several variations of instruction on how to administer the test are in use. Consistent use of one protocol will increase confidence in application and interpretation. To avoid embarrassment, explain it as a 'test of memory'. This will quickly engender some pride in those elderly successfully answering questions. Those unable to answer often display no embarrassment at their inability. As with all aspects of assessing the elderly at home, an honest non-threatening approach quickly builds a therapeutic relationship.

The MMSE result can be interpreted in terms of deficits in certain areas of testing (e.g. recall, orientation, etc.) or as an overall score. Allowance should be made for acute illnesses (fever, hyperglycaemia, confusion, etc.) that temporarily impair cerebral function. A score of 25 or greater is taken as normal. A score of 19–24 indicates possible cognitive impairment requiring further investigation. A score of 18 or less indicates cognitive impairment. Having arrived at a score that indicates possible or definite cognitive impairment, it is important to look for a likely cause. Alzeheimer's dementia and the multi-infarct dementia due to cerebrovascular disease are the most common types. Risk factors for cerebrovascular disease are assessed throughout the 75+ Health Assessment so they may have implications in the management of dementia (see Chapter 15).

Abbreviated Mental Test Score

The Hodkinson's Abbreviated Mental Test Score (AMTS) uses only 10 questions but does not yield as much information as the MMSE (see 'Bibliography and further reading'). It remains quicker to use and arguably functions just as well as a screening tool. Either test can be used but both depend on clinical interpretation before decisions are made about further investigation or management.

Mood/depression

The disorder of mood most frequently encountered in the elderly population is depression. While clinical depression, defined according to DSM criteria, is less common among the elderly than younger adults, the prevalence of depressive symptoms increases with age. It is estimated that around 1% of older people in the community suffer major depression and that 20–30% of community-dwelling elderly experience depressive symptoms. However, by its nature of causing withdrawal and despondency, depressed patients may not be obvious to GPs. Depressed people tend to stay at home and ruminate and not present to GPs with their mood disorder. In many cases depressive symptoms in the elderly are unrecognised and depression is therefore untreated.

Assessment and classification of depression in older people can be difficult; older people manifest fewer of the somatic symptoms of depression and depressive symptoms may be masked by co-morbidities. There are, however, several depression rating scales that are useful methods of screening for depression and are validated for use with older people. The Geriatric Depression Scale (GDS) originated in 1983 as a scale to measure depressive symptoms in an elderly population. The questions focus on sad mood, lack of energy, agitation and social withdrawal. Higher scores reflect more depression. The GDS originally consisted of 30 items but was later shortened to provide a more concise 15-item scale. Ease of comprehension is an important consideration when deciding upon a depression screening scale for the elderly. The GDS 15 essentially has a format where questions do not rely on the participant's memory. 'Are you', 'do you' and 'how often' form the question structure, placing emphasis on the recognition of 'now' and removing demand from memory function. The questions cover the symptoms of depression that

Box 4.7 Folstein Mini-Mental State Examination

ORIENTATION

1. What is the:		Points	2. Where are we?		Points
Year	_______	1	Country	_______	1
Season	_______	1	State/Territory	_______	1
Date	_______	1	Town/City	_______	1
Day	_______	1	Suburb (Street no.)	_______	1
Month	_______	1	Address (Street name)	_______	1

REGISTRATION

3. Name three objects, taking one second to say each. Then ask the patient all three after you have said them (TREE, CLOCK, BOAT). Give one point for each correct answer. Repeat the answers until the patient learns all three. _______ 3

ATTENTION AND CALCULATION

4. Serial sevens: Give one point for each correct answer. Stop after five answers.

OR if this is too hard

5. Spell WORLD backwards. (One mark for each letter in correct order.) _______ 5

RECALL

6. Ask for names of three objects learned in Q. 3. Give one point for each correct answer. _______ 3

LANGUAGE

7. Point to a pencil and a watch. Have the patient name them as you point. _______ 2
8. Have the patient repeat 'No ifs ands or buts'. _______ 1
9. Have the patient follow a three-stage command: 'Take a paper in your right hand. Fold the paper in half. Put the paper on the floor.' _______ 3
10. Have the patient read and obey the following: 'Close your eyes.' _______ 1
11. Have the patient write a sentence of his or her own choice. (The sentence should contain a subject and an object, and should make sense. Ignore spelling errors when scoring.) _______ 1
12. Have the patient copy the design printed over page. (Give one point if all sides and angles are preserved and if the intersecting sides form a diamond shape.) _______ 1

TOTAL _______ 30

Source: M. Folstein, S. Folstein & P. McHugh (1975), '"Mini-Mental State": a practical method of grading the cognitive state of patients for the clinician', *Journal of Psychiatric Research*, 12, pp. 189–98.

are predominant in the elderly and do not rely on somatic symptoms of depression (see Box 4.8).

A score of 3 or greater on the GDS 15 detects all cases of depression (100% sensitivity). However, only 20% of people will have depression (20% specificity) and another 50% will have depressive symptoms. As higher scores are recorded the likelihood of real depression increases (increasing specificity). Depressive symptoms may require drug treatment or psychotherapy or no treatment at all.

Box 4.8 Geriatric Depression Scale

15 questions, Yes/No answer to each question.

	YES	NO
Are you basically satisfied with life?	☐ 0	☐ 1
Have you dropped many of your activities and interests?	☐ 1	☐ 0
Do you feel that your life is empty?	☐ 1	☐ 0
Do you often get bored?	☐ 1	☐ 0
Are you in good spirits most of the time?	☐ 0	☐ 1
Are you afraid that something bad is going to happen to you?	☐ 1	☐ 0
Do you feel happy most of the time?	☐ 0	☐ 1
Do you often feel helpless?	☐ 1	☐ 0
Do you prefer to stay at home, rather than going out and doing new things?	☐ 1	☐ 0
Do you feel that you have more problems with memory than most?	☐ 1	☐ 0
Do you feel that it is wonderful to be alive now?	☐ 0	☐ 1
Do you feel worthless the way you are now?	☐ 1	☐ 0
Do you feel full of energy?	☐ 0	☐ 1
Do you feel that your situation is hopeless?	☐ 1	☐ 0
Do you feel that most people are better off than you are?	☐ 1	☐ 0

Source: J. I. Sheikh & J. A. Yesavage (1986), 'Geriatric Depression Scale (GDS): Recent evidence and development of a shorter version', *Clinical Gerontologist*, 5, pp. 165–73.

Depression remains a common problem in this age group and decisions about psychotherapy or medication with antidepressants require careful clinical appraisal and follow-up. Also, since depression can be a side effect of other therapies (e.g. β-blocker medication), a thorough clinical assessment and medication review is the foundation of therapy (see also Chapter 9).

Social

Social and community services

Social ties have long been recognised as important to the health of older people. There are several dimensions to social health. *Social function* refers to the individual and includes aspects such as those measured by the Social Functioning scale of the Short Form-36. *Social networks* have been defined as the linkages among groups of people, and the size of these networks tends to decrease as people age. *Social support* is the interactive process through which emotional, instrumental and informational aid is received from one's social network, regardless of the size or density of that network. *Instrumental support* includes services such as help with shopping, food preparation and personal care. *Formal services* may provide assistance in the form of health care, activities of daily living, or need for expressive and informational support; these services may be purchased through either the public or private sector. In some cases formal services fulfil needs for support that cannot be provided by family or friends (see also Chapter 7).

There are many scales available for measuring social aspects of health for older people. The Duke's Social Support Instrument is one example of a brief scale (11 items) that can be used in clinical practice and that has been validated for use with Australian elderly (see Box 4.9).

Box 4.9 Duke's Social Support Instrument

1. How many persons in this area, within one hour's travel, do you feel you can depend on or feel very close to? Do not include people in your own family.
   0 persons = 1 point
   1–2 persons = 2 points
   > 2 persons = 3 points
2. How many times during the past week did you spend some time with someone who does not live with you? (For example, you went to see them or they came to visit you, or you went out together?)
   No times = 1 point
   1–2 times = 2 points
   > 2 times = 3 points
3. How many times during the past week did you talk to someone—friends, relatives or others—on the telephone? (Either they called you, or you called them.)
   None–1 time = 1 point
   2–5 times = 2 points
   > 5 times = 3 points
4. About how many times in the past week did you go to meetings of social clubs, religious meetings or other groups that you belong to?
   None–1 time = 1 point
   2–5 times = 2 points
   > 5 times = 3 points
5. Does it seem that your family and friends (that is, people who are important to you) understand you?
   1 — never = 1 point
   2 — hardly ever = 1 points
   3 — some of the time = 2 points
   4 — most of the time = 3 points
   5 — all of the time = 3 points
6. Do you feel useful to your family and friends?
   1 — never = 1 point
   2 — hardly ever = 1 points
   3 — some of the time = 2 points
   4 — most of the time = 3 points
   5 — all of the time = 3 points
7. Do you know what is going on with your family and friends?
   1 — never = 1 point
   2 — hardly ever = 1 points
   3 — some of the time = 2 points
   4 — most of the time = 3 points
   5 — all of the time = 3 points
8. When you are talking with your family and friends, do you feel you are being listened to?
   1 — never = 1 point
   2 — hardly ever = 1 points

Box continues

Box 4.9 *continued*

3 — some of the time = 2 points
4 — most of the time = 3 points
5 — all of the time = 3 points

9. Do you feel you have a definite role/place in your family and among your friends?
   1 — never = 1 point
   2 — hardly ever = 1 points
   3 — some of the time = 2 points
   4 — most of the time = 3 points
   5 — all of the time = 3 points

10. Can you talk about your deepest problems with at least some of your family and friends?
   1 — never = 1 point
   2 — hardly ever = 1 points
   3 — some of the time = 2 points
   4 — most of the time = 3 points
   5 — all of the time = 3 points

11. How satisfied are you with the kinds of relationships you have with your family and friends?
   1 — extremely dissatisfied = 1 point
   2 — very dissatisfied = 1 points
   3 — somewhat dissatisfied = 2 points
   4 — mostly satisfied = 3 points
   5 — always satisfied = 3 points

Points for each question are added. A score of 23 or less is considered to be low, but in general the relationship between social support is monotonic, with better health outcomes for each increase in social support score.

Source: H. G. Koenig, R. E. Westlund, L. K. George, D. C. Hughes, D. G. Blazer & C. Hybels (1993), 'Abbreviating the Duke Social Support Index for use in chronically ill elderly individuals', *Psychosomatics*, 34, pp. 61–9.

Other questions to consider are:

- Does this person live alone or with partner or children?
- Do she have support available from neighbours, friends or nearby family?
- Is she in the role of carer, or cared for or is it a mutually supportive role?

Sometimes one partner is physically disabled and the other has impaired cognition. Even if support is adequate at present, it may change suddenly with illness or absence of a carer. Apart from human contact, does she have phone numbers or an alarm system for emergencies? Loneliness is a frequent problem and, if found, social suggestions can be made which may be taken up. Some of this age group are gainfully employed at work.

Community services currently in use or needed should be reviewed. This will depend on knowing what is available locally and what transport arrangements are possible. If the elderly person no longer drives, has she a taxi concession voucher? Fitness to drive and to hold a driver's licence needs to be sought, particularly in reference to Mini-Mental State/dementia. We can afford to be definite about a person's need to surrender her licence. For every upset patient disqualified from driving, there are five grateful relatives who realise that the decision is right.

Physical activities

The health benefits of exercise for the elderly are far-reaching. They include prevention of disease, such as osteoporosis, diabetes, hypertension, ischaemic heart disease and stroke; prevention of problems such as constipation, incontinence and deep vein thrombosis; and having a positive impact on loneliness and depression. Strength training has also been shown to be effective in reducing falls when provided in the context of multiple risk factor intervention and to improve gait and balance.

Even light exercise such as walking, gardening and Tai Chi has value in primary prevention of heart disease and death and in improving balance and preventing falls. Exercise is also an important part of maintaining the social network, and physical, social and productive activities have been strongly correlated.

Subsequent general practitioner consultation

A joint consultation with the patient, partner or carer and nurse/allied health professional who visited is the most effective way to interpret the 75+ Health Assessment data. This is an essential part of the 75+ Health Assessment process in Australia to allow the assessment to be claimed on Medicare.

Measurement of BP, pulse rate and rhythm can be left to this consultation. Consistency of method of blood pressure measurement in the consulting room has greater validity as it is on this that clinical trial evidence is based. Other aspects of physical examination will be directed to the problems highlighted by the home visit. Incontinence may require pelvic examination, urine culture or referral for a gynaecological opinion.

Immunisation status should be entered into the practice recall system after administration of required vaccinations.

Data collected at the home visit needs to be interpreted clinically. Some is in the form of 'scores' (e.g. Folstein, ANSI), some subjective impressions of deficits and some objective observations (e.g. medication on hand, state of the back door steps, etc.). Interpretation of this information should be made in consultation with your patient. What problems have been detected? Are they amenable to change? Does change depend on altered prescriptions (easy to do) or are they lifestyle changes centred around exercise, diet or alcohol? These changes will require considerable effort by the patient and an agreed process of change needs to be negotiated.

The usefulness of 75+ Health Assessments depends on the GP's ability to clinically interpret the data that are collected in a thorough home assessment of the functional abilities of the individual.

Bibliography and further reading

Bush, L. A., Horenkamp, N., Morley, J. E. & Spiro, A, 3rd. (1996), 'D-E-N-T-A-L: a rapid self-administered screening instrument to promote referrals for further evaluation in older adults', *Journal of the American Geriatric Society*, 44(8), pp. 979–81.

Byles, J. (2000), 'A thorough going over: evidence for health assessments for older people', *Australian and New Zealand Journal of Public Health*, 24(2), pp. 117–23.

Ewing, J. A. (1984), 'Detecting alcoholism. The CAGE questionnaire', *Journal of the American Medical Association*, 252(14), pp. 1905–7.

Fryback, D. G., Martin, P. A., Klein, R. & Klein, B. E. K., et al. (1993), 'Short questionnaires about visual function to proxy for best-corrected visual acuity', *Investigative Opthalmology and Visual Science*, 34, p. 1422.

Goodger, B., Byles, J. E., Higginbotham, H. N. H. & Mishra, G. (1999), 'Assessment of a brief scale to measure social support among older people', *Australian and New Zealand Journal of Public Health*, 23(3), pp. 260–5.

Hodkinson, H. M. (1972), 'Evaluation of a mental test score for assessment of mental impairment in the elderly', *Age and Ageing*, 1, pp. 233–8.

Hunt, S. M., McKenna, S. P., McEwen. J., Williams. J. & Papp, E. (1981), 'The Nottingham Health Profile: subjective health status and medical consultations', *Social Science and Medicine [A]*, 15(3 Pt 1), pp. 221–9.

Koenig, H. G., Westlund, R. E., George, L. K., Hughes, D. C., Blazer, D. G. & Hybels, C. (1993), 'Abbreviating the Duke Social Support Index for use in chronically ill elderly individuals', *Psychosomatics*, 34(16), pp. 61–9.

Saunders, J. B., Aasland, O. G., Babor, T. F., de la Fuente, J. R. & Grant, M. (1993), 'Development of the Alcohol Use Disorders Identification Test (AUDIT): WHO Collaborative Project on Early Detection of Persons with Harmful Alcohol Consumption–II', *Addiction*, 88(6), pp. 791–804.

Stewart, A. L. & Kamberg, C. J. (1992), 'Physical functioning measures', in Stewart, A. L. & Ware Jnr, J. E. (eds), *Measuring Functioning and Well Being: the Medical Outcomes Study Approach*, Duke University Press, Durham, North Carolina, pp. 86–101.

Stuck, A. E., Siu, A. L., Wieland, G. D., Adams, J. & Rubenstein, L. Z. (1993), 'Comprehensive Geriatric Assessment: a meta-analysis of controlled trials', *Lancet*, 342, pp. 1032–6.

Tinetti, M. E. & Ginter, S. F. (1988), 'Identifying mobility dysfunctions in elderly patients. Standard neuromuscular examination or direct assessment?', *Journal of the American Medical Association*, 259, pp. 1190–3.

Tinetti, M. E., Richman, D. & Powell, L. (1990), 'Falls efficacy as a measure of fear of falling', *Journal of Gerontology*, 45, pp. 239–43.

van Haastregt, J. C. M., Diederiks, J. P. M., van Rossum, E., de Witte, L. P. & Crebolder, H. F. J. M. (2000), 'Effects of preventive home visits to elderly people living in the community: systematic review', *British Medical Journal*, 320, pp. 754–8.

Ware, J. E., Snow, K. K., Kosinski, M. & Gandek, B. (1993), *SF36 Health Survey Manual and Interpretation Guide*, New England Medical Center, The Health Institute, Boston.

Williamson, J., Stokoe, I., Gray, S., Fisher, M., Smith, A., McGhee, A. & Stephenson, E. (1964), 'Old people at home: their unreported needs', *Lancet*, 1, pp. 1117–20.

Chapter 5

Prescribing drugs for the elderly: Pitfalls

DAVID T. LOWENTHAL, SAMIR ARRAY, JORGE RUIZ, JOEL RICH and JOHN R. MEULEMAN

Introduction

Iatrogenic illness is often caused by a lack of physician sensitivity to how medications act in the elderly and where standard dosages go far beyond the acceptable levels given to younger adults. The three cases presented in this chapter exemplify iatrogenic errors of commission. They are followed by questions with discussions.

Case 1

An 88-year-old male (weight 75 kg, serum creatinine 1.4 mmol/dL) has a long history of seizures controlled with phenytoin and a year ago had an uncomplicated myocardial infarction. His current medications include phenytoin 300 mg daily, isosorbide dinitrate 20 mg tid and metoprolol 50 mg bid. His mood has been low and he has anhedonia. You diagnose depression and start imipramine 50 mg at bedtime, with an increase to 100 mg qhs after 1 week. One month later his mood is somewhat better but he complains of an unsteady gait and occasional urinary incontinence. You refer him to a urologist who diagnoses benign prostatic hypertrophy (BPH). Because of his age and cardiac history the urologist feels that prostate surgery is too risky, so he starts the patient on doxazosin at night and refers the patient back to you. When you next see the patient the incontinence is somewhat better but he is now using a cane because of dizziness. He also complains of heartburn. His neurological examination is normal. You check his phenytoin level, which is 15 µg/mL (normal therapeutic range 10–20 µg/mL).

Why did he develop incontinence?

There are many types of incontinence: functional incontinence, where the patient cannot get up from a chair quickly enough to get to the bathroom on time and then will lose his bladder control; stress, as in pelvic muscle weakness, often encountered by multiparous women who when they sneeze or cough are doing some form of Valsalva manoeuvre and lose control; urge as in an infection or inflammatory and irritative process that may affect the bladder; or urinary outlet obstruction as in Case 1.

What type of incontinence does he probably have?

The patient described probably has outlet obstruction due to the BPH exacerbated by imipramine, a secondary amine for the treatment of his depression. He developed the incontinence because of an iatrogenic error. The types of incontinence that he has are multiple, as is often seen in elderly men and women. Selective serotonin reuptake inhibitor (SSRI) antidepressants such as fluoxetine or paroxetine or sertraline do not possess anticholinergic activity sufficient to exacerbate outlet obstruction. Metoprolol can contribute to depression and should have been discontinued. The SSRI do not apparently cause depression and the standard approved dosage has produced a therapeutic plasma concentration.

Why has he developed heartburn?
The heartburn is most likely related to a relaxation or weakness of the lower oesophageal sphincter. It could very well be related to smooth muscle relaxation due to his age but exacerbated by isosorbide dinitrate and/or doxazosin (a peripheral α-blocking drug), both smooth muscle relaxants.

Which drugs might be contributing to his dizziness?
Doxazosin can cause venous pooling and a decrease in preload and cardiac output resulting in orthostatic disease. This can also be a problem with isosorbide dinitrate and when combined with doxazosin clearly adds insult to injury. A reduction in the dosage of isosorbide to 20 mg once or twice a day with long-acting isosorbide mononitrate can be substituted.

You defer starting any new medicines for his dizziness or heartburn and decide to see the patient again in 2 weeks. When he returns he states he is more unsteady. On examination he now has signs of ataxia. What test will you order?

Ataxia is one of the later signs and symptoms of phenytoin intoxication. The first manifestation is nystagmus and that is equated with a plasma concentration between 20 and 30 μg/mL. Ataxia usually presents with a concentration greater than 30 μg/mL. The next test to be ordered is a plasma concentration.

What over-the-counter medicine could be contributing to his unsteadiness?
Since the patient is complaining of dyspepsia and because cimetidine is available over the counter in American pharmacies, the patient acts on the advice of his friends. At the intermediate care centre where he lives, he demands to have tagamet or cimetidine purchased over the counter. This is in a low dosage yet still has the capacity to inhibit hepatic microsomal enzyme metabolising systems which acts now to inhibit the metabolism of phenytoin which rises in concentration and has a significant pharmacodynamic effect to produce ataxia. In all likelihood the nystagmus was not a problem, as he did not seek any medical help for it.

Causes

Overmedication in the elderly can occur secondarily to any of the mechanisms shown in Table 5.1.

Overlooking age related pharmacokinetic-pharmacodynamic changes

Multiple pharmacokinetic changes (what the body does to the drug) are associated with ageing and have been reviewed extensively (see Table 5.2). Absorption is essentially preserved in the elderly.

Table 5.1 Causes of overmedication in the elderly (Case 1)

Physiologic changes with age	Pharmacological implications of these changes
Age related changes in pharmacokinetics and pharmacodynamics	Increased doses and/or frequent dosing intervals for elderly individuals See Table 5.2
Drug interactions	Enhancement of pharmacological effects (i.e. cimetidine potentiating phenytoin, theophylline and warfarin)
Use of inappropriate drugs	Appropriate diagnosis, but wrong medication (i.e. amitriptyline, long-acting benzodiazepines, propoxyphene or dipyridamole)
Inappropriate diagnostic process	Appropriate medication, but wrong diagnosis (i.e. treating delirium with sedatives or antipsychotics ignoring the aetiology)

Table 5.2 Age related pharmacokinetic changes (Cases 1 and 2)

Kinetic changes with age	Effects of these changes
Absorption	Preserved in the elderly
Distribution	
Serum albumin	Reduced
Body fat	Increased
Lean body mass	Reduced
Clearance	
Liver	Reduced liver size Reduced hepatic blood flow
Kidneys	Reduced GFR Reduced renal plasma flow Reduced reabsorptive capacity Reduced tubular function

Distribution

In the elderly, distribution is affected on two levels. An age related reduction in the level of serum albumin results in reduced protein binding of acidic organic compounds such as phenytoin, barbiturates, salicylates, sulfonamides and increased free fraction. This is especially important for highly protein bound drugs, such as phenytoin. These drugs can cause higher total serum concentrations and expose the patients to overmedication if physicians increase the dosage of phenytoin. In the elderly there is also an increase in total body fat and a reduction in lean body mass and total body water. The implications of these changes are that lipophilic drugs such as tricyclic antidepressants, lidocaine and psychotropics will have an increased volume of distribution in older persons and result in prolonged half-lives in these individuals. The opposite phenomenon occurs with polar drugs such as digoxin or aminoglycosides.

Clearance

The liver and kidneys are the major organs involved in this process. In the former case a reduction in liver size and hepatic blood flow can reduce the clearance of drugs that undergo extensive liver metabolism such as antidepressant tricyclics, theophylline and psychotropics. There is also an apparent impairment of oxidative reactions determined by the microsomal system in the liver, and ageing affects the metabolism of drugs such as lidocaine, phenytoin and barbiturates. Conjugative processes (glucuronidation, acetylation) involved in the metabolism of drugs such as acetaminophen seem to be preserved in the elderly.

In the case of renal function there is an age related decrease in glomerular filtration rate (GFR), renal plasma flow, reabsorptive capacity and tubular function. Drugs such as digoxin and aminoglycosides are predominantly eliminated through the kidneys, and impairments in renal function due to ageing can result in overmedication if GFR is not taken into consideration.

Pharmacodynamic responses (what the drug does to the body) have been defined in elderly individuals for drugs such as glyburide (glibenclamide), warfarin, benzodiazepines and tricyclic antidepressants. In the elderly, similar drug levels to those in younger persons can result in enhanced pharmacological actions.

Drug interactions

The concomitant use of certain drugs can result in an enhancement of the pharmacological action of another drug. This can result in dangerous overmedication. The best known example is cimetidine, a potent inhibitor of cytochrome P450 known to potentiate the pharmacological effect of drugs such as phenytoin, propranolol, tricyclic antidepressants, benzodiazepine, theophylline and warfarin. The elderly are particularly at risk given the high frequency of polypharmacy in this population.

Use of inappropriate drugs

Given their high profile incidence of adverse drug reactions, ineffectiveness and potentially dangerous drug interactions, there are medications that should be avoided in elderly patients. Examples include drugs such as amitriptyline, long-acting benzodiazepines, indomethacin, propoxyphene and dipyridamole. Elderly patients frequently self-medicate with over-the-counter medications that often are not indicated. These drugs can cause dangerous adverse reactions directly as part of their pharmacological action or indirectly through drug interactions.

Examples are non-steroidal anti-inflammatory drugs (NSAIDs)—such as ibuprofen, naproxen and aspirin, which can cause gastritis and gastrointestinal bleeding—or antihistamines, such as diphenhydramine, which can cause anticholinergic effects in frail elderly persons. These effects include urinary retention, tachycardia and/or orthostatic hypotension. Finally, antacids can bind digoxin, iron or tetracycline and can result in decreased absorption and lessened pharmacodynamic activity.

Inappropriate diagnostic process

Often a drug is prescribed without an appropriate diagnosis of the condition for which the drugs are used. For example, the use of benzodiazepines to treat anxiety or agitation in a hospitalised elderly patient ignores a basic diagnostic work-up for delirium that may include a drug induced reaction (see Chapter 16). These reactions include severe hyponatremia due to NSAIDs, tricyclics and chlorpropamide and can lead to misdiagnosis and overmedication in elderly patients.

Table 5.3 Complications of overmedication (Cases 1 and 2)

Results of polypharmacy	Manifestation of polypharmacy
Adverse drug reactions	Typical presentations in the elderly: falls, urinary incontinence, failure to thrive, delirium, dementia
Increased drug costs	Increased budget to purchase more medication Hospitalisation. More drugs and more overmedication Impairment of function
Use of inappropriate drugs	Appropriate diagnosis, but wrong medication, (i.e. amitriptyline, long-acting benzodiazepines, propoxyphene or dipyridamole)
Non-compliance	Afraid of adverse drug reactions Apparent lack of therapeutic effect results in the physician increasing doses and/or intervals

Complications

The dangers of overmedication are multiple and include the following among the most important (Table 5.3).

Adverse drug reactions

Overmedication of elderly individuals will have as its most immediate consequence the development of adverse drug reactions (ADRs) that will break the delicate balance that allows a frail elderly individual to function. Once this balance is disrupted it can result in increased morbidity and mortality. ADRs in the elderly can present in atypical ways, manifested by impairments of daily living activities such as impaired mobility, falls, urinary incontinence, failure to thrive, delirium and cognitive decline. A potentially critical problem is the use of drugs to treat ADRs, resulting again in a vicious circle of overmedication and polypharmacy.

Increased drug costs

Cost considerations are an important problem in the new era of cost containment and managed care. Overmedication will directly increase drug costs when a drug is used in greater doses and frequency in excess of what is recommended. Overmedication indirectly raises drug costs when it results in ADR, causing hospitalisation and impairment of functionality.

Non-compliance

Overmedication can cause unintended non-compliance when associated with ADRs. Non-compliance is probably not very frequent in elderly patients, but lack of consideration of appropriate prescribing can be a cause of overmedication by encouraging patients to discontinue drugs because of fear of side effects.

Settings

With inpatient care a large number of elderly patients receive sedative and hypnotic drugs that frequently result in ADRs. The incidence of adverse drug reactions increases with age in hospitalised elderly persons, with some reduction in incidence in patients over 70 years old. A significant number of elderly patients in nursing homes receive drugs on an as-needed (PRN) basis that results in a large number of unnecessary prescriptions and no appropriate indications or diagnoses. A particularly important problem in nursing homes is excessive use of psychotropic medications. In the US, the 1987 OBRA legislation aimed to reduce the use of such drugs in the elderly population in nursing homes because of the evidence of overmedication in this age group.

Elderly persons in the community are characterised by more frequent use of drugs associated with drug interactions. Drugs such as barbiturates, digoxin, cardiovascular medications, diuretics, analgesics, laxatives and sedatives are most frequently prescribed to elderly persons.

The patient in Case 1 has had multiple complications of overmedication, including adverse drug reactions. The best way of preventing this is to have a primary caregiver trained in geriatrics as well as clinical pharmacology who can write medications, monitor drug therapy and avoid drug disease interactions with careful attention.

Case 2

An 80-year-old woman (weight 60 kg, serum creatinine 1.5 mmol/dL) is hospitalised for the onset of atrial fibrillation. She has a past history of a severe anxiety disorder. She is started on digoxin 0.25 mg qd (to control her ventricular response) and Coumadin (warfarin) 5 mg qd and restarted on Valium (diazepam) 5 mg tid, which she had used effectively until it was stopped 5 years ago. When you see her in your office 2 weeks after discharge her pulse is 68 but she complains of a lack of energy. On her next visit a month later you note she has lost 2.2 kg and is mentally not as sharp as previously. Her affect is flat and she admits to a low mood. You start her on Zoloft (sertraline) 50 mg qd, but when she returns 4 weeks later she complains of nausea. She has lost another 2.7 kg and is even less interactive. Her complete blood examination is normal, her renal function is unchanged, her urinalysis shows 8-10 wbc and her INR is 2.3.

Why is she nauseated?
Her serum digoxin concentration has not been monitored; her dosage is rather high in relation to her age and renal function. The digoxin has achieved its pharmacodynamic effect (to slow the ventricular response) even though she is still fibrillating. The ventricular response has been brought under good control. The sertraline can certainly produce nausea and anorexia.

Which of her drugs may be causing her decline in function?
There is a high possibility that it is the diazepam, which is metabolically altered by the liver to produce active metabolites that are probably accumulating and contributing to her depressed mood as well as profound loss of energy and a decrease in fluid intake.

What other drugs commonly affect mental function in the aged?
Besides sertraline and diazepam in her regimen, digoxin may cause some alterations in brain white matter that can contribute to her decline.

How would the pharmacokinetic changes of ageing affect your drug dosing in this patient?
The most appropriate ways to improve drug prescriptions for the elderly are shown in Box 5.1. Some of these methods are discussed below.

Box 5.1 Preventing overmedication in the elderly (Cases 1, 2 and 3)

- Diagnose appropriately.
- Choose the right medication.
- Choose the right dose based on principles of geriatric pharmacology.
- Monitor drug therapy.
- Use the lowest effective dose and least frequent dosing interval of a medication.
- Establish realistic treatment goals.
- Obtain a complete drug history.
- Consider non-drug alternatives.
- Simplify drug regimens.
- Consider the high prevalence of cognitive decline with ageing.
- Determine the appropriate duration of treatment.
- Avoid drug–disease interactions.

Diagnose appropriately

The most important preventive aspect of overmedication is to appropriately diagnose the conditions for which the drugs are being prescribed. Misdiagnosis of hypertension by relying on a single measurement in the office can result in aggressive treatment producing a very dangerous hypoperfusion and subsequent exacerbation of angina or the development of stroke in an elderly patient with borderline cerebral blood flow.

Choose the right medication

As mentioned earlier, there are multiple medications that should definitely be restricted in elderly individuals due to their profile of adverse reactions and inefficacy. In the case of elderly individuals the selection of a drug must be dictated by a good side effect profile, especially excluding those drugs that are associated with cognitive function impairment.

Choose the right dose based on principles of geriatric pharmacology

Dosing errors with elderly individuals are caused by ignorance of geriatric pharmacokinetics and pharmacodynamics. Education of physicians in training, primary care physicians, nurse practitioners and physician assistants is essential.

Monitor drug therapy

Pharmacotherapy is a dynamic process and as such does not end with the prescription of a medication. The practitioner must be involved in a continuous process of re-evaluation and attention to the development of an ADR in elderly patients. The practitioner must also decide when to reduce the dose of medication or, even better, to discontinue a drug if it is one associated with an ADR or is ineffective. Therapeutic drug monitoring is limited for a handful of drugs but can be a very useful alternative in avoiding overmedication in some elderly patients. However, therapeutic decisions should be based on good clinical judgment and not on the artificial numerical limits of published therapeutic ranges.

Lowest effective dose and least frequent dosing interval

The aphorism 'Start low, go slow' should be a dictum for physicians treating elderly patients. Body weight decreases with ageing and one study revealed that older patients who weighed less than 50 kg received mg per kg doses that were substantially higher than those who weighed more than 90 kg.

Establish realistic treatment goals

Often physicians accede to the demands of elderly patients and use medications even when they are not indicated, or they increase doses due to lack of pharmacological effect. An adequate discussion with each elderly patient about the nature of the treated disease is imperative and will ensure that the patient understands the benefits and limitations of drug therapy.

Obtain a complete drug history

Primary care physicians serve a vital role in this area. Often one of the major determinants of overmedication in the elderly is the use of several different drugs prescribed by multiple physicians. These drugs are sometimes dispensed by multiple pharmacies without any consideration of possible drug interactions or overmedication. The primary care physician should oversee the overall drug therapy of her patient and constantly inquire about new medications being introduced. This includes prescription drugs as well as over-the-counter drugs.

Consider non-drug alternatives

In many cases medical conditions can be managed with non-pharmacological modalities. Classic examples are the use of low sugar diets for type II diabetes mellitus or lifestyle modifications that include a low salt diet, exercise and avoidance of smoking and alcohol in the treatment of hypertension.

Simplify drug regimens

Simplified regimens help lower the possibility of polypharmacy and potential drug interactions that can result in overmedication. Use of once-daily medications will not only assure better compliance but will also prevent the development of overmedication. Restriction of the use of as-needed medications (PRN) and automatic renewals should be discouraged.

Consider the high prevalence of cognitive decline with ageing

The presence of cognitive decline in patients will emphasise the need for more aggressive education of elderly patients and their caregivers concerning the use of medication and the possibility of side effects due to overdose. It is especially worth noting the possibility of overmedication causing drug induced cognitive impairment.

Determine the appropriate duration of treatment

Determination of the appropriate duration of treatment is especially important in the case of short courses of treatment, such as antibiotics or analgesics for acute pain followed by physical therapy.

Avoid drug–disease interactions

In addition to normal age related changes, elderly individuals will have a higher prevalence of multiple chronic medical conditions that will influence pharmacokinetics and pharmacodynamics. Such medical conditions will undoubtedly affect the delicate homeostasis of elderly persons and possibly result in overmedication and adverse drug reactions. Conditions such as congestive heart failure, dehydration and renal failure will cause further impairment of renal blood flow and GFR. Further readjustment of dosage regimens for elderly patients suffering from these conditions will be required.

You adjust her medication regimen and she improves

The digoxin was discontinued to see if her ventricular rate increased. If necessary she can receive digoxin 0.125 mg every other day. The diazepam has been gradually discontinued. The sertraline can be gradually tapered to a lower dose and replaced with fluoxetine (Paxil) which has some energising effects as well as an antidepressant action. You repeat the urinalysis and order a urine culture. It demonstrates greater than 10^5 *E. coli*. The question that comes up is whether this asymptomatic bacteruria should be treated. An asymptomatic urinary tract infection in the absence of clear-cut anatomical obstruction or hydronephrosis and/or diabetes can be managed conservatively by increasing fluid administration and making sure that the perianal area has been cleaned adequately. The lack of energy in elderly patients may be indicative of an underlying illness such as a urinary tract infection.

Pharmacokinetics

Because digoxin is absorbed through passive diffusion there is no age related decrease in the absorption of digoxin. However, the bioavailability of the different formulations of the drug (between 40% and 100%) has strongly contributed to the variable relationship between dose and plasma or serum drug concentration (PSDC) in different populations. Furthermore, the concomitant use of laxatives and antacids, medications that are commonly used by the elderly, can also substantially impair the absorption of digoxin and result in variable PSDC. One important pharmacokinetic effect that influences the use of digoxin levels in therapeutic drug monitoring (TDM) is the recognised deterioration of glomerular filtration that leads to a decreased clearance of digoxin and toxicity when elderly individuals receive the same doses given to younger persons. Reduced digoxin clearance in elderly individuals has been shown to correspond with decreased kidney function. A reduction in the plasma clearance of digoxin in older individuals (mean age 81 years) has been demonstrated in mild congestive heart failure.

The reduction in lean body mass with age can result in a reduced volume of distribution for digoxin but will not have any influence on the PSDC at steady state. Calculated digoxin clearance by pharmacokinetic formulas based on the GFR are a poor predictor of serum digoxin levels in the elderly. The reason for this is not completely clear; however, one possible explanation points to the contribution of renal tubular secretion since it is also affected by ageing, extra-renal routes of metabolite elimination that are not routinely assayed and that in some cases are responsible for toxicity even with therapeutic levels. Disease states that are highly prevalent in the elderly population, such as thyroid disease and congestive heart failure, contribute also. Their contribution is due to their effect on renal function that causes variable PSDCs. The frequency of polypharmacy in the elderly and the use of multiple drugs that interact with digoxin (such as quinidine, amiodarone, antacids, antibiotics, warfarin, phenobarbital, levodopa, calcium channel blockers, etc.) can modify the pharmacokinetics of a drug because of their intervention in several different processes. These findings stress the need for a more liberal use of digoxin PSDCs given the multiple pharmacokinetic changes that affect digoxin in the older population.

Pharmacodynamics

Most of the data on altered pharmacodynamic response with age are based on animal studies. One study described the increased sensitivity of rat myocardium to digoxin due to a reduction in Na^+K^+-ATPase. Another found a reduction in Na^+K^+-ATPase with ageing in rats. Yet another study demonstrated an age related alteration in pharmacodynamics that included increased sensitivity of the aged myocardium to cardiac glycosides in rats. These findings suggest an increased sensitivity of digoxin independent of other disease states in the elderly. However, evidence in support of an abnormal pharmacodynamic response is not compelling and the conclusion is that there is little evidence of an age related alteration in the inotropic response to digoxin in humans.

Perhaps more important in the elderly are other concomitant conditions, such as abnormal homeostatic mechanisms, that contribute to an enhanced sensitivity to digoxin. Another important pharmacodynamic consideration is the interaction of electrolytes and hormones as illustrated by digoxin. Diuretic induced hypokalemia in elderly patients causes increased sensitivity to digoxin by increasing myocardial uptake, and binding and promoting tubular secretion. Serum magnesium may decrease and serum calcium may increase, resulting in arrhythmia, all of which are reduced by diuretics. On the other hand, thyroid hormone increases the amount of Na^+K^+-ATPase on the cell membrane, which results in a diminished sensitivity to digoxin in hyperthyroid patients even with levels within the therapeutic range. The presentation of hyperthyroidism in the elderly is atypical and often the only clue may be a lack of response to digoxin or atrial fibrillation.

Conditions such as fever, infections and other causes of increased sympathetic activity are associated with diminished sensitivity to digoxin. Important drug interactions can influence the use of digoxin and among them quinidine, verapamil and amiodarone can cause an increase in digoxin PSDC. Drugs such as antacids, cholestyramine and rifampicin can cause reduced drug levels. Based on this information we suggest that the use of digoxin PSDC in the elderly is fundamentally influenced by altered pharmacokinetics, although pharmacodynamic responses cannot be ignored completely.

Therapeutic drug monitoring

Although the elderly experience multiple age related pharmacokinetic changes, there is no evidence in the literature that recommends a distinct therapeutic range or sampling time for this population. Given a digoxin half-life of approximately 40 hours, the steady state concentration occurs at approximately 8 days. This would be the best time to obtain the sample unless toxicity is suspected. In that case the level can be drawn any time. The time of the day most appropriate for sampling is at least 6 hours after digoxin is given (ideally 11–12 hours) and always before the next dose is taken. This is because the digoxin levels peak 1 hour after administration. The therapeutic range is usually 0.5–2.0 ng/mL. Of course these levels are somehow arbitrary and do not necessarily correlate with therapeutic effect or toxicity.

The other important aspect is how often to monitor digoxin PSDC. The answer is not straightforward. The futility of ordering routine periodic digoxin PSDC has been demonstrated in a study of elderly nursing home patients (mean age 83 years). The use of digoxin PSDC should be mandatory any time an elderly patient presents with symptoms that are not clearly explained by the underlying disease and are suggestive of drug toxicity, such as new arrhythmias or gastrointestinal and/or neuropsychiatric symptoms. Digoxin PSDC should also be used if a new potentially interacting drug is introduced or if there is evidence of impaired kidney function. On the other hand, the frequency of variable and atypical presentations of digoxin toxicity in the elderly should encourage physicians to be more aggressive in their use of PSDC in this population. An important caveat is that the correlation between therapeutic levels and pharmacological action is not as precise as was once believed. Digoxin levels in a therapeutic range have been described as unreliable when used to control rapid ventricular rates in a group of patients with chronic atrial fibrillation. One patient subgroup required levels of 2–5 ng/mL to control ventricular response, whereas subtherapeutic levels achieved rate control in still another subgroup of patients. Another study proved underdigitalisation in 16 of 38 elderly patients with digoxin levels in the therapeutic range.

Although nothing can substitute for a careful clinical evaluation complemented by electrocardiograms and electrolyte determinations, digoxin PSDC can be an especially useful tool in managing geriatric patients.

PSDC and toxicity

Multiple age related changes in pharmacokinetics, polypharmacy and impaired homeostatic mechanisms are probably responsible for the higher frequency of digoxin toxicity in the elderly. The critical presentation of toxicity in the elderly is extremely variable and lacks specificity. Arrhythmias that are manifestations of digoxin toxicity are frequently preceded by extracardiac events. Symptoms of toxicity such as nausea, vomiting and anorexia can also be manifestations of congestive heart failure or toxicity caused by concomitant medications. A confounding problem in the elderly is the high incidence of neuropsychiatric manifestations, such as confusion, disorientation or delirium. A correlation has been demonstrated between diverse symptoms of digoxin toxicity (such as arrhythmias) and levels above the therapeutic range. However, many other studies do not show a correlation between digoxin PSDC and such manifestations with a significant overlap. One recent study found that of 58 patients with digoxin levels above 3 ng/mL obtained at steady state, 14 did not show any evidence of digoxin toxicity.

Theophylline

Theophylline is another drug that, despite being used for many years, is still surrounded by multiple unresolved issues. This drug lost popularity when β-adrenergic and atropine-like agents used by inhalation became available. Inhalation allows many of the undesirable systemic effects of these drugs to be avoided while maintaining the therapeutic efficacy and multiple side effects have made it only a second or third line medication in the treatment of COPD and asthma.

Pharmacokinetics

Theophylline is metabolised through oxidative pathways by hepatic microsomal enzymes (80–90%) and excreted unchanged through the kidneys (10%). Studies regarding the clearance of theophylline in the elderly are contradictory. Some authors report an impairment of theophylline disposition while others report no change. Part of the problem is the variety of patients included in these studies, ranging from healthy volunteers to critically ill patients. Another important factor is that decreased protein binding in the elderly may be responsible for an augmentation of the theophylline clearance that compensates for any age related reduction in the metabolism of the drug. The effects of smoking cannot be discounted either. Smoking enhances the clearance of theophylline by inducing hepatic microsomal enzymes. In a study of COPD patients, no difference was found in the theophylline clearance of both elderly smokers and middle-aged smokers and improved clearance in elderly non-smokers.

Drug interactions are also very important factors that influence both the pharmacokinetics of theophylline and the eventual determination of PSDCs in the elderly. Cimetidine, erythromycin and allopurinol can decrease theophylline clearance and cause lower PSDCs, whereas barbiturates, rifampicin and phenytoin have the opposite effect.

Pharmacodynamics

Information on the pharmacodynamics of theophylline in the elderly is scarce. A group of 10 elderly non-smoker patients with COPD (mean age 63 years) was used to demonstrate that at the same theophylline concentrations as younger asthmatics, the percentage change in FEV_1 was dramatically reduced in the older group. This can be explained by the greater degree of baseline airway obstruction in the elderly group and the more remarkable irreversible changes in the respiratory tree, including loss of lung elasticity with age. This results in an increased functional residual capacity and residual volume.

Therapeutic drug monitoring

It is widely accepted in the literature that the therapeutic range of theophylline is 10–20 µg/mL. A study of patients with asthma and COPD (mean age 68 years; range 32–84 years) divided the patients into two groups for study: one group received doses of aminophylline aimed at a PSDC of 10 µg/mL, the other group at the higher rate. A significant improvement in the FEV_1 and FVC was found in the group with the higher theophylline PSDC. Another study of a group of COPD patients (mean age 61 years; range 3–73 years) demonstrated a meaningful improvement in physiological end-points in the subgroup that attained theophylline concentrations as high as 18.3 µg/mL. These studies show that elderly patients do not respond to theophylline PSDC as strongly as younger individuals. This suggests that elderly patients would need a theophylline PSDC approaching the upper limit of 20 µg/mL.

On the other hand, studies on younger populations suggest a reduction in therapeutic range. In young asthmatics there was a lack of significant improvement in the FEV_1 when the serum level surpassed 15 µg/mL. More recent evidence comes from studies that targeted theophylline concentrations of 10 µg/mL and 20 µg/mL in two subgroups that predominantly included asthmatics (average age 38 years). These studies showed no evidence of additional clinical benefit at a PSDC of 20 µg/mL and at the same time an increased incidence of side effects. The poor tolerance of elderly COPD patients to theophylline and the possibility of an inferior response when higher theophylline levels were attained has been highlighted in a study that challenged the notion of the 10–20 µg/mL range for this age group. Furthermore, theophylline is no longer the only drug used in the treatment of COPD in this group. Another argument is the theoretical possibility that the lower amounts of albumin with ageing might cause reduced binding and increased clearance of the free fraction of the drug, which would result in a reduction in total theophylline PSDC. Based on these facts we are inclined to agree with other authors who suggest a level of 8–12 µg/mL as adequate and safer for most elderly patients. However, for some elderly patients the conventional therapeutic range of 10–20 µg/mL might be necessary and appropriate depending on the overall clinical status of the patient. Yet more studies in this field are necessary.

The half-life of theophylline will vary widely depending on the individual, smoking status, type of preparation and route of administration.

Plasma or serum drug concentration and toxicity

There is a dramatic increase in manifestations of theophylline toxicity when the level of 20 µg/mL is exceeded. Elderly patients are considered more prone to developing theophylline toxicity. Elderly patients have been shown to have a significantly greater risk of life-threatening events due to toxic theophylline levels than do younger patients. Patients over 75 years old have a 16.7-fold greater risk of life-threatening events than do patients younger than 25 years old despite comparable median serum concentrations of theophylline.

Theophylline induced seizures may be potentially fatal in the elderly. Factors such as prior neurological damage, hypoxia and cerebral vasoconstriction lower the theophylline PSDC at which seizures develop in the elderly and in some cases can even occur at therapeutic levels in this age group.

Theophylline has also been associated with cardiac arrhythmias. Multifocal atrial tachycardia

(MAT) is a frequent arrhythmia that occurs during theophylline use and can also occur at therapeutic levels. However, MAT disappears when levels decrease in elderly individuals. Other types of arrhythmias are also associated with a theophyline PSDC within the therapeutic range. Congestive heart failure or liver disease can cause an elevated theophylline PSDC and potentially adverse drug reactions.

These studies exemplify the possibility of fatal theophylline PSDC toxicity in the elderly population, even with levels within the therapeutic range, and emphasise the need for careful clinical evaluation of each patient as well as recognise the limitations of PSDC in the diagnosis of toxicity without appropriate clinical judgment.

Aminoglycosides

Elderly patients are more susceptible to infections not only because of age associated immune dysfunction, but also because of the increased frequency and severity of chronic illnesses that impair the ability to fight infections. Elderly patients in particular are at a higher risk of developing sepsis and have greater morbidity and mortality from it. Serious gram-negative bacillary infections that are common in the elderly require systemic antibiotics with a broad spectrum of activity (e.g. cephalosporins, fluoroquinolones and aminoglycosides).

It is important to monitor aminoglycoside serum concentrations due to their lower therapeutic index, the occurrence of clinically significant toxicity at a high frequency, great interindividual pharmacokinetic differences and the need to maximise the dose to improve survival rates.

Pharmacokinetics

Aminoglycosides are usually administered parenterally through intermittent intravenous infusion and in a few cases are administered intramuscularly to ensure 100% bioavailability. The aminoglycosides are almost completely excreted from the body by renal clearance, predominately by glomerular filtration but with some participation by tubular reabsorption. The correlation between creatinine clearance and aminoglycoside elimination is fairly precise and allows clinicians to calculate adequate doses for patients with impaired GFR.

In elderly individuals (age range 60–79 years) with normal creatinine clearance the pharmacokinetics of amikacin (an aminoglycoside), gentamicin and tobramycin were not influenced by age. This suggests that aminoglycoside doses do not need to be modified in elderly individuals with preserved renal function. Gentamicin clearance has been shown to be dependent on creatinine clearance in a group of 49 elderly patients with impaired renal function, but age was excluded as an independent factor influencing the pharmacokinetics of the drug.

Pharmacodynamics

The pharmacodynamics of aminoglycosides have not been studied satisfactorily and most studies refer to animals. They show that homeostatic mechanisms, such as reduced injury threshold and reduced capacity for cellular regeneration, are implicated in the increased risk of aminoglycoside toxicity in aged animals.

PSDC and toxicity

The concomitant use of loop diuretics for the treatment of congestive heart failure can also contribute to a higher incidence of aminoglycoside ototoxicity in older individuals. Finally, plasma concentrations seem to have no effect on the occurrence of ototoxicity. This is because aminoglycosides bind to the organ of Corti and are eliminated from the endolymph and perilymph very slowly.

Phenytoin

Seizures occur more frequently with ageing. In the elderly population the aetiology predominantly includes cerebrovascular disease and brain tumours. Phenytoin has been used to treat partial and generalised tonic-clonic seizures in older persons. Aspects of phenytoin PSDC in the management of seizures and epilepsy in the elderly are reviewed below.

Pharmacokinetics

Phenytoin is absorbed slowly and incompletely orally. There is some evidence of impaired absorption of phenytoin with ageing. The drug is almost 0% bound to proteins and its major route of metabolism is by hepatic microsomal enzymes to inactive metabolites. An increase in phenytoin clearance is evident in people over 65 years old, but after correcting for protein binding, no difference in clearance due to age is demonstrated.

In one study there was no significant change in phenytoin metabolism in elderly patients. However, another study demonstrated a decline in the rate of drug metabolism in patients 60–79 years old with normal albumin levels when compared to a group of subjects aged 20–59 years. They recommended a reduction in the phenytoin doses given to elderly patients. These discrepancies in phenytoin metabolism are probably due to the effects of protein binding that is usually reduced in the elderly and to the striking variability in the characteristics of the elderly population.

Phenytoin follows first-order kinetics at lower doses but at higher doses the drug follows zero-order kinetics. This means that an elevated phenytoin, PSDC, is caused by very small increases in drug concentrations, causing potential toxicity.

Drugs such as cimetidine, allopurinol, omeprazole and sulfonamides can cause inhibition of the metabolism of phenytoin and, in turn, carbamazepine and rifampicin stimulate phenytoin metabolism and reduce phenytoin concentrations in blood when used concomitantly. Liver disease is most commonly associated with the impairment of phenytoin metabolism and requires more careful TDM.

Pharmacodynamics

Lower concentrations of phenytoin can suppress seizure activity in older mice. There are no studies that show altered pharmacodynamics with ageing. Such studies would be extremely difficult to perform given the unpredictable nature of seizure activity, multiple aetiologies and great variability of phenytoin PSDC. However, impaired homeostatic mechanisms in the elderly can predispose them to increased neurotoxicity when exposed to higher phenytoin concentrations.

Therapeutic drug monitoring

The main reason to monitor phenytoin PSDC routinely is to detect significant increases in drug concentrations when higher dosages are used, caused by the known zero-order kinetics of the drug at higher levels and the potential for toxicity. The attainment of a target concentration is not the main objective given the possibility of good seizure control at therapeutic levels, levels below and levels above the established therapeutic range.

In reality the therapeutic level is where seizure control is obtained without side effects, even if the level is above or below the standard range. A randomised prospective study of 79 patients (mean age 26 years) found no difference between a group in which a subtherapeutic level was corrected by a physician by readjusting the doses to attain the therapeutic range, and a group in which the subtherapeutic level was maintained. This study supports the notion that increased doses of phenytoin in patients with good seizure control despite a subtherapeutic PSDC should be discouraged.

Another consideration in the TDM of phenytoin in the elderly is the marked variability in serum phenytoin concentrations. It is recommended that nursing home patients who receive phenytoin therapy should have periodic phenytoin PSDCs done even in the absence of signs for phenytoin toxicity.

The free concentration is the pharmacologically active moiety. In the case of phenytoin, total drug concentrations are measured routinely and usually provide a reliable index of the free concentration in most epileptic patients. However, the determination of the unbound phenytoin would benefit those patients in whom decreased phenytoin binding is expected, as in hepatic or renal disease, patients taking drugs that displace phenytoin from its albumin binding, and patients with hypoalbuminaemia. These are all conditions in which the free fraction is likely to increase. Age per se is not an indication for the measurement of free phenytoin levels and, in all populations, changes in protein binding are more important determinants of the need to use such levels.

The half-life of phenytoin is between 7 and 42 hours after oral administrations and between 10 and 15 hours after intravenous administrations, but these are rough estimates given the extreme variability of the half-life. The time for blood collection at steady state is much more difficult to predict due to the saturation kinetics of the drug and the large interindividual variability of phenytoin. One strategy is to wait several days or to obtain multiple PSDCs at weekly intervals. Another is to obtain multiple PSDCs over consecutive days and when the levels do not change any more, that is probably the steady state concentration. Once in the steady state the PSDC can be sampled any time. Nomograms and Bayesian forecasting can help reduce the number of PSDCs and avoid multiple drug determinations. The guidelines for the therapeutic range are 10–20 μg/mL, but this is only a reference to help avoid toxicity due to rapid changes in phenytoin concentrations when the doses are increased.

PSDC and toxicity

The saturation kinetics of phenytoin sometimes pose serious problems when PSDCs are in the upper limit. Minor changes in dosage can result in remarkable elevations of PSDC and lead to the potential for adverse effects. Nystagmus, ataxia, dysarthria, drowsiness, tremor, confusion and psychiatric disturbances are some of the symptoms associated with phenytoin PSDC. Nystagmus is probably the first sign to appear, often while the phenytoin PSDC is in the therapeutic range. The frequency and severity of other toxic effects are also rising at continuously higher levels. High phenytoin concentrations are also associated with neurotoxicity in the long term and in some cases with a paradoxical exacerbation of seizures. Unfortunately, few studies have systematically studied the relationship between phenytoin PSDCs and adverse effects in the elderly. Due to the age related decrease in albumin concentrations and a reduction in affinity of albumin receptor and binding sites, there is a stronger possibility of toxicity at low phenytoin serum levels in elderly epileptics. On the other hand, due to the high prevalence in the elderly of neurological conditions such as cerebrovascular disease, dementia or Parkinson's disease, this population may be more vulnerable to the adverse effects of phenytoin mainly in the form of neurotoxic effects, such as cognitive deficits or ataxia.

Case 3

A 75-year-old female (weight 75 kg, serum creatinine 1.3 mmol/dL) presents as a new patient with the chief complaint of new onset oedema and worsening hypertension as measured by her home BP cuff. Her past history is positive only for hypertension and gradually worsening arthritis. She claims to be fully compliant with her atenolol 50 mg qd, which is the only therapeutic agent she takes. She has a local general practitioner but is concerned about her oedema and wants to obtain a second opinion. On examination she has 2 + oedema of her feet and her BP is 166/100 mm Hg.

What additional current medication history should you ask?
Because she has untreated arthritis it is necessary to know what medication is possibly controlling her pain that could produce hypertension and oedema. She admits to buying over-the-counter non-prescribed NSAIDs—that is, ibuprofen 200 mg and taking it 3 times daily. You decide to stop the atenolol and start diltiazem cd (controlled dissolution) 120 mg qd. She returns 3 weeks later and her BP is 160/98. She feels fine except for the persistent oedema.

On her next visit her BP is 148/88. She is recovering from an upper respiratory tract infection for which her local doctor treated her. Her oedema persists although it is somewhat improved. You prescribe furosemide 20 mg qd. She misses her appointment in 2 weeks and then returns on an urgent basis 3 weeks later with the history of a near syncopal episode and an increasing feeling of weakness. She is orthostatic and her BP on standing after 5 minutes is 118/70. On examination she has no oedema.

What additional medication history should you ask?
'Did you in fact buy the diltiazem cd and are you in fact taking it?' The patient is honest and candid and says that it costs too much and she did not buy it. This is often a problem in the elderly who are on a fixed income where a prescription drug plan is not part of their health insurance. In the US, President George W. Bush thinks he will have a prescription drug plan for the elderly. Cost is a very important issue in the area of patient compliance.

Overmedication can cause unintended non-compliance when associated with adverse drug reactions. Non-compliance is probably not frequent in elderly patients but lack of consideration of appropriate prescribing can be a cause of overmedication. This may result in unnecessary adverse effects and lead to discontinuation and non-compliance. Finally, the excessive cost of some medications may prevent the patient from purchasing the medication and therefore from receiving the intended therapeutic benefits.

Her doctor provides her with samples of controlled release diltiazem 120 mg to be taken daily. The medication that she is taking for her upper respiratory tract infection is checked and found to contain phenylpropanolamine which acts as vasoconstrictor and can cause a rise in blood pressure. Furosemide (Lasix) is a potent loop-blocking diuretic and can cause a fall in BP if the urinary response is profound, as in this patient. Her oedema was improved and she has lost 1.8 kg since her last visit. She is told not to take any more diuretic and reminded that the NSAID, which she has been warned not to take any more, is more likely to cause oedema and a rise in BP. A diuretic should not have been prescribed for the oedema but a more careful line of questioning would have been more appropriate to find out what else she is taking without the physician's knowledge—that is, self-medication, which can contribute to her constellation of additional problems and not be totally iatrogenic.

The practising physician should heed the warning 'start low and go slow' when considering therapeutics in the elderly. Start with as low a dose as possible and increase very gradually, keeping in mind the physiological changes that occur with increasing age impacting on liver function, renal function and the peripheral vascular flexibility to respond to drugs which act directly on it. The response can be blunted and a delayed reaction may be met with untoward consequences, such as profound hypotension in the elderly resulting in an impaired orthostatic reaction. Therapeutic drug monitoring in the elderly—that is, plasma concentrations—may not be as valuable as in younger people. Therapeutic drug monitoring is done on very few drugs, but in some cases is very useful in the elderly. Examples are digoxin (clearance decreases with age and declining renal function), carbamazapine (to check if the patient is compliant and within therapeutic range) and aminoglycosides (nephrotoxicity is more pronounced in the elderly due to declining renal function). The interpretation of data must consider the distinct conditions such as body size, age, renal and hepatic function, dosing intervals and interacting drugs of a patient population being treated.

Bibliography and further reading

Antal, E. J., Kramer, P. A., Mercik, S. A., Chapron, D. J. & Lawson, I. R. (1981), 'Theophylline pharmacokinetics in advanced age', *British Journal of Clinical Pharmacology*, 12, pp. 637–45.

Aronson, J. K. & Hardman, M. (1992), 'ABC of monitoring drug therapy: Digoxin', *British Medical Journal*, 305, pp. 1149–52.

Avorn, J. & Monane, M. (1992), 'Documenting, understanding and fixing psychoactive drug use in the nursing home', *Annual Review of Gerontology Geriatrics*, 12, pp. 163–82.

Bauer, L. A. & Blouin, R. A. (1981), 'Influence of age on theophylline clearance in patients with chronic obstructive pulmonary disease', *Clinical Pharmacokinetics*, 6, pp. 469–74.

Beller, G. A., Smith, T. W., Abelmann, W. H., Haber, E. & Hood, W. B. (1971), 'Digitalis intoxication. A prospective clinical study with serum level concentrations', *New England Journal of Medicine*, 18, pp. 989–97.

Campion, E. W., Avorn, J., Reder, V. A. & Olins, N. J. (1987), 'Overmedication of the low weight elderly', *Archives of Internal Medicine*, 147, pp. 945–7.

Caranasos, G. J., Stewart, R. B. & Cluff, L. E. (1974), 'Drug-related illness leading to hospitalization', *Journal of the American Medical Association*, 228, pp. 713–17.

Dobbs, R. J., O'Neill, J. A., Desmukh, A. A., Nicholson, P. W. & Bobbs, S. M. (1991), 'Serum concentration monitoring of cardiac glycosides. How helpful is it for adjusting dosage regimens?', *Clinical Pharmacokinetics*, 20, pp. 175–93.

Doherty, J. E. & Perkins, W. A. (1966), 'Digoxin metabolism in hypo- and hyperthyroidism: Studies with tritriated digoxin in thyroid disease', *Annals of Internal Medicine*, 64, pp. 489–507.

Hayes, M. J., Langman, M. J. S. & Short, A. H. (1975), 'Changes in drug metabolism with increasing age: 2. Phenytoin clearance and protein binding', *British*

Journal of Clinical Pharmacology, 2, pp. 73–9.

Hunt, S. N., Jusko, W. J. & Yurchak, A. M. (1976), 'Effect of smoking of theophylline disposition', *Clinical Pharmacology and Therapeutics*, 19, pp. 546–51.

Inouye, S. K. (1994), 'The dilemma of delirium: Clinical and research controversies regarding diagnosis and evaluations of delirium in hospitalized elderly patients', *American Journal of Medicine*, 97, pp. 278–88.

Koren, G. & Soldin, S. J. (1987), 'Cardiac glycosides', *Clinics in Laboratory Medicine*, 7, pp. 587–606.

Lowenthal, D. T. & Nadeau, S. E. (1994), 'Drug induced dementia', *Southern Medical Journal*, 84(5 Suppl. 1), pp. S24–31.

Nolan, P. E. & Mooradian, A. D. (1993), 'Digoxin', in Bressler, R. & Katz, M. D. (eds), *Geriatric Pharmacology*, McGraw-Hill Inc, New York, pp. 151–63.

Ouslander, J. (1981), 'Drug therapy in the elderly', *Annals of Internal Medicine*, 95, pp. 711–22.

Owens, N. J., Fretwell, M. D., Willey, C. & Murphy, S. (1994), 'Distinguishing between the fit and the frail elderly, and optimizing pharmacotherapy', *Drugs and Aging*, 4, pp. 47–55.

Ruiz, J. G., Array, S. & Lowenthal, D. T. (1996a), 'Avoiding overmedication of elderly patients', *American Journal of Therapeutics*, 3, pp. 784–8.

Ruiz, J. G., Array, S. & Lowenthal, D. T. (1996b), 'Therapeutic drug monitoring in the elderly', *American Journal of Therapeutics*, 3, pp. 839–60.

Ruiz, J. G. & Lowenthal, D. T. (1995), 'Geriatric pharmacology', in Munson, P. L., Meuller, R. A. & Breese, G. R. (eds), *Principles of Pharmacology. Basic Concepts and Clinical Applications*, Chapman and Hall, New York, pp. 1717–26.

Part II

Healthy ageing

Chapter 6

Health promotion and ageing

ALEX KALACHE and SHEEL M. PANDYA

Introduction

Health promotion is 'the process of enabling people to increase control over, and to improve, their health' (Ottawa Charter, 1986). It established itself as an important force within the 'New Public Health' movement. Recent developments in health promotion and public health have been rapid and concurrent with paradigm shifts in medicine and health policy in the 20th century. With these shifts, health promotion has developed both independently and in relation to the New Public Health movement.

Public health is a social and political concept aimed at improving health, prolonging life and improving the quality of life among whole populations through health promotion, disease prevention and other forms of health intervention. The distinction between public health and the 'new' public health movement has been cited in the literature to emphasise significantly different approaches to the description and analysis of the determinants of health and the methods of solving public health problems. This New Public Health is distinguished by its basis in a comprehensive understanding of the ways in which lifestyles and living conditions determine health status and a recognition of the need to mobilise resources and create sound programs, policies and services which result in supportive environments for health.

Public health went through profound changes during the 20th century. In the 19th century, public health mainly directed interventions at environmental infrastructures that affected health. By the early part of the 20th century, the focus shifted towards individual health, with the development of comprehensive vaccination and immunisation programs. However, during the second part of the 20th century, the focus of public health shifted back to the more traditional 19th century approaches, including concerns for structure, environment and ecology. Clinical medicine broadened its focus to include, like public health, concerns for lifestyles and health behaviours. Patients became more informed consumers of health services and more involved in the diagnosis and treatment of disease.

Health promotion has emerged as a unifying concept, bringing together many separate fields of study. It forms an important part of health services in most developed nations and, increasingly, in the developing world. Since the late 1980s it has been the subject of a growing number of professional training courses and academic activities. In recent years, there has been a plea for more evidence based health promotion action—that is, justification of health promotion programs on the basis of research information on their effectiveness in achieving predetermined outcomes. However, health promotion is not the only area under scrutiny in the health sector. There seems to be greater attention on outcomes and evidence of effectiveness within the health sector worldwide.

This chapter gives an overview of health promotion and ageing by providing, first, a brief description of health promotion, its origins and World Health Organization (WHO) related activities. Second, it gives a summary on ageing and health, its definition and the perspective adopted by WHO in the mid-1990s. Finally, the chapter highlights the life-course perspective, describes health promotion in old age, provides examples of health promotion programs for older persons and effective means of health promotion.

Background on health promotion

The term 'health promotion' first appeared in 1974 when the Canadian Minister of National Health and Welfare, Marc Lalonde, published *A New Perspective on the Health of Canadians*. In this report, Lalonde introduced the idea that health and disease are determined by four distinct elements: lifestyle or behavioural factors, supportive environments, biogenetic characteristics and the health services system. The fundamental message in this report is that critical improvements within the environment and in individual lifestyles could lead to a significant reduction in morbidity and premature death. The Lalonde report led to a series of WHO initiatives, beginning with the Alma Ata declaration in 1977.

Alma Ata was an important landmark in the declaration of WHO policy. The principal thrust of this declaration was that primary health care was to be the basis of national health care systems in developing and developed countries alike. It also incorporated a commitment to societal participation and intersectoral action. There are three prevailing principles in this declaration. The first is to secure a more equitable distribution of health care among different geographic and social groups of the population. The second is to use health care technologies that are acceptable and appropriate from a social, medical and economic point of view. The third and final principle is that individual citizens and communities must be made more aware of the factors influencing their own health and that people must be empowered to further influence those factors.

By the early 1980s, some basic tenets in the development of a health promotion movement had emerged, including: (1) cultural specificity; (2) food, shelter and income as the basic resources for health; and (3) information and knowledge about health factors, appropriate skills for health and supportive environments to enhance health and opportunities for healthier choices are necessary. In 1984, the WHO European Regional Office (HP-EURO) launched a formal program on health promotion with the new vision of health promotion combining both environmental and lifestyle approaches. In 1986, HP-EURO organised the first international conference on health promotion in Ottawa, Canada, in collaboration with the Canadian Public Health Association and the Canadian Ministry of Health. The result of this conference was The Ottawa Charter for Health Promotion (see Box 6.1). The Charter identified three basic mechanisms for health promotion: advocacy for health; enabling all people to achieve their full health potential; and mediating between the different interests in society in pursuit of health. These are supported by five principal strategies for action which provide a useful framework for health promotion action.

The Ottawa Charter for Health Promotion delineated important prerequisites for health, including peace, shelter, education, food, income, a stable ecosystem, sustainable resources, social justice and equity. Improvement in health requires a secure foundation in these basic requisites.

Through the Charter, a firm commitment to health promotion was expressed. The platform provided by it has been progressively built on with international conferences in Adelaide, Australia (1988), which focused on healthy public policy; Sundsvall, Sweden (1991), where the emphasis was on supportive environments for health; Jakarta,

Box 6.1 The Ottawa Charter for Health Promotion

Health promotion strategy means:
- building healthy public policy
- creating supportive environments
- strengthening community action
- developing personal skills
- reorienting health services

A commitment to health promotion refers to:
- political commitment to health and equity in all sectors
- counteraction of the effects of harmful products, environments and living conditions
- response to the health gap within and between societies
- acknowledgment of people as the main health resource
- reorientation of health services towards health promotion, sharing power with people themselves
- recognition of health and its maintenance as a major social investment and challenge

Indonesia (1997), whose theme was 'new players for a new era—leading health promotion into the 21st century'; and Mexico City, Mexico (2000), which focused on equity in health. The Jakarta Declaration on Leading Health Promotion in the 21st Century confirmed that the strategies for action outlined in the Ottawa Charter are relevant for all countries. Furthermore, over time, several key factors with the purpose of lifting the health status of people, improving their quality of life and providing cost-effective solutions to health problems have been clarified. Since then, evidence has been gathered which indicates that:

- comprehensive approaches using all five strategies (see Box 6.1) stated in the Ottawa Charter are required;
- certain 'settings', including schools, workplaces, cities and local communities offer opportune environments for effective health promotion work;
- individuals, particularly those who are most affected by health issues, need to be at the heart of health promotion action programs and decision-making processes to ensure maximum effectiveness;
- equitable access to education and information is essential in achieving effective participation and the empowerment of people and communities; and
- health promotion is a key 'investment'—an essential element of social and economic development.

A declaration made at the Fourth International Conference on Health Promotion in Jakarta called for new players to form novel partnerships in the development of health promotion strategies and to adopt an evidence based approach to policy and practice. The Jakarta Declaration identifies five priorities:

1. Promote social responsibility for health.
2. Increase investments for health development.
3. Expand partnerships for health promotion.
4. Increase community capacity and empower the individual.
5. Secure an infrastructure for health promotion.

Definition of health promotion

Health promotion has been defined in a myriad of ways. The approach taken and parameters surrounding health promotion are sometimes determined by the social context of the organisation defining it. However, at the very simplest level, health promotion is a strategy for promoting the health of whole populations. Health promotion consists of a range of interventions that lead to improvement, maintenance and prevention of decline in health status. Over time, as more and more evidence on the influence of the broad determinants or prerequisites for health has become available, the definition of health promotion has broadened to more explicitly recognising the determinants of health. Therefore, health promotion can now be defined as 'the process of enabling people to exert control over the determinants of health and thereby improve their health' (WHO,

1998). Health promotion has been described here as a process. The purpose of this is to strengthen the skills and capabilities of individuals to take action and the capacities of groups and communities to act collectively to exert control over the determinants of health, including individual health behaviours and use of health services. It has been proposed that effective health promotion strategies include four main components (see Figure 6.1):

1. *Health education*—the process of supplying information that promotes health through conventional and innovative ways.
2. *Disease prevention*—using interventions for early diagnosis or prevention of specific diseases with a special focus on the control of risk factors.
3. *Health maintenance*—using treatment interventions to prevent the decline in health status, particularly in vulnerable populations, and to promote wellbeing.
4. *Healthy public policy*—influencing policy makers to develop healthy public policy interventions or creating a supportive climate for the development of policy (e.g. public transport policy, education policy, advertising regulations).

The more these four elements are implemented in a comprehensive way, the greater the impact of health promotion and commitment to healthy public policy.

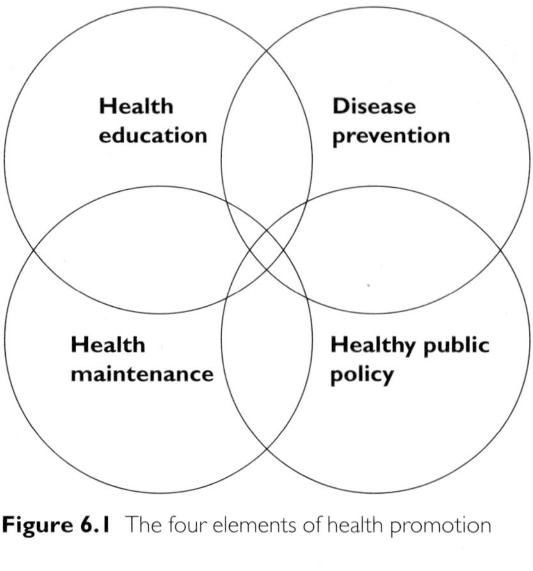

Figure 6.1 The four elements of health promotion

Definition of ageing

Ageing can be defined as the process of progressive change in the biological, psychological and social structure of individuals. For statistical purposes, 'the aged' are commonly placed into specific groups, e.g. 60 years and over, depending on cultural and personal perceptions of ageing. However, ageing is a lifelong process, which begins before we are born and continues throughout life. Ageing is associated with health unless there is sickness or disability and the majority of healthy ageing individuals are testimony to this. However, as people age, their risk of disease and disability increases. This risk may subside or often be avoided altogether. While heredity may impact on the risk of disease and disability, lifestyle and behaviour, living conditions and environmental factors are paramount as they strongly affect the presence of disease and disability as well. It may be possible for individuals to maintain their everyday functions and further prevent a decline in disability through healthy lifestyles and supportive environments over a lifespan. Therefore, health promotion and ageing involve efforts to provide the best possible environment (social and physical) for human development as early as possible, the adoption of healthy habits at an early stage in life and the maintenance of those habits throughout the lifespan. This notion has been coined by the term 'healthy ageing/active ageing' which has been actively promoted by WHO, Age Concern and the European Union.

WHO perspective on ageing

Life expectancy rose sharply in the 20th century and is expected to continue to rise in both developed and developing countries. At present, there are approximately 590 million people in the world aged 60 years and above, and this figure is expected to increase to around 1.2 billion by 2025. Older people, particularly the very old, aged 80 and over, are the fastest growing segment of the population and most of this growth is taking place in developing countries, such that, by 2025, approximately three-quarters of older persons will be residing in the developing world. The elderly population growth in the developed world is expected to increase only marginally compared to that in developing countries, but will still represent a significant increase as a percentage of the population. The timing, rapidity and effects of population ageing are, and will continue to be, very different in the developed world compared to developing countries. For example, in France, it took 115 years for the proportion of the elderly population to increase from 7% to 17%. In contrast, it is expected that the same doubling of the elderly population will take 27 years in China—that is, four times more rapidly. The gradual evolution of population ageing in developed countries was largely due to improved living standards and conditions since the Industrial Revolution. This phenomenon is now occurring much more rapidly in developing countries because of improved living conditions (in some countries), disease prevention (such as immunisation) and a rapid decline in fertility.

WHO's interest in the health care of older persons dates back to 1955 but it was only in 1974 that the Expert Committee's meeting report on ageing was conveyed. In 1979, the World Health Assembly adopted its first resolution, which was targeted to the health care of older persons. This led to the establishment of The Global Programme on Health of the Elderly (HEE) in 1980. The objective of the Programme was 'to support the continuous evolution and adaptation of technologies and approaches aimed at protecting and promoting the health of elderly people'.

WHO prepared a policy paper for the 1982 World Assembly on Aging, which was convened by the United Nations. This paper provided the basis for the Vienna International Plan of Action on Aging that was adopted by the World Assembly on Aging and became the framework for WHO activities aimed at older persons between 1982 and 1987. The Plan of Action outlines goals and policy recommendations for the international community, governments and other institutions and society at large to meet the challenge of an ageing population. It encouraged Member States to develop demographic and health profiles; formulate programs for community based health care for older persons, with a special focus on health promotion and self-health care; and to advocate issues related to the health of older persons with scientific and professional organisations.

In January 1995, a proposal was submitted to the 95th session of the Executive Board with the interest of developing a more integrated program on Ageing and Health, one that focuses not just on diseases, but also on the long-term developmental processes that have resulted in disease. This proposal called for a reorientation and renaming of the HEE Programme to become a new, integrated Programme on Ageing and Health (AHE). The purpose of the Programme was not only to promote health in old age, but also to promote health and wellbeing throughout the lifespan. This approach is designed to attain the highest possible level of quality of life for the longest period of time for the largest contingent of people. The Programme built on seven perspectives:

1. life-course perspective
2. health promotion perspective
3. cohort perspective
4. cultural perspective
5. gender perspective
6. intergenerational perspective
7. ethical perspective

Furthermore, the Programme included the following key components: information strengthening, information dissemination, advocacy, informed research, training and policy development.

Recent changes in organisation at WHO have led to the establishment of the Health Promotion/Non-Communicable Disease Prevention and Surveillance Department (HPS), which is part of the Non-Communicable Disease and Mental Health (NMH) Cluster. The HPS Department is divided into four areas, including a group that focuses on The Life-Course. The purpose of this group is to continue to emphasise the life-course perspective, a concept vitalised by AHE, and the importance of healthy lifestyles and supportive environments over a lifespan.

To draw attention to the challenges and opportunities of an ageing population, the United Nations designated 1999 as the International Year of Older Persons. This provided WHO with a platform to promote the importance of healthy and active ageing programs and policies throughout the world, while working with multiple partners to provide initiative and support for the organisation of events and activities that promote active ageing.

WHO celebrated ageing with the Global Embrace, a worldwide 24 hour walk event organised under the leadership of WHO on 2 October 1999 and the largest health promotion activity for older persons ever held. Over 3000 cities in 96 countries and all continents participated in this event. It is estimated that over 2 million people, both young and old, walked along beaches, country roads, in parks and stadiums, as they celebrated active ageing. Involving both young and older persons in this event is a reminder that today's adults are tomorrow's older persons. Families and friends, community organisers, local and international celebrities and the like joined together in expressing their solidarity and support for active ageing. The worldwide walk event began in the Pacific (Fiji, New Zealand, New Caledonia) and continued across Australia, Japan, Korea, China, the Philippines, India, the Middle East, Africa, many parts of Europe and culminated in the Americas. The global embrace walk event launched the global movement for active ageing, which was conceived by WHO. It is a network of individuals and organisations interested in moving policies and practice towards active ageing. The purpose of the global movement is to provide an arena in which interested parties can share and exchange ideas about model programs and policies that promote active ageing.

As a global agency on health, WHO has taken a leadership role on the issue of global ageing by adopting the life-course perspective on achieving healthy/active ageing and ensuring the attainment of the best possible quality of life, for as many people as possible, for the longest period of time. There is much an individual can do to remain healthy in later life, including adopting a healthier lifestyle and remaining active in society.

The life-course perspective

Health and activity in older age are a summary of the living conditions and actions of an individual over an entire lifespan. Health promotion over a lifespan involves the adoption of healthy lifestyles and behaviours, which can play a critical role in how individuals age, the extent of disability and quality of life. This conceptual approach presents individuals with the opportunity to impact on how they age by adopting healthier behaviours and lifestyles early on and by adapting to age associated changes. However, for individuals to do this, society must adopt a more positive view of ageing and support such individuals through legislative efforts and accessibility and availability of services. There are many factors, including economic, social and environmental conditions, that influence health and ageing and may not be modifiable by the individual. In a living environment that is supportive, an individual who has experienced a significant loss in any given functional capacity may continue to live independently, while another individual with the same degree of functional loss, but living in a less than supportive environment, will experience a loss of independence.

It is particularly useful to introduce the concept of physical functional capacity within a life-course, as seen in Figure 6.2. Our functional capacity, in relation to a number of biological functions—such as ventilatory capacity, muscle strength and cardiovascular output—increases throughout childhood and reaches a peak in early adulthood. This peak is typically followed by a decline. How quickly this decline occurs is largely determined by factors related to adult lifestyles, such as smoking, alcohol consumption, lack of physical activity and inadequate diet. For example, the natural decline in cardiac function can be hastened by smoking, leaving an individual with a functional capacity level lower than would normally be expected for their age. The gradient may become so steep as to result in premature disability. However, the acceleration in decline may be reversed at any age. For example, smoking cessation and small increases in the level of exercise can significantly reduce the risk of developing coronary heart disease.

It is also important to consider factors such as education, poverty, harmful living and working conditions that can affect the functional capacity of an individual later in life.

The slope of the decline is influenced at any stage of one's life by both individual and public

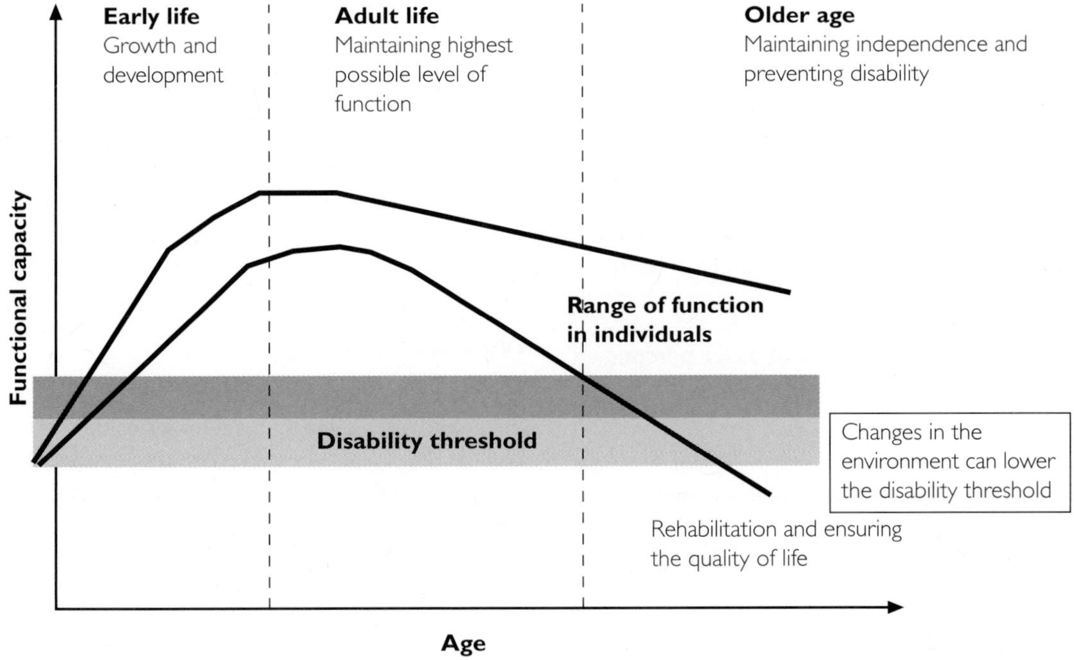

Figure 6.2 A life-course perspective for maintenance of the highest possible level of functional capacity

policy measures. Positive individual measures include smoking cessation, healthy eating or a balanced diet high in fibre and low in total fat, physical activity and lifelong learning. Policy measures may include increasing legislation and taxation to control tobacco use and consumer awareness about the relationship between good nutrition and health.

For individuals who become disabled, rehabilitation programs and further adaptation to the environment may reduce the extent of disability. Quality of life should be a major consideration throughout the life-course, particularly for those people whose functional capacity can no longer be maintained. Providing support to these vulnerable people, through formal or informal means, should be one of the main goals of policies for an ageing population. Furthermore, environmental changes, including adequate public transport in urban areas, elevators placed in apartment and office buildings, and ramps that make places more accessible can lower the disability threshold and ensure more independence in old age. Therefore, it is important to note that the 'disability threshold' in Figure 6.2 is not rigidly defined.

Health promotion in old age

Although the conceptual framework surrounding the life-course calls for the adoption of healthier lifestyles and behaviours early in life, health can be promoted at any point over the life-course, particularly in old age. There is evidence in the literature that age 50 marks a period of life during which the benefits of physical activity programs, for instance, are particularly relevant. Furthermore, in a recent population based study, Glass et al. (1999) found that social and productive activities that involve little or no enhancement of fitness lower the risk of all cause mortality as much as fitness activities do. The authors suggest that activity may confer survival benefits through psychosocial pathways and therefore such social and productive activities may complement physical exercise programs and serve as alternative interventions for frail older persons.

Effective health promotion interventions for older persons requires the recognition that ageing is a process (not a disease) and older persons have special characteristics, as seen in Box 6.2. With ageing, there is a progressive decline in the ability to respond to stressors in the environment, which may lead to functional impairment. The ageing process can be impacted upon by extrinsic factors associated with lifestyle, environmental conditions and disease. However, the effects of ageing—including decline in functional capacity, disease and disability and loss of adaptability—can be dealt with in a positive way through health promotion interventions that are relevant to older persons.

Box 6.2 Characteristics of older persons that impact on health promotion programs

- Heterogeneity
- Increased risk of disease and/or disability
- Multiple pathologies often present
- Iatrogenic problems common and frequently not recognised
- Social deficits
- Low adaptability to changes
- Premature intervention may trigger dependency
- Negative stereotypes created by society towards older persons

Health promotion programs for older persons

The majority of health promotion programs that exist for older persons fall into one of the following categories: physical activity, healthy nutrition, prevention of frailty or injury (including falls), smoking cessation, chronic disease management, socialisation and empowerment, immunisation, holistic wellbeing and health promotion in primary care.

Physical activity

There is a high prevalence of certain non-communicable diseases among people over the age of 60, including cardiovascular disease, cancer, osteoporosis, arthritis and diabetes, as well as health problems resulting from injuries and falls. There is now a wealth of data demonstrating the benefits of physical activity in diminishing the risk of and/or ameliorating these diseases and delaying a decline in function in both healthy and chronically ill older persons, while the risks of physical activity have been found to be modest. Physical activity is also considered a significant factor in improving musculoskeletal and mental health. Substantial evidence also shows that physical activity can increase average life expectancy by as much as two years.

Nutrition

Nutrition is an important aspect of healthful behaviour and a major component of the general wellbeing of individuals over the course of a lifetime (see Chapter 30). However, the process of ageing is accompanied by various economic, physiologic and social changes that may compromise nutritional status and that affect the need for several essential nutrients. Therefore, it is important that nutrition programs, as well as nutritional guidelines, be established to serve as an important educational reference for older persons.

Falls

Falls are common in the elderly, often causing considerable morbidity and mortality. As individuals age, there is a loss in balance function through loss of sensory elements, the ability to integrate information and issue motor commands. In addition, certain non-communicable diseases that are common in older persons lead to further deterioration in balance function in some individuals. Therefore, both prevention and rehabilitation play an important role in helping older persons reduce the extent and/or impact of injury and falls.

Smoking

Older persons who continue to smoke are at a greater risk of death, stroke, heart attack and cataracts and are more likely to be disabled by respiratory problems. Research has shown that giving up smoking after the age of 65 reduces the risk of cardiovascular disease and improves breathlessness. Educational efforts made by medical practitioners regarding the health risks of smoking have contributed to smoking cessation rates of approximately 15% in the general population and are considered one of the most cost-effective existing health promotion activities.

Chronic disease management

Healthy ageing over a life-course is important; however, the reality of growing old is an increased susceptibility to different chronic illnesses. Therefore, it is important that there are effective chronic disease management programs so that older persons, in particular, can learn to live with specific disease and become actively involved in their management.

Empowerment

With the growth of the population, the theme of empowerment has emerged as an issue of great importance. The contribution of older persons is often undermined or underestimated. Older persons are a great resource to society, not a burden, as they are often regarded. Therefore, it is important that programs that encourage the active involvement of older persons be established.

Immunisation

Research has shown that both healthy older persons and those older persons with underlying medical conditions are at risk for the serious complications of influenza and would benefit from vaccination. Therefore, immunisation programs for the prevention of viruses like influenza would be beneficial to the growing older population.

Holistic wellbeing

Nowadays, more health promotion programs are becoming more holistic—that is, address more biomedical, mental, social and spiritual aspects of healthy/active ageing. In this way, importance is given to the entirety of a person's wellbeing, not just one's physical health.

Health promotion in primary health care

The emergence of community based primary health care programs is considered to be one way of improving the health of the community, especially the older population. Many such programs aim to empower the older population and promote equity and access, while meeting the major principles of primary health care. Primary health care workers—including physicians, nurses and other health care professionals—can play an instrumental role in promoting health over the life-course, particularly in old age. Such professionals have the knowledge and expertise to inform, educate and advise people of ways of maintaining healthy lifestyles and further encouraging them to assume control of their own health by becoming informed consumers. Furthermore, primary care professionals can help people navigate their health by acting as a reference and mediator of knowledge that others may obtain from outside sources, including publications and sources on the Internet. Primary health care workers can also act as important advocates by not only disseminating information regarding the benefits of healthy lifestyles, but also by appealing to policy makers about appropriate environmental and social changes which would encourage people to live healthily and actively in society. Therefore, primary health care professionals can play an integral role in promoting health over a lifespan and among older persons, and impacting on policy.

Effective health promotion for older persons

Many health promotion programs specifically designed for older persons clearly show not only the positive health benefit for those concerned, but also the affirmative, contributory effect on society as a whole when this population is empowered to take control of their health. Instead of regarding older persons as a burden, programs and policies should be formulated to acknowledge, value and enhance their potential and active involvement in many formal and informal, social and economic roles, past, present and future.

However, to provide evidence for effectiveness and to further impact on and influence policy, health promotion programs for older persons, like other health promotion interventions, must be planned on the basis of a thorough assessment of the evidence from epidemiological, behavioural and social research, which show reasonable linkages between the short-term impact of interventions and the changes that ensue in the determinants of health and in health outcomes.

Health promotion programs should be informed by established theory, which is related to the type of intervention planned. There are many theories and models which are often used to provide guidance in program development and implementation and which can be adapted to fit most health promotion interventions. Also, the program should be of sufficient size, duration and sophistication to be detected among other pervasive societal issues.

It is important to establish the necessary conditions for successful implementation of a health promotion program. For instance, this could include ensuring that there is sufficient public and political awareness of an issue and the need for action, developing capacity for the delivery of a program through training of health personnel or securing the resources needed for the implementation and sustenance of a program.

Challenges ahead

An ageing population that is not healthy could easily become a drain on societal resources. This problem is magnified in developing countries because population ageing is occurring much more rapidly in these areas than in the developed world within a context of limited or even scarce resources.

Appropriate evaluation of health promotion programs poses a significant challenge. Evaluation is necessary in assessing the impact of particular health promotion interventions. The ability to influence policy makers depends on the ability to demonstrate the effectiveness of various health promotion programs. A considerable amount of progress is being made in understanding the complexity of health promotion and in the corresponding need for effective measures and in evaluating research designs which reflect the challenges of health promotion assessment. It is important to foster and develop evaluation designs which combine the positive aspects of different research methodologies, both qualitative and quantitative, in ways which are relevant to the stage of development of a particular program. Above all, it is important that evaluation of health promotion programs be tailored to suit the type of activity and circumstances of programs.

There is a pressing need for intersectoral action, as was formally declared in the Alma Ata declaration, in health promotion. It is necessary that public and private, governmental and non-governmental agencies and organisations work together in promoting health through advocacy, effective programming and policy. Health departments, organisations and professionals need to work in collaboration with other parties, including individuals and organisations involved in recreation and sport, transportation, advocacy groups, faith organisations, community groups and others to encourage healthy lifestyles among older people.

The impact of a healthy ageing population is seen in older persons being active and therefore productive for a longer period of time, thereby reducing health and social care costs. Health promotion programs and policies should ensure that older persons can remain active, that those who want to have paid work have the opportunity to do so, and that a positive and active image of ageing is created and promoted through society. After all, within or outside the work force the vast majority of older persons are contributors to society. And those who are not, due to ill health and frailty, need to be supported and have their individual health protected and promoted.

Bibliography and further reading

Blumberg, J. (1997), 'Nutritional needs of seniors', *Journal of American College of Nutrition*, 16(6), pp. 517–23.

Bunton, R. & Macdonald, G. (eds) (1992), *Health Promotion: Disciplines and Diversity*, Routledge, London, pp. 1–240.

Ebrahim, S. & Kalache, A. (eds) (1996), *Epidemiology of*

Old Age, BMJ Publishing Group, London, Chapter 16, pp. 153–61.

Glass, T. A., Mendes de Leon, C., Marottoli, R. A. & Berkman, L. F. (1999), 'Population based study of social and productive activities as predictors of survival among elderly Americans', *British Medical Journal*, 319, pp. 478–83.

Higgins, M. W., Enright, P. L. et al. (1993), 'Smoking and lung function in elderly men and women. The Cardiovascular Health Study', *Journal of the American Medical Association*, 269, pp. 2741–8.

Lalonde, M. (1999), 'A new perspective on the health of Canadians', Ottawa Information, Canada.

Nay, R. (1997), 'The 60 and Better Program: A primary health care program for the aged', *Contemporary Nursing*, 6(1), pp. 8–14.

Nicol, K. L. (1998), 'Ten-year durability and success of an organized program to increase influenza and pneumococcal vaccination rates among high-risk adults', *American Journal of Medicine*, 105(5), pp. 385–92.

Nutbeam, D. (1998), 'Evaluating health promotion—progress, problems and solution', *Health Promotion International*, 13(1), pp. 27–44.

Nutbeam, D. & Harris, E. (1999), *Theory in a Nutshell: A Guide to Health Promotion Theory*, McGraw-Hill Australia, Sydney.

Paffenbarger Jnr, R. S., Kampert, J. B., Lee, I. M. et al. (1994), 'Changes in physical activity and other lifestyle patterns influencing longevity', *Medical Sciences and Sports*, 26, pp. 857–65.

Schoenfelder, D. P. & Van Why, K. (1997), 'A fall prevention educational program for community dwelling seniors', *Public Health Nursing*, 14(6), pp. 383–90.

Stewart, A. L., Mills, K. M. et al. (1998), 'Evaluation of CHAMPS, a physical activity promotion program for older adults', *Annals of Behavior Medicine*, 19(4), pp. 353–61.

'The Evidence of Health Promotion Effectiveness, Shaping Public Health in a New Europe', Report for the European Commission by the International Union for Health Promotion and Education, Parts 1 and 2, 1999.

United Nations Population Division (1999), *World Population Prospects: The 1998 Revision*, United Nations Department of Economic and Social Affairs, http://www.popin.org/pop1998/8.htm.

US Department of Commerce (1993), 'An Aging World II', *International Population Reports*, Washington, DC.

Vetter, N. J. & Ford, D. (1990), 'Smoking prevention among people aged 60 and over: A randomized controlled trial', *Age and Ageing*, 19, pp. 164–8.

World Health Organization (1978), The Alma Ata Declaration, WHO, Geneva.

World Health Organization (1986), The Ottawa Charter, Adopted at the International Conference on Health Promotion (17–21 November 1986, Ottawa, Ontario, Canada), WHO, Geneva.

World Health Organization (1997), Jakarta Declaration, WHO, Geneva.

World Health Organization (1998), Health Promotion Glossary, WHO, Geneva, reference: WHO/HPR/HEP/98.1.

World Health Organization (1999), Life Course Perspective, WHO, Geneva.

Chapter 7

Home care—back to the future?

L. J. MYKYTA

Introduction

Aged care, and health care of all types, began at home. Operations were done on kitchen tables long before operating theatres or even hospitals existed. Nor should we forget that hospitals have always been dangerous places for patients. The high death rates following surgery and childbirth in the late 19th century led to a common fear that admission to hospital was tantamount to a sentence of death.

Home care has always been the dominant mode of aged care. The institutional forms, again, had less than illustrious origins. It can be fairly argued that modern geriatric medicine began in the UK. It is easy to forget that British geriatrics was built on the heritage of the Poor Law system, which offered care of a sort to the needy aged, unfortunate enough to have no other means of support. There are some lingering similarities between the modern residential facility and a 19th century workhouse.

Both health care and aged care were strongly influenced by the deinstitutionalisation movement from the middle of the 20th century, which resulted in major advances in the care and management of the mentally ill, the chronically ill and disabled, and the aged. It also added a social and humanitarian rationale that could subsequently be exploited by economic rationalists.

Factors shaping the system

Ageing of the population

The net effect of population ageing is that the growth in the potential (and actual) target populations of the various care and support services greatly outstrips the rate of increase in resources, and this is virtually regardless of the wealth of the nations concerned.

Population ageing is usually accompanied by other demographic changes that have an impact on the capacity of the newly shaped population to respond to various social needs. Among these changes are rising ages at marriage; changes in family size, type, function and mobility; urbanisation; altered employment practices; and altered living arrangements.

Regardless of social and welfare structures and provisions, there is virtually no nation in the world that can maintain its dependent populations without some form of self-funding—for example, in the form of long-term care insurance.

The burden of care is also increasingly shifted to the informal sector, essentially the family.

Escalating costs of care

Costs of care are progressively escalating for a variety of reasons, including the emergence of new technology, and improved salaries and conditions of workers among many other factors, which can be loosely described as the infrastructure costs of maintaining the system.

The changing role of the hospital

Rising cost has been one of the main factors that have determined the current role of the hospital within the wider system of care.

Until quite recently, we expected our hospitals to be the source of many services that we needed, when we needed them, for as long as we needed them, including:

- health promotion
- prevention
- cure
- amelioration
- rehabilitation and convalescence
- asylum, support
- palliation, comfort.

Narrowing of hospital role

Rising costs and new methods of funding of hospitals, such as casemix based funding, have resulted in a narrowing of the hospital's role into a limited range of acute health care and the shifting of all other activities into different sorts of institutions or what is euphemistically described as 'the community'.

Responses

This narrowing of the hospital role, usually accompanied by a decrease in size, has resulted in a number of responses:

- more day, ambulatory or outpatient activity
- more short stay procedures
- shorter stay, early discharge for all medical and surgical conditions
- shift of routine outpatient activity to the private or non-hospital sector
- shift of routine procedures from public to private hospitals
- shift of uncomplicated acute medical cases, rehabilitation and convalescence to home based care.

Needs

The needs that emerge as a result of these trends include:

- development of different types of inpatient facilities
- strengthening of the community/home care sector
- integrating hospitals with all regional services to create a better continuum of care.

Emergence of the consumer and the claiming of 'rights'

This is the age of information. The consumer is better educated and better informed, as well as being more aware of his rights than previously. Consumer rights have been increasingly recognised and institutionalised in all jurisdictions.

Increasingly, users of services believe that having their preferences met is a right that must be met by their country's health and welfare system, particularly when they are making a major financial contribution through taxation or insurance. Much of the new consumerism is couched in the language of rights. Most of the rights being claimed are not true rights in any legal or moral sense, but reflect demands and wishes stated in a more compelling way.

Home care and community care is easy to 'sell'. It is virtually everyone's preference to remain in the comfort of his own home, among family, friends and neighbours, regardless of circumstances.

It is also common for people to promise those nearest and dearest to them that they will never abandon them or commit them to an institution.

Competing ideologies

In the fields of disability and aged care, there is a tendency to denigrate the 'medical model' and to hold the medical profession responsible for all past injustices suffered by disabled people. The home and the community are presented as arenas where the consumer holds sway, unlike hospitals and residential facilities.

Unforeseen effects of government policy

Deinstitutionalisation

Goffman, a sociologist writing in the 1960s, introduced the term 'total institution', which he defined as 'a place of residence and work where a large number of like-situated individuals, cut off from the wider society for an appreciable period of time, together lead an enclosed, formally administered round of life'. He went on to describe the four main characteristics of a 'total institution':

- *Batch living* describes a situation where 'each phase of the member's daily activity is carried on in the immediate company of a large batch of others, all of whom are treated alike, and are required to do the same thing together'. It is the antithesis to individual living.
- *Binary management* refers to the existence of two groups, the managers and the managed. Management is characteristically bureaucratic, with formal rules, regulations and schedules that allow for little free time.
- *The inmate role* involves a loss of role and individual identity and privacy and the acquisition of a new and depersonalised identity as a cipher with few personal possessions. This can lead to adjustments that may range from withdrawal to rebelliousness.
- *The institutional perspective,* where Goffman was describing a perception of the prisons and mental institutions of his day, although subsequent scholars have suggested that 'his aim was to set up a model against which reality could be measured, rather than to describe reality itself'.

Goffman's views were very influential, and contributed to dramatic changes in the way that long-stay psychiatric patients were managed throughout the world.

Initially, the impetus behind this movement came from concern about the poor conditions and lifestyle of residents in large institutions. In more recent times, economic imperatives have taken over as the most compelling factor.

In Australia, the Nursing Homes and Hostels Review (1986) set out the principles of the Commonwealth government's Aged Care Reform Strategy. These principles included:

- Aged and disabled people should as far as possible be supported in their own homes, in their own communities.
- Aged and disabled people should be supported by residential services only where other support systems are not appropriate to meet their needs.

It is evident that the authors of the Reform Strategy assumed that there was a progression of care and that residential care was both a last resort and a less desirable alternative than community care.

The progression could be envisaged as:

- independent unsupported living
- community supported living
- low level residential care
- high level residential care.

In practice, it becomes quite evident that this orderly progression does not occur, and that there is little qualitative difference in characteristics between people who enter residential care and those who receive long-term care in the community. In many countries, residential care is no longer even considered as an option, whatever the level of disability for young people with disability.

There is a prevalent belief that community based care is inevitably and invariably cheaper than the residential or institutional alternative.

The question that arises is: 'Cheaper for whom?' All forms of community and home based care shift a burden of responsibility and cost on to the informal sector, predominantly the immediate family of the care recipient. This informal input is rarely costed and translated into financial terms.

While the shift to the community and home care is to be applauded, governments have often failed to recognise that major shifts in policy and direction have to be funded, essentially with new money, as the needs of the hospital and residential sector do not diminish to enable a transfer of finance.

The scope of home care

Virtually any type of care or support can be provided in any environment (see Table 7.1).

While all activities can be undertaken in any setting, there are very good reasons for retaining the whole system and determining the most appropriate setting on the basis of outcomes for the users and for the funders of services. The outcome factors to be considered include safety and efficacy, user satisfaction, effectiveness and efficiency.

Table 7.1 The scope of home care

	Inpatient residential	Ambulatory centre based	Home based
Primary care	++[(a)]	+++++	+++
Acute medical care	+++++	++	++++
Convalescence	+++++	++	+++++
Rehabilitation	+++++	++++	++++
Long stay	+++++	++	+++++
Respite	+++++	+++	+++++
Crisis care	+++++	++	+++

(*a*) + = Ease and practicability of undertaking each case.

The feasibility of home care

The questions that must be asked (and answered) for any potential target population are:

- Can the same level (intensity) of care be provided in the home/community as in institutional/residential care?
- Can the same or better health outcomes be achieved?
- Can the same quality of care be achieved and maintained, and for whom?
- Can the same levels of safety be achieved for the client and the carers?
- Can the quality of life of clients and carers be equalled or improved?
- Can this be achieved without increasing carer burden and stress?
- Can cost be lower or equal to residential/institutional care?

Care of any intensity can be provided in the community, but home care will not always be the best option in terms of quality and the social and emotional needs of clients and carers. A range of options will have to continue to be offered, and informed choices will still need to be made to ensure optimal outcomes for clients and carers. These options will only be realistic if they are realistically funded.

Choosing a care option

The entry into any form or level of care should always be on the basis of comprehensive assessment. The assessor(s), ideally an interdisciplinary team, must be capable of fulfilling the following obligations:

- accurate diagnosis of all significant problems, and precise definition of disability and dependency
- prognosis: recognition of *preventive, remedial* and *rehabilitation potential*
- determination of intellectual capacity and mental illness, including decision-making competence
- identification of the social support network, carer stress
- identification of the patient's and family's perceptions of needs and possible solutions
- formulation of a management plan that can be offered to the patient, the family and referrers
- information, communication with patients, family and referrers
- assistance with access to the most appropriate alternative care options
- continuing surveillance and review
- awareness of comparative need and ability to set priorities.

The decision to seek external assistance or admission into residential care is triggered by a number of factors, including:

- physical deterioration
- mental deterioration
- bereavement, loss of social support
- loneliness
- insecurity, fear for the future
- external pressure
- dissatisfaction with current home or living arrangements.

These reasons must be understood if our responses are to be appropriate and effective.

In aged care, external pressure is often applied by families out of concern for their relatives, and these concerns must be addressed, rather than dismissed. They must be offered explanation and reassurance rather than a seemingly arbitrary dismissal of what they perceive are major risks.

The decision about the selection of the appropriate form of care is determined by a number of medical and non-medical factors.

Health related factors

- *Dependency level* Dependency is a measure of the assistance required from other people and can be accurately quantified in accordance with a number of conventions.
- *The interval of care need* If intervention is required at predictable intervals and for relatively short periods, it is easy to provide community support. If care is required frequently, urgently and at unpredictable intervals, it becomes extremely difficult.
- *Intensity of care* If a number of persons are involved in care provision, or if regular intensive care is provided, it becomes difficult, and costly, to deploy sufficient community resources.
- *Complexity of care* There are some levels of care —for example, respirator management—that virtually mandate continuing care in a hospital-type setting.

Personal attributes

The individual's determination and drive to independence can override most difficulties.

Social factors

The strength of a person's family support system is the most valuable asset in aged care, but the presence of a severely disabled elderly person also puts great stress on a household, and it becomes necessary to consider the needs of the caregivers as well as the patient.

Environmental factors

At times the quality of the living environment will impact on the decision. For example, a severely disabled, wheelchair bound person cannot live successfully in a multilevel house without costly modification and adaptation.

Implications for residential care facilities

It must be apparent from Table 7.1 that residential facilities will progressively be dealing with more physically and, particularly, mentally disabled residents, who will require higher and more skilled levels of care. In many countries residential facilities are difficult to distinguish from hospitals. This has obvious implications for staffing and the physical environment.

Hospital-in-the-home (HIH)

Many activities that have in the past been considered the exclusive domain of inpatient facilities are being successfully shifted into the community. These include acute care, rehabilitation and palliative care.

Drivers

The drivers of these moves include:

- legislated change
- patient preference
- improvement in housing standards
- new technologies which make HIH possible
- long waiting lists for elective surgery
- concerns about the overall cost of inpatient hospital care and, arguably,
- better health outcomes.

Potential benefits of home based programs

For selected patients, most notably disabled old people, home based programs offer many advantages, including:

- the comfort of being in one's own home, familiar cuisine
- least disruption of normal relationships, greater convenience for carers

- safety:
  - lower infection rates (there is a very markedly decreased risk of nosocomial infection)
  - fewer adverse events
  - less opportunity for iatrogenic complications
  - avoidance of the complications of bed rest
- maintenance of autonomy and independence.

For the hospital a home care program allows:

- flexibility, ability to offer choices and options
- avoidance of admission or reduction in length of stay (LOS) for selected conditions
- reduction in waiting lists for particular conditions and generally
- improved hospital throughput.

For general practitioners there are opportunities and incentives to become involved in more acute levels of care and to work with a multidisciplinary team.

Characteristics of successful programs

Capacity to provide intensive levels of care in a cost effective manner

This implies availability of diverse categories of workers to ensure that the cheapest (least trained, least qualified) worker capable of undertaking a given task to a required standard is utilised. Economies of scale are important. It is more cost effective to deploy staff who are already in the field than to call out a worker to undertake a single task, or small number of tasks. By and large, unless volume of work permits, it is more cost effective to utilise a home care agency than to provide intensive home care on a hospital outreach basis.

Case management

Utilisation of case managers, who are identifiable key contacts/workers, is of prime importance. The ability to contact a familiar person who has the capacity and authority to initiate change and respond to concerns, at any time, is the single factor most frequently cited by patients and carers as the greatest source of satisfaction with home care programs.

It is extremely important to focus on the provision of social and emotional support to carers, regardless of how much actual patient care they are expected to provide.

Appropriate technology

The care provider should have access to all necessary equipment and, particularly, to high level information and communication systems.

Clinical discipline

A home care episode should be considered as no different to an inpatient admission. There should be a limited, manageable number of cases per case manager (comparable to a hospital unit). Targets should be set for 'lengths of stay', similar to those that would apply for the same condition in an inpatient facility, and following management protocols appropriate to the type of care being provided, whatever the care setting. At the completion of the episode, the patient should be formally discharged from the program.

Management of the interfaces

Effective management of the interface between inpatient facilities and the community includes discharge planning, and documented clinical communication between all of the involved parties, which includes the patient and his family, hospital staff, community care staff and the patient's general practitioner. It is useful for these communications to be formalised as management plans and service agreements.

Patients and carers are greatly disturbed by transitions that do not go smoothly, particularly what they perceive as precipitate discharge from hospital.

Medico-legal considerations

Medico-legal issues are specific to jurisdictions, but there are some common issues that need to be considered.

A decision that is based on the intent to improve the quality of care and quality of life would generally be seen as in the best interests of the patient. The decision to opt for HIH in preference to inpatient care should be based on these grounds, rather than on some imperative to clear hospital beds at all costs. The overriding consideration must be that it is medically appropriate for the patient to be managed at home. All Occupational Health and Safety requirements must be met. Ideally, the patient should be given the opportunity to choose from a range of realistic options in line with the principles of informed consent.

As in any other form of health care, it is essential to ensure full documentation of care plans, service agreements, contracts, consents, etc. It is advisable to develop and adhere to prepared protocols. It is also extremely important to ensure that there is a good communication strategy in place. Much patient satisfaction in health care is based on the quality of communication rather than on actual care, which patients may find difficult to evaluate.

All staff involved in the program must be appropriately qualified, trained and experienced, and there must be systems in place for clinical decision making, supervision and support.

Patient selection criteria

- There must be a suitable home to stay in or return to. At times this may be the home of a relative, rather than the patient's own home.
- The availability of a carer at home is a desirable but not obligatory requirement, provided that all necessary basic and instrumental activities of daily living can be supported, and appropriate monitoring strategies are in place.
- There should be a telephone line for communication and monitoring available.
- The patient or legal guardian is able to comprehend and give an informed consent to participation in the program.
- The patient must be medically stable, and all investigations and interventions should be complete. Protocols and criteria for patient selection are now available for a number of conditions. These specify exactly what 'medically stable' implies in terms of physiological state, and disease activity indicators.
- Management according to the relevant condition specific protocol is feasible and appropriate.
- The patient should have the option of admission or readmission as necessary.
- The patient's general practitioner or other clearly designated medical practitioner accepts the medical responsibility for patient care.

The continued move towards home and community care is as inevitable as the tide. This will require us to ensure that we understand and are equipped to play a chosen role in the care system. It will also call on a level of co-ordination that we have never achieved before.

Bibliography and further reading

AARP Foundation website: http://research.aarp.org/health/index.html This site is the American Association of Retired Persons Research Centre on Health and Long Term Care. There are a number of research and review papers relevant to the topic.

Hughes, S. L., Weaver, F. M., Giobbie-Hurder, A., Manheim, L. et al. (2000), 'Effectiveness of team-managed home-based primary care. A randomized multicenter trial', *Journal of the American Medical Association*, 284, pp. 2877–85. Also available at: http://jama.ama-assn.org/issues/v284n22/abs/joc00629.html

Joint Commission on Accreditation of Healthcare Organizations website: http://www.jcaho.org/mainmenu.html There is a section on accreditation of Home Care organisations.

Monk, A. & Cox, C. (eds) (1991), *Home Care for the Elderly. An International Perspective*, Auburn House, New York; Westport, CT; London.

Sheps, S. B., Reid, R. J., Barer, M. L., Krueger, H. et al. (2000), 'Hospital downsizing and trends in health care use among elderly people in British Columbia', *Canadian Medical Association Journal*, 163, pp. 397–401. Also available at: http://www.cma.ca/cmaj/vol163/issue-4/0397.htm

Spratt, J. S., Hawley, R. L. & Hoye, R. E. (eds) (1997), *Home Health Care. Principles and Practices*, GR/St Lucie Press, Delray Beach, FL.

Chapter 8

Sexual function and the older adult

FRAN E. KAISER

Introduction

Sexual function in the older adult is neither an oxymoron nor a passing historical comment. Although the first sexual 'revolution' in the 20th century was regarded as the province of the young and healthy, the second revolution, bridging into the 21st century, belongs to older adults. This second revolution is in its infancy for both men and women. As our global society continues to age, quality of life issues become increasingly important, and among these issues, sexuality and sexual function have become increasingly important. Sexuality can be described as a quality or state that includes sexual desire (libido), arousal, function, activity and satisfaction. However, sexuality goes beyond these descriptors. Intimacy, affection, connection and self-pleasure are also important factors that go beyond the usual measures of sexual activity. Sense of self, interaction with others and the ethnic, environmental and societal cohort in which an individual exists will have an impact on the sexuality of that person. Unfortunately, the majority of studies published on sexual function with ageing measure intercourse as the sole defining issue. Since women generally tend to surpass males in surviving to older ages, this has often been reported as decreased sexual function with age in women. Clearly for both women and men, one does have to factor in changes engendered by partner availability and function, environmental issues (privacy/opportunity) as well as self or partner illness.

In data that examined sexual interest and behaviour in a group of 80 to 102-year-old men and women, touching and caressing as well as masturbation were important means of sexual expression. Since many of these individuals were not partnered, coital activity was less common than other modalities of expression. Predictors of sexual activity that lasts into older adulthood included the level of sexual interest, enjoyment and activity that occurred in younger years. In addition to barriers to optimal function related to partner availability and partner and/or self-health issues, the overlay of physiological/pathologic alterations in sex drive, erectile dysfunction in males or dyspareunia in females may hamper capability.

From the early days of Kinsey, over 50 years ago, sexual function in older adults has been measured as coital frequency and, according to this parameter, both men and women have decreased activity with age. At all reported ages over 60 in the literature of the past few decades, a higher percentile of men reported sexual activity and moderate to strong sexual interest than did women. In the Duke longitudinal study of ageing, the most common reasons for alteration in sexual activity/interest was erectile dysfunction in men, and in women the death, illness or lack of performance ability of a partner. By age 85 there are 39 men for every 100 women, further denoting the disadvantage of measuring sexual intercourse as the parameter of function.

In highly healthy men over the age of 80, 29% were having intercourse weekly, and 38.8% of unmarried males were sexually active. A British study of a stratified random sample of 1000 adults aged 18 to 75 found 49.6% of men noted the actual frequency of intercourse met their desired frequency, while 66.2% of women were satisfied with the frequency of intercourse. In addition, 25.4% of women and 48.9% of men responded that the frequency was less than desired. Unfortunately, few data related to the prevalence of masturbation have been captured, although data that are available suggest that about two-thirds of men over age 65 and nearly 30% of women over 65 practise masturbatory activity at least monthly.

It is also clear that despite environmental barriers, such as institutional living, sexual interest does not cease. In institutional settings assessing capability of assent and the importance of privacy are paramount in providing a setting for what is one of the most important quality of life issues that a person can have.

Changes in the sexual response cycle with ageing

Masters and Johnson studies of the sexual response cycle remain the standard of physiological data on sexuality and have been supported by myriad findings in self-reported surveys (see Table 8.1). It has become clear that libido in both men and women is at least in part regulated by testosterone. Testosterone tends to have an impact on general energy and feelings of wellbeing for both genders. Low testosterone levels in women have been found to correlate with reduction in the frequency of intercourse. In a study of women over the age of 60, circulating free testosterone showed a positive correlation with sexual desire. In men, ageing is associated with a decrease in circulated testosterone and, more importantly, 'bioavailable' or weakly bound testosterone decreases with age (see Table 8.2). Bioavailable testosterone is testosterone that is not bound to sex hormone-binding globulin (non-SHBG bound). This appears to be a better correlate of clinical evidence of hypogonadism (see below). Data have also shown a strong correlation of bioavailable testosterone and libido in men.

Table 8.1 Sexual response cycle changes with ageing

Phase	Men	Women
Desire/libido	Variable: none to ↓	Variable: none to ↓
Excitement/arousal	Delayed erection, ↓ scrotal vasocongestion, ↓ testicular elevation, ↓ pre-ejaculatory secretion	Slower response, ↓ genital vasocongestion, ↓ lubrication
Climax/orgasm	Shorter duration, ↓ prostatic and urethral contractions, ↓ ejaculatory force	↓ frequency of orgasms, weaker uterine/vaginal contractions
Resolution	Rapid detumescence Longer refractory period	More rapid return to pre-stimulatory state

Note:
↓ = decreased.

Table 8.2 Alterations in sex hormones in the ageing male

	Age 50–70	Age > 70
Testosterone	None or slight ↓	↓↓
Bioavailable testosterone	About a 50% ↓	70% ↓↓
Free testosterone	20% ↓	40% ↓↓
SHBG	None or ↑	↑
LH	None or slight ↑	None or ↑
FSH	↑	↑

Note:
↓ = decreased.
↓↓ = markedly decreased.
↑ = increased.

The excitement phase—a combination of visual, auditory and olfactory sensations, memories and other emotional stimuli as well as physical stimuli—is triggered by, or in turn triggers, neurotransmitters that await elucidation. Muscle tension that is engendered by both men and women during the excitement/arousal phase tends to be less than seen in younger years. Orgasm tends to be shorter in duration for both men and women; women do retain multiorgasmic capacity. Urethral and prostatic contractions are fewer, and ejaculatory force less in the older male, and weaker and fewer vaginal/uterine contractions may occur in older women. In some women uterine contractions may be painful.

Issues in the ageing male

Erectile dysfunction (impotence), the inability to get or maintain an erection sufficient for intercourse in at least 50% of attempts, has a prevalence that can range from 55–95% of men over the age of 70, and is clearly an issue of great concern to the ageing male. It is important to note that erectile dysfunction can occur in the face of normal sexual desire, drive, and orgasmic and ejaculatory capability. It is also important to remember that erectile dysfunction is not considered normative ageing, just as hypertension that increases in prevalence with age is not considered normal, but represents underlying pathology.

A greater prevalence of erectile dysfunction tends to occur in individuals with diabetes or other co-morbid conditions that accelerate atherosclerosis, as vascular disease is the number one aetiology of erectile dysfunction (see Figure 8.1). In the Massachusetts Male Aging Study that examined a younger cohort of men aged 40–70, erectile dysfunction has an overall prevalence of 52%, with the overwhelmingly predominant aetiology of vascular disease being the primary cause. It has also been shown that the non-invasive measurement of abnormal penile brachial pressure indices can predict the occurrence of a major vascular event such as myocardial infarction and stroke in an asymptomatic patient. A prospective study has

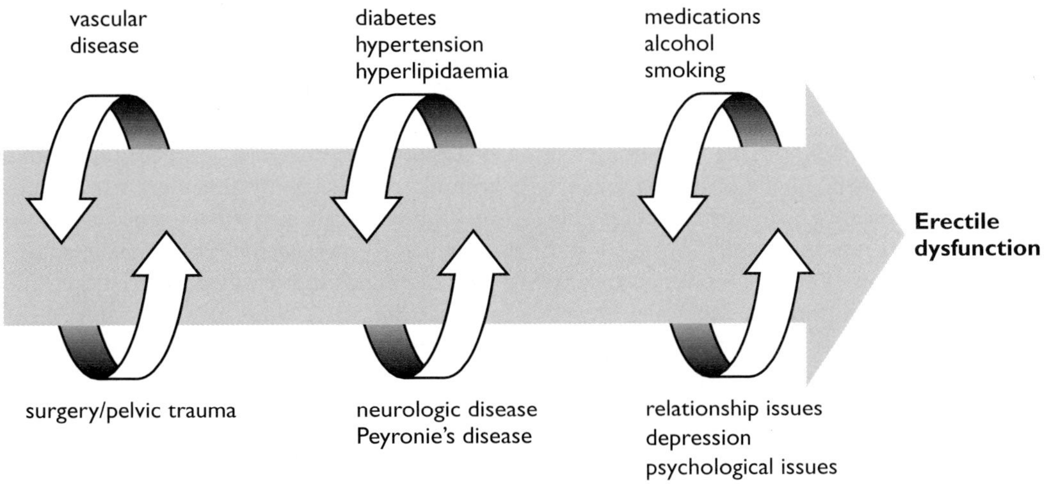

Figure 8.1 Risk factors for erectile dysfunction

noted that within 2 years of the diagnosis of abnormal penile brachial pressure indices, 23% of males will have a myocardial infarction, stroke or both, compared with 4.5% of men with normal penile pressure indices. This may be even more predictive than ankle arm index as a harbinger of cardiovascular risk.

Erectile dysfunction may occur as a result of inadequate arterial filling, excessive venous outflow, or a combination of these factors. Venous leak syndrome (penile 'varicosities'), and changes in the fibre concentration and content of the tunica albuginea that may further impair veno-occlusive properties, can also contribute to erectile dysfunction. In addition, there has been the suggestion that venous leaks may also result from local ischaemia and thus be associated with arterial atherosclerotic change. Peyronie's disease, the presence of bands or plaques in the penis that can result in severe curvature of the penis, may make intercourse difficult.

It has become apparent that neurotransmitters affect erectile function, and in turn alter or may be altered by the presence of disease states such as atherosclerosis. Nitric oxide from neural and endothelial sources activates cyclic guanosine monophosphase (cyclic GMP), resulting in vasodilatation due to smooth muscle relaxation. Nitric oxide is one of many neurotransmitters implicated in erectile control, with others still to be discovered. Neurologic function is also important as sympathetic, parasympathetic and motor nerves supply the penis. At the level of S2–S4, sacral parasympathetics mediate 'reflexogenic' erections that are erections occurring as a result of local stimulation. This 'reflex arc' explains why partial erections may be seen in individuals who have cord lesions, if this area is intact. Sympathetic activation tends to result in detumescence. Stroke, temporal lobe epilepsy and cord lesions are all associated with erectile dysfunction. Vascular and neuropathic change due to pelvic trauma, including bicycle riding (which is a cause of pelvic trauma), have received attention in the past few years. Endocrine and metabolic disorders—such as hypo- or hyperthyroidism, Cushing's disease and hyperprolactinaemia, albeit relatively rare in older males—can be associated with dysfunction. Diabetes, of course, due to the alterations in nitric oxide, acceleration of atherosclerosis and autonomic as well as peripheral neuropathy, is associated with a high prevalence of men with erectile difficulties.

Hypogonadism

The occurrence of hypogonadism is not a rare finding in older men. Hypogonadism is present in about one-third of men over the age of 50 who have erectile dysfunction. However, as previously noted, hypogonadism is by far more commonly linked to alterations in libido than alterations in erectile function. There may be an individual threshold effect, however, or a level of bioavailable testosterone below which not only does desire decrease but also erectile capability diminishes. In the New Mexico Aging Process Study, a longitudinal cohort study of men aged 61–87 at entry into the study with a follow-up as long as 15 years, noted a decrease in total testosterone levels of 100 ng/dL per decade. The change in hormones with ageing in the male has come to be associated with clinical symptomatology. In addition to decrease or loss of libido, hypogonadism can exist with increased risk of osteoporosis, loss of muscle strength, decrease in wellbeing and energy, anaemia and impaired cognition, especially visual spatial tasks. The ADAM (Androgen Deficiency in the Aging Male) is a validated screening questionnaire for hypogonadism (see Box 8.1). In the absence of depression, a male answering 'yes' to either question 1 or 7 or any 3 other questions meant there was a high likelihood of hypogonadism. The questionnaire has 88% sensitivity and 60% specificity.

Medication remains another important contributor to erectile dysfunction, with numerous medications such as antihypertensives (nearly all categories—especially β-blockers and diuretics), with α-blockers and angiotensin receptor blockers causing far less difficulty. Most antidepressants, including selective serotonin reuptake inhibitors (SSRIs), are also associated with erectile dysfunction, as are some H-2 receptor antagonists (especially cimetidine), other testosterone antagonists or drugs blocking testosterone synthesis (such as spironolactone), and ketoconazole, and also commonly used drugs such

Box 8.1 St Louis University ADAM (Androgen Deficiency in Aging Males) Questionnaire

#/Alias/
Name____________________
Date of birth____________________
(month/day/year)

1. Do you have a decrease in libido (sex drive)?
2. Do you have a lack of energy?
3. Do you have a decrease in strength or endurance?
4. Have you lost height?
5. Have you noticed a decreased 'enjoyment of life'?
6. Are you sad and/or grumpy?
7. Are your erections less strong?
8. Have you noted a recent deterioration in your ability to play sports?
9. Are you falling asleep after dinner?
10. Has there been a recent deterioration in your work performance?

Note: An affirmative response to either question 1 or 7 is considered a positive response. An affirmative response to any 3 questions can be considered a positive response and an indication to assess further for hypogonadism, in the absence of depression.

Source: Adapted from J. E. Morley, E. Charlton, P. Patrick, F. E. Kaiser, P. Cadeau, D. McCready, H. M. Perry III (2000), 'Validation of a screening questionnaire for androgen deficiency in aging males', *Metabolism*, 49, pp. 1239–42.

as alcohol. Although there are a variety of medications implicated in causing erectile dysfunction, the conditions for which they are given may also contribute to dysfunction—for example, depression and many of the therapies used to treat it can, on their own, result in erectile dysfunction. Instead of changing an effective drug regimen the patient is on, it is often easier to consider therapy for erectile dysfunction. It is important then to remind patients who are being started on antihypertensive medication, for example, to discuss any sexual difficulty they may find while on medication, but not to stop that medication. It is easier to treat erectile dysfunction than a stroke that may ensue from lack of adequately controlled blood pressure!

Depression has been reported to be present in 8–33% of patients with erectile dysfunction, and it is important to note that this can form a vicious cycle; depression can cause erectile dysfunction and erectile dysfunction can cause depression. All patients should be screened for depression with validated tools, such as the Yesavage Geriatric Depression scale or other well documented assessments, such as the Beck or Hamilton Depression inventory. Probably the more common psychological issue is performance anxiety or fear of failure that may deter activity. In addition, relationship issues are important components of sexual function and esteem. It is vital to have a discussion with the partner, as even if a good therapeutic outcome is achieved in treatment of erectile dysfunction, if the partner is unwilling or unable to participate in a sexual relationship, this may be an obstacle to optimal success for that couple. It is important to assess the level of communication that exists between partners, and help keep expectations realistic.

Evaluation

Probably the simplest way to evaluate a patient is to begin with a history. Using a single question—'Is there any problem with your ability to have sex?'—is a good opening with the patient and helps create an atmosphere where the patient knows you are willing to discuss this issue. Sensitivity to cultural/ethnic issues is imperative. It is important to distinguish issues related to loss of desire or drive, or ejaculatory issues, from erectile dysfunction. Assessing the type of disorder and the situation in which it may occur will also be helpful. A description of marked curvature of the penis when flaccid or erect may suggest Peyronie's disease. The presence of early morning erections is not helpful in distinguishing organic from psychogenic disorders, as this may occur in the presence of organic aetiologies. It is important to elicit not only what medications have been prescribed for the patient but also what over-the-counter medications are being taken. The use of over-the-counter cold remedies with α-agonist activity may be the culprit. Using the opportunity of the patient presenting for care should also drive assessment for other diseases such as diabetes, cardiovascular risk factors, past surgeries or trauma. Screening for depression, discussing relationship/emotional issues and gaining the partner's perspective are also helpful. Physical examination should encompass evaluation of secondary male sexual characteristics, neurological exam (both peripheral and autonomic assessment, such as heart rate variability with respiration), pulses (especially those in the lower extremity) and an examination for the presence of penile bands or plaques. Orthostatic change on blood pressure may suggest autonomic dysfunction in a diabetic, or autonomic alteration with age. The ADAM questionnaire may facilitate finding those in whom laboratory assessment of testosterone and bioavailable testosterone are most appropriate. Consideration of thyroid hormone assessment should be undertaken, as clinical evaluation of hypo- or hyperthyroidism is often difficult in older adults. Penile brachial pressure indices taken in the resting and post-exercise states (bicycling legs in the air for 3–5 minutes) may indicate risk of vascular events. However, there are other modalities, such as colour coded duplex ultrasonography, that provide greater sensitivity, but at far greater cost. Response (or the lack thereof) to a test dose of intracavernosal alprostadil or 'tri-mix'—a non-FDA approved combination of papaverine, phentolamine and alprostadil—does not indicate presence or absence of a vascular aetiology of erectile dysfunction, as anxiety can mitigate against a tumescent response.

Treatment options

The patient should be the primary driver of choosing an option that matches risk–benefit ratios, lifestyle choice and the patient's (and hopefully partner's) goals. Some men wish to have an intervention in altering their erectile function, others may decide they do not desire a change in their erectile capability. Underlying disorders that are out of control—such as glycaemic control in a diabetic, hypertension or hyperlipidaemia—should be optimised. Sildenafil (Viagra) has become the treatment option of choice because of ease of administration as an oral agent. This medication is a selective, but not specific, inhibitor of type 5 phosphodiesterase, with some inhibition of both type 3 and 6. As such, this drug is contraindicated in individuals on nitrates, whether they use them intermittently or regularly. Arrhythmias, transient ischaemic episodes, stroke and changes in colour vision diplopia have been reported as adverse events. The 50 mg dose has a half-life of 4 hours and a mean duration of effect on rigidity of 11.2 minutes, and may be somewhat less efficacious in those with diabetes.

Yohimbine, an oral α-antagonist, does not appear to be more effective than placebo in randomised controlled studies, and adverse effects include hypertension, tachycardia, insomnia, dizziness and nausea. The advent of drugs such as apomorphine, a dopaminergic CNS stimulant (which may improve erections but is associated with nausea), and new generations of more specific phosphodiesterase inhibitors may offer additional oral therapies.

Another modality is vacuum devices, an effective therapeutic option for many patients, especially for those who enjoy good communication with their partner. When pumped, the vacuum device causes a negative pressure to be generated that draws blood into the penis. Then a band or ring is placed at the base of the penis, the tube is removed, then the ring removed after 30 minutes. Adverse effects associated with vacuum device include haematomas, reduction in penile tip temperature, impairment of ejaculation, and penile reddening or cyanosis.

Administration of alprostadil either transurethrally or intracavernosally by injection can also result in erectile improvement. Improved erections resulting in the ability to have sexual activity occur in about 65% of men with intraurethral alprostadil and 94% of those using intracavernosal injections. Both modalities of alprostadil administration can be associated with penile burning or aching sensations, haematomas, and rarely with hypotension, dizziness or priapism. Intracavernosal penile injections with papaverine, phentolamine and alprostadil are not approved for use in the US.

Intracavernosal therapy should not be used in men on anticoagulants, those with poor manual dexterity (unless their partner is willing to perform the injections) or in those with Peyronie's disease.

Surgical intervention with penile prosthesis implantation has become a lesser priority choice for many men, but remains a viable option for those in whom medical therapy has failed or those who weigh the risks and benefits and choose this due to lifestyle priorities. Infection, device failure and scarring of the corpora cavernosa are some adverse events that may occur.

It has become clear that many options are available and will become increasingly available for those interested in restoring erectile function, and it is incumbent on all health care providers to assess and offer assistance in this area.

Issues in the older woman

The loss of oestrogen following the menopause (the cessation of menses for at least 12 months) results in effects on many organs and body functions, with increased risk of cardiovascular disease, osteoporosis, change in vocal range, mood lability, sleep alterations and a host of other symptoms. This section will focus on those changes affecting sexuality function. However, the mix of emotion, libido and organ responsiveness is understood far less in women than in men. Lesbian sexual activity and ageing is also poorly studied, but in the sparse literature that exists the major cause of sexual inactivity appears to be lack of a partner. Lack of a partner or a partner whose illness or inability to get or maintain erections may have a major impact on function as well as self-esteem issues for some women. Oestrogen plays a major role in urogenital, breast and uterine integrity. Many of the changes impacting on sexual function relate to changes resulting in urogenital atrophy (see Figure 8.2). These vulvovaginal changes tend to occur gradually, and do not necessarily dissipate over time, but in fact worsen without therapy. Vaginal dryness, soreness and dyspareunia may occur in 10–40% of postmenopausal women. Over time painful intercourse will reduce desire. Symptoms may also include itching, burning and incontinence. The sexual response cycle is altered with age in women (see Table 8.1). Loss of vaginal lubrication can lead to dyspareunia (vaginal pain on intercourse), vaginal trauma and bleeding. In the absence of oestrogen, lactobacilli that maintain a normal vaginal pH of 4.5–5 are absent, and without the presence of lactobacilli and a normal pH, the protection against *Escherichia coli* and other coliform organisms is lost.

Urogenital atrophy

⇩

vaginal dryness
vaginal bleeding
labial/mons irritation/itching/burning
urge incontinence—frequency, nocturia, dysuria
dyspareunia
urinary tract infections

Figure 8.2 Symptoms of urogenital atrophy

Urethral closing pressure diminishes with thinning of the urethral epithelium secondary to oestrogen deficiency. Urethral prolapse may occur with loss of adequate collagen-supporting endopelvic fascia. With both menopause and age, the prevalence of stress (the loss of urine with increased intra-abdominal pressure such as occurs with laughter, coughing, etc.) as well as urge incontinence, with the loss of small amounts of urine, increases. Incontinence certainly provides no enhancement to sexual function. These symptoms are readily reversible with oestrogen administration. Localised application of oestrogen via suppository, cream or intravaginal oestrogen ring (ESTring) may provide greater alleviation of symptoms than is seen with systemic administration of oestrogen. It is important to note that localised administration may not mitigate against a systemic effect occurring, and even with this method of administration, risk–benefit must be carefully weighed on an individual basis. If there is an absolute contraindication to oestrogen use, then water soluble lubricants may provide relief for vaginal dryness. Vaginal elasticity is reduced after the loss of oestrogen, and may be a source of discomfort that might even require progressive vaginal dilatation.

Hot flushes per se may have an impact on sexual function. Hot flushes may occur for years following the menopause. Described as heat or flushing of the face, accompanied by sweats, palpitations, chills, shivering and anxiety, this can even be brought on by body contact, and thus be disruptive to efforts at intimacy. While hot flushes respond to oestrogen in a dose response fashion, resolution of hot flushes does not occur immediately with oestrogen administration, and it may in fact take up to 12 weeks to eliminate symptoms. Oestrogen replacement also seems to enhance mood, although it is unclear whether this is a reflection of the improvement in vasomotor symptoms. Progesterone is also effective in reducing hot flushes, but spotting or bleeding, mood changes and bloating may make sole use of progesterone less than ideal. It is important to note that for any woman taking oestrogen who has an intact uterus, progesterone must be utilised to avoid endometrial hyperplasia or worse. Clonidine has been utilised as an alternative therapeutic option in those who cannot take oestrogen. Clonidine is effective in diminishing hot flushes in women with breast cancer on tamoxifen, when the hot flushes are related to tamoxifen administration.

Libido in women is clearly related to androgen, and more specifically, testosterone. Testosterone concentrations do fall in women following the menopause, and even in postmenopausal women undergoing oophorectomy. The administration of testosterone in women is associated with increased arousal, desire and frequency of sexual fantasies. Testosterone also improves the sense of wellbeing and energy levels. However, the long-term risk of testosterone administration, especially on cardiovascular risk in women, as well as the most appropriate form of administration remain to be clarified. It is important to note that oral testosterone that has been used in the US—whether it is combined with oestrogen (such as Estratest) or not—represents 17 α-alkylated testosterone which can be associated with hepatic dysfunction.

The impact of vascular changes on sexual function in women is not as clear cut as the impact of atherosclerosis and its risk factors are for erectile dysfunction in men. While atherosclerotic changes can result in diminution of clitoral engorgement, or even sensation, and may contribute to loss of vaginal lubrication and clitoral sensation, it is also clear that sexual function is not just a blood flow issue for women. Medication plays a role in sexual abilities, but far less is known about the impact of medications, both prescription and over-the-counter, on female sexual function. Antihypertensive agents may reduce vaginal lubrication, monoamine oxidase inhibitors may decrease arousal, and amphetamines, diazepams and SSRIs may produce anorgasmia. Little assessment on a systematic basis of drug impact on female sexual function seems to be the usual state, rather than the exception.

Evaluation

As for a man experiencing sexual dysfunction, a woman should be asked whether there is any difficulty in her ability to have sex, again to create a milieu where she can feel a level of comfort in discussing these issues. This discussion is especially useful in the setting of postmenopausal counselling, or counselling at any later age, because assessment surrounding the issues of the menopause and beyond generally does not occur for women. The discussion should be considered with the same tone as assessing risk of heart disease, osteoporosis and other later life events. Again, the type of problem, medical issues or symptoms relative to the menopause, or the impact of another disease state, should be considered. Screening for depression is often useful, and a discussion of stressors and relationship issues should be undertaken.

A new classification by a consensus panel on female sexual dysfunction has been put forward:

1. Sexual desire disorders:
   - Hypoactive sexual desire disorder
   - Sexual aversion disorder
2. Sexual arousal disorder
3. Orgasmic disorder
4. Sexual pain disorders:
   - Dyspareunia
   - Vaginismus
   - Other sexual pain disorders.

These terms are further defined in Box 8.2.

Box 8.2 Definitions of female sexual dysfunction

Definitions

hypoactive sexual desire disorder the persistent or recurrent deficiency/absence of sexual fantasies/thoughts and/or desire for, or receptivity to, sexual activity, which causes personal distress

sexual arousal disorder the persistent or recurrent inability to maintain sufficient sexual excitement, causing personal distress, which can be expressed as a lack of subjective excitement, or lack of genital (lubrication/swelling) or other somatic responses

orgasmic disorder the persistent or recurrent difficulty, delay or absence of attaining orgasm following sufficient sexual stimulation and arousal, which causes personal distress

Sexual pain disorders

Dyspareunia is recurrent or persistent genital pain associated with sexual intercourse.

Vaginismus is the recurrent or persistent involuntary spasm of the musculature of the outer third of the vagina that interferes with vaginal penetration, which causes personal distress.

Non-coital sexual pain disorder is the recurrent or persistent genital pain induced by non-coital sexual stimulation.

Note: Each can be further subdefined as A: lifelong versus acquired; B: generalised versus situational; and C: aetiological origin (organic, psychogenic, mixed, unknown).

Source: Adapted from R. Basson et al. (2000), 'Report of the International Consensus Development Conference on Female Sexual Dysfunction: Definitions and Classification', *The Journal of Urology*, 163, pp. 888–93.

The issue of hypoactive desire can be assessed by evaluating for a history of sexual abuse and depression, and obtaining testosterone and bioavailable testosterone levels (non-sex hormone binding globulin bound testosterone that correlates extremely well with libido). Relationship issues and sexual techniques used by the patient and/or the partner may need to be addressed. Orgasmic issues should be probed to find out whether the problem is primary or secondary, and whether there is a relationship to any medication. Counselling and techniques such as learning to masturbate to orgasm (self-pleasuring) may be helpful. Issues such as pain, whether dyspareunia or vaginismus, should be carefully evaluated. The use of oestrogen or water soluble lubricants, vaginal dilators and relaxation techniques have been effective for many women.

A frank discussion between patient and health provider, as well with the patient's partner, and the willingness to explore avenues of assistance and education can greatly improve the sexual quality of life for women as they age.

Bibliography and further reading

Anonymous (1992), 'Drugs that cause sexual dysfunction: An update', *The Medical Letter on Drugs and Therapeutics*, 34, pp. 73–8.

Ansong, K. S., Lewis, C., Jenkins, P. et al. (1998), 'Help seeking decisions among men with impotence', *Urology*, 52, pp. 834–7.

Carrier, S., Brock, G. & Kour, N. W. (1993), 'The pathophysiology of erectile dysfunction', *Urology*, 42, pp. 468–81.

Condra, M., Morales, A., Surridge, D. et al. (1986), 'The unreliability of nocturnal penile tumescence as an outcome measurement in the treatment of organic impotence', *The Journal of Urology*, 135, pp. 280–2.

Dennestein, L., Smith, A. M. A., Morse, C. A. & Burger, H. G. (1994), 'Sexuality and the menopause', *Journal of Psychosomatic Obstetrics and Gynecology*, 15, pp. 59–66.

Feldman, H. A., Goldstein, I., Hatzichristou, D. G., Krane, R. J. & McKinlay, J. B. (1994), 'Impotence and its medical and psychological correlates: Results of the Massachusetts Male Aging Study', *The Journal of Urology*, 151, pp. 54–61.

Glatt, A. E., Zinner, S. H. & McCormack, W. M. (1990), 'The prevalence of dyspareunia', *Obstetrics and Gynecology*, 75, pp. 433–6.

Goldstein, I., Lue, T. F., Padmanathan, H. et al. for the Sildenafil Study Group (1998), 'Oral sildenafil in the treatment of erectile dysfunction', *The New England Journal of Medicine*, 338, pp. 1397–404.

Greendale, G. A., Hogan, P. & Shumaker, S. (1996), 'For the Postmenopausal Oestrogen/Progestin Interventions (PEPI) Trial Investigations sexual functioning in postmenopausal women: The Postmenopausal Oestrogen/Progestin Interventions (PEPI) Trial', *The Journal of Women's Health*, 5, pp. 445–56.

Hermann, H. C., Chang, G., Klugherz, B. D. & Mahoney, P. D. (2000), 'Hemodynamic effects of sildenafil in men with severe coronary artery disease', *The New England Journal of Medicine*, 345, pp. 1622–6.

Kaiser, F. E. (1996), 'Sexuality in the elderly', *The Urologic Clinics of North America*, 23, pp. 99–109.

McCoy, N. L. & Davidson, J. M. (1985), 'A longitudinal study of the effects of menopause on sexuality', *Maturitas*, 7, pp. 203–12.

Morales, A., Johnston, B., Heaton, J. P. & Lundie, M. (1997), 'Testosterone supplementation for hypogonadal impotence: Assessment of biochemical measures and therapeutic outcomes', *The Journal of Urology*, 157, pp. 849–54.

Morley, J. E., Charlton, E., Patrick, P., Kaiser, F. E., Cadeau, P., McCready, D. & Perry III, H. M. (2000), 'Validation of a screening questionnaire for androgen deficiency in aging males', *Metabolism*, 49, pp. 1239–42.

Nusbaum, M. R., Gamble, G., Skinner, H. & Heiman, J. (2000), 'The high prevalence of sexual concerns among women seeking routine gynecologic care', *The Journal of Family Practice*, 49, pp. 229–32.

Pandya, K. J., Raubertas, R. F., Flynn, P. J., Hynes, H. E., Rosenbluth, R. J., Kirshner, J. J., Pierce, I., Dragalin, V. & Morrow, G. R. (2000), 'Oral clonidine in postmenopausal patients with breast cancer experiencing tamoxifen-induced hot flashes: A University of Rochester cancer center community clinical oncology program study', *Annals of Internal Medicine*, 132, pp. 788–93.

Rendell, M. S., Rajfer, J. Wicker, P. A. et al. (1999), 'Sildenafil for treatment of erectile dysfunction in men with diabetes', *Journal of the American Medical Association*, 281, pp. 421–6.

Roughan, P. A., Kaiser, F. E. & Morley, J. E. (1993), 'Sexuality and the older woman', *Clinics in Geriatric Medicine*, 9, pp. 87–106.

Vinik, A. & Richardson, D. (1998), 'Erectile dysfunction in diabetes', *Diabetes Reviews*, 6, pp. 16–33.

White, C. B. (1992), 'Sexual interest, attitudes, knowledge and sexual history in relation to sexual behavior in institutionalized elderly', *Archives of Sexual Behavior*, 11, pp. 11–21.

Part III

Psychiatric and behavioural issues

Chapter 9
Common psychiatric disorders

WILLIAM M. H. GOH and ROHAN S. DHILLON

Introduction

Many elderly people with psychiatric disorders have grown old with them. Others remain relatively well until the effects of advancing years and misfortunes of life eventually exceed their ability to cope. The accumulative effects of the physical and psychosocial stressors associated with ageing make psychiatric disorders in the elderly unique.

It is well established that the precise diagnosis and treatment of psychiatric disorders in the elderly may not be a simple matter and may require special knowledge because of possible differences in clinical presentation, pathogenesis and pathophysiology of mental disorders in the elderly. Complicating factors in elderly patients that need to be considered are the presence of co-existing chronic medical diseases, physical disabilities, the use of multiple medications and increased susceptibility to cognitive impairment.

Although ageing itself does not imply pathologic decline in emotional balance or deterioration in mental health, growing old is accompanied by a gradual reduction in the adaptive reserves of all vital organs, including the brain. Elderly people have survived many physical and psychosocial stresses from their life experiences. These include genetic influences, diseases, accidents, nutritional imbalances and self-abuse, such as alcohol excesses, cigarette smoking and illicit drug use.

Psychosocial changes in old age

The sensitivity of the elderly patient's higher cognitive functions to chemicals and to physical and psychosocial stressors predispose them to be more vulnerable to psychiatric disorders, especially acute brain syndromes. The ageing body leads to changes in the body image. The elderly patient experiences diminished hearing, impaired vision, reduced reaction time and decline in physical health. These changes are experienced as losses that have to be addressed.

Old people are more likely to lose their spouses and friends as they age. Other losses that elderly people commonly encounter include changes in their psychosocial environment. These include voluntary retirement or involuntary loss of job, which leads to reduced income, loss of social status, loss of personal prestige and social interaction that normally occurs at the workplace. Often homes are lost because of decreased income or due to the inability of older people to maintain them. When older people move to a residential facility for the elderly, they may lose their sense of privacy as well. Above all, older people have little potential or opportunity to improve their circumstances.

Bereavement and depression

It is important to be aware that elderly people frequently devote a considerable amount of energy and time to attending to the adjustment and resolution of these losses. Loss is a predominant theme in their emotional life, and the prospect of their own death is an issue that the elderly will inevitably need to address. Consequently, grief and bereavement are major issues that colour the emotional life of elderly people.

As part of their reaction to the loss of loved ones, some grieving elderly people present with symptoms characteristic of a major depressive episode. Both grief and depression may manifest as sadness, tearfulness, withdrawal from interpersonal contact, insomnia, poor appetite and weight loss. Bereaved people generally regard their sadness and associated symptoms as normal. Some bereaved elderly people may seek medical help not for their depressed mood but for the relief of associated symptoms such as insomnia, poor appetite or weight loss.

Psychiatric assessment

Elderly people are reluctant to complain of emotional or memory problems, and when they do their relatives or even family doctors may put these down to the normal effects of ageing. Occasionally, relatives may see their complaints as the elderly person 'being difficult'.

Psychiatric history taking and mental status examination of the elderly should follow the same format as that utilised in assessing the young adult. The patient should be seen alone even if there is clear evidence of cognitive impairment so that a positive doctor–patient relationship can be established. If cognitive impairment interferes with history taking, an independent history should be obtained from a family member or from significant others.

A comprehensive psychiatric history will identify the precipitating, predisposing and perpetuating factors associated with the psychiatric disorder, and will contribute to the diagnostic, therapeutic and prognostic formulations. A detailed medical history is required as psychiatric disorders in the elderly often occur co-morbidly with physical illnesses, and any management plan needs to take this into consideration.

Assessment at home can often reveal much about the elderly patient that an assessment in the doctor's room or in hospital cannot. A home visit may reveal if there is a lack of food, a presence of alcohol dependence, or excessive security measures installed by a paranoid person against imagined persecutors. Self-neglect is usually easily observed at home. Warning signs of psychiatric disturbance in the elderly are:

- self-neglect
- sudden onset of confusion
- self-harm behaviour
- persistent somatic complaints
- repeated complaints by family, neighbours or police
- exhaustion of carers.

Family members may report self-harm behaviour or the patient may present with symptoms of self-inflicted injuries. Persistent somatic complaints in the absence of organic disease should alert the doctor to a probable psychiatric disorder. Repeated complaints by family, friends, neighbours or the police are frequently indicative of a psychotic illness or an organic brain disorder. Exhaustion of carers frequently indicates that some underlying psychiatric disorder has been missed.

Depressive disorders

The most common psychiatric disorder in the elderly besides dementia is depression. Yet depression in the elderly is an underdiagnosed and undertreated disorder. In the elderly, depression often occurs as a co-morbid disorder associated with other diseases.

The symptoms of depression are more distressing to the patient and cause more disability than most physical diseases, such as hypertension, diabetes or arthritis. Moreover, depression has a high mortality rate, as there is a strong link between depression and suicide. Consequently, all depressed elderly patients require accurate diagnosis and appropriate treatment.

Epidemiology

Community based surveys reveal that clinically significant depressive symptoms occur in 8–16% of the elderly, with the prevalence of major depressive disorders occurring in 1–3%. However, measuring the true prevalence of depression in older people is inherently difficult because of medical and social influences that may obscure its detection.

Depression is more common in elderly people who consult general practitioners. In the primary care setting the prevalence of depressive symptoms is between 11% and 29%, and of major depressive disorders between 5% and 17%. Among elderly people in nursing homes and in institutional settings, the prevalence of depressive symptoms is 40%, with 24% suffering diagnosable major depressive disorders.

The reason for the discrepancy between prevalence of depression in the community, in primary care setting and in residential settings is unclear. It might be that elderly people who suffer from depression are more likely to consult their medical practitioners and are more likely to be admitted to residential care facilities. It is probable too that elderly people who are admitted to residential settings experience depression due to a variety of losses, including their homes, friends, independence and privacy.

Aetiology

Depression is higher in elderly women than in elderly men, and tends to be associated with loss of role and self-esteem. In elderly men marital conflicts and chronic ill health are significant factors contributing to their depression. Those elderly people with a past history of alcohol dependence have an increased risk of depression. There is also consistent evidence that a family history of depression is a risk factor.

Physical diseases and medical treatment are significantly associated with depression. For example, the prevalence rates for depression associated with neurodegenerative disorders, such as dementia, Parkinson's disease and stroke, are between 30% and 60%, probably due to changes in brain monoamines. In addition, elderly people may not cope well with physical diseases and so become depressed.

Brain imaging studies reveal that cortical tissue density in a depressed group of elderly patients is more similar to a group of demented patients than to normal controls. Monoaminergic function in depression has been studied and it is now accepted that decreases in serotonin, dopamine and noradrenaline are implicated in the genesis of depression.

There are few recent studies that examine psychological or personality factors in old age depression. Low self-esteem, history of unresolved loss of a loved one early in life, and childhood sexual or physical abuse are common in patients with depression. The premorbid personality of elderly patients with depression is more likely to show dependent, obsessive compulsive and histrionic features.

Foremost among the psychosocial factors that precipitate depression is bereavement. Other social factors implicated in the onset of depression include loneliness, limited social interaction, poverty, deaths or accidents among relatives and friends, and conflicts with family or close friends.

Clinical presentation

The elderly patient may complain of feeling depressed but often presents with sleeplessness, loss of energy, loss of enjoyment or aches and pains. Any of the clinical symptoms of depression can lead the elderly to seek medical attention. Many elderly people present with the classical symptoms seen in younger adults (see Box 9.1).

Although older people may present with the classical symptoms of major depressive episodes seen in younger adults, there are significant differences.

1. *Masked depression* Occasionally there is an absence of the usual symptoms of depressed mood and the elderly patient may present with a smiling facade. Searching for other signs and

Box 9.1 DSM-IV criteria for major depression

Five (or more) of the following symptoms have been present during the same 2 week period nearly every day. At least one of the symptoms is either: (1) a depressed mood or (2) loss of interest or pleasure.

1. Depressed mood most of the day
2. Diminished interest or pleasure in normal activities
3. Significant weight loss or weight gain or change in appetite
4. Insomnia or hypersomnia
5. Psychomotor agitation or retardation
6. Fatigue or loss of energy
7. Feelings of worthlessness or excessive guilt
8. Diminished ability to think or concentrate
9. Recurrent thoughts of death, suicidal thoughts or attempts

Source: American Psychiatric Association (1994), *The Diagnostic and Statistical Manual of Mental Disorders*, 4th edn, APA, Washington.

symptoms may then uncover the underlying depression.

2. *Agitated depression* Agitation may be the predominant symptom and is manifested by increased activity, restless pacing and incessant hand wringing. Increase in anxiety is 15–20 times more common in elderly patients with depression.
3. *Somatic symptoms* Elderly patients may present with persistent pain or other somatic symptoms, especially fatigue, which may mask the underlying depression.
4. *Pseudodementia* Subjective memory difficulty may be the major presenting symptom of the elderly patient with depression. In contrast to patients with dementia, those with pseudodementia are unwilling to attempt cognitive assessment.
5. *Behavioural disturbances* In some elderly patients with cognitive impairment associated with depression, behavioural disturbances may be the major presenting symptoms.
6. *Overlapping physical illness* Anorexia, weight loss, anergia and insomnia which accompany physical illnesses may mask an underlying depressive disorder.

The elderly are more likely to suffer from prominent depressive cognition with negative thoughts of self, the world and the future. Compared to the young, they are less likely to complain of suicidal ideation or make suicide gestures, but more likely to complete suicide.

Improving detection of depression in the elderly

The detection of depression in the elderly requires special skills and experience. Up to 50% of elderly patients with depression are missed in the primary setting. It may be exceedingly difficult to differentiate the neurovegetative and somatic symptoms from the depressive disorder in people with established physical illness.

Also depressed mood is often absent or masked in older people with depression. It has been suggested that it is more informative to consider the cognitive aspects of depression in the elderly. Anhedonia (loss of the capacity to enjoy), Beck's triad (negative views of the world, self and the future), and marked hopelessness are particularly diagnostic of a major depressive episode.

There are a number of clinical scales for aiding diagnosis of depression in the elderly. The most useful screening instrument is the Geriatric Depression Scale (GDS: Yesavage et al. 1983), which is a 30 item scale for self-completion. This has been shortened to a 15 item version. For the general physician the 4 item GDS scale is adequate (see Box 9.2).

Suicide in the elderly

Depression in the elderly causes not only morbidity but also mortality. The elderly patient with depression is more likely to suicide than a younger patient, so suicide prevention is a major goal when managing depression in elderly patients.

Loneliness and social isolation are major factors that contribute to the elderly committing

Box 9.2 Geriatric Depression Scale (GDS 4 item)

1. Are you basically satisfied with your life?	Yes/**No**
2. Do you feel that your life is empty?	**Yes**/No
3. Are you afraid that something bad is going to happen to you?	**Yes**/No
4. Do you feel happy most of the time?	Yes/**No**

Answers indicating depression are in bold type and score 1 point.

0	No depression
1	Uncertain
2–4	Probably depression present

suicide. The pattern of an elderly man living alone, suffering from depression and from chronic ill health, possibly recently abusing alcohol, and expressing feelings of hopelessness should indicate an extremely high risk for suicide. It is sobering to note that many patients who completed suicide had consulted medical practitioners in the recent past. Suicide in the elderly is covered comprehensively in Chapter 10.

Investigations

Severe depressive illness can cause metabolic imbalances in the elderly, which compound their depression, and consequently they should be investigated. In addition, investigations are necessary for detecting any medical condition causing depression.

These investigations include:

1. *ESR and full blood count* Anaemia can cause anergia and lethargy. Chronic infections can lead to the patient developing depression.
2. *Serum electrolytes* Metabolic imbalances can cause restlessness, agitation and confusion.
3. *Vitamin B_{12} and folate* Both low serum vitamin B_{12} and folate can cause depression. Depression with accompanying anorexia contribute to dietary deficiency in vitamin B_{12} and folate, which further compounds the depression.
4. *Thyroid function tests* Both low or high thyroxine levels can cause depression.
5. *Chest X-ray* Carcinoma, chronic chest infection and cardiac failure can cause depression.
6. *Neuroendocrine* Dexamethasone suppression test (DST) was originally reported as a highly sensitive and specific test for melancholia. Relatively high rates of DST non-suppression in elderly patients with depression have been reported.
7. *Brain imaging* Computerised axial tomography or computerised tomography (CT) scan reveals enlarged ventricles. Magnetic resonance imaging (MRI) reveals both white matter hyperintensities and lesions of subcortical grey nuclei. Positron emission tomography (PET) and single photon emission computerised tomography (SPECT) reveal reduced anterior frontal and anterior temporal blood flow and an increase in occipital cortex flow.
8. *Others* Positive finding in syphilis serology can be associated with depression. Electroencephalogram (EEG) reveals decreases in slow-wave sleep, total rapid eye movements (REM) sleep and REM latency. Although raised platelet monoamine oxidase (MAO) was found in elderly people with depression, it is now thought to be probably genetically determined and a non-specific marker for psychopathology in general.

Treatment

Depression in the elderly responds well to pharmacotherapy, and this is the first option, especially when the depression is severe and has obvious 'biological' signs. When depression appears to be reactive to recent psychosocial stressors, there is no clear guideline as to when to use medication. Some reactive depressions respond to psychotherapy or environmental changes. If they are too severe or are resistant to psychological approaches, antidepressants should be prescribed. It has been shown that when antidepressants and psychotherapy are used in combination a better outcome ensues. Electroconvulsive therapy (ECT) is another very effective treatment, usually given by psychiatrists in a hospital setting.

Drug treatment

There is no evidence that any class of antidepressant is more efficacious than the others. All antidepressants produce about 50–60% improvement rate, compared to placebo which gives 30–40% improvement. The choice of first line antidepressant should depend on the clinician's experience and familiarity with the particular drug. In choosing any antidepressant, the factors that need to be considered are its efficacy, its side effects profile, safety, potential drug interaction, the presence of co-morbid psychiatric or medical conditions, suicide risk and the patient's previous response to antidepressants.

The classes of antidepressants in current use include those listed in Table 9.1.

Selective serotonin reuptake inhibitors are effective, safe and well tolerated by the elderly. They have fewer and milder side effects than TCAs; in particular, they do not have anticholinergic activity or disturb cardiac function, an important consideration in the elderly. They are increasingly being viewed as a first choice antidepressant for the elderly. Their side effects include nausea, agitation, sleep disturbance, headache and sexual dysfunction. Nefazodone has a profile similar to SSRIs and causes drowsiness as well. A serotonergic syndrome characterised by myoclonus, agitation, tremor and hypertension has been described.

Venlafaxine is reported to be efficacious in severe depression and has been used with some success in treatment resistant depression. It has a short half-life, few side effects and few drug interactions. It is found to be safe for the elderly. Increased blood pressure has been reported with its use.

Table 9.1 Classes of antidepressants

Antidepressant	Dosage
1. Selective serotonin reuptake inhibitors (SSRIs)	
Sertraline (Zoloft)	25–200 mg once daily
Paroxetine (Aropax)	10–40 mg once daily
Fluoxetine (Prozac, Lovan, Zactin, Erocap)	10–40 mg once daily
Citalopram (Cipramil)	10–60 mg once daily
Fluvoxamine (Luvox)	50–200 mg once daily
2. Serotonin (5HT2) antagonist	
Nefazodone (Serzone)	200–600 mg divided doses
3. Serotonin and noradrenaline reuptake inhibitors (SNRIs)	
Venlafaxine (Efexor)	75–375 mg divided doses
4. Reversible inhibitors of monoamine oxidase-A (RIMA)	
Moclobemide (Aurorix)	300–600 mg divided doses
5. Heterocyclics	
Mianserin (Tolvon, Lumin, Lerivon)	30–90 mg divided doses
6. Tricyclic antidepressants (TCAs)	
Amitriptyline (Tryptanol, Endep, Tryptine)	
Imipramine (Tofranil, Melipramine)	Use low dose
Dothiepin (Dothep, Prothiaden)	10–50 mg in evening
Doxepin (Sinequan, Deptran)	
Clomipramine (Anafranil, Placil)	
Trimipramine (Surmontil)	
Desipramine (Pertofran)	Higher dose can be used
Nortriptyline (Allegron, Nortab)	100–250 mg divided doses
7. Monoamine oxidase inhibitors (MAOIs)	
Phenelzine (Nardil)	15–45 mg divided dose
Tranylcypromine (Parnate)	10–30 mg divided dose

Moclobemide is also a safe antidepressant in the elderly. It is non-sedating and it does not have the same side effect profile as the older monoamine oxidase inhibitors. Therefore dietary restriction is not necessary.

Mianserin has no cardiotoxicity and has been used effectively in the elderly. It has few side effects and its safety in medically ill patients has been established. However, drowsiness and increased confusion have limited its use in the elderly.

Tricyclic antidepressants, proven to be efficacious in treating depression in the elderly since 1960s, are considerably cheaper than the newer agents. Unfortunately, elderly patients are more likely to experience side effects.

The side effects of TCAs are:

- *Anticholinergic:* memory problems, confusion, urinary retention, blurred vision, worsening of glaucoma, constipation, dry mouth.
- *Antihistaminic:* drowsiness, sedation, weight gain.
- *Anti-adrenergic:* orthostatic hypotension, dizziness, falls.
- *Others:* cardiotoxicity, lowered seizure threshold, sexual dysfunction.

The secondary amines series, nortriptyline and desipramine, have far fewer side effects and could be used in higher doses in the elderly. Nortriptyline has been reported to be effective in post-stroke depression.

Monoamine oxidase inhibitors have to be used with considerable care because of their interactions with tyramine-rich foods and other medication. They have a role in depression that is unresponsive to other antidepressants, and in depression with atypical, phobic, hypochondriacal and hysterical features.

Psychological treatment

Psychological treatment not only treats the depression but also prevents its recurrence. Psychological treatment promotes coping and helps resolve life stresses, such as bereavement, other recent losses and family conflicts. There is a great diversity of available psychological treatments. The most commonly used ones in depression are:

- cognitive behavioural therapy (CBT)
- interpersonal therapy (IPT)
- supportive psychotherapy and counselling.

Cognitive behavioural therapy emphasises how negative cognitions mediate feelings and behaviour and aims to modify this thought process. Depressed patients tend to think negatively about themselves, the world around them and their future. These negative thoughts are believed to aggravate and perpetuate depression. The patient is taught to identify this automatic negative thought pattern, challenge the negative thoughts and alter them. Psychiatrists, psychologists and other mental health practitioners practise CBT.

In interpersonal therapy patients are taught to objectively evaluate their interactions with others and to become aware of how they isolate themselves, which contributes to or aggravates depression. People with depression tend to be more easily upset by the comments of others because of their negative self-evaluation and low self-esteem. They may feel personally criticised when no criticism was intended. IPT is designed to address this through clarification of feeling states, testing perceptions, improvement of interpersonal communication and development of interpersonal skills.

Supportive psychotherapy and counselling are therapeutic techniques utilised by a helping professional to ameliorate the distress and suffering of a depressed patient and to help the patient cope with psychosocial stressors. Psychoeducation helps the patient develop insight and an understanding of the illness and focuses on strategies to help recovery.

Electroconvulsive therapy

This is a highly effective (70–80% response rate) and safe treatment for depression in the elderly. There is evidence that older people with depression may have a better response to ECT than younger patients. It is a treatment of choice for depressed elderly patients who are acutely suicidal, who have stopped eating and drinking, and in depression with psychomotor retardation or psychotic features. ECT is usually given by psychiatrists in hospitals with equipment capable of stimulus dose monitoring, metering out an accurate amount of electricity. Some patients develop cognitive impairment, such as confusion and amnesia. Permanent brain damage does not occur. However, patients with underlying brain pathology may develop delirium.

Psychotic depression

Feelings of guilt, hopelessness and low self-esteem may develop to delusional intensity in psychotic depression. Mood congruent psychotic features include delusions or hallucinations whose content is entirely consistent with the typical depressive themes of personal inadequacy, guilt, disease or nihilism. On the other hand, mood incongruent psychotic features include persecutory delusions, thought insertion or delusions of control.

When psychotic symptoms are present, antipsychotic medication should be used in addition to antidepressants. ECT is a very effective treatment for psychotic depression in the elderly. These patients need referral to a psychiatrist.

Manic episodes

Although manic and hypomanic episodes may appear in old age, they are less frequent than depression. The patient, family and doctor may fail to recognise the hypomanic phase of a bipolar disorder, as it may be ascribed to the irritability, aggressiveness and poor judgment of old age. The hypomanic episode is characterised by the presence of these symptoms:

- inflated self-esteem and grandiosity
- increased energy and decreased need for sleep
- pressure of speech and flight of ideas
- distractability
- increase in goal directed activity or psychomotor agitation
- excessive involvement in pleasurable activities (e.g. spending sprees, sexual indiscretions, or foolish business investments).

The treatment of bipolar disorder includes the use of mood stabilisers, such as lithium carbonate 750–1250 mg daily in divided doses, carbamazepine 400–1200 mg daily in divided doses, or sodium valproate 1000–2000 mg daily in divided doses. The therapeutic range of serum levels should be adhered to. For tranquillisation before mood stabilisers exert their full effects, low dose major tranquillisers or clonazepam can be used.

Prognosis

The prognosis for a first episode depression in old age is much better than that in younger adults. Over 60% of elderly people with depression recover completely after an episode of depression, although many later relapse. For recurrent depression the prognosis is much poorer, with a relapse rate of over 80%. In the long term only 20–25% will remain completely well. The outcome is determined to a substantial extent by adequacy of treatment.

There is increased mortality associated with depression in the elderly. Death through suicide is higher, and death through diseases not related directly to depression itself, such as from vascular disease and chest infections, show an increase. Physical illness is a major factor contributing to a poor prognosis. The severity of depression and presence of cognitive impairment are also poor prognostic signs.

Dementia and delirium

Dementia (Chapter 15) and delirium (Chapter 16) frequently come to psychiatric attention because of behavioural and psychological symptoms.

At some stage during the course of the illness, behavioural complications will affect 90% of patients with dementia. These behavioural symptoms include agitation, wandering, screaming and aggression. These problems are among the most distressing symptoms to the patients and to their carers. They undermine self-care ability and social interactions. Often, the inability to control these symptoms results in the elderly being placed in institutions, and frequently leads to overmedication.

Psychological symptoms include depression, anxiety and psychosis. Significant depression occurs in about 25% of patients with dementia. Psychosis occurs in 25% and manifests as delusions, hallucinations and illusions.

Prevalence

The prevalence of dementia among people aged over 65 is 6–8% in the community and in people over 80 is 25–30%. In residential and nursing homes the prevalence is over 80%.

Dementia includes:

- Alzheimer's disease: 60–70%
- vascular dementia: 10–20% (vascular dementia occurs co-morbidly with Alzheimer's disease in 20%)
- dementia with Lewy bodies: 20–25%
- other causes include alcoholism, Pick's disease, Creutzfeldt-Jakob dementia, Huntington's disease and Parkinson's disease.

The prevalence of delirium is 20–30% among elderly patients admitted to general hospitals. Ten to fifteen per cent of elderly patients develop delirium following general surgery, and 50% develop it after surgery for hip fracture.

Clinical presentation

The characteristic clinical feature of dementia is the presence of cognitive deficits sufficient to cause functional impairment. Cognitive deficits include impairment in memory, language, recognition and executive functions, such as planning. It may be difficult to differentiate between dementia and depression (see Table 9.2).

In its early stages the most accurate method of identifying any dementia is by interviewing the patient's closest relative. Delirium is characterised by clouded sensorium (impaired attention, thinking and awareness of surrounding); disorientation in place, person and time; memory losses; and language disturbance. Visual illusions and hallucinations are common.

In the elderly, it is a more frequent prodrome to physical illnesses than pain, fever or tachycardia. Delirium can occur in chronic dementia and tends to aggravate dementia. Delirium in the elderly often heralds the onset of dementia within the next 3 years. It is essential that delirium be delineated early in the diagnostic process (see Table 9.3).

Aetiology

There are multiple risk factors in dementia; the two main ones are advancing years and family history. If there is a family history of Alzheimer's disease, the incidence is increased two- to fourfold. Genetic studies reveal that the presence of apolipoprotein

Table 9.2 Features of dementia and depression

Depression with pseudodementia	Dementia
Acute onset	Insidious onset
Symptoms of short duration	Symptoms of long duration
Rapid progression	Slow progression
Depressed mood prominent	Affect apathetic
Family history of depression	Patient unaware or minimises memory deficits
Patient unwilling to do tests	Patient struggles with tests
Recent and remote memory loss similar	Recent memory loss greater
Orientation intact, no aphasia or apraxia	Disoriented, presence of aphasia and apraxia

Table 9.3 Features of delirium and dementia

Delirium	Dementia
Sudden onset	Insidious (unless vascular)
Short duration (days or weeks)	Chronic (months to years)
Reversible	Irreversible
Affect aroused or fearful	Affect apathetic
Pronounced disorientation early	Disorientation later in illness
Fluctuating course	Steady (vascular step-wise) deterioration
Clouded consciousness	Consciousness not affected

E4 (ApoE-ε4) allele in chromosome 19 increases the probability that the dementia is Alzheimer's disease. The most common neuropathological features of Alzheimer's disease are amyloid plaques, neurofibrillary tangles, neuronal loss, and cortical and central atrophy.

The most common causes of delirium in the elderly include:

- infection of urinary tract, chest, skin and ear
- cardiac failure
- cerebrovascular ischaemia
- iatrogenic causes, primarily the use of medication, especially anticholinergics and tricyclic antidepressants
- alcohol and drug withdrawal.

Treatment

Reversible dementia accounts for 2% of all cases and treatment should address the underlying cause. Reversible dementia includes:

- hypothyroidism
- vitamin B_{12} and folate deficiency
- communicating hydrocephalus
- slow growing operable cerebral tumour
- hyperparathyroidism
- renal failure, electrolyte imbalances, syphilis, HIV infection, heavy metal poisoning.

Treatable symptoms such as depression, anxiety and psychosis should be addressed. When using antidepressants the SSRIs, venlafaxine or moclobemide are preferred to the tricyclic antidepressants, due to their side effects. When antipsychotic medication is necessary the use of atypical antipsychotics such as olanzapine, risperidone, quetiapine or clozapine is recommended. These neuroleptics, as well as sodium valproate and low dose haloperidol, are also useful in reducing agitated, aggressive and violent behaviour. However, wherever possible, behavioural and interpersonal strategies should be used to modify difficult behaviour.

Acetylcholinesterase inhibitors such as tacrine and donepezil have been used with some success in the management of Alzheimer's disease. They are more effective in the early stage of the illness. Tacrine has a high incidence of side effects.

Carers of patients with dementia are usually spouses who are old themselves. It has been shown that about 50% are depressed due to the hardships of looking after the patients. They need support and often require treatment for their depression.

For vascular dementia, anticlotting agents can be used to minimise further infarcts. In dementia with Lewy bodies, neuroleptics are contraindicated as they aggravate the disorder.

With delirium the underlying cause should be treated. Tranquillisation is often necessary to settle agitation. For this purpose low-dose haloperidol or atypical antipsychotics can be useful. Nursing support is an essential component of effective management.

Course and prognosis

Alzheimer's disease progresses inexorably until death within 7 years from the time of onset of the disease. Vascular dementia deteriorates in a stepwise fashion. In the final phases, patients are severely dysphasic and dyspraxic, they fail to recognise family members, have limited mobility, are doubly incontinent, and require total nursing care.

Delirium has an acute onset, usually hours or a few days. The duration of the disorder is brief. It runs a fluctuating course, being worse at night, and is potentially reversible. It ends in resolution or death.

Anxiety and other psychiatric disorders

Anxiety disorders

Anxiety disorders are the most frequent and least studied psychiatric illnesses in the elderly. The elderly tend to under-report their anxiety problems. The signs and symptoms in the elderly appear less severe than those in the younger age group. However, the effects of anxiety disorders are in most cases more debilitating.

The prevalence of anxiety disorders in people over 65 years old in the community is 19.7%. This consists of:

- phobia (agoraphobia, social phobia, specific phobia): 10–15%
- panic disorder: 0.5–1%
- generalised anxiety disorder: 2–8%
- obsessive compulsive disorder: 2–3%
- post-traumatic stress disorder: 5–11%.

Anxiety is often secondary to depression, or co-exists with it and is frequently not diagnosed. In the elderly it is often a response to frightening physical illnesses. Phobias, particularly agoraphobia, are over-represented, in part due to the older person's feelings of fear of leaving the security and safety of home during illness or trauma. Panic disorder is sometimes difficult to distinguish from medical conditions, such as paroxysmal nocturnal dyspnoea, cardiac arrhythmia or irritable bowel syndrome. Late onset anxiety may herald the onset of dementia.

Treatment is essentially similar to that in the younger age group. Both anxiolytic drugs and psychosocial therapy can be used effectively. Anxiolytic agents include SSRIs, venlafaxine, buspirone, or atypical antipsychotics in low doses. Benzodiazepines can also be used but dependence may rapidly occur.

Psychosocial therapy includes environmental changes, relaxation exercises, slow breathing, cognitive behavioural therapy and psychotherapy. The response to treatment in the elderly is as good as for the younger age group. There is little data regarding the course or prognosis of anxiety disorders in the elderly.

Somatoform disorders

The prevalence of somatoform disorders in the elderly is 0.1%. Somatoform disorders characterised by physical symptoms in the absence of organic disease are much harder to identify in the elderly because of the frequent presence of actual medical illnesses. More than 80% of elderly people have at least one chronic disease, such as arthritis or cardiovascular disease.

Somatoform disorders in the elderly are difficult to manage. Frequent medical examinations are necessary in order not to miss actual medical diseases. However, intensive investigations are to be avoided. It would help to gradually influence the patient to reattribute the symptoms to psychosocial stressors.

Alcohol and drug use disorders

The lifetime prevalence of alcohol dependence in people over 65 years old for men is 14% and 1.5% for women. It is often associated with depression, medical illnesses, accidents and suicide.

Alcohol use disorder in the elderly is often unrecognised. It is sometimes detected when withdrawal symptoms occur after abrupt cessation of alcohol intake when the elderly patient is admitted to hospital or when access to alcohol is not possible for other reasons. Falls, confusion, self-neglect, poor hygiene and medical illness may be the presenting complaints. In the later stages the patient may present with organic brain disorders, such as Wernicke's encephalopathy or Korsakoff's psychosis.

Illicit drug use disorder is extremely rare in old age. Drug abuse in the elderly almost always involves prescription drugs. The common drugs of abuse include sedative-hypnotics, anxiolytics and analgesics.

Frequent requests for these drugs should raise a high index of suspicion of dependence. Withdrawal symptoms occur when the supply is suddenly terminated. Preventative measures, such as taking great care when prescribing these medicines, is essential in suspicious circumstances. It is difficult to wean the elderly off these drugs.

Personality disorders

The prevalence of personality disorders in the elderly is unknown. These are disorders with an onset in adolescence or early adulthood, and continue into old age. Late onset emergent personality disorders may occur but are rare.

Some personality difficulties come to attention in old age when the elderly person is less able to cope with physical hardships or increased psychosocial stressors. Personality problems that develop for the first time in old age may be due to organic brain damage, and is termed an organic personality disorder.

Schizophrenia and other psychoses

These are conditions in which there is gross impairment of reality testing: the patient incorrectly evaluates the accuracy of his or her perception and thoughts and makes incorrect interpretation of external reality. Direct evidence of psychotic behaviour is the presence of delusions, hallucinations, thought disorder or disorganised inappropriate behaviour.

Psychosis in the elderly can be divided into 'organic' and 'functional' psychosis, based on aetiology. Organic psychoses include delirium, dementia, psychoses due to medical disorders, and alcohol and drug induced psychosis. Functional psychoses include schizophrenia, delusional disorder (or paranoid disorder), and psychoses associated with mania and depression. Acute transient psychotic episodes are uncommon in late life.

Epidemiology

Community surveys reveal the incidence of schizophrenia to be about 1% in the general population. Schizophrenia usually begins in late adolescence or young adulthood and persists throughout life. By the time patients with schizophrenia reach old age, 20% show no active symptoms, 30% show a residual type of schizophrenia, and others show varying degrees of impairment.

Less than 10% of patients treated for schizophrenia are over 65 years of age. It is suggested that late onset schizophrenia is a distinct subgroup of schizophrenia with a prevalence rate of 10–26 per 100 000 and a preponderance of female patients.

Aetiology

Schizophrenia is a neurodevelopmental disorder of the brain. The major brain areas involved are the limbic system, the frontal cortex and the basal ganglia. In schizophrenia these areas have too much dopaminergic and serotonergic activity. GABAergic and glutamatergic neurotransmission have also been implicated.

Studies strongly implicate a genetic component. The likelihood of a person developing the disorder correlates with the closeness of the relationship with a patient with schizophrenia (see Table 9.4).

Predisposing factors associated with schizophrenia include prenatal exposure to viral infection, winter births and any factor leading to foetal hypoxia.

The evidence for psychosocial factors acting as aetiological agents is extremely weak. There is evidence, however, that schizophrenic relapses are precipitated by family interaction with high expressed emotion, characterised by criticism, hostility and over-involvement.

Late onset schizophrenia is characterised by paranoid symptoms, and schizoid or paranoid traits in premorbid personality. Negative symptoms are less prominent, and partition delusions appear to be a pathognomonic feature. As the disorder manifests in late life after many years of relative mental stability, it is proposed to be a neurodegenerative disorder of the brain.

Clinical presentation

Schizophrenia is clinically differentiated from delusional disorder by the presence of bizarre symptoms, prominent hallucinations and disorder in form of thought. The symptoms of schizophrenia are often divided into positive and negative symptoms.

Positive symptoms are:

- delusions
- hallucinations
- formal thought disorder
- inappropriate affect
- disorganised behaviour.

Table 9.4 Prevalence of schizophrenia in the family

Population	Prevalence (%)
General population	1.0
Sibling of a schizophrenic patient	8.0
Child with one schizophrenic parent	12.0
Dizygotic twin of a schizophrenic patient	12.0
Child of two schizophrenic parents	40.0
Monozygotic twin of a schizophrenic patient	47.0

Negative symptoms are:

- blunted affect
- poverty of speech and thought
- impaired volition
- anhedonia
- social withdrawal.

Treatment

Antipsychotic drugs, sometimes referred to as neuroleptics, are the most effective symptomatic treatment for schizophrenia and their continued use prevents relapses. Psychosocial interventions discussed subsequently are also used to augment clinical improvement.

Drug treatment

Antipsychotic drugs are divided into conventional or typical and newer or atypical antipsychotics. With the elderly a practical principle for drug treatment is to start low and go slow to avoid unpleasant side effects.

Typical antipsychotics

Typical antipsychotics block dopamine-D2 receptors. Although they have proven antipsychotic activities, they do not treat negative symptoms and have side effects of considerable significance for the elderly patients. These side effects are:

- anticholinergic: confusion, memory problems, blurred vision, constipation, dizziness, postural hypotension, falls, drowsiness, etc.
- extapyramidal: dyskinesia, dystonia, Parkinson's symptoms
- tardive dyskinesia
- neuroleptic malignant syndrome: characterised by hyperpyrexia, muscular rigidity, autonomic instability, altered mental status, with rhabdomyolysis, acute renal failure and raised creatine phosphokinase level
- raised serum prolactin level.

Typical antipsychotics in common use are listed in Table 9.5. Table 9.6 lists the depot antipsychotics in common use when compliance is a major problem.

Table 9.5 Antipsychotic drugs in common use

Class	Drug	Dose (mg)
Phenothiazines	Chlorpromazine	25–1000 mg
	Thioridazine	25–500 mg
	Trifluoperazine	2–30 mg
Butyrophenones	Haloperidol	1.5–20 mg
Thioxanthines	Flupenthixol	6–18 mg
Diphenylbutyl	Pimozide	2–10 mg

Table 9.6 Depot antipsychotics in common use

Antipsychotics	Dose
Fluphenazine decanoate	6.25–25 mg per month
Haloperidol decanoate	12.5–25 mg per month
Flupenthixol decanoate	5–20 mg every 2–4 weeks
Zuclopenthixol decanoate	50–100 mg every 2–4 weeks

Atypical antipsychotics

Atypical antipsychotics block dopamine-D2 and serotonin-5HT2 receptors. Dopamine-D3 and D4 have also been identified as important targets for the newer antipsychotics. They treat both negative and positive symptoms. They have fewer side effects than the typical antipsychotics and are increasingly used as the first line antipsychotics for the elderly.

Atypical antipsychotics are listed in Table 9.7.

Psychosocial treatment

It is important to show compassion to these patients, who believe that their delusions and hallucinations are real and therefore respond to them. An emotionally arousing discussion is best avoided. Psychosocial treatments include psychoeducation, cognitive behavioural therapy, social skills training and family therapy.

Psychoeducation aims at providing information about the nature and treatment of schizophrenia and soliciting the patient's co-operation in managing the disorder. Cognitive behavioural therapy aims at modifying the patient's experience of delusions and hallucinations and responses to them. Social skills training aims at helping patients to improve self-care, interaction with others, and adjustment to

Table 9.7 Atypical antipsychotics

Antipsychotic	Dose	Comment
Clozapine	200–400 mg daily	Most efficacious but most dangerous; 1% develop agranulocytosis. Requires blood count weekly for 6 months and then fortnightly
Olanzapine	2.5–20 mg daily	Well accepted by patients; weight gain, drowsiness
Risperidone	0.5–4 mg daily	Only atypical antipsychotic that elevates serum prolactin levels
Quetiapine	75–150 mg daily	Headaches, drowsiness, dizziness

living in the community. As families are often carers, they benefit from psychoeducation and training in communication.

Prognosis

Long-term follow-up of schizophrenia shows that about 20–30% of patients lead normal lives, are relatively independent, working full-time, and raising families. Twenty to thirty per cent continue having moderate symptoms. Forty to sixty per cent are significantly impaired. The suicide rate is 10 times that in the general population. The prevalence of drug and alcohol dependence is as high as 90%.

The characteristic course of schizophrenia is one of relapses and remissions. Each exacerbation results in the patient not returning to baseline function. Deterioration continues for an average of 5 years when most patients reach a plateau. Elderly patients with early onset schizophrenia are often seen in this state.

Bibliography and further reading

American Psychiatric Association (1994), *Diagnostic and Statistical Manual of Mental Disorders*, 4th edn, DSM-IV, APA, Washington.

Ames, D., Flynn, E., Tuckwell, V. et al. (1994), 'Diagnosis of psychiatric disorder in elderly, general and geriatric hospital patients: AGECAT and DSM-III-R compared', *International Journal of Geriatric Psychiatry*, 9, pp. 627–33.

Cooper, B. (1993), 'Principles of service provision in old age psychiatry', in Jacoby, R. & Oppenheimer, C. (eds), *Psychiatry in the Elderly*, Oxford University Press, New York, pp. 274–300.

Copeland, J. R. M., Davidson, I. A., Dewey, M. E. et al. (1992), 'Alzheimer's disease, other dementia, depression and pseudodementia: Prevalence, incidence and three-year outcome in Liverpool', *British Journal of Psychiatry*, 161, pp. 230–9.

Hassett, A. (1999), 'A descriptive study of first presentation psychosis in old age', *Australian and New Zealand Journal of Psychiatry*, 33, pp. 814–23.

Howard, R., Almeida, O. & Levy, R. (1994), 'Phenomenology, demography and diagnosis in late paraphrenia', *Psychological Medicine*, 24, pp. 397–410.

Howard, R., Rabins, P. V. & Castle, D. J. (1999), *Late Onset Schizophrenia*, Chapter 10, Wrightson Biomedical Publishing Ltd, Petersfield, UK, and Philadelphia, US, pp. 127–38.

Katona, C. L. E. (1994), *Depression in Old Age*, Chapter 3, John Wiley & Sons, Chichester, pp. 29–41.

Roth, M. & Kay, D. W. K. (1998), 'Late paraphrenia: A variant of schizophrenia manifesting in late life or an organic clinical syndrome? A review of the literature', *International Journal of Geriatric Psychiatry*, 13, pp. 775–84.

Shader, R. I. & Kennedy, M. D. (1995), 'Psychopharmacology', Chapter 49, 'Geriatric psychiatry', in Kaplan, H. I. & Sadock, B. J., *Comprehensive Textbook of Psychiatry*, 6th edn, Wilkins & Wilkins, Baltimore, MD, pp. 2603–16.

Stewart, J. T. (1991), 'Diagnosing and treating depression in the hospitalised elderly', *Geriatrics*, 46, pp. 64–72.

Yesavage, J. A., Brink, T. L., Rose, T. L. & Lum, O. (1983), 'Development and validation of a geriatric depression screen scale: A preliminary report', *Journal of Psychiatric Research*, 17, pp. 37–49.

Chapter 10

The suicidal patient and other psychiatric emergencies

ROHAN S. DHILLON and WILLIAM M. H. GOH

Introduction

Psychiatric emergencies are acute disturbances of affect, mood, cognition or behaviour that require immediate intervention to avert serious outcomes. Psychiatric emergencies range from risk situations caused by intense personal distress, acute anxiety, suicidal or violent intentions, or self-neglect, to situations where others are placed at risk by the patient.

Deinstitutionalisation, a phenomenon of the latter part of the last century, has led to many severely and persistently mentally ill older people being inadequately cared for in the community. They form a significant portion of the urban homeless, and frequently use hospital emergency departments as their major source of care. Medical practitioners are often called to attend to emergency situations involving them.

Elderly people who complain of suicide ideation, make suicide attempts, suffer delusions or hallucinations, or have behavioural or cognitive disturbances are easily recognised by the medical practitioner as having psychiatric disorders. The challenge lies in identifying the more subtle presentation of psychiatric problems masquerading as organic diseases.

In an emergency, the primary clinical task is to anticipate and contain the acute situation, thereafter aiming to treat the underlying cause in a definitive manner. As access to psychiatric services is not always immediately available, it is important that general practitioners have an awareness and understanding of these emergency presentations, including approaches to management.

Causes of psychiatric emergencies

In the elderly, common psychiatric emergencies involve patients who are confused (delirium and dementia), aggressive, depressed and suicidal or psychotic. Emergency situations also occur in the so-called neurotic states, such as acute anxiety, panic disorder, grief and adjustment reactions, and substance misuse problems, especially with alcohol (see Box 10.1). Sometimes the elderly person with 'physical problems' for which there is a psychological basis (somatisation) or with occult physical disorders which present as vague psychological symptoms can create a challenge for the general practitioner; failure to recognise

Box 10.1 Types of psychiatric emergencies

Risk to a patient's safety

- Deliberate self-harm (as a result of personality disorder, delusional beliefs or poor coping skills)
- Suicidal intentions (with plans and preparations, especially if concealed from others)
- Chaotic behaviour (during intense anxiety, panic, psychosis, delirium)

Risk to a patient's health and wellbeing

- The patient stops drinking or eating (depressive stupor, delusion of being poisoned, catatonia and acute mania)
- The patient becomes exhausted and dehydrated (manic or catatonic excitement)
- Self-neglect (depression, dementia, chronic schizophrenia)
- Substance intoxication/withdrawal states (especially alcohol)
- Physically ill and refusing treatment
- Amnesic and confusional states
- Dissociative and fugue states (epilepsy, head injury, cerebrovascular accident)

Risk to others

- To family (due to depressive or paranoid delusions)
- To other patients in nursing homes, aged care facilities (due to confusional states, anxiety states, psychosis and other mental disorders)
- To the general public (due to paranoid or persecutory delusions or passivity symptoms such as delusions of being controlled by a specific person)

this problem at the early stage could have serious consequences.

Assessment of psychiatric emergencies

Preparing for the assessment

The setting of the assessment is important. There should be a safe and suitably equipped room available for interviewing the patient. In an emotionally charged situation, it could help put both the patient and the examiner at ease.

It is important before seeing the patient to collect all the information already available. This should include previous case records, interviews with family members or carers and other general practitioners who might be known to the patient. If relevant, case managers and support agencies should also be contacted as part of the assessment process (see Box 10.2).

Box 10.2 Information before interview

- Nature of previous psychiatric contact
- Recent contact with psychiatric services
- Contact with other services
- Any recent changes in contact
- Any problems associated with her contacts, such as violence, substance misuse or self-harm

Assessment interview

You should introduce yourself and anyone present when starting the acute assessment. You should ask the patient's permission for any third party to be present, unless the risk of violence necessitates that the elderly patient is not seen alone. It is very important in the early part of the interview to let the patient know that you understand her anxieties and that the aims of the interview or examination are to get to the bottom of her problems.

It is useful to begin the interview by letting the patient talk uninterruptedly for a few minutes. This helps you gain useful information about her mental state while demonstrating a willingness to listen. A structured interview ensures that important information is not omitted. Although history should focus on the main current problems and the possible precipitants, and identify the patient's expectations, the other routine key areas of inquiry should not be omitted. Overall, the interview should be focused so that it deals with the current crisis.

History taking

History taking is all-important when assessing an emergency situation in the elderly. It is often necessary to corroborate the story with a carer or relative. Often it is not the patient who is the complainant, and a clear understanding of the reasons for the consultation must be gained. Timing of symptoms or changes in behaviour, collateral life events, presence of physical symptoms, previous medical problems and previous psychiatric problems are essential basic information which is relevant in most cases.

A family history of psychiatric disorders gives clues to a genetic predisposition to later life illnesses. An indication of the patient's psychological adaptation to old age and previous personality is helpful when separating mental illness from behavioural idiosyncrasy. Understanding about the patient's support networks, family relationships, previous work history, sociability, interests and recreational substance use, especially alcohol, gives information about the patient's lifestyle and experience.

Mental state examination

Developing a mental illness can reduce an elderly person's ability to undertake the basic activities of daily living. The initial encounter may reveal if the patient is sad or happy, anxious or confused. Disorientation can be observed by watching the patient's reaction to her surroundings. Speech may be fast or slow, jumbled and obscure, or clear and precise. The detection of irritability, depression, hostility, fear, feeling of worthlessness, guilt and possibly incongruous happiness would indicate the presence of major depressive disorders.

Inappropriateness of affect is usually seen in psychotic disorders, mania or organic brain syndromes. Looking for abnormal thought processes means detecting, for instance, paranoia, delusions, false perceptions and irrational obsessions.

Cognitive functions are assessed by simple memory tests, determining orientation and testing concentration, such as recounting the months of the year backwards. Asking the patient the meaning of proverbs can test abstract thinking.

Physical examination

A full physical examination, especially focusing on the neurological system, is usually necessary in emergency presentations. Physical causes of mental disorders could be easily missed if a physical examination is not conducted.

Further investigations

Associated physical illnesses may be responsible for changes in mental state and may require specific tests to be undertaken, including blood count, electrolytes, liver and renal function tests, thyroid function test and urinalysis. Other tests, such as brain imaging, electroencephalogram, electrocardiogram and chest X-rays are indicated when specific pathology is suspected.

Management

When there is a clear psychiatric reason for the emergency, referral to the nearest hospital with psychiatric cover is often warranted. The need for compulsory admission of a patient to hospital, including whether or not to involve the police, ambulance or acute mobile mental health team, is dictated by the clinical situation and an understanding of the issues of safety and dangerousness (see Box 10.3).

After an initial assessment, the presence or absence of psychiatric illness, including underlying

Box 10.3 Factors associated with urgent treatment and/or admission

1. Severity of illness
2. Ability to care for self (is there evidence of neglect or emaciation?)
3. Risk of self-harm
4. Risk of harming others
5. Availability of supports
6. Level of insight
7. Need for supervision (e.g. with medication)
8. Need to clarify the diagnosis/severity of illness

physical problems, may remain uncertain. In such cases, further assessment is required and whether this can occur on an outpatient or inpatient basis is decided. Again, the way to proceed is dictated by the clinical situation and whether the emergency concerns have resolved through an intervention.

Explanations, reassurance and support, simple behavioural techniques (e.g. anxiety management) and crisis intervention techniques can all be useful and most general practitioners should make themselves familiar with them. Any relevant concurrent physical illness should be treated.

Not all individuals who present with psychiatric emergencies require ongoing psychiatric treatment and follow-up. Depending on the specific problem, some patients can be directed to other resources, including social workers, Drug and Alcohol Services, self-help groups and voluntary organisations.

Improved consultation–liaison between primary care and specialised services, especially mental health, should be encouraged. All general practitioners should be encouraged to establish access to a psychiatrist whom they can contact for advice in an emergency situation. If available, it might be useful to acquire a good doctor's handbook, which contains valuable guidelines on the management of particular problems, such as deliberate self-harm and substance misuse.

The suicidal patient

Despite the fact that suicide prevention is a major focus of health policy in most Western countries, suicide in the elderly remains a neglected area that receives little interest and research attention. The notion that suicides in the elderly are rational acts in response to irreversible, understandable situations such as intolerable pain or terminal conditions is not supported in clinical research. Suicidal behaviour in the elderly is undertaken with greater intent and lethality than in younger age groups. General practitioners play a vital role in the recognition and prevention of suicide in this age group.

Managing a suicidal crisis can be a very stressful experience for even the most experienced clinician. Even when risk factors are taken into account, it is not possible to accurately predict whether a person will commit suicide in the next 24 hours, especially in an emergency situation.

Despite this, a sound and logical approach will help to reduce morbidity and mortality in this group. It is very important to note that demographic risk factors merely serve as an estimation of the overall probability that someone will eventually die from suicide. They do not predict the acuteness of risk.

Epidemiology

In the geriatric population, males aged 75 and over have the highest suicide rates in most industrialised countries. Recent trends have shown a decline in suicide rates among elderly men compared to the 25- to 34-year-old group, which have risen approximately 30%, and a rise of about 50% in the 15- to 24-year-old male group. Despite this, the overall rates of suicide in elderly men are still higher than in any other male age group.

Female suicide rates have shown a similar overall decrease during the last decade. However, elderly women retain the highest rates of suicide throughout their lifespan. The ratio of male to female elderly suicide deaths remains around 3:1. Cross-cultural differences clearly influence suicide rates. Elderly first generation immigrants have lower suicide rates than the Indigenous elderly population.

The method of suicide employed varies over time, with age, gender and sociocultural factors. In general, elderly men adopt more violent methods (hanging, firearms) than elderly females (self-poisoning), which possibly explains the gender differences in suicide rates.

Aetiology of elderly suicides

The concept of suicidal behaviour as a distinct neurobiological entity has received little attention in the elderly. The most consistent finding in the biology of suicidal behaviour suggests dysregulation of the serotonergic systems in the brain.

Social factors and illness factors have received greater attention in the research of suicides in the elderly. Loneliness and social isolation are major factors that contribute to the elderly committing suicide. The role of bereavement appears to be a significant factor contributing to suicide in the elderly, especially in males. The first year of widowhood seems to be a vulnerable period. Marriage appears to be a protective factor.

Most studies of suicide in the elderly cite mental illness as a significant contributing factor. Major depression was diagnosed in about 50% of cases with other mood disorders (e.g. alcohol related) accounting for between 10% and 20%. Non-affective psychoses and addictive disorders were less commonly diagnosed in elderly suicides.

Primary substance use disorders account for a smaller proportion of suicides in the elderly. However, the role of substance misuse, especially alcohol, should not be underestimated as a contributing factor to elderly suicides.

The role of personality factors in elderly suicides has not been studied to any major extent. However, certain character traits—especially the cognitive propensity to perceive problems in dichotomous, black and white terms, a rigidly defined self-concept and diminished behavioural repertoire—decreases an elderly person's capacity to adapt to loss or change.

Physical illness

There is a large body of research demonstrating physical ill health as a major antecedent in elderly suicides. Some studies have reported that medical illness directly contributes to elderly suicides in around 60–70% of cases. This association is more significant in male elderly suicides compared to females, thus suggesting gender differences in coping with such age-normative stressors.

A number of specific neurological and systemic disorders have been linked with an increased risk of suicide in the elderly. These include multiple sclerosis, epilepsy, Huntington's chorea, head injury, peptic ulcer and rheumatoid arthritis. However, the association of cancer with suicide has yielded equivocal findings. The studies showing a significant relationship between cancer and suicide were conducted when the symptom of pain was present.

Sometimes hypochondriacal and other somatic symptoms may mask an underlying depressive illness. Such a symptom profile in the elderly may be a greater marker of suicidal tendencies than in the young.

Assessment

Risk factors

An act of suicide is a complex phenomenon involving multiple psychological, physical and social factors operating at a crucial point in an elderly person's life. Risk assessments performed by the general practitioner need to reflect these varied antecedents. A so-called typical high-risk elderly individual may be a male, living alone through a recent bereavement, who has a co-existent painful, chronic health problem. Such a person may have made a previous suicide attempt and be currently depressed (see Box 10.4).

The main problem with using risk factors is reflected in the high rate of false positive prediction of suicide. No risk assessment tool with adequate sensitivity and specificity has been developed in the elderly. For the general practitioner, a thorough clinical interview and mental state examination remains the best means of identifying suicidal risk in the elderly.

Detecting suicidal risk in the elderly is a greater challenge for the general practitioner than detecting it in the young because of factors related to the differences in the verbalisation of such threats in the elderly. Of note is the commonly reported fact that

Box 10.4 Risk factors for elderly suicides

- Older age
- Male gender
- Living alone
- Bereavement (especially in men)
- Depression (especially with feelings of hopelessness)
- Alcohol misuse
- Previous suicide attempt
- Vulnerable personality traits
- Chronic physical ill health (especially with pain)
- Family history of suicide

40–70% of elderly suicides have seen their general practitioner in the 30 days preceding their death.

Suicidality

Asking about suicide does not put the thought in an individual. Suicidality can be assessed by initially asking general questions (e.g. 'Does it seem that life is not worth living?'). Then proceed to more direct questions (e.g. 'Have you thought of harming or killing yourself?'). Follow up these questions with a discussion about alternative strategies for solving the person's problems. If appropriate to the situation, seek an agreement that if suicidal ideas are to recur again, the person will first seek help (see Box 10.5).

Box 10.5 Assessment of suicidality

1. Consider the person's risk factors
2. Ask about feelings of hopelessness
3. Ask about any plans of suicide
4. Evaluate the context of any suicidal act and its meaning to the individual
5. Ask about access to firearms and other means
6. Clarify the problem that the suicidal act attempts to solve
7. Diagnose the underlying mental disorder
8. Diagnose the physical disorder
9. Document past suicidal behaviour
10. Assess the extent of social supports

Suicidal intent

It is often useful to ask the person to describe what happened in the days leading up to a suicide attempt. This will help in understanding the context in which the attempt occurred and the meaning of the act. Clarifying whether the attempt was impulsive or planned has important implications for the seriousness of the person's actions. It is important to ask whether the person expected to die or intended another outcome.

The influence of substances like alcohol in the suicide attempt also has important implications in assessing the intent involved. In general, an impulsive suicide attempt in the context of alcohol intoxication is less significant than a planned attempt occurring without the influences of disinhibiting substances like alcohol. Strong intent to die is usually implied when a suicide note is written.

Lethality

Assess the lethality of the act by noting the means, the situation in which it occurred, and whether others were nearby so that the chances of discovery would have been high. Ask about access to firearms and other means. It is important to note that the lethality of the act may not correlate with the intent.

Other factors

Other factors that need to be considered include recent psychosocial factors, psychiatric disorders, physical disorders and social supports. Suicidal acts are usually attempts at solving problems in a person's life. Clarifying the precipitating problem is the first step in trying to solve it. Listening to a person describe her problem will itself provide some relief. Use learnt counselling and structured problem-solving techniques to help the person resolve the crisis.

Management

1. Treat the physical sequelae of the suicide attempt. The person might require referral to hospital for inpatient treatment.
2. Establish a therapeutic alliance. Listening to the person, being sensitive to verbal and non-verbal cues, and having an empathic style will promote open communication.
3. Ensure the person's safety. Before deciding that a person is safe to be home, ensure an agreement is reached that the person is no longer suicidal. If suicidal thoughts should recur, there is a clear plan on how the person can seek help (see Box 10.6).
4. Mobilise social supports. Any safety contract will usually require the co-operation of family members or other close supports. A plan that has the agreement of everybody concerned is more likely to succeed and all participants will share some responsibility for its implementation.

5. Diagnose and treat the underlying mental illness. In the immediate aftermath of a suicide attempt, explain the nature, causes, treatment and prognosis of the underlying condition to the person and her carers. This might give the person a sense of control and help to restore hope.
6. It is important to deal with your own and others' emotional reactions. Suicidal behaviour evokes strong feelings in those close to the patient and in those who treat them. Monitor counter-transference feelings to ensure that such feelings do not distort your judgment. Common reactions include denial of the seriousness of the attempt through colluding with the patient's dismissiveness of the attempt, anger and distancing (e.g. labelling suicidal thoughts as manipulative and attention seeking), and rescue fantasies that may only reinforce a person's feelings of helplessness.

Box 10.6 Criteria for allowing a suicidal patient to remain at home

- The person no longer feels suicidal
- His or her mental condition is stable
- The person is able to promise to seek help before self-harming if suicidal ideas recur
- The person is neither intoxicated, delirious nor psychotic
- Firearms have been removed from the home
- Acute problems have been identified and steps taken to begin to address them
- Treatment has been arranged for underlying psychiatric problems
- The clinician feels confident that the person will not follow through with the plan
- Social supports have been contacted and there is general agreement with the plan

When a patient commits suicide

Sometimes, despite our best efforts at prevention, there are some people who will commit suicide. It has been estimated that, on average, general practitioners will lose a patient by suicide around once every 6 years.

In the aftermath of a suicide of a patient under your care, it is advisable to contact the family and to offer to meet them. Encourage discussion and ventilation of feelings. Acknowledge that the grieving process after a suicide may be particularly painful, with conflicting emotions of sadness, guilt, shame and anger. Consider attending the funeral. Contrary to what you might expect, families are generally grateful for your attendance and are unlikely to be critical.

An audit of the case should be conducted with a group of colleagues. The focus should be on a supportive review and what can be learnt rather than 'what went wrong'. It is important to seek the support of a colleague at this time.

The acutely anxious elderly patient

Acute anxiety in the elderly carries a high risk of impulsive behaviour, which may result in harm to self and others and must be regarded as a psychiatric emergency. Anxiety may be generalised and pervasive, or present in acute and discrete episodes.

Extreme forms of anxiety can occur in primary and secondary anxiety disorders and concomitantly with other psychiatric disorders. Very often, anxiety symptoms in the elderly are secondary to depression. The prevalence of general anxiety states among people aged over 65 in the community is approximately 4% (10% for phobias).

Causes of anxiety

Stressful life events or the onset of physical disorders can exacerbate anxiety states in the elderly and heighten feelings of insecurity. Neglecting the consequences of frightening physical illness, such as falls, may very often cause significant anxiety. Elderly people require a psychiatric assessment after hip fractures, falls, crime or unexpected illnesses to ensure that anxiety symptoms, such as agoraphobia, are not present. Failure to do so may cause the condition to become chronic and difficult to treat. Untreated anxiety states in the elderly can have serious consequences, including death from suicide.

Anxiety caused by a specific organic factor is referred to as an organic anxiety disorder or a secondary anxiety disorder. Medications, substance abuse (both ingestion and withdrawal) and medical and neurological illnesses may cause secondary anxiety syndromes. Certain medications (e.g. sympathomimetic agents, the theophyllines and thyroid) are potentially anxiogenic.

Medical and neurological disorders can sometimes cause pathological anxiety. Anxiety can be caused by endocrine conditions (e.g. pheochromocytoma and thyroid dysfunction) and neurological disorders, such as subarachnoid haemorrhage, tumours in the vicinity of the third ventricle and seizures. Patients with organic anxiety states can be differentiated from patients with primary psychiatric disorders or adjustment reactions by careful scrutiny of their histories and careful physical examination.

Manifestation of anxiety

As anxiety states for the first time in the elderly are rare, the task of the general practitioner in the acute setting is to exclude medical emergencies that can mimic acute anxiety. Panic disorder is sometimes difficult to distinguish from medical conditions such as paroxysmal nocturnal dyspnoea and cardiac dysrhythmias (see Table 10.1).

Late onset anxiety may also be a sign of early dementia. For example, a patient with dementia may become extremely distressed when faced with a difficult task. The patient may have a 'catastrophic reaction' as a result of her cognitive impairment. The clinician needs to rule out other psychiatric disorders, such as dementia, delirium, psychotic disorders or mood disorders, before diagnosing an anxiety disorder.

Management of acute anxiety

Checking an elderly person's cognitive state is an important task to perform when managing anxiety states. It will help guide treatment strategies as normal anxiety management techniques may not work so well in the presence of cognitive difficulties. In such cases, using low dose major tranquillisers rather than benzodiazepines may also be necessary.

Table 10.1 Medical emergencies that may mimic acute anxiety

Type of emergency	Presentation
Vascular	Angina pectoris, myocardial infarction, cardiac arrhythmias, acute cardiac failure of any cause
Respiratory	Acute bronchospasm of any cause, pulmonary embolism, pneumothorax, pneumonia
Toxins	Acute ingestion of directly or indirectly acting sympathomimetic agents, withdrawal from CNS depressants
Metabolic emergencies	Hypoglycaemia, electrolyte disturbances, thyrotoxic crisis
Others	Temporal lobe epilepsy, anaphylaxis, vertigo, severe anaemia

An adequate psychiatric history and mental state assessment will help the examiner rule out other causes of anxiety in the elderly, such as depression. If depression is present, treat this first before addressing the anxiety symptoms specifically. Most antidepressants are also anxiolytics, especially at higher doses. The newer agents, like the serotonin reuptake inhibitors, are safer in the elderly than the older tricyclic antidepressants.

Once acute medical emergencies have been reasonably excluded, reassure the patient that the anxiety state or experience, although severe and uncomfortable, is not life-threatening. If the patient is able, initially attempt controlled breathing exercises (not with a paper bag). Explain to the person that if the anxiety state does not settle or is acutely unbearable, pharmacological intervention is an option.

In the acute setting, benzodiazepines are the medication of choice. Lorazepam at 1–5 mg can be given sublingually, which can provide symptomatic relief within minutes. If lorazepam is not available, intramuscular clonazepam (0.5–4 mg) is a suitable alternative. Because of its long half-life, presence of active metabolites and its erratic absorption, intramuscular diazepam is not recommended.

Psychosis in the elderly

Psychotic symptoms can sometimes result in emergency presentations, especially when elderly individuals are suicidal, threatening aggression or not caring for themselves. Command auditory hallucinations telling a person to harm themselves or others is a particularly serious situation which warrants urgent intervention. Acting on such commands is not uncommon, especially if the hallucinations are persistent with no respite.

Schizophrenia and delusional disorders

Persecutory delusions are a common cause of aggressive impulses in the elderly. This is especially so when cognitive impairment affecting judgment (as in a dementia) is also present. Suicide is another noted risk in a persecuted elderly individual because of the extreme fear experienced with anxiety and the sense of isolation and desperation. Delusions of reference and influence sometimes cause an elderly person significant distress because of the false belief that she is being talked about and that random events such as accidents have been designed to harm or influence her. Incorporating other individuals in her delusional system, especially if they are known to the person, is a significant risk factor for homicidal actions. It is important to ask about suicidal and/or homicidal ideation or fantasies in any elderly patient who is deemed psychotic.

Somatic delusions and visual or tactile hallucinations in the elderly can potentially lead to dangerous behaviours, including self-mutilation, especially when they believe their body is infested by worms or parasites which they can sometimes see crawling under their skin. Self-mutilation could also occur when psychotic individuals attempt to remove electronic devices they falsely believe are implanted in their body. Somatic delusions that trigger suicidal actions usually involve having cancer or a decaying body. When such delusions are present, a depressive illness could exist co-morbidly.

Catatonic excitement is a hypermetabolic state and a psychiatric emergency. The patient's activity and speech may be excessive, driven and purposeless. Patients in this state may be violent. Before pharmacologic and electroconvulsive therapy, these patients usually died from acute hyperthermia. Catatonic excitement may be caused by organic conditions and manic psychosis.

Depression and bipolar disorder

Elderly patients with major depressive disorders may have difficulties in initiating and maintaining purposeful and goal directed activities. The loss of interest in themselves and the environment could result in extreme states of self-neglect. Such patients do not look after their physical health or take their medications properly. This is particularly serious if they are on treatment for potentially life-threatening illnesses such as diabetes or heart diseases.

Depressive stupor is a state of dramatic motor inactivity in which patients may, if untreated and if it is in its extreme form, be immobile for days or weeks at a time. Patients may be unable to initiate eating, drinking or elimination functions, which places them at acute risk from various medical complications, including dehydration and septicaemia from infected bedsores.

In manic states, grandiose delusions could cause an elderly individual to act in a dangerous or self-damaging fashion. In such a situation, the person could believe she is indestructible and act in a risky way or spend money excessively to the detriment of her financial state of affairs. Sexual indiscretions sometimes occur with or without consent when a person is manic and psychotic.

Management

The management of psychiatric emergencies related to psychosis is dictated by clinical circumstances. Issues of safety and/or dangerousness dictate whether the patient can be managed in her home situation or require hospitalisation. It is the job of the general practitioner to clarify the cause of the psychosis, whether acute or chronic, organic or functional.

Once the aetiology has been clarified, treatment can be initiated with antipsychotic medication as described in Chapter 9. Sometimes treatment involves re-establishing previous medication(s) the patient has recently ceased and monitoring compliance. Once the emergency has passed, the general practitioner should monitor the patient's clinical state closely and liaise with mental health services if required.

Iatrogenic factors

Complications of antipsychotic treatment

Antipsychotic medications used in the treatment of psychotic disorders in the elderly can themselves result in serious life-threatening complications. The older high potency traditional agents like haloperidol and related medications are more likely to cause these problems than the newer atypical antipsychotics such as risperidone, olanzapine and quetiapine (see Box 10.7).

Box 10.7 Complications seen with antipsychotic treatment

1. Extrapyramidal syndromes
   (a) Acute dystonic reactions
   (b) Drug induced parkinsonism
   (c) Akathisia
   (d) Neuroleptic induced catatonia
2. Tardive dyskinesia
3. Neuroleptic malignant syndrome
4. Anticholinergic delirium
5. Others

Extrapyramidal syndromes

Extrapyramidal syndromes result from the blockade of dopamine receptors in the basal ganglia. Acute dystonic reactions involve sudden tonic contractions of the muscles of the tongue, neck (torticollis), back (opisthotonos), mouth and eyes (oculogyric crises). As well as being very frightening, such reactions can be dangerous if the patient's airway is compromised. These patients can be effectively treated with benztropine (1–2 mg intramuscularly) or diphenhydramine (25–50 mg intramuscularly or intravenously).

Drug induced parkinsonism can be a distressing experience and the akinesia can be mistaken as a drug induced depression. If possible, the antipsychotic dose should be reduced or the patient switched to a newer agent. Alternatively, use benztropine 0.5–4 mg orally daily or benzhexol 2–5 mg orally 3 times a day.

Akathisia is a severe sense of agitation, which may be experienced in the limbs or as mental perturbation. Short-term measures for treating akathisia include propranolol 20–40 mg orally, 3–4 times a day. Alternatively, diazepam 2–5 mg orally, 3–4 times a day, can be effective. Benztropine is sometimes used (0.5–4 mg orally) but is less effective for akathisia.

Neuroleptic induced catatonia is characterised by symptoms of withdrawal, mutism and motor abnormalities, including rigidity, immobility and waxy flexibility. It should be treated by temporarily discontinuing antipsychotic therapy and, on resolution, changing to a different class of antipsychotic. Amantadine administered in an oral dose of 100 mg 3 times a day may be helpful.

Tardive dyskinesia

Tardive dyskinesia is a late onset movement disorder, a complex syndrome of involuntary hyperkinetic movements characterised by fasciculations of the tongue (sometimes the earliest symptom), lingual-facial hyperkinesia (persistent involuntary chewing, lip smacking or grimacing movements) and choreoathetoid movements of the extremities and trunk (sometimes involving the respiratory muscles). Anxiety increases the abnormal movements, which then disappear in sleep. They can interfere with speaking and eating and are socially stigmatising.

Atypical antipsychotic medications (risperidone, olanzapine, quetiapine) should be considered in elderly patients even if they are stabilised on typical antipsychotic medications. Clozapine is the treatment of choice for established tardive dyskinesia when all other measures fail and the symptoms are quite distressing for the patient. Such patients require referral to specialised psychiatric services.

Neuroleptic malignant syndrome

Neuroleptic malignant syndrome is a rare but potentially fatal adverse effect of antipsychotic treatment which can develop at any time during treatment. The full syndrome is thought to occur in 0.5–1% of those on traditional antipsychotic medication. Onset of the full-blown syndrome is rapid over 1–2 days after a period of gradual progressive rigidity.

It is characterised by high temperature, muscle rigidity and altered consciousness. Other features can include neutrophilia, raised creatine kinase, autonomic instability and occasionally haemorrhagic tendency. Milder variants of the full syndrome are thought to occur with both newer and traditional antipsychotics.

Treatment involves immediate discontinuation of antipsychotic medication and support of respiratory, renal and cardiovascular functioning and possible treatment with dantrolene or bromocriptine. Immediate referral to the nearest general hospital is essential to reduce the risk of permanent morbidity and mortality, especially in the elderly.

Anticholinergic delirium

A life-threatening anticholinergic delirium can sometimes occur in the elderly as a direct result of treatment with a combination of drugs, including antipsychotics, anticholinergic agents used to treat parkinsonian side effects of antipsychotics, and the inappropriate use of medications from other classes, such as the tricyclic antidepressants. Mild anticholinergic symptoms include blurred vision, dry mouth, urinary retention (especially in elderly men with prostate enlargement) and constipation. Toxic anticholinergic symptoms include restless agitation, confusion, disorientation, hallucinations (especially visual) and delusions, with accompanying signs of facial flushing, dry skin, dilation of the pupils, tachycardia, decreased bowel sounds and urinary retention.

Anticholinergic toxicity is a particularly insidious risk of polypharmacy as it may occur in the elderly without obvious physiological signs. Clinicians must be aware of elderly patients developing psychotic symptoms caused by additional or different medications in the patient's treatment plan and be suspicious of an anticholinergic delirium if the patient appears confused.

Other emergencies

Other emergencies related to antipsychotic therapy in the elderly include orthostatic hypotension (falls) from adrenergic blockage and potentially life-threatening ventricular arrhythmias with electrocardiographic abnormalities (i.e. T wave changes and QT prolongation) and with cardiac repolarisation abnormalities.

Finally, agranulocytosis (especially with clozapine therapy) and ophthalmological complications like pigmentary retinopathy (especially associated with thioridazine in doses greater than 800 mg/day), lens and corneal pigmentation, and worsening of narrow angle glaucoma secondary to anticholinergic effects can occur.

Complications of antidepressant treatment

Serotonin syndrome

Serotonin syndrome is a potentially life-threatening complication when the selective serotonin reuptake inhibitors (SSRIs) are prescribed with other medications or preparations with serotonergic effects. The clinical features of a serotonin syndrome include abdominal cramps, agitation, diarrhoea, myoclonus, tremulousness, coma, tachycardia, hypotension, confusion, disorientation, profuse sweating and hyperpyrexia and can be a medical emergency, especially in the elderly who are frail.

Sometimes it may be difficult to distinguish between the clinical features of depression, adverse effects of SSRIs, SSRI discontinuation effects and the potentially life-threatening serotonin syndrome. Elderly patients should be referred for a psychiatric opinion if a serotonin syndrome is suspected.

Sometimes this syndrome occurs when there is an inadequate drug-free interval in changing antidepressant medications. Rarely, it is an idiosyncratic reaction. Preparations like St John's Wort, bought over the counter, can trigger this syndrome when used concurrently with an SSRI.

The syndrome usually settles when the SSRI is stopped and/or the interacting medication is ceased. If the serotonin syndrome is severe or does not settle quickly with the above measures, immediate referral to an emergency department is required.

Hypertensive crises

Hypertensive crises can occur when patients on the irreversible non-selective monoamine oxidase inhibitors consume foodstuffs containing large quantities of tyramine or other amines. All patients on monoamine oxidase inhibitors (MAOIs) should be warned about dietary restrictions and given a list of foods high in tyramine that must not be consumed. Pethidine can interact with MAOIs to produce hyperpyrexia, hypertension or hypotension, and prolonged coma. This combination should be avoided and the MAOI ceased one week before any elective surgery. However, the potential problems with anaesthesia need to be balanced against the necessity for an antidepressant.

Personality disorders and substance use disorders

Personality disorders

Individuals with personality disorders usually still have the same problems when they reach old age. Personality problems (e.g. antisocial behaviour) that develop for the first time in the elderly are likely to be due to organic brain disease (e.g. frontal lobe dementia). Some personality disorders may emerge only in old age when older persons are less mobile, have to face physical problems or lose major support networks through the death of spouses or family members. This is especially so for obsessional, narcissistic and dependent individuals.

Aggressive and behavioural problems attributable to personality dysfunction are usually situational, impulsive and directed to known individuals. Management strategies are pragmatic and social. The role of medications is usually limited except in cases of personality changes brought on by physical disorders. Any central nervous system traumatic injury or disease has the potential to cause a change in personality and is referred to as an 'organic personality syndrome'.

Organic personality disorders

Typical injury or lesions associated with personality change are head trauma, complex partial seizures (temporal lobe seizures), brain tumours, multiple sclerosis, dementias and strokes. Mild cognitive impairment may or may not be present in secondary personality disorders. However, global cognitive deficits are highly suggestive of dementias.

Lesions in the orbital region of the frontal lobes can cause varying degrees of disinhibition, ranging from mild irritability to frank aggression. Such elderly patients, often described as 'pseudopsychopathic', behave inappropriately and exhibit poor impulse control. Lesions to the convex portions of the frontal lobes can cause apathy and abulia. Such patients lack motivation and are sometimes incorrectly labelled as being depressed. The term 'pseudodepressed' is sometimes used to describe these individuals.

Treatment of the organic personality syndrome is aimed at amelioration of the specific organic factor judged to be aetiologic in each case. Behavioural problems may be controlled by medications like anticonvulsant mood stabilisers. Target symptoms like irritability, mood lability, impulsiveness and disinhibition resulting from brain pathology in the elderly might respond to an empirical trial of sodium valproate or carbamazepine used at anticonvulsant doses.

Alcohol use disorder

Estimates of the prevalence of alcohol abuse in the elderly community setting range from 3% to 3.7%, especially in men over the age of 65. Alcoholism in the elderly is sometimes hidden and unrecognised by the general practitioner. It is sometimes a marker for depression in the elderly and is related to issues such as dealing with loss, coping with physical illness and facing an uncertain and lonely future.

Elderly alcoholics have a high risk of physical and psychological morbidity and mortality. The acute consumption of alcohol is known to impair cognitive function, and its chronic use is associated with dementia. Organic brain syndromes, including withdrawal delirium, carries a high risk of mortality in the elderly if untreated. Depression and suicide is a significant risk in those elderly with alcohol misuse problems.

Management may include attempts to lessen the feelings of loneliness and isolation. The general practitioner might have to look at options such as referring the person to social or group activities or specifically to a detoxification program run by Drug and Alcohol Services. Anxieties and sources of distress also need to be formally addressed by the general practitioner.

Other drugs of misuse

Intoxication and withdrawal syndromes related to other substances besides alcohol can be a major factor in causing self-destructive or dangerous behaviour in the elderly. Although relatively little attention has been given to these problems in the elderly, some recent studies suggest that it could affect as many as 14–25% of elderly outpatients presenting with co-morbid psychiatric disorders. For the most part, the use of 'street drugs' is not a major problem in the elderly.

Addiction to hypnotics and anxiolytics is not uncommon in the elderly and can result in similar problems to those seen with alcohol abuse/dependence. It is usually difficult to wean elderly people off these medications. Cessation might require professional help. If at all possible, prescribing such medications on a regular basis should be avoided. Sometimes the abuse of over-the-counter addictive medication, such as antihistamines and decongestants containing amphetamines, can result in behavioural problems in the elderly. A detailed history of medication and substance use with collateral information might alert the general practitioner to such problems.

When an elderly person refuses treatment

A serious problem sometimes noted in the elderly is when essential treatment is refused without a rational reason. Exploring the causes behind these actions is important before various intervention strategies are explored and implemented. As compulsory treatment can be given only in hospital, admission is sometimes the only option.

Situations where compulsory treatment is warranted include:

- dementia with acute untreated physical illness (e.g. urinary tract infection)
- dementia with danger to self (such as nocturnal wandering in winter) when all reasonable alternatives (such as a night sitter service) have failed
- delirium (due to whatever cause) and disturbed behaviour
- seriously physically ill with an acute psychiatric disorder
- persecutory delusions and very distressed or dangerous to others
- severely depressed and deluded or suicidal (e.g. depressive stupor)
- refusal to eat or drink resulting in dehydration (e.g. catatonia).

If there is any doubt over whether an elderly patient requires compulsory admission, advice should be sought from a psychiatric colleague or the local mental health service.

Conclusion

Despite the frequency with which psychiatric emergencies are encountered in the geriatric population, the literature is relatively sparse, with little systemic research on areas of clinical interest relevant to general practice.

Psychiatric emergencies in the elderly can arise from a variety of causes. Physical factors are just as likely as psychological ones to result in an emergency situation in the elderly. Early recognition and management of the potential causes of such emergencies in the elderly can avert serious consequences, including the death of the patient.

Having the knowledge to assess and investigate these presentations is essential before intervention strategies are implemented. If the cause of the psychiatric emergency is unclear despite a thorough assessment, admission to hospital should be considered, even under detention, to allow further monitoring of the situation. Managing such emergencies should also involve making changes relevant to the patient and her environment in order to prevent further episodes.

Bibliography and further reading

Brown, Tom (1998), 'Psychiatric emergencies', *Advances in Psychiatric Treatment*, 4, pp. 270–6.

Cattell, Howard (2000), 'Suicide in the elderly', *Advances in Psychiatric Treatment*, 6, pp. 102–8.

Craig, T. K. J. & Boordman, A. P. (1998), 'Common mental health problems in primary care', in Davies, T. & Craig, T. K. J. (eds), *ABC of Mental Health*, BMJ Books, London, pp. 5–8.

Davies, John (1999), 'A manual of mental health care in general practice', *Commonwealth Department of Health and Aged Care*, 3, pp. 25–32.

Harris, G. T. & Rice, M. E. (1997), 'Risk appraisal and management of violent behaviour', *Psychiatric Services*, 48, pp. 1168–76.

Macdonald, A. J. D. (1998), 'Mental health in old age', in Davies & Craig, op. cit., pp. 46–50.

Pilowsky, L. S., Ring, H., Shine, P. J., Battersby, M. & Lader, M. (1992), 'Rapid tranquillisation: A survey of emergency prescribing in a general psychiatric hospital', *British Journal of Psychiatry*, pp. 831–5.

Ramirez, A. & House, A. (1998), 'Common mental health problems in hospital', in Davies & Craig, op. cit., pp. 9–11.

Shader, R. I. (1994), 'Assessment and treatment of suicide risk', in Shader, R. I. (ed.), *Manual of Psychiatric Therapeutics*, 2nd edn, Little Brown and Co., Boston, pp. 159–66.

Shader, R. I. & Greenblatt, D. J. (1994), 'Approaches to the treatment of anxiety states', in Shader, op. cit., pp. 275–98.

Teifion, Davies (1998), 'Risk management in mental health', in Davies & Craig, op. cit., pp. 75–8.

Thienhaus, O. J. & Piasecki, M. (1997), 'Assessment of suicide risk', *Psychiatric Services*, 48, pp. 293–4.

Thienhaus, O. J. & Piasecki, M. (1998), 'Assessment of psychiatric patients: Risk of violence towards others', *Psychiatric Services*, 49, pp. 1129–47.

Wescott, R. (1994), 'Emergencies, crises and violence', in Pullen, I., Wilkinson, G., Wright, A. & Pereira Gray, D. (eds), *Psychiatry and General Practice Today*, Royal College of General Practitioners, London, pp. 170–9.

Zerrin, Atakan & Teifion, Davies (1998), 'Mental health emergencies', in Davies & Craig, op. cit., pp. 12–14.

Chapter 11
Grief and bereavement

PAULA BRINDLEY, BETTE EMERY and JOSE PEREIRA

Introduction

Grief and bereavement care is a critical component in the health care continuum of all patients, including the elderly. It should not be regarded as an 'add on', but rather as an integral part of the care we provide. Grief and bereavement are integral and inevitable parts of the universal human experience. The death of a loved one is an experience that can simultaneously significantly impact on a person's physical, psychological, emotional, spiritual and social state and functioning. The manifestation of grief encompasses a range of feelings and behaviours that in many instances mirror those of other psychiatric illnesses. Therefore, adequate and effective bereavement care requires an understanding of the phenomenon of grief, a systematic assessment of its effects upon the patient and a customised management protocol. A working knowledge of the processes, tasks and responses involved in the experience is required. Recognising the factors that may affect it and the risk factors for poor bereavement outcome allows the physician to more realistically assess whether this is normal or complicated grief. An accurate assessment will facilitate a more precise and appropriate management aimed at lessening the patient's discomfort and pain of the loss, and enhance his long-term wellbeing.

Definitions

Definitions and terms relating to grief and bereavement are numerous and consensus among researchers and theorists as to their usage is sometimes lacking. Health care professionals and patients may use various terms related to grief and bereavement care interchangeably. Below is a list of practical definitions of the terms that are often used. These definitions will apply to this chapter.

- *Bereavement* Bereavement is the loss of a close or loved person.
- *Bereavement reactions* These are the psychological, physiological or behavioural reactions to that loss.
- *Grief* Grief is the normal idiosyncratic response to the loss of someone or something precious. This response is based upon an individual's unique situation and circumstance. It is commonly viewed as a lengthy process, composed of a number of components and reactions.

In essence, grief is the psychological and emotional reaction to bereavement. Despite the subtle differences between 'bereavement reactions' and 'grief', these two terms are often used interchangeably.

- *Mourning* Mourning refers to the social expression of grief performed after a death. It allows others to recognise that a person is bereaved and it includes rituals and behaviours that are specific to each culture and religion. Wakes, wearing black clothing, wailing and lamentations are some examples of these rituals and expressions.

Classification of grief

Attempts are often made to differentiate between 'normal' bereavement reactions and grief and complicated or 'abnormal' reactions. However, bereavement reactions and grief encompass a wide range of responses and people vary greatly in their manifestations and expressions of these reactions. It is complex and can be viewed from many different perspectives. Given the large range of reactions, their intensities, duration, perspectives and the personal circumstances of the bereaved, compartmentalising bereavement reactions and grief into 'normal' or 'abnormal' ('complicated') can be difficult and even somewhat artificial. Nevertheless, a working conceptual framework will facilitate the care of bereaved patients and assist in identifying those at risk of complicated grief and those in need of specialised help. In establishing such a framework, a review of the phases of 'normal' grief responses, the normal reactions associated with them, the duration of grief, the models and the tasks of the bereavement process as well as the factors that affect the process is required.

Normal grief

Timing of normal grief

Anticipatory grief

Where the loss is anticipated, as in the case of a terminally ill relative or friend, grief may begin before the actual death. The expression of anticipatory grief is considered valuable as it allows for some of the grief to take place prior to the death. As it is believed by some bereavement experts to lessen the severity of the grief response following the death, a strong case can be made for ensuring that both terminally ill patients and their families are informed in an honest and sensitive manner of the patient's prognosis. An individual who is grieving the impending loss of his own or someone else's life invariably exhibits the same grief reactions—for example, anxiety, anger, sadness, etc.—as those of a bereaved person after a death has occurred.

It should be noted that a relative may show relief when the anticipated death occurs and few, if any, of the typical manifestations of acute grief. However, this doesn't necessarily mean that the person will not experience the grief. Rather it may be delayed by weeks or months as he slowly adjusts to his changed world.

Acute or post-mortem grief

This refers to the grief following the death and is what most people mean when they speak of grief, mourning or being bereaved. The loss may be unexpected and sudden or may be anticipated. The immediate reaction to the death varies considerably. It often begins immediately or within hours, but its onset may sometimes be delayed. The spectrum of possible reactions are discussed and listed in the following section. The duration of the grief, too, is variable.

Chronic phase of normal grief

Following the anticipatory or acute reactions, there follows a period, ranging from months to years, that is characterised by reducing symptoms of acute grief. However, these symptoms may wax and wane in nature, intensity and duration and may be precipitated by events or times that remind the bereaved of their loved ones. Events such as birthdays, family celebrations and religious times (such as Christmas) may all remind the bereaved of their loved ones and elicit a return or aggravation of grief and bereavement reactions.

Normal grief and bereavement reactions

Normal grief and bereavement reactions encompass a myriad of reactions and responses. These include physical, cognitive (thoughts), emotional (feelings), spiritual and behavioural responses. The wide spectrum of possible responses is listed in Box 11.1. Patients do not present with all the responses listed but rather a combination of them. Furthermore, all the responses are not necessarily experienced at the same time: they may present at different times. Responses may also recur in time and wax and wane in intensity. The responses listed in Box 11.1 are generally all normal responses. However, they may become abnormal if they are pervasive, excessive and interfere with personal and social functioning, especially in the long term.

Box 11.1 Grief and bereavement reactions

Feelings (emotions)

- Sadness, possibly expressed through crying
- Anger with self, God or health care profession
- Guilt or self-reproach
- Anxiety about future
- Awareness of one's own mortality
- Loneliness and/or aloneness
- Fear
- Apathy
- Shock
- Numbness
- Yearning
- Relief
- Remorse
- Freedom/emancipation

Thoughts (cognition)

- Disbelief
- Confusion
- Inability to concentrate
- Absentmindedness or forgetfulness
- Difficulty making decisions
- Making hasty decisions
- Preoccupation
- Decreased confidence or self-worth
- Ruminating about illness process or deceased
- Awareness of presence of deceased
- Continual questioning
- Panic

Physical symptoms

- Hollowness or emptiness in the stomach
- Nausea
- Tightness in chest
- Sense heart is breaking
- Irregular heart beat
- Breathlessness
- Lump in throat
- Decreased libido
- Dry mouth
- Muscle weakness
- Fatigue
- Listlessness/restlessness
- Digestive problems
- Abdominal pain
- Constipation or diarrhoea
- Headaches
- Rashes
- Aches and pains
- Sleep disturbances, including early morning wakening

Behaviours

- Social withdrawal
- Avoidance of reminders of deceased
- Searching for deceased
- Calling out for deceased
- Sighing
- Over-activity
- Inertia
- Sleeping or other numbing activities, including the abuse of alcohol or drugs
- Seeking out objects, places or activities associated with the diseased

Spiritual

- Searching for meaning
- Anger at God
- Questioning of God
- Re-evaluation of faith
- Increased participation in or withdrawal from church
- Contemplation
- Meditation
- Feeling of being distant from God
- Desperate prayers

Note: These responses have been arbitrarily separated into categories. Some responses may be mutual to more than one category.

Societal taboos regarding loss and death may prevent a grieving person from realising that he is experiencing something that is perfectly normal. Consequently the bereaved may feel isolated and unable to talk about his experience and carries the added fear that he is not coping, is failing or even going 'mad'.

People have been known to question whether or not they are really grieving if some emotions or reactions are absent. This particularly applies to the feelings of shock and anger. It must be stressed that the absence of shock or anger does not exclude or minimise grief and the bereavement process. Shock may be absent, for example, if death is expected, whether by illness or by advanced age. Patients may still be grieving even without a shock response.

Duration of grief

This is probably both the question most often asked and the hardest one to answer. It is not possible to clearly demarcate a point where the grieving process ends. Often grief does not fully resolve or permanently disappear. Many argue that grief never ends, it just gets easier over time. The length of time is indeterminable, especially given the complexity of grief and the individuality of the persons involved. Grief is a process that can fluctuate over time and will depend upon a unique constellation of factors that will determine the length and mode of the mourning responses. The bereaved may have various grief related feelings, symptoms and behaviour throughout life. Memories may last a lifetime. A bereaved person may experience elements of acute grief every time he hears his spouse's name or sees her photograph. The process of 'letting go' of the relationship may take a long time.

Theorists do agree that there are certain times when grief is particularly hard and the bereaved person appears to have regressed. Approximately 3 months after the death is when the reality—that the deceased person is not going to come back—manifests. This may coincide with family and friends returning to their own routines, thereby reducing the amount of support that the bereaved person receives. Birthdays, holiday celebrations, anniversaries and family occasions are times that commonly cause increased reactions, regardless of the length of time since the death occurred. Anxiety around such upcoming events can be the catalyst for increased grief and the reason why the bereaved person is coming to seek help.

Giving patients exact timelines on the duration of grief may be problematic. When the bereaved person finds himself falling short of the suggested time limit, grief may be aggravated.

The duration may be affected by the same factors that affect the grief response. These include individual traits and cultural and societal influences. In 'Anglo-Saxon' cultures the bereaved may be expected to return to work in a few weeks and to establish equilibrium within a few months. This may cause distress. It has been observed that one predictor of the duration and severity of grief may be the intensity of the initial distress. The length of grief can be shaped by the suddenness of the death. If death occurs without warning, shock and disbelief may last for a long time, while in anticipated death, the mourning process is likely to have already begun by the time death occurs.

The bereavement process, models and tasks

A plethora of models from a variety of theoretical and philosophical frameworks have been developed to understand the bereavement and grief process and to assist the bereaved in 'working through' their grief and adjusting to the loss of a loved one. Theorists—including Freud, Linderman, Parkes, Bowlby, Worden, Kubler-Ross, Marris and Schneider—have described the process in terms of phases, stages, tasks or themes. There are some common threads among these models. Parkes, for example, describes a model that includes the following phases:

1. disbelief, alarm and unreality;
2. searching, anger, guilt, pining and yearning;
3. isolation and withdrawal;
4. loneliness;
5. mitigation; and
6. socialisation, new identity and reinvestment.

Bowlby's framework consists of a first phase of numbing, followed by yearning and searching, disorganisation and despair and, finally, reorganisation. A detailed description of these theories is beyond the scope of this chapter and readers are referred to materials listed in the bibliography for more details.

Pragmatically, one may construct a model that draws upon the main common threads of the theorists. Such a model may consist of three main phases. Shock and disbelief characterise the first phase. Feelings of numbness and blunting predominate and denial may sometimes occur. The funeral, gathering friends and other rites may help survivors to accept the loss and facilitate passage through this stage. If the death is unexpected this phase may be magnified or prolonged. The next phase is ushered in when the death is acknowledged, both intellectually and emotionally. In this second phase a range of grief responses are experienced. These include a range of feelings, physical symptoms, behaviours, thoughts and spiritual responses (see Box 11.1). Thoughts of the deceased may preoccupy the survivor. Occasionally, some survivors may adopt some traits of the deceased. These may be related to the final illness, such as pain or a particular admired mannerism. Acute episodes of discomfort, sometimes referred to as 'pangs of grief', may be experienced. These can occur in waves and last from several minutes to a few hours. Disorganisation and despair can be experienced in the latter parts of this phase. As time passes, the intensity and the frequency of the pangs of grief diminish, and social withdrawal and introversion may occur. The grieving process can become arrested at this point, resulting in constant rumination and pervasive questioning.

The final phase is one of relative adjustment. The bereaved recognises the extent of the loss and that grieving has been accomplished, and begins to re-establish new relationships. Attention shifts to life without the deceased. It is often suggested that the hallmark of the adjustment is that survivors recognise that they can return to work, resume their previous roles, make new friendships, develop new interests, experience pleasure and seek companionship and love. However, this can be challenged and some authors suggest that there are no specific hallmarks to characterise this phase. The saying 'you really don't get over it, you get used to it' encapsulates it best. Memories of the deceased can be recalled without significant sadness and new relationships can be formed without guilt. Sometimes the normal grieving process may lead to emotional and psychological growth.

Most grief models suggest that there are a number of tasks which the bereaved have to complete in order to achieve relative resolution. A compilation of these tasks is presented in Box 11.2. In essence, the main task in the initial shock phase is to accept the reality of the loss. In the intermediate phase, the main task is to experience the pain of grief and to adjust to an environment from which the deceased is absent. The main task in the resolution phase is to emotionally relocate the deceased to an important, but not central, place in

Box 11.2 Tasks of bereavement

- Regulate the emotions to enable safety in experiencing and limiting the emotional and physical pain of loss.
- Accept the reality of the loss.
- Accept and experience the many emotions of grief.
- Experience the pain of separation.
- Develop or maintain hope that the pain of loss can be endured.
- Maintain a sense of personal worth.
- Accommodate lowered energy levels associated with the acute phase of grief.
- Find and utilise some means of support.
- Adjust to changed roles, responsibilities and an environment without the deceased.
- Develop new skills needed for altered lifestyle.
- Keep existing relationships intact to ensure family and social continuity.
- Identify and resolve secondary losses and unfinished business.
- Develop perspectives that will provide insights into both the positive and negative aspects of the loss.
- Emancipate energy from the past.
- Reinvest energy into the present and future.
- Transform the pain of loss into a fuller sense of being.

the bereaved person's life. In other words, the person needs to 'move on'.

It is important to note that while some of the tasks may have been attempted and even have been completed within the first year of bereavement, others may take many years to be completed. Some may never be achieved. If the physician uses this list of criteria alone and inflexibly as a guideline, incompletion of these tasks may be erroneously viewed as an indicator of abnormal or complicated grief.

Although these models may be helpful as frameworks, there is a real danger in rigidly applying any single theory or model to bereaved individuals to try and explain what might be happening to them. These models are general guidelines that describe an overlapping and fluid process that varies from person to person. The responses, phases and processes ebb and flow over time and do not always occur in ordered sequential patterns. They appear to overlap and even recur.

The effectiveness of a healthcare professional's care depends on these theories and models being applied in combination with an awareness of the individual's particular needs, experiences or realities and an environment that provides the bereaved with presence, acceptance, hope, empathy, assurance, accurate information and a skilled assessment.

Factors that influence the bereavement process

A person's bereavement process is influenced by many factors. Gender, age, society, support structures, culture and religion are important influences. Each impacts on what the person sees as normal or acceptable grief and mourning practices. However, it is important not to make assumptions about how someone may grieve, or expect total agreement within individuals or families on what they consider to be helpful or necessary in their healing. The elderly may cling to more traditional ways of grieving, whereas younger people may consider these outdated and unimportant. The main factors are listed in Box 11.3.

Box 11.3 Factors affecting the bereavement process

- Cultural influences
- Religious influences
- Societal influences
- The unique nature and meaning of the loss
- The significance and individual qualities of the lost relationship
- The roles that the deceased occupied in the family/social system of the bereaved
- Coping behaviours
- Personality and level of maturity and intelligence
- Mental health
- Past experience with death
- Sex role conditioning
- Age of the bereaved
- Characteristics of the deceased
- Amount of unfinished business
- Perception of the deceased's fulfilment in life
- Circumstances surrounding the death
- Timeliness of the death
- Perception of preventability
- Sudden versus unexpected death
- Length of illness prior to the death
- Duration and level of anticipatory grief and involvement with the deceased
- Number, type and quality of secondary losses
- Presence of concurrent stresses or crises
- Available support systems and their perception as valuable
- Funerary rituals
- Use of drugs, including sedatives, anxiolytics, over-the-counter formulations and alcohol
- Physical health, including exercise

Gender differences

Gender differences in the expression of grief have been noted by several theorists. They suggest that women are usually more emotionally expressive and interactive (i.e. talk about it), whereas men tend to be more action oriented in dealing with their grief. Lieberman (1990) looked at bereavement patterns of 600 widows and 100 widowers over a 6 year period. Although he found some marked differences—specifically in how each gender used support, sought remarriage and thought about their vulnerability and mortality—both experienced the same intensity of devastating loneliness.

Men predominantly may try to remain 'the strong one', not openly expressing their feelings, appearing less likely to cry, talk or think about their grief. Generally they appear to be more reluctant to seek the support or help of others. Such males may prefer to discuss other health related problems of a more physical nature. Males may also assume the full responsibility of the bereaved state and depend totally upon themselves. In particular, widowers describe grief as being 'lost with no compass or direction'. Observations suggest that men tend to cope more frequently in the following ways than widows:

- remain silent;
- engage in solitary mourning;
- take physical or legal action;
- become immersed in activity or work; and
- exhibit addictive and aggressive behaviour.

Elderly widowers are considered by many grief theorists to be a higher risk for suicide than widows.

In contrast women appear to be more communicative and exhibit a wider range of emotions. They tend to seek and accept help more often and feel more comfortable in a support group. However, these are generalities only. It can be argued that in societies where women have adopted the more masculine work model, they are often forced to take a more masculine approach to their grief. Therefore, when assessing a person's grief, one needs to be cautious of stereotyping grief by gender. Patients may be expressing their grief through a unique blend of the two.

Grief and bereavement in the elderly

The grief of the elderly is sometimes erroneously described as less intense and prolonged and less likely to be associated with increased drinking, health concerns, depression or anxiety. Seniors may face more losses than individuals at other phases of the life cycle. Intense loneliness may occur. Bereavement reactions may, therefore, be profound for highly impaired seniors who lose a spouse they depended upon for daily functions or who was their sole source of companionship.

The needs of confused elderly people in dealing with bereavement have often been ignored. Repeated explanations and involvement in important events, such as the funeral and visiting the grave, have been shown to reduce the confused elderly person's repetitious questions about the whereabouts of the dead person.

Abnormal or complicated grief

In the absence of objective criteria to determine when a normal bereavement and grief process becomes abnormal or complicated, it is not easy to adequately define abnormal or complicated grief as an outcome. A variety of different terms used to describe a grief process that doesn't follow a normal path includes abnormal, atypical, absent, chronic, converted, delayed, distorted, morbid, pathological and unresolved grief. Each term has particular characteristics, although some have overlapping meanings. Wolfelt (1991) prefers to use the more hopeful term 'complicated grief', as it implies that skilled interventions could 'uncomplicate' it.

Grieving may be judged to be abnormal when it is more severe and long-lasting than one might expect, or when there seems to be avoidance or denial in acknowledging the loss and the resultant reactions. The bereaved person may be unable to return to their pre-loss level of functioning. In complicated grief, customary coping strategies are absent, distorted or ineffective. Complicated grief can take several forms, ranging from absent or delayed grief to excessively intense and prolonged grief. Grief responses in complicated grief may not resolve with time. Depressive symptoms may predominate. It may involve extreme anger or guilt. The latter may be characterised by continuing guilty ruminations and self-blame. Anger is likely if the bereaved was very dependent on the deceased or if there is a sense of desertion. Aspects of normal grieving may become distorted and intensified to reach psychotic proportions. Hearing a fleeting, transient voice of a deceased person may be normal; however, persistent, intrusive auditory hallucinations are not normal. While denial of certain aspects of the death may be normal, denial that includes the belief that a dead person is still alive is not normal. To compound the difficulty in making the diagnosis of complicated grief, duration of grief is not always a reliable indicator.

Establishing what the loss means to the patient is a good place to begin. Knowing the patient's attitudes to death and mourning can provide valuable clues to the appropriateness of their grief behaviour. It is also helpful to have a working knowledge of the factors that can confound or complicate the bereavement process.

Risk factors for a poor outcome of bereavement

A number of risk factors that predispose to unresolved grief have been identified. These are listed in Box 11.4. The assessment of risk factors should be routine in those family members who are closest to the deceased or terminally ill patient. When assessing for the presence of these, clinicians are advised to look for the severity rather than only the number of factors as they relate to the bereaved.

Box 11.4 Risk factors for poor outcome of bereavement

- High initial distress with depressive symptoms
- Sudden and unexpected death
- Death of a young person
- Elderly male widower
- Caring for the deceased for over 6 months
- Inhibited grief
- Lack of perceived and real social support
- Poor response to previous losses
- History of psychiatric illness, especially depression
- Lack of opportunities for new interests
- Stress from other life crises
- Inability to carry out valued religious rituals
- Multiple prior bereavements
- Low self-esteem of bereaved person
- High dependency on the deceased
- If child dies first
- Multiple losses

Differentiating between bereavement and major depressive disorder

The most frequent and potentially significant complication of bereavement is depressive symptoms. However, the relationship between grief and depression is complex. It is complicated by its numerous symptom similarities. These include sadness, restlessness, fatigue, anhedonia and insomnia, among others. The sadness of grief can closely resemble the sadness associated with a major depressive episode. Although depressive symptoms associated with bereavement are common, loss of a loved one may precipitate depressive episodes in vulnerable individuals. Depressive syndromes, even in the context of bereavement, deserve attention and evaluation. They may herald a disabling illness. At least one-third of people who manifest a depressive syndrome within a few months of their loss continue to be depressed a full year later. These people may experience medical morbidity, psychosocial disability and suicidal ideation. In general, the more severe the depressive symptoms and the more the bereaved person has a positive family or personal history of major depressive disorder, the more likely it is that a major depression is evolving.

The diagnosis of major depressive disorder is generally not given unless the symptoms are still present 2 months after the loss. DSM-IV Criteria (*The Diagnostic and Statistical Manual*, Fourth Edition) state that if the depressive symptoms begin within 2 months of the loss of a loved one and cease after 2 months, they are generally considered to be the result of the bereavement, unless they are associated with marked functional impairment and include morbid preoccupation with worthlessness, suicide ideation, psychotic symptoms or psychomotor retardation. It is becoming generally accepted that evidence of a major depression extending beyond 2 months after the loss warrants consideration for treatment, the caveat being that many normal grief and bereavement responses last longer than 2 months. One such example is guilt, which may continue for an inordinate period of time in cases where the survivor feels responsible for the death due to their action or inaction. One must also take into account particular aspects and extenuating circumstances of the loss. Worden

(1982) suggests that loss of self-esteem commonly found in most cases of clinical depression is not evident in people who have lost someone. They do not respect themselves less as a result of the loss or, if they do, it tends to be for a brief period of time.

Assessing and caring for the bereaved

All elderly patients who have experienced the loss of someone close to them should be assessed for symptoms and signs of complicated grief.

The physician needs to tailor any proposed interventions to specific grief reactions. Not everyone responds to a major loss in a similar predictable way. Therefore it is important to try and appreciate the idiosyncratic nature of the loss, including the circumstances surrounding it, and the meaning which the bereaved apply to their loss.

It is best to avoid assumptions regarding a person's belief system, understanding of death or the afterlife and preferable to find out what they consider significant or important. This needs to be done sensitively. When asking these types of questions, what is considered acceptable language or questions in one culture may be taboo in another. Seeking understanding of another's loss builds a bridge of compassion.

Assessment of grief and bereavement requires a multidimensional approach. Areas that need to be assessed in the bereaved person include:

- emotional and cognitive responses of the individual;
- their coping strategies;
- the extent of continuing relationship with the deceased;
- changes in functioning (personal, social and in the workplace if applicable);
- support structures (personal, social, religious, etc.);
- alterations in existing relationships;
- forming relationships; and
- changes in identity.

Box 11.5 lists some key questions that can facilitate the assessment process. These questions may alert caregivers to what may be abnormal in both the person's expression of grief and their means of coping. They may also provide clues regarding what would be most helpful to the bereaved person. During the assessment, clinicians should look for the presence or absence of factors that may predict a poor outcome (see Box 11.5).

Clinicians should allow sufficient time for the initial visit of a bereaved patient to be able to listen

Box 11.5 Some key questions when assessing bereaved persons

Note: The sequence in which these questions are asked needs to be individualised.

- How are you doing?
- Tell me about the circumstances around his/her death. What happened? (If the clinician was not involved in the event.)
- Do you need more information about the event?
- How is your daily life affected?
- What are you feeling?
- Which of these feelings or problems bother you the most?
- What are the things you miss the most about your loved one?
- What are the things you don't miss about your loved one?
- What are your supports?
- What do you feel you need?
- Are you feeling angry?
- Are you sleeping/eating?
- Of all the problems you are experiencing, which is the worst?
- In the past when you have experienced difficult circumstances, what has helped you get through those difficult times?
- Are you taking any over-the-counter medications for any problem you are experiencing?
- Have you started drinking alcohol or have you increased the number of glasses of alcohol you would normally drink?
- Do you have any questions?
- Would it be helpful to have regular follow-up visits with me?

with compassion and understanding and be sensitive to the uniqueness of the individual's experience.

Patients should be assisted in recognising and expressing their emotions and the ways they are coping, or might cope, with them. Their expressions of guilt, anger and sadness should be accepted and validated. In regularly scheduled sessions, grieving people are encouraged to talk about their feelings of loss and about the person who has died. Many bereaved people have difficulty in recognising and expressing angry or ambivalent feelings towards a deceased person, and they must be reassured that these feelings are normal. They may have many questions regarding the exact details of the illness and the nature of the death. Repeated explanations often help in their need to understand and accept what has happened.

The death of a loved one can cause the bereaved to be concerned about their own mortality. They may become focused on physical symptoms and see it as an omen of impending serious health problems. They may also experience catastrophic thinking and worry constantly about further losses or tragedies. It is important to take their symptoms seriously and, following a physical examination, allay their concerns wherever possible. Bereaved persons should be cautioned against effecting major changes (home, job, relationship), particularly within the first year following the death. Elderly widowers are at particular risk for health problems and suicide. Paying particular attention to both the spoken and unspoken may help to identify potential problems before they become serious.

People who are isolated, or perceive themselves to be isolated, have a more difficult time. They need to be reconnected with support networks to reduce the feelings of isolation. For some people a regular appointment with their primary physician can provide a sense of being connected.

Bereaved patients should be provided with information regarding grief and available resources, including local services and resources, such as support groups. They should be encouraged to take good physical care of themselves, including having sufficient food and sleep.

During follow-up visits, clinicians must continue to provide ongoing acceptance and a safe place in which the bereaved can express his emotions and to tell and retell the story of the death. The small positive changes and successes of daily living should be recognised. Clinicians should encourage and demonstrate understanding and acceptance for the expression of feelings of relief, joy and energy surges that may occur shortly after the death occurs.

Most bereaved persons recover from their loss without requiring specialised services. In the majority of cases, the support of family and friends, and time, are all that are required for successful bereavement. Professionals from a variety of disciplines—including the clergy, nurses, social workers and physicians—provide the support, reassurance and information they require. Supportive care by listening and validating the experience is often all that is required.

Sometimes a combination of formal psychotherapy and pharmacological interventions are required to facilitate the grieving process, particularly in patients at risk for complicated grief and those with intractable or prolonged symptoms. When grief is complicated by a major depressive episode, psychotherapeutic techniques and medications may be required. Antidepressant treatment may ameliorate depression without impeding the grieving process. Effective treatment facilitates adaptive processes and prevents the distortion–coping interference brought on by depression. Treating anxiety or sleeplessness pharmacologically is controversial. A mild sedative to induce sleep may be useful in some situations, but antidepressant medication or anti-anxiety agents are rarely indicated in normal grief and may cause significant adverse effects, particularly in the elderly.

Some individuals may need to be referred to more specialised treatment settings. Specialised counselling should be targeted at those with severe complicated grief and bereavement reactions. Severe or intractable prolonged depressive symptoms, concrete suicidal ideation, drug or alcohol abuse or exacerbation of other medical and psychiatric problems may be some of the reasons for referral.

As a final note, it is important to recognise that to conduct grief therapy, clinicians must be comfortable in dealing with issues of death and dying, and must be able to handle patients' intense emotional reactions of sadness, anger and guilt.

Conclusion

The provision of appropriate bereavement related care and support is an ongoing task in the care of the elderly. When assessing a patient's grief one needs to remember that the elderly are particularly vulnerable to simultaneous multiple losses that include not only the death of spouses, relatives and friends, but also retirement, changed income, health issues, increased dependency and changing roles.

Bibliography and further reading

Katz, L. & Chochinov, H. M. (1998), 'The spectrum of grief in palliative care', in Bruera, E. & Portenoy, R. K. (eds), *Topics in Palliative Care*, Vol. 2, Oxford University Press, New York, pp. 295–310.

Lieberman, M. (1996), *Doors Close, Doors Open: Widows Grieving and Growing*, G. P. Putman's Sons, New York.

O'Toole, D. (1995), *Bridging the Bereavement Gap. Manual for the Preparation and Programming of Hospice Bereavement Services*, Lapeer Hospice, Michigan, USA.

Rando, T. A. (1984), *Grief, Dying and Death: Clinical Interventions for Caregivers*, Research Press Company, Illinois.

Rando, T. A. (1993), *Treatment of Complicated Mourning*, Research Press Company, Illinois.

Raphael, B. (1982), *The Anatomy of Bereavement*, Basic Books, Inc., New York.

Staudacher, C. (1994), *Men and Grief*, New Harbinger Publications Inc., Oakland, CA.

Wolfelt, A. D. (1991), 'Towards an understanding of complicated grief: A comprehensive overview', *American Journal of Hospice and Palliative Care*, 2, pp. 28–30.

Worden, J. W. (1982), *Grief Counselling and Grief Therapy*, Tavistock Publications, London.

Chapter 12

The violent patient

ROHAN S. DHILLON and WILLIAM M. H. GOH

Introduction

Violent behaviour per se is not necessarily a medical or psychiatric problem, although there is evidence that psychiatric patients are more likely to commit violent and other criminal acts. The elderly are more likely to be the victims of violent behaviour rather than the perpetrators. Consequently, there has been little investigation of this population as perpetrators of violence.

While not as common or personally threatening as in younger populations, violent or aggressive behaviour in the elderly can have devastating consequences for the individuals themselves, their families, their caregivers and for society in general.

Most medical practitioners might believe they have adequate knowledge about violence and aggression among elderly patients in various settings. However, understanding and controlling violent behaviour in the elderly can be quite a complex and challenging exercise for the general practitioner. If one can understand the complex social and neurobiological causes of violent behaviour in the elderly, including the various aetiologies, it sets the stage for appropriate clinical treatment to be initiated wherever possible.

The concept of violence

The concept of violence might be familiar to most medical practitioners but a clear definition is usually lacking. It is this factor that complicates most of the research findings in the area of violence in general. Numerous attempts have been made in the literature to define and measure aggression, anger, hostility, irritability, agitation and violence. The first step is to define common clinical terms like violence, aggression and agitation.

Violence can be defined as exertion of any physical force so as to injure or abuse another person or thing. Aggression refers to a hostile action or threat directed towards others that may be verbal, physical, vocal or sexual. Agitation manifests as excessive motor activity associated with a feeling of inner tension that is usually unproductive and repetitive (e.g. pacing, fidgeting and wringing hands).

Agitation and violence in the form of aggression are frequent behaviour manifestations of psychiatric and related medical conditions in the elderly. Agitation and aggressive impulses are usually precursors to the act of violence. Actual infliction of physical harm is commonly regarded as separating violence from these entities. Aggression can be viewed as a dimensional construct, which cuts across categorical constructs. It manifests phenomenologically in a variety of ways (see Table 12.1).

In the geriatric population, the infliction of harm may be forestalled because of the feebleness of the perpetrator. This feebleness may be counterbalanced by the fact that victims such as spouses, carers or fellow nursing home residents are often elderly and are themselves too feeble to defend themselves.

Table 12.1 Aggression: variable phenomenology

Type of violence	Presentation
Verbal	Loud noises, shouting, cursing, vague or specific threats
Physical (objects)	Slamming doors, throwing clothes/food/objects, breaking objects/furniture/windows, defacing/marking, setting fires
Physical (self)	Picking/scratching, hitting/pinching, pulling hair, head banging, hitting/punching objects/walls, cutting, burning, throwing self onto the floor/into objects
Physical (others)	Threatening gestures, hitting, kicking, biting, spitting and using weapons against

Source: Adapted from J. M. Silver & S. C. Yudofsky (1991), 'The Overt Aggression Scale: Overview and guiding principles', *Journal of Neuropsychiatry and Clinical Neurosciences*, 3, pp. S22–9.

Epidemiology

Past research on violence has neglected the study of the geriatric population. This is especially important because it is well documented that the number of older patients will increase quite substantially in the next few decades. This will likely translate into greater episodes of violence among the elderly population.

Aggression and violent incidents are among the most common causes of referral to psychogeriatric services. They are the most frequent causes for admission to a nursing home or hospital. This has considerable implications for general practitioners who are involved in the care of elderly patients in the community.

Violence in the general population shows a strong association with young adults, especially males, thus suggesting that older age exerts an effect in reducing the potential for violence. The fate of the violent young in middle to late adult life has not been well studied.

Among the young, violent and aggressive behaviour occurs significantly more frequently in individuals with serious mental illness such as schizophrenia and major affective disorders with or without substance misuse problems. Unlike in the young, neuropsychiatric conditions associated with cognitive impairment are the major causes of violent behaviour in the elderly. Among geriatric patients, aggressive behaviour has usually been found to increase with age and with the severity of dementia in both hospitalised and community populations.

The association of violence with male gender persists in the elderly. The patient's spouse is the frequent victim in these cases. Elderly patients who live with families are more likely to be violent than those who live alone. Under-reporting of violence may result from failure to apprehend the very elderly who are obviously infirm and demented.

The dramatic changes in patterns of institutionalisation in the past few decades have meant that a significant number of elderly psychiatric patients reside in rest homes, adult homes and nursing homes. The patient mix of those above 65 years of age in these residential settings has a high potential for violence. Most of these patients have significant physical morbidity as well.

Causes of violence

The causes of violence in the elderly reflect complex biological and sociological processes. Even though most can be related to specific neuropsychiatric disorders, a significant proportion do not meet syndrome criteria for any specific medical or psychiatric disorders. Such cases can still prove to be very difficult to treat. Non-aetiological classification of violence can sometimes be a useful first step in identifying the specific causes of violence in particular patients.

Classification

The nosology of violence in the elderly can be divided into three aspects, namely:

1. medically related (i.e. symptom of an identifiable disease process)
2. impulsive (i.e. explosive and irrational)
3. premeditated (i.e. cold blooded and rational).

Violence can also be classified in the following way:

1. offensive (e.g. intrudes into another person's space)
2. defensive (e.g. response to challenge or perceived challenge)
3. dominant (e.g. non-violent but threatening behaviour).

Rather than focusing immediately on a diagnosis, understanding the nosology of the violence gives the clinician some clues about the context and underlying motivation behind a patient's actions. Impulsive, unprovoked acts of violence in the elderly that are non-goal directed usually result from cognitive impairment as seen in delirium, dementia or other cerebral pathology. Premeditated, offensive violent behaviour that is goal directed is more suggestive of mental illnesses, such as psychotic disorders or personality difficulties, where there is some intactness of cognitive functioning. In the case of psychotic disorders, the elderly person might be responding to persecutory delusions and/or command auditory hallucinations.

Table 12.2 Clinical risk factors for violence in the elderly

Aetiological factor	Clinical presentation
Psychological	Anxiety or fears for personal safety (attack as a means of defence) Anger or arguments Feelings of being overwhelmed or inability to cope Learnt behaviour History of physical/emotional abuse Catastrophic reactions
Organic	Intoxication with alcohol or illicit drugs Side effects of medication (sedation, disorientation, akathisia, and disinhibition) Inadequate control of symptoms (e.g. pain, constipation) Delirium/dementia (cognitive difficulties)
Psychotic	Delusions of persecution Command hallucinations to harm others Depressive or nihilistic delusions and intense suicidal ideation

Risk factors

The risk factors associated with violence in the elderly are tabulated in Table 12.2. None of these factors is definitive; they are the subject of continuing research. The presence of multiple factors in an elderly person can be considered a warning that violence is an imminent outcome.

Psychiatric causes

It is important to note that not all aggressive elderly persons are psychiatrically ill. However, a large proportion of aggressive elderly patients will require a thorough medical and psychiatric evaluation and possibly referral to an emergency department. Physical morbidity is a greater cause of aggression in the elderly than is the case in the young.

There are four major psychiatric syndromes that may provoke aggression in the elderly. These are:

1. delirium and other organic brain syndromes, like dementia
2. psychotic disorders
3. alcohol and substance intoxication or withdrawal
4. personality and related anxiety disorders.

Each of the above categories may have a number of different causes or appear in any combination as the cause of violent behaviour. There are some basic questions, which a clinician needs to answer to help in the assessment of a potentially aggressive or violent patient:

1. What is the context of the aggressive behaviour?
Decide if it is unprovoked (aggressive) or provoked (defensive).

2. What is the diagnosis of the patient?
Determine if the patient suffers from depression, brain injury, delirium or dementia.

3. Are concurrent medications exacerbating the aggression?
Find out if the patient is using benzodiazepines, stimulants or decongestants.

In the elderly, a medical history is important not only because of the possible direct effect of a medical condition in causing violence, but because of the effect of concurrent medical conditions on proposed treatment. Medication being prescribed for medical conditions, especially if it has anticholinergic properties, can sometimes precipitate a delirium.

Disorders in the elderly associated with violence

Psychiatric disorders in the elderly associated with violence are listed in Table 12.3.

Assessment

Dealing with physical aggression in the elderly should begin with an analysis of the circumstances in which it occurs. It is simplistic to believe that there is no pattern to the violence and that the elderly perpetrator could be violent at any time. Such statements, which appear to blame the victim or find fault with the caregivers, should be avoided.

Comprehensive assessment of the violent elderly patient is affected by the urgency of the situation. Some of the important things to consider first are the resources available, the vulnerability of potential victims and the placement of the patient within the spectrum of care. The prevention of violent incidents has two main components—preparation and prediction.

Preparation

Preparation requires a clinician to be constantly aware of potential risks and hazards to personal safety and the safety of others like carers, family

Table 12.3 Psychiatric disorders in the elderly associated with violence

Classification	Clinical disorder
Organic brain disorders	Delirium Dementia (Alzheimer's disease, vascular, others) Organic mood disorder Organic personality disorder
Neurodegenerative disorders	Huntington's disease Parkinson's disease Multiple sclerosis
Other CNS disorders	Traumatic brain injury Brain tumour CNS infections Cerebrovascular accidents
Mood disorders	Mania Depression Mixed affective states Substance facilitated (e.g. alcohol)
Personality disorders	Antisocial/borderline/narcissistic Chronic impulse control problems
Psychotic disorders	Schizophrenia Paranoid states
Other psychiatric disorders	Anxiety disorders Substance abuse/dependence/withdrawal

members, other nursing home patients and health care providers like nurses or nurses aides. Environmental settings where elderly patients reside should be open to a degree, pleasant and relaxing. Dead ends, blind spots and potential weapons should be avoided if possible when designing residential or nursing homes for the elderly. Overcrowding of such homes can sometimes be a factor in violent behaviours because of the case mix. All staff and carers should receive training in personal safety and emergency procedures.

General practitioners visiting such facilities, or doing house visits, should have some training in these procedures. Dealing with emergencies in the community can be difficult. Just as for medical emergencies, the ability of the lone general practitioner to manage a situation may be limited. The priority is to be able to raise the alarm and obtain assistance without delay. A general practitioner without knowledge or training in mental health emergencies and facing an unfamiliar clinical situation could be a recipe for disaster.

Prediction

Prediction requires awareness of the risks posed by a specific patient or situation. A short-term predictor of violent behaviour depends on recognising the early warning signs in elderly patients. Any threats of violence should be taken seriously in the first place. Worsening of symptoms, especially delusions or hallucinations that focus on individuals, can sometimes be predictive. Other warning signs will vary from patient to patient and may not be reliable. These include changes or extremes of behaviour (shouting or whispering), outward signs of inner tension (pacing, slamming doors, sweating, clenched fists) and repetition of previous behaviour patterns associated with violence (see Box 12.1).

Long-term prediction of violent behaviour is generally poorly understood. The best long-term predictor of a person's propensity for violence is a past history of violent behaviour. A general practitioner working with the elderly should in all cases make attempts to understand her patient's past history and problems. The knowledge of a patient's pattern of behaviour and what triggers violence is of greatest importance in preventing future episodes of violence.

Box 12.1 Predicting violence in the elderly

- Verbalised threats of violence
- Worsening of symptoms, especially delusions or hallucinations
- Signs of increasing tension, such as pacing and clenching of fists
- Alcohol or substance intoxication
- Carrying of weapons
- Past history of violence
- Agitation, wandering and isolation

Behaviour that may indicate the potential for aggression in the elderly includes wandering, agitation and isolation.

Wandering is common in dementia and can take several forms. Aimless wandering by the patient is often the result of boredom. In sundowning wandering, the patient becomes increasingly confused and disoriented late in the afternoon. When darkness and lack of visual cues induce spatial disorientation, the elderly person may experience an increase in the level of anxiety and confusion. Nocturnal wandering is due to poor sensory functioning, associated with dim lighting and misinterpretation of shadows and sounds.

Agitation is characterised by pacing, wringing of hands, fiddling, responding to real or imagined threats. The restless elderly person tends to be unable to concentrate on a particular task or participates in an activity that may result in the patient becoming frustrated, anxious or angry. Agitation occasionally manifests as the so-called catastrophic reaction, which is an intense and explosive emotional response to stress or to the possibility of task failure. This reaction may occur whenever the patient is placed in an unfamiliar environment, or when bathed, dressed or toileted.

Elderly patients who isolate themselves may respond aggressively when approached to engage in an activity or require a nursing intervention such as toileting and feeding. Since many different underlying causes lead to the final common pathway of aggression, the various aetiologies will need to be explored in a systematic fashion.

When in a difficult situation that is escalating, call for help, as there is no place for heroics. Pointers to impending aggression or violence include signs of increasing anxiety and tension (e.g. clenching and unclenching fists, tensing of torso and biceps, excessive working of masseters and tightness of the mouth), worsening verbal abuse and increasing physical activity.

Mental state examination

Mental state examination should commence on contact with the patient. Make note of the patient's general appearance, grooming, motor activity and behaviour. Evaluate the sensorium of the patient, assessing whether a delirium is present. If possible, clinically assess the intelligence of the patient, thus formulating the type of level at which interactions may proceed. It is important to note the mood and emotional state of the patient and whether reality testing is intact. Assessment of the patient's insight and judgment as well as your rapport with them will help in planning the next level of intervention.

Special note should be taken of the features of drug and alcohol intoxication or withdrawal. Evaluation of cognitive function is an important part of the assessment of the elderly violent patient. Rating scales such as the Mini-Mental Status Examination (MMSE) might provide clues to the person's cognitive status if the situation allows for such an intervention.

Physical examination

A physical examination is essential, especially if medical causes for the violent behaviour are suspected. This should only be attempted if the patient has settled through the above measures or after she has been sedated with medication. Several authorities recommend batteries of blood tests for possible causes of dementia and delirium. The utility of these tests in the acute setting has not been fully established in the elderly.

Other investigations, such as computerised tomography or magnetic resonance imaging of the head, could provide information about the medical causes of violence as well as influence treatment decisions.

Achieving co-operation from the violent patient for such examinations may be difficult. If sedation is necessary for the examination, the risks versus the benefits have to be weighed up by the clinician. Usually in this situation, the general practitioner needs to refer a patient to a general hospital for more intensive review.

Management

A primary consideration in dealing with emergencies like violence is the safety of all concerned. Actions taken in good faith to avert a serious consequence are sanctioned by common law and do not require recourse to the *Mental Health Act*. Compulsory admission to hospital for continued treatment might need to be considered at a later time.

The principles of dealing with violence have mostly been derived from clinical experience and have not been statistically validated. Familiarity with local resources and with methods for gaining access to resources is as important as clinical skill in the treatment of the violent elderly.

The setting and placement where violence occurs might require some assessment by the clinician. Within institutions like nursing or residential homes and hospitals, the case mix must be looked at from time to time for its violence potential. If possible, the able-bodied demented should be separated from the vulnerable feeble. If there is an option, potentially violent individuals should be given a single room. Empty space is often the most effective straitjacket for preventing violence.

The first step in the assessment process is to obtain an unobstructed access to the elderly patient who is acting aggressively or has been violent. Ensure the surrounding environment is safe by removing any objects that could be used as weapons.

If the patient is in a residential home or nursing home setting, ask onlookers to leave, as large numbers of people can create a frightening and stimulating environment for the aggressor and themselves be potential victims of further violence. It is very important for the general practitioner to have help at hand as well as an escape route when dealing with a potentially volatile elderly patient.

Threats of violence can often be successfully managed by intervention at the verbal level where rapport and psychodynamic issues are important considerations. Occasionally physical restraints or seclusion are necessary. Chemical restraints are often useful. Finally, aftercare issues also need attention.

Verbal intervention

In the initial instance when in the presence of a threatening individual, it is important not to rush but to allow the patient to calm down. In other words, think quickly but act slowly. Do not take any abuse from the patient personally. Maintain a non-aggressive stance and avoid counterthreats. Treat the elderly patient in a humane and respectful manner. Talking in a calm and authoritative manner might be enough to defuse a potentially volatile situation. Listen carefully to what the patient has to say and set limits in a non-aggressive manner. Most patients can be 'talked down' with time. Engaging them in conversation allows them to ventilate their anger and frustration therapeutically.

Without promising anything concrete, try to reassure the patient that you are taking each request or demand seriously. Do not refuse any request or demand outright. If appropriate to the situation (e.g. if a weapon is brandished, or if the patient is restlessly pacing or verbally abusive), admit to the patient your anxiety, fear and difficulties, concentrating on those circumstances. The patient's identification of similar feelings within themselves might defuse a potentially dangerous situation.

Physical restraint

From a medicolegal point of view, physical intervention in an emergency setting is acceptable in order to prevent harm to either the patient or others, to prevent damage to property, or for the administration of necessary treatment. It is best to leave physical restraints to those who are trained to handle them. However, there are times when this help is not available and the medical practitioner has to take decisive actions.

If the general practitioner is contemplating physical restraint, there should be at least five suitably trained people other than the clinician present. Each person should control a limb, leaving the remaining person to control the head. Sometimes throwing a blanket over a particularly aggressive elderly patient before jumping her can reduce the amount of force that is needed. The general practitioner should only attempt the above in the right setting and when suitably trained people are available. Attempting such an intervention in the elderly is not without its problems because of the frailness of the old. Rapid access to medical services and resuscitation equipment (by ambulance if necessary) should be arranged prior to contemplating physical restraint and rapid tranquillisation with psychotropic medication.

If physical intervention, as described above, is needed, ensure the patient is thoroughly restrained. Injecting a struggling patient risks inadvertent intra-arterial injection causing necrosis, or damage to nerves or other soft tissue injuries. Depending on the seriousness of the sedation required, the choice should be between the intramuscular or intravenous route. The violent patient should be restrained until he shows some signs of sedation. Further doses might be required.

Medication

Medication has an important role to play in the controlling of aggressive or potentially violent behaviours. A meta-analysis of several double blind, placebo controlled trials of various drugs in dementia have shown their effectiveness for symptoms such as agitation, combativeness, hostility and unco-operativeness. No medication has ever been officially approved or indicated for use in the treatment of violence. The use of drugs to control violent behaviour is basically empirical, even if theoretically linked to concepts that the behaviour is a manifestation of conditions like psychosis, epilepsy, mood disorder or disordered serotonin activity.

Frequent complaints of overmedication of disturbed patients in nursing homes are mainly directed at antipsychotics being used as chemical restraints. Medications should only be used for well defined indications.

Normal ageing changes can affect dosage requirements. Ageing changes that can affect the pharmacokinetics of psychotropic drugs involve reductions in serum albumin; reduced drug clearance by the liver and kidney; increased α-acid glycoprotein; and increase in the proportion of body weights due to fat. Most of these changes constitute indications for dosage reduction of psychotropic medication. The best advice is to start low and go slow. This advice would be difficult to follow in emergency situations involving violence. The limitations to using drugs in the elderly are often set by concurrent illness and potential drug interactions. Falls and drowsiness are important considerations.

General principles in the use of psychopharmacological agents for violence in the elderly are as follows:

- Use medication dose relevant to the clinical 'metaphor'.
- Start low and go slow.
- Assess target symptoms.
- Be alert to response and signs of toxicity.
- Increase dose only after reasonable trial at previous dose.
- If effective, continue for weeks to months, taper and re-evaluate.
- If ineffective, taper and re-evaluate; consider a second agent.
- Remember that medication does not always work.

Patients who accept oral tranquillisation should be allowed to calm down in a quiet room. Sedated patients should be placed in a recovery position and their heart rate, respiration and blood pressure closely monitored. The aftercare of such patients (i.e. whether they remain or are transported to hospital) is dependent on the seriousness of the incident and the underlying cause of the violent or aggressive episode.

In some situations, the clinician might need to do a screening physical examination to rule out life-threatening causes of aggression (cerebral events) once the patient is sedated. Primary conditions or underlying illnesses should be treated once the acute situation is under control.

Antipsychotics

The traditional antipsychotics, such as haloperidol, have been widely studied and shown to be helpful in the management of aggression associated with psychosis of any aetiology. Haloperidol is especially useful in the acute setting of violence when given intramuscularly. Low doses are mainly used in the elderly who are particularly sensitive to side effects such as akathisia and parkinsonism. Other traditional antipsychotics, such as chlorpromazine and thioridazine, are quite sedative but cause anticholinergic side effects and prolongation of the QT interval, which actually exacerbate confusion or cause hypertension. They have a greater tendency to reduce seizure threshold than haloperidol.

Beyond the actual episode, atypical antipsychotics are slowly gaining appeal (risperidone, olanzapine and clozapine). However, they have not been studied in a controlled fashion. Empirical evidence suggests their usefulness in aggression and they are better tolerated in the elderly because of a more attractive side effect profile. Risperidone has been used at doses of 0.5–2 mg in the elderly. Olanzapine is particularly sedating in the elderly at doses of 2.5–10 mg. Clozapine is quite sedating but limited to treatment of refractory-schizophrenic states, mainly because of the risk of agranulocytosis.

Benzodiazepines

These drugs are particularly useful in aggression associated with disordered anxiety states, for acute sedation and aggression related to extrapyramidal side effects. They are also useful in alcohol withdrawal (delirium tremens). Their choice is related to their shorter half-life and simpler metabolism. Lorazepam and oxazepam are commonly used in the elderly.

Because of their anticonvulsant properties, the benzodiazepines are protective against the epileptogenic potential of antipsychotics. Antipsychotics protect against benzodiazepine provoked disinhibition. Depending on the urgency of the situation, the intramuscular route is a safer option in the elderly than the intravenous route. Precaution should be taken to avoid injuries due to confusion, falls or inco-ordination. For this reason, a combined dose enough to induce sedation is recommended.

α-adrenergic blockers

Choices here involve propranolol, metoprolol and pindolol. They are useful in organic brain diseases but can take up to 2 months to have a full effect. The dose needs to be gradually increased, although dose–response relationships have not been symptomatically studied. Therefore there is a variable effective dose in the elderly. Selective β1-adrenergic blockers like metoprolol cause more cardiovascular side effects than pindolol, which is a non-selective β-adrenergic blocker. Approximate doses in the elderly are propranolol 10 mg bid and pindolol 10 mg/day. Side effects can be lethargy, depression, confusion, respiratory suppression, hypotension and bradycardia.

Buspirone

Buspirone (5-HT1A agonist) is an anxiolytic with antidepressant properties that has a primary usefulness in the elderly for treating aggression associated with anxiety and depression, which is intermixed. There is limited controlled data available. The usual starting dose is 5–10 mg. In the elderly, the dose is gradually titrated up to a maintenance dose of 30 mg a day or until a therapeutic effect is achieved.

Antidepressants

The use of antidepressants is based on the theoretical model of serotonergic dysregulation in impulsive aggression. Only open trials of their use in aggressive patients have demonstrated their usefulness. Their main purpose is to treat mood related aggression and irritability, with a role in impulsive aggression. Trazadone has the most data available, and should be started at 25–50 mg/day in the elderly. Side effects are usually sedation and hypertension. Data on other selective serotonin reuptake inhibitors (SSRIs) are limited. SSRIs that have been tried include fluoxetine and citalopram.

Mood stabilisers

Mood stabilisers are not prototypic anti-aggressive drugs. They are used for impulse control and assaultative tendencies in clinical practice.

Lithium carbonate has been shown in open trials to have anti-aggressive properties associated with mood disturbance. Use low doses in the elderly because of lithium's neurocognitive side effects. Aim for blood levels around 0.5 to 0.8 mmol/L in the elderly.

Anticonvulsants have not been studied in double blind, placebo controlled conditions. Most data is available on carbamazepine and, to a lesser extent, on sodium valproate. These drugs may lower aggression in a broad spectrum of disorders such as seizure disorders, mood disorders and brain injured with EEG abnormalities, and are a useful adjunct to antipsychotics.

The mechanism of anti-aggressive actions of anticonvulsant mood stabilisers is unknown. Most reported trials are of their use as adjuvant treatment. It is possible that some of the beneficial effects depend on pharmacologic and pharmacokinetic interactions with concomitant medication like antipsychotics. Anticonvulsants should be used with caution in the elderly because of drug–drug interactions and potential haematological side effects.

Carbamazepine use in manic states and episodic violence associated with complex partial seizures led to its consideration for other forms of violence. Some see its usefulness in demented individuals who are disinhibited, impulsive, potentially aggressive or resistive during care. A similar role has been suggested for sodium valproate even though studies are lacking.

Cholinergic agents

These agents are now being increasingly used in the treatment of aggression/agitation in dementia. Their mechanism of action is possibly through an effect in improving cognitive functioning or slowing its decline. Their potential for anti-aggression has not yet been established and therefore they should only be used with some caution. Tacrine (tetrahydroaminoacridine) is such an agent.

Rapid tranquillisation

Rapid tranquillisation is the short-term use of drugs to control potentially destructive behaviour. It should only be used when other non-pharmacological methods have failed. It is important first to try to persuade the patient to take the necessary medication orally or intramuscularly.

Controlled trials of drugs for emergency situations involving violence have not been done. Most experts like Yudofsky and colleagues, based on their clinical experience, suggest initial use of haloperidol 1 mg by mouth or 0.5 mg intravenously, repeated every hour until the control of aggression is achieved. If lorazepam is used, they suggest 1–2 mg by mouth or intravenously, repeated every hour until the patient is calm. Combinations of low doses of haloperidol and lorazepam can also be used for emergency sedation.

The following are guidelines to the parental use of psychopharmacological agents in the management of violence in the elderly:

- Use a 'butterfly' cannula in a large vein.
- Administer intravenous drugs slowly.
- Ensure resuscitation equipment is available.
- If antipsychotic drugs are used, have antimuscarinic drugs available in case of acute dystonias.
- If benzodiazepines are used, have flumazenil available in case of respiratory depression (give 200 μg intravenously over 15 seconds if respiration rate falls below 10 breaths/min).
- Use lower doses in older patients not previously exposed to the drug, patients intoxicated with drugs and alcohol, patients with an organic disorder (delirium).
- Avoid intramuscular chlorpromazine (risk of hypotension and crystallisation in tissues).
- Avoid longer-acting antipsychotic drugs (including zuclopenthixol acetate) in patients not previously exposed to them.
- Avoid antipsychotics in patients with heart disease (use benzodiazepines alone).

Doses require titration based on clinical response and the likely aetiology of the aggression. A combination of an antipsychotic (e.g. haloperidol 2.5–5 mg) and a benzodiazepine (e.g. lorazepam 1–2 mg) is a safer option than either agent alone. Lower benzodiazepine doses will decrease the risk of respiratory depression while lower doses of antipsychotics diminish the potential for cardiac irregularities.

Aftercare

Once a violent patient has been brought under control, further hospitalisation will usually be necessary in order to assess and treat the underlying cause of the aggression. Immediate management should include a thorough physical and neurological examination. This will then serve as a guide to further laboratory and other physical investigations. With the exclusion of an acute medical emergency, an understanding of events leading up to and immediately preceding the violent episode may be of assistance in planning further management.

Treating the injuries

Any physical injuries sustained during the incident to the patient, staff or others should be examined and treated.

Recording the incident

The details of the incident should be carefully recorded and reported to the appropriate authority. Staff involved in the incident may require help in recording the incident.

Involving the police

The police should always be informed if a criminal offence has been committed, or a weapon has been used. This is especially so if the evaluation does not uncover psychiatric or medical causes for the violence. The general practitioner should use his discretion when deciding whether or not to involve the police. Clinicians have a duty of care to inform the police (or the intended victim) if they believe a specific person, place or institution is at risk from a particular patient.

Debriefing

Everyone involved in a violent or distressing incident, including the patient and any onlookers, may suffer psychological distress. All staff involved in the incident, including the general practitioner, should assemble a day or two later to discuss the incident, support each other and glean any lessons that may be learnt. Ample time should be allowed for all involved to talk about the incident. The patient might require specific psychological counselling and treatment at a later date.

Pharmacotherapy for the long-term management of violent behaviour is highly dependent on the individual patient's underlying clinical problem. The theoretical rationale for the use of pharmacotherapy in managing aggression and violence should follow psychobehavioural metaphor of aggression.

Conclusion

The violent elderly patient presents numerous clinical challenges for the general practitioner working in the community. Management of the potentially aggressive elderly individual needs to be proactive rather than reactive. Even though violence has not been previously recognised as a major problem in the elderly, increased survival rates of the elderly as well as the present social climate makes this type of patient a more significant problem for all health care providers working in the community.

When violence occurs in the elderly it needs to be understood from a biopsychosocial perspective. Assessment should also include understanding the coping resources and deficits of the violent individual. Sometimes an elderly individual engages in violent actions in response to direct and indirect stimuli from her surrounding environment. The environment, including physical and interpersonal factors like relationship to caregivers, should be part of the assessment process. Others factors to consider include cognitive and sensory impairment, language difficulties, recent changes in health and functional status, loss of independence and support network, cultural factors and somatic complaints like pain and constipation.

Non-pharmacological interventions can prove to be just as important as the use of medication in dealing with violent/aggressive behaviours in the elderly. The use of pharmacotherapy in this population will need to take into account concomitant medical illness and potential drug–drug interactions as well as the physiological changes of ageing which affect drug metabolism.

Safer psychotropic medications, which make a significant difference in the area of safety and efficiency, have come onto the market recently. Further systematic evaluations will need to occur before these drugs can be safely recommended as a treatment of choice for aggressive/violent behaviour in the elderly.

Bibliography and further reading

Birkett, P. (1997), 'Violence in geropsychiatry', *Psychiatric Annals*, 27(11), pp. 752–6.

Craig, T. K. J. & Boordman, A. P. (1998), 'Common mental health problems in primary care', in Davies, T. & Craig, T. K. J. (eds), *ABC of Mental Health*, BMJ Books, London, pp. 5–8.

Davies, T. (1998), 'Risk management in mental health', in Davies & Craig, op. cit., pp. 75–8.

Harris, G. T. & Rice, M. E. (1997), 'Risk appraisal and management of violent behaviour', *Psychiatric Services*, 48, pp. 1165–76.

Hughes, D. H. (1998), 'Pharmacologic management of the chronically aggressive psychiatric patient', *Psychiatric Annals*, 28(7), pp. 367–77.

Kalunian, D. A., Binder, R. L. & McNiel, D. E. (1990), 'Violence by geriatric patients who need psychiatric hospitalisation', *Journal of Clinical Psychiatry*, 51(8), pp. 340–3.

Macdonald, A. J. D. (1998), 'Mental health in old age', in Davies & Craig, op. cit., pp. 46–50.

Macpherson, R., Anstee, B. & Dix, R. (1996), 'Guidelines for the management of acutely disturbed patients', *Advances in Psychiatric Treatment*, 2, pp. 194–201.

Nilsson, K., Palmstierna, T. & Wistedt, B. (1998), 'Aggressive behaviour in hospitalised psychogeriatric patients', *Acta Psychiatrica Scandinavica*, 78, pp. 172–5.

Pabis, D. J. & Stanislav, S. W. (1996), 'Pharmacotherapy of aggressive behaviour', *The Annals of Pharmacotherapy*, 30, pp. 278–87.

Patel, V. (1993), 'Aggressive behaviour in elderly people with dementia: A review', *International Journal of Geriatric Psychiatry*, 8, pp. 457–72.

Pilowsky, L. S., Ring, H., Shine, P. J., Battersby, M. & Lader, M. (1992), 'Rapid tranquillisation: A survey of emergency prescribing in a General Psychiatric Hospital', *British Journal of Psychiatry*, 60, pp. 831–5.

Shah, A.V. (1992), 'Violence and psychogeriatric inpatients', *International Journal of Geriatric Psychiatry*, 7, pp. 39–44.

Teri, L. & Logsdon, R. (1990), 'Assessment and management of behavioural disturbances in Alzheimer's disease clients', *Comprehensive Therapy*, 16, pp. 36–42.

Thienhaus, O. J. & Piasecki, M. (1998), 'Assessment of psychiatric patients' risk of violence toward others', *Psychiatric Services*, 49, pp. 1129–47.

Turpin, J. P. (1983), 'The violent patient: A strategy for management and diagnosis', *Hospital and Community Psychiatry*, 34(1), pp. 37–9.

Westcott, R. (1996), 'Emergencies, crisis and violence', in Pullen, I., Wilkinson, G., Wright, A. & Pereira Gray, D. (eds), *Psychiatry and General Practice Today*, Royal College of General Practitioners, London, pp. 170–6.

Yudofsky, S. C., Silver, J. M. & Hales, R. E. (1990), 'Pharmacologic management of aggression in the elderly', *Journal of Clinical Psychiatry*, 51[10, suppl.], pp. 22–8.

Part IV

Neurological conditions

Chapter 13
Falls

KEITH D. HILL, JENNIFER A. SCHWARZ and JANE SIMS

Introduction

Falls among older people are often a sign of underlying health problems, many of which can improve with a range of management options to minimise future risk of falling. This chapter aims to highlight the important role of the medical practitioner in the early identification of risk of falling, and provide a framework for effectively managing the identified risk factors, if possible, prior to the first fall.

The overarching theme of this chapter is that many falls and falls-related injuries among older people are preventable. Falls should not be ascribed merely due to ageing, although it is true that there is deterioration in function in each of the component systems that contribute to effective balance with increasing age. This deterioration, though, is small relative to the capacity of the system, and of itself does not explain the marked increase in falls seen in older age. Instead, the primary contribution to this increase is disease affecting one or more components of the balance system.

A number of definitions of falls have been used but the most common definition is from the Kellogg International Working Group on Prevention of Falls by the Elderly, which defined a fall as 'any event which results in a person coming to rest inadvertently on the ground or other lower level, and other than as a consequence of the following: sustaining a violent blow, loss of consciousness, sudden onset of paralysis such as stroke, or an epileptic seizure'. The circumstances of a fall can give some indication as to the possible causes and management strategies, and should form a key component of the subjective assessment of someone who has experienced a fall. These will be discussed in greater detail in the section on clinical tests.

Costs associated with falls need to be considered in terms of costs to the individual, the family and support network, and to the health system generally. To an older person, falls can cause injury, reduced mobility, reduced confidence, pain, and a range of stresses, including concerns about continuing to live independently in the community. Falls have been noted as a major factor in up to 40% of nursing home admissions. To the family and support network of an older person who falls, there are also considerable stresses. These include concerns about many of the above factors, as well as concern about the likelihood of future falls and injuries. At times, these issues can cause tensions between the older person and the family/support network. The medical practitioner needs to be sensitive to these issues and ensure that the older person and his family/support network have the necessary support and information to facilitate their discussion of these issues. Involvement of other health professionals, such as social workers, who are experienced in counselling and are familiar with the range of services available to help minimise risk and assist in independent living may be useful.

While many of the costs of falls to the older person and his family/support network are somewhat intangible, aspects of the costs associated with falls on the health system have been quantified. Estimates from the United States indicate that falls by older people account for nearly 8% of the total lifetime economic cost associated with all unintentional injuries. Furthermore, almost US$10 billion is spent annually on health expenditures associated with osteoporosis, much of which is for the management of fall-related fractures. Falls also account for 5% of hospitalisations for people aged 65 years or older in the United States. In addition to these direct costs, other costs include outpatient therapy, home services such as meals on wheels, home maintenance, and home nursing, medical care and medications.

Aetiology and epidemiology

Approximately one in three people aged greater than 65 years living in the community fall one or more times in a 12-month period, increasing with age to one in two for those aged greater than 90 years. Between 10% and 15% of falls in older people cause serious injuries requiring hospitalisations, with 4–6% of these being fractures. Fractured neck of femur constitutes one-quarter of these fractures, although this proportion increases with age. In almost all cases of hip fracture, the fracture is caused by the impact with the floor surface. Hip fractures are associated with relatively poor prognosis in older people, with 20% dying within 12 months of fracture, and less than half returning to the pre-fracture level of function on a range of functional measures at 12 months post fracture. Less serious injuries, including lacerations, bruising, shock and sprains, occur more commonly after a fall.

Self-reporting of falls is considered to underestimate the true rate of falls. Studies that have compared recall of falls over a 12-month period with a falls diary and telephone call follow-up method have identified that the latter method results in at least 10% more reported falls. Up to 25% of fallers seek medical attention for their falls, either through hospital admission, emergency department presentation, or attendance to the medical practitioner. These generally are for those falls causing more serious injury. A number of reasons other than severity of the injury associated with the fall may influence whether an older person reports a fall or increasing unsteadiness to his medical practitioner. These include having the perception that nothing can be done about preventing falls, and in some cases, the faller will be concerned that by reporting these incidents, the medical practitioner and/or family may consider this a sign of not coping at home, which may prompt consideration of the need to move to supported accommodation. Both of these circumstances could potentially deter falls' reporting.

As well as the physical consequences of a fall, there are often psychological effects that can be undetected but which can, over time, result in reduced confidence in mobility, reduced activity level, and ultimately, an increased falls risk. Loss of confidence in mobility, or fear of falling, has been reported in 30% of a sample of community dwelling older people, and to severely limit activity level in 7%. When compared to a number of other fears, including fear of robbery, fear of forgetting an appointment, fear of financial problems and fear of losing a cherished item, fear of falling was the greatest fear reported by a sample of older people. These figures highlight that medical practitioners need to be vigilant in identifying the presence of fear of falling, often by noting changes in behaviour and activity, and to encourage strategies to overcome the loss of confidence.

Commonly, falls are classified as being due to extrinsic or intrinsic risk factors.

Extrinsic and intrinsic falls risk factors

Extrinsic falls risk factors include any aspects of the environment that may have contributed to the fall.

Examples include uneven footpaths, poor lighting, slippery or wet surfaces, poorly defined steps and kerbs, and cords or loose mats across floor surfaces. Also included under the broad category of extrinsic falls are those related to a high-risk activity, where a fall would not be an unexpected outcome. Examples include climbing onto a chair on a table to change a light globe, or clearing gutters on a ladder on a windy day. Where there is a strong element of extrinsic factors associated with a fall, the underlying message is that the fall may have been avoided if the environmental risk factor were not present, or the high-risk activity was modified to reduce the risk (e.g. using a step ladder to change a light globe).

Intrinsic falls risk factors include:

- the age-related decline in all components of the balance system
- abnormality in any of the components of the balance system, which may include:
  - acute medical conditions, such as labyrinthitis, urinary tract infection, or delirium
  - chronic medical conditions, such as cataracts, glaucoma, postural hypotension, stroke, Parkinson's disease or osteoarthritis
- medications that can affect the balance system, including psychotropic medications.

Abnormality affecting the balance system accounts for the greatest proportion of intrinsic falls, making a comprehensive examination of the balance system a key component of the assessment process.

While syncopal episodes may result in a fall, they are considered a discrete medical diagnosis in their own right and warrant a comprehensive review by a cardiologist. Diagnosis and management of syncopal episodes are reviewed in detail in Chapter 25.

A number of studies based on self-report of falls have estimated that approximately 50% of all falls are primarily associated with extrinsic factors, although intrinsic falls risk factors become more common with increasing age. Studies that have investigated more thoroughly for intrinsic falls risk factors have indicated that the rate of falls due to extrinsic falls risk factors may be substantially lower. In many falls there is a combination of both intrinsic and extrinsic factors evident, and part of the assessment needs to identify the relative importance of both.

Many falls risk factors have been identified for community dwelling older people. The presence of one or more previous falls has been highlighted as a key risk factor for subsequent falls. Other intrinsic falls risk factors include:

- female gender
- increased age
- multiple medications (more than four medications)
- specific types of medications (e.g. psychotropics, antidepressants)
- chronic medical conditions (mentioned above)
- reduced mobility or assistance with activities of daily living
- low level of physical activity
- reduced muscle strength
- impaired balance and unsteadiness in gait
- impaired vision (acuity and contrast sensitivity)
- dizziness
- cognitive impairment
- psychological dysfunction (anxiety and depression).

The presence of any one of these risk factors increases an individual's risk of having a fall. Furthermore, there is a cumulative effect, so that the risk of falling becomes magnified the more risk factors an individual has.

Pathophysiology

The balance system is a complex integrated system, comprising a number of integrated elements, each of which needs to function effectively for efficient balance to be achieved. Abnormality can occur in one, or commonly, in several of the components of the balance system, which compromises the ability to institute effective balance reactions in instances when balance is threatened. If effective balance reactions cannot be instituted when balance is threatened, a fall will occur. The balance system can be considered broadly in terms of three main component systems: the sensory systems, the motor system, and the integrative/executive system.

The sensory systems

The three sensory systems critical to effective balance are the visual, somatosensory and vestibular systems. Each provides unique although complementary sensory information about the body's alignment, position and movement through space, which is integrated centrally continuously. Vision provides the most important sensory input and can compensate to a degree for deficits in the other two sensory modalities.

The *visual system* provides key information about the body relative to its environment. Although the main aspect of vision assessed regularly in older people is visual acuity, there are other common visual functions at least as important in terms of balance. These include contrast sensitivity, dark adaptation, depth perception and visual fields. Abnormality can impact upon any one or more of these functions. Older people with impaired vision should undergo a comprehensive ophthalmological review. Furthermore, older people should have their vision reviewed at least every 2 years. Common visual abnormalities associated with increased likelihood of falling include:

- cataract
- age-related macular degeneration
- glaucoma.

Early detection of abnormality in some cases can be linked to early intervention and greater likelihood of successful treatment: for example, in the case of cataracts, extraction will markedly improve visual contrast sensitivity. Another important aspect of vision is the use of corrective lenses. Many older people require different lenses for distance and near vision. This can be cumbersome and a decision not to carry both glasses when they go out may result in some older people not wearing their distance glasses to optimise vision when walking outdoors on various terrains. This may compromise their early identification of environmental obstacles to be negotiated. Another commonly described visual factor in falls is the wearing of bifocal glasses when on stairs and kerbs. Although there is limited research evidence linking these, unless care is taken and the head tilted at an appropriate angle to enable vision through the distance component of the glasses, misjudgment of step and kerb edges can occur, resulting in a fall.

The *somatosensory system* provides sensory information for balance about the relative positions of joints (i.e. joint angles/proprioception), the body alignment over the base of support and weight distribution over the base of support. Intact somatosensory input requires effective functioning of the joint, muscle and other somatosensory receptors, as well as efficient conduction of the sensory information centrally. Common abnormalities causing somatosensory dysfunction in older people and which can increase an individual's risk of falling include:

- peripheral neuropathy
- arthritic degeneration of joint surfaces, particularly in the cervical spine.

In particular, potential causes of peripheral neuropathy should be explored, with special consideration given to treatable entities such as vitamin B_{12} or folate deficiency, alcohol-nutritional deficiency, or toxic drug-related polyneuropathies.

The *vestibular system* comprises three components: a bilateral peripheral sensory apparatus, a central processor and a mechanism for motor output. The peripheral vestibular system lies within the inner ear, and consists of three semicircular canals and two associated otolith organs. Information from the periphery is sent via the vestibular nerve to central structures located in the brain stem and cerebellum. Motor output from the central vestibular system is to the ocular motor nuclei and the spinal cord, and serves two important reflexes that play key roles in the maintenance of balance. The vestibulo-ocular reflex (VOR) generates eye movements that allow visual fixation on an object while the head is moving. An abnormal VOR can result in sensations of dizziness and vertigo, as well as impaired balance due to the degradation in visual acuity that occurs during head motion. In addition, the vestibulo-spinal reflex (VSR) is intricately involved in maintaining postural stability when the head is moving, and disruption of this reflex can result in impaired balance and a subsequently higher risk of falls.

Lesions of the vestibular system can result from peripheral inner ear abnormality or central dysfunction. Common abnormalities involving the vestibular system that can increase a person's risk of falling include:

- benign paroxysmal positional vertigo (BPPV)
- vestibular neuronitis/labyrinthitis
- Menière's disease
- acoustic neuroma
- traumatic brain injury
- stroke.

A number of drugs, including aminoglycosides and frusemide, may also damage the vestibular system and impair balance abilities.

Vertigo (see Chapter 19) is a common symptom associated with unilateral vestibular abnormality. It should be noted that in cases of bilateral vestibular abnormality, such as can occur in a small proportion of cases of gentamicin (aminoglycoside) toxicity, vertigo is not a presenting symptom, although balance performance can be markedly impaired.

A detailed otological examination is often necessary to diagnose the cause of vestibular dysfunction. This is important, both in terms of informing the patient of the prognosis and possible time course of the abnormality, as well as informing him of the choice of treatment. These options are discussed in greater detail in Chapter 19.

The motor system

The motor or output system includes the neural connections to the muscles and joints that are responsible for implementing an effective balance response. It is important to note that effective balance reactions often require lower limb, trunk and upper limb activity. Therefore, abnormality of the arm (e.g. a fractured humerus requiring sling support) will limit effective balance responses.

Key components of an effective motor response include rapid reaction time (motor component), ability to achieve fast and large torque (strength) in key muscle groups, and adequate flexibility in the joints being moved for the balance response. Musculoskeletal diseases are common with increasing age and include:

- arthritis
- osteoporosis
- osteomalacia
- proximal myopathies
- foot disorders.

Importantly, a number of these not only increase the risk of falls but also the risk of serious injury such as fractures after a fall. However, with a comprehensive management program, a number of these problems can at least be stabilised, if not improved.

Central processing/executive system

Central processing of sensory input occurs at multiple levels, including the cerebellum, brain stem and motor and sensory cortex. Motor planning occurs in the frontal lobe. Central processing of sensory information occurs continuously, providing an 'on-line' monitoring of the body's equilibrium within the base of support. Some stereotyped balance strategies have been reported, including:

- an ankle strategy, which involves initial response in the ankle muscles to save balance, usually associated with small range perturbations (e.g. stepping on a rock)
- a hip strategy, which involves substantial hip and trunk movement prior to distal muscle activation to save balance, and is usually seen with larger amplitude perturbations or on narrow or compliant support surfaces (e.g. walking on a beam)
- a stepping strategy, which involves taking a step to regain balance within a newly defined base of support.

Each of these balance strategies can be modified by cortical control, often in response to environmental constraints. While these balance strategies have been well documented in research settings, they are often seen in combination in clinical assessment. Older people have been shown to demonstrate less consistency in their balance strategy response to small perturbations in force platform studies. In some cases where abnormality has markedly compromised balance responses to a perturbation, a 'timber response' is observed, where there is no attempt by the person to respond to the perturbation and a fall would occur.

Central processing can be impaired by a number of diseases, increasing the risk of falls. These include:

- dementia
- stroke
- Parkinson's disease
- multiple sclerosis.

Clinical tests

The assessment procedures described below can be applied to older people who have experienced falls, or those presenting who may be considered at risk of falls. There will be occasions when reviewing a patient for reasons other than the issue of increasing unsteadiness or near falls will alert the medical practitioner to the need to undertake similar subjective and objective examinations, with the aim of primary prevention. Early identification of falls risk or falls-related injury risk and development of a targeted management plan reduces the likelihood of development of secondary problems, such as fear of falling and reduced activity level, and increases the likelihood that interventions will be successful.

Subjective examination

The subjective examination should commence with a review of the circumstances of any falls or near falls. Particular questions should target:

- time and date of the fall/s
- circumstances of the fall/s, including location and direction of the fall (forwards, backwards or to the side), if there was any environmental factor involved, any preceding symptoms such as palpitations or dizziness, and whether there was any loss of consciousness. It should be noted that frequently the cause of the fall is rationalised by statements such as 'I must have tripped'. These need to be explored to identify the significance of any environmental obstacle
- consequences of the fall/s, including any injuries, loss of confidence or change in activity level
- where there has been more than one fall, if there are any common elements about the falls, such as always in one direction, when turning or when standing up from a chair.

Responses to the falls questions may provide some foundation for guiding the objective assessment. Examples of some common falls circumstances and the possible causes are listed in Table 13.1.

Table 13.1 Common circumstances of falls and possible causes to be considered in the medical examination

Circumstance of fall	Possible causes to be considered in the assessment
At night	Is there a night light? Were glasses worn when up at night? Are any medications taken prior to bed, especially sedatives or drugs predisposing to postural hypotension? Are there incontinence issues?
Turning	Is there any dizziness associated with turning? Is there any evidence of unilateral paresis? Are there any signs of Parkinson's disease or syndrome, especially if associated with gait festination?
Loss of consciousness	Was the head knocked in the fall? Are there any cardiac factors, such as arrhythmias, postural hypotension or aortic stenosis? Are there any neurological causes (e.g. epilepsy)?
Associated with lightheadedness	Is there any postural drop in blood pressure (measure lying, and standing up to 2 minutes)? Is there any dizziness?
'Furniture walking'	Is there one or more causes for impaired balance? Is there a need for a walking aid? Is fear of falling present?

Objective assessment

The immediate concern in the medical assessment of an older person presenting after a fall is to identify the extent and nature of injuries sustained. These may include fractures, sprains, strains, bruises and lacerations. Presence of shock needs to be excluded.

If no serious injury has been sustained, or once the acute nature of the injuries has settled, a comprehensive examination is necessary to identify potential intrinsic falls risk factors that contributed to the fall. Following a detailed history and review of medication (both prescribed and over the counter), a general physical examination needs to be performed with emphasis on the neurological, musculoskeletal and cardiovascular systems. Romberg's Test, described in Table 13.2, is a test of the dorsal column (posterior column), which carries vibration sense, position sense and a proportion of light touch. It is important that vibration

Table 13.2 Simple measures of balance and mobility, and criterion scores

Test	Equipment required	Method of assessment[(a)]	Normative range of scores and age range[(b)]
1. Functional reach	Tape measure on wall at shoulder height	Standing with feet comfortably apart, dominant arm straight out in front. Read the distance at the knuckles, then ask the patient to reach as far forward as possible, and note the distance at the knuckles. The difference is the functional reach (cm).	Sample: age 70–87 years Males: > 31 cm Females: > 23 cm
2. Timed 'up and go' test	Standard height chair with arms, 3 m walkway area, stopwatch	The person is seated, and on the command 'go' he stands, walks at his comfortable speed (using normal walking aid) 3 m, turns, returns to the chair and sits down. The full process is timed (seconds).	Sample: men and women aged 70–84 years < 10 seconds
3. Step test	7.5 cm (3 inch) block or step, stopwatch	Standing facing the block, feet 5 cm from the block. The person is asked to step one foot fully on, then off the block as many times as possible in 15 seconds. Then the test is repeated for the opposite leg.	Sample: men and women, mean age 72.5 years (SD = 4) > 14 steps/15 seconds with either leg
4. Walking speed (6 m walk)	Corridor area, 6 m distance marked. Start the walk 1 m before the start of measurement area.	Instruct the person to walk to the end of the corridor at his comfortable walking speed without stopping or talking. Record the time taken to walk the 6 m (seconds). Divide the time into 360 to derive speed in metres/minute.	Sample: 60–80 years of age > 60 m/min
5. Romberg's Test	Nil	Standing with the feet together, ask the person to balance and to close his eyes.	A small increase in postural sway is normal, although a moderate increase in sway or overbalancing is abnormal.
6. Heel–toe walking	Nil	Ask the person to walk heel to toe for a distance of 2 m.	High-level task: healthy older person can perform without stepping out of the line of progression.

(*a*) No hand support is allowed with any of these test procedures except for the use of a walking aid in the timed 'up and go' test.

(*b*) Criterion measures are calculated as one standard deviation from the mean for a healthy group of older people (sample as described).

sense be tested using a tuning fork with a frequency of 128 Hz. A positive Romberg's sign is often mistaken as a sign of cerebellar disease. This is not so. It is also vital to check for postural hypotension, measuring lying and standing blood pressure at 1 and 2 minutes.

Clinical measures of balance and mobility

A number of simple tests of balance and mobility can be performed quickly and with minimal equipment within a medical examination office. Examples are listed in Table 13.2, with reference to how the test is performed and an anticipated range of scores that may be considered within normal limits for an older population. Scores falling outside the range indicated suggest the need for comprehensive assessment to identify the causes of reduced performance. Whenever observing performance on any of these tasks, practitioners should position themselves so they can steady the person being assessed if he overbalances. It should be noted that a reduction in performance occurs with increased age so that scores need to be adjusted for those younger or older than the sample described. Many of the tests are useful in not only providing baseline information about a person's performance but also for monitoring change in performance (improvement or deterioration) over time.

Fear of falling

Loss of confidence in mobility, or fear of falling, is a common but frequently poorly recognised consequence of falls. In fact, fear of falling can be present even when a fall has not occurred. Questioning about loss of confidence should be part of a routine subjective assessment of the older person at risk of falls or who has had a fall. It is important to note that fear of falling can be situation specific, so that the person may report no fear of falling within his own home but may have high levels of fear of falling as soon as he goes out the front door. Therefore, questioning should go beyond merely asking 'are you afraid of falling?'. Standardised questionnaires can be used to objectively quantify fear of falling, such as the Falls Efficacy Scale, the Modified Falls Efficacy Scale (Box 13.1) and the Activities and Balance Confidence Scale.

Dizziness

Dizziness is a common health problem for older people, with over 20% reporting one or more episodes in a 12-month period. Central or peripheral vestibular dysfunction, or a combination of both, are often the cause and can also be associated with reduced balance performance and falls. The Hallpike manoeuvre is an essential component of a falls assessment for a person complaining of true vertigo.

The Hallpike manoeuvre is conducted to identify the effect of inducing endolymph flow in the posterior semicircular canal of the vestibular apparatus. To perform the Hallpike manoeuvre, the patient is positioned in long sitting on the plinth (sitting with legs outstretched on the plinth at the same height as the hips). Then, as he is lowered quickly into the supine position, the head is rotated to one side and extended by the examiner. The patient is instructed to keep his eyes open if possible so that the examiner can identify the presence of nystagmus. Allow a short rest if symptoms develop. The patient is then raised to the starting position (long sitting looking straight ahead) with a quick movement. A Hallpike manoeuvre is positive if the patient develops nystagmus and vertigo in any part of the manoeuvre. The test is repeated rotating the head to the opposite side. A common cause of a positive Hallpike manoeuvre is benign paroxysmal positional vertigo (BPPV). In BPPV, the Hallpike manoeuvre is positive, although there is a short latency between commencing the manoeuvre and commencement of signs and symptoms, and the symptoms will settle with rest. The affected labyrinth is the one on the side to which the head is rotated.

The assessment and management of the older person with dizziness is reported in detail in Chapter 19. Importantly, a range of management procedures, including particle repositioning, desensitising exercises and balance exercises, have been shown to be effective in the management of dizziness from a range of causes.

Diagnosis

When an older person presents to the medical practitioner following a fall, undertaking the range of

Box 13.1 The Modified Falls Efficacy Scale

On a scale of 0–10, how confident are you that you can do each of these activities without falling? A score of 0 means 'not confident/not sure at all', 5 means 'fairly confident/fairly sure', and 10 means 'completely confident/completely sure'.

Activity	0 (Not confident at all)	1	2	3	4	5 (Fairly confident)	6	7	8	9	10 (Completely confident)
1. Get dressed and undressed											
2. Prepare a simple meal											
3. Take a bath or a shower											
4. Get in/out of a chair											
5. Get in/out of bed											
6. Answer the door or telephone											
7. Walk around the inside of your house											
8. Reach into cabinets or closet											
9. Light housekeeping											
10. Simple shopping											
11. Using public transport											
12. Crossing roads											
13. Light gardening or hanging out the washing[(a)]											
14. Using front or rear steps at home											

(*a*) Rate most commonly performed of these activities.

Note: If you have stopped doing the activity at least partly because of being afraid of falling, score a 0. If you have stopped an activity purely because of a physical problem, leave that item blank.

Adapted from Tinetti et al. 1990 and Hill et al. 1996.

assessment procedures will often identify one or more intrinsic factors contributing to the fall/s. In more complex cases, further investigations or referral to other specialists may be required to confirm diagnosis. The specialists who may be involved include geriatricians, neurologists, cardiologists, rheumatologists, and ear, nose and throat surgeons. A variety of specific tests may be required, which include blood tests, radiological studies, Holter monitoring and vestibular function testing.

An indication of the broad range of major contributory factors to falls identified in a specialist falls clinic for older people are shown in Table 13.3. Many new diagnoses were identified by the falls clinic process, despite most referrals being from general practitioners. This highlights the need to consider additional referral or assessment where the diagnosis or cause of falls/unsteadiness may not be clear.

Treatment

As discussed above, the aetiology of falls is extensive and therefore a variety of measures need to be instituted to address specific aetiology entities. Especially in older people, the consequences of falls, such as injuries, are significant.

Medical management

Components of the medical management program include optimising medical conditions, reviewing medications, patient and carer education, and consideration of behaviour modification if fear of falling is evident. Given the multifactorial nature of falls, there is often a need to refer the older person for management by other health professionals.

The medical practitioner also has a pivotal role in co-ordinating management of acute injuries and subsequent morbidity associated with falls. Management of acute soft tissue injuries should include rest and intermittent ice packs. Following the acute stage, heat can be quite effective in reducing pain, swelling and stiffness. Physiotherapy referral for heat therapy, mobilisation and exercise may speed recovery of function.

Falls are even more common in older people in residential aged-care facilities than in the community. It is important that the same approach to assessment and management of falls and falls risk factors be considered for the older person in residential aged-care settings as for frailer older people in the community.

Physiotherapy management

The physiotherapist can provide a range of management options for the older person at risk of falling or who is experiencing falls. Management will be determined by the assessment findings but may include:

1. Exercise. A range of exercise types may be provided, including balance, strength, cardiovascular fitness and flexibility exercises. These may be undertaken supervised by the physiotherapist (particularly for those at moderate risk), as home programs or as part of a group-based program. Exercises may be land based or include hydrotherapy. Exercises should be tailored to the individual's needs based on the assessment findings.

Table 13.3 Major factors contributing to falls for older people referred to a specialist falls clinic

Major factor	Number (%) of patients
Neurological	
• Degenerative (Alzheimer's disease, Parkinson's disease, progressive supranuclear palsy)	55 (36.9%)
• Stroke	25 (16.8%)
• Visual/aural (cataract, glaucoma, Menière's disease, vestibular neuritis, BPPV)	24 (16.1%)
• Other	14 (9.4%)
Musculoskeletal (osteoarthritis, osteoporosis, rheumatoid arthritis)	40 (26.9%)
Drugs	17 (11.4%)
Psychological (fear of falling, anxiety syndromes)	17 (11.4%)
Cardiac (postural hypotension, arrhythmias)	13 (8.7%)

Note: People may have more than one factor, resulting in a column total greater than 100%.
Source: Hill et al. 1994.

2. Functional retraining, including transfers and gait re-education. This may include an emphasis on confidence during walking, mobility on different surfaces and mobility during dual-task conditions.
3. Walking aid prescription and education. The provision of a walking aid will increase an individual's stability. A walking frame provides considerably greater support than a walking stick, although it impedes the natural gait pattern more, and is a problem where steps need to be negotiated or objects need to be carried. Careful selection of the appropriate walking aid is required, and instruction regarding correct height and pattern of use are critical if the walking aid is to improve stability. Consideration should be given to a physiotherapy exercise program to improve stability whenever a decision is made to introduce a walking aid.
4. If the person reports difficulty getting up from the floor after a fall, the physiotherapist should consider whether practising getting down onto the floor and then practising methods of rising from the floor is indicated. Where the older person can be trained to rise from the floor, increased confidence in general mobility is also often achieved.
5. The physiotherapist may also be involved in the management of injuries associated with falls. A range of pain-relieving modalities are available, often associated with improved resolution of bruising, inflammation, and muscle and ligament strains. These include transcutaneous electrical nerve stimulation, ultrasound, interferential stimulation and heat packs. In addition, joint and soft tissue mobilisation and specific exercise regimens are often indicated to ensure maximal recovery of function. If the physiotherapist is involved in the management of injuries associated with a fall, it is critical that the causes of the fall and ways to reduce the likelihood of future falls are closely investigated and incorporated into the treatment plan.

Occupational therapy management

An occupational therapy management program for an older person at risk of falling will address the individual's functional capacity within his environmental domains. This may include modifications within the home and surrounding yard, as well as giving consideration to means of transport, access to shops and buildings, and other public places. Consideration of activities undertaken by the older person and the relative falls risk associated with these need to be discussed. If activities have been reduced, the occupational therapist may need to consider strategies to facilitate re-engagement in these, with a particular focus on community and leisure activities. In cases where there is a high risk associated with specific activities, the focus may be on achieving increased caution or modification of those activities that place the older person at greatest risk.

Nursing management

In a number of settings, including domiciliary care and many medical practices, the nurse may be a key person to identify falls risk at an early stage. Particularly in the domiciliary setting, the nurse may also be able to encourage ongoing compliance with medical and allied health management plans on a regular basis.

Psychological management

Fear of falling is the most common psychological problem associated with falls. Mild fear of falling is quite appropriate where there is some level of balance impairment and this will often lessen with a physical approach in an exercise program. A walking aid may be used in the short term to help improve confidence and maintain activity level, especially outdoors walking. Severe fear of falling, or fear of falling that does not lessen with a physical approach, is best considered as a phobia and treated with a behaviour modification program. This may require referral to a clinical psychologist.

Podiatry management

Feet and footwear provide the basis for effective interaction with the support surface and are critical at times when balance is threatened. Specific feet and footwear problems should be referred to a podiatrist.

Injury minimisation

It is unrealistic to expect to prevent all falls. It is therefore important to consider strategies to reduce injuries also. Some injuries (e.g. hypothermia, dehydration and pressure sores) can occur after a 'long lie' on the floor after a fall. Personal alarm systems worn at all times can enable an older person to summon assistance promptly. Appropriate footwear, which fits well, has a broad heel, firm patterned sole and preferably ankle support will also aid stability.

Treating osteoporosis/osteomalacia with vitamin D_3, calcium supplementation, oestrogens and bisphosphonates decreases the likelihood of a fracture (see Chapter 55). For those with evidence of osteoporosis, a management plan incorporating strategies to enhance bone strength, as well as improving effectiveness of balance responses and minimising environmental risk, is likely to be most effective. Another innovative approach to reduce hip fractures is the use of hip protectors. These are specially designed underwear that have energy-absorbing or -dissipating inserts over both hips. In nursing home studies, these have been shown to reduce the rate of hip fractures by 50%. The role of hip protectors in fitter older people is still being investigated. The major problem with hip protectors at present is the limited compliance of older people considered 'at risk' of falls in wearing the garments.

Prognosis

Falls and falls-related injuries are often an indicator of a complex interaction between both intrinsic and extrinsic falls risk factors. Prognosis will vary depending upon a range of issues, including early identification of risk, early implementation of targeted management programs, and number and type of intrinsic falls risk factors present. However, there is increasing evidence from well-conducted, randomised controlled trials that a number of single and multiple intervention approaches can be effective in reducing falls rates among older people in the community setting. These approaches include:

- exercise:
  - a home-based exercise program provided by a physiotherapist after a comprehensive assessment, the exercises being tailored to the individual's needs, and incorporating balance and strengthening exercises, with the physiotherapist visiting four times in a 6-month period
  - a tai chi program
  - group exercise programs, which incorporate balance, strength, cardiovascular and flexibility exercises
- home assessment by an occupational therapist, including home hazard assessment and modification, as well as advice on changing behaviours to minimise future falls risk
- medication reviews, particularly with a focus on reduction of psychotropic medication use.

There is also evidence that falls-related injuries can be reduced with vitamin D_3 and calcium supplementation.

Older people with more complex presentation, or those who do not respond to initial management options, may benefit from a comprehensive review and management plan by a multidisciplinary team with specific skills in falls prevention. These specialist falls clinics usually involve a comprehensive assessment by medical specialists/geriatricians, physiotherapists, occupational therapists and nursing staff. One study involving a limited multidisciplinary approach (medical and occupational therapy assessment and management) demonstrated a significant reduction in falls in a sample of older people presenting to emergency departments following a fall.

In some cases, despite comprehensive assessment and management programs, falls continue to occur. Hip protectors have been shown to reduce hip fracture rates in at-risk older people.

Conclusion

Falls and their consequences present a complex issue, which requires a strong focus on early identification of risk and early implementation of a targeted management program. This often also requires involving the multidisciplinary team in the assessment and management process. There is increasing evidence that these approaches can reduce the magnitude of the problems of falls and falls-related injuries in older people.

Bibliography and further reading

Alexander, N. (1994), 'Postural control in older adults', *Journal of the American Geriatrics Society*, 42, pp. 93–108.

Campbell, A. (1997), 'Preventing falls by dealing with the causes', *The Medical Journal of Australia*, 167, pp. 407–8.

Duncan, P., Weiner, K., Chandler, J. & Studenski, S. (1990), 'Functional reach: a new clinical measure of balance', *Journal of Gerontology*, 45, pp. M192–7.

Gillespie, L., Gillespie, W., Cumming, R., Lamb, S. & Rowe, B. (1998), *Interventions to reduce the incidence of falling in the elderly (Cochrane review)*, update software, The Cochrane Library, Oxford.

Hill, K. D., Dwyer, J., Schwarz, J. & Helme, R. (1994), 'A Falls and Balance Clinic for the elderly', *Physiotherapy Canada*, 45, pp. 20–7.

Hill, K., Schwarz, J., Kalogeropoulos, A. & Gibson, S. (1996), 'Fear of falling revisited', *Archives of Physical Medicine and Rehabilitation*, 77, pp. 1025–9.

Hill, K., Schwarz, J., Flicker, L. & Carroll, S. (1999), 'Falls among healthy community dwelling older women: a prospective study of frequency, circumstances, consequences and prediction accuracy', *Australian and New Zealand Journal of Public Health*, 23, pp. 41–8.

Hill, K., Schwarz, J., Smith, R., Gilsenan, B. & Bull, K. (2001), 'Falls: their impact on older people, assessment and prevention strategies', in Cluning, T. (ed.), *Practical Approaches to Community Care*, Ausmed Publications, Melbourne.

Kellogg International Working Group on Prevention of Falls by the Elderly (1987), 'The prevention of falls in later life', *Danish Medical Bulletin*, 34 (suppl. 4), pp. 1–24.

Kendig, H., Helme, R., Teshuva, K., Osborne, D., Flicker, L. & Browning, C. (1996), *Health Status of Older People project: preliminary findings from a survey of the health and lifestyles of older Australians*, Victorian Health Promotion Foundation, Melbourne.

King, M. & Tinetti, M. (1995), 'Falls in community-dwelling older persons', *Journal of the American Geriatrics Society*, 43, pp. 1146–54.

King, M. & Tinetti, M. (1996), 'A multifactorial approach to reducing injurious falls', *Clinics in Geriatric Medicine*, 12, pp. 745–59.

Lord, S., Ward, J., Williams, P. & Strudwick, M. (1995), 'The effect of a 12-month exercise trial on balance, strength, and falls in older women: a randomised controlled trial', *Journal of the American Geriatrics Society*, 43, pp. 1198–206.

Nevitt, M. (1997), 'Falls in the elderly: risk factors and prevention', in Masdeu, J., Sudarsky, L. & Wolfson, L. (eds), *Gait Disorders of Aging: Falls and Therapeutic Strategies*, Lippincott-Raven, Philadelphia.

Ostrosky, K., VanSwearingen, J., Burdett, R. & Gee, Z. (1994), 'A comparison of gait characteristics in young and old subjects', *Physical Therapy*, 74, pp. 637–46.

Norton, R. (1999), 'Professional practice update: preventing falls and fall-related injuries among older people', *Australasian Journal on Ageing*, 18, pp. 160–6.

Podsiadlo, D. & Richardson, S. (1991), 'The timed "Up & Go": a test of basic functional mobility for frail elderly persons', *Journal of the American Geriatrics Society*, 39, pp. 142–8.

Powell, L. & Myers, A. (1995), 'The Activities-specific Balance Confidence (ABC) Scale', *Journal of Gerontology*, 50A, pp. M28–34.

Schwarz, J. (1995), 'Falls in the elderly: management and prevention in general practice', *Modern Medicine in Australia*, May, pp. 89–95.

Tinetti, M., Richman, D. & Powell, L. (1990), 'Falls efficacy as a measure of fear of falling', *Journal of Gerontology*, 45, pp. P239–43.

Tinetti, M., Baker, D., McAvay, G., Claus, E., Garrett, P., Gottschalk, M., Koch, M., Trainor, K. & Horwitz, R. (1994), 'A multifactorial intervention to reduce the risk of falling among elderly people living in the community', *The New England Journal of Medicine*, 331, pp. 821–7.

Walker, J. & Howland, J. (1991), 'Falls and fear of falling among elderly persons living in the community: occupational therapy interventions', *American Journal of Occupational Therapy*, 45, pp. 119–22.

Chapter 14
Neurodegenerative conditions

MARGARET BULLING

Parkinson's disease

Introduction

Parkinson's disease (PD) is one of a group of neurodegenerative disorders characterised by selective and premature decay of functionally related populations of neurons. It is believed environmental insults, such as infection or neurotoxins, partially deplete selected neuronal populations and, together with age related degeneration, result in further neuronal loss, leading to clinical disease.

It is important to distinguish between PD and parkinsonism. James Parkinson first described parkinson's disease in 1817 in his *Essay on the Shaking Palsy*. His account gives this definition: 'Involuntary tremulous motion, with lessened muscular power, in parts not in action and even when supported; with a propensity to bend the trunk forward, and to pass from walking to a running pace, the senses and intellect being uninjured.'

The presence of 2 out of 3 of the cardinal motor signs of tremor, rigidity and bradykinesia in conjunction with a robust response to an adequate dose of levodopa are considered necessary for the diagnosis of PD and to distinguish it from other causes of parkinsonism. Parkinsonism is a clinical syndrome defined by the presence of tremor, rigidity and bradykinesia and the aetiology includes a variety of causes, listed in Box 14.1. Parkinson's disease accounts for approximately 75% of cases of parkinsonism. In parkinsonism other than PD and some cases of drug induced parkinsonism which are fully reversible, treatment response is generally poor and progression of the disease is more rapid.

Box 14.1 Causes of parkinsonism

- Parkinson's disease
- Drug induced parkinsonism
- Progressive supranuclear palsy
- Vascular parkinsonism—small, shuffling steps, relatively broad base, 'lower half parkinsonism'
- Multiple system atrophy
  - Striatonigral degeneration
  - Olivopontocerebellar atrophy
  - Shy-Drager syndrome
- Diffuse Lewy body disease
- Corticobasal degeneration
- Wilson's disease

Aetiology and epidemiology

Parkinson's disease occurs in all ethnic groups. There is a slight preponderance of males. The prevalence of PD is 3% over 65 years and increases exponentially with age between 65 and 90 years.

It is probably not one disease but several, with common clinical, pathological and possibly biological end points. Discovery of the neurotoxin 1-methyl-4-phenyl-1,2,3,6-tetrahydropyridine (MPTP) to induce nigral cell death spawned broad interest in potential environmental factors in aetiology. This concept is further supported by the ability of various toxins to cause symptomatic forms of parkinsonism. The rural environment has generally been associated with increased risk and there may be a relationship with the use of pesticides, herbicides and exposure to well water.

There is increasing evidence of the importance of genetic factors in PD. A family history of PD is a strong predictor of an increased risk of disease and there are high rates of concordance among monozygotic twins when one twin has young onset disease. A small number of multigenerational families have been reported; these families often have atypical features such as young onset, rapid course to death, predominant rigidity and dementia.

Two distinct mutations in the α-synuclein gene located on chromosome 4q which are associated with an autosomal dominant form of PD have been identified. α-synuclein is a highly conserved, abundant protein of unknown function that is expressed mainly in presynaptic nerve terminals. Another group of families with an autosomal dominant inheritance has been described with linkage to chromosome 2p13. An autosomal recessive form of neuronal degeneration involving the pars compacta of the substantia nigra and locus coeruleus without Lewy body formation causes a substantial proportion of young onset PD. This disorder is associated with mutations on the long arm of chromosome 6. The protein produced by this mutation, parkin, is homologous with the ubiquitin family of proteins involved in the pathogenesis of several neurodegenerative diseases.

It is hoped that investigation of the genetic basis of familial PD will help elucidate the mechanisms of cell death involved and provide insight into the mechanisms of cell death of the much more common sporadic form of the disease, and so lead to developments in treatments and the possibility of prevention.

Smoking has consistently been associated with a reduced risk of Parkinson's disease although this may be restricted to those with a relatively young age of onset of the disease.

Pathophysiology

The pathology of PD involves cell degeneration and loss of pigmented, dopaminergic neurons in the brain stem, particularly the substantia nigra. It is generally believed that at least 80% of the neurons in the substantia nigra need to be lost before PD becomes clinically manifest. Other pigmented brain stem neurons are also involved, including the noradrenergic locus coeruleus. There is a reduction in dopamine in the caudate and putamen due to the cell loss in the substantia nigra. The degenerating pigmented brain stem nuclei contain Lewy bodies. These are eosinophilic hyaline inclusion bodies. Lewy bodies are not specific to PD and may be found in small numbers in other neurodegenerative diseases, such as diffuse Lewy body disease in which Lewy bodies are found in the cortex as well as in the basal ganglia.

Clinical features

Bradykinesia may be assessed by the patient tapping the index finger and thumb and by foot tapping. Patients will often have difficulty with getting out of a chair, initiating gait, turning in bed and fine motor tasks, such as doing up buttons and handwriting.

Tremor should be assessed with the patient at rest, while performing an activity and while maintaining a posture. It may be made worse when the patient is stressed or asked to do a task involving concentration or a motor task with the contralateral extremity.

Rigidity usually begins unilaterally and often has a cogwheel quality best seen at the wrists. It is detected by flexing and extending each extremity and the neck. Reduced arm swing is evidence of increased rigidity.

Balance should be assessed with the 'pull test' (the patient should be able to maintain balance while being pulled backwards). The examiner stands behind the patient and pulls her towards him by a brief pull on both shoulders. Findings on the pull test are abnormal (the patient is unable to recover unaided) only in the later stages of PD.

The gait may be small stepped and shuffling with a stooped posture, and multiple steps may be needed for turning.

Evaluation of eye movements, particularly the speed of vertical and horizontal saccades (quick eye movements between two stimuli), helps exclude other parkinsonian disorders, which are discussed below. Elderly patients with PD may have age related limited upward gaze and convergence.

Diagnosis

Patients with PD usually present after the age of 50 years with motor complaints, such as tremor at rest, micrographia, slowness or poverty of movement, or stiffness. Typically the onset is insidious and progression is slow, initially affecting one limb and then spreading to the others. Asymmetric involvement usually persists. Tremor, usually at rest, increases in periods of anxiety and disappears during sleep or motor actions. The hands are preferentially affected, but with more advanced disease the legs, chin and head may be involved. It is classically described as pill-rolling. Postural tremor, which usually occurs while the patient maintains a posture such as extension of the upper extremities, should be differentiated from essential tremor, which is slowly progressive and not associated with akinesia or rigidity. Decreased associated movements, slowness when walking, reduced speech volume and monotony may occur relatively early in the disease. Depression may antedate or coincide with motor symptoms.

As the disease progresses, patients will often exhibit a masked facies and decreased eye blinking. Postural instability is usually a late sign and is more common in the elderly. Postural reflexes become lost and the patient tends to fall either forwards (propulsion) or backwards (retropulsion). Short or shuffling steps, instability and falls occur. Sialorrhoea secondary to dysphagia develops because of autonomic involvement. Autonomic disturbances such as orthostatic hypotension, constipation, dysphagia and urinary bladder dysfunction are usually a late feature of PD. Sleep is often disrupted and patients may experience cramps and paraesthesia.

Dementia is usually a late manifestation and is associated with an older age of onset of PD and predominant bradykinesia and rigidity. There is slowness of information processing and deficits in visuospatial discrimination, frontal lobe executive function and memory retrieval. Psychosis with visual hallucinations and paranoia is more common in elderly, demented and depressed patients.

The diagnosis of PD is predominantly a clinical one and a number of guidelines are available. Errors in diagnosis are not infrequent. In an autopsy series of 100 patients with a clinical diagnosis of PD made by a neurologist, only 76% had typical Lewy bodies, the pathologic hallmark of PD.

Akinesia and rigidity are almost universal in PD and a tremor ultimately develops in about 75% of patients. Classical tremor is highly suggestive of PD or drug induced parkinsonism, since it rarely occurs in other parkinsonian disorders. Virtually all PD patients have a good or excellent response to levodopa preparations. The diagnosis of PD is highly probable when a patient presents with a slowly progressive akinesia with either the classical pill-rolling rest tremor or rigidity, excellent and sustained response to levodopa, asymmetric parkinsonism at onset, and absence of unusual features such as brisk reflexes, extensor plantar responses and cerebellar signs. Likewise, orthostatic hypotension is not usually seen in early PD.

The challenge in diagnosing PD is to distinguish it from essential tremor and other forms of parkinsonism.

Box 14.2 Characteristic features of Parkinson's disease

- Progressive onset and slow progression of asymmetric akinesia
- Excellent and sustained levodopa response
- Either classical pill-rolling rest tremor or rigidity

Box 14.3 Features suggestive of an alternative diagnosis

Motor

- Early instability and falls
- Rapid disease progression
- Absent, poor or waning response to levodopa
- Pyramidal signs
- Cerebellar signs
- Early dysarthria and/or dysphagia

Oculomotor

- Supranuclear gaze palsy, slowing of saccades, difficulty initiating saccades

Cognitive and behavioural

- Early dementia
- Visual hallucinations not treatment induced
- Apraxia
- Sensory or visual neglect, cortical disturbances

Autonomic

- Early autonomic failure unrelated to treatment (orthostatic hypotension, impotence or urinary disturbances)

Box 14.4 Differential diagnosis of PD

- Essential tremor
- Drug induced parkinsonism (drugs: phenothiazines, e.g. prochlorperazine; butyrophenones, e.g. haloperidol)
- Progressive supranuclear palsy
- Vascular parkinsonism
- Multiple system atrophy
- Diffuse Lewy body disease
- Corticobasal degeneration
- Wilson's disease

Essential tremor is characterised by a postural tremor that remains stable or dampens with action and resolves at rest. In severe cases the tremor may occur in all positions. The tremor is usually bilateral and symmetric and an autosomal dominant pattern of inheritance is often found.

Drug induced parkinsonism is an important differential diagnosis. It is most commonly due to neuroleptics. Phenothiazines (including prochlorperazine), butyrophenones and thioxanthenes block D2 and D3 dopamine receptors. Other drugs which can cause drug induced parkinsonism include metoclopramide, methyldopa, reserpine, verapamil, flunarizine, lovastatin, amiodarone and various anticonvulsants. The frequency of parkinsonism in patients taking neuroleptics is approximately 20–40%. Possible risk factors include advanced age, female gender and genetic predisposition. Most cases resolve within weeks of stopping the medication.

Suggestive clinical features for drug induced parkinsonism include subacute, bilateral onset and progression of symptoms, early presence of postural tremor and concurrent choreoathetoid dyskinesias, especially of the face and mouth. Drug induced parkinsonism is a risk factor for the later development of PD. If parkinsonism persists following drug withdrawal, one has to consider the possibility that the medication has uncovered latent disease.

Progressive supranuclear palsy is most commonly misdiagnosed as PD early in the course of the illness. It presents as an akinetic-rigid syndrome. Postural instability tends to occur soon after onset and rest tremor is rare. Characteristics that differentiate progressive supranuclear palsy from PD include abnormalities of ocular motility, including supranuclear vertical gaze palsy, upright posture with tendency to fall backwards, pseudobulbar emotionality (characterised by inappropriate laughing and crying) and axial and limb dystonia. Patients with progressive supranuclear palsy may respond to levodopa early in the illness but the effect diminishes as the disease progresses and motor fluctuations are rare.

In vascular parkinsonism individuals develop parkinsonian signs after an acute infarct in the caudate, putamen, globus pallidus or brain stem. In addition, vascular events can cause gait disorders that may be confused with Parkinson's disease. The lower half of the body is predominantly involved and patients often have small, shuffling steps. Clues to suggest a vascular cause include a long history of hypertension, a step-wise or lack of progression of the disorder, poor response to levodopa, and other clinical signs such as aphasia and hemiparesis.

Multiple system atrophy as a diagnostic label encompasses the older terminology of olivopontocerebellar atrophy, striatonigral degeneration and Shy-Drager syndrome. This syndrome is characterised by parkinsonism (without tremor), ataxia and autonomic failure.

Diffuse Lewy body disease is characterised by progressive dementia, fluctuations in cognitive function, well formed visual hallucinations and parkinsonian signs. Rest tremor is less frequent than bradykinesia and rigidity. Other associated features include syncope, repeated falls and neuroleptic sensitivity. These patients are often given neuroleptics because of visual hallucinations although they are particularly sensitive to the adverse effects of these drugs and have an increased mortality when exposed to them.

Corticobasal degeneration presents in the 50s or 60s as a progressive, akinetic-rigid syndrome characterised by unilateral coarse tremor, bradykinesia, marked rigidity and limb apraxia. The apraxic limb (usually an arm) is held in a fixed, dystonic posture, with wrist flexed and fingers extended. Forced grasping and alien involuntary movements are less common but, when they occur, are findings that differentiate corticobasal degeneration from PD. Other signs include cognitive disturbances, postural instability, athetosis, myoclonus, cortical sensory loss, hyperreflexia, pseudobulbar palsy and supranuclear gaze palsy. The gait or balance disturbance is often a late finding.

Wilson's disease is a rare autosomal recessive disease that causes symptoms as a result of abnormal accumulation of copper in various organs, especially the brain and liver. Central nervous system symptoms include tremor, at rest or with action, dysarthria, dystonia, rigidity and bradykinesia. Psychiatric symptoms can occur at onset, usually in the first three decades of life. Consequently, Wilson's disease is not an important differential diagnosis of PD in later life.

The United Kingdom Parkinson's Disease Society has developed an algorithm to aid the diagnosis of PD (see Box 14.5).

Computerised tomography and magnetic resonance imaging of the brain may help to exclude other diagnoses, such as vascular disease and normal-pressure hydrocephalus. Laboratory testing is not usually needed to diagnose PD except to rule out hypothyroidism and Wilson's disease in patients younger than 50 years.

Box 14.5 UK Parkinson's Disease Society Brain Bank Diagnostic Criteria

Step 1 Diagnosis of parkinsonian Syndrome

- Bradykinesia (slowness of initiation of voluntary movement with progressive reduction in speed and amplitude of repetitive actions)
- At least one of the following:
  - Muscular rigidity
  - 4–6 Hz rest tremor
  - Postural instability not caused by primary visual, vestibular, cerebellar or proprioceptive dysfunction

Step 2 Exclusion Criteria for PD

- Parkinsonism due to identifiable causes, such as stroke, head injury, encephalitis, neuroleptic exposure, hydrocephalus or brain tumour
- Oculogyric crises
- Sustained remissions
- Supranuclear gaze palsy
- Cerebellar signs
- Early severe autonomic insufficiency
- Early severe dementia
- Poor response to large doses of levodopa

Step 3 Supportive Criteria for PD

- Three or more required for diagnosis of definite PD
  - Unilateral onset
  - Rest tremor present
  - Progressive signs and symptoms
  - Persistent asymmetry affective side of onset
  - Excellent early response to levodopa with persistence for > 5 years
  - Levodopa induced dyskinesia
  - Clinical course of > 10 years

Treatment

Prevention

None of the currently available treatments for PD have been proven to slow progression. It was previously believed that the selective monoamine oxidase B (MAO-B) inhibitor selegilene delayed the onset of disability requiring therapy with levodopa by slowing the progression of the disease. Selegilene is a monoamine oxidase B inhibitor that prolongs the action of dopamine at the synapse. It is now thought that much of this effect was due to the amelioration of symptoms. An additional issue is whether selegilene is associated with increased mortality in PD patients. The Parkinson's Disease Research Group of the United Kingdom reported a significantly higher mortality rate on selegilene and levodopa compared to patients on levodopa alone in an open, prospective, long-term trial. Many issues have been raised regarding the methodology and results of this study and it is not currently possible to arrive at a firm conclusion regarding selegilene's effect on mortality rates in PD.

Symptomatic therapy

Early

In older patients the focus is on providing adequate symptomatic benefit in the near term with the fewest possible side effects. Symptomatic therapy is introduced when a patient experiences functional disability. Patients should be examined and observed performing activities such as writing, buttoning, drinking, feeding, speaking, arising from a chair and walking.

Anticholinergic agents, amantadine and selegilene provide only mild to moderate benefit. In older patients anticholinergic medications and amantidine are usually avoided because of cognitive side effects.

Levodopa remains the most effective treatment for PD. Most patients experience a good response on a daily levodopa dose of 400 to 600 mg/d for 3 to 5 years or more.

Levodopa is always combined with a dopa decarboxylase inhibitor to reduce peripheral side effects and enhance absorption.

If disability is due to bradykinesia, rigidity, decreased dexterity, soft speech or shuffling gait, either levodopa or a dopamine agonist should be introduced. The medication should be started at a low dose, slowly escalated and titrated to control symptoms. In younger patients many clinicians elect to use a dopamine agonist (e.g. bromocriptine 2.5 mg 3 times a day) as initial therapy and add levodopa when the dopamine agonist no longer provides adequate symptomatic control. There is some evidence that this is associated with a lower incidence of dyskinesias and fluctuations long-term.

For older individuals and demented patients who may be prone to the side effects from dopamine agonists and those likely to require treatment for a few years, a dopamine agonist is not used and levodopa is the primary symptomatic therapy.

The controlled release formulation of levodopa and dopa decarboxylase inhibitor has been demonstrated to provide significantly greater long-term improvement in activities of daily living than immediate release levodopa/carbidopa. If no improvement in bradykinesia or rigidity is apparent after several weeks of therapy at adequate dosage, then the diagnosis should be reviewed and other causes of Parkinsonism should be considered.

Later

Motor fluctuations occur in approximately 50% of patients after 5 years of levodopa therapy and 70% among those treated for 15 years. As PD progresses, fewer dopamine neurons are available to store and release dopamine derived from levodopa. Motor fluctuations are the consequence of diminishing dopamine neuron storage capacity such that the clinical response begins to fluctuate more and more closely in concert with plasma levodopa levels. As the disease progresses, failing endogenous synthesis and capacity to store dopamine in presynaptic neurons and post-synaptic changes contribute to the shorter duration of levodopa effect.

'Wearing off' is the perception of loss of mobility or dexterity, usually over a period of minutes, related to the timing of medications. Wearing off can be managed by more frequent doses of standard levodopa, controlled release levodopa (lower bioavailability often requires an increase in total dosage), addition of a dopamine agonist and drugs designed to extend the duration of response to levodopa, dopamine or both. These include the MAO-B antagonist selegilene and the catechol O-methyl transferase (COMT) inhibitors. COMT inhibitors decrease peripheral levodopa metabolism and prolong its half-life, making more levodopa available. They smooth serum levodopa fluctuations and augment and extend the clinical response to levodopa, reducing off time (when the patient is immobile and rigid). Increased dyskinesias and hallucinations may require a reduction in the dose of levodopa. Unfortunately, problems with hepatic toxicity have limited the usefulness of some of these agents.

Dyskinesia is initially related to peak dose plasma levodopa levels and is termed 'peak dose dyskinesia'. Square wave dyskinesias persist throughout the response to an individual dose. Peak dose and square wave dyskinesias may improve in response to a lower dose of levodopa.

Diphasic dyskinesias particularly affect the lower body, at the onset or end of the response to medication. This pattern occurs during the period when plasma levodopa levels are rising and falling through a window, above which the movements lessen and below which off symptoms recur. Because these motor fluctuations do not seem to correlate with plasma levodopa levels, increasing emphasis is usually placed on dopamine agonist therapy. Disabling dyskinesias are often resistant to currently available treatments.

Dystonic posturing of a limb is usually due to a low level of dopaminergic stimulation, typically occurring in off periods.

Treatment of motor fluctuations is aided by correlating specific symptoms with the levodopa dosing cycle and maintaining plasma levels within a therapeutic window. This may require frequent smaller dosing of the standard preparation as often as every 2 hours or conversion to the controlled release formulation. Conversion to the controlled release tablet, however, delays intestinal absorption and may produce a delay in morning response, prolong peak dose dyskinesia and potentiate dyskinesia later in the day. A dose of the standard preparation on waking, in addition to the controlled release preparation, helps to ameliorate the delay in morning response.

Apomorphine is indicated when levodopa responses become erratic and marred by fluctuations in motor responses, on–off oscillations (rapid and unpredictable fluctuations) and dyskinesias. It can be administered either as a subcutaneous 'rescue' injection or continuous infusion. Apomorphine appears to have an antagonistic effect on the side effects of levodopa, such as dyskinesia and nausea, and has a low incidence of neuropsychiatric problems. Timed injections of apomorphine may help specific symptoms such as off-period pain, belching, screaming, constipation, nocturia, restless legs syndrome, dystonias, erectile incompetence and post-surgical state in selected patients.

Rapid and unpredictable fluctuations (on–off effects with the patient changing from immobile and rigid to mobile and dyskinetic) develop as the response to levodopa becomes less graded, with small changes in concentration producing large changes in response. At this stage, there is an important contribution of pharmacokinetic factors—for example, delayed gastric emptying may cause delayed onset of effect or dose failure.

Approaches to improve the absorption of levodopa, including cisapride and restriction of dietary protein, have also been used.

When the patient has an inadequate response to the peak effect of levodopa, it is important to review the accuracy of the diagnosis and to ask whether the target symptoms are typically levodopa resistant. Levodopa resistant symptoms can sometimes worsen paradoxically in response to higher doses of levodopa or dopamine agonists (e.g. on-period freezing of gait, falling or dysarthria). A cautious trial of a lower dose of these agents should be considered.

Psychiatric disturbances

Depression is very common in PD but treatment poses some challenges. Elderly patients are more susceptible to the anticholinergic effects of the tricyclic antidepressants. There is also a theoretical concern about the use of selective serotonin reuptake inhibitors because of their potential to worsen parkinsonism and to interact adversely with selegilene.

If visual hallucinations develop it is important to rule out a systemic illness such as a concurrent infection or a metabolic disturbance. The drugs with low ratios of therapeutic to toxic effects should then be eliminated. These include anticholinergic drugs, amantidine and selegilene. The dose of the dopamine agonist and then levodopa should be reduced to a minimum.

If hallucinations are mild, infrequent and not threatening, one can then monitor the patient. In the case of more severe hallucinations or psychosis, the use of an atypical neuroleptic agent is indicated. Clozapine, at daily doses of 45 mg or less, significantly improves drug induced psychosis without worsening parkinsonism. The major limitation of clozapine is the necessity of weekly blood counts because of the 1–2% incidence of neutropenia. Olanzapine is effective in the suppression of hallucinosis but in larger dosage increments may increase motor disability. These agents may increase parkinsonism although this is unusual when used in low dosage. Generally, there is no justification for drug holidays as they may be associated with substantial morbidity.

Autonomic disturbances

Prolonged gastrointestinal transit time is seen in more than 80% of patients and constipation is described in 60% of patients. Biopsy reveals diminished dopaminergic neurons in the myenteric plexus of the colon and Lewy bodies in the peripheral autonomic ganglia and the interomediolateral cell column of the spinal cord. Constipation may be initially treated by gradually increasing the potency of the therapy and discontinuing anticholinergic agents. Other measures include increasing the dietary intake of fibre, fluids and increasing physical activity as well as the sequential addition of stool softeners, lactulose, laxatives and enemas (see Chapter 35). Cisapride may also be used to treat constipation and also delay gastric emptying.

Urinary frequency, urgency and nocturia are usually due to detrusor hyperactivity and may respond to anticholinergic medication such as oxybutynin 5–30 mg/d. If this approach is unsuccessful then urologic evaluation may be required.

Orthostatic hypotension increases with age and severity of PD. Symptoms include lightheadedness, initial dizziness when standing, fatigue and pain across the back of the shoulders and neck. Simple treatments include the withdrawal of antihypertensive drugs, increasing fluid and salt intake and compression stockings. If these measures are not sufficient, volume expansion with fludrocortisone may be helpful.

Excessive sweating is most often a function of plasma levodopa fluctuations and is often seen with peak dose dyskinesia when dyskinesia develops as the serum levodopa concentration peaks. Levodopa dosage adjustment to lower peak plasma levodopa levels and the addition of a dopamine agonist may be helpful.

Sleep disorders

Sleep problems are common in PD. Cramping, particularly in the side worst affected with PD, may result from wearing off from levodopa. Bedtime dosing of a sustained release preparation may be helpful.

All anti-PD medications (with the exception of selegilene) can produce sleepiness but it is most often due to dopamine agonists. If medication reduction cannot be accomplished, selegilene 5 mg at breakfast and lunch may be helpful.

Non-pharmacologic management strategies

Education is critical in the development of a positive attitude towards PD and offers the patient a degree of control in managing PD. Parkinson's disease societies provide information and support for patients and families and organise education and management tips.

After an intensive rehabilitation program, PD patients show improvement in mobility, grip strength and flexibility. However, they return to baseline after 6 months if a regular exercise program is not continued.

If freezing (sudden immobility while walking) occurs at the initiation of walking or when walking through narrow spaces, visual cues such as lines on the floor may be beneficial. A home safety evaluation by an occupational therapist can provide recommendations for a safe environment in the home to help maintain the PD patient's independence. Devices such as handrails, flexible shower hoses, bath boards, dressing aids, emergency call systems and special clothing can make life more manageable for both the caregiver and the patient. Speech therapy can assist in the management of dysarthria and dysphagia.

Surgical therapy and restorative therapy

Surgery is reserved for disabling, medically refractory problems. The introduction of magnetic resonance imaging and the use of microelectrode recording techniques have improved the safety and accuracy of functional neurosurgical procedures.

Interventions at the ventrointermediate thalamic nucleus provide approximately 80% reduction in contralateral tremor. Disabling akinesia is not improved, although rigidity may decrease and levodopa induced dyskinesias may also improve. However, this may not be accompanied by improvement in activities of daily living. Ablative procedures are still associated with a risk of permanent complications, particularly when bilateral lesions are created surgically.

Pallidotomy (involving a lesion of the globus pallidus) is associated with an improvement of 80% or more in contralateral drug induced dyskinesias and significant reductions in contralateral akinesia, rigidity and tremor. These benefits translate into improvements in activities of daily living, although the improvements in gait and postural symptoms may be relatively short-lived.

Long-term electrical stimulation through implanted deep brain electrodes is being studied as a potentially reversible and adjustable treatment method and appears to provide good control of tremor. The mechanism of action is probably inhibition of the neurons around the electrode tip. Bilateral stimulation can be applied without the high morbidity associated with bilateral destructive lesions. Unfortunately, akinesia is not alleviated.

Prognosis

PD generally progresses gradually and has a prolonged course, although the rate of progression is very variable. Over time most patients have increasing difficulty with speech, eating, washing, dressing and mobility as the disease progresses. A number of studies have shown that with current treatment PD does not shorten life expectancy.

Progressive supranuclear palsy

Introduction

The first clinicopathologic description of progressive supranuclear palsy (PSP) dates from 1963 when Richardson reported a series of eight cases of parkinsonism in combination with supranuclear palsy. PSP is also referred to as Steele-Richardson-Olszewski syndrome.

Aetiology and epidemiology

Progressive supranuclear palsy is the most common form of degenerative parkinsonism after Parkinson's disease. The average annual incidence rate is estimated to be 5.3 new cases per 100 000 person-years for ages 50 to 99; it increases steeply with age from 1.7 at 50 to 59 years to 14.7 at 80 to 99 years and is consistently higher in men. However, these incidence figures are probably an underestimate since it takes at least half of the disease course to diagnose a case and many PSP patients die with other diagnoses. In data from the United Kingdom Parkinson's Disease Brain Bank, 6% of 100 prospectively followed patients dying with the clinical diagnosis of Parkinson's disease actually had PSP at autopsy, and 58% of 24 patients with pathologically confirmed PSP died with a diagnosis of Parkinson's disease.

The presence of tau protein in neurofibrillary tangles suggests a possible involvement of tau in the pathogenesis of PSP. Recent case control studies with sporadic PSP suggest that PSP is a recessive disorder in linkage disequilibrium with the tau A0/A0 genotype. Possible aetiological mechanisms include the presence of abnormalities of the tau gene leading to the formation of abnormal tau proteins and development of neurofibrillary tangles and decreased neurotrophic factors promoting accelerated neuronal necrosis and apoptosis.

Pathophysiology

PSP is characterised by abundant neurofibrillary tangles formed by aggregated tau protein and/or neurophil threads in areas of the basal ganglia and brain stem. There is accompanying neuronal loss and gliosis. Macroscopically there is marked dilatation of the third ventricle and volume loss of the periaqueductal area of the midbrain.

Clinical tests

Supranuclear ophthalmoplegia is the most important clinical sign for the diagnosis of PSP. The eye movements are examined to command and pursuit and the oculocephalic movements are tested by having the patient fix on an object held at arm's length in front of her and then moving her head up and down and from side to side. Usually movements to command are more affected than those to pursuit and, by definition, the oculocephalic movements are preserved. Downward gaze palsy has to be present for the gaze palsy to be significant because upward gaze palsy can occur in Parkinson's disease, other neurologic illnesses and some normal elderly individuals.

Clinical features

The onset of this condition is typically in the seventh decade and can be very difficult to diagnose in the early stages. Falls are a common presenting feature and more than half of patients with PSP have repeated falls during the first year of symptom onset. Patients often pivot and fall backwards when turning. Patients present with:

- early postural instability and falls;
- a peculiar wide based, slow and unsteady gait;
- supranuclear vertical gaze palsy followed by horizontal gaze abnormalities;
- Parkinsonism characterised by symmetric bradykinesia;
- axial more than limb rigidity not benefiting from levodopa therapy;
- early dysarthria and dysphagia;
- frontal-type cognitive disturbances.

The cardinal feature of the disorder is the supranuclear gaze disturbance. This preferentially affects saccadic eye movements, particularly downward gaze. Slowing of saccades and decreased saccade amplitude may precede the supranuclear gaze palsy in PSP patients.

Symmetric bradykinesia, rigidity and tremor are seen in some patients. The akinesia and rigidity are greater proximally than distally. Rigidity is typically lead-pipe throughout the range of movement rather than cogwheel, and affects axial extensor muscles more than appendicular musculature, in contrast to Parkinson's disease. Nuchal rigidity is present in approximately 50% of cases covered by axial rigidity. Tremor is not a feature. Pyramidal signs eventually occur in one-third of patients. Limb dystonia, blepharospasm and oromandibular dystonia are common dystonic manifestations of PSP.

Gait is always abnormal in PSP and is usually affected in the early stages. PSP patients have a stiff, broad based gait with an ataxic quality. In contrast to PD patients, these patients often have preserved arm swing when walking. Slowness, shortness of stride, shuffling, festinating, freezing and postural instability are other features of PSP gait.

There is early slurring of speech because of spastic dysarthria, and speech can be slow with a strained, strangled quality. Dysphagia also occurs early and tends to progress. Approximately 50% of patients report dysphagia by 5 years (see Chapter 32).

Patients with PSP usually exhibit early frontal lobe problems, including cognitive slowing, apathy, impairment of abstract thought, decreased verbal fluency, concrete thought and difficulty with planning and problem solving.

Diagnosis

The National Institute of Neurological Disorders and Stroke (NINDS) and the Society for PSP (SPSP) have developed a set of diagnostic criteria. Probable PSP requires the presence of a gradually progressive disorder with onset at age 40 or later, vertical supranuclear gaze palsy, prominent postural instability and falls in the first year of onset.

Computerised tomography and magnetic resonance imaging may show atrophy of the midbrain and the region around the third ventricle in more than one half of PSP patients. Imaging may also exclude other diagnoses such as corticobasal degeneration (asymmetric atrophy in the parietal area), multiple system atrophy (atrophy of the pons, middle cerebellar peduncles and cerebellum or altered signal intensity in the putamen), multi-infarct states, hydrocephalus or tumours.

The differential diagnosis of PSP includes the conditions listed in Box 14.7. In Parkinson's disease the parkinsonian signs are usually asymmetric. Multiple system atrophy is usually differentiated by the presence of severe autonomic signs, cerebellar disturbance with normal cognition and behaviour. Corticobasal degeneration is characterised by asymmetric onset, unilateral ideomotor apraxia, unilateral cortical sensory signs, unilateral visual neglect and severe unilateral dystonia.

Box 14.6 NINDS-SPSP Clinical Criteria for Probable PSP

- Gradually progressive disorder
- Onset at age 40 years or later
- Vertical supranuclear ophthalmoparesis (either severe upward or any downward gaze abnormalities)
- Prominent postural instability with falls within first year of symptom onset

Box 14.7 Differential diagnosis of progressive supranuclear palsy

- Parkinson's disease
- Multiple system atrophy
- Corticobasal degeneration
- Creutzfeldt-Jakob disease
- Diffuse Lewy body disease
- Pick's disease
- Multi-infarct state

Treatment

Although levodopa in combination with carbidopa is widely used in the early stages of PSP, the benefit is always mild and brief. The response to dopamine agonists has been similar with increased adverse effects. Nevertheless, in the absence of more effective treatment, these therapies should be tried when slowness or rigidity is present.

Anticholinergics and amantidine are minimally effective in PSP, even less than levodopa. Physostigmine, a cholinesterase inhibitor, improves long-term verbal memory and visuospatial attention slightly, but worsens gait. In a study of 12 cases of autopsy confirmed PSP, use of anti-parkinsonian medications and other neurotransmitter replacement therapies were largely ineffective and caused frequent adverse effects.

Low dose amitriptyline may significantly improve severe motor dysfunction in PSP. Dosing must be individualised for optimal response and minimal toxicity. Amitriptyline has also been reported to improve the emotional incontinence. Non-pharmacological management includes the use of prisms for gaze palsy. Speech therapy may assist by providing alternative means of communication and assist the dysphagic patient by teaching safer swallowing techniques and monitoring the patient for the need for feeding gastrostomy.

Weighted and wheeled walking frames serve as counterbalance against falls and are more stable than conventional walking frames.

Prognosis

The median survival time from symptom onset is estimated to be 5.6 years (range 2–16.6 years). The onset of falls during the first year, early dysphagia and incontinence predicts a shorter survival time.

Motor neuron disease

Introduction

Motor neuron disease (MND) is a devastating, neurodegenerative disease affecting pyramidal neurons of the corticospinal tract (upper motor neurons), brain stem motor nerve nuclei and spinal cord anterior horn cells (lower motor neurons). It results in progressive muscle weakness and wasting, usually accompanied by pathologically brisk reflexes, eventually involving the limb, bulbar and respiratory muscles. The term amyotrophic lateral sclerosis (ALS) is widely used interchangeably with MND, although ALS is strictly the combination of upper and lower motor neuron degeneration. Both terms are used to encompass limb and bulbar onset forms of the disease.

Aetiology and epidemiology

The annual incidence of MND is between 1 and 2 per 100 000, with a clear male predominance. In most studies, the mean age of onset is between 55 and 60 years. The age specific incidence rises steeply with age, reaching 1 in 10 000 per year between the ages of 65 and 85 years. The disease is sporadic in 90% of cases but about 10% are familial, usually with an autosomal dominant mode of inheritance.

Multiple different gene products can set the scene for motor neuron degeneration. More than 60 different mutations have been described in about 250 pedigrees of familial motor neuron disease. One of the most important findings has been that mutations in the gene on chromosome 21 encoding the enzyme copper/zinc superoxide dismutase underlie 20% of familial cases of motor neuron disease and 2% of all cases. Another form of familial motor neuron syndrome occurs in X-linked bulbospinal atrophy (Kennedy's disease). This mutation in the androgen receptor gene causes a progressive atrophy of limb and bulbar muscles as well as gynaecomastia and testicular atrophy.

A number of hypotheses have been formulated to explain the aetiology of MND. It has been postulated to be an autoimmune disease; however, immunotherapy has proved unsuccessful thus far. An alternative hypothesis explains damage to the motor neurons in MND by excessive formation of free radicals. This hypothesis is supported by the discovery of an association between familial MND and mutations in the copper-zinc superoxide dismutase gene on chromosome 21. A causative role of superoxide dismutase dysfunction has not been firmly established; nevertheless, therapeutic trials with antioxidants in MND are being considered. A further hypothesis involves glutamate. Glutamate is the principal excitatory neurotransmitter in the brain and spinal cord. Excessive activation of glutamate receptors mediates neuronal injury or death. The glutamate hypothesis offers opportunities for pharmacotherapy and new drugs have been developed using this theoretical basis.

Pathophysiology

Motor neuron disease causes progressive injury and cell death of lower motor neuron groups in the spinal cord and brain stem and usually of upper motor neurons in the motor cortex. The precise cause of the neurodegenerative process remains unknown. The selectivity of the disease process for the motor system is now recognised to be relative rather than absolute. Motor neuron disease is now regarded as a multisystem disease in which the motor neurons tend to be affected earliest and most severely.

Clinical tests

Those affected typically develop a combination of upper and lower motor neuron signs with progressive muscle weakness and wasting usually accompanied by pathologically brisk reflexes, eventually involving the limb and bulbar muscles. Lower motor neuron signs include fasciculations, atrophy and weakness. Fasciculations may be seen in the tongue, around the shoulders, in the thighs and calves. The patient should be undressed completely to examine for fasciculations and the muscles completely relaxed. The patient should sit forward to aid examination of the shoulders from behind. Muscle atrophy may be difficult to assess in elderly persons but asymmetrical wasting is more likely to be pathological. Bulbar palsy is manifest by fasciculations of the tongue, wasting and weakness. Fasciculations and wasting are best observed with the tongue resting in the floor of the mouth.

Clinical features of diseased upper motor neurons are spasticity, clonus, brisk tendon reflexes and extensor plantar responses. Pseudobulbar palsy due to bilateral upper motor neuron lesions affecting the bulbar muscles is characterised by a brisk jaw jerk, a small, stiff tongue which moves slowly and 'Donald Duck' speech.

Motor neuron disease may also be associated with frontal lobe dementia and aphasia characterised by word-finding difficulties. The aphasia may be masked by dysarthria and missed if not specifically examined.

Diagnosis

The predominant symptom of motor neuron disease is weakness. The sensory system is clinically spared. The presence of abnormalities of both lower and upper motor neurons should be established. About a third of patients will present with symptoms of a bulbar or pseudobulbar palsy, a third with weakness of the upper limbs, and the remaining third with symptoms and signs in the lower limbs. Clinical variants of the disease may affect purely the lower motor neurons (progressive muscular atrophy) or the upper motor neurons (primary lateral sclerosis). A notable feature of MND is the sparing of the oculomotor cranial nerve neurons and the bowel and bladder sphincters until very late in the illness.

Creatine kinase is often raised by up to 3–4 times the normal level. Nerve conduction studies and electromyography help to localise the pathological process and demonstrate evidence of widespread denervation of anterior horn cell origin without motor nerve conduction block.

In the differential diagnosis of MND it is important to consider spinal cord lesions, in particular cervical myelopathy. The combination of a spastic paraparesis and lower motor neuron signs in the upper limbs should always lead to close scrutiny of the spinal cord. Magnetic resonance imaging is indicated to exclude compression or infiltration of the spinal cord. Multiple cerebrovascular accidents may also need to be considered, although a pure motor syndrome is unlikely. Inclusion body myositis preferentially involves the quadriceps and finger flexors. Muscle biopsy may be helpful when electromyography is either equivocal or suggestive of a myopathic process.

Pure motor neuropathies such as the late manifestations of poliomyelitis, diabetic amyotrophy and multifocal motor demyelinating neuropathy also need to be considered. Multifocal motor demyelinating neuropathy is an acquired immune mediated neuropathy characterised by slowly progressive asymmetrical predominantly distal weakness. Antiganglioside antibodies may be present. Electrophysiologic testing reveals multifocal motor demyelinating features and persistent, localised, partial motor conduction block. Most patients show marked improvement in strength after treatment with intravenous human immunoglobulin or cyclophosphamide. In chronic inflammatory demyelinating neuropathy there are symmetrical signs and there may be sensory symptoms. Raised cerebrospinal fluid protein and prolonged nerve conduction studies may be demonstrated. Steroids and other immunomodulatory treatments should be considered.

The Scottish Motor Neuron Disease Association analysed how commonly a diagnosis of MND had been made erroneously. Eight per cent of those on their Register were false positives: half had treatable diseases, which ranged from common disorders, such as cervical spondylotic myeloradiculopathy to rare disorders such as multifocal motor neuropathy. Three principal reasons led to diagnostic revision: radiological and neurophysiological investigations, a failure to progress, or the development of atypical clinical features. Comorbidity can complicate the presentation, in particular: cerebrovascular disease causing bulbar signs and spinal degenerative disease causing fasciculations.

Box 14.8 Differential diagnosis of motor neuron disease

- Spinal cord pathology, especially cervical myelopathy
- Multiple cerebrovascular accidents
- Inclusion body myositis
- Chronic inflammatory demyelinating neuropathy
- Pure motor neuropathies, e.g.:
  - multifocal motor neuropathy
  - diabetic amyotrophy
  - late manifestations of poliomyelitis

Treatment

Riluzole is a sodium channel blocker that inhibits the release of glutamate and has several other potentially neuroprotective effects. It became the first drug approved for use in MND after studies demonstrated a modest effect in prolonging survival (by about 3 months after 18 months administration). The decision to begin treatment with riluzole should include a careful discussion with the patient, balancing the substantial cost of the drug against the modest change in survival and lack of any demonstrated functional benefit.

A small trial of N-acetylcysteine (an antioxidant) found a non-significant improvement in survival in patients whose disease symptoms started in the limb muscles. Insulin-like growth factor 1, a neurotrophic factor, has produced a positive effect in slowing disease progression, but this result was not replicated in a second trial.

Baclofen can be useful for pain due to muscle cramps and stiffness related to spasticity. Sialorrhoea can be treated with amytriptyline or unilateral parotid gland radiotherapy. Emotional lability may respond to amitriptyline or selective serotonin reuptake inhibitors.

Speech pathologists can assist with the provision of appropriate communication aids, assessment and management of swallowing difficulties. Weight loss of 10% or more denotes nutritional risk and is a good indicator that alternate feeding routes should be explored. Percutaneous endoscopic gastrostomy (PEG) feeding has been shown to maintain weight and significantly improve survival. In many cases patients may continue to eat what they enjoy and can still manage orally, while the feeding tube reduces the burden of eating for kilojoules.

The physiotherapist can instruct the patient and family in proper exercise techniques, safe and efficient transfers and prescribe assisting devices such as sticks, walking frames and ankle foot orthoses. Occupational therapy interventions include upper extremity bracing and provision of adaptive equipment such as large handled eating utensils, velcro fasteners for dressing, reaching devices and bathroom equipment. A wheelchair is eventually required for mobility for almost all patients and appropriate prescription should include planning for future modifications.

When skeletal and respiratory weakness rather than bulbar muscle weakness predominates, non-invasive ventilation can be used to manage hypoventilation. Chest wall and diaphragmatic weakness can cause significant distress. A history of specific respiratory symptoms and symptoms of hypoventilation (poor sleep, daytime somnolence, morning headache) should be sought as early indications of respiratory compromise. The aim should be to provide symptomatic relief, enhancing quality of life rather than prolonging it. Non-invasive positive pressure ventilation avoids tracheostomy, and has been shown to improve survival and respiratory symptoms. When bulbar weakness predominates and becomes severe, complications can only be prevented by permanent placement of an indwelling tracheostomy tube.

Terminal care often involves alleviating distress from respiratory failure and hospice services can prove invaluable. Oral, subcutaneous or intravenous morphine may be indicated to relieve dyspnoea, anxiety, pain or other distress.

Motor neuron disease associations provide information, advice and practical support to patients and their carers. Patients should be given the contact details for their local organisation.

Prognosis

The disease course is one of progressive weakness, atrophy, spasticity, dysarthria, dysphagia and respiratory failure due to weakness of the ventilatory muscles. The average 5 year survival rate is 30%.

Multiple system atrophy

Introduction

Multiple system atrophy (MSA) describes a group of degenerative syndromes with overlapping clinical and pathological manifestations. The conditions covered by this term are striatonigral degeneration, olivopontocerebellar atrophy and Shy-Drager syndrome. The three major clinical manifestations are parkinsonism, ataxia and autonomic failure.

Aetiology and epidemiology

Of the three subtypes constituting MSA, only olivopontocerebellar atrophy occurs clearly on a familial basis, with most kindreds showing an autosomal dominant inheritance. Both sexes are affected and symptoms begin typically in middle age but may appear in later life.

Pathophysiology

The different clinical subtypes are associated with varying degrees of pathologic change. Loss of cells relating to parkinsonism occurs in the substantia nigra zona compacta. Striatal cell loss occurs in the putamen, external globus pallidus and the locus coeruleus. Cases with prominent ataxia show marked loss of pontine nuclei and the middle cerebellar peduncle. Pathways related to autonomic functioning that are affected include the interomediolateral cell column of the spinal cord and the dorsal motor nucleus of the vagus nerve.

Clinical tests

The relative ineffectiveness of anti-parkinsonian medications and the presence of pyramidal signs can be useful in establishing a diagnosis of MSA versus Parkinson's disease. Autonomic testing may be helpful in distinguishing between MSA and Parkinson's disease, although the sensitivity and specificity are less than ideal. These tests include tilt table testing of blood pressure and heart rate response.

Diagnosis

Parkinsonism is demonstrated in approximately 90% of patients with MSA. Bradykinesia and rigidity are the most notable features. Tremor occurs in about two-thirds of patients, although it is not usually pill-rolling.

Extraocular movement abnormalities are common, particularly abnormal pursuit movements. Pyramidal findings, including brisk reflexes, and upgoing plantars occur in two-thirds of patients. Ataxia occurs in about one half of patients, often initially in the lower limbs.

Autonomic failure may lead to orthostatic hypotension, dysphagia, constipation, faecal incontinence, urinary incontinence, urinary retention, impotence and hyperhidrosis or hypohidrosis. Frontal lobe dysfunction may result in deficits in abstract reasoning, learning and memory, visuospatial and executive functions.

Magnetic resonance imaging shows pontine and cerebellar atrophy in olivopontocerebellar atrophy.

Treatment

Anti-parkinsonian medications should be attempted because a mild response is not infrequently present, particularly early in the course of the illness. Levodopa is usually tried first. Patients who fail to respond to levodopa occasionally respond to a dopamine receptor agonist.

Orthostatic hypotension may be managed by a number of means, including sleeping with the head elevated, caffeine-containing beverages after meals, support stockings, indomethacin, fludrocortisone, intranasal desmopressin and ephedrine. Physical and occupational therapy may provide benefit in activities of daily living.

Prognosis

The disease course is unfortunately one of gradually progressive disability over years or decades.

Bibliography and further reading

Bennett, D. A., Beckett, L. A., Murray, A. M. et al. (1996), 'Prevalence of parkinsonian signs and associated mortality in a community population of older people', *New England Journal of Medicine*, 334(2), pp. 71–6.

Compston, D. A. S. (1999), 'Motor neuron disease and its management', *Journal of the Royal College of Physicians of London*, 33, pp. 212–18.

Davenport, R. J., Swingler, R. J., Chancellor, A. M. & Warlow, C. P. (1996), 'Avoiding false positive diagnoses of motor neuron disease: Lessons from the Scottish Motor Neuron Disease Register', *Journal of Neurology, Neurosurgery and Psychiatry*, 60(2), pp. 147–51.

Francis, K., Bach, J. R. & DeLisa, J. (1999), 'Evaluation and rehabilitation of patients with adult motor neuron disease', *Archives of Physical Medicine and Rehabilitation*, 80, pp. 951–63.

Lang, A. E. & Lozano, A. M. (1998a), 'Parkinson's disease. First of two parts', *New England Journal of Medicine*, 339(15), pp. 1044–53.

Lang, A. E. & Lozano, A. M. (1998b), 'Parkinson's disease. Second of two parts', *New England Journal of Medicine*, 339(16), pp. 1130–43.

Litvan, I. (1998), 'Progressive supranuclear palsy revisited', *Acta Neurologica Scandinavica*, 98, pp. 73–84.

Litvan, I. & Hutton, M. (1998), 'Clinical and genetic

aspects of progressive supranuclear palsy', *Journal of Geriatric Psychiatry and Neurology*, 11, pp. 107–14.

The Parkinson Study Group (1999), 'Low dose clozapine for the treatment of drug-induced psychosis in Parkinson's disease', *New England Journal of Medicine*, 340(10), pp. 757–63.

Schapira, A. H. V. (1999), 'Parkinson's disease', *British Medical Journal*, 318(7179), pp. 311–14.

Shaw, P. J. (1999), 'Motor neurone disease', *British Medical Journal*, 318(7191), pp. 1118–21.

Stern, M. B. & Hurtig, H. I. (1999), 'Parkinson's disease and Parkinsonian syndromes', *Medical Clinics of North America*, 83(2).

Stoessl, A. J. & Rivest, J. (1999), 'Differential diagnosis of Parkinsonism', *Canadian Journal of Neurological Science*, 26 (Suppl.), pp. 2-S1–S4.

Chapter 15

Dementia and Alzheimer's disease

JANE HECKER

Introduction

With an ageing population, Alzheimer's disease (AD) and the other neurodegenerative conditions have an increasing medical, social and economic impact. Approximately 5% of people aged over 65 have some form of dementia, with the incidence increasing exponentially with age. The advent of drug therapy for AD increases the importance of accurate assessment and diagnosis to distinguish the diseases causing the dementia syndrome.

Alzheimer's disease

Alzheimer's disease, the most common cause of dementia, accounts for approximately 60% of dementia in Australia.

Neuropathology

While we still lack a clear understanding of the cause of AD, the typical neuropathological changes are now well recognised (Figure 15.1). These include:

- neuronal degeneration
- reduced synapse density
- senile plaques (extracellular deposits of β-amyloid protein) (Figure 15.2)
- neurofibrillary tangles (intracellular deposits of the fibrillary protein tau, thought to interfere with cellular metabolism) (Figure 15.3).

A definitive diagnosis of AD has traditionally relied on neuropathological changes in the setting of an appropriate clinical history, as a 'gold standard'. The situation in practice is more complex, however, as the neuropathological assay techniques and the significance of different neuropathological lesions are still debated. Microscopically evident brain changes, notably neurofibrillary tangles and amyloid plaques, have long been recognised as occurring in AD. Neurofibrillary tangles are intraneuronal structures containing paired helical filaments of hyperphosphorylated protein, tau. The diagnostic and prognostic meaning of the diverse morphology of amyloid plaques remains controversial. The most important form is the neuritic plaque that is composed of a central core of β-amyloid and a reactive outer zone with fibrillary, cellular and inflammatory material. The β-amyloid, the core of the senile

Light micrographs of human brain in Alzheimer's dementia

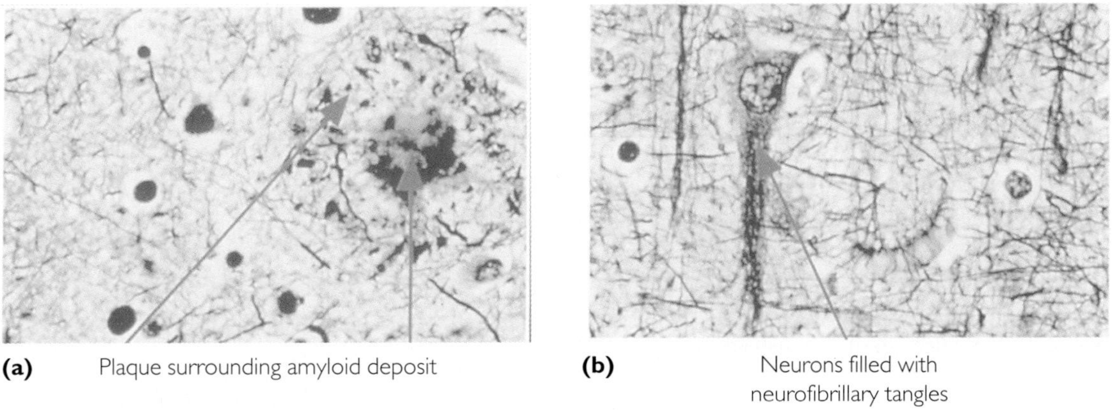

Figure 15.1 (a) and (b) GAUTHIER SCIENCE PHOTO LIBRARY (1996)

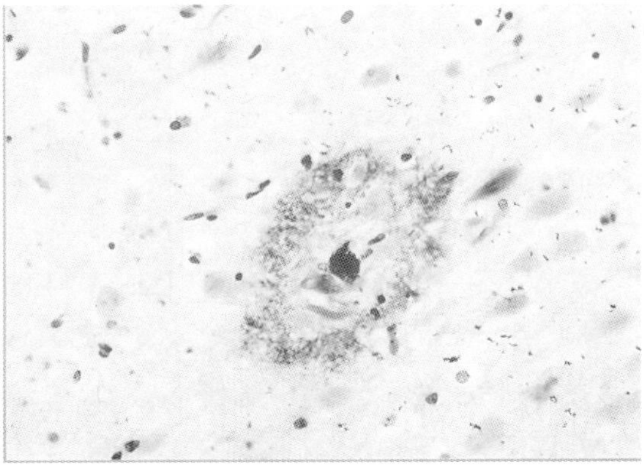

Figure 15.2 Neuropathology of Alzheimer's disease—neuritic plaque GAUTHIER (1996) DR J RICHARDSON

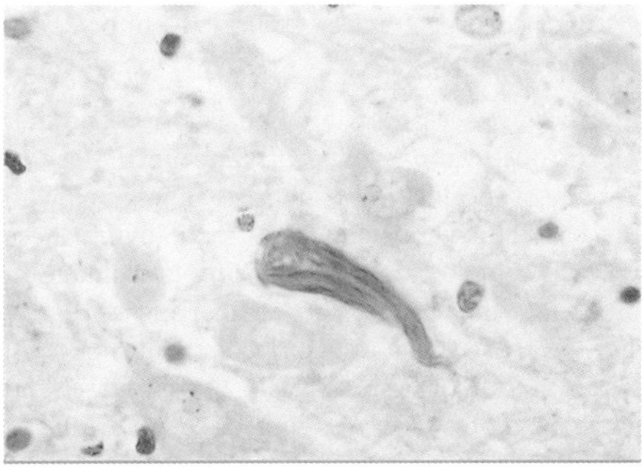

Figure 15.3 Neuropathology of Alzheimer's disease—neurofibrillary tangle

plaque, is known to be composed of a 42–43 amino acid peptide, the β-amyloid peptide. This peptide is cleaved from the larger molecule, amyloid precursor protein (APP).

Although there is increasing knowledge regarding the precise molecular nature and aetiology of AD pathology, two fundamental findings limit the diagnostic value of neuropathological findings. The neuropathological hallmarks are not unique to AD, also being present in normal ageing and other neurodegenerative diseases. Because these features are not pathognomonic of AD and, in particular, because of the overlap with normal ageing, the emphasis in AD diagnosis has been on quantifying the changes in supporting or confirming a clinical diagnosis. Amyloid appears to have a key role in AD but not all studies have shown correlation between the amyloid burden, total plaque count and dementia severity.

Plaque and tangle numbers are counted per light microscope field, with the density of these pathological features calculated for relevant brain regions. The described criteria are currently considered most favourably, although expert opinion varies regarding the most appropriate criteria. Progressive amyloid deposits occur in three stages: diffuse patchy deposits in the basal neocortex (stage A), more intensely stained plaque-like deposits spreading into the adjacent neocortex and hippocampus (stage B), and widespread through the cortical areas (stage C). The evolution and distribution patterns of the amyloid deposits are independent of the neurofibrillary changes. These include neurofibrillary tangles, neuropil threads and components of neuritic plaques which develop symmetrically in both hemispheres with significant morphological variation.

The first neurofibrillary changes develop in the transentorhinal region of the medial temporal lobe, spreading to the hippocampus and eventually the neocortex. This sequence of changes in distribution is subject to only minor interindividual variation and can be used to distinguish six stages in the evolution of lesions:

- transentorhinal stages I and II—clinically silent
- limbic stages III and IV—initial clinical symptoms and
- the neocortical stages V and VI—fully developed AD.

These observations are consistent with other recent observations that correlate linear loss of volume of specific hippocampal brain regions with the clinical severity of AD. Accompanying these volume changes are an increasing percentage of neurons with neurofibrillary change and a progressive decrease in neuron numbers. The neuronal losses appear to be linear with the temporal and clinical progression of AD, with loss of up to 90% of neurons in some hippocampal regions over the course of the disease.

The variety of AD risk factors and pathological correlates at the anatomical, cellular and molecular level support the view that a range of different mechanisms may contribute to the characteristic features of the clinical disease process. The concept that AD represents a convergence syndrome has implications for treatment, suggesting that a number of therapies directed at controlling different factors may be useful and that patients may respond differently to individual therapies.

Risk factors

Age

Age is clearly the most important risk factor for AD. The prevalence of AD rises exponentially until at least age 90. The prevalence of the disease doubles every 5 years after age 60, with 1% of individuals suffering AD at age 60 to greater than 25% affected at age 85 (Figures 15.4 and 15.5).

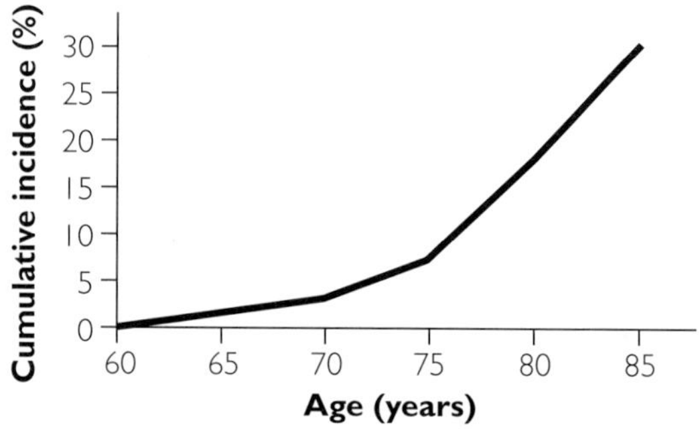

Figure 15.4 Lifetime risk of Alzheimer's disease

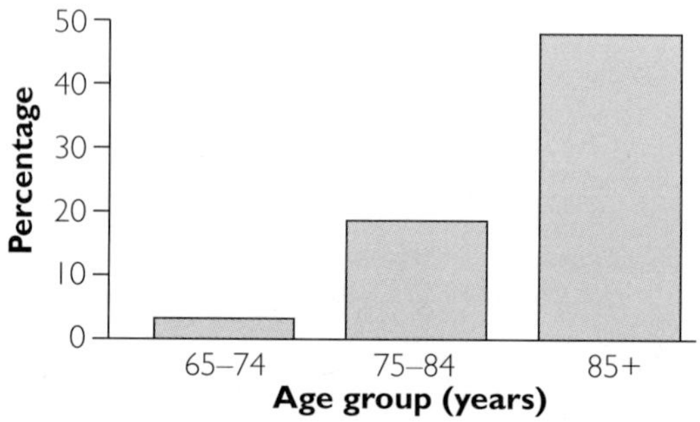

Figure 15.5 Prevalence of Alzheimer's disease according to age group in population

Genetic factors

About 50% of people with AD have a history of dementia in at least one first degree relative. A family history of AD in a first degree relative increases the relative risk of AD threefold.

A number of autosomal dominant genetic mutations (present on chromosomes 21, 14 and 1) account for about 50% of the rare early onset familial forms of AD. Mutations in the amyloid precursor protein (APP) gene on chromosome 21 were the first mutations related to early onset AD and account for 10–20% of familial AD. Individuals with Down's syndrome (trisomy 21) frequently develop the neuropathological changes of AD at a young age. Two presenilin genes, PS1 (accounting for 50%) and PS2 (rare), are also associated with early onset familial AD. Genetic testing is best performed at a recognised centre and as part of an approved research project. As known mutations do not account for all cases of early onset AD, negative screening results for these mutations would not exclude a genetic cause of the disease.

In over 90% of patients there is no clear autosomal inheritance and AD develops in a sporadic late onset pattern. An important recent discovery was the link between a polymorphism of the apolipoprotein E (apo E) gene (a cholesterol-carrying protein), located on chromosome 19 and risk of late onset sporadic AD. The ε4 allele of ApoE is associated with AD. It is found in 20–30% of the general population and in 45–60% of patients with AD. The homozygous genotype, ApoE-ε4/ε4, is found in 12–15% of patients with AD, but in only 2–3% of the general population. ApoE-ε4 correlates with an increased risk of AD, decreased age of onset, increased senile plaque density and reduced cholinergic neuron density. The mechanism of this increased risk is not yet clear. It is important to remember that ApoE-ε4 is a risk factor only, and the presence of this allele alone is neither necessary nor sufficient for the development of AD.

Currently there is considerable debate on the clinical usefulness of ApoE genotyping. The suggestion that it may increase diagnostic accuracy in patients presenting with cognitive impairment is not universally accepted. It is generally agreed that ApoE genotyping is not recommended in asymptomatic individuals with or without a family history of AD. At present, the predictive value of such testing is uncertain, as the exact significance of an ApoE-ε4 allele in asymptomatic individuals has not been confirmed. Currently there is no proven preventative treatment intervention, and the social and ethical consequences are potentially detrimental. ApoE is an area of considerable ongoing research. It may prove of value in differentiating subtypes of AD and in predicting responsiveness to future drug treatments. Other genetic risk factor genes are likely and the search for these genes continues.

Gender

Epidemiological studies have established that female sex is an independent risk factor for AD, even allowing for the increased proportion of women in the older at-risk population. Hormonal factors may relate to the explanation for this finding. The significant reduction in AD prevalence in women who have received hormone replacement therapy from menopause (relative risk reduction of approximately 50%) supports this theory.

Trauma

Head trauma has been reported as a risk factor for AD in several but not all studies.

Toxins

Epidemiological studies have not identified an environmental toxin which contributes to the development of AD. Aluminium has been shown to be neurotoxic but any link with AD is not proven.

Vascular disease

The recent European systolic hypertension study showed a link between untreated systolic hypertension and dementia, including AD. Other vascular disease, such as previous myocardial infarction, increases the risk of probable AD fivefold. Neuroradiological studies indicate that white matter abnormalities consistent with vascular damage to the brain occur in 15–30% of neurologically intact elderly, 30–60% of patients with AD and most patients with 'multi-infarct' dementia. Furthermore,

Box 15.1 Risk and protective factors for Alzheimer's disease

Risk factors
- Age
- Apolipoprotein ε4
- Family history of dementia
- Down's syndrome
- Head trauma
- Systolic arterial hypertension

Protective factors
- Apolipoprotein ε2
- High education
- Use of oestrogens
- Use of anti-inflammatory drugs

the high incidence of the ApoE-ε4 allele in patients with coronary heart disease strengthens the concept of a relationship between vascular diseases and AD.

The development of clinical symptoms in AD may be viewed as a threshold effect. The brain has a considerable reserve and it is likely that the process of brain cell loss continues for years before clinical presentation with cognitive impairment. A diagrammatic representation showing potential factors affecting this process is shown in Figure 15.6.

Clinical assessment

Dementia is a constellation of characteristic symptoms and signs with a number of specific causes, the most common of which is AD. When considering the patient's symptoms, the clinician must first diagnose the syndrome by differentiating dementia from other syndromes with similar symptoms—for example, delirium, amnesia and depression. Having diagnosed dementia, it is important to make a specific disease diagnosis by analysing the constellation of symptoms and performing appropriate further investigation (Box 15.2).

Characteristic features of Alzheimer's disease

Alzheimer's disease is the most common cause of dementia, accounting for approximately 60% of dementia in Australia. The cardinal feature is memory loss. In addition, there is impairment of cortical cognitive functions, which can include:

- aphasia (loss or impairment of language caused by brain dysfunction)
- apraxia (inability to execute learnt movements to command)
- agnosia (inability to recognise or associate meaning with a sensory perception)
- acalculia (inability to perform arithmetic calculations)
- agraphia (inability to write)
- alexia (inability to read).

Defects in executive function may involve impairments in problem solving, planning and

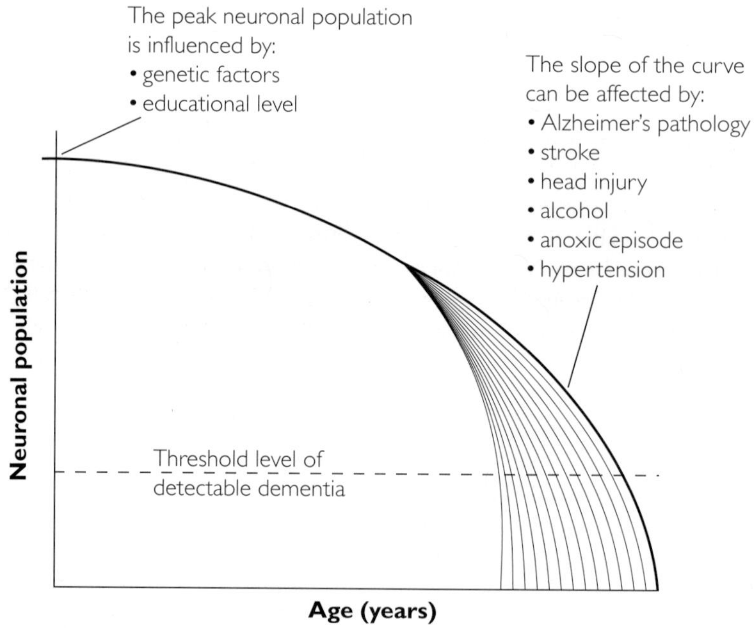

Figure 15.6 Factors affecting the age of clinical presentation with cognitive impairment. A lower peak neuronal population or a steeper slope of decline of the neuronal population will result in detectable dementia being reached at an earlier age APA (1994); HECKER (1997)

Box 15.2 DSM-IV criteria for dementia

- Memory impairment
- One of:
  - Aphasia (impaired comprehension, naming, reading, writing)
  - Apraxia (inability to perform certain movements on command or imitation)
  - Agnosia (inability to recognise familiar objects)
  - Disturbance in executive function (impaired planning, organisation, abstraction and attention)
- Impairment in occupational or social functioning
- Decline from previous level of functioning
- Deficits not occurring exclusively in the course of a delirium

Source: American Psychiatric Association (1994), *The Diagnostic and Statistical Manual*, 4th edition; J. Hecker (1997), 'What's new in dementia?', *Modern Medicine of Australia*, August, pp. 30–45.

organisation, judgment and insight. Changes in behaviour, personality and mood are also features of Alzheimer's disease and frequently cause most concern to relatives and carers.

The onset of symptoms is insidious, with a gradual and progressive loss of memory and other cognitive abilities.

Memory loss is invariable and is often the most prominent symptom and the earliest feature of the disease. Memory loss is most pronounced for *recent* events, with better retained recall of distant memories. In practice a patient will often recall precise details of childhood or early adulthood but be unable to recall events of the previous day or details of a conversation 5 minutes before. Patients with AD have difficulty registering new memory traces, unlike in age associated memory loss which is a problem of retrieval only. Patients with retrieval problems perform better with prompted recognition tasks whereas those with AD perform poorly despite prompting. Characteristic of AD memory loss is a rapid 'rate of forgetting'. Neuropsychological tests of delayed recall are thought to be most useful in detecting the significance of memory loss at an early stage and predicting rate of decline to AD. Patients with AD frequently have limited insight into the significance of their problems and tend to justify and dismiss their symptoms.

Impairment of language is characteristic of AD but is subtle in early disease. Word-finding difficulty (nominal dysphasia) can be detected in conversation or by asking the patient to name items in the environment. The difficulty of this task can be increased by asking for item names followed by parts of the item—for example, watch (face, winder, strap, buckle) or jacket (collar, lapel, cuff). Brief object-naming tests (often pictures of items) can be used for formal testing. The fluency of speech is impaired with repetition, rambling or loss of train of thought. Comprehension is also affected as disease progresses; initially patients experience difficulty following more complex concepts.

Apraxia, the presence of impairments in skilled motor activities, may also form part of the constellation of deficits present in early AD. Screening would exclude motor, sensory or co-ordination deficits as the primary problem. The earliest signs of dyspraxia include subtle changes in dress, with the normally immaculately presented patient appearing a little dishevelled. As the disease progresses, more prompting and later physical help is required to complete this task. Increasing difficulties present with personal hygiene and other household skills, including the ability to work household gadgets and equipment. In assessing apraxia patients can be asked to perform a pantomime (e.g. 'show me how you would use a key') or use an actual object ('comb your hair'). Similarly, patients can be asked to copy the examiner in this task. Patients can be tested in the home setting by an occupational therapist, who tests performance in a wide variety of tasks required for independent living.

Impairment in the ability to recognise objects is known as agnosia. When testing this domain it is important to exclude confounding problems with sensory impairment (blindness, hearing loss, parasthesia or loss of joint position sense) or aphasia. Patients can be asked to identify objects visually, by touch (e.g. recognise a coin with the eyes closed) and by sound. Visuospatial skills can be evaluated by asking patients to copy geometric figures (e.g.

intersecting pentagons or a cube). Drawing a clock-face is another useful brief screening test utilising visuospatial skills. Correct placement and spacing of the numbers can be assessed as well as accurate placement of the hands to show a nominated time (e.g. 2.45).

Geographical disorientation is a common and disabling problem. Patients initially lose the ability to orientate in an unfamiliar environment, and confusion and disorientation in a new holiday location is a common presenting symptom in the early stages of the disease. Progressively becoming lost in familiar places can result in wandering, often causing carers considerable anxiety. Finally, having difficulty finding their way in their own home can result in inability to locate the toilet.

Assessment of higher intellectual skills or executive function—including abstract thought, problem solving, planning and organisation—should be included as part of the cognitive screening. Judgment and insight are best assessed by obtaining an independent history from the family followed by discussion with the patient. Verbal fluency, involving the ability to categorise and list items, is a useful screening tool shown to be sensitive to diagnosis in the early stages of AD. Patients are asked to list as many items in a category (e.g. animals) as possible in a limited time, usually 1 minute (Table 15.1).

Behavioural and psychological symptoms are common in AD and often change in nature and severity at different stages of the disease. Early in the illness, subtle changes in personality can be sought by inquiry from family. Increase in anxiety or irritability or reduced perception of the needs of others can often be identified as one of the earliest signs of the disease. Depressive symptoms are common early in the course of the disease when insight is relatively well preserved (see discussion under 'Differential diagnosis'). Neuropsychiatric symptoms, including delusions and hallucinations, are more common later in the disease course.

Medical assessment process

The standard criteria established for the diagnosis of AD are the DSM-IV and the NINCDS-ADRDA criteria (Box 15.3). The important features of these guidelines include:

Table 15.1 Cognitive domains tested in assessing dementia

Domain	Test
Memory	Recall of a name and address Recall of recent events (check with informant) Recall of a 10 word list (delayed recall after distractor tasks)
Language	Comprehension—follow increasingly complex commands Object naming—name parts of watch (band, buckle, winder, hands) or jacket (lapel, collar, sleeve, pocket) Verbal fluency—list 10 fruits, flowers, etc.
Praxis	Bimanual pantomime (e.g. 'Show me how you would slice a loaf of bread.') Fold a piece of paper and place in envelope
Visuospatial	Draw clock and place the hands at, e.g. 2.45 Copy geometric figures, e.g. cube
Attention and concentration	Repeat sequence of numbers forwards or backwards List months of the year backwards
Calculation	Serial 7 subtraction Change calculation
Judgment/reasoning/ abstract thought	Explaining word similarities and differences (e.g. cabbage/cauliflower, mistake/lie) Proverb interpretation Hypothetical situation (e.g. water leak)

Box 15.3 NINCDS-ADRDA criteria for AD: Summary

Definite AD
- Clinical criteria for probable AD
- Histopathology of AD by biopsy or autopsy

Probable AD
- Dementia by history and neuropsychological testing
- Progressive deficits in memory and one other area of cognition
- No disturbance of consciousness
- Onset between 40 and 90
- Absence of systemic or other brain disorder causing dementia

Possible AD
- Dementia with variations in onset or course
- Presence of systemic or other brain disorder
- Single progressive cognitive deficit

- an *acquired* decline in cognitive function
- defects in at least two cognitive domains (e.g. memory, orientation, language, visuospatial function, perception, praxis and executive function)
- a deficit sufficient to have an impact on occupational or social function
- absence of a delirium, psychiatric or systemic disorder accounting for the symptoms
- *insidious* onset and *progressive* decline.

Utilising these criteria as guidelines, the diagnosis is a clinical judgment based on a careful clinical assessment (Box 15.4). This should include:

- a careful history, substantiated by a reliable informant
- physical examination, in particular a thorough neurological examination
- objective cognitive assessment (dementia can be hidden behind a well preserved social façade unless formal cognitive testing is performed)
- laboratory investigations (biochemistry, complete blood picture, erythrocyte sedimentation rate, thyroid function, vitamin B_{12} and folate, and infective screens if relevant)

Box 15.4 Diagnostic evaluation

History (reliable informant)
- General medical (include vascular risk factors)
- Neurological history
- Neuropsychiatric history
- Mode of symptom onset, pattern of cognitive impairment
- Drugs, nutrition, alcohol
- Family history

Examination
- Particularly neurological examination

Objective cognitive assessment

Laboratory investigations

Routine
- Complete blood picture
- Biochemistry
- Thyroid function
- Serum vitamin B_{12}
- Syphilis serology

Optional
- Erythrocyte sedimentation rate
- Serum folate
- HIV screen
- Chest X-ray
- Urinalysis
- Toxicology screen
- Lumbar puncture
- Electroencephalogram

Neuroimaging
- CT or MRI scan
- Optional: functional scan (e.g. SPECT)

- brain imaging (CT or MRI scan) to detect unsuspected cerebrovascular lesions and to exclude rare (approximately 1%) treatable abnormalities (Figure 15.7).

While a definitive diagnosis of the dementia type requires neuropathological examination, autopsy studies suggest that with the above approach a clinical diagnosis is 85–90% accurate in skilled hands. Early diagnostic tools for AD are being actively sought. Brain imaging techniques include the detection of selective medial temporal

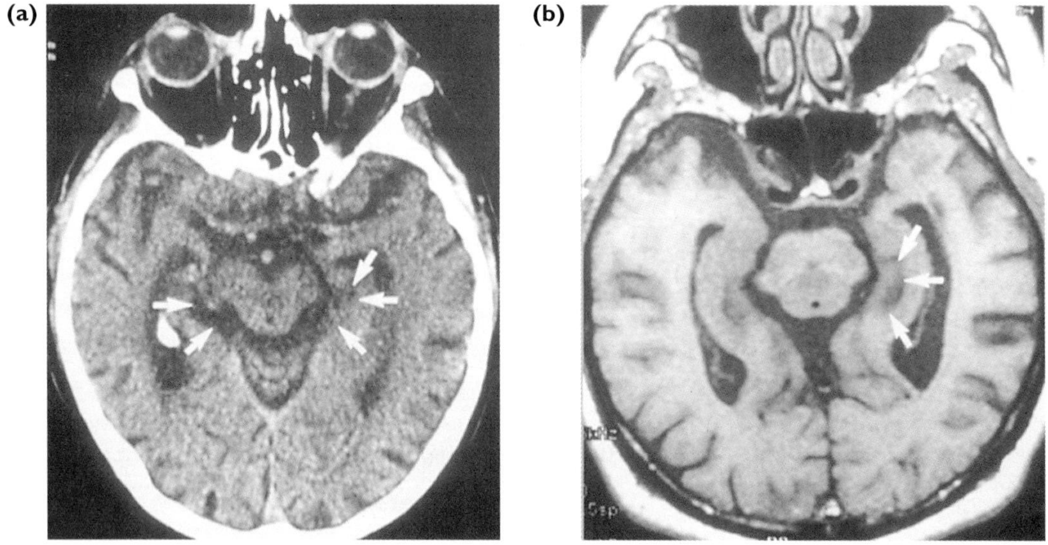

Figure 15.7 **(a)** CT head scan showing hippocampal atrophy; **(b)** MRI scan showing hippocampal and medial temporal lobe atrophy GAUTHIER, SMITH AND JOBST, DR S FONTAINE

lobe atrophy assessed by a CT scan orientated to the temporal lobe. Small reductions in cortical brain volume can be assessed by computerised measurement of serial CT or MRI scans. Functional brain scans have been developed to show changes in cerebral blood flow (SPECT scan) and the finding of bilateral posterior temporoparietal hypoperfusion, characteristic of AD, may increase diagnostic accuracy (Figure 15.8). In all brain scan techniques, however, there is overlap between normal ageing, age associated memory impairment and dementia, making accurate differentiation problematic. Biological markers for AD (e.g. CSF markers based on components of the neuropathological lesions, amyloid and tau proteins) are being developed. As yet no investigative technique in routine clinical practice can provide a definitive diagnosis.

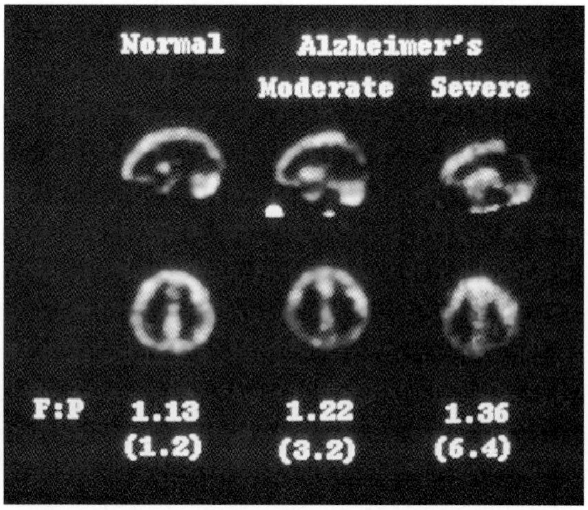

Figure 15.8 SPECT scans showing bilateral temporoparietal reduction in cerebral perfusion in moderate and severe Alzheimer's disease compared to normal

Brief screening instruments are useful for assessing the degree of cognitive impairment as they provide quick, objective and repeatable information. Two suitable instruments include the Abbreviated Mental Test Score (AMTS), and the Mini-Mental State Examination (MMSE). The AMTS is a brief 10 point scale where a score of less than 8 is indicative of cognitive impairment and should prompt further cognitive examination and investigations. The most commonly used instrument in clinical practice is the Mini-Mental State Examination (Folstein et al. 1975) (Box 15.5). The MMSE is a more detailed instrument, testing more cognitive domains, with scoring out of a maximum 30 points. This screening tool usually takes about 10 minutes to complete. As with all cognitive assessment tools, it is important to carefully follow instructions for the conduct of the test and scoring rules (see Box 15.5). Results must be interpreted in the context of the patient's educational and cultural background and other medical problems, particularly visual and hearing impairment. Most patients with dementia score below 25, but no cut-off point is definitive and some patients with low intellectual ability or education level also score below this. Patients with high intellectual and educational background can score above 25 with a clear diagnosis of dementia. Patients with early dementia, particularly those previously higher performing individuals, often require more detailed and complex testing to detect early changes in cognition. Test scores in themselves do not establish a diagnosis of dementia, nor do they determine the cause of the dementing illness.

Box 15.5 Mini-Mental State Examination (MMSE)

Maximum score	Score	
		Orientation
5	( )	What is the (year) (season) (date) (day) (month)? *One point for each correct response.*
5	( )	Where are we: (state) (country) (town or city) (hospital) (floor)? *One point for each correct response.*
		Registration
3	( )	Name 3 common objects (e.g. apple, table, penny) *One point for each correct response at the first attempt.* *Count trials and record. Trials:*
		Attention and calculation
5	( )	Serial 7s, backwards. One point for each correct response. *Stop after 5 answers.* Alternatively, spell 'WORLD' backwards. *One point for each correct response.*
		Recall
3	( )	*Ask for the 3 objects repeated above.* *One point for each correct response.*
		Language
2	( )	Name a pencil and a watch.
1	( )	Repeat the following: 'No ifs, ands, or buts.'
3	( )	Follow a 3-stage command: 'Take a paper in your right hand, fold it in half, and put it on the floor.' *One point for each part correctly executed.*
1	( )	Read and obey the following: CLOSE YOUR EYES
1	( )	Write a sentence.
1	( )	Copy the following design.
Maximum total 30	Total score ____	

Source: M. F. Folstein, S. E. Folstein & P. R. McHugh (1975), '"Mini-Mental State": A practical method for grading the cognitive state of patients for the clinician', *Journal of Psychiatry Research*, 12, pp. 189–98. Reprinted with permission.

The MMSE also has a role in assessing and quantifying disease severity. Patients with mild AD usually score 18–25, moderate dementia 10–17 and severe dementia below 10. Correlation between functional performance and score on the MMSE has been demonstrated.

Detailed neuropsychological assessment, which can be performed at specialist centres, can sometimes provide valuable additional information. This type of assessment uses detailed standardised objective testing of individual cognitive domains assessed in comparison to age matched normal ranges. Characteristic patterns of impairment can be recognised. See Box 15.6 for when to refer to a specialist or memory unit.

There are a number of advantages in diagnosing AD as early as possible. These include the following.

- Acknowledging and explaining symptoms by careful assessment and diagnosis allows discussion and sharing of concerns and distress rather than denial. Both patients and their families are usually aware of some problems and often fear the worst.
- Time for adjustment and education about the disease allows family and carers to respond appropriately. Similarly, it allows doctors to approach issues proactively rather than reacting to crisis.
- It allows the increasing number of drug treatment options to be considered. Failure to detect and diagnose AD will deprive substantial numbers of patients of effective therapies.
- It can delay institutionalisation.
- Patients and their carers have the time and ability to plan lifestyle and legal issues (e.g. legal documents, such as wills and enduring powers of attorney, and advance directives).
- A diagnosis is required to enable provision of community services to help support people in their desired lifestyle.
- Education, counselling and support can help patients and their families cope with difficulties and maximise function and quality of life.
- There is time to look at safety issues, including driving licence retention, drug compliance and home safety.
- It reduces caregiver stress.
- It can lead to involvement in research—epidemiological and drug treatment trials.

Box 15.6 When to refer to specialist/ memory unit

- Diagnostic uncertainty:
  - Atypical or complicated presentation or disease course
  - Early/mild impairment
  - Very high or low premorbid education/ intellect
  - Disease onset at young age
- Difficult to distinguish between depression and dementia (which can co-exist)
- Unexpected or rapidly deteriorating course
- Advice on newly available drug treatments
- Interest in new clinical drug trials
- Advice on testamentary capacity, driving ability or occupational competency
- Management of resistant behavioural and psychological symptoms
- Patient or family request a specialist opinion

The general practitioner often holds the key to early diagnosis. It is easy to fail to recognise cognitive impairment in routine clinical practice. Patients with Alzheimer's disease retain social skills and can sustain social conversation, masking the extent of their cognitive deficits. Patients often have limited insight, thereby denying or dismissing problems as memory loss 'no worse than for others my age'. It can be difficult to challenge this assumption and undertake objective testing. The earliest signs of dementia are subtle and show considerable overlap with normality or age associated memory loss. Early pointers are listed in Box 15.7.

If the screening cognitive instrument suggests cognitive impairment, further investigation should be conducted (Figure 15.9). The clinician must decide:

- Is the cognitive impairment due to dementia? (Exclude age associated memory loss, depression or other psychiatric conditions, delirium, drugs with a central action.)

Box 15.7 Historical pointers to dementia

- Forgetting recent events, despite prompting
- Failure to attend appointments
- Frequent repetition of statements, stories or questions
- Frequent lost or misplaced items
- Increasing number of lists and reminder notes at home
- Repetitive telephone calls to family or general practitioner
- Problems with drug compliance
- Losing track in a conversation; word-finding difficulty
- Difficulty understanding conversation or following the story in a book or on television
- Confusion with time, e.g. day, date, time of day
- Becoming lost, unable to find the way
- Difficulty handling money or paying bills
- Difficulty working gadgets, planning or preparing meals, performing practical tasks
- Neglect of personal care, home maintenance or nutrition
- Withdrawal from previous community and social activities (poor work performance if employed)
- Difficulty coping with new events or change to routine

- If the problem is dementia, what is the disease specific diagnosis?
- Are there any reversible or remediable causative or contributory factors?

Differential diagnosis

The differential diagnosis of disorders causing cognitive impairment includes:

- decline in memory (age associated memory impairment)
- delirium
- depression
- drugs.

Age associated memory impairment

Distinguishing between normal ageing and early dementia can be difficult. With advancing age, there is sometimes slowing of cognitive processing and impairment of short-term memory (Figure 15.10). This is labelled age associated memory impairment or mild cognitive impairment. Individuals with mild cognitive impairment have a higher than average chance of developing dementia in the future. Twelve to fifteen per cent of these patients per year decline to dementia compared to 2% of those with 'normal' cognitive function. There is some debate about whether this group of patients all develop progressive decline if followed long enough; however, current studies do not support this theory. Features that help distinguish the memory loss of early AD include:

- significant decline in the acquisition of new information (learning across repeat trials)
- impaired delayed recall (rapid rate of forgetting)
- failure of memory retrieval despite prompting
- significant impact on daily activities
- associated impairment of other cognitive modalities.

A useful diagnostic tool when there is doubt is repeated cognitive testing and assessment over time (every 6–12 months). At present we are unable to predict at what point and which individuals will undergo progressive cognitive decline. Research is under way to develop tests that may help to make this distinction. Prediction of decline may be of clinical importance in the future, as preventative drug therapy for AD becomes available. Current treatment trials, using cholinesterase inhibitors and antioxidants in this group with mild impairment, are under way overseas.

Depression

Many psychological disorders—including depression, anxiety, mania, schizophrenia and hysteria—can mimic dementia. These conditions are frequently called pseudodementias and are often treatable. Depression is the most common of the pseudodementias and can be difficult to distinguish from dementia (see Box 15.8). Depression can present with similar symptoms, including:

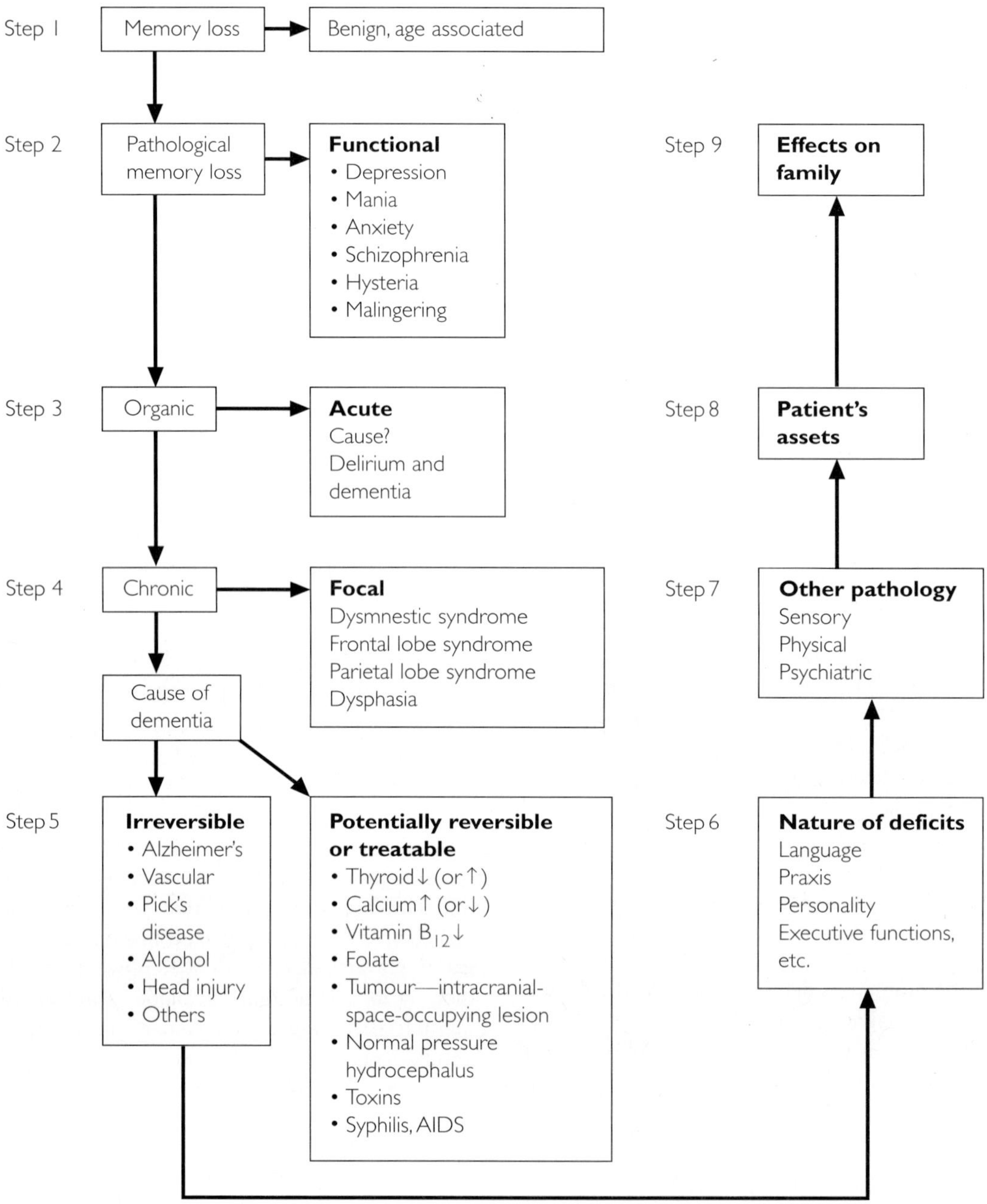

Figure 15.9 Nine-step decision tree for assessing a person with memory loss BRODATY (1999)

- memory loss
- poor concentration
- reduced interest and initiation of activities (apathy and neglect)
- changes in psychomotor activity
- sleep disturbance
- fatigue
- changes in eating habits or weight.

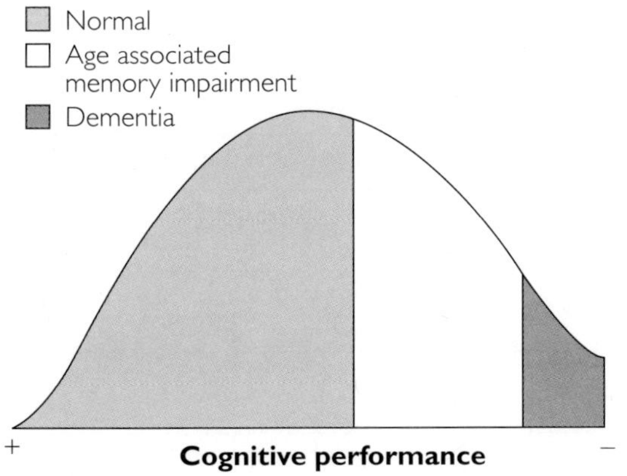

Figure 15.10 The distribution of cognitive function from normal through age associated memory impairment to dementia in individuals aged over 65 HECKER (1997)

Depression is less likely to result in cortical deficits (e.g. aphasia, apraxia and agnosia). In pseudodementia or 'reversible dementia', cognitive impairment improves with the successful treatment of depression. If in doubt, a trial of antidepressant therapy is indicated. Many elderly patients who respond to antidepressant therapy subsequently develop the progressive impairment of dementia. Of those patients presenting with a late life depressive episode associated with cognitive features, there is a 50% chance of a dementia diagnosis over the next 5 years. Features that help to distinguish depression and dementia are documented in Table 15.2.

The apathy and neglect occurring in some patients with early dementia can mimic depression. Depression is also a common concomitant diagnosis

Box 15.8 Geriatric Depression Scale

15 questions, Yes/No answer to each question.

	YES	NO
Are you basically satisfied with life?	☐ 0	☐ 1
Have you dropped many of your activities and interests?	☐ 1	☐ 0
Do you feel that your life is empty?	☐ 1	☐ 0
Do you often get bored?	☐ 1	☐ 0
Are you in good spirits most of the time?	☐ 0	☐ 1
Are you afraid that something bad is going to happen to you?	☐ 1	☐ 0
Do you feel happy most of the time?	☐ 0	☐ 1
Do you often feel helpless?	☐ 1	☐ 0
Do you prefer to stay at home, rather than going out and doing new things	☐ 1	☐ 0
Do you feel that you have more problems with memory than most?	☐ 1	☐ 0
Do you feel that it is wonderful to be alive now?	☐ 0	☐ 1
Do you feel worthless the way you are now?	☐ 1	☐ 0
Do you feel full of energy?	☐ 0	☐ 1
Do you feel that your situation is hopeless?	☐ 1	☐ 0
Do you feel that most people are better off than you are?	☐ 1	☐ 0

Table 15.2 Depression versus dementia

Clinical features	Depression with cognitive impairment	Dementia
Onset	Rapid	Insidious
Duration	Initial quicker descent and then plateaus	Slow progressive decline
Mood	Diurnal variation, pervasive depression	Fluctuating from apathy to irritability
Intellectual function	Many complaints; 'don't know' answers	Minimises or rationalises errors or failures
Memory loss	Recent and remote	Greatest for recent events
Self-image	Poor	Normal
Associated symptoms	Anxiety, insomnia	Rare; sometimes anorexia, insomnia or unco-operativeness
Reason for consultation	Self-referral	Brought by family or friend
Past/family history	Psychiatric history or family/personal problems	Family history of dementia not uncommon

in patients with AD, usually in the early stages of dementia, when insight is retained. Present in up to 40% of patients with AD, depression is generally underrecognised and undertreated. Depression is frequently an associated feature of vascular dementia.

Appropriate treatment should be instituted, including supportive counselling and, if necessary, antidepressant drug therapy. The choice of pharmacological agent should take into account the side effect profile of different drugs: drugs with anticholinergic effect (such as tricyclic antidepressants) can increase confusion and are best avoided. The selective serotonin reuptake inhibitors (SSRIs) with relatively short half-lives and minimal anticholinergic, adrenergic and histaminic side effects are a good choice.

Delirium and drugs

Delirium is characterised by a history of symptoms of rapid onset and short duration with clouding of consciousness (i.e. reduced awareness and fluctuating alertness). Other features commonly associated with delirium include motor restlessness, hallucinations (especially visual) and sleep disturbance. A specific cause is often although not always detected, particularly infective episodes (chest and urine are common) and centrally acting drugs. There are a large number of medications that exhibit anticholinergic properties and this group is particularly likely to precipitate cognitive decline or delirium. Studies have shown that 50% of cases of 'reversible dementia' are due to depression or drug intoxication. In managing older patients with cognitive impairment it is always important to consider iatrogenic illness. Older patients with reduced brain reserve are often extremely sensitive to centrally acting agents, including antipsychotics, benzodiazepines, antidepressants, anticholinergics, anti-parkinsonian drugs and antihistamines. Resultant cognitive impairment may present as a chronic rather than an acute brain syndrome, and improvement following drug withdrawal may take weeks. The co-existence of delirium and dementia is common and an acute confusional episode on hospitalisation (either with a medical illness or postoperatively) is a frequent initial sign of what is often an underlying dementia. Diagnostic features of delirium are listed in Box 15.9.

Box 15.9 Diagnostic criteria for delirium

- Disturbance of consciousness with change in cognition that is not better accounted for by a dementia
- Develops over hours to days
- Fluctuates during the course of the day
- Impaired ability to focus, sustain or shift attention
- Impaired cognition (memory, orientation, language) or perceptual disturbance (misinterpretation, illusions, hallucinations)
- Associated with sleep-wake cycle, psychomotor, emotional or EEG disturbance
- Evidence that the disturbance is caused by a general medical condition, substance intoxication or withdrawal or multiple aetiologies

Source: Modified from American Psychiatric Association (1994), *The Diagnostic and Statistical Manual*, 4th edition.

Box 15.10 Differential diagnosis of Alzheimer's disease

1. Vascular dementia
2. Diffuse Lewy body disease
3. Frontal lobe dementia (including Pick's disease)
4. Focal cortical atrophy syndromes
5. Parkinson's disease with dementia
6. Subcortical dementias, e.g.:
   - Progressive supranuclear palsy
   - Multisystem atrophy
   - Corticobasal degeneration
   - Huntington's disease
7. Normal pressure hydrocephalus
8. Prion diseases, e.g. Creutzfeldt-Jakob disease
9. Post-traumatic, toxic or anoxic encephalopathies
10. Progressive multifocal leucoencephalopathy
11. Chronic CNS infection
12. Multiple sclerosis, motor neuron disease

Differential diagnosis of diseases causing dementia

Although AD accounts for approximately 60% of dementia, with the advent of new drug therapies it is increasingly important to make an accurate disease specific diagnosis. Other dementias to be differentiated from AD are shown in Box 15.10. Determining the true prevalence rates of the dementias is difficult because there are relatively few studies where patients are followed closely through clinical assessment to autopsy. Secondly, many cases of dementia show neuropathological criteria or features of more than one dementing disease—for example, mixed AD and vascular dementia.

Vascular dementia

The contribution of cerebrovascular disease to dementia has been debated in recent years. Vascular dementia has replaced the previous term, 'multi-infarct' dementia, because it is recognised that a range of cerebrovascular disorders cause dementia. These include strategically placed single cerebral infarcts, multiple larger vessel infarcts or small vessel lacunes, haemorrhagic lesions (including subdural or subarachnoid haemorrhage), global or watershed ischaemia (e.g. resulting from cerebral hypoxia) and extensive subcortical and periventricular white matter lesions (known by various names, including Binswanger's disease and subcortical arteriosclerotic encephalopathy).

Distinguishing between AD and vascular dementia (particularly with cortical signs) can be difficult. Both stroke and AD are common in older people and often coincide. A stroke may be the added event that overcomes the compensatory capacity of a brain already compromised by the plaques and tangles of AD.

Newly established guidelines for the diagnosis of vascular dementia are listed in Box 15.11.

A temporal relationship can be difficult to establish, particularly in small vessel disease where there is often no history of discrete events. Such patients are likely to meet the diagnosis of possible, rather than probable, vascular dementia.

The clinical features of vascular dementia can be very diverse and may involve cortical deficits

Box 15.11 NINDS-AIREN Criteria for the Diagnosis of Vascular Dementia

- Dementia involving memory loss and impairment of other cognitive functions interfering with daily functioning
- Cerebrovascular disease as documented by a combination of history, neurological examination and/or brain imaging
- Evidence that the above features are related, e.g.:
  - Temporal relationship between stroke and dementia
  - Abrupt or stepwise deterioration in mental function or a fluctuating course
  - Specific brain imaging findings indicating damage to regions important for higher cerebral function
- Supportive clinical features:
  - History of cerebrovascular risk factors (e.g. hypertension, diabetes mellitus, cardiac disease, hypercholesterolaemia, smoking)
  - Early appearance of gait disturbance or frequent falls
  - Early appearance of urinary incontinence not explained by urological disease
  - Frontal lobe or extrapyramidal features
  - Pseudobulbar features with or without emotional incontinence

(related to the site of cortical infarction) similar to those found in AD. Alternatively, a subcortical dementia pattern is seen with small vessel disease affecting the deeper white matter (subcortical structures include the basal ganglia, thalamus, brain stem and frontal lobe projections to these regions). Features of subcortical dementia include memory loss (usually a retrieval defect aided by prompts rather than a learning deficit associated with AD), slowed cognitive processing, impairment of problem solving and judgment, and behavioural features, including apathy and depression. Other commonly associated features include gait disturbance (small step or apraxic gait similar to a parkinsonian gait), rigidity, bradykinesia, unsteadiness and frequent falls, urinary urgency and incontinence, pseudobulbar palsy, emotional incontinence and psychomotor retardation. These features can make distinction from Parkinson's disease (see Chapter 14) very difficult. Small vessel cerebrovascular disease does not usually produce a parkinsonian tremor and responds poorly to levodopa.

The aetiology and clinical significance of white matter changes remain unclear. These changes are found as periventricular hypodensity (leucoaraiosis) on CT scans or bright areas (called periventricular white matter hyperintensities) in T2-weighted MRI images. They are associated with increasing age and with a history of stroke and hypertension. Although these changes are often interpreted as evidence of ischaemic disease, they are also found in 30% of 'normal elderly' and 50% of neuropathologically proven AD and do not always correlate with significant cognitive impairment.

The consequences of a diagnosis of vascular dementia are a less predictable prognosis than AD (where steady decline is characteristic) and implications regarding treatment options. Secondary prevention measures for vascular disease should be instituted. These include aspirin or alternative antiplatelet therapy, careful management of hypertension, diabetes or other vascular risk factors. Current trials are under way with the cholinesterase inhibitors (both donepezil and rivastigmine) to establish their role as primary therapy for vascular dementia. As vascular dementia is mixed with AD in many cases, a trial of cholinesterase inhibitor therapy should not be ruled out.

Diffuse Lewy body disease

Improvements in immunochemical staining methods have resulted in increased recognition of another primary dementia known as diffuse Lewy body disease (DLBD) (Chapter 14). Lewy bodies (rounded eosinophilic inclusions in brain cells, composed of altered neurofilament, ubiquitin) have classically been found in the basal ganglia in association with Parkinson's disease. The presence, in DLBD, of more diffuse Lewy bodies throughout the cerebral cortex is thought to be a factor in up to 20% of dementia cases. Cortical Lewy bodies may be found either alone or in association with AD

Box 15.12 Diagnostic criteria for dementia with Lewy bodies (DLB)

- Progressive cognitive decline interfering with social or occupational functioning; memory loss may not be an early feature
- One (possible DLB) or two (probable DLB) of:
  - fluctuating cognition with pronounced variations in attention and alertness
  - recurrent visual hallucinations
  - spontaneous motor features of parkinsonism

Source: Modified from I. G. McKeith, D. Galasko & K. Kosaka (1996), 'Consensus guidelines for the clinical and pathological diagnosis of dementia with Lewy bodies (DLB): Report of the consortium on DLB international workshop', *Neurology*, 47, pp. 1113–24.

pathology and DLBD probably represents an overlap syndrome between AD and Parkinson's disease (Box 15.12).

The clinical features that help distinguish DLBD include fluctuating cognitive state (can be mistaken for acute brain syndrome), prominent neuropsychiatric features (in particular clearly formed visual hallucinations, often of small people or animals) present at an early stage of illness, and extrapyramidal features (rigidity, slowness and poverty of movement, and gait impairment). The typical pattern of cognitive impairment differs from AD in that an attentional deficit is prominent, visuospatial perception is significantly impaired, and memory and orientation are better preserved than is typical of AD.

The clinical course tends to be shorter and more fluctuant than AD and can in a small percentage of patients be very rapidly progressive. Other features that can be associated include episodes of sudden collapse or transient loss of consciousness, and falls. The parkinsonian features in DLBD often respond to levodopa therapy in those patients with motor symptoms causing a clinically significant deficit. Importantly, these patients are characterised by increased sensitivity to antipsychotic agents, even small doses of which may provoke a dramatic decline in cognitive and motor function. This is likely to be the result of the prominent cholinergic deficit in this disease. Antipsychotic therapy should be avoided if possible, but if essential, low doses of one of the new atypical antipsychotics with minimal extrapyramidal side effects, such as olanzapine, are preferable. A clinical drug trial with the cholinesterase inhibitor, rivastigmine, showed a significantly positive outcome on the neuropsychiatric and behavioural symptoms, together with the attentional deficit and cognitive impairment. The parkinsonian features were not adversely affected with this therapy.

Parkinsonian findings are not unique to DLBD and they also occur in subcortical vascular disease (see above), the later stages of AD and other secondary degenerative dementias such as Parkinson's disease, progressive supranuclear palsy and multisystem atrophy. Clinical differentiation of these conditions is sometimes difficult, even in the most experienced hands.

Frontal lobe dementia

Pick's disease is a primary degenerative dementia affecting the frontal and temporal lobes. More recently the term 'frontal lobe dementia' has been used to describe cases with similar clinical features but an absence of classic Pick bodies on neuropathological examination. Pick bodies are argyrophilic inclusions in neuronal cell bodies found in the neocortex and hippocampus. Neuronal degeneration in the frontal lobes results in defects in 'executive' function (problem solving, judgment, abstract thought and insight) and associated behavioural disturbance, frequently social disinhibition and personal neglect. The clinical importance of this dementia is the difficulty in detection using traditional cognitive assessment tools (such as the MMSE) which do not effectively test frontal lobe function. A history from relatives or other contacts can produce vital clues to poor performance in domestic and social settings. Because this dementia often develops before retirement age, performance in the occupational sphere is often a problem. Subtypes of frontal lobe syndrome can be identified, depending on the area of the frontal lobe affected:

- medial—apathy, lack of spontaneity, lack of initiative, dullness and slowness

- orbito-basal—disinhibition, fatuous jocularity, lack of control; and
- lateral convexity—impairment of planning, executive functions, organisation and abstract conceptualisation.

Other characteristic features of frontal dementia include evidence of language difficulties, often leading to mutism (Box 15.13). In some cases the dementia is accompanied by signs of motor neuron disease. The onset is relatively early and as many as 50% of cases are familial with an autosomal dominant pedigree. Neuroimaging can reveal selective frontal lobe atrophy or hypoperfusion (SPECT).

Focal syndromes

Dysmnestic (impaired memory) syndromes cause loss of short-term memory with sparing of other intellectual functions. Causes can include alcohol (Korsakoff's psychosis), herpes simplex encephalitis, carbon monoxide poisoning, focal temporal lobe atrophy, sclerosis or infarction.

Primary progressive aphasia is a focal atrophy syndrome usually presenting with impairment of verbal fluency with marked word-finding deficit. Typically this focal onset usually progresses to a more global dementing pattern with time. Vascular or degenerative lesions in the dominant parietal lobe (angular gyrus syndrome) can result in aphasia, alexia, agraphia, acalculia, right–left disorientation, finger agnosia and construction difficulties. Non-dominant parietal lesions may produce abnormalities in dressing, visuospatial orientation and constructional deficits.

Box 15.13 Diagnostic criteria for frontotemporal dementia

Behaviour disorder
- Insidious onset and slow progression
- Early loss of personal and social awareness
- Early signs of disinhibition
- Mental rigidity and inflexibility
- Hyperorality, stereotyped and perseverative behaviours

Affective symptoms
- Depression, anxiety
- Somatic preoccupations
- Emotional unconcern, amimia

Speech disorder
- Reduction and stereotypy of speech
- Echolalia and perseveration

Physical signs
- Early primitive reflexes and incontinence
- Late akinesia, rigidity, tremor

Source: Modified from A. Brun, B. England, D. M. Mann et al. (1994), 'The Lund and Manchester Groups. Clinical and neuropathological criteria for frontotemporal dementia (consensus statement)', *Neurology, Neurosurgery and Psychiatry*, 57, pp. 416–18.

Dementia management

Breaking the news

Informing patients and families of a feared diagnosis requires sensitivity and attention to the responses and wishes of both the patient and his relatives. Opinion varies about the benefits and potential harm of imparting this information to the patient and every situation should be judged individually. A discussion with the patient about his memory loss can help judge his level of insight and concern regarding a serious diagnosis. Explaining that a brain disease rather than the ageing process is responsible for the symptoms can leave the discussion open for further questions. In some situations it can be reasonable not to provide a specific name for the disease. An independent interview with the family can provide the opportunity for more frank discussion, particularly if the patient has more advanced dementia. Counselling should include discussion about the nature of the disease, the expected symptoms, treatment options and practical advice about management, including legal issues.

Drug treatments for Alzheimer's disease

The availability of new drug treatments for AD has increased the importance of making an early and accurate diagnosis (Figure 15.11). Interest in the cholinergic approaches to treatment of AD was based on the observed loss of cholinergic neurons in the nucleus basalis together with their cortical projections. Studies showed the predominant although not the only neurotransmitter deficit in AD is acetylcholine. Acetylcholine has an important role in memory function and other areas of cognitive and behavioural function. Cholinesterase inhibitors are the only drugs currently marketed as symptomatic therapy for AD. These drugs work by preventing the breakdown of acetylcholine in the synapse, thereby improving cholinergic neurotransmission (Figure 15.12).

What drugs are available?

The first cholinesterase inhibitor developed was tacrine (Cognex), which is little used as a result of problems with hepatotoxicity and poor gastrointestinal tolerance. A number of other cholinesterase inhibitors with improved side effect profiles are now available or under development (Box 15.14). The first of these, donepezil (Aricept), was marketed in Australia in March 1998 and has greatly improved tolerance. Rivastigmine (Exelon), launched in July 2000, is a carbamate cholinesterase inhibitor with a similar improved side effect profile. Neither of these drugs produces hepatotoxicity. They have both been approved for PBS subsidy in Australia from February 2001 under authority conditions. These include a specialist (consultant physician or psychiatrist) diagnosis of Alzheimer's disease of mild to moderately severe degree, with provision of the MMSE score at treatment baseline (or Alzheimer's Disease Assessment Scale Cognitive score (ADAS-cog) for patients with an MMSE score > 25). Initial authority is for 6 months with repeat authority dependent on improvement of 2 points on the MMSE score or 4 points on the ADAS-cog between 3 and 6 months after treatment initiation. Patients on these drugs prior to 1 December 2000 are allowed continuing authority until severe dementia.

Other cholinergic drugs are likely to follow on to the market in the near future. Galantamine, a cholinesterase inhibitor with additional nicotinic

Box 15.14 Potential Alzheimer's disease treatments

Cholinesterase inhibitors

- Tacrine (Cognex)
- Donepezil (Aricept)
- Rivastigmine (Exelon)
- Galantamine (Reminyl)

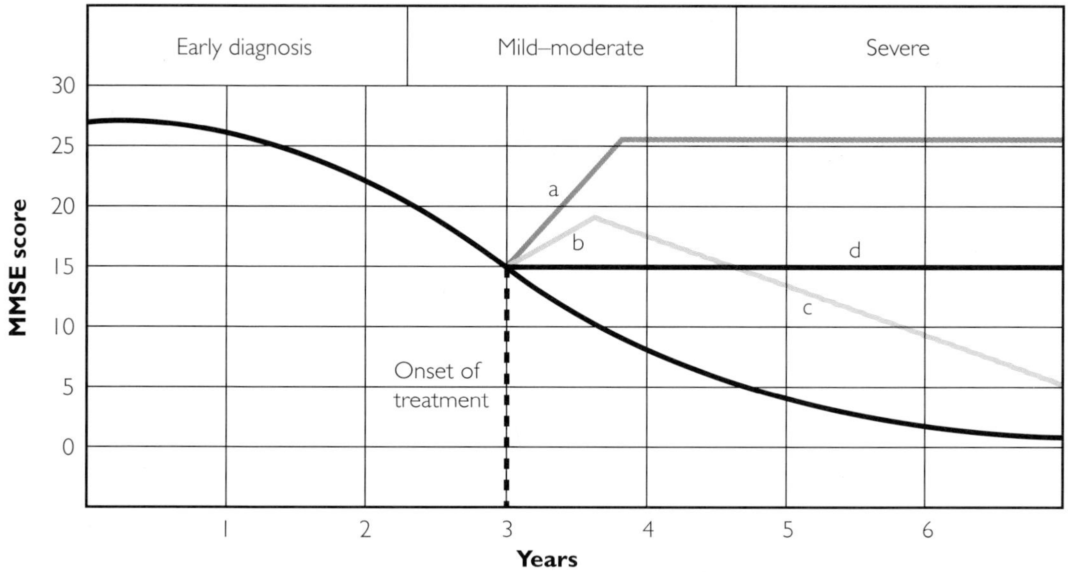

Figure 15.11 Hypothetical treatment responses in Alzheimer's disease: (a) cure, (b) symptomatic improvement, followed by (c) parallel decline and (d) stabilisation of progression GAUTHIER (1996)

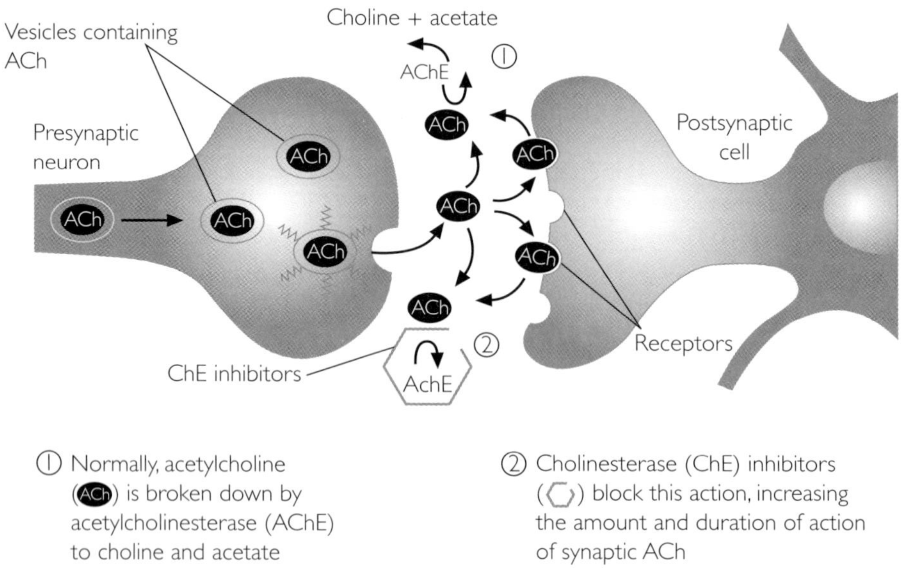

Figure 15.12 Current therapeutic approaches—cholinesterase inhibitors. Diagrammatic representation of mechanism of action

modulatory effects, is also in the marketing pipeline and is available overseas. As yet there are no direct double-blind comparative studies to compare the efficacy of these drugs, although at least one such clinical trial is planned in the near future.

What benefit can be expected?

Treatment with the cholinesterase inhibitors may improve symptoms or stabilise decline, resulting in a gain of 6–12 months, but cannot halt or reverse progression of the disease (Figure 15.13).

It has been suggested that cholinesterase inhibitors may slow the progression of the disease by altering the rate of cognitive decline, but this has not been proven. Studies suggest a modest benefit in 60–70% of patients treated with cholinesterase inhibitors. About 20% of these patients demonstrate a more significant response, but the characteristics of this subgroup are unknown.

The benefits of treatment with cholinesterase inhibitors may be apparent in various areas, including:

- activities of daily living (particularly initiation of tasks)
- behaviour: improvement in neuropsychiatric features (delusions and hallucinations), apathy and agitation or more subtle improvements in mood and behaviour early in the disease course ('cognitive engagement')
- cognition: concentration, alertness, memory, language, problem solving.

These benefits result in improved quality of life for both patients and their families.

Who should be treated?

The new cholinesterase inhibitors are indicated for patients with a clear diagnosis of AD that is at a mild to moderately severe stage. Recent clinical trial results with donepezil (presented but not published) suggest patients with moderately severe AD may gain even more benefit than those with early disease. There is no indication to treat patients with age associated memory loss or mild cognitive impairment alone, but clinical trials to test whether these drugs may delay diagnosis of dementia in this group are under way. A large study treating diffuse Lewy body dementia with rivastigmine has shown positive results on cognition and attention together with significant improvements in the neuropsychiatric symptoms (hallucinations and delusions) and other behavioural features of the disease. There was no increase in the parkinsonian features. This

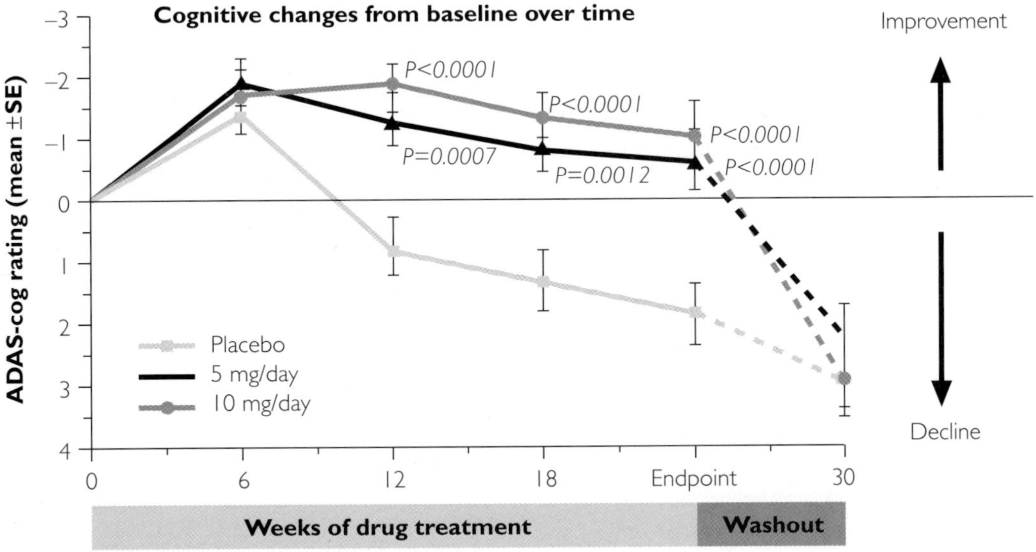

Figure 15.13 Response to donepezil (5 mg and 10 mg doses) versus placebo—measured on the Alzheimer's Disease Assessment Scale; 24 week double-blind placebo controlled clinical trial, followed by 6 week single-blind washout phase

ROGERS ET AL.

response fits with the known marked cholinergic deficit in this disease. There are studies currently under way to assess the value of cholinesterase inhibitors in patients with vascular dementia. There is no evidence of benefit in other rarer forms of dementia at this stage.

When should treatment be commenced?

After a diagnosis of AD or DLBD is established, treatment can be commenced as soon as benefit is sought. Anecdotal experience suggests that quality of life can be improved with treatment at the early stages of AD when cognitive impairment is mild and behavioural problems are less common. If the suggestion of a positive effect on disease progression is clearly established, treatment should obviously be commenced at diagnosis. There is no evidence these drugs are beneficial for memory loss alone, prior to a diagnosis of dementia.

Potential side effects

Donepezil is well tolerated by most patients. The incidence of expected cholinergic side effects is low, with nausea and diarrhoea being the most common problems. Commence with 5 mg donepezil daily for the first month to minimise side effects, with an increase following this to 10 mg daily if the lower dose is well tolerated (Box 15.15). Some patients develop agitation, hallucinations or unpleasant dreams, which often resolve if the drug is administered in the morning or the dose is reduced; if necessary, these symptoms reverse on drug cessation.

Rivastigmine requires twice daily dosing. The recommended dose schedule commences with 1.5 mg capsules twice daily, increasing gradually through 3 mg bid, 4.5 mg bid to a maximum dose of 6 mg bid. It is aimed to titrate to the highest well tolerated dose at monthly intervals. It is important rivastigmine is taken with food to improve tolerability. Side effects include expected cholinergic gastrointestinal symptoms and weight loss. Studies suggest a higher rate of gastrointestinal side effects with rivastigmine during the dose titration phase, but this improves when the optimal dose is established for maintenance treatment.

It is important to remember that drugs with anticholinergic action will oppose the effects of the cholinesterase inhibitors and are best avoided in AD because they exacerbate the cholinergic deficit. The cholinesterase inhibitors also enhance the effect of any other cholinomimetic drugs and this can be important in relation to some drugs used during anaesthesia.

Box 15.15 Donepezil (Aricept)

- Indication—symptomatic treatment of mild to moderate dementia of Alzheimer's type
- Commence with 5 mg per day—clinically effective dose
- Optional increase to 10 mg per day after 4–6 weeks
- Single daily dose
- Take with a glass of liquid, relationship to food unimportant
- No requirement for biochemical monitoring
- No dose alteration for renal, hepatic impairment
- No known drug interaction except with other cholinomimetics or anticholinergic drugs
- Review at 3 and 6 months to assess efficacy and side effects

How long should treatment be continued?

Benefit appears to be maintained while therapy continues, but earlier studies suggest loss of treatment effect within 6 weeks when treatment is discontinued. Information from extension studies, where all patients receive active treatment in open label fashion following the initial randomised protocol, are now available for more than 4 years' treatment duration. Double-blind placebo controlled scientific studies have not exceeded 12 months' duration. If treatment benefit is doubted, an effective clinical test is a brief (2–6 weeks) treatment withdrawal trial; treatment can be reinstituted if deterioration occurs (Figure 15.14).

Assessment of the treatment effect should include discussion with the patient and the caregiver or informant as well as an objective test of cognition (MMSE) and function in daily activities.

There is no current evidence to support the use of cholinesterase inhibitors in severe dementia. There is no documented clinical trial evidence to support treatment duration with cholinesterase inhibitors or to document results on treatment withdrawal at later stages of the disease. The anecdotal experience suggests it is reasonable to withdraw therapy when patients require high level (nursing home) residential care (after allowing 1–2 months for stabilisation in the new environment). Some patients do experience a relatively sharp decline in either functional performance or behaviour when treatment is withdrawn, even at this level of dementia severity. For these individuals, therapy can be recommenced but not under the authority for subsidised treatment currently.

Other putative cognitive enhancers?

A number of drugs are reputed to have cognitive-enhancing effects.

Ginkgo biloba

Ginkgo biloba, a derivative of the leaf of the Chinese maidenhair plant, is sold in health food shops. There are a couple of well conducted studies that have supported a very small positive effect on cognitive function. The active ingredient tested (EGb716) is contained in varying quantities in differing preparations of this drug.

Antioxidants

Antioxidants have long been postulated as effective in a number of degenerative diseases associated with ageing. There are no studies showing a benefit on cognitive function, but one large study suggested a positive effect of vitamin E (1000 IU twice daily) or selegiline on the rates of death, time to institutionalisation, and loss of basic daily living activities.

Folate

Recent studies in several sites have shown a correlation between AD, high serum homocysteine levels and low serum folate. As yet, there is no evidence that high homocysteine or low folate is causative in AD, as opposed to a consequence or association of AD. No treatment studies have been conducted, nor can treatment implications be drawn from the evidence to date. Further research in this area may lead to promising therapeutic advances.

Other agents

A number of other agents are being tested in large international studies for potential benefits on disease progression. These include anti-inflammatory drugs,

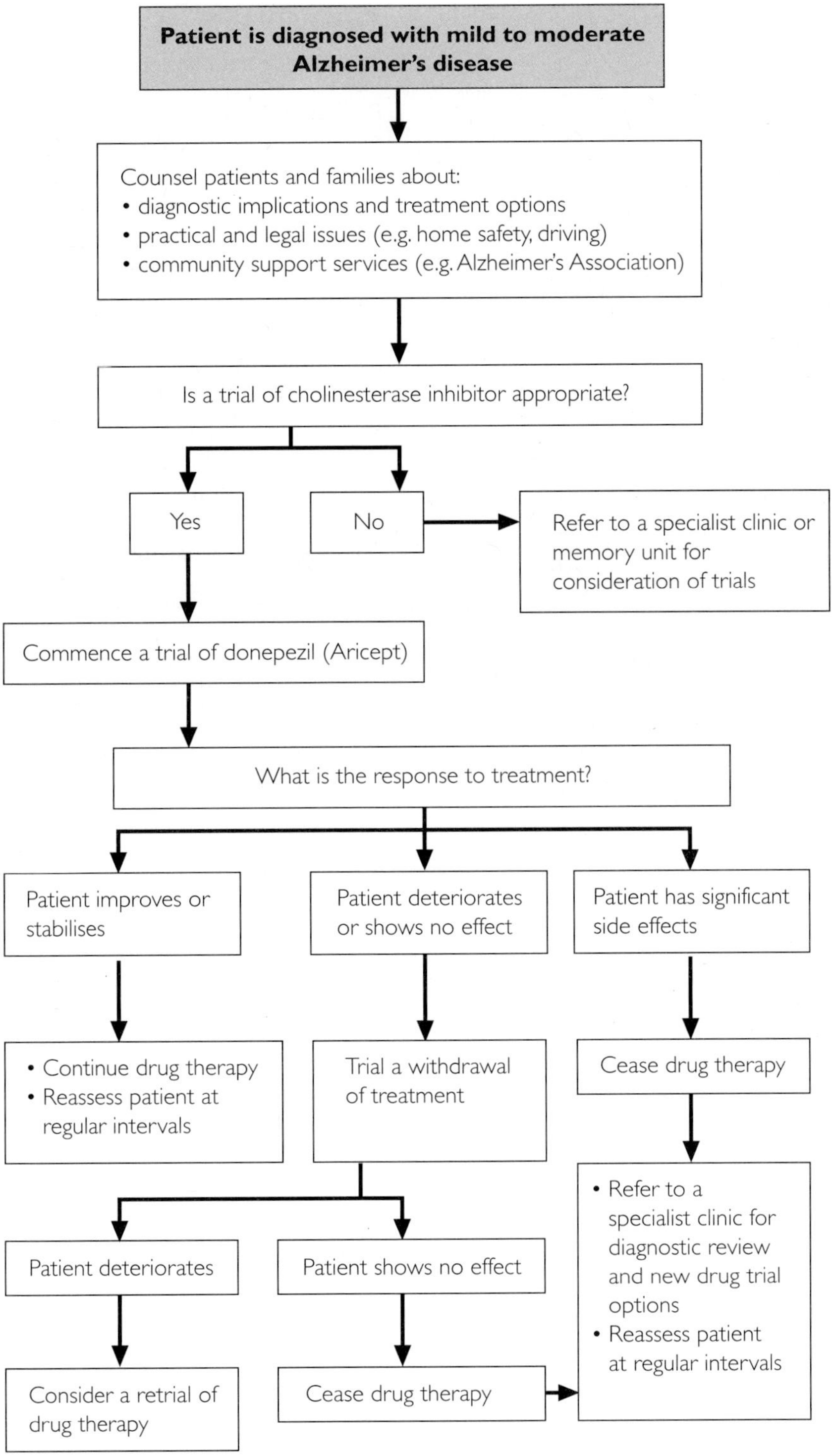

Figure 15.14 Pharmacological therapy for Alzheimer's disease BRODATY (1999)

oestrogens, metabolic enhancers and neurotrophic agents (Table 15.3).

Disease prevention

Unfortunately, there is no current evidence to support the use of any pharmacologic agent in the role of AD prevention, but research is under way in the area. A number of studies are being conducted worldwide in patients with memory loss or mild cognitive impairment to test agents that may delay the onset of AD. Drugs under investigation for disease prevention include cholinesterase inhibitors, anti-inflammatory agents, antioxidants (including vitamin E) and oestrogens (in women). Drug treatments and genetic manipulation aimed at the underlying pathogenic mechanisms, including γ- and β-secretase inhibitors designed to prevent the amyloidogenic processing of APP, are being developed.

Hypertension appears to be emerging as a risk factor for AD. A recent large study showed a significant reduction in the prevalence of AD in those patients (over age 65) whose systolic hypertension was treated when compared with the untreated placebo group, both followed for a 5 year period. Attention to other modifying vascular risk factors may have a role in AD as well as vascular dementia.

Practical and legal issues

Testamentary capacity

Patients with an early diagnosis of AD who retain testamentary capacity can organise appropriate provisions for a will, enduring power of attorney (management of finances and assets), enduring power of guardianship (management of treatment and lifestyle decisions) and advance directives. It is important that these documents be brought to the attention of patients at the time of the diagnosis, before legal capacity is lost and guardianship board involvement is required. Capacity is a legal concept and is decision specific, requiring assessment of the ability to understand the relevant information and appreciate the consequence of decisions.

Driving licence retention

Assessment of driving is a difficult issue that faces all medical practitioners at times. It is a legal requirement to report patients whose physical or mental impairment is likely to affect driving safety. It is advisable to perform brief cognitive screening when medical certification of fitness to drive is required in older patients. Objective evidence of possible cognitive impairment can be followed with

Table 15.3 Potential AD treatments under trial in Australia (current or previous)

Drug	Type	Company
Tacrine (Cognex)	Acetylcholinesterase inhibitor (acridine)	Parke-Davis
Lazabemide (1993)	MAOI-B	Hoffman-La Roche
E2020 (donepezil, Aricept)	Acetylcholinesterase inhibitor (piperidine)	Eisai
Milameline	M_1 muscarinic agonist	Hoechst Marion Roussel
202026 (Memric)	M_1 muscarinic agonist	Smith Kline Beecham
Galantamine (reminyl)	Acetylcholinesterase inhibitor	Janssen Cilag
Lazabemide (1997)	MAOI-B	Protodigm
Celecoxib	NSAID (cyclo oxygenase II inhibitor)	Searle
DHEA	Neurosteroid	Cromedica
Talsaclidine	M_1 muscarinic agonist	Boehringer Ingelheim
Neotrofin (AIT-082)	Nerve growth factor	Neotherapeutics

Source: J. Hecker (1998), 'Alzheimer's disease: The advent of effective therapy', *Australian and New Zealand Journal of Medicine*, 28, pp. 765–71.

more detailed assessment and diagnosis.

When a diagnosis of AD is established, it is important to discuss driving ability with the patient and family. In a large number of patients, it is effective to explain the many ways in which AD can affect driving performance, and to encourage self-restriction and appropriate voluntary licence relinquishment. It is useful to discuss this issue at an early stage, when insight is better maintained. This will allow time for patients to accept the loss of driving and to plan alternative arrangements.

Studies have suggested that patients with moderate and severe dementia are clearly unsafe on the road. However, the situation is very variable in mild dementia and many patients are safe drivers in the early stages of AD. Mandatory licence suspension on diagnosis (which is not required in Australia) seems to be unnecessarily harsh, but the Austroads guidelines for Australian practitioners do not provide clear guidelines on how to assess risk in the clinical setting. A clear relationship between cognitive tests and road performance has not been demonstrated. Questioning family about driving habits and recent accidents can be useful. In situations of doubt or a lack of patient co-operation, an on-road driving assessment, preferably conducted by a skilled assessor (such as an occupational therapist), can provide objective evidence and relieve the doctor of having to take the punitive role.

Activities of daily living

Practical advice on maximising function may help on a wide range of issues, including:

- aids for memory and orientation
- simple, regular routines
- drug compliance
- home safety
- communication hints
- suitable diversional activities
- financial planning, including the availability of disability or carer's pensions
- appropriate structuring of the home environment
- access to community support groups and services (e.g. Alzheimer's Association).

A balance is necessary between stimulation to enhance and maintain function and provide enjoyment and overwhelming with excessive activities or tasks that lead to frustration. In dementia, patients lose skills in the reverse order to which they were acquired (Figure 15.15) and this knowledge can be used to therapeutic advantage by

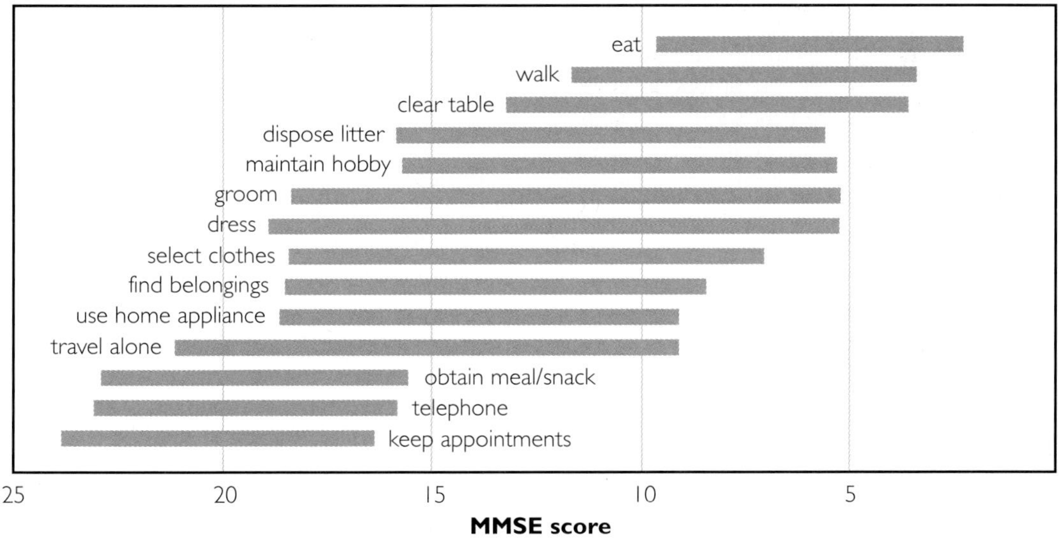

Figure 15.15 Progression of impairment in activities of daily living over time using the MMSE objective test of cognition GAUTHIER (1996).

focusing on retained skills. Creative solutions can often be found to daily problems if you remember that adapting the environment is easier than attempting to change the patient. Creating a sense of usefulness and achievement can be a challenge for patients with dementia; however, the disease does not remove the need for a sense of importance and mastery.

In the more advanced stages of the disease, advice about nutrition and the management of continence and personal care may be of help.

Superimposed medical problems

From a medical perspective, it is important to consider, detect and treat any superimposed medical problems or drug induced iatrogenic problems that may be compounding disability. This is particularly relevant if there has been recent unexplained cognitive decline, superimposed delirium or new behavioural problems. A proactive approach of scheduling regular reviews with the patient and family at intervals of 3–6 months will allow problems to be detected at an early stage and preventative strategies to be instituted.

Comprehensive care-giver training delays admission

The carer is the second victim in AD, and the stress associated with the caregiving role can result in medical and psychological morbidity associated with increased use of health services. Appropriate education, counselling and support (Box 15.16), together with adequate provision of respite services, can improve carer health and delay the requirement for residential care (Figure 15.16). Referral to support groups, such as the Alzheimer's Association, lends support to the medical practitioner's input. In Australia, doctors, patients or their families can contact the Alzheimer's Association on the national toll-free HelpLine, 1800 639 331.

Box 15.16 Caregiver support

- Education (diagnosis, implications, prognosis, treatment)
- Counselling support (grief)
- Community resources
  - Alzheimer's Association
  - In home services
  - Respite
  - Support services for behaviour management
- Guidance on practical issues
  - Memory aids
  - Home safety
  - Driving licence
  - Legal issues
  - Advance directives
  - Continence management
  - Advice on behaviour management strategies

Managing behavioural and psychological symptoms of dementia (BPSD)

Changes in personality and behaviour are commonly associated with AD, often becoming significant in the moderate and severe stages of dementia. There is great individual variation in the occurrence and severity of behavioural symptoms, but they are often extremely disruptive to patients and caregivers in both home and residential care settings, resulting in reduced quality of life and increased costs of care. More common problem behaviours include those listed in Box 15.17.

A thorough assessment should include identification of the specific problem behaviour, documentation of relevant antecedents and consequences, and a careful search for any medical illness, physical symptoms or iatrogenic factors (drug side effects or interactions) that may be contributing. Non-pharmacological approaches (including environmental interventions) should be tried before resorting to drug therapy (Box 15.18).

Pharmacological therapy should be reserved for drug responsive symptoms of at least moderate severity that are disturbing to the patient or caregivers. Antipsychotic medication is the most effective in the treatment of psychotic symptoms (delusions and hallucinations), agitation and aggression (Chapter 12). When choosing a therapeutic agent, consideration should be given to the

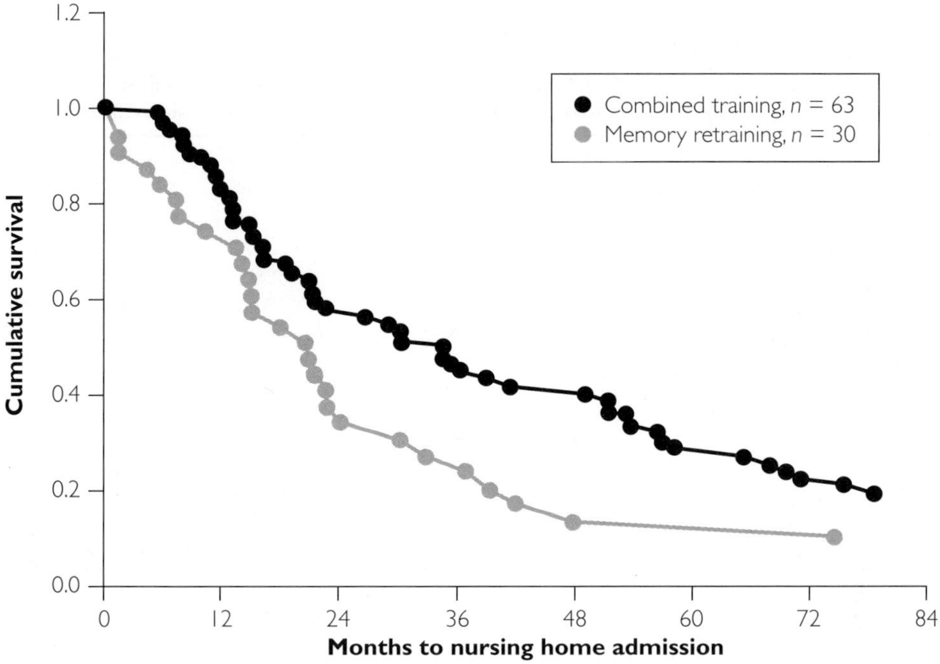

Figure 15.16 Kaplan-Meier survival curve for nursing home admission comparing combined care-giver training groups (immediate and wait list) with a memory retraining group BRODATY (1999)

Box 15.17 Behaviour problems in AD

- Delusional ideation (e.g. paranoia)
- Agitation/restlessness
- Activity disturbance:
  - Wandering/pacing
  - Purposeless or inappropriate activity
  - Apathy, loss of initiative
- Irritability/aggression/catastrophic reaction
- Demanding, attention-seeking behaviour (repetitive questions, clinging behaviours)
- Anxiety, phobias (e.g. fear of being left alone)
- Sleep disturbance (altered diurnal rhythm)
- Hallucinations
- Mood disturbance (e.g. depression, withdrawal)

Box 15.18 Behavioural problems: Treatment strategies

- Behaviour management is a challenge!
- Assessment of behaviour antecedents and consequences
- Explanation, support and counselling for carers—family and professional
- Exploration of potential behavioural or environmental manipulation
- Drug treatment as a last resort for specific target symptoms (agitation, aggression, psychotic features)

side effect profile of individual drugs (Table 15.4). In general, elderly patients with dementia are more sensitive to centrally acting drugs, and the dosages of medication required are significantly lower (Box 15.19). It is important to begin treatment with a low dose and to increase the dose slowly. Regular review of both efficacy and any potential adverse effects is important. In general, if antipsychotic treatment is required, use of a potent antipsychotic with minimal anticholinergic action, in low dose, is the preferred option (e.g. haloperidol 0.5 mg once or twice daily).

Patients with diffuse Lewy body dementia often

Table 15.4 Pharmacotherapy of BPSSD

Symptoms	Pharmaco-therapeutic options	Starting dose	Dose adjustment	Usual daily dose	Major side effects
Aggression[a]	*Antipsychotics*				
	Haloperidol	0.25–1.5 mg	0.25–0.5mg every 5–10 days	0.25–5 mg	Parkinsonism, akathisia
	Thioridazine	10 mg	10–20 mg every 5–10 days	10–100 mg/day	Postural hypotension, sedation, falls (and fractures), anticholinergic side effects,[c] tardive dyskinesia, neuroleptic malignant syndrome
	Risperidone	0.25–0.5 mg	0.5 mg	0.5–2 mg	Insomnia, agitation, extrapyramidal and orthostatic hypotension
	Olanzapine	5 mg	5 mg	5–15 mg	Drowsiness, weight gain, orthostatic hypotension
	Anticonvulsants				
	Carbamazepine[b]	100–200 mg	100–200 mg every 5–10 days	200–1200 mg	Blurred vision, headache, rash, blood dyscrasia, hyponatraemia, liver enzyme abnormality
	Sodium valproate[b]	125 mg twice a day	250 mg	250–1500 mg	Gastrointestinal, drowsiness, haematological
Anxiety	*Short-acting benzodiazepines*				
	Lorazepam	0.5 mg	0.5–1 mg every 3 days	0.5–5 mg	Sedation, dizziness, unsteadiness, weakness
	Oxazepam	7.5 mg	7.5 mg every 3 days	7.5–45 mg	Sedation, falls, confusion
	Azaspirodecanediones				
	Buspirone	5 mg 3 times a day	5 mg	10 mg 3 times a day	Dizziness, headache, drowsiness, nausea
Delusions and hallucinations	*Antipsychotics*	As above			
Depression	*SSRIs*				
	Sertraline	50 mg	50 mg	50–200 mg	Male sexual dysfunction, nausea/vomiting, diarrhoea, dry mouth
	Paroxetine	10 mg	10 mg	10–40 mg	Headaches, nausea/vomiting, sedation, dry mouth, potent inhibitor of cytochrome P-450 (check drug interations)
	Citalopram	10–20 mg	10–20 mg	20–40 mg	Nausea, dry mouth, somnolence, sweating, tremor, diarrhoea

Table 15.4 *continued*

Symptoms	Pharmaco-therapeutic options	Starting dose	Dose adjustment	Usual daily dose	Major side effects
	Fluvoxamine	25–50 mg	50 mg	50–300 mg	
	Fluoxetine	5–20 mg	5–20 mg every 14–21 days	5–40 mg	Agitation, anxiety, dyskinesia, inhibits cytochrome P-450 (check drug interactions), insomnia, anorexia
	SNRIs				
	Venlafaxine	37.5 mg twice a day	37.5 mg	75–375 mg	Dizziness, dry mouth, insomnia, nervousness, somnolence
	Atypical antidepressants				
	Nefazodone	50 mg	50 mg	200–600 mg	Somnolence, asthenia, headache, confusion
	Trazadone	25–50 mg	50 mg	50–300 mg	Sedation, orthostasis, priapism
	Cyclic antidepressants				
	Desipramine[b]	25–50 mg	25 mg every 2–3 days	75–200 mg	Sedation, anticholinergic side effects[c]
	Nortriptyline[b]	25 mg	25 mg every 2–3 days	75–125 mg	
	Mianserin	20 mg	10–20 mg	60–120 mg	Sedation, anticholinergic side effects[c]
	Reversible MAO inhibitors				
	Moclobemide	150 mg	150 mg	300–600 mg	Drug interactions, nausea, headache, insomnia, confusion
	MAO inhibitors				
	Phenelzine	15 mg	15 mg every 2–3 days	15–60 mg	Drug and food interactions, postural hypotension, confusion, anticholinergic side effects[c]
	Tranylcypromine	10 mg	10 mg every 2–3 days	10–40 mg	Tranylcypromine has a stimulant action
Insomnia	*Intermediate or short-acting benzodiazepines*				
	Temazepam	10 mg	10 mg	10–20 mg	
	Oxazepam	15 mg	15 mg	15–30 mg	Sedation, falls, confusion
	Lorazepam	0.5 mg	0.5–1 mg every 3 days	0.5–5 mg	
Screaming	*Antipsychotics*	As above			
	SSRIs	As above			

(continues)

Table 15.4 *continued*

Symptoms	Pharmaco-therapeutic options	Starting dose	Dose adjustment	Usual daily dose	Major side effects
Sexual disinhibition	Antipsychotics	As above			
	Medroxyprogesterone (promising, but needs further study)				

Note: Non-pharmacological strategies should be tried first, if possible. All medications should be checked for drug interactions, indications and contraindications before prescribing. Caution is always required, as individuals may vary in their sensitivity to different medications.
(*a*) Other drugs reported for treatment of aggression include serotonergic agonists, SSRIs, propranolol, lithium.
(*b*) Monitoring of serum levels available (NB: nortriptyline has a narrow therapeutic window).
(*c*) Blurred vision, urinary retention, constipation, dry mouth.

Source: H. Brodaty (1999), *Managing Alzheimer's Disease in Primary Care*, Science Press Ltd, London.

Box 15.19 Behavioural management: Drug treatment principles

- Start with a low dose.
- Increase slowly.
- Monitor for side effects.
- Regularly review drugs.
- *Remember:* Elderly patients with cognitive impairment are extremely sensitive to centrally acting drugs.
- Results of antipsychotic treatment:
  - 30% improve
  - 30% no change
  - 30% worse
- Depression:
  - commonly associated with AD
  - often reactive and responds to support therapy—if drug treatment is necessary, the newer antidepressants (e.g. SSRIs) are less likely to increase cognitive impairment

respond very poorly to antipsychotics, deteriorating in both mobility and cognition. It is preferable to avoid the use of neuroleptics in this group. The newer antipsychotic drugs, such as risperidone and olanzapine, appear to be at least as effective as conventional neuroleptics but with fewer undesirable side effects, particularly on the extrapyramidal system. These agents are used routinely in other countries, but are not currently subsidised in Australia for behaviour management in dementia (Figure 15.17).

Prognosis

An estimate of the pattern and speed of progression is an important component of the clinical assessment of AD in clinical practice, in order to advise families on resources required through the early, intermediate and late stages. Many factors, including education level, age, occupation (work, active or passive retirement), will influence our ability to determine the time of onset of dementia. Different aspects of the disease process, including cognitive, behavioural and functional, may progress at different rates in individual patients. The tools we use to measure disease progression can be dependent on preservation of different cognitive domains—for example, the MMSE score is language dependent. Institutionalisation in residential care is usually more dependent on functional and behavioural problems rather than cognitive impairment.

The 50% survival rate for patients with AD is 8 years, compared to 6.7 years for vascular dementia. Lewy body dementia often has a more rapid progression with a range of 3–8 years.

The rate of progression of AD is not linear. Early in the disease there is often a relative plateau, followed by a sharp decline and finally a phase of apparent gradual deterioration when a floor effect is noted with most change scales (Figure 15.18). Research studies suggest an average decline of approximately 3–4 points per year on the MMSE scale, although this instrument was not developed to demonstrate change.

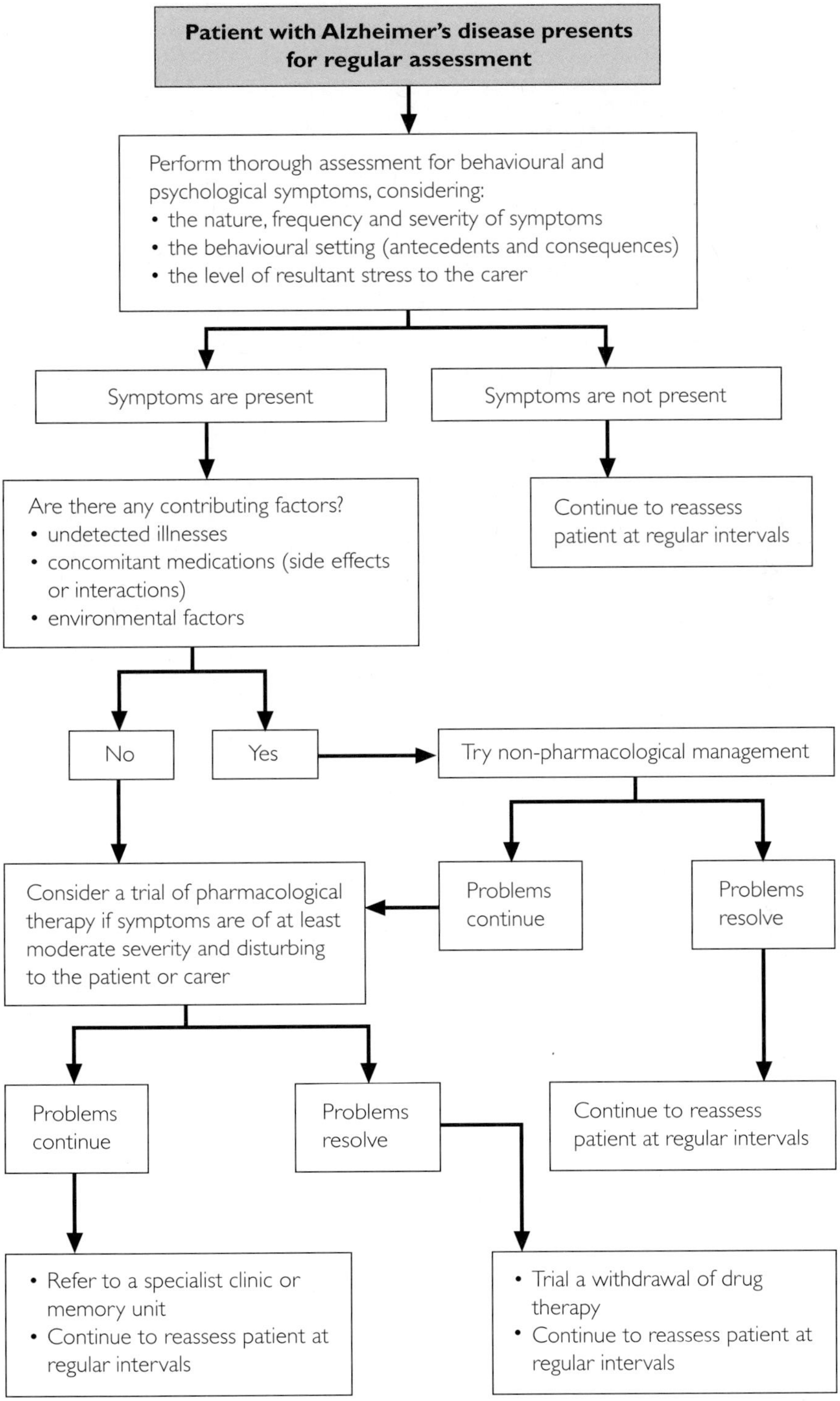

Figure 15.17 Managing psychological and behavioural symptoms BRODATY (1999)

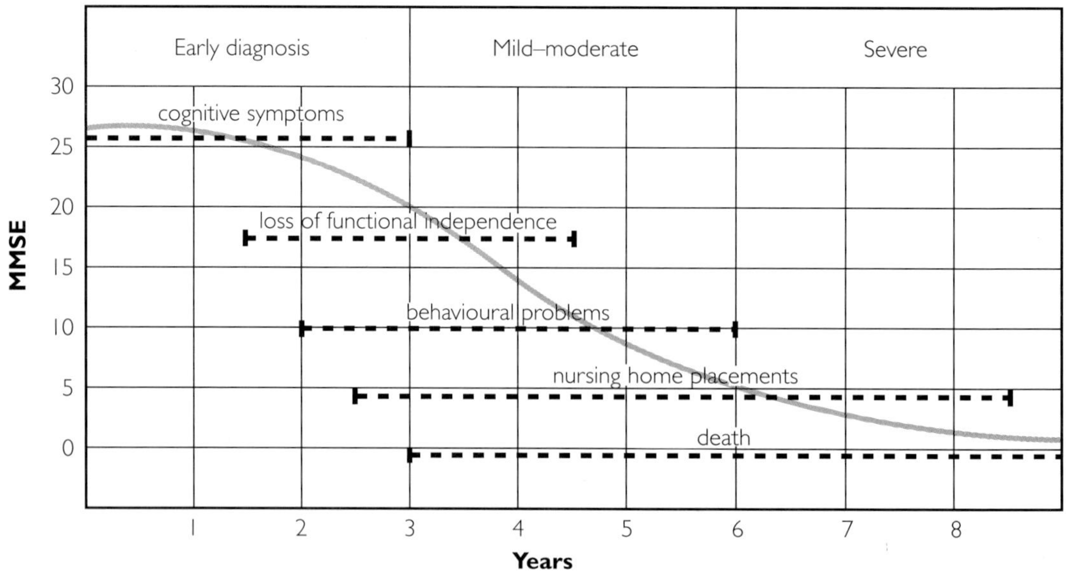

Figure 15.18 Natural history of Alzheimer's disease GAUTHIER (1996)

A number of factors have been identified as relevant to prognosis. Early age at onset of symptoms has been correlated with rapid progression and shorter survival but not all studies confirm this suggestion. For any level of assessed disease severity, the underlying pathology is more advanced in patients with higher educational levels, resulting in a shorter duration of diagnosed disease. The better accepted features associated with a bad prognosis are the presence of myoclonus, extrapyramidal signs and neuropsychiatric symptoms. This may relate in part to newly recognised dementia syndromes—for example, Lewy body disease. Frontal lobe deficits have also been associated with a worse prognosis in many studies. Similarly, patients with marked dysphasia or dyspraxia have been shown to deteriorate more rapidly in some studies. These problems may be markers of disease severity.

The difficult issues facing patients and carers vary with stage of the illness. Depressive features are common in early AD whereas significant behavioural problems (e.g. agitation, paranoia) are more common as the disease advances (Figure 15.19). Early in the course of the illness discussions centre around legal and financial planning, relinquishing work and/or driving. Support for the patient is important, particularly if insight is retained. Later in the disease, dependence increases with associated increasing stress for the family and caregivers. Practical issues arising at home include safety, wandering, urinary incontinence, disturbance of sleeping and eating patterns—all of which need to be addressed. Counselling, support and respite should be provided for the family. In the later stages of the illness, dependence in the basic living activities—including walking, toileting and feeding—increases. Counselling regarding residential care options and relinquishing care is required. Finally, in the terminal stages of AD, decisions are required regarding the level of medical intervention and palliative approach to management.

Conclusion

General practitioners are in a unique position to detect and diagnose dementia. Regular review is necessary in this chronic, progressive disease to assess cognition, functional performance in daily living activities, and behavioural and psychological symptoms associated with dementia. Ongoing medical management should include careful detection and treatment of intercurrent illness, and attention to

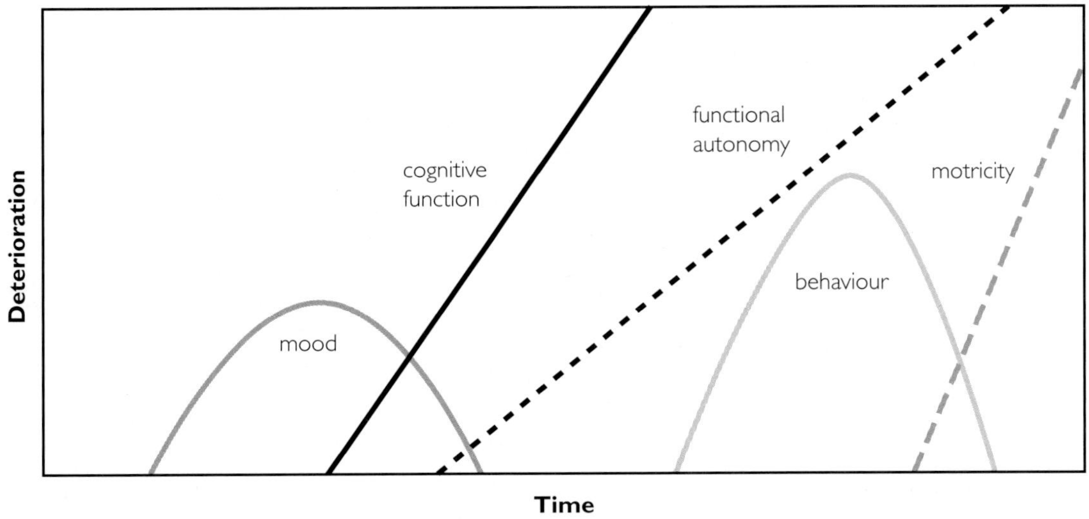

Figure 15.19 Symptomatic domains of typical Alzheimer's disease over time GAUTHIER (1996)

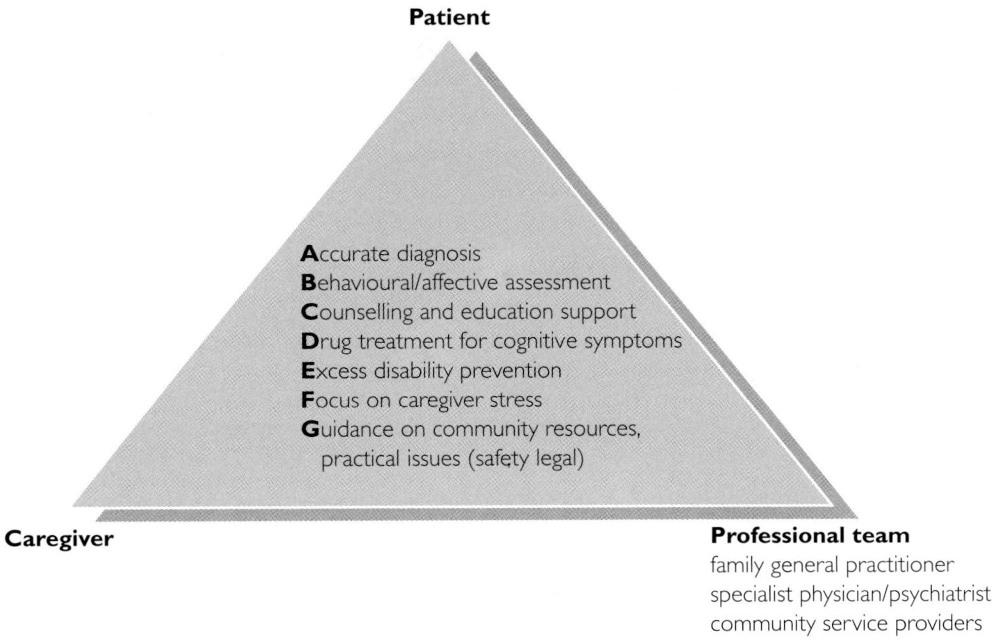

Figure 15.20 Management plan for Alzheimer's disease

drug compliance, side effects and interactions. The burden of care may be eased and residential care delayed with continuing counselling support, referral to community support services and monitoring of carer stress. Effective long-term management requires liaison with other professionals, including specialist geriatricians and psychogeriatricians, community health teams, aged care assessment teams and other community service providers, such as domiciliary care, Meals on Wheels and home nurses. Management plans (Figure 15.20) require continual monitoring and re-evaluation, a process that is best done in partnership with the patient, family and community or residential care providers.

Bibliography and further reading

Ancill, R. J., Holliday, S. G., Thorpe, L. & Rabheru, K. (2000), *Treating Dementia: Cognition and Beyond*, Canadian Academic Press, Vancouver.

Brodaty, H. (1999), *Managing Alzheimer's Disease in Primary Care*, Science Press Ltd, London.

Brodaty, H., Gresham, M. & Luscombe, G. (1997), 'The Prince Henry Hospital dementia care-givers' training programme', *International Journal of Geriatric Psychiatry*, 12, pp. 183–92.

Brodaty, H. & Sachdev, P. S. (1997), 'Drugs for the prevention and treatment of Alzheimer's disease', *The Medical Journal of Australia*, 167, pp. 447–52.

Brun, A., England, B., Mann, D. M. A. et al. (1994), 'The Lund and Manchester Groups. Clinical and neuropathological criteria for fronto-temporal dementia (consensus statement)', *Neurology, Neurosurgery and Psychiatry*, 57, pp. 416–18.

Burns, A., Rossor, M., Hecker, J. et al. (1999), 'The effects of donepezil in Alzheimer's disease—results from a multi-national trial', *Dementia and Geriatric Cognitive Disorders*, 10, pp. 237–44.

Cummings, J. L. (1995), 'Dementia: the failing brain', *Lancet*, 345, pp. 1481–4.

Gauthier, S. (1996), *Clinical Diagnosis and Management of Alzheimer's Disease*, Martin Dunitz, London.

Gauthier, S., Burns, A. & Petit, W. J. (1997), *Alzheimer's Disease in Primary Care*, Martin Dunitz, London.

Geldmacher, D. S. & Whitehouse, P. J. (1996), 'Evaluation of dementia', *The New England Journal of Medicine*, 335, pp. 330–6.

Harvey, R. J., Fox, N. C. & Rossor, M. N. (1999), *Dementia Handbook*, Martin Dunitz, London.

Hecker, J. (1997), 'What's new in dementia?', *Modern Medicine of Australia*, August, pp. 30–45.

Hecker, J. (1998), 'Alzheimer's disease: the advent of effective therapy', *Australian and New Zealand Journal of Medicine*, 28, pp. 765–71.

International Psychogeriatric Association, Finkel, S. (ed.) (1998), *Behavioural and Psychological Symptoms of Dementia (BPSD)* educational pack, seven modules. Gardiner-Caldwell Communications, http://www.vermeulen.net/bpsd/home.htm.

Jorm, A. F. (1997), 'Alzheimer's disease: risk and protection', *The Medical Journal of Australia*, 167, pp. 443–6.

Lundberg, C., Johansson, K., Ball, K. et al. (1997), 'Dementia and driving: an attempt at consensus', *Alzheimer's Disease and Associated Disorders*, 11(1), pp. 28–37.

McKeith, I. G. (1998), 'Dementia with Lewy bodies: clinical and pathological diagnosis', *Alzheimer's Reports*, 1(2), pp. 83–7.

Molloy, D. W., Darzins, P. & Strang, D. (1999), *Capacity to Decide*, New Grange Press, Ontario.

National Institute on Aging/Alzheimer's Association Working Group (1996), 'Apolipoprotein E genotyping in Alzheimer's Disease (consensus statement)', *Lancet*, 347, pp. 1091–5.

Panegyres, P., Goldblatt, J., Walpole, I. et al. (2000), 'Genetic testing for Alzheimer's disease', *The Medical Journal of Australia*, 172, pp. 339–43.

Pesiah, C. & Brodaty, H. (1994), 'Practical guidelines for the treatment of behavioural complications of dementia', *The Medical Journal of Australia*, 161, pp. 558–63.

Report of an International Psychogeriatric Association Special Meeting Work Group under the co-sponsorship of Alzheimer's Disease International, the European Federation of Neurological Societies, the World Health Organization and the World Psychiatric Association, Reisberg, B. & Burns, A. (ed.) (1997), 'Diagnosis of Alzheimer's Disease', *International Psychogeriatrics*, 9 (Suppl. 1), pp. 1–327.

Roman, G. C., Tatemichi, T. K., Erkinjuntti, T. et al (1993), 'Vascular dementia: diagnostic criteria for research studies (Report of the NINDS-AIREN International Workshop)', *Neurology*, 43, pp. 250–7.

Rosler, M., Anand, R., Cicin-Sain, A., Gauthier, S. et al. (1999), 'Efficacy and safety of rivastigmine in patients with Alzheimer's disease: international randomised controlled trial', *British Medical Journal*, 318, pp. 663–8.

Sano, M., Ernesto, C., Thomas, R. G. et al. (1997), 'A controlled trial of selegiline, alpha-tocopherol, or both as treatment for Alzheimer's disease. The Alzheimer's Disease Co-operative Study', *The New England Journal of Medicine*, 336, pp. 1216–22.

Small, G. W., Rabins, P. V., Barry, P. P. et al. (1997), 'Diagnosis and treatment of Alzheimer's disease and related disorders. Consensus statement of the American Association for Geriatric Psychiatry, the Alzheimer's Association, and the American Geriatrics Society', *Journal of the American Medical Association*, 278, pp. 1363–71.

Chapter 16

Confusional states

SHELLEY ANN DE LA VEGA

Definition

Delirium is a syndrome of acute confusion marked by periods of waxing and waning levels of consciousness, altered psychomotor behaviour, and perceptual impairment. *The Diagnosis and Statistical Manual*, Revised Third Edition (DSM-III-R), focuses on four key features:

1. acute change in mental status with fluctuating course
2. inattention
3. disorganised thinking and
4. altered level of consciousness.

The diagnosis requires features 1 and 2, plus either 3 or 4.

Symptoms

The symptoms of delirium are varied in their onset, clinical presentation and duration. Patients may present insidiously in a course of weeks as a result of polypharmacy or drug interactions; within a few days as a result of, for example, an infection such as pneumonia; or suddenly from alcohol withdrawal. Symptoms may last for a few days to a few months after hospital discharge. An observational cohort study of 432 patients over the age of 65 (Rudberg, Pompei, Foreman et al. 1997) showed variations in time course, with delirium on single or multiple days.

There are three types of delirium, based on the level of psychomotor disturbance:

1. Hyperactive delirium is marked by agitation, verbal outbursts, delusional thought processes, visual hallucinations and poor sleep. Patients in hospital may pull out their intravenous lines, 'escape' from bed and refuse medical care. These patients may perceive the staff as threatening, and may be physically violent.
2. Hypoactive delirium is marked by increased sleep and lethargy.
3. In the mixed type of delirium, periods of hyperactivity are punctuated by periods of hypoactivity. A study of 325 patients in a general hospital identified a 15% incidence of hyperactive delirium, 19% hypoactive and 52% mixed type (Liptzin & Levkoff 1992).

Differential diagnosis

Clinicians may find it difficult to distinguish delirium from other forms of cognitive impairment. Differential diagnosis of the acutely confused older patient includes:

- dementia
- manic disorder
- acute paranoid disorders
- delusional depression
- acute psychotic episodes of schizophrenia.

A careful clinical history provided by family members and caregivers will help narrow down the diagnosis. A sudden change in behaviour and personality, and the absence of a prior psychiatric history, usually points to the diagnosis of delirium. It is also important to ask for a history of intellectual impairment, psychologically traumatic events, and possible suicidal ingestion of toxic substances. In contrast to schizophrenia, patients with delirium and visual hallucinations will not have auditory hallucinations and prominent delusions.

Disorientation, impaired memory and inability to learn new information are features that are common in both delirium and dementia. Table 16.1 lists useful points of differentiation.

Aetiology

The progressive decline in the physiological ability to cope with external and internal stresses (homeostenosis) predisposes the older patient to the syndrome of delirium. As such, causes are cumulative and multifactorial. An underlying history of dementia (Chapter 15) is the most significant risk factor for the development of delirium. Delirium is a frequent cause of admission to hospital and may also develop during hospitalisation for other illnesses. Age over 80 years and male sex are independent risk factors for the development of delirium in hospitalised patients. It is a common complication of acute myocardial infarction among patients aged 90 years and older. Intermittent episodes of delirium have been described to occur with various types of arrhythmias. Other causes include infection, pain, drugs, sleep and sensory deprivation, surgery and metabolic abnormalities. Table 16.2 lists the aetiological factors in delirium.

A nested case control study of non-cardiac surgery patients by Marcantonio (1994) at the Brigham and Women's Hospital, Boston, revealed that delirium was positively associated with exposure to meperidine (odds ratio (OR): 2.7; 95% confidence interval (CI): 1.3–5.5) and to benzodiazepines (OR: 3.0; 95% CI: 1.3–6.8). In an earlier prospective study of orthopaedic patients at the same institution, Rogers et al. (1989) revealed a 26% incidence of postoperative delirium in the 46 patients studied. Drugs such as scopolamine, flurazepam and propranolol were associated with a relative risk (RR) for delirium of 11.7 ($p = 0.0028$).

The anticholinergic syndrome is one of the most common causes of drug induced delirium. Drugs that can cause the syndrome include antipsychotics, anti-parkinsonian agents and tricyclic antidepressants. Symptoms of peripheral anticholinergic toxicity (e.g. dry mouth, urinary retention, constipation, ileus, increased intraocular pressure and cardiac dysrhythmias) accompany the CNS symptoms. Table 16.3 lists common drugs associated with delirium in the elderly.

Table 16.1 Differentiating delirium from dementia

Delirium	Dementia
Acute onset	Gradual onset
Lasts for a few hours	Lasts for years
Mental status fluctuates through the day	Mental status declines within months or years
Attention span is impaired	Normal attention span in early stages
Incoherent, rambling speech	Coherent language with word-finding difficulty
Identifiable organic factor or illness	Relatively healthy physical state

Table 16.2 Aetiological factors

	Diagnostic possibility	Caveat
1.	*Infection* Pneumonia, urinary tract infection, cellulitis	May occur in the absence of fever or organ related symptoms
2.	*Drugs* Long-acting benzodiazepines, meperidine, propanolol, scopolamine, H-2 receptor blockers	Drugs with anticholinergic activity Drugs with decreased clearance
3.	*Withdrawal states* Alcohol, benzodiazepines, meprobamate	Daily intake of small amounts of alcohol may cause dependence in older patients
4.	*Hypoperfusion* Congestive heart failure, blood loss, arrhythmias	Tachycardia may be absent
5.	*Hypoxaemia* Pneumonia, COPD exacerbation	May occur in the absence of cough, fever
6.	*Pain* Postoperative, faecal impaction, urinary retention, fracture	Severely demented patients may not be able to verbalise pain
7.	*Malignancy* Paraneoplastic phenomenon, pain	
8.	*Electrolyte abnormalities* Sodium, calcium, magnesium, potassium	May point to a history of neglect or abuse
9.	*Endocrine problems* Hypo- and hyperthyroidism, hypo- and hyperglycaemia	Atypical presentation common
10.	*Sensory deprivation*	
11.	*Sleep deprivation*	
12.	*Physical restraints*	A vicious cycle

Table 16.3 Drugs commonly associated with delirium

	Drug class	Common offending agent
1.	Analgesics	Codeine, meperidine, indomethacin
2.	Antihypertensives	Clonidine, methyldopa, propranolol
3.	Antihistamines	Diphenhydramine
4.	Steroids	
5.	H-2 blockers	Cimetidine
6.	Antimicrobial agents	Isoniazid, gentamicin
7.	Anti-parkinsonian agents	Bromocriptine, l-dopa, carbidopa
8.	Digitalis	
9.	Psychotropics	Antipsychotics, tricyclics, lithium

Prognosis

A recent multicentre study on patients with delirium by Inouye et al. (1998) describes an increased risk of death, nursing home discharge and functional decline even after controlling for age, gender, dementia, severity of illness and functional status. In this study, delirium was present on admission in 12% of 727 patients. At hospital discharge, new nursing home placement was associated with an adjusted OR for delirium of 3.0 (95% CI: 1.4–6.2). Death or new nursing home placement was associated with an adjusted OR for delirium of 2.1 (95% CI: 1.1–4.0). At 3 month follow-up, new nursing home placement occurred in 13% of 600 patients (adjusted OR for delirium 3.0; 95% CI: 1.5–6.0). Francis and Kapoor (1992) reported a trend towards progressive cognitive decline among patients with delirium ($p = 0.023$). Patients with hypoactive delirium were sicker on admission, had the longest hospital stay and were predisposed to develop decubitus ulcers (O'Keefe & Lavan 1999). Hyperactive delirium also predisposes patients to falls and fractures. Postoperative orthopaedic patients in the study by Rogers (1989) revealed that delirium in this subgroup of patients was associated with increased postoperative complications ($p = 0.01$), decline in postoperative mood ($p = 0.06$) and delay in improvement of function 6 months after discharge ($t = 6.43, p < 0.001$).

Medical management

Early recognition of delirium and treatment of its underlying medical cause is the cornerstone of delirium management. A complete medical history should highlight the onset and progression of symptoms. A past medical history of significant medical, psychiatric or dementing illness should be confirmed with relatives or caregivers. A complete list of medications must include over-the-counter drugs. Questions on possible alcohol abuse or drug dependence are essential.

The physical examination should include a description of the patient's mental status. Nutritional status (Chapter 30) may be recorded through the body mass index (kg/m^2) and compared to established cut-off levels. A thorough evaluation of possible systemic illness, orthostatic blood pressure measurement and a complete neurologic examination should be performed.

Routine laboratory tests should include a complete blood count, electrolytes, thyroid stimulating hormone, urinalysis, electrocardiagraph and chest radiograph. Tests for reversible causes of dementia, including syphilis serology and serum vitamin B_{12} levels, may be requested if indicated. A cranial CT scan is recommended if one is considering acute cerebrovascular haemorrhage or subdural haematoma. Otherwise, the emphasis should be on looking for medical causes outside the brain that are reversible and amenable to medical treatment. Careful consultation with family members may help focus the extent and aggressiveness of diagnostic tests and medical care.

Non-pharmacological management includes discontinuation of drugs that may contribute to delirium, especially if no clear indication exists. Frequent reorientation of patients to their surroundings by a familiar face is recommended. Other helpful measures are providing patients with eyeglasses and a hearing aid if they use these, and comfortable lighting and soothing music. A gentle but firm touch may help minimise the use of restraints. Family members or caregivers should be allowed to stay in the patient's room 24 hours a day.

In the presence of severe agitation, hallucinations and combativeness, it is important to ensure that there is no risk to the patient and to staff members. Specific drug treatment aimed at sedation may be appropriate in such situations. Antipsychotic agents with minimal anticholinergic effects that are useful include haloperidol (0.5–2.0 mg per day), risperidone (0.25–2.0 mg/day) and olanzapine (2.5–10 mg/day). Benzodiazepines are reserved for the management of alcohol and sedative withdrawal. Doses of these drugs should be tapered as soon as symptoms improve. When necessary, short-acting benzodiazepines are preferred. When delirium occurs in a patient taking psychotropic drugs, discontinuation of the offending agent is advised.

Delirium is not always reversible, and may persist, especially in patients with pre-existing dementia. Donepezil (2.5–5 mg/day), a cholinesterase inhibitor used in Alzheimer's disease, may be useful (Wengel et al. 1998). The use of physical restraints is best minimised, as it may cause more harm. Table 16.4 lists the most commonly used drugs for behavioural management.

Nutrition

The acutely confused patient is subject to malnutrition and dehydration due to poor oral intake. It is important to make sure that at mealtimes adequate food is consumed. Monitoring the nutritional status is a valuable adjunct to therapy. Sometimes, oral feeding is withheld for fear of aspiration, especially in the drowsy hypoactive delirious state. Feeding by

Table 16.4 Antipsychotic drugs that may be used for delirium

Drug	Dose	Comments
Haloperidol	0.5–2.0 mg/day po or IV, IM	Extrapyramidal symptoms (EPS)
Risperidone	0.25–2.0 mg/day po	Less EPS than haloperidol; sedating
Olanzapine	2.5–10 mg/day po	Sedating
Quetiapine	25–200 mg/day po	Orthostatic hypotension

nasogastric tube may be started if a pattern of poor intake is established. Strict aspiration precautions should be maintained by nursing staff and care-givers.

Rehabilitation

Rapid deconditioning accompanies the state of prolonged delirium. The use of antipsychotic medications and physical restraints contribute to prolonged debilitation. Early referral to a physiatrist (rehabilitation medicine specialist) is essential. Passive range of motion exercises and frequent repositioning every two hours may be initiated in order to prevent decubitus ulcers, dependent oedema and atelectasis in the bed-bound elderly. Ambulatory physical therapy, including gait and balance exercises, are essential.

Prevention

As more studies on delirium become available, the reversible risk factors for delirium will be identified, especially in the hospitalised and perioperative patient. Prevention is multifaceted and demands a great deal of creativity from the medical staff. Primary prevention entails identification of individuals with pre-existing dementia, a recognised risk factor for delirium; avoidance of medications with known anticholinergic activity; minimisation of polypharmacy; and minimisation of sensory deprivation. Secondary prevention consists of early recognition and management of delirium. Tertiary prevention involves early rehabilitation, minimisation of physical restraints, and adequate nutrition. Box 16.1 lists some useful tips that may help minimise the occurrence of delirium.

Box 16.1 Tips on minimising delirium in hospitalised patients

1. Identify patients with underlying dementia or multisensory deficits.
2. Frequently reorient patients to place, time and reason for hospitalisation.
3. Provide the hearing impaired with a hearing aid, the visually impaired with eyeglasses.
4. Make sure the patient receives a comforting touch and a friendly smile from a familiar face.
5. Minimise polypharmacy.
6. Minimise use of long-acting benzodiazepines for sedation.
7. Avoid meperidine use for perioperative pain management.
8. Monitor and correct electrolyte and glucose abnormalities.
9. Ensure early mobilisation.
10. Avoid physical restraints.
11. Have low lighting and soft music in the room.

Bibliography and further reading

Cole, M. G., Primeau, F. J. & Elie, L. M. (1998), 'Delirium: Prevention, treatment, and outcome studies', *Journal of Geriatric Psychiatry and Neurology*, 11(3), pp. 126–37; discussion pp. 157–8.

Djernes, J. K., Gulmann, N. C., Abelskov, K. E., Juul-Nielsen, S. & Sorensen, L. (1998), 'Psychopathologic and functional outcome in the treatment of elderly inpatients with depressive disorders, dementia, delirium and psychoses', *International Psychogeriatrics*, 10(1), pp. 71–83.

Fearon, M. P. & LaPalio, L. (1992), 'Complete heart block presenting as intermittent delirium: Case report and review of the literature on cardiac disease in the elderly', *Journal of the American Geriatrics Society*, 40(5), pp. 507–9.

Fisher, B. W. & Flowerdew, J. (1995), 'A simple model for predicting postoperative delirium in older patients undergoing elective orthopedic surgery', *Journal of the American Geriatrics Society*, 43(2), pp. 175–8.

Francis, J. & Kapoor, W. N. (1992), 'Prognosis after hospital discharge of older patients with delirium', *Journal of the American Geriatrics Society*, 40(6), pp. 601–6.

Inouye, S. K., Rushing, J. T., Foreman, M. D., Palmer, R. M. & Pompei, P. (1998), 'Does delirium contribute to poor hospital outcomes? A three-site epidemiologic study', *Journal of General Internal Medicine*, 13(4), pp. 234–42.

Inouye, S. K., Bogardus Jnr, S. T., Charpentier, P. A., Leo-Summers, L., Acampora, D., Holford, T. R. & Cooney Jnr, L. M. (1999), 'A multicomponent intervention to prevent delirium in hospitalized older patients', *The New England Journal of Medicine*, 340(9), pp. 669–76.

Liptzin, B. & Levkoff, S. E. (1992), 'An empirical study of delirium subtypes', *British Journal of Psychiatry*, 161, pp. 843–5.

Lynch, E. P., Lazor, M. A., Gellis, J. E., Orav, J., Goldman, L. & Marcantonio, E. R. (1998), 'The impact of postoperative pain on the development of postoperative delirium', *Anesthesia and Analgesia*, 86(4), pp. 781–5.

Malone, M. L., Rosen, L. B. & Goodwin, J. S. (1998), 'Complications of acute myocardial infarction in patients > or = 90 years of age', *American Journal of Cardiology*, 81(5), pp. 638–41.

Marcantonio, E. R., Juarez, G., Goldman, L., Mangione, C. M., Ludwig, L. E., Lind, L., Katz, N., Cook, E. F., Orav, E. J. & Lee, T. H. (1994), 'The relationship of postoperative delirium with psychoactive medications', *Journal of the American Medical Association*, 272(19), pp. 1518–22.

Marcantonio, E. R., Goldman, L., Mangione, C. M., Ludwig, L. E., Muraca, B., Haslauer, C. M., Donaldson, M. C., Whittemore, A. D., Sugarbaker, D. J., Poss, R. et al. (1994), 'A clinical prediction rule for delirium after elective noncardiac surgery', *Journal of the American Medical Association*, 271(2), pp. 134–9.

Marcantonio, E. R., Goldman, L., Orav, E. J., Cook, E. F. & Lee, T. H. (1998), 'The association of intraoperative factors with the development of postoperative delirium', *The American Journal of Medicine*, 105(5), pp. 380–4.

O'Keeffe, S. T. & Lavan, J. N. (1999), 'Clinical significance of delirium subtypes in older people', *Age and Ageing*, 28(2), pp. 115–19.

Rogers, M. P., Liang, M. H., Daltroy, L. H., Eaton, H., Peteet, J., Wright, E. & Albert, M. (1989), 'Delirium after elective orthopedic surgery: Risk factors and natural history', *International Journal of Psychiatry in Medicine*, 19(2), pp. 109–21.

Rudberg, M. A., Pompei, P., Foreman, M. D., Ross, R. E. & Cassel, C. K. (1997), 'The natural history of delirium in older hospitalized patients: A syndrome of heterogeneity', *Age and Ageing*, 26(3), pp. 169–74.

Salzman, C. (1992), *Clinical Geriatric Psychopharmacology*, 2nd Edn, Williams & Wilkins, Baltimore.

Wengel, S. P., Roccaforte, W. H. & Burke, W. J. (1998), 'Donepezil improves symptoms of delirium in dementia: Implications for future research', *Journal of Geriatric Psychiatry and Neurology*, 11(3), pp. 159–61.

Williams-Russo, P., Sharrock, N. E., Mattis, S., Szatrowski, T. P. & Charlson, M. E. (1995), 'Cognitive effects after epidural vs. general anesthesia in older adults. A randomized trial', *Journal of the American Medical Association*, 274(1), pp. 44–50.

Zarate Jnr, C. A., Baldessarini, R. J., Siegel, A. J., Nakamura, A., McDonald, J., Muir-Hutchinson, L. A., Cherkerzian, T. & Tohen, M. (1997), 'Risperidone in the elderly: A pharmacoepidemiologic study', *The Journal of Clinical Psychiatry*, 58(7), pp. 311–17.

Chapter 17

Cerebrovascular events

JAMES F. TOOLE and ETERI BIBILEISHVILI

Introduction

Clinical expression of cerebrovascular diseases is most common among those aged 65 or older, but the main causes—atherosclerosis and hypertension—begin in young adulthood. In Western nations cerebral infarction is usually the result of atherosclerosis and accounts for more than 80% of strokes, while intracerebral haemorrhage accounts for only 10–15%. In some Oriental nations, such as Japan, the reverse is true. The risk of having stroke is higher in men than in women and greater for blacks than whites of comparable age and sex.

Surprisingly, the 30-day case fatality rate for cerebral infarction has not declined over a 45-year period in Rochester, Minnesota, despite aggressive risk factor reduction programs, new diagnostic techniques and earlier intervention. Mortality is greater for haemorrhage than infarction.

Hypertension is the most potent of the modifiable risk factors for reduction of ischaemic and haemorrhagic stroke. As has been shown by the Framingham study, risk for stroke among people with blood pressure consistently > 160/95 mmHg was 3.1 times as likely for men and 2.9 for women compared to normotensives. Approximately 10–30% of all strokes are lacunar infarctions, the underlying cause of which is occlusion resulting from hypertensive changes in the muscularis of the penetrating arteries which are 100–400 μm in diameter.

The second major risk factor is atherosclerosis. It is a patchy process disseminated throughout the cerebrovascular bed. Caucasians are more commonly affected and it is twice as frequent in men as women of the same age. Other controllable risk factors are atrial fibrillation, valvular heart disease, coronary artery disease and congestive heart failure.

Transient ischaemic attack (TIA) is considered by many to be a modifiable risk factor. It occurs most often after age 50, is more common in whites than blacks, and men are affected twice as frequently as women. Some consider TIAs to be a form of stroke, while others believe that they are a risk factor. No matter which, TIA is an important indicator of the patient at high risk for subsequent development of an ischaemic stroke.

Diabetes mellitus can involve the cerebral arteries and microangiopathy is a serious complication.

Studies investigating a relationship between stroke and obesity are equivocal, as are those of elevated blood lipid levels. In addition to being carcinogenic, tobacco use promotes arterial vasoconstriction, hypercoagulation and reduces cerebral blood flow.

The relationship between alcohol and stroke remains equivocal. To drink more than 1 oz of 100% alcohol daily even diluted to taste as beer, wine or whisky is associated with elevated risk of stroke. On the other hand, the evidence suggests that light drinking reduces risk.

Sickle cell anaemia, a disease prevalent in blacks, increases stroke incidence.

Pathophysiology

The brain cannot store oxygen or glucose, so it is extremely sensitive to deprivation of blood supply. In ischaemia some cortical cell function ceases within 20 seconds and undergoes irreversible changes within 3 hours. On the other hand, less evolved portions have a greater tolerance. For instance, neurons of the medulla oblongata can function normally for about 20 minutes during hypoxia and may be restored to function after some hours.

The brain is protected from oscillations in blood pressure and flow by its autoregulatory capacity which sustains cerebral blood flow at the same level within mean arterial pressures ranging between 60 and 180 mmHg. Arterial blood pressure is cyclical during a 24-hour period. Its level increases during daytime activities and declines during sleep. These normal fluctuations in systemic blood pressure, when associated with atherosclerosis, can result in critical hypoperfusion. Despite short-lived systemic elevations and reductions, pressure in the arteriolar-capillary network of the brain normally remains constant, because if arterial blood pressure increases, the cerebral arterioles constrict to maintain constant pressure.

Cerebrovascular insufficiency develops when there is discrepancy between the metabolic needs of brain tissue and the supply of blood containing oxygen and other nutrients. Many processes are the result of morphological changes in the arteries, such as occlusion, deformation, compression, anomalies or malformations. Furthermore, fluctuations in haemodynamics, changes in rheological properties of the blood (increased viscosity and coagulation), functional disturbances of intracerebral arteries like persistent spasm, insufficiency of autoregulation and defective collateral circulation are contributing causes. For those interested in detailed consideration of the physiology and pathophysiology of cerebral circulation, we have supplied references at the end of this chapter.

Atherosclerosis

Atherosclerosis predominantly damages the intima of large and medium sized arteries, although small arteries can also be affected. It begins as lipid deposits in young adults, children and even infants, and remains asymptomatic until growing plaque affects blood flow or ulcerates and embolises to the organ it irrigates.

Plaques are most often found at bifurcations, curvatures, angulations and branching points of an artery. Lipids and cholesterol accumulate in the intima that cause proliferation of smooth-muscle cells and connective tissue surrounding the deposit. The plaque increases in size and becomes well vascularised by newly formed vessels from the media. If ulceration of the intimal surface of the plaque occurs, these penetrating vessels may rupture and bleed into the plaque. The ulcerated surface initiates adhesion of platelets which causes thrombus formation, which in turn increases the thickness of the plaque, further reducing the lumen. Moreover, thrombus may break loose into the bloodstream as a thromboembolus to distal arteries. At the same time the arterial wall underlying the plaque atrophies and bulges, resulting in segmental dilatation which causes narrow and dilated segments. These segments change the normally laminar blood flow to a turbulent stream which, in turn, damages new segments of the endothelial wall, inducing further platelet aggregation and accelerating the process.

Atherosclerosis concomitant with hypertension leads to manifestation of the disease at a younger age because hypertension itself increases endothelial permeability and induces thickening of the intima.

Hypertension

In hypertension, the pressure sustained for months and years causes structural changes in the vessels, especially in arterioles, which lose their capacity to dilate and constrict in response to fluctuations in systemic pressure. When this happens, capillary permeability increases, allowing exudation of plasma and erythrodiapedesis. In addition, hypertension causes the walls of the arteries to be necrotised, and increased pressure results in rupture and haemorrhage.

Hypotension

In normal individuals reduction in systemic blood pressure is accompanied by dilatation of the cerebral arteries and arterioles with maximum compensation at about 60 mmHg, below which syncope usually results. Patients with atherosclerosis and hypertension have diminished cerebral autoregulation and so may experience syncope at levels tolerated by normal persons. When systemic blood pressure drops rapidly, cerebral vascular insufficiency may be produced, whereas gradually developing hypotension may have no effect.

Embolism

Infarction can be a result of occlusion of the cerebral artery by an embolus. Such cardiac diseases as rheumatic endocarditis, bacterial endocarditis, myocardial infarction, congenital heart disease and cardiac surgery may be the source for clot emboli which lodge in cerebral arteries. Clots may also form in pulmonary veins and embolise to the brain. Very rarely they originate in the veins of the systemic circulation (thrombophlebitis of the limbs) and travel from the right into the left atrium through a patent foramen ovale.

Embolism occurs more often in the carotid system than in the vertebral-basilar, because the middle cerebral artery is a direct continuation of the internal carotid artery. Therefore, the vast majority of intracranial emboli lodge in the cerebral hemisphere, affecting predominantly the cerebral cortex and subcortical ganglia.

In older patients cerebral embolism is more often caused by emboli made up of cholesterol crystals which are particles dislodged from atheromatous plaques situated on the carotid and vertebral-basilar arteries and arch of the aorta. Air, fat, solid foreign bodies, and tumor emboli circulating in the bloodstream can move to the brain.

Vasospasm

Being a vasospastic disease involving the arteriolar bed, migraine is an unusual cause for ischaemic stroke, most of which occur in posterior cerebral circulation.

Haematologic abnormalities

Blood flow and cerebral oxygen delivery depend on rheologic properties of the blood. Increased viscosity reduces flow velocity and volume, particularly at the capillary level. Therefore, increased haematocrit is an important risk factor for stroke.

Disorders that change the balance between the coagulation and fibrinolytic systems lead to thrombus formation, which may cause stroke. Most important are antithrombin III, protein C, protein S, tissue plasminogen activator deficiency, hypoplasminogenaemia and hyperfibrinogenaemia. Quantitative and qualitative changes of blood cells may lead to increased viscosity or accelerated coagulation. Patients with sickle cell anaemia have abnormal haemoglobin HbSS, which distorts erythrocytic morphology to create the 'sickle' shape. Sickled erythrocytes lose their pliability and tend to adhere to endothelium and clog small capillaries and venules.

Decreased blood flow

Decreased blood flow results in a zone of non-homogeneous brain tissue with a dense core of infarction and a graduated surrounding penumbra of functionally alive but inactive neurons and glia, showing no electrical activity. It is this penumbra with reversible injury that determines stroke outcome because of the ability of these cells to regain function. Therefore, the time elapsed before reperfusion is a critical issue.

Oedema

Oedema is a very threatening complication of stroke. Oedema causing swelling of infarcted segments can increase intracranial pressure and result in compression of adjacent structures and death.

Oedema can be cytotoxic or vasogenic. Cytotoxic oedema, due to intracellular uptake of water, develops shortly after stroke and gradually progresses to a maximum in 2 or 3 days. During ischaemia the permeability of the cell membranes increases and intracellular accumulation of sodium, calcium and chloride ions and degradation products causes influx of water. Vasogenic oedema is associated with disruption of the blood–brain barrier that occurs 3–6 hours after the onset.

Transient ischaemic attack (TIA)

Transient ischaemic attack (TIA) is a focal cerebrovascular event from which the patient recovers completely within 24 hours. Most last no more than 15 minutes, and when they are so brief they leave no abnormal findings on imaging studies. When they persist for many hours, infarcts may become visible even if clinical symptoms resolve within 24 hours, resulting in cerebral infarction with transient symptoms (CITS).

TIAs of less than 30 minutes are most often caused by microemboli, consisting of platelets or cholesterol crystals which travel easily through the large vessels and lodge in the microcirculatory arterial bed. On the other hand, blood clots from the heart valves are usually bigger and lodge in larger arteries where they can produce TIAs of longer duration or CITS.

Vasospasm associated with hypertension and migraine can manifest as TIA, as also can complication of the use of oral contraceptives or street drugs. Sometimes rapid rotation or extension of the head (as when someone looks directly overhead or to the side while reversing in a car) may be associated with a feeling of imbalance or lightheadedness, especially in persons with cervical spondylosis. In such cases one vertebral artery may be hypoplastic, and compression of the normal one during rotation or extension may lead to vertebral-basilar insufficiency.

Lesions of the subclavian artery may invert the normal pressure gradients, resulting in reversed flow through the vertebral artery and thereby diverting blood from brain to arm (see Figure 17.1). In such cases repetitive arm exercise that increases muscle blood flow can cause brain stem ischaemia that subsides as soon as exercise ceases. The portion of the subclavian artery proximal to the origin of the left vertebral artery is the most common site for obstructive lesions. Ultrasound can display this reversed direction of flow. Most are asymptomatic and only those with transient ischaemia clearly precipitated by limb exercise should be remediated.

Other unusual conditions—such as dissection, vasculitis, vasculopathy, systemic lupus erythaematous and Takayasu's arteritis—may produce TIA.

Clinical features

About half of TIAs persist less than 5 minutes, 25% an hour, and only the remaining 25% may continue up to 24 hours. All definitions of TIAs limit their duration to 24 hours. Therefore the examination is usually normal by the time the patient is brought to be examined and the only method for making the diagnosis is the patient's history and the lack of residual neurological deficit.

Clinically TIAs are the symptoms and signs caused by loss of function in the ischaemic segment of brain tissue. When the carotid artery perfusing the cerebral hemisphere is involved, about half experience loss of strength in a hand or foot or the entire side of the body, including the face (see Box 17.1).

Forty per cent of patients experience visual disturbances, such as transient blurring, greying, fogging of vision, with a 'shade' descending over the eye, or even blindness because the ipsilateral ophthalmic artery perfusing the retina is involved. Dysphasia, apraxia and confusion may occur if the dominant hemisphere is involved. Others may describe loss of feeling such as occurs with local anaesthesia. Rarely does a person notice only weakness or numbness of several fingers of the hand (because of its extensive cortical representation).

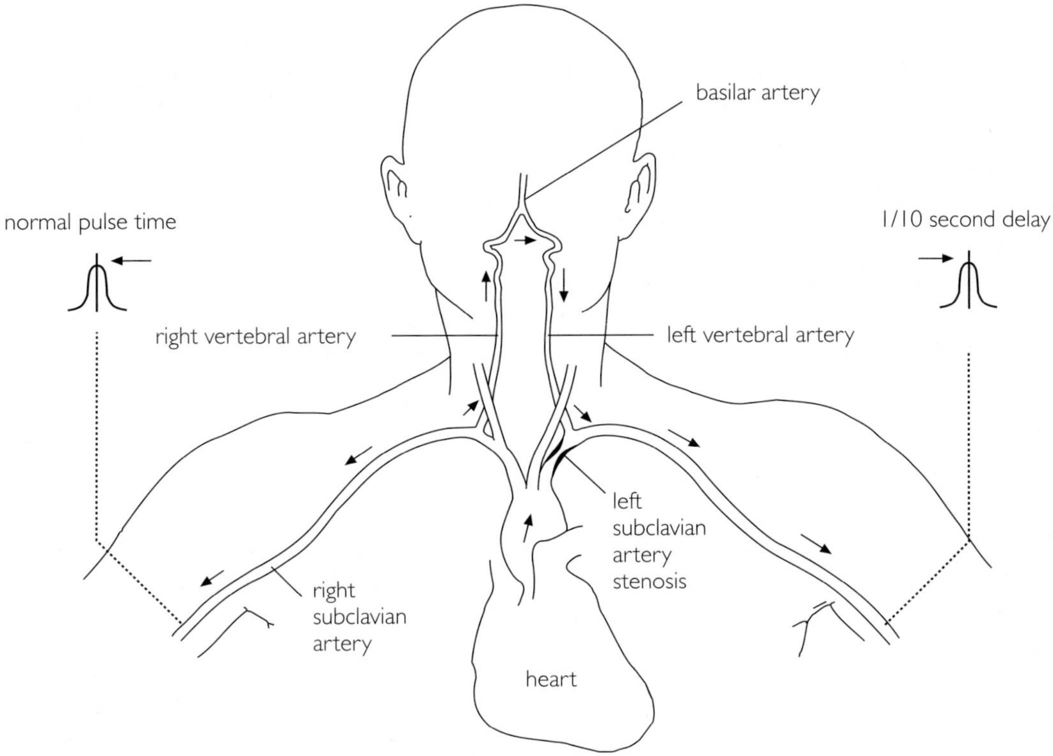

Figure 17.1 Stenosis of the left subclavian artery results in reversed flow through the left vertebral artery which can lead to symptoms and signs of vertebral-basilar insufficiency. The usual physical finding is reduced arterial pressure and a bruit at the subclavian-vertebral junction

Box 17.1 Symptoms and signs suggestive of carotid distribution TIA

- Contralateral paresis or paralysis
- Contralateral paresthesias or numbness
- Ipsilateral transient blurring of vision or amaurosis fugax
- Ipsilateral headache
- Dominant hemisphere:
  - Dysphasia
  - Apraxia
  - Confusion
- Non-dominant hemisphere:
  - Lack of awareness
  - Inattention

Brief involuntary shaking of the arm or leg is a very unusual representation of TIAs.

A particularly troubling problem is limbic system TIA which manifests with episodic behavioural abnormality or amnesia. Some patients are referred to a physician because of transient memory lapses, others with temporary behavioural changes, but many are unaware of illness because of inattention associated with non-dominant hemisphere lesions.

TIA in the vertebral-basilar territory produces many different symptoms (see Box 17.2). The patient can experience vertigo, nausea, vomiting, dystaxia, homonymous visual field loss, cortical blindness or diplopia. If the branches to the upper spinal cord and lower brain stem are involved, a person can have weakness or paralysis of four extremities (drop attacks) with or without loss of consciousness, dysarthria or dysphagia. If small branches to cochlea are affected, an attack may manifest as sudden deafness.

Box 17.2 Symptoms and signs suggestive of vertebral-basilar distribution TIA

Sudden onset

- Unilateral or bilateral weakness or numbness
- Weakness or paralysis of legs or all four extremities (drop attack)
- Diplopia
- Homonymous visual field deficit
- Blindness of cortical type
- Dystaxia
- Dysarthria and dysphagia
- Vertigo, nausea, vomiting
- Decreased hearing or deafness
- Occipital headache
- Lightheadedness, confusion or coma

Differential diagnosis

The essential elements for diagnosis of TIA are:

- sudden loss of function localised to a specific vascular distribution
- restoration of function within 24 hours.

Sometimes it is difficult to differentiate TIA from migraine, syncope, epilepsy, Menière's syndrome and other disorders. For example, focal convulsions can be accompanied by short-lived focal neurologic deficit (postictal Todd's paralysis). Menière's syndrome may simulate TIA in the vertebral-basilar territory. Furthermore, migraine is a paroxysmal disorder with an aura such as visual disturbances, vertigo, dysarthria or ataxia followed by headache of varied intensity which can simulate TIA. In some cases the young age of the patient and family history of migraine help in decisions regarding aetiology.

Evaluation

Disappointingly only about 20% of infarctions are preceded by TIAs. If an event suggestive of TIA has occurred within the past week, the patient must receive an immediate diagnostic evaluation and then management appropriate to the probable aetiology, because such patients represent a high risk group for recurrent TIA or infarction.

Most important is auscultation for bruits, which are likely to be present in patients with carotid artery stenosis or subclavian steal. ECG, CT, MRI, magnetic resonance angiography (MRA) and transoesophageal echocardiography are very helpful for differential diagnosis in specific cases.

Ultrasound can evaluate the degree of stenosis, describe the content of plàques and even detect microemboli. The correlation among ultrasound, magnetic resonance angiography and arteriography is inexact. Stenosis determined by measurement of flow velocity abnormalities on Doppler ultrasound may equate to a lesser degree of stenosis using arteriography. Therefore duplex ultrasound or MRA should be used whenever possible. If a stenosis exceeding 70% is present, the patient should be considered for surgical management.

Management

Platelet-inhibiting agents, such as aspirin (ASA), reduce the occurrence of myocardial infarction and ischaemic stroke. The mechanism of action is based on irreversible acetylation of platelet cyclooxygenase and inhibition of thromboxane A_2 (TXA_2), resulting in decreased platelet aggregation.

The dose of ASA for preventing TIA or stroke has not been fully defined. On one hand, 25 mg dosage decreases the risk of adverse effects, such as gastrointestinal bleeding and haemorrhagic stroke. On the other hand, there are advocates for doses as high as 1500 mg daily. Both regimens have similar therapeutic effects.

Ticlopidine (Ticlid) can be offered to patients with TIA or ischaemic stroke in dosage of 250 mg twice daily if refractory to ASA in high doses or allergic to it. The complications are agranulocytosis, diarrhoea and cutaneous allergy. Clopidogrel (Plavix) is slightly more effective than aspirin and safer than ticlopidine, but requires periodic blood counts and liver function studies. Dipyridamole inhibits uptake of adenosine and is a weak phosphodiesterase inhibitor. The recommended dose of this drug is 50 mg 3 or 4 times per day, and in combination with ASA, could become the safest, most effective and widely used medication for prevention of adverse reactions. It is packaged as aspirin 25 mg and dipyridamole 200 mg (Aggrenox) and does not result in gastrointestinal bleeding or liver dysfunction.

Ischaemic stroke

A variety of pathologic conditions can lead to inadequate blood supply to the brain or any of its component parts, but the pathology common to all is lack of sufficient oxygen and/or other nutrients for normal neuronal function. These include plugging of arteries or arterioles by inflammation, atherosclerosis and emboli, hypercoagulability, vasospasm or hypoperfusion due to low blood pressure.

Ischaemic stroke can develop without warning or be preceded by one or more TIAs. The symptoms and signs depend upon the involved vessels.

Carotid system

Each common carotid artery divides into the internal and external carotid arteries behind the angle of the jaw (see Figure 17.2). Just distal to the bifurcation the internal carotid artery is the bulbous carotid sinus, a common site for atherosclerotic plaques. The cervical internal carotid artery has no branches and traverses the skull through the carotid canal in the petrous part of the temporal bone. Then the internal carotid artery penetrates the dura mater and enters the subarachnoid space above the sella turcica. At this level it gives rise to the ophthalmic, posterior communicating and anterior choroidal arteries before dividing into the anterior and middle cerebral arteries.

In 90% of cases, internal carotid artery stenosis or occlusion occurs in the extracranial part of the vessel, and for these the likely cause for stroke is embolic debris. One-third of the infarctions that patients experience in this territory are preceded by one or more TIAs, probably the result of microemboli.

The typical internal carotid artery syndrome consists of a combination of ipsilateral visual symptoms and contralateral motor or sensory deficit. Temporary loss of vision is often interpreted by patients as 'spots', 'blackout' or 'blurred vision'. Rarely is this loss permanent. Contralateral motor

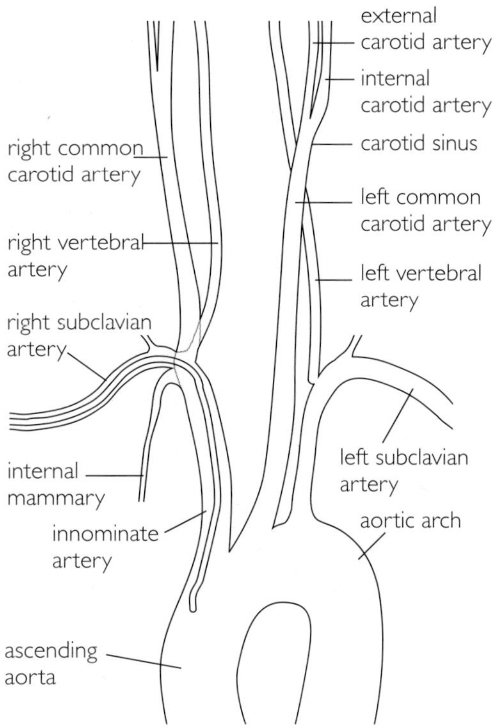

Figure 17.2 Normal aortic arch and great vessels. The common carotid divides into the external and internal carotid at the angle of the mandible. The vertebral arteries arise from the subclavians

deficit may be represented by mono (usually arm) or hemiparesis or hemiplegia. Sensory phenomena may manifest as paresthesias or numbness of the opposite extremities (usually hand or arm) and/or side of the face. If the dominant hemisphere is involved, difficulties with speech and comprehension often occur. Unilateral occlusion of the internal carotid artery can be silent or expressed as middle cerebral artery syndrome because it is the direct continuation of the carotid. If collateral supply from the external carotid, opposite carotid and vertebral-basilar system is sufficient, there may be no signs or symptoms. If, however, the other carotid becomes involved, there may be bilateral hemispheric infarction.

Middle cerebral artery syndrome

About one-quarter of patients with middle cerebral artery stenosis due to atherosclerosis have TIAs because complete recovery is possible if the collateral arterial support is adequate. In some cases of embolic occlusion, the clot disintegrates rapidly or moves to the distal branches and the artery recanalises, restoring function. Atherosclerosis of the middle cerebral artery also occurs, and if there is occlusion at or near its origin, the infarction is devastating and includes the internal capsule and the extensive parts of the cerebral cortex and white matter, causing massive oedema, contralateral hemiplegia, hemianaesthesia and hemianopia. The dominant hemisphere is associated with (Broca's) aphasia; non-dominant lesions produce lack of initiative and anosognosia (failure to recognise the left half of space and body).

Distal blockage of the middle cerebral artery (MCA) causes motor and sensory disturbances of cortical type (deficit will be more prominent in the opposite side of the face and upper extremity) associated with the other signs mentioned above. In some cases the symptoms and signs may include only weakness and numbness of a few fingers and motor aphasia. Infarction of the superior temporal gyrus of the dominant hemisphere may result in receptive (Wernicke's) aphasia. Posterior temporal lesions are associated with upper quadrantanopia. Posterior parietal lesions produce lower visual quadrantanopia.

It can be difficult to differentiate the internal carotid from middle cerebral artery lesions but, as a rule, deficits of the latter are more severe and abrupt than those of the internal carotid artery.

Anterior cerebral artery distribution

The anterior cerebral artery gives rise to numerous deep penetrating branches to the basal ganglia and cortical branches supplying two-thirds of the medial surface of the hemisphere. When the two anterior cerebral arteries reach the midline just above the optic chiasm, they are joined together by the anterior communicating artery. This is a highly important but variable anastomosis which helps to complete the circle of Willis anteriorly (see Figure 17.3).

The signs and symptoms resulting from occlusion of the anterior cerebral artery depend on the location of the obstruction and the collateral anastomoses. For example, blockage of the anterior cerebral artery distally may be asymptomatic. Infarction in the anterior cerebral artery territory only is unusual. The most prominent syndrome includes paralysis of the opposite lower limb with sensory loss, grasp and sucking reflexes, apraxia, aphasia, intellectual deterioration and loss of sphincter control. If both anterior cerebral arteries arise from a common stem, bilateral occlusion may develop with devastating effects.

Vertebral-basilar system

See Figure 17.4. The vertebral arteries arise from the subclavian arteries (in about 5% of persons the left arises directly from the arch of aorta). At the level of the sixth cervical vertebra they enter the bony canal formed by the foramina of the transverse processes of the cervical vertebrae, through which they ascend to the axis (C2), wrap around the posterior arch of the atlas (C1), and finally enter the skull through the foramen magnum. Ascending along the ventro-lateral part of the medulla oblongata, the vertebral artery gives rise to the anterior median spinal artery, numerous unnamed perforating branches, and the posterior inferior cerebellar artery. At the junction between the medulla and pons the two vertebral arteries join to form a single basilar artery.

During rotatory movements of the head upon the neck in normal persons, the blood flow through one vertebral artery may be decreased, and that through the other increased, so that flow through the basilar artery remains constant. However, if one vertebral artery is occluded, such movements can produce temporary disturbances in vertebral-basilar circulation. The vertebral arteries can be stenosed by osteophytes of the cervical vertebrae and this may result in symptoms of brain stem ischaemia during movements of the head upon the neck.

The vertebral-basilar system supplies the upper cervical spinal cord, brain stem, cerebellum, thalamus and occipital lobes of the cerebral hemisphere. Stenosis or occlusion of one or both vertebral arteries leads to a variety of symptoms and signs. Unlike the internal carotid artery, the vertebral artery anastomoses with its opposite artery and

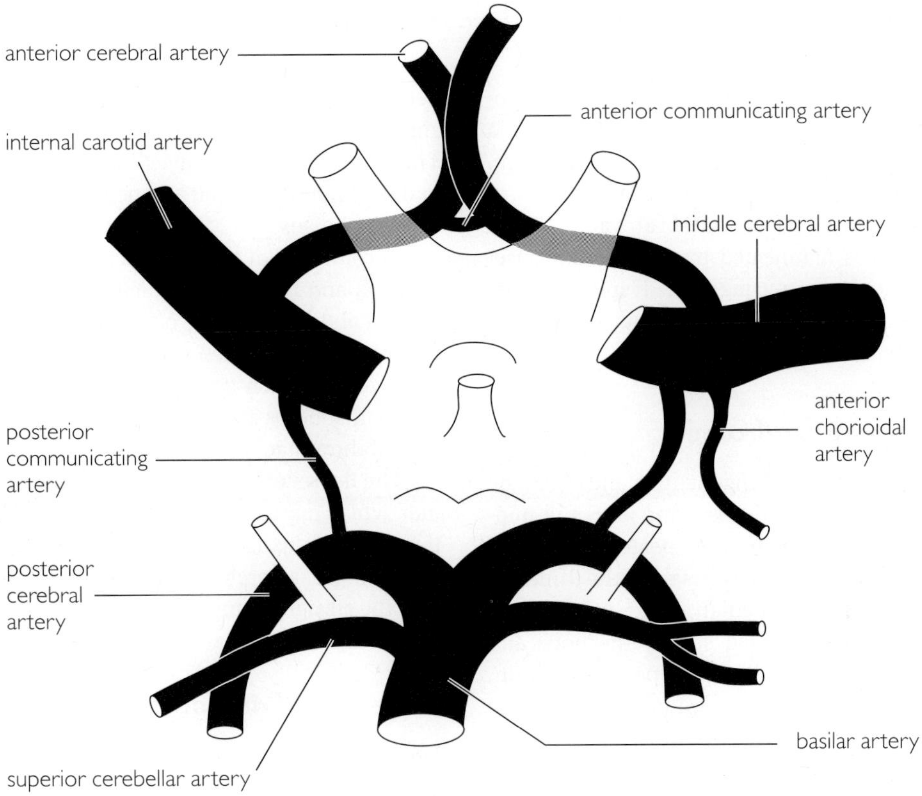

Figure 17.3 Circle of Willis

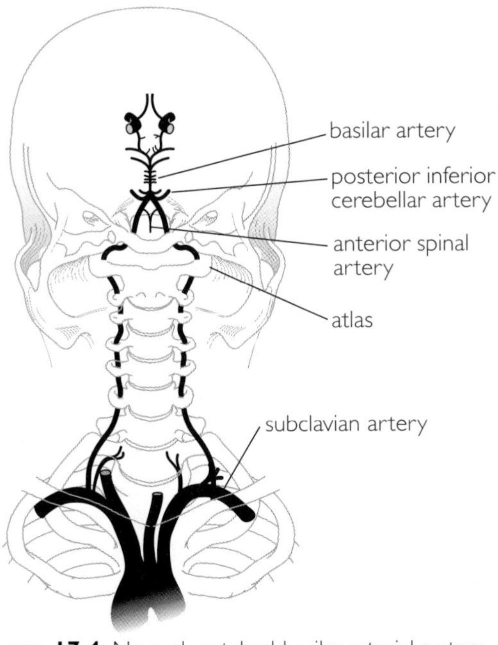

Figure 17.4 Normal vertebral-basilar arterial system

occipital branches of the external carotid artery, allowing blood flow to circumvent vertebral artery occlusion.

In the posterior circulation about half the patients experience TIA before they have an infarction. Motor and sensory deficits are represented by paresis/paralysis and loss of sensation or paresthesias in any combination of extremities. Loss of vision may appear as a segmental homonymous deficit or blindness. Vertigo can present with or without nausea and deafness. Dystaxia, imbalance and intention tremor point to cerebellum involvement.

Ten cranial nerves and the long ascending and descending tracts traverse the brain stem. Cranial nerve involvement (peripheral paresis or paralysis) on one side and hemiparesis/hemiparalysis and/or hemianaesthesias due to long tract lesions on the other (crossed syndromes) are pathognomonic of brain stem abnormality, as are dysarthria, dysphagia, nystagmus and diplopia. Occipital headache is a premonitory symptom in 60% of cases.

Posterior inferior cerebellar artery (PICA) syndrome

PICA originates from the vertebral artery and supplies the lateral wedge-shaped area of the medulla and part of the surface of the cerebellar hemisphere. Infarction in this territory occurs as the result of the direct PICA (10%) or vertebral artery (75%) occlusion and is manifested by the sudden onset of vertigo, deafness, nystagmus, dysphagia, dysarthria, ataxia, nausea and vomiting. Consciousness remains intact.

Basilar artery syndrome

Formed at the junction of the medulla and pons, the basilar artery ends where the pons joins the midbrain by dividing into the two posterior cerebral arteries. The basilar gives rise to the anterior inferior cerebellar, paramedian, short and long circumferential arteries which supply the pons and superior cerebellar supplying upper cerebellum, midbrain and thalamus. Its terminal branches—the posterior cerebral arteries—supply the occipital lobes. Infarction in the territory of the basilar artery is distinctive and includes coma, quadriplegia, ophthalmoplegia, pinpoint or unreactive pupils, decerebrate rigidity and tachypnea.

Cerebellar infarction

Stenosis or occlusion of any of the arteries which supply the cerebellum may lead to oedema with secondary brain stem compression. There develops increased intracranial pressure which should alert the physician to oedema with compression of the brain stem by a swollen cerebellum.

Posterior cerebral artery (PCA)

Occlusion of one PCA usually leads to homonymous hemianopia, while both cause cortical blindness (vision is lost but pupils respond to light). Blockage of the thalamogeniculate branch is represented by the thalamic syndrome, in which pain and temperature perception are reduced and replaced by a particular discomfort (anaesthesia dolorosa).

Venous system

The brain is drained by the superficial and deep venous systems which in turn empty into the dural sinuses and thence into the internal jugular veins. The superficial veins collect blood from the cortex and the underlying white matter and empty into the venous sinuses.

Thrombosis of the superficial veins may cause seizures and neurologic deficit, which depends on the site and extent of the oedema and haemorrhage caused by the occluded veins. Rupture of the superficial veins, which transit the subdural space from the hemispheres to the venous sinuses, results in the subdural haematoma.

The deep venous system drains the periventricular white matter, corpus striatum, thalamus and the choroid plexuses. Blood from this region drains into the great cerebral vein of Galen and thence into the straight sinus.

Differential diagnosis

Because of the large number of structures supplied by the vertebral-basilar system, many diseases can mimic the signs and symptoms of vascular disorder. Aneurysms, meningiomas, cerebellar neoplasm, migraine, episodic hypotension, hypoglycaemia, cardiac dysrhythmias and Menière's syndrome may all present with symptoms and signs suggesting vascular insufficiency.

Lacunar infarctions

Lacunar infarctions occur when penetrating arteries and arterioles supplying the basal ganglia, internal capsule, thalamus and brain stem are occluded. These arteries are especially susceptible to degenerative changes caused by hypertension and diabetes. Cranial CT shows lesions no more than 2 cm in diameter. Lacunes (holes) increase in incidence with age. Usually the clinical presentation consists of unilateral motor or sensory deficit. Multiple lacunes can cause cognitive impairment which impairs a stroke victim's private and social life and accounts for 25% of dementias.

Clinical management

Arterial blood pressure, lipid levels and blood coagulation should be controlled; atherosclerosis, cardiac disorders, coronary artery disease, heart failure and dysrhythmias should be treated.

If the physician suspects brain ischaemia or infarction, emergency transportation to a medical centre for appropriate examinations, tests and therapy is required. Emergency neurovascular and cardiac examinations, CT or MRI of the brain, blood count, prothrombin time, blood glucose and urinalysis must be performed.

In carotid distribution lesions, duplex ultrasound or MRA is essential for making decisions concerning surgical intervention. Within the first 6 hours after ischaemic stroke onset, only 50% of infarctions are visible on cranial CT, but it can identify haemorrhage in 95% of cases. MRI is much more sensitive than CT for lacunar infarctions. Magnetic resonance diffusion-weighted imaging (DWI) can detect and localise an ischaemic region within minutes after onset. Cerebral infarction is demonstrated on standard MRI within 24 hours of onset (see Figure 17.5).

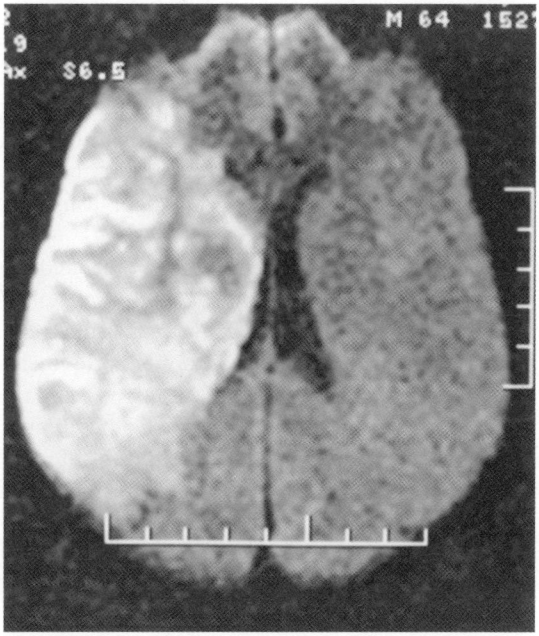

Figure 17.5 MRI. A massive MCA ischaemic infarction with effacement of the right lateral ventricle by oedema

When a patient has cerebral ischaemia for more than 3 hours, treatment is the same, whether it is a TIA or infarction; if less than 3 hours, tissue plasminogen activator (t-PA) derived from endothelial cells should be considered. It activates the fibrinolytic system by converting plasminogen to plasmin, which lyses fibrin. t-PA must be administered intravenously within 3 hours of onset. Blood circulation, respiratory function, urine excretion and electrolyte balance should be maintained. Careful monitoring is necessary and surgical intervention may be considered. In the acute stage of infarction, arterial blood pressure levels of 150–160/100 mmHg are acceptable and do not need correction. Oral diuretics (thiazide or furosemide) or β-adrenergic blockers may be used. If blood pressure exceeds 200 mmHg systolic and 110 mmHg diastolic, labetalol or diazoxide should be administered.

Oedema of some degree accompanies cerebral infarction, and mannitol, furosemide or ethacrynic acid may be useful. For progressing infarction, consider the use of subcutaneous low-molecular-weight heparin or intravenous heparin. For patients with cardioembolic infarction when the risk of haemorrhagic transformation is increased, most delay the use of anticoagulants until the infarct has stabilised. Aspirin in daily doses of 325 mg in the acute phase of ischaemic stroke is recommended for the protection from cardiac and venous clots if the patient can swallow them.

Cerebral haemorrhage

Haemorrhage is divided into bleeding into the brain parenchyma—cerebral haemorrhage—or haemorrhage into the subarachnoid space surrounding the brain. Non-traumatic intracerebral haemorrhage accounts for about 15% of all strokes. In all age groups hypertension is the most common cause because chronic sustained high blood pressure leads to arteriolar lipohyalinosis and fibrinoid necrosis, which weaken the vessel wall and cause its eventual rupture. In most cases haemorrhage originates in parenchymal arteries which perfuse the brain.

Ischaemic infarction can be transformed into haemorrhage because of weakening of arterial and venous wall in the infarcted tissue. Haemophilia, leukaemia, thrombocytopenic purpura, polycythemia and sickle cell disease can cause a massive cerebral haemorrhage. Anticoagulants or thrombolytic agents, given as a treatment for myocardial or ischaemic brain infarction, increase the risk of bleeding as do brain neoplasm and metastases.

The symptoms, signs and outcome depend on the size and location of the haematoma. Lobar haematomas are larger than those in the basal ganglia but usually have a better prognosis. Haematoma situated in the putamen, caudate nucleus or external capsule may have a favourable outcome, but if associated with rupture into the ventricular system or oedema of such degree that it causes herniation and brain stem compression, the chances for survival decrease dramatically.

Intracerebral haemorrhage usually occurs between the ages of 50 and 75 years, and men are affected more frequently than women. The ictus almost always begins during daytime activities. The clinical picture consists of focal symptoms and signs resulting from the loss of function of the brain region in which the bleeding occurs and general symptoms and signs—headache, nausea, vomiting and impaired consciousness due to increased intracranial pressure. If the vessel becomes spastic or a blood clot acts as a tampon, bleeding stops sooner, the haemorrhage remains small, and symptoms of increased intracranial pressure may not occur. This is especially true in the elderly because atrophy of the brain, so often present in this age group, provides additional space into which the haematoma can expand.

Lobar cerebral haemorrhages are located in the supratentorial white matter and usually have a better prognosis than other intracerebral bleedings. Because they are more superficially situated, irritation of grey matter may initiate seizures.

Thalamic haemorrhage usually begins with contralateral hemisensory loss. If the adjacent internal capsule is affected, contralateral paresis or paralysis occurs. If haemorrhage extends to the third ventricle, blood leaks into it, and a clot blocks the aqueduct of Sylvius, obstructive hydrocephalus develops. Extension to the dorsal midbrain leads to miosis and deviation of the eyes downwards and inwards (the converged eyes looking at the tip of the nose). A lesion in the dominant thalamus may lead to aphasia; in non-dominant, to anosognosia and neglect. Prognosis is directly related to the size of the haematoma.

Pontine haemorrhage, as a rule, is associated with sudden, deep coma without preceding symptoms or signs. In contrast to hemispheric lesions, it is characterised by deviation of the eyes and head away from the side of the lesion.

The triad of ataxia, ipsilateral gaze palsy and ipsilateral VII nerve palsy is pathognomonic of cerebellar haemorrhage which may rupture into the fourth ventricle or into the posterior fossa, causing bloody subarachnoid fluid. Swelling of the cerebellum leads to herniation of the tonsils into the foramen magnum, causing brain stem compression. Therefore prompt recognition of cerebellar haemorrhage is important for emergency surgical decompression or insertion of a ventricular drain.

Diagnosis

Infarction usually occurs in the morning or during sleep (the patient wakes up with developed symptoms and signs), after one or more episodes of TIAs; cerebral haemorrhage, on the other hand, develops without warning during daytime activities. Papilloedema, retinal haemorrhages and signs of meningeal irritation are associated with haemorrhage and not with infarction.

Sometimes differentiation between haemorrhage and infarction by history and examination is impossible, but CT (see Figure 17.6) or MRI of cerebral haematoma is easily identified as a dense homogeneous mass, sometimes with a surrounding ring of reduced density consisting of ischaemic tissue and oedema that displaces structures from their normal positions.

It is important to remember that if brain haemorrhage occurs, there is no medical treatment with which to stop it. It is necessary to keep patients as quiet as possible in the hope that the haemorrhage will stop spontaneously. Ventilation and blood pressure must be controlled at once. Blood pressure should be monitored, and its reduction, especially in hypertensive patients, is recommended if the systolic pressure exceeds 200 mmHg and diastolic

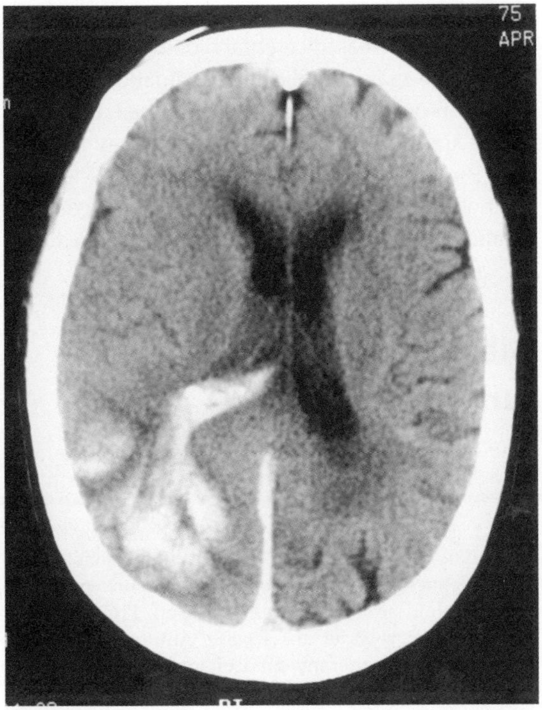

Figure 17.6 CT. Large right occipital lobe intraparenchymal haemorrhage with ventricular extension

110 mmHg. For this purpose nitroprusside or labetalol may be used. For promoting venous drainage, the head of the bed should be elevated to 15–30° above the horizontal. Corticosteroids and osmotic agents, such as mannitol and glycerol, may help control intracranial pressure, but if there are evolving signs of increasing intracranial pressure and brain stem compression, surgical intervention is the only effective choice.

Location of the haematoma plays a key role when surgery is considered. Lesions in the non-dominant hemisphere, in the poles of dominant hemisphere or in the cerebellum may be evacuated, but haematomas in the internal capsule or thalamus should be left alone. Although surgery has higher risks and complication rates in the elderly, age alone is not a contraindication to surgical treatment. Unfortunately, patients with large haemorrhages usually die before treatment can be initiated. Medical treatment with complete bed rest is the best management for patients with small and moderate sized (2–4 cm) haematomas.

Subarachnoid haemorrhage

Subarachnoid haemorrhage (SAH) in the majority of cases is a result of ruptured aneurysm or cerebrovascular malformation. Usually it occurs in the middle decades of life, more often in women than men. The most common cause for subarachnoid haemorrhage in the elderly is iatrogenic, as a result of taking warfarin and other anticoagulants. Head trauma causing subdural haematoma should always be considered because of the increased tendency to fall and to be confused or amnestic after the fall.

Primary SAH develops when blood leaks into the subarachnoid space from a ruptured artery or vein. If it extends from an intracranial haemorrhage through the parenchyma to the surface of the brain or into the ventricles, it is called secondary. In most cases SAH strikes instantaneously; in others headaches, giddiness, diplopia, blurred vision or neck stiffness precede the onset. The clinical picture depends on the site of the rupture, the quantity of blood leaked into the subarachnoid space, and the rate at which it accumulates. The patient's level of consciousness varies from normal to deeply comatose. If patients are conscious, they may think that something has struck them on the head or they may feel something 'pop' or snap inside their skull. They describe this headache as more severe than any other they have had before. Ache begins focally in any part of the head and then rapidly becomes generalised and radiates into the neck. Nausea and vomiting are common, caused by a sudden increase in intracranial pressure. Bilateral extensor plantar reflexes (Babinski signs) are present within an hour of the onset. Resistance to neck flexion rapidly develops. Papilloedema or haemorrhages in the retina may be present within an hour of the ictus. If convulsions are to occur, they usually take place at the time of the ictus or immediately thereafter. Patients with subarachnoid haemorrhage are not paralysed and usually do not have focal neurologic signs because blood is released quickly into the cerebrospinal fluid. Although constriction of the ruptured vessel is lifesaving, spasm of the neighbouring or distant arteries which usually accompanies SAH can produce focal neurologic signs, cerebral infarction, cerebral oedema and lead to a bad outcome.

Differential diagnosis

If the patient's complaints are confined to headache and nuchal resistance, meningitis, migraine, sinusitis, allergy and cervical radiculopathy may be diagnosed incorrectly. Clouded consciousness with papilloedema and retinal haemorrhages may suggest hypertensive encephalopathy. Patients with headache, impaired consciousness and signs of irritated meninges should undergo CT at once to identify the presence of blood in the subarachnoid space and to detect associated intracerebral or intraventricular blood and source of bleeding. CT is more specific for detecting acute SAH than MRI in the first 2–3 days. Thereafter blood may be dispersed and CT will become negative. In contrast, MRI may become positive. If there are no neuroimaging abnormalities or transtentorial or transforaminal herniation, a diagnostic spinal puncture and examination of the CSF should be performed. If the CSF contains blood, a traumatic lumbar puncture should always be considered.

Treatment

Patients should be transported at once to a specialised centre where surgical treatment is available. Surgical intervention cannot be performed if MRI and conventional contrast arteriography reveal no aneurysm, neoplasm and other abnormalities. Surgery should be avoided in patients who are *in extremis* or have other disease that precludes surgery. For patients who are managed medically, bed rest is indicated for a period of 4 weeks after SAH. Headaches may be controlled by codeine. Blood pressure should be sustained at levels just sufficient for coronary, renal and cerebral perfusion (to reduce the risk of rebleeding). For normotensive patients a systolic level of 100 mmHg is recommended, while for hypertensive persons it can be higher. To control elevated intracranial pressure dehydration using dexamethasone (6–10 mg every 6 hours), mannitol or glycerol is recommended. Nimodipine can be used for prevention of vasospasm which usually develops between the 4th and 17th day. Intracranial pressure should be carefully monitored. If it is greatly elevated, additional vasodilatation and increased cerebral blood flow caused by nimodipine may complicate the situation. Epsilon-aminocapronic acid infusion can be used, but initial effects appear 48 hours later and this may increase the risk of thrombotic complications. When the haemorrhage is caused by the use of anticoagulants, vitamin K should be immediately administered.

Bibliography and further reading

Adams, Harold P. et al. (1994), 'Guidelines for the management of patients with acute ischaemic stroke', *Circulation*, 90, pp. 1588–98.

Adams, Harold P. et al. (1996), 'Guidelines for thrombolytic therapy for acute stroke: a supplement to the guidelines for the management of patients with acute ischaemic stroke', *Circulation*, 94, pp. 1167–81.

Albers, Gregory W. et al. (1998), 'Antithrombotic and thrombolytic therapy for ischaemic stroke', *Chest*, 114, pp. 683S–98S.

Alberts, M. J. et al. (2000), 'Recommendations for the establishment of primary stroke centers', *Journal of the American Medical Association*, 283, pp. 3102–9.

Awad, A. (1992), *Cerebrovascular Occlusive Disease and Brain Ischaemia*, American Association of Neurological Surgeons, United States.

Haley Jnr, E. C. (1997), 'Myths regarding the NINDS rt-PA Stroke Trial: setting the record straight', *Annals of Emergency Medicine*, 30(5), pp. 676–82.

Hossman, K. A. (1988), 'Pathophysiology of cerebral infarction', in Vinken, P. J., Bruyn, G. W. & Klawans, H. L. (eds), *Handbook of Clinical Neurology*, Elsevier Science Publishers, Amsterdam and New York, pp. 107–53.

Karanjia, P. N. et al. (1997), 'Validation of the ACAS TIA/stroke algorithm', *Neurology*, 48, pp. 346–51.

'Post stroke rehabilitation' (1995), in *Clinical Practice Guideline* Number 16, US Department of Health and Human Services, AHCPR Publication No. 95-0662.

Semple, Peter F. & Sacco, Ralph L. (eds) (1999), *An Atlas of Stroke*, The Panthenon Publishing Group, New York.

The National Institute of Neurological Disorders and Stroke rt-PA Stroke Study Group (1995), 'Tissue plasminogen activator for acute ischaemic stroke', *The New England Journal of Medicine*, 333, pp. 1581–7.

Toole, James F. (ed.) (1999), *Cerebrovascular Disorders*, Lippincott Williams & Wilkins, Philadelphia, PA.

Welch, K. M. A., Caplan, Louis R., Reis, Donald J., Siesjö, Bo K. & Weir, Bryce (eds) (1997), *Cerebrovascular Diseases*, Academic Press, London.

Part V

ENT and eye conditions

Chapter 18

Hearing impairment and tinnitus

PETER-JOHN WORMALD

Introduction

Hearing is one of the most important faculties for the ageing person. The ageing person is often able to compensate for loss of mobility by still interacting with friends and family. However, loss of hearing leads to isolation of the person, even in a room full of people. Such isolation can have very detrimental consequences, with the person feeling abandoned and alone in the world as a direct consequence of not being able to hear and interact. This can result in social withdrawal and depression.

Prevalence of hearing loss in the elderly

Hearing loss is a very common condition in the ageing patient. The incidence of deafness in the 65 to 74 year age group is 12%, in the 75–84 year age group 16% and in the 84+ age group 30%. About three-quarters of these patients will use a hearing aid for their deafness. This high prevalence is due to the interaction of the ageing process and noise which causes damage to the hair cells of the organ of Corti (the hearing organ in the cochlea). Sound waves stimulate the basilar membrane and movement of this membrane stimulates hair cells. These hair cells connect to neurones that transmit electrical impulses to the brain where the noise is heard. Loss of hair cells causes a sensorineural hearing loss.

Aetiology of hearing loss

Presbycusis (hearing loss due to ageing)

The most common causes of hearing loss are presbycusis and wax impaction. Wax impaction is easily remediable and its management is described below. Presbycusis occurs due to hair cell loss and damage in the cochlea. This is due to constant lifelong exposure to noise and sounds that causes hair cell loss predominantly in the basal turn of the cochlea (higher frequencies). Consequently the patient develops the classic high frequency hearing loss of ageing (presbycusis). The classic audiogram has a ski-slope appearance (see Figure 18.1) with preservation of the low frequencies and loss of the high frequencies. Preservation of the low tones results in the person being able to hear that they are being spoken to, but loss of the high frequencies results in the inability to clearly make out the words. While the volume is contained in the low frequencies, the clues for word recognition (the consonants) are in the high frequencies. Background noise will also aggravate this situation, as the noise tends to mask the higher frequencies and decrease the person's ability to discriminate the words.

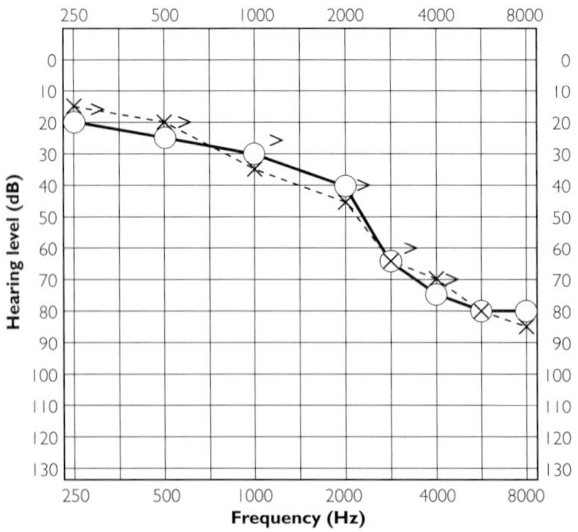

Figure 18.1 Classic ski-sloped audiogram associated with presbycusis

Tinnitus

Tinnitus is commonly associated with sensorineural hearing loss. The usual cause for the tinnitus is the loss of hair cells. The outer hair cells in the organ of Corti are inhibitory and allow accurate discrimination of the tone by inhibiting hair cells adjacent to those stimulated by the tone. The hair cell loss of presbycusis occurs mostly among the outer hair cells. The loss of the inhibitory role of the outer hair cells causes the residual hair cells to generate a noise, which is perceived by the patient as tinnitus.

Tinnitus is extremely common in the general population, with up to 20% of the population experiencing tinnitus at some point in their lives. As tinnitus is caused by hair cell damage, treatment is difficult. One of the most effective measures for tinnitus in patients with a hearing loss is to provide a hearing aid. Not only will the aid amplify the spoken word but it will also amplify the background noise and thereby mask the tinnitus. An alternative therapy is to teach the patient to focus on other sounds, thus obliterating the tinnitus from the consciousness—so-called tinnitus retraining. This is a multidisciplinary approach that requires input from the ENT surgeon, audiologist and psychologist.

Wax

Wax impaction is a very common cause of hearing loss. The impacted wax prevents the sound waves from striking the tympanic membrane, resulting in a conductive hearing loss (Figure 18.2). The easiest way to remove wax is to syringe the external canal (see 'Obtaining a view' below).

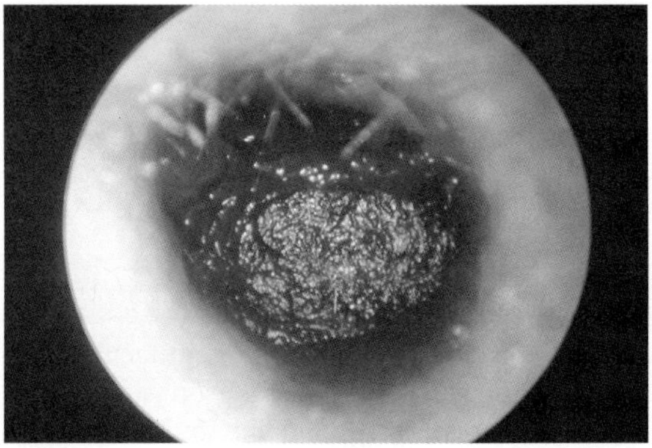

Figure 18.2 Wax in the external auditory canal obscuring the view of the tympanic membrane

Chronic suppurative otitis media (CSOM)

CSOM is less common but still an important cause of hearing loss. CSOM may either be active or inactive. Active CSOM presents with a discharging ear and hearing loss, while inactive CSOM will only present with hearing loss. CSOM can be classified into mucosal or squamous disease. Mucosal disease usually presents with a perforation in the pars tensa (Figure 18.3), while squamous disease (also called cholesteatoma) usually presents with a retraction/perforation in the pars flaccida. It is important to recognise CSOM because mucosal disease can be remedied by simple surgery and squamous disease is potentially dangerous and needs to be surgically removed.

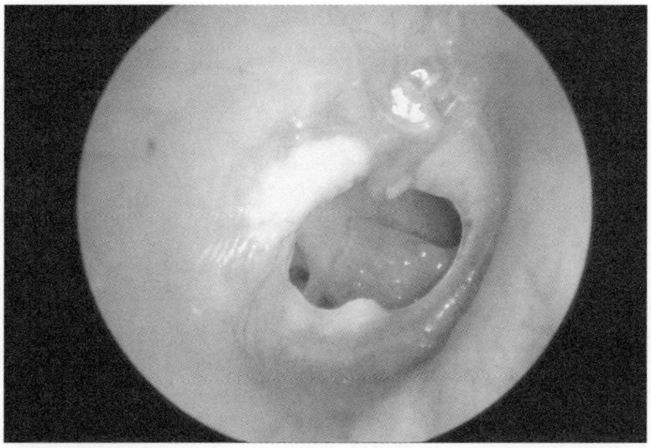

Figure 18.3 Perforation of the pars tensa of the tympanic membrane resulting in a conductive deafness

Retrocochlear causes of hearing loss

Acoustic neuroma is an uncommon but important cause of hearing loss and is found in relation to the vestibular nerve in the internal auditory meatus and/or cerebello-pontine angle. The acoustic neuroma (or vestibular Schwannoma) is a benign Schwann cell tumour that is found on the inferior vestibular nerve. It may cause hearing loss by pressure on the cochlear nerve. The clue to this diagnosis is the discrepancy in the hearing between the two ears. An acoustic neuroma should always be considered in patients with asymmetric hearing loss without an obvious cause for such asymmetry. Figure 18.4 illustrates a small acoustic neuroma in the internal auditory meatus on an MRI scan. Figure 18.5 shows the typical asymmetrical hearing loss on

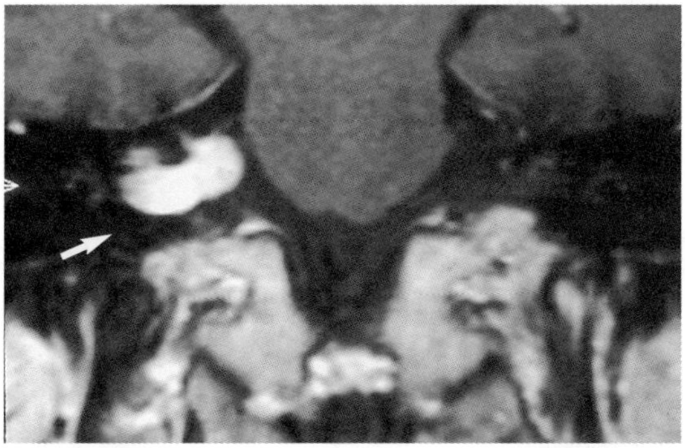

Figure 18.4 MRI scan of the cerebro-pontine angle showing a small acoustic neuroma (arrow). Gadolinium has been given and the neuroma lights up white on the MRI scan

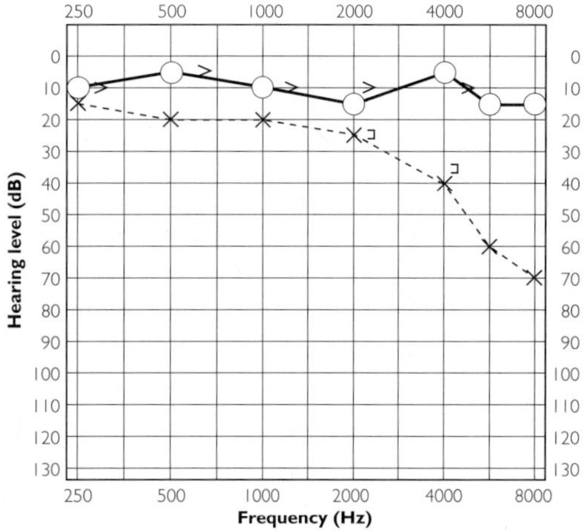

Figure 18.5 Audiogram showing the classic asymmetric sensorineural hearing loss associated with an acoustic neuroma

audiological assessment found in patients with an acoustic neuroma.

Practical management of hearing loss

History

When taking a history from a patient complaining of hearing loss and/or tinnitus, the following information is relevant:

- the duration and progression of the hearing loss
- the severity and whether it is unilateral or bilateral
- whether the hearing loss has been associated with any significant events, such as treatment with intravenous drugs or a significant head injury
- whether there are associated symptoms such as tinnitus and dizziness (should the patient have tinnitus, the side/s, severity and duration must be ascertained; should the patient have dizziness, please see Chapter 19 on dizziness for its assessment and management)
- whether otalgia (the pain felt in the region of the ear) and/or otorrhoea were present—these would normally indicate an infective cause for the hearing loss

- possible predisposing conditions, such as a history of noise exposure.

Obtaining a view

The practitioner cannot make a diagnosis if the tympanic membrane cannot be examined. If a patient has an otological symptom it is mandatory for the eardrum to be examined. If a view cannot be obtained, the patient should be referred to a specialist so that the eardrum can be examined and the appropriate treatment given. Wax is the most common substance obstructing the external auditory canal. The easiest way to remove wax is to syringe the external canal with lukewarm water. The equipment required is a 20 mL or larger syringe with the soft (silastic) part of an 18 gauge intravenous cannula firmly attached to the end of the syringe. You must make sure that the cannula is very firmly attached to the syringe in order to avoid the cannula being shot down the external canal as pressure is generated in the syringe barrel. Sterile water that has been warmed to 37°C should be used. A rule of thumb is that if the water feels slightly warm to the back of the hand it should be around 37°C. The saline is placed in a receiver and liquid soap added. The soap decreases the surface tension of the water and allows the water to ingress into the wax and thereby soften it. If the wax is impacted or solidly occludes the external canal, tilt the patient's head to the opposite side and fill the external canal with soapy water. Then the patient pushes the tragus in and out of the ear canal in a so-called squidging motion for about 20 minutes. This softens the wax and facilitates syringing. Should residual wax remain, you may need to repeat this process. For very serious cases of impaction, you may need to send the patient home with soapy warm water to squidge overnight and instruct her to return the next day for repeated syringing.

For the syringing process, in addition to the syringe and intravenous cannula, you need an adequate headlight, a receiver dish and warm soapy water. The first principle is to view the obstructing wax plug with an auroscope and establish where the wax does not touch the side wall of the ear canal. Straighten the external canal by pulling the ear postero-superiorly. With the headlight illuminating the canal, aim the cannula at the gap between the wax and the canal wall. Bounce the water off the canal wall so that water pressure is generated behind the wax ball and causes its extrusion (Figure 18.6).

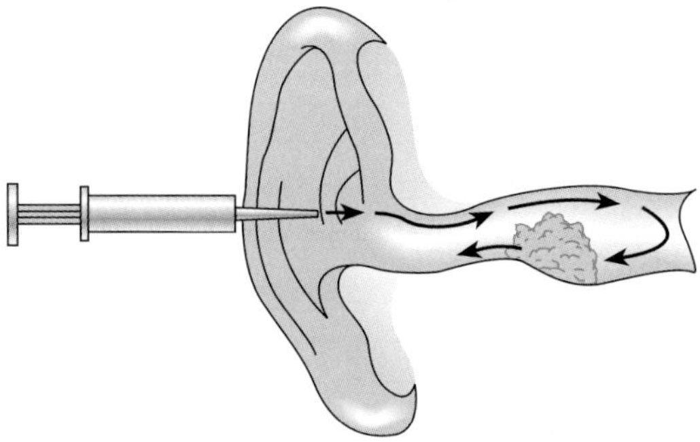

Note: *For extrusion to occur, the stream of water needs to be bounced off the wall of the ear canal so that water pressure is built up behind the wax.*

Figure 18.6 Stream of water bounced off the wall of the external auditory canal in order to generate water pressure behind the wax plug to produce its extrusion

The principles of otoscopy

The first step is to straighten the ear canal by pulling the pinna in a postero-superior direction. Place the largest speculum available on the otoscope and gently slide it into the external canal. Achieve orientation by actively seeking the handle of the malleus, light reflex and lateral process of the malleus (Figure 18.7). The normal drum can vary in its appearance from translucent (Figure 18.7) to

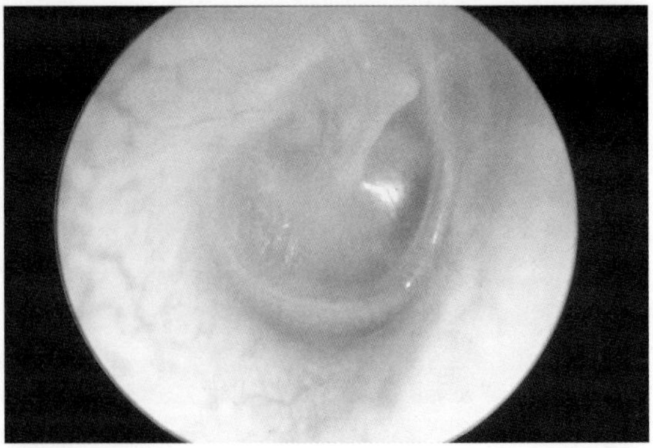

Figure 18.7 Normal tympanic membrane with handle of malleus visible. The tympanic membrane appears pearly grey and translucent

opaque (Figure 18.8). White plaques on the drum (tympanosclerosis) (Figure 18.9) represent calcium deposits in the drum which indicate previous infections in the middle ear. It is important to be able to recognise normality, otherwise pathology cannot be diagnosed. Chronic suppurative otitis media usually presents with a history of hearing loss and discharge from the ear. The tympanic membrane will often have a perforation visible (Figure 18.3). These patients should be referred to an ENT surgeon for further management.

Hearing tests and audiology

A clinical test of hearing can be performed to assess hearing by using your voice at various intensities to ascertain in a gross manner the degree of hearing loss. With the patient facing forward, stand opposite the ear to be tested. Place a finger over the tragus of the non-test ear and push this in and out during the testing procedure. This masks the non-test ear and prevents the patient using this ear to hear the tested sounds. Then whisper a combination of letters and numbers, keeping an arm's length from the tested ear. Use numbers and letters such as 9b and 7e. If the patient is able to score greater than 50% correct then the hearing will usually be within normal range. This technique will usually test the lower frequencies more accurately than the higher frequencies. If the patient cannot hear a soft conversational voice at arm's length than there is a moderate hearing loss present in the tested ear. If both ears have moderate or worse hearing, the patient would probably benefit from using a hearing aid and formal assessment is necessary.

Formal audiological assessment is performed by an audiologist in a soundproof booth. The classic audiological picture of presbycusis is a ski-sloped audiogram with greater hearing loss in the higher frequencies than in the lower frequencies. The higher frequencies in the basal turn of the cochlea appear to be more susceptible to the combination of noise and the ageing process (Figure 18.1).

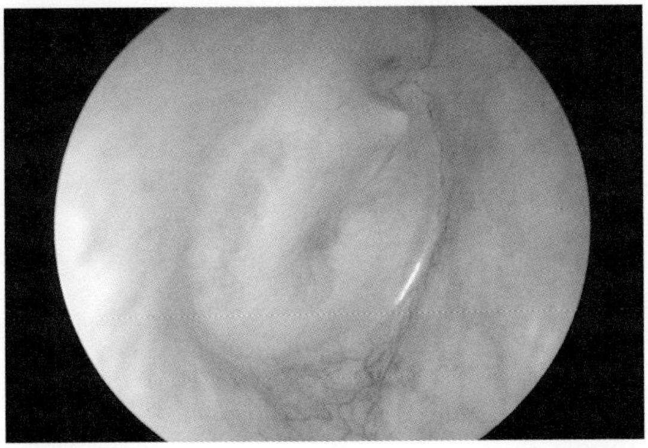

Figure 18.8 Normal tympanic membrane with diffuse thickening of the drum, resulting in an opaque appearance of the drum

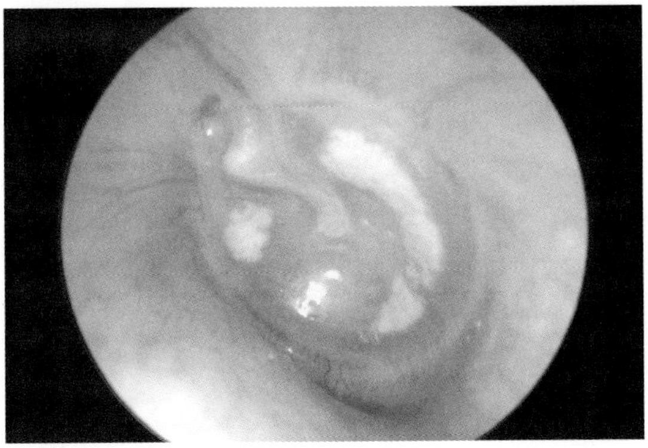

Figure 18.9 White calcified plaques visible in the tympanic membrane. These plaques are the result of previous middle ear infections

Hearing aids

Hearing aids remain the most effective means of treating hearing loss in the elderly. Patients with normal hearing in the lower frequencies of either one or both ears would not normally benefit from a hearing aid. When the lower frequencies are affected in both ears, the patient would benefit from a hearing aid. In the hearing aid, amplification can be adjusted so that the higher frequencies are amplified more than the lower frequencies. This allows the amplification of each frequency to be matched to the frequencies lost in each patient. One of the benefits of a hearing aid is the ability of the aid to amplify background noise. This background noise tends to mask the tinnitus of the patient and is often the most effective way of managing the tinnitus. Properly trained personnel should be involved in the testing, prescription and fitting (including adjustment) of hearing aids to ensure the most suitable aid is provided. This will ensure that the patient receives maximum benefit from the hearing aid.

Bibliography and further reading

Havlik, R. J. (1986), 'Ageing in the eighties, impaired senses for sound and light in persons age 65 years and over', NCHS Advancedata no. 125.

Wormald, P. J. & Browning, G. G. (1996), *Otoscopy: A Structured Approach*, Arnold, London.

Chapter 19

Dizziness and lightheadedness

PETER-JOHN WORMALD

Introduction

The words 'dizziness' and 'lightheadedness' may sound similar and, in fact, lay people may interchange them to describe their symptoms. In the medical fraternity, dizziness is defined as rotatory vertigo. This is the sensation of either the room or the patient spinning, an hallucination of movement. Lightheadedness, in contrast, is the feeling of 'floating', 'unsteadiness' or 'lack of security while standing or walking'. In the elderly lightheadedness is common, as the process of ageing affects the sensory inputs into the brain and this results in the feeling of 'lightheadedness'. If this distinction can be made early in the consultation, the further direction of both the history and examination will be clearer, with a diagnosis more likely to be achieved.

How balance is maintained

Balance is maintained by a complex interaction between the senses, vestibular system and the brain. The important senses are the proprioceptive sensors and visual stimulation. The proprioceptive senses in the neck and shoulders and, to a lesser extent, in the rest of the body deliver constant messages to the brain about the position of the head and its relation to the rest of the body. The vision sends messages regarding the body's interaction with the environment. If these sensory inputs are perceived as abnormal by the brain during car and boat rides, motion sickness and a feeling of unsteadiness may result. These sensory inputs are correlated to the continuous information from each vestibular apparatus by the cerebellum (see Figure 19.1). Disturbance from the sensory inputs usually results in lightheadedness or unsteadiness without rotatory vertigo. If patients have arthritis of the neck, proprioceptive information may be disrupted and the cerebellum may recognise this altered information: the patient may feel lightheaded or unsteady.

Acute disruption of the vestibular systems results in a severe dizziness or rotatory vertigo as the role of the vestibular apparatus is more substantial than the other sensory inputs. The analogy to explain this is to liken the vestibular apparatus to an airplane with two engines. When both engines are working equally, the pilot is in control and the plane is flying level and steady. But if one engine develops a fault and cuts out, the airplane is all over

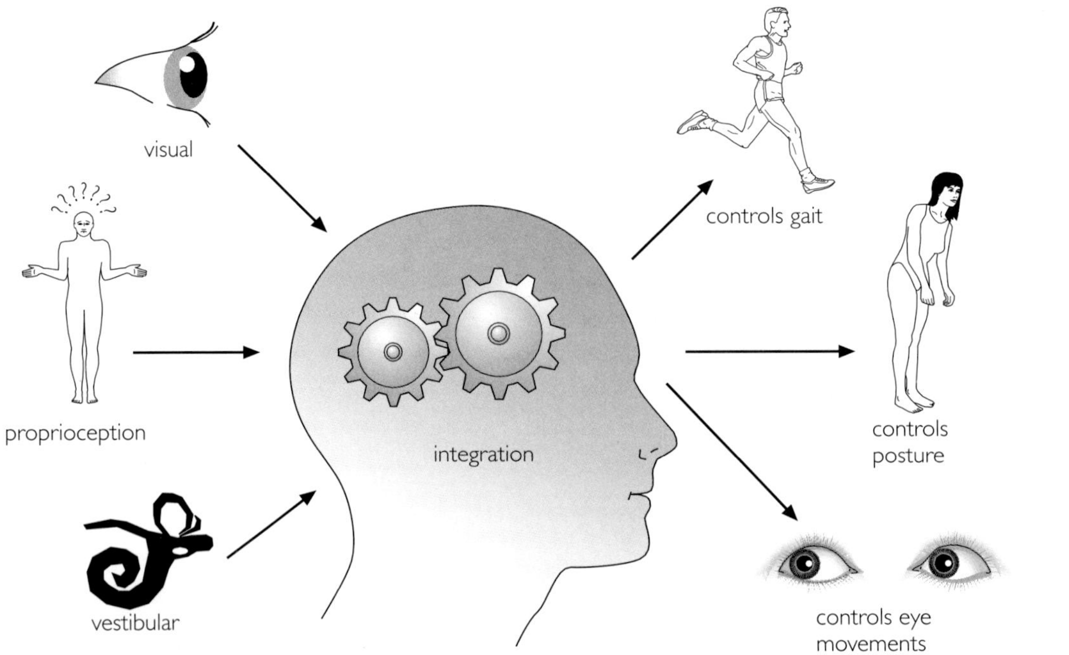

Figure 19.1 The integration of the various sensory inputs into the brain allows the brain to control posture, gait and eye movements (nystagmus)

the sky as the pilot struggles to regain the plane's equilibrium and bring it on a steady course (see Figure 19.2). Eventually the pilot learns to compensate for the loss of the engine and regains control. Steady flight resumes. In the patient who suddenly loses one vestibular apparatus, the same inability to control balance occurs and the patient is acutely dizzy. Before the sensation of dizziness resolves, compensation for this loss needs to occur. To further explain this analogy one must understand that the vestibular apparatus has a constant electrical discharge telling the brain where the head is in space. Should one of these apparati suddenly cease to function, the brain is unable to interpret the mismatched information and the patient becomes acutely dizzy with rotatory vertigo. However, as time passes, the brain will be able to compensate for the loss of vestibular input and the patient will slowly regain his equilibrium. In the clinical setting vestibular neuronitis or vestibular failure from an infarct or embolus would present in this way. These patients classically give a history of one attack of severe prostrating vertigo that lasts days before slowly resolving. However, it is more common for the labyrinth to have intermittent dysfunction. This occurs in conditions in which the electrical discharge is altered intermittently, such as occurs when the particles in the posterior canal move in benign paroxysmal positional vertigo (BPPV) and when cochlea hydrops (increased pressure within the inner ear) develops in Menière's syndrome. The ability of the patient to compensate is reduced by the fluctuating electrical activity generated by the vestibular system.

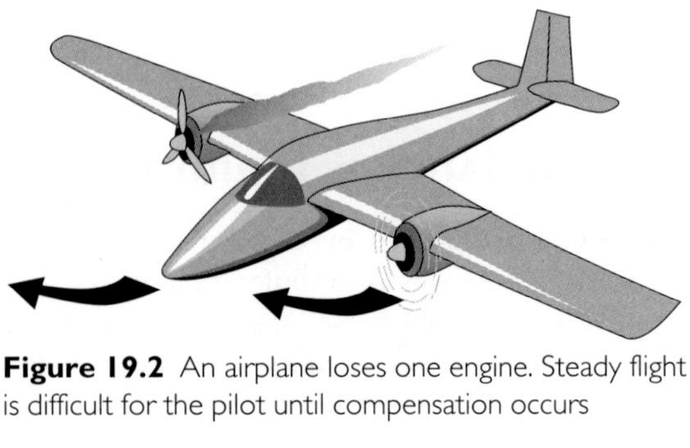

Figure 19.2 An airplane loses one engine. Steady flight is difficult for the pilot until compensation occurs

Dizziness or lightheadedness?

This is the central question for the general practitioner. The differentiating factor in dizziness and lightheadedness is the presence of rotatory vertigo. Rotatory vertigo indicates true dizziness. There are two major causes of rotatory vertigo. The most common cause is loss of function of a vestibular apparatus. However, infarcts or haemorrhages in the brain stem or brain tissue may also produce rotatory vertigo. The differentiating factors are the presence of nystagmus, associated otological symptoms or associated neurological symptoms or signs. Patients who have a peripheral (vestibular or ear) cause for their rotatory vertigo will have horizontal nystagmus present when they feel dizzy. They will often have associated ear symptoms such as hearing loss, tinnitus or ear fullness. Dizziness from the central nervous system may have changing or vertical nystagmus but it is extremely rare without other focal neurological signs, such as abnormalities of gait, diplopia, dysphagia or sensory or motor disturbance.

Dizziness

Common causes of peripheral vertigo (dizziness)

The most common causes of peripheral (true rotatory) vertigo are benign paroxysmal positional vertigo (BPPV), Menière's syndrome, vestibular neuronitis and labyrinthine fistula.

Benign paroxysmal positional vertigo (BPPV)

The aetiology of BPPV is uncertain and most cases have no discernible cause. The pathology is thought to be free otoconia (crystals) drifting in a gravity dependent fashion in the posterior semicircular canal (PSCC). Head injuries have been implicated and are thought to loosen otoconia in the PSCC. When the PSCC is placed in a position (by head movement) that allows the gravity to move the otoconia, the patient experiences acute transitory (about 10–30 seconds) vertigo. The Dix-Hallpike test is used to place the PSCC in a gravity dependant position (see Figure 19.3). The vertigo reoccurs every time the head is placed in this position but fatigues after each repetition. The patient will classically say that he feels dizzy in bed, especially when he rolls to one side or the other. Another common complaint is that the dizziness is brought on by looking up when placing a book on a high shelf or hanging up the washing. Hearing loss and tinnitus may be coincidental findings but are not caused by the otoconia. Treatment is by performing Epley's manoeuvre or by habituation exercises, such as the Brandt-Daroff exercise routine. Epley's manoeuvre is intended to manoeuvre the PSSC in such a manner that the crystals drop out of the PSSC. The patient is usually asked not to lie flat for 48 hours to prevent the crystals from drifting back into the canal. The Brandt-Daroff exercise routine allows for habituation of the PSCC and compensation. The patient is asked to sit on the edge of the bed and turn his head 45° to the left. The patient lies down on his right side with the back of his head touching the bed. Dizziness usually occurs and the patient waits until this resolves. The patient sits upright, then turns his head to the right (45°) and lies down on his left side with his head touching the bed. This process is repeated for about 10 minutes and at least 3 times a day. BPPV is often self-limiting and may improve spontaneously over months or years.

Menière's syndrome

Menière's syndrome consists of episodic rotatory vertigo (usually associated with nausea and vomiting), fluctuating hearing loss and tinnitus. The

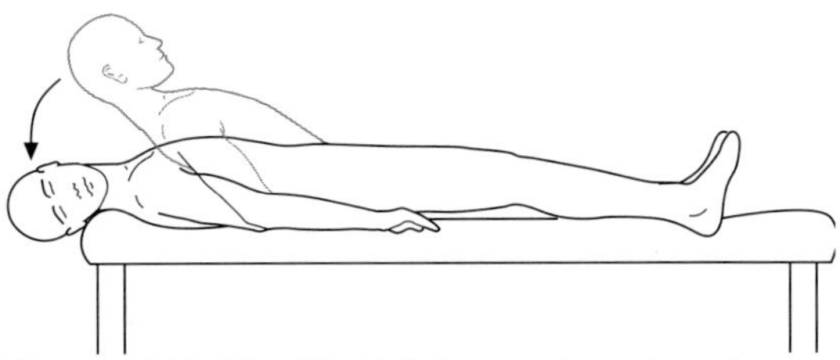

Figure 19.3 The Dix-Hallpike test is used to demonstrate benign paroxysmal positional vertigo (BPPV). The patient's head is turned 45° before it is lowered over the end of the bed. This is first done to the right then repeated to the left to allow testing of both vestibular systems

syndrome is thought to be caused by endolymphatic hydrops (increased pressure of the endolymph in the inner ear). Classically the patient will feel a fullness develop in the ear (aura) and this will be followed by prostrating vertigo, nausea and often vomiting. The patient is aware that the tinnitus is often aggravated by the episode. The dizzy spell is also often associated with a hearing loss. The hearing loss usually resolves over the next few days. The vertigo typically lasts for about 20 minutes but the patient will usually feel unwell for the whole day. Attacks can occur at any frequency but usually range from one a month to one a week. Medical treatment consists of restricting the salt in the diet, vasodilators (such as β-histadine), diuretics or labyrinthine sedatives (such as stemetil). Should medical treatment fail, surgical treatment may be necessary. The least invasive treatment consists of instilling gentamycin into the middle ear to cause a chemical labyrinthectomy (this can cause hearing loss in about 30% of patients). Other surgical procedures include endolymphatic sac decompression (an attempt to prevent pressure from building in the inner ear), labyrinthectomy (surgically destroying the balance and hearing) or vestibular nerve section.

Vestibular neuronitis

This condition presents with sudden onset acute rotatory vertigo associated with nausea and vomiting. It is usually severe and the patient is prostrated. Nystagmus is present and this indicates acute vestibular failure. The cause is uncertain but in most cases there is a preceding history of an upper respiratory tract infection in the previous weeks. This raises the possibility of a viral inflammation of the vestibular nerve. The patient will slowly improve over subsequent days as central compensation occurs. As the patient improves, so the nystagmus will resolve. The patient's hearing needs to be tested and should be normal for his age. If the hearing is affected then there is involvement of the labyrinth and not the vestibular nerve and the patient does not have vestibular neuronitis. The patient should be referred to an ENT surgeon for assessment. Treatment is supportive with encouragement and help in mobilising the patient as rapidly as possible. Early mobilisation improves the patient's ability to compensate and regain equilibrium.

Labyrinthine fistula

Labyrinthine fistula is an abnormal communication between the membranous labyrinth and the middle ear with a leakage of fluid from the inner to the middle ear. The most common causes are head trauma with temporal bone fractures, erosion of the labyrinth by cholesteatoma or spontaneous rupture of the round or oval window usually following straining when lifting heavy objects or coughing. The dizziness is usually associated with fluctuating hearing levels and may be positional in nature. Diagnosis is usually made by suspicion of such a leak on history associated with a positive fistula test. The fistula test requires the pressure in the external canal to be raised and lowered. The change in pressure is transmitted to the inner ear by the fistula and produces a burst of dizziness, often with visible nystagmus. Surgical repair may be required if the leak is persistent.

Common causes of central vertigo (dizziness)

The most common causes of central vertigo are tumours (such as brain tumours and acoustic neuroma), vascular incidents in the vertebrobasilar area, and atypical migraine.

Brain tumours

Brain tumours are an uncommon cause of vertigo. Of the brain tumours acoustic neuroma (or, more correctly termed, vestibular schwannoma) is one of the more common tumours to cause dizziness (see Figure 19.4). It usually presents with unilateral sensorineural hearing loss, tinnitus and dizziness (which may be rotatory in nature). All patients who present with dizziness and have a significant unilateral sensorineural hearing loss should have this tumour excluded by MRI scanning. The tumour is benign and can be treated either by stereo-tactic radiotherapy or by surgical removal. Other tumours that involve the brain stem and/or cerebellum usually produce unsteadiness and lightheadedness,

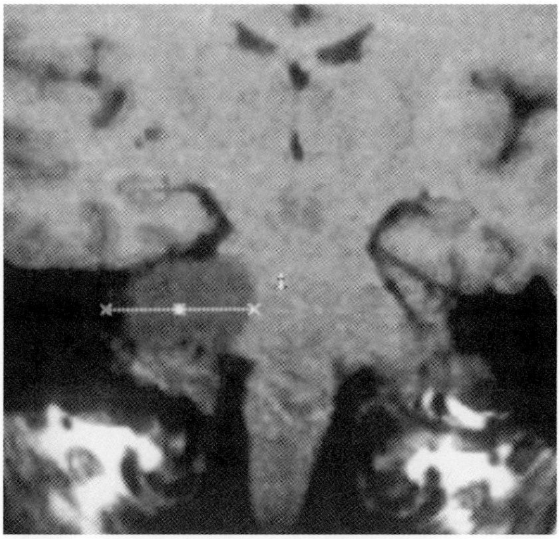

Figure 19.4 MRI scan through the cerebro-pontine angle demonstrating a small acoustic neuroma. The tumour is indicated by the dotted line joining the Xs

although they may produce rotatory vertigo on rare occasions.

Vascular incidents in the vertebrobasilar system

A vascular incident in the vertebrobasilar system may produce vertigo but it is rare for it to be present without associated neurological features. The most common associated neurological features are abnormalities of gait, dysphagia, dysarthria, diplopia, motor or sensory abnormalities or cranial nerve deficits.

Atypical migraine

Migraine can cause vertigo but usually occurs in younger patients. The vertigo may present as an aura which is often followed by a headache. It may present in a fluctuating manner and mimic peripheral vertigo of vestibular origin. One of the distinguishing features is the lack of associated auditory symptoms. Antimigraine therapy can be effective in treating both the dizziness and the headache.

Lightheadedness

The most common causes of lightheadedness are cervical arthritis and visual problems.

This is often termed 'multisensory lightheadedness' or 'disequilibrium' and is common in the elderly. It occurs most often on walking and is due to disrupted sensory inputs from the cervical spine and eyes. The mismatch when the brain compares the sensory information with the vestibular information results in the brain interpreting the information incorrectly and the patient feeling unsteady.

It is also important to consider postural hypotension as a possible cause of lightheadedness. This is relatively common in elderly patients, especially those on antihypertensive medication. Lightheadedness is present when the patient changes position from lying to sitting or from sitting to standing.

The treatment of lightheadedness is to give the patient a vestibular exercise program that will improve his ability to compensate and thereby match up the sensory, visual and vestibular inputs. In patients with chronic unsteadiness individually designed exercise programs are of more benefit than general exercise programs.

Making a diagnosis

In the majority of patients the diagnosis will be made from the history. If a diagnosis is not made after the history is complete, it is unlikely to be made after the examination. The central question that needs to be answered is whether the patient's symptom is one of true dizziness (vertigo) or lightheadedness/disequilibrium. Once this is established you can concentrate on the most common diagnosis in each of these groups. The examination will in most cases be normal but it is important to establish that the patient's hearing and middle ears are normal. A full neurological examination is needed to exclude significant intracranial causes. Gait and balance should be evaluated. Balance is tested by the Romberg test and BPPV can be excluded by the Dix-Hallpike test (see Figure 19.3). The patient needs to be referred to an ear nose and throat specialist if there is any hearing loss, tinnitus or probable vestibular cause for the dizziness. Patients in whom the diagnosis is unclear also need referral.

Bibliography and further reading

Brandt, T. & Daroff, R. B. (1980), 'Physical therapy for benign paroxysmal positioning vertigo', *Acta Otolaryngoicall,* 106, pp. 484–5.

Epley, J. M. (1995), 'Positional vertigo related to semicircular canalithiasis', *Otolaryngology—Head and Neck Surgery*, 112, pp. 154–61.

Waterston, J. (2000), 'Dizziness', *The Medical Journal of Australia*, 172, pp. 506–11.

Chapter 20

Visual impairment and cataracts

NICHOLAS P. STRONG

Introduction

Poor vision is a frequently encountered handicap in the elderly. The aims of this chapter are to:

- outline the causes for poor vision in the elderly: aetiology and pathophysiology
- explain how to assess visual function in the elderly
- explain how to detect treatable causes of poor vision in a general medical setting
- outline the treatment of ophthalmic presentations
- describe the rehabilitative measures that can be undertaken in patients who have irreversible visual loss.

In addition to loss of visual acuity, elderly patients may suffer other forms of visual handicap. These include loss of all or part of the field of vision and double vision deriving from loss of binocular co-ordination of the two eyes.

Aetiology, epidemiology and pathophysiology

Impaired vision

It is useful to consider the causes of visual impairment in a structured manner, starting with the patient's glasses first, then the eyelids, the optical components of the eye (cornea, lens and vitreous), the retina and the visual neural pathway in turn.

Box 20.1 Common causes of impaired vision

The most common causes of impaired vision in the elderly are:

- uncorrected refractive error
- cataract
- age-related maculopathy
- retinal vascular occlusion (venous or arterial occlusion)
- cerebrovascular accident

Uncorrected refractive error

This is a common cause of visual handicap in the elderly, especially in underprivileged, ill or confused patients. When patients are admitted to hospital it is common for their glasses to be left at home. Most elderly patients will require glasses to read small print. Many patients who have undergone cataract surgery may not see well without glasses.

Problems with the ocular adnexae

Involutional changes in the ocular adnexae may give rise to visual difficulty.

Lower eyelids

Laxity of the lower eyelids may give rise to either ectropion or entropion. Ectropion is an out-turning of the lower lid, including the lower lacrimal punctum (Figure 20.3). This results in failure of tear drainage, causing a watering eye. This in turn often leads to a secondary chronic conjunctivitis and the conjunctiva of the lower lid becoming exposed, swollen and injected.

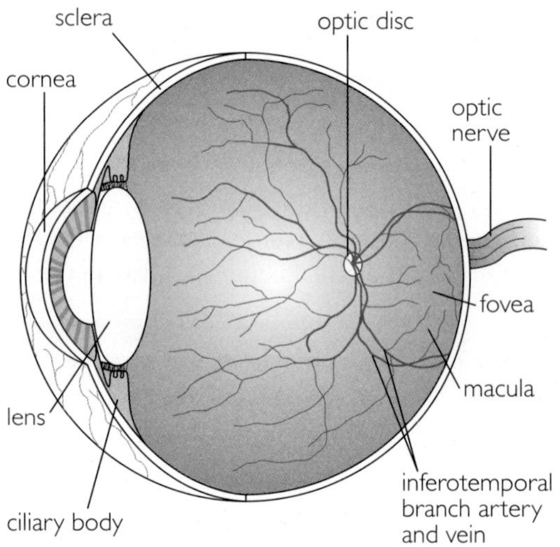

Figure 20.1 Basic ocular anatomy. Light passes through the cornea and lens to reach the retina. The macula is the zone that lies within the retinal vascular arcades (superotemporal and inferotemporal branch retinal arteries and veins). The most central part of the macula is the fovea. If the optics of the eye are normal then it is foveal function that determines visual acuity. If the fovea is damaged by a disease process, such as macula degeneration or vascular occlusion, then visual acuity will be impaired

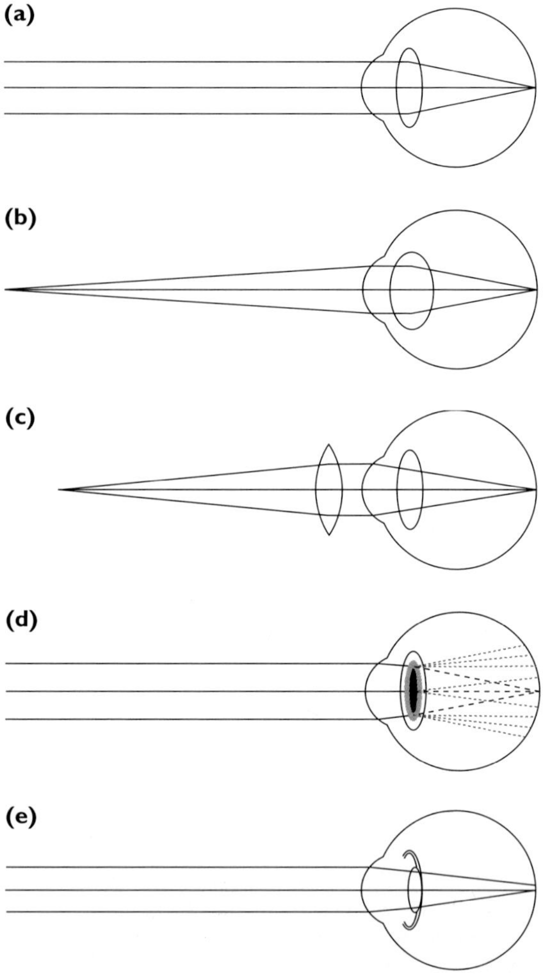

Figure 20.2 (a) Distance vision. Parallel light rays from an object at far distance are focused on to the retina. Note that this refraction is performed partly by the cornea (65%) and partly by the crystalline lens (35%). **(b)** Close vision. A near object produces divergent light rays. A young person can accommodate (change the shape of the crystalline lens) to bring the image into focus. **(c)** Presbyopia. In order to focus divergent light rays from a near object most older patients (and also patients who have had cataract surgery) require glasses. This is because the crystalline lens has hardened with age and will no longer change shape to allow accommodation. **(d)** Cataract. Light is blocked and/or scattered by opacity within the crystalline lens. **(e)** Pseudophakia. The natural (crystalline) lens has been replaced by an intraocular lens.

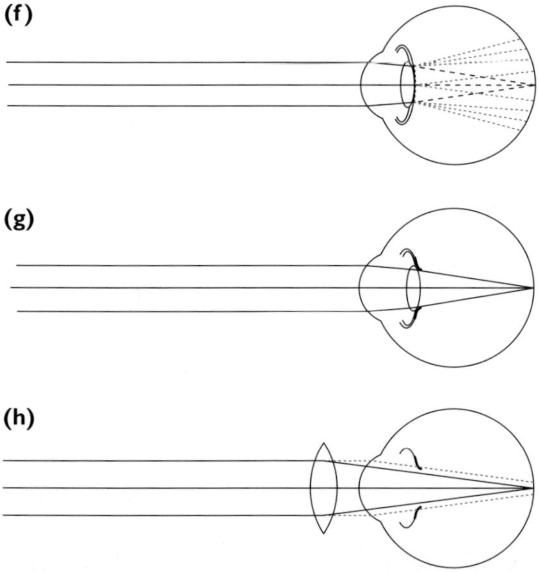

Figure 20.2 (f) Posterior lens capsule thickening (secondary cataract). Again light is blocked or scattered. **(g)** Posterior capsule thickening. This can be divided by YAG laser capsulotomy, thus restoring the optics. **(h)** Aphakia. Some patients who have had cataract surgery may not have had an intraocular lens inserted. This is uncommon in Western countries but is encountered frequently in the developing world due to the cost of intraocular lenses. In most cases these patients will be very out of focus (dotted line) and will need very thick glasses (or a contact lens) in order to see clearly

In entropion, overriding of the orbicularis muscle over the underlying tarsus causes the lid to turn inwards (Figure 20.4). This brings the lashes into contact with the cornea, giving rise to an uncomfortable eye. There may be blepharospasm and reading may be difficult, as looking down encourages contact between the lashes and the cornea. It is surprisingly easy to overlook this condition.

In trichiasis the lids are in a normal position but some of the lashes are misdirected and ingrowing (Figure 20.5). This usually derives from longstanding chronic lid disease, frequently associated with rosacea.

Upper eyelid: Ptosis

The most common cause of ptosis in the elderly is involutional dehiscence of the levator tendon from the tarsal plate of the upper lid (Figure 20.6). This is characterised by a loss of the upper lid crease and the development of a deep sulcus under the upper orbital margin. Less common causes of ptosis include ocular myaesthenia, chronic progressive external ophthalmoplegia and myotonica dystrophica. Unilateral ptosis may arise as part of a Horner's syndrome or a third nerve palsy.

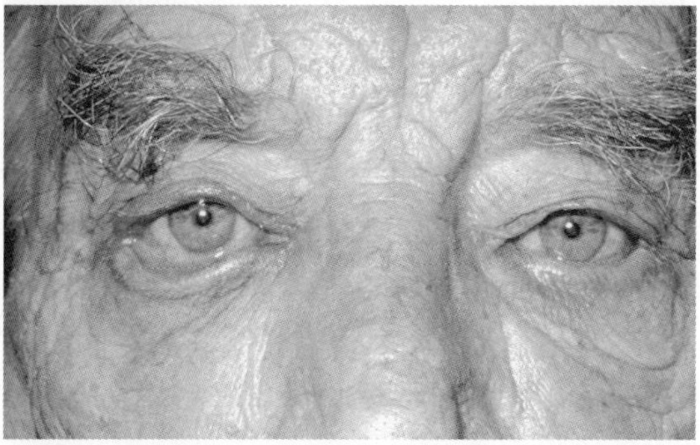

Figure 20.3 Ectropion. The lid is sagging outwards, giving rise to conjunctival exposure and inflammation

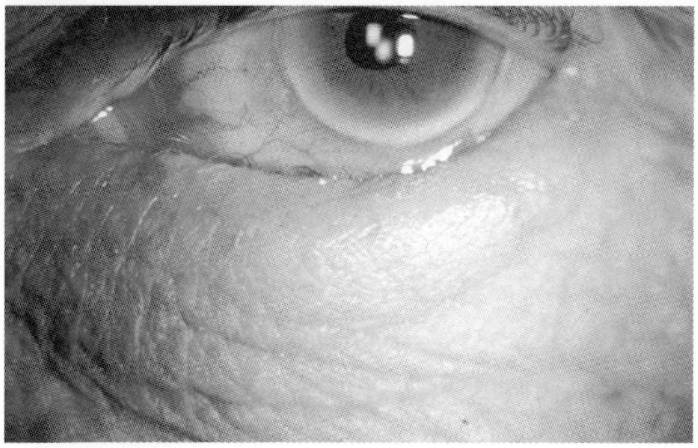

Figure 20.4 Entropion. The entire lid has rolled inwards and the lashes are rubbing on the cornea

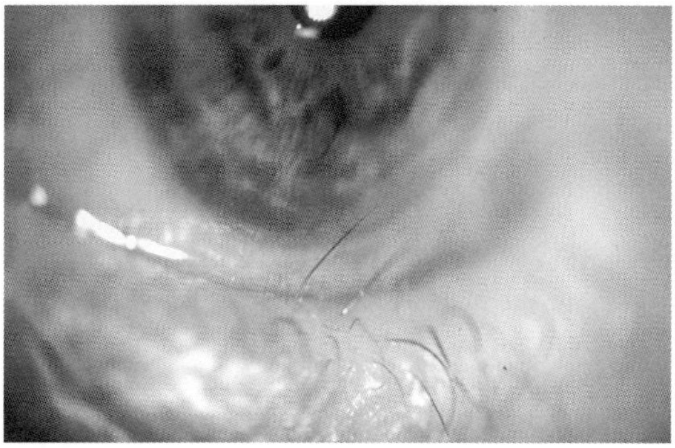

Figure 20.5 Trichiasis. The lid is in a relatively normal position but the eyelashes are misdirected and touching the cornea, in this case secondary to ocular pemphigoid

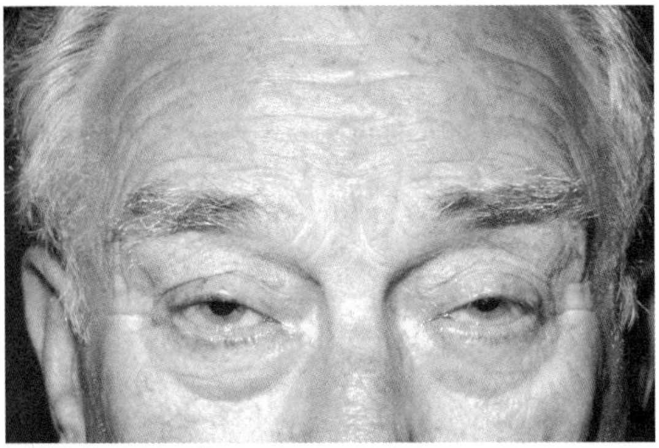

Figure 20.6 Ptosis. This shows the most common form of ptosis, that due to age-related levator dehiscence. The levator muscle is gradually losing its attachment to the tarsal plate of the upper lid. Note the loss of the upper lid crease so that a large proportion of the upper tarsus is visible

Lacrimal problems

Poor tear production may give rise to ocular surface discomfort, blepharospasm and photophobia, often accompanied by difficulty reading. There is a strong association with rheumatoid arthritis and Sjögren's syndrome.

Corneal diseases

A range of disease processes may damage the cornea. The most common of these is Fuch's endothelial dystrophy. This is characterised by progressive loss of corneal endothelial cells, which results in the cornea becoming oedematous and losing transparency.

Other diseases of the cornea are generally characterised by infective or inflammatory episodes that lead to visual loss through corneal scarring. These include:

- *Herpes simplex keratitis* This can take two forms. The first is epithelial, in the form of a 'dendritic ulcer'. This is characterised by a red, painful photophobic eye with a foreign body sensation. Alternatively, it can involve the corneal stroma, giving rise to corneal oedema and eventual scarring.
- *Corneal melting* (usually in association with rheumatoid arthritis).
- *Corneal bacterial infections* These usually occur in debilitated patients, or in patients in whom the cornea is exposed, such as by Bell's palsy.

Cataract

Cataract is the most common treatable cause for visual loss in the elderly (see Figure 20.7). Prevalence increases with age. Other risk factors include diabetes and other metabolic disorders, inflammatory eye disease (uveitis) and racial origin. Cataract is more prevalent in Afro-Caribbean and Asian patients.

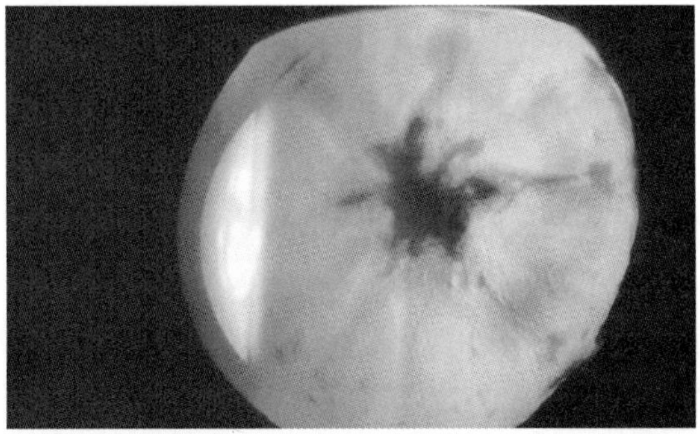

Figure 20.7 Cataract. Here the lens opacity is seen against the red reflex. This view is possible by viewing the eye with an ophthalmoscope from a distance of 20–50 cm

Posterior capsule thickening

Patients who have had cataract surgery may develop thickening of the posterior lens capsule months or years later, a condition sometimes called 'secondary cataract' (Figure 20.8). This complication is quite common, affecting 5–10% of eyes after cataract surgery, and is very easily treated by YAG laser capsulotomy (Figure 20.2(g)).

Vitreous haemorrhage

This is an uncommon presentation. There are a number of possible causes (see Table 20.1).

Retinal diseases

In the elderly the common retinal causes of poor vision are age-related maculopathy, retinal vein

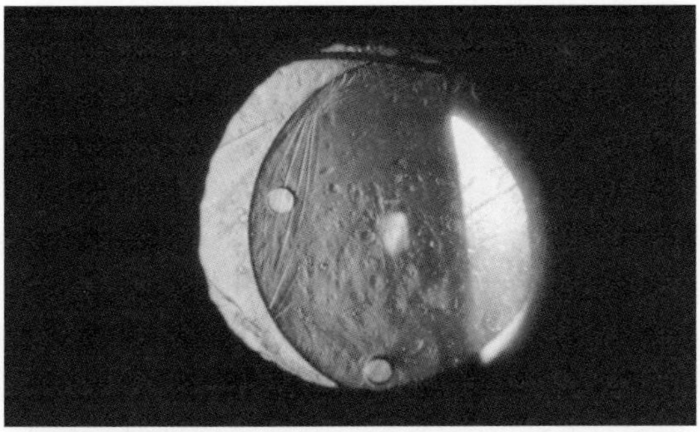

Figure 20.8 Posterior capsule thickening. Again this can be seen easily against the red reflex with an ophthalmoscope, in which cases the lens epithelial 'pearls' will appear as black dots. In this photograph the eye has been dilated and the edge of the intraocular lens can be seen

Table 20.1 Causes of vitreous haemorrhage

Disease	Mechanism	Systemic association
Proliferative diabetic retinopathy	Tearing of neovascular fronds arising from retinal surface	Diabetes
Retinal tear	Vitreous traction upon retina	None
Age-related maculopathy	'Break-through' bleeding from subretinal neovascular membrane	None
Macroaneurysm	Rupture of aneurysm	Hypertension
Neovascular response to retinal branch vein occlusion	Similar mechanism to proliferative diabetic retinopathy	Hypertension

occlusion, retinal embolism, diabetic retinopathy and ischaemic optic neuropathy.

Age-related maculopathy (ARMD)

ARMD is the most common irreversible cause of visual loss in the developed world. The term 'ARMD' covers a heterogeneous group of diseases of the choroid, retinal pigment epithelium and retina, all of which have increasing prevalence with age, rising to at least 10% in the over 80s. Prevalence is highest in patients of European origin and least in Afro-Caribbean patients.

The most useful classification as far as treatment, prognosis and functional effect are concerned is into 'wet' and 'dry' types.

'Wet' ARMD is characterised by a relatively sudden onset of visual loss. In the early stages the vision is often distorted with central blurring. As it progresses, a central scotoma develops. Visual acuity often falls below 6/60 (20/200) in the affected eye. Both eyes may eventually be affected; once one eye has suffered visual loss the risk of involvement of the second eye is about 7% per annum.

Ophthalmoscopy may reveal macular haemorrhage, exudates or disciform scarring.

A small proportion of patients presenting with 'wet' ARMD may benefit from treatment with an Argon laser. These patients are most likely to be those with a short history of visual loss (weeks rather than months) and visual acuity of better than 6/24.

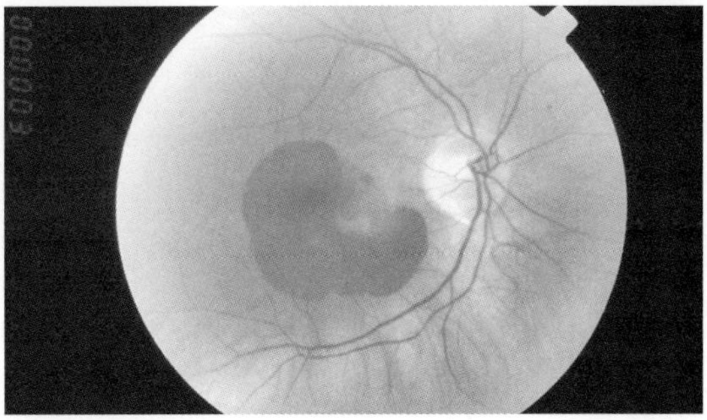

Figure 20.9 Recent presentation of 'wet' age-related macular degeneration (ARMD). In this case there is a large macular haemorrhage

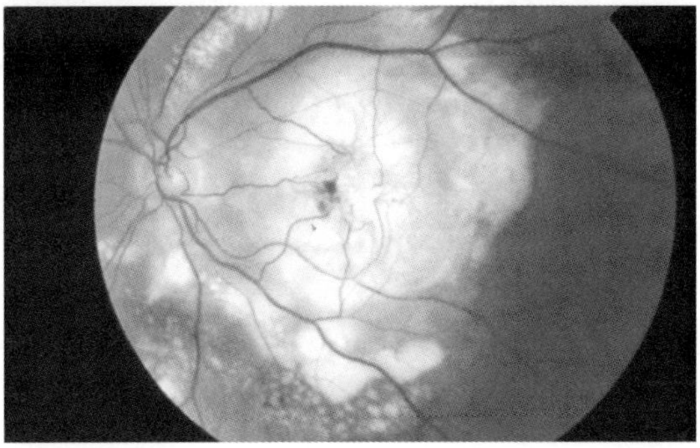

Figure 20.10 Late stage of 'wet' ARMD. A pale scar has formed and central vision has been lost. This appearance is often referred to as 'disciform degeneration'

'Dry' ARMD is of much slower onset. It progresses relentlessly but vision may be only moderately affected for many years. It is more common in short-sighted individuals. It is characterised by gradual changes in the architecture of the central retina with the formation of pigment clumps and atrophic patches within the retina.

Retinal vascular events

These may be arterial or venous. Arterial occlusions may be classified into those involving:

- the entire central retinal artery (CRAO); or
- a branch artery (RBAO).

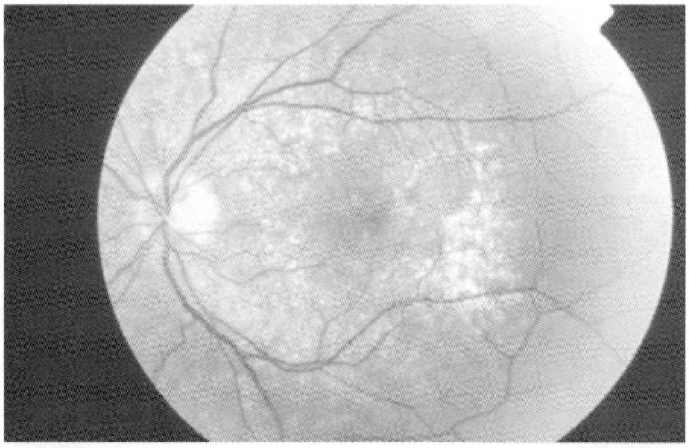

Figure 20.11 Early 'dry' macular change. Scattered yellowish lesions are called drusen. Drusen are hyaline bodies that form under the retina and are very common. These should not be confused with the retinal exudates associated with diabetes or other retinal vascular diseases (Figures 20.18 and 20.19)

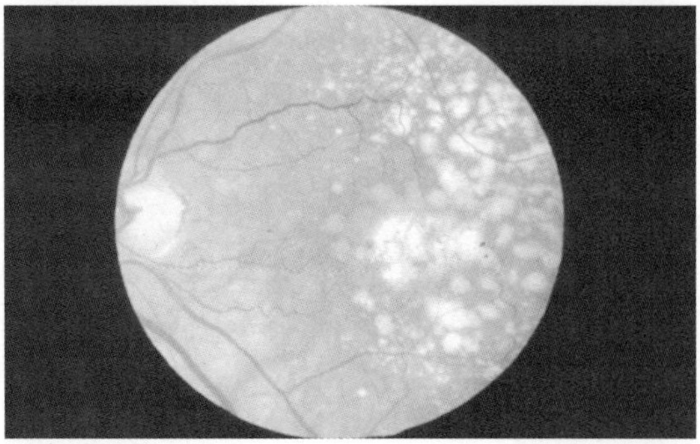

Figure 20.12 Moderate 'dry' ARMD. This photograph shows pale drusen and some disturbance of the central macula where pigment clumping and early atrophic change are evident

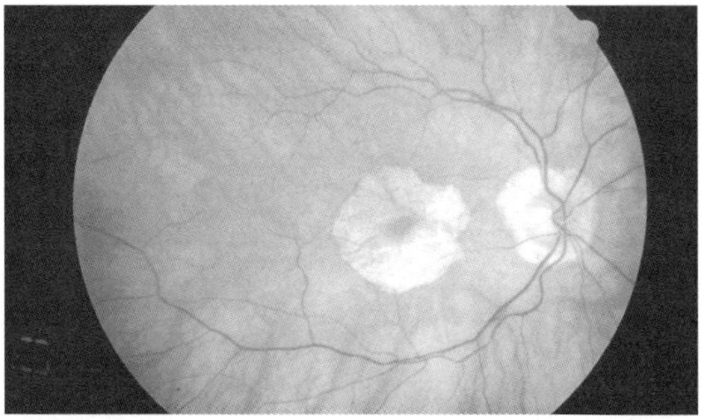

Figure 20.13 Advanced 'dry' ARMD. This patient does not have many drusen but the central retina has become atrophic. The central visual field has been lost

Most cases of central arterial occlusion are embolic in origin, deriving either from large vessel atherosclerosis or in association with atrial fibrillation. However, CRAO may be a manifestation of giant cell arteritis. Essentially all *branch* artery occlusions in the elderly are embolic in nature.

Vein occlusions are more common than arterial events. Again the occlusion may be central (CRVO) or a branch vein only (BRVO). There is an association with hypertension and possibly diabetes.

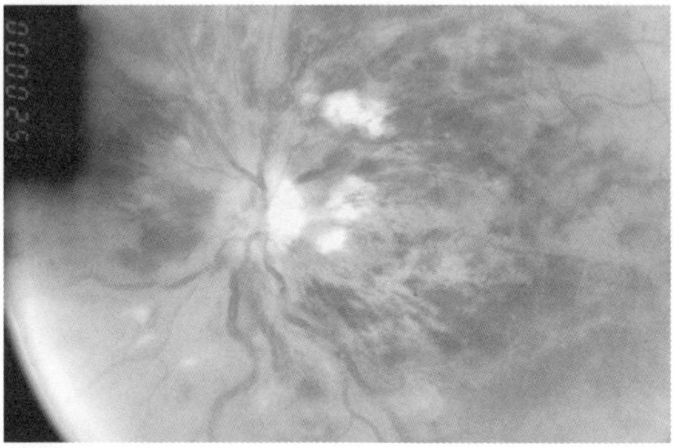

Figure 20.14 Central retinal vein occlusion (CRVO). This is characterised by widespread retinal haemorrhages. A CRVO may vary in severity from mild (i.e. only a few small haemorrhages and little effect on vision) to severe, as in this example. This demonstrates a CRVO with a severe degree of occlusion which has resulted in marked retinal ischaemia (see Figure 20.32) and in the vision falling to hand movement detection only

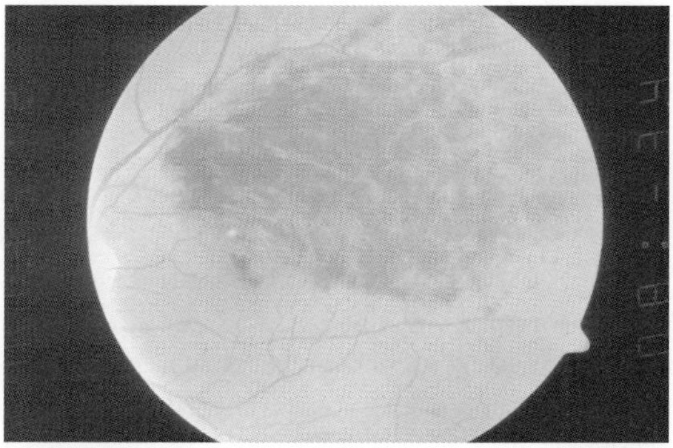

Figure 20.15 Branch retinal vein occlusion (BRVO). This shows an occlusion of the superotemporal retinal branch vein. The rest of the retinal vascular tree is unaffected

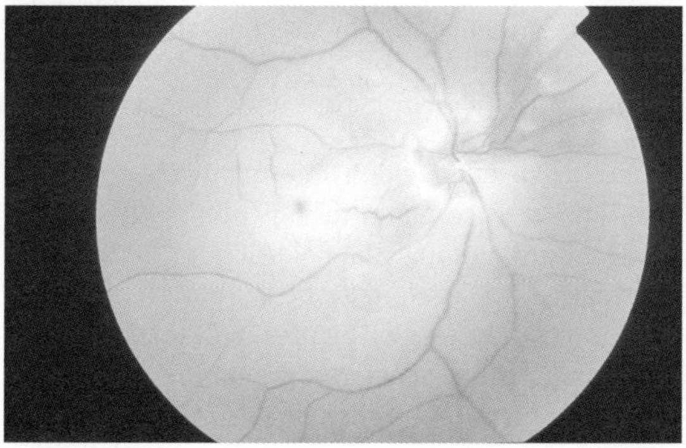

Figure 20.16 Central retinal artery occlusion (CRAO). This is shown by a pale swollen ischaemic retina with a 'cherry red spot' at the fovea. This may be the presenting sign for giant cell arteritis

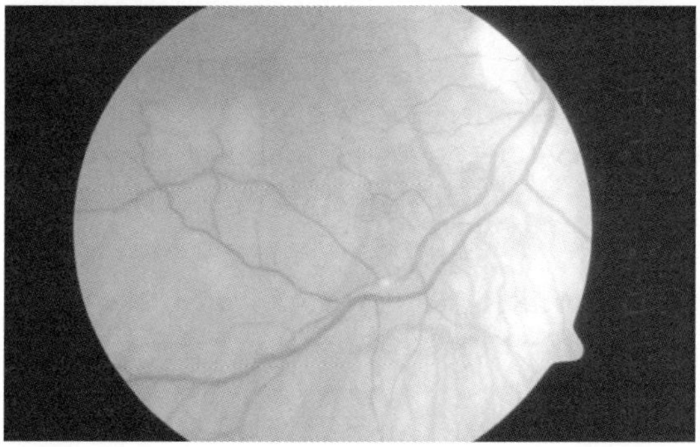

Figure 20.17 Embolic branch retinal artery occlusion (BRAO). The embolus can be seen where the inferotemporal branch retinal artery divides. This is a crystalline cholesterol embolus which is not completely occluding the arteriole, so the retina is not as ischaemic as in the example of a CRAO (see Figure 20.16)

Diabetic retinopathy

Visual loss in diabetes may arise from proliferative retinopathy or from diabetic maculopathy. Most elderly diabetic patients have late onset (type II) diabetes. Proliferative retinopathy is relatively uncommon in these patients, whereas diabetic maculopathy is a frequent complication and may already be established at presentation.

Proliferative diabetic retinopathy is characterised by new vessels forming on the retinal surface or optic disc, which if left untreated may lead to vitreous haemorrhage and eventually to tractional retinal detachment. Diabetic maculopathy

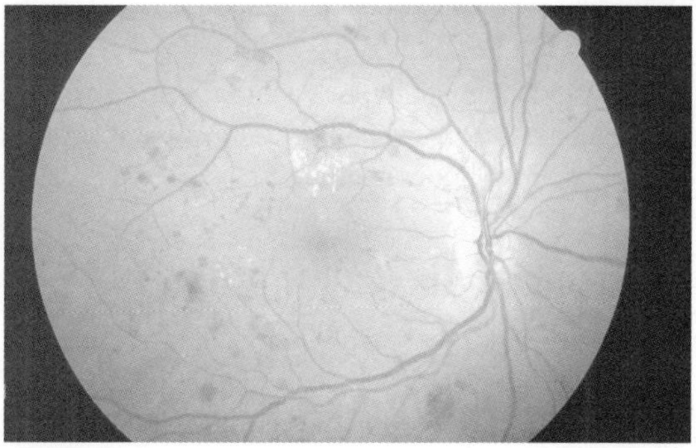

Figure 20.18 Background diabetic retinopathy. Scattered small haemorrhages, microaneurysms and exudates but no macular oedema or new vessels. Visual acuity is normal

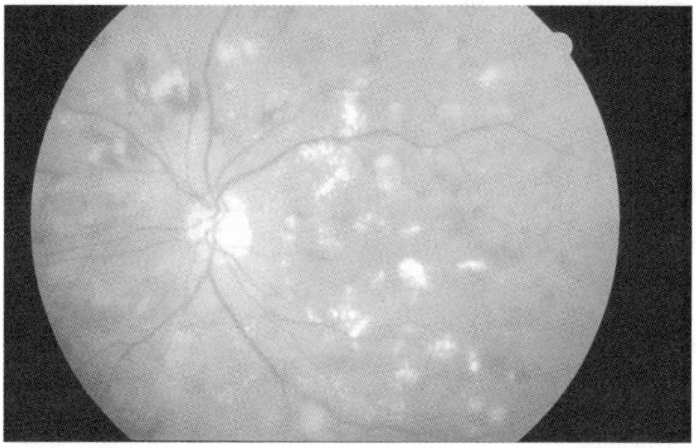

Figure 20.19 Diabetic maculopathy. There is extensive macular oedema and exudate formation. The exudates derive from protein leakage through an incompetent vascular endothelium. Note that these exudates are more clearly defined in appearance than retinal drusen, and have a different pattern of distribution. Patients with this degree of maculopathy require laser treatment

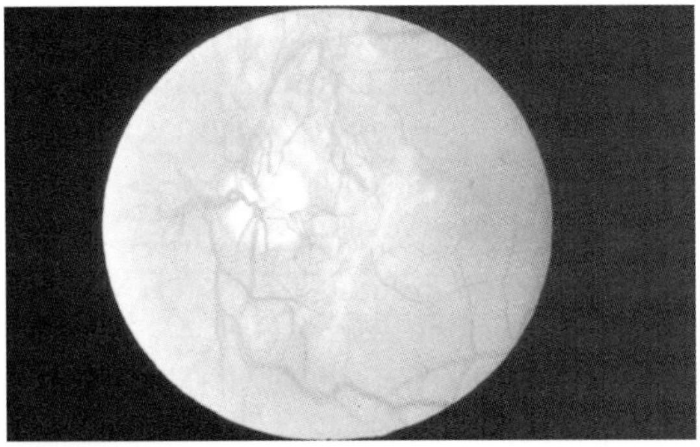

Figure 20.20 Proliferative retinopathy. There are new vessels growing from the disc and adjacent vessels. These may tear and produce vitreous haemorrhage, or become organised, resulting in extensive scarring, contracture and eventual tractional retinal detachment

is characterised by macular oedema, haemorrhages and exudates, and gives rise to a gradual loss of acuity, especially for reading.

Ischaemic optic neuropathy

Closely related to glaucoma, ischaemic optic neuropathy derives from loss of the small vessel blood supply to the optic nerve and nerve head. It may arise due to generalised atherosclerosis, systemic hypertension, arteritis (such as giant cell arteritis) or in association with diabetes (see Chapter 21).

Retinal detachment

This tends to present in middle life but may occur in the elderly. It is characterised by sudden flashes and floaters followed by a progressive field defect and then loss of visual acuity. It can be difficult to recognise on direct ophthalmoscopy, but upon careful examination it may be possible to determine that the retina is ballooned forwards from its normal position.

In the early stages of retinal detachment only the peripheral retina is involved and the visual acuity may be normal ('macula-on'). If the macula is detached at presentation then vision will be markedly impaired ('macula-off'). Macula-on retinal detachment requires urgent surgical intervention to prevent the detachment progressing to detach the macula, whereas if the macula is detached surgery may be deferred for a number of days.

Lesions of the visual pathway

Space-occupying lesions

It is uncommon for a patient with an intracranial mass to present on account of visual symptoms. Nevertheless patients may present with visual loss secondary to:

- pituitary adenoma
- anterior communicating aneurysm
- meningioma
- parasellar metastasis (most frequently breast)
- cerebral metastasis (breast, bronchus, bowel).

Cerebral infarction

A cerebrovascular event may give rise to visual loss. The most common form is homonymous loss of the contralateral visual field (Figure 20.27(a)). If only part of the occipital lobe is infarcted, a quadrantinopia may result (Figure 20.27(c)). In some individuals the macula representation within the calcerine sulcus is supplied by the anterior cerebral artery and may be spared even when both occipital lobes are infarcted, sparing a small area of central field. These patients may have normal acuity but be very handicapped due to the small field of view.

Infarction of the parietal or temporal lobes may give rise to acquired disorders of higher visual processing, such as dyslexia. These patients may have normal acuity for single letters but be unable to understand the meaning of words or phrases (see Chapter 15).

Less common causes of visual problems in the elderly

Glaucoma

See Chapter 21.

Inherited disorders

There are many genetic diseases that may not present symptomatically until later life. All are

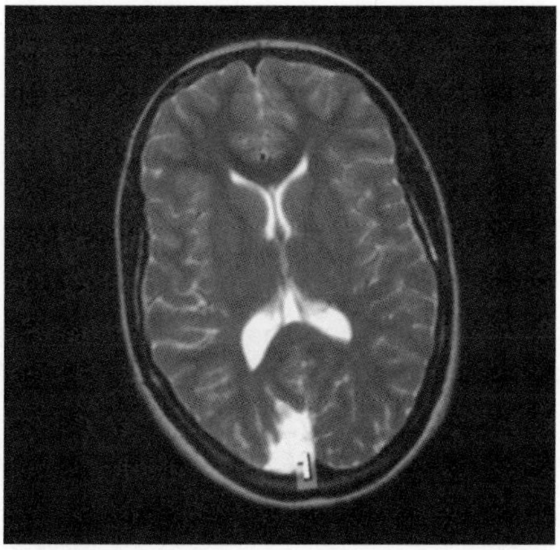

Figure 20.21 MRI of the head showing an infarction of the right occipital cortex. This has given rise to a left homonymous hemianopia (see Figure 20.27(a))

relatively rare. An example is the patient with autosomal dominant retinitis pigmentosa who may have a long history of night blindness but who does not suffer significant visual handicap in daylight conditions until retirement age.

Uveitis

Uveitis may be acute or chronic. Acute uveitis presents primarily on account of pain, photophobia, ocular injection and visual blurring. Most patients will have presented to an ophthalmology department earlier in life and will be known to have uveitis that is either ideopathic or associated with ankylosing spondylitis. Patients with chronic uveitis often have fewer symptoms and signs and may present on account of visual loss only, usually deriving from a secondary complication of the uveitis such as cataract or glaucoma. Again most presentations are idiopathic but there may be an underlying systemic inflammatory disease, most commonly sarcoid.

Patients presenting with ophthalmic herpes zoster are at risk of developing a secondary uveitis. This occurs within a few months of the onset of the disease and these patients should be referred for specialist examination.

The large majority of patients with uveitis do not suffer irreversible visual loss, but there is an increased prevalence of cataract and glaucoma in these patients.

Scleritis

This is a rare disease usually characterised by pain, injection and eventually by melting of the sclera. Systemic associations include rheumatoid arthritis and Wegener's granulomatosis.

Double vision

Double vision (diplopia) is a common symptom in the elderly. When a patient reports this symptom a distinction must be made between 'true' diplopia, in which there is separation of the images from the two eyes, and 'monocular' diplopia, a sensation that the image seen through one (or both) eyes is 'double'. True diplopia is abolished by covering one or other eyes, whereas monocular diplopia persists even when the other eye is covered.

Monocular diplopia may be due to uncorrected refractive error or to early cataract, especially of the 'water cleft' type (Figures 20.7 and 20.29).

True diplopia is perceived because the two eyes are no longer aligned for some or all directions of gaze (strabismus). This may be due to the breakdown of a longstanding latent squint or due to a newly acquired problem.

Breakdown of a longstanding latent squint is characterised by intermittent symptoms, usually when tired or after drinking alcohol. The patient can usually control the double vision with effort, but can no longer do so as easily as when she was younger. It is often possible to restore control of the latent squint by incorporating prism into the patient's glasses.

The more common causes of acquired strabismus in the elderly are:

- sixth nerve palsy
- fourth nerve palsy
- third nerve palsy
- chronic progressive external ophthalmoplegia (CPEO)
- thyroid eye disease.

Sixth, fourth and third nerve palsies are usually due to microvascular disease, especially in association with diabetes and hypertension. The majority resolve spontaneously. However, if there is no improvement after 4–6 months, recovery is unlikely. In these circumstances restoration of single vision requires the use of prisms (only practicable if the angle is small), strabismus surgery or occlusion of one eye. Third nerve palsies are the most likely presentation to be associated with more serious underlying pathology, such as an aneurysm or other mass lesion.

CPEO is characterised by a gradual loss of range of eye movement, especially upwards. It is relentlessly progressive and often associated with other evidence of brain stem dysfunction and other signs of neurodegenerative disease (see Chapter 15).

Clinical tests and procedures

History

Assessment of visual loss in the elderly should always start with a history. However, it should be borne in mind that history taking in elderly patients with visual problems can sometimes be misleading. In particular the following should be noted:

1. Patients may not volunteer that they need their glasses to see properly. Always ask about spectacles before testing the vision.
2. One of the most common causes of 'sudden' visual loss in the elderly is unilateral cataract or other pathology that has developed or been present over many months. Unilateral cataract often goes unnoticed by an elderly patient until some event such as rubbing the other eye draws it to her attention.
3. Loss of one hemifield secondary to cerebral infarction is often described by the patient as loss of vision of the eye on the affected side.
4. Many patients complaining of 'double vision' are not describing true diplopia—that is, double vision due to having developed a squint. Often this symptom derives from *monocular* diplopia secondary to uncorrected refractive error or early cataract.

Painful or painless?

Most visual loss is painless. The most common causes include cataract, ARMD, retinal vascular occlusions and stroke.

Mild to moderate ocular surface discomfort may indicate an external eye disease problem such as dry eye syndrome, entropion or trichiasis (Figures 20.3 and 20.4).

Painful visual loss is relatively uncommon. Possible causes include acute glaucoma, rubeotic glaucoma, anterior uveitis, corneal infections (bacterial and viral) and scleritis. All of these are likely to result in a red eye. Painful visual loss in which the eye is not red is unlikely to be due to an ophthalmic cause.

Headache associated with visual loss may be due to giant cell arteritis, aneurysm or pituitary apoplexy.

Sudden or gradual visual loss?

As noted above a history of rapid visual loss may be misleading, especially for monocular visual loss. Visual impairment over many months is usually due to cataract or 'dry' ARMD. Visual loss over a few weeks may be indicative of 'wet' ARMD, especially if accompanied by a history of distortion of central vision. Sudden loss is consistent with a retinal vascular event (CRAO, CRVO) or cerebral event.

Causes of sudden painless visual loss are:

- central/branch retinal vein occlusion
- central/branch retinal artery occlusion
- subretinal haemorrhage secondary to 'wet' ARMD
- cerebrovascular accident
- vitreous haemorrhage
- retinal detachment.

Causes of gradual visual loss are:

- cataract
- posterior capsule thickening
- both 'wet' and 'dry' ARMD
- diabetic maculopathy.

Examination

This account presumes that the patient is being examined by a general physician rather than an ophthalmologist, and that the examining doctor has access to the following equipment:

- distance vision test chart (Snellen chart or equivalent) (Figure 20.22)

- near vision test type (Figure 20.23)
- red/white pins for field examination
- direct ophthalmoloscope

but does not have more sophisticated devices such as a slit-lamp or indirect ophthalmoscope.

Testing visual acuity

Always ask the patient whether she wears glasses, and whether these are for near, distance or both. In order for the assessment of visual function to be meaningful, it is essential that poor vision that is simply due to refractive error is not mistaken for evidence of acquired visual loss. Note that confused or ill patients may have lost their glasses or mixed up their near and distance prescriptions.

Distance vision should be tested at 6 m (20 ft). Each eye should be tested separately.

Near vision is assessed as the smallest test type that can be read at 30 cm.

If there is any doubt as to whether a patient has appropriate glasses then the patient should be referred for refraction to an optometric service in the first instance.

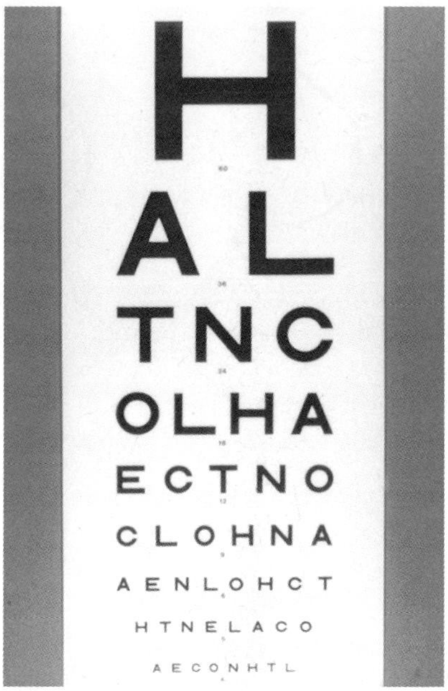

Figure 20.22 Snellen type. The visual acuity is expressed as the viewing distance as numerator (usually 6 m) over the smallest line read as denominator. On this chart the lines are marked 60, 36, 24, 18, 12, 9, 6, 5 and 4. Thus if the patient can only read to the fourth line (OHLA), then the acuity is 6/18

N 14

The office was furnished in sombre good taste that was relieved by a pair of bronze puppies on the chimney-piece. A low trolley of steel and white enamel alone distinguished the place from a hundred thousand modern American reception-rooms; that and the clinical smell. A bowl of roses stood beside the telephone; their scent contended with the carbolic, but did not prevail.

muse waxes over iron sawn ream vows

N 18

The two weak points in our age are its want of principle and its want of profile. Chin a little higher dear. Style largely depends on the way the chin is worn. They are worn very high just at present.

nice women rave cocoa essence

N 24

It is always right that a man should be able to render a reason for the faith that is within him.

sincere omen sour voice over

Figure 20.23 Near test type. This comes in a range of type sizes, usually N5 (the smallest) to N36

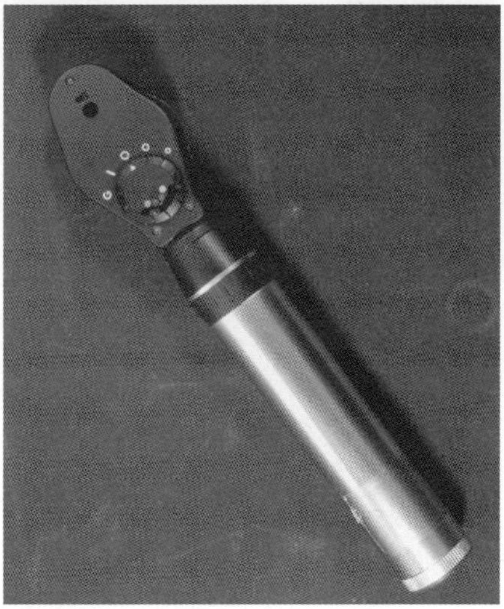

Figure 20.24 Ophthalmoscope. This can be employed to examine the anterior segment as well as the retina (see text)

Field of vision

In this context the purpose of visual field examination is to detect gross field loss such as that arising from occipital infarction. Specialist field-testing equipment is required in order to detect lesser degrees of field loss deriving from causes such as

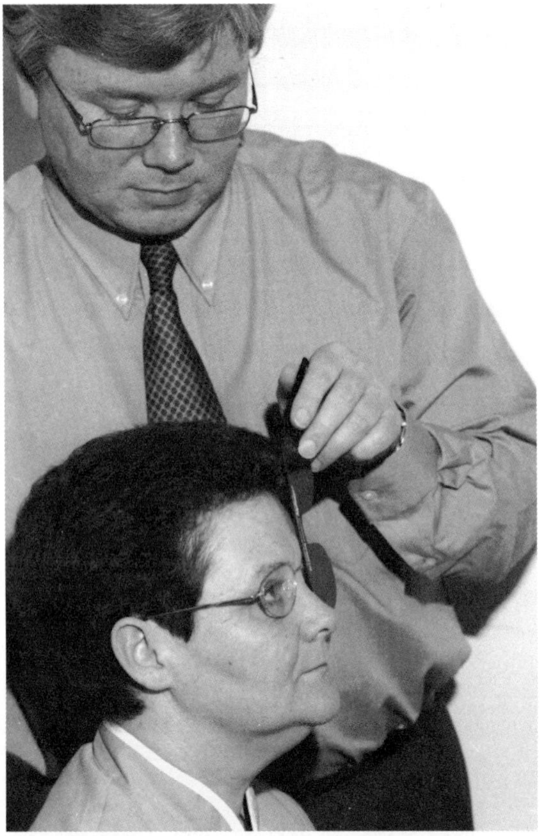

Figure 20.25 Testing the distance vision of a patient. Each eye should be tested separately. The other eye should be covered carefully as patients may unintentionally 'cheat' by looking past the cover when the eye with the poorer vision is being tested

glaucoma. Testing is best with a white or red tipped pin, but finger waving is often surprisingly effective. The patient should be instructed to look at the examiner's nose while the pin or a wiggling finger is advanced from the periphery. The patient is instructed to report the moment the target is seen. The test should be performed both above and below the horizontal meridian and attention paid to whether there is a field defect that respects either the vertical midline (indicating a chiasmatic or cerebral lesion) or the horizontal meridian (indicative of a hemispheric vascular occlusion or glaucoma) (Figure 20.15).

The optic nerve fibres from each eye partly decussate in the optic chiasm. The fibres serving the nasal retina (thus the temporal visual field) of one eye cross over and join the fibres from the temporal retina which serve the corresponding area of the visual field of the other eye (i.e. nasal visual field) (Figure 20.26). Thus if a field defect is found to respect the vertical midline in both eyes the lesion must lie in the proximal visual pathway, at the optic chiasm, optic radiations or cerebral cortex.

Chiasmatic lesions (usually pituitary tumours) tend to compress the crossing fibres from each eye, so typically produce a bitemporal field defect (Figure 20.27(b)). Note that it is necessary to test each eye separately to detect this form of field defect.

Infarction of the optic radiations or occipital cortex interrupts the uncrossed fibres from the ipsilateral eye and the crossed fibres from the contralateral eye, and so gives rise to homonymous (identical) field loss in each eye (Figure 20.27(a)).

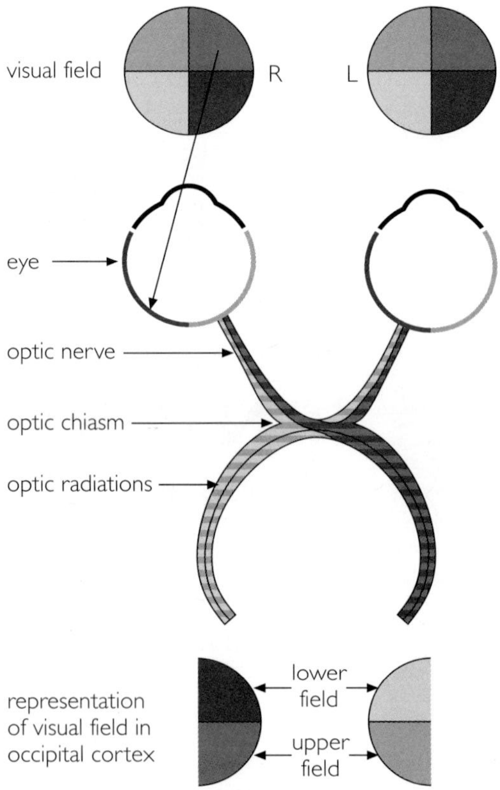

Figure 20.26 Visual pathway. The image of the left visual hemifield falls on the temporal retina of the right eye and nasal retina of the left eye, and is transmitted to the right visual (occipital) cortex

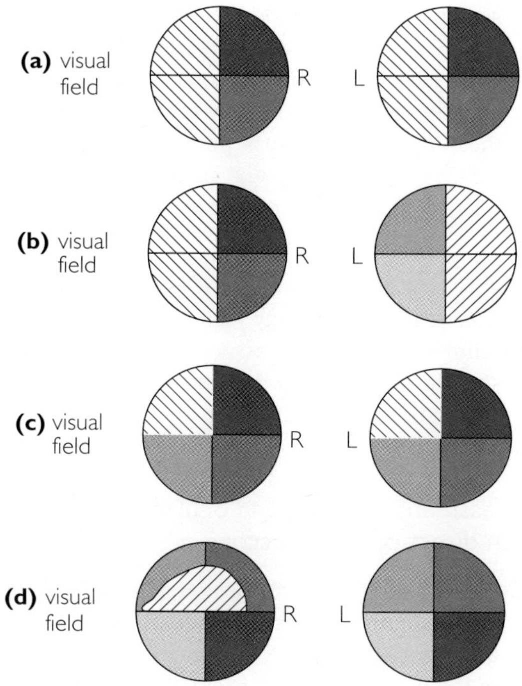

Figure 20.27 Field defects. **(a)** Left homonymous hemianopia secondary to infarction of the entire visual (occipital) cortex of the right hemisphere. **(b)** Bitemporal field loss arising from compression of the optic chiasm by a tumour (usually pituitary). **(c)** Quadrantic field loss deriving from partial infarction of the occipital cortex. This is quite common and is easily missed. Visual acuity is usually normal. **(d)** Altitudinal field defect respecting the horizontal but not the vertical midline. This tends to be due to ophthalmic disease such as glaucoma, retinal vascular occlusion or ischaemic optic neuropathy

Homonymous field loss is evident even when the patient is tested with both eyes open.

The vascular supply to the retina is split into arcades above and below the horizontal midline (Figures 20.1 and 20.11). Thus interruption of one arcade (either arterial or venous) may produce a field defect respecting the horizontal midline (Figures 20.27(d) and 20.15).

Field loss respecting the horizontal meridian is also common due to optic atrophy caused by glaucoma or ischaemic optic neuropathy.

Retinal detachment is characterised by a progressive loss of visual field of one eye which does not respect either vertical or horizontal meridia.

Relative afferent pupillary defect (RAPD)

This is an important test of retinal and optic nerve function that is often misunderstood and thus poorly performed. The purpose of the test is to determine how well each eye can drive the pupillary light reflex. To perform the test a bright light should be shone at one eye and then *rapidly* transferred to the other eye (Figure 20.28). If there is gross retinal dysfunction in one eye only (advanced ARMD, CRAO, total retinal detachment, etc.) or a significant unilateral optic nerve lesion (ischaemic optic neuropathy, gross glaucomatous damage), then the pupils of both eyes will be seen to dilate

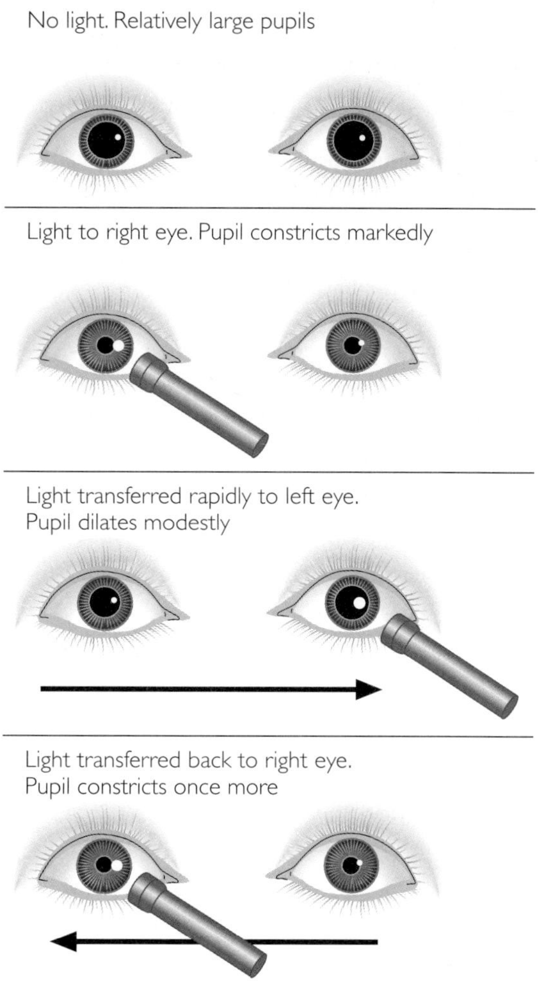

Figure 20.28 How to perform a test for a relative afferent pupillary defect (see text)

when the light is transferred to the affected eye. The most common error in performing this test is to assume that any constriction of the pupil to a light shone into the eye (without rapid transfer from previously shining it into the other eye) equates to an absence of a RAPD. If there is any sight in an eye then constriction will occur; the purpose of the test is to detect a *relative* defect in the reflex arc driven from one eye as compared to the other.

Causes of visual loss with marked RAPD (assuming other eye healthy) are:

- central retinal artery occlusion
- ischaemic optic neuropathy
- total/subtotal retinal detachment
- severe central retinal vein occlusion
- advanced glaucoma
- large intraocular melanoma.

Causes of visual loss with little of no RAPD are:

- cataract and capsule thickening
- both 'wet' and 'dry' ARMD
- mild to moderate central retinal vein occlusion
- branch retinal vein occlusion
- branch retinal artery occlusion.

Anterior segment examination

The direct ophthalmoscope may be used as an illuminated magnifying glass to examine the anterior segment of the eye. This is achieved by setting the ophthalmoscope to about +20 diopters. This can be achieved by focusing the ophthalmoscope on the back of your other hand until the hairs can be seen from about 5 cm, at which setting the anterior structures of the eye can be examined from a similar distance. Using this technique it may be possible to detect corneal ulceration, corneal foreign bodies, trichiasis or cataract (against the red reflex).

Pupil dilatation

This is an essential element of the assessment of many ocular presentations. It is often omitted by non-specialists on account of a perceived risk of precipitating angle closure glaucoma. In respect of this it should be understood that:

- a predisposition to angle closure is rare
- such patients are almost all very hypermetropic (glasses very thick in the middle) so that patients who are myopic or have a low prescription are highly unlikely to be at risk and
- the rare patient who is predisposed to angle closure will most likely angle close spontaneously at some future date in any case.

The risk of angle closure is low. Against this small risk of angle closure must be set the risk of missing treatable pathology such as cataract, retinal detachment or arteritic associated CRAO, or of missing signs associated with systemic disease such as embolism or retinopathy due to hypertension or diabetes.

Assessment of optics and ocular fundus with direct ophthalmoscopy

The direct ophthalmoscope is a useful tool for assessing not only the retina and optic disc but also the anterior segment.

In the elderly the pupil is small (senile miosis) and there is often some minor lens opacity. These make ophthalmoscopy through the undilated pupil at best difficult and frequently impossible, *and dilatation is recommended.*

Examination should take account of the following:

Optics of the eye

Optical defects may arise within the cornea, lens or vitreous but the only common presentation is cataract. This may take a number of forms that have a different appearance on ophthalmoscopy.

Examination technique Holding the ophthalmoscope to your eye, look at the red reflex from arm's length. Rack the ophthalmoscope's lens until you are focused on the reflex through the pupil. Lens opacities will appear as black spots, radial spokes or a nuclear ring (Figures 20.7 and 20.29).

Optic disc and macula

The optic disc of an elderly patient will appear cupped relative to younger patients, and disc cupping is *not* necessarily diagnostic of glaucoma. Small yellow lesions are often seen and may be interpreted as exudates and thus be indicative of

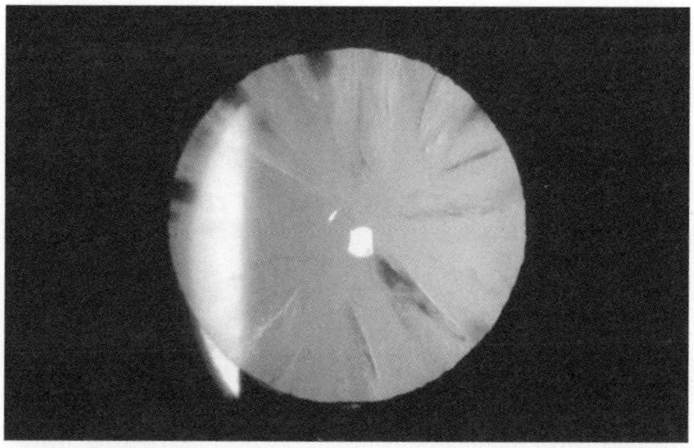

Figure 20.29 Water cleft lens opacity viewed against the red reflex. This cataract is less dense than the previous example (see Figure 20.7) and is typical of the type that gives rise to symptoms of monocular diplopia. This image can be seen with a direct ophthalmoscope used at 20–50 cm

diabetes or other vascular problems. However, these lesions are more commonly retinal drusen. Drusen are hyaline bodies that lie just under the retina. They have an association with ARMD but are not in themselves clinically significant (Figures 20.11 and 20.12). True exudates are rarely seen in the absence of retinal haemorrhages (see Box 20.3).

Box 20.2 Causes of no red reflex

- Dense cataract (the only common cause)
- Vitreous haemorrhage
- Total retinal detachment
- Large intraocular melanoma

Box 20.3 Causes of retinal haemorrhages

Small widely scattered haemorrhages
- Diabetes
- Venous occlusion (central or major branch retinal vein occlusion)
- Hypertension
- Blood dyscrasias such as thrombocytopenia, anaemia and leukaemia

Localised haemorrhage
- 'Wet' age-related macular degeneration
- Retinal branch vein occlusion
- Macroaneurysm

Examination technique Ask the patient to look at a specific object across the room. Approach along an axis on the horizontal plane of the eye about 15° temporal to the line of fixation. This should bring you close to the disc, then follow a major vessel back. The fovea lies 1.5–2 disc diameters lateral and centered a little lower than the centre of the optic disc.

Investigations in ophthalmology

Investigations into the ocular causes of visual dysfunction are generally ordered and interpreted by ophthalmic specialists. They include the following:

- *Formal field testing: Automated perimetry* Mostly employed in testing for field loss associated with glaucoma, this also has a role in the assessment of visual field loss from other sources, especially intracranial mass lesion, such as pituitary tumours.
- *Fluoroscein angiography and related angiographic techniques* The passage of intravenously administered fluoroscein through the retinal and choroidal vasculature can be monitored photographically. This technique has applications in the diagnosis and assessment of diabetes, ARMD, vascular occlusion and retinal vasculitis.
- *Ophthalmic ultrasound* This is used primarily when the optics of the eye are impaired by cataract or vitreous haemorrhage. Most useful for detecting retinal detachment, intraocular melanoma and gross ARMD when no direct view is possible.

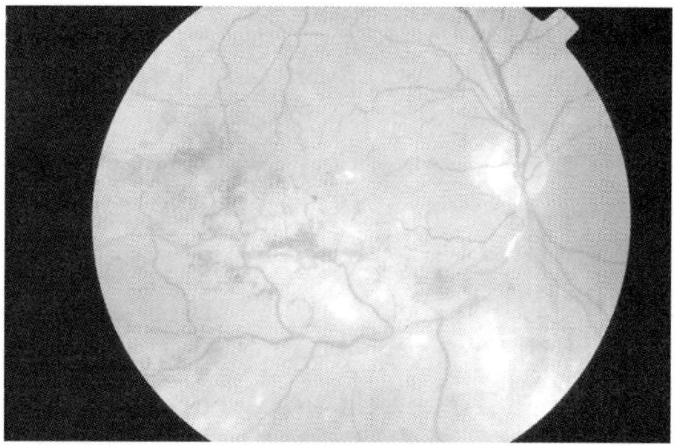

Figure 20.30 Inferior temporal branch vein occlusion right eye

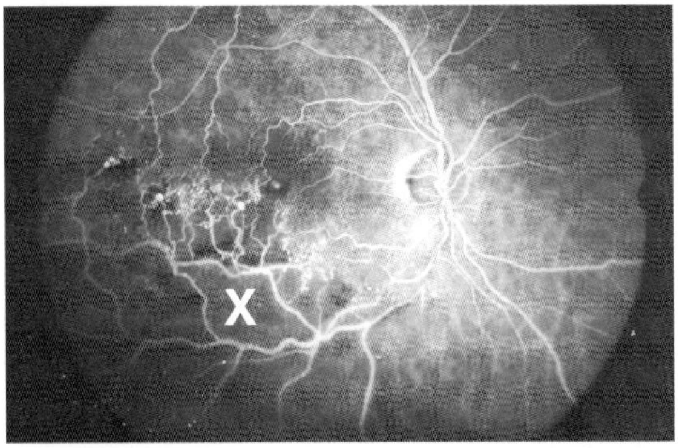

Figure 20.31 Fluoroscein angiogram of the same eye. This demonstrates a zone of poor perfusion in the zone of the inferotemporal retina served by the occluded vessel (X). This is characterised by the major vessels appearing more prominent but there is a loss of capillary circulation so the area between these vessels appears dark

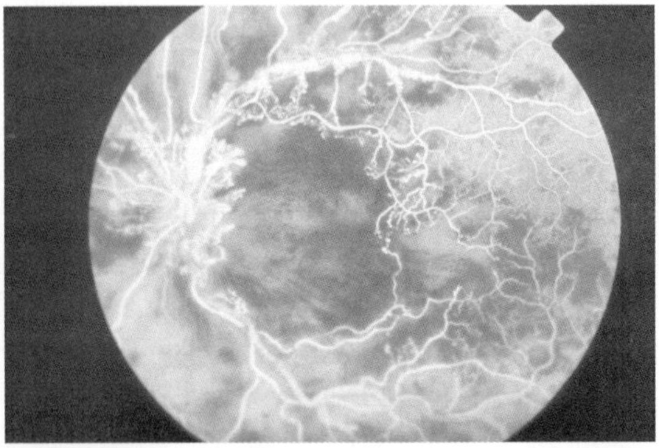

Figure 20.32 Fluoroscein angiogram of the same eye as in Figure 20.17. Note widespread loss of capillary perfusion

Diagnosis

Most diagnoses in ophthalmology are arrived at on the basis of clinical examination rather than systemic investigation. It is not appropriate for most specialist investigations (such as angiography) to be ordered by general physicians.

Treatment and prognosis

Uncorrected refractive error

The importance of ensuring that an elderly patient has appropriate glasses cannot be overemphasised. Refraction (testing for glasses) should be one of the first steps in the assessment of a patient with gradual painless loss of vision.

Problems with the ocular adnexae

Eyelids

Involutional changes in the ocular adnexae (ectropion, entropion, ptosis secondary to levator dehiscence) are easily managed by means of local anaesthetic oculoplastic procedures. A useful short-term management of an uncomfortable entropion is to use tape between the lower lid and upper cheek to prevent the lid from turning in until a definitive surgical repair can be performed (Figure 20.33).

Lacrimal problems

Poor tear production may be augmented by topical tear substitutes. Hypromellose has been largely superseded by polyvinyl alcohol preparations and other polymers. As a general rule the more viscous preparations are more effective at relieving discomfort but they may interfere with vision. In severely dry eyes, such as may arise in association with rheumatoid arthritis, it may be necessary to occlude the lacrimal punctae with silicon plugs or by cautery.

Corneal disease

A cornea that has become opaque due to Fuch's dystrophy or scarring secondary to bacterial or viral infection may be replaced by transplantation.

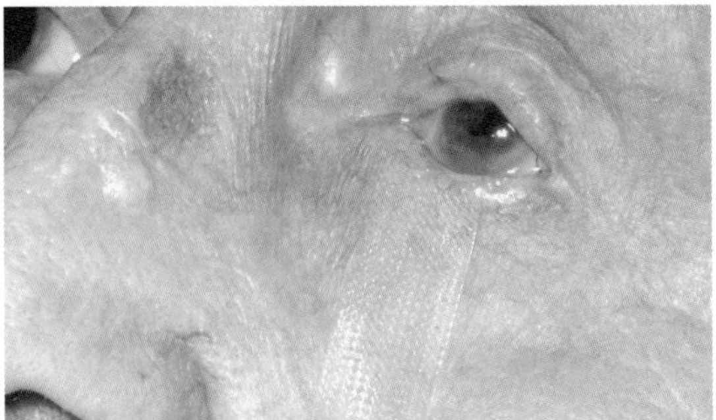

Figure 20.33 Temporary control of an entropion by taping the skin of the lower lid to the cheek

Unlike many other organs, tissue matching is not obligatory although it may be undertaken for some high-risk grafts. Some patients with a lesser degree of corneal damage may see better with contact lenses rather than glasses.

Cataract

Cataract is the commonest treatable ophthalmic presentation and the condition with the greatest potential for effective treatment and rehabilitation.

Most surgery in the developed world is now conducted by phacoemulsification through a small wound, usually under local anaesthesia. Most patients can be managed as day admissions, and rehabilitation is rapid. Age and infirmity should not be regarded as a reason not to refer for surgery, as there are almost no absolute contraindications to local anaesthetic cataract surgery in co-operative patients. However, patients suffering dementia may require a general anaesthetic which may be contra-indicated if the patient is grossly unfit.

Vitreous haemorrhage

The management of vitreous haemorrhage depends upon the diagnosis of the underlying cause. If it is believed that the cause of the haemorrhage does not require immediate intervention (RBVO, ARMD) then the blood may be left to clear, which may take many months. The only alternative is surgical vitrectomy which may be indicated if the haemorrhage is secondary to retinal detachment or proliferative diabetic retinopathy.

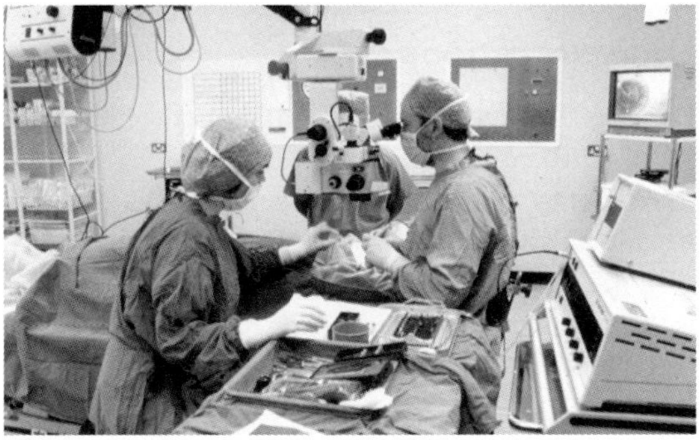

Figure 20.34 Cataract surgery. The procedure takes place under an operating microscope. The phacoemulsification machine is in the right foreground. Above and beyond it an image of the eye can be seen on a CCTV connected to the microscope

Age-related maculopathy (ARMD)

A small proportion of patients presenting with 'wet' ARMD may benefit from laser therapy. There are new techniques under development that may widen the clinical indications for intervention. Nevertheless, it seems likely that it will remain that the large majority of patients presenting with ARMD will not have treatable disease and the principal thrust of management should be towards rehabilitation with low vision aids and modification of home circumstances as appropriate.

A small proportion of patients presenting with 'wet' ARMD may benefit from treatment with an Argon laser. These patients are most likely to be those with a short history of visual loss (weeks rather than months) and visual acuity of better than 6/24.

There are new surgical and laser treatments under development which may allow treatment of further groups of patients with 'wet' ARMD who are not suitable for argon laser therapy. It is possible to excise the membrane surgically but the surgery is technically difficult and laborious. Alternatively, photodynamic therapy employs a photoactivated drug which is injected intravenously and activated as it passes through the neovascular complex by laser light directed through the pupil. The activated drug induces occlusion of the capillaries within the neovascular complex and the overlying retina. The intention is that the retinal vessels are less sensitive to the effect of the drug and recover, whereas the capillaries of the neovascular complex are permanently occluded. The disadvantages of this treatment are that it is very expensive and may need to be repeated several times before becoming fully effective.

'Dry' ARMD is of much slower onset. It progresses relentlessly but vision may be only moderately affected for many years. It is more common in short-sighted individuals. It is characterised by gradual changes in the architecture of the central retina with pigment clumping and atrophic patches within the retina.

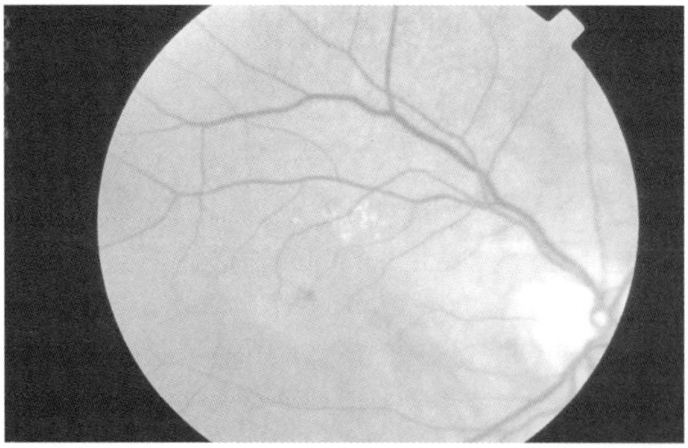

Figure 20.35 Age-related macular degeneration (ARMD). This patient presented with distortion of vision and moderately reduced visual acuity. There is a small parafoveal haemorrhage and subretinal fluid is present

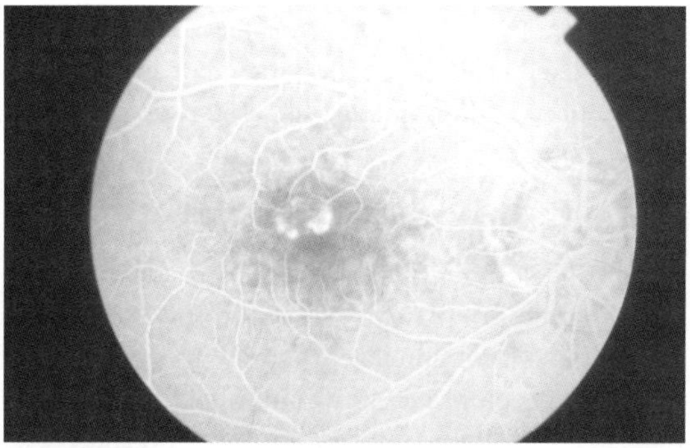

Figure 20.36 Angiogram of the same patient. This shows a fibrovascular membrane adjacent to the fovea (this is the intense white area of fluorescence adjacent to the fovea). The natural history of such lesions is that most progress to cause substantial loss of central vision

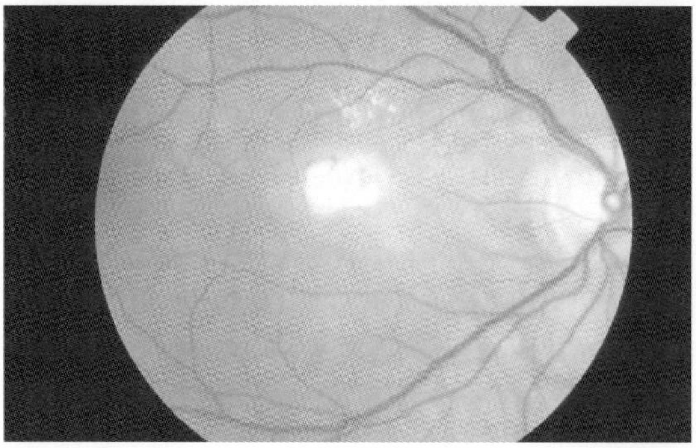

Figure 20.37 ARMD after laser treatment. The lesion has been treated with intense argon laser burns, giving a small paramacular scar

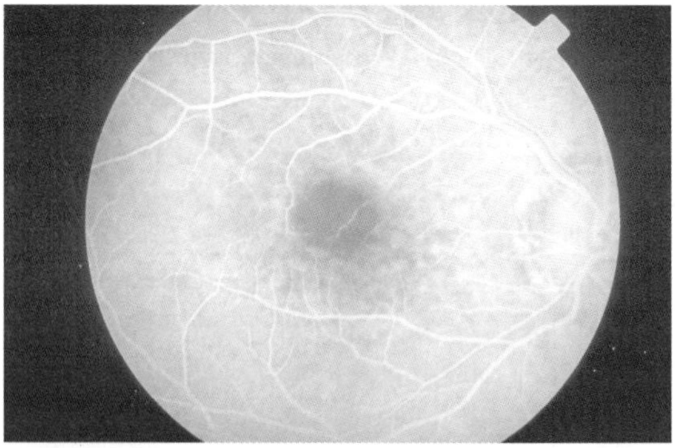

Figure 20.38 Angiogram after laser treatment. The membrane has been obliterated (now appears as dark area). Unfortunately, the recurrence rate is quite high

Vascular diseases affecting the eye

Ischaemic optic neuropathy and arterial occlusions rarely benefit from direct intervention, but any underlying treatable disease such as atrial fibrillation or giant cell arteritis must be treated appropriately. Patients with embolic disease should be treated with an antiplatelet agent unless contraindicated.

The visual loss arising from CRVO is difficult to reverse with treatment; however, treatment may be required if secondary glaucoma arises (see Chapter 21). Some patients with branch vein occlusion do benefit from laser therapy to reverse the visual loss from secondary macular oedema.

Systemic hypertension associated with a vein occlusion should be treated.

Diabetic retinopathy

Patients with proliferative diabetic retinopathy require urgent laser therapy.

Patients with mild to moderate diabetic maculopathy also require laser treatment to conserve visual function, but if maculopathy is gross and established then it is unlikely to be amenable to treatment.

Cerebral infarction

These patients should be managed as with all patients presenting with evidence of cerebrovascular disease (see Chapter 17).

Retinal detachment

Any patients suspected of having a retinal detachment should be referred for specialist advice. Most retinal detachments are managed surgically under a general anaesthetic but local anaesthesia is often feasible if general anaesthesia is contraindicated.

Management of other causes of visual loss

Uveitis and scleritis require treatment with immunosuppressives, usually steroids in the first instance. Mild to moderate uveitis may respond to topical or locally injected steroid, but severe uveitis and scleritis generally require systemic immunosuppressive therapy.

Double vision

It is often possible to restore control of a longstanding latent squint by incorporating prism into the patient's glasses. Similarly, it is frequently possible to use prisms to manage squints that are likely to resolve with time, such as a mild to moderate sixth nerve palsy. The amount of conventional prism that can be incorporated into glasses is limited by the increase in weight of the spectacles. An alternative is a Fresnel prism, which is very light but may be rejected by patients as it degrades the retinal image and thus reduces acuity slightly (Figure 20.39).

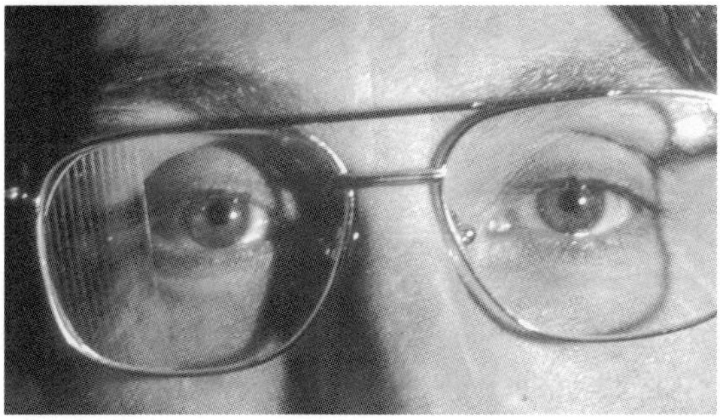

Figure 20.39 Management of a squint with prism. This patient has a partial right sixth nerve palsy. This is limiting abduction of the right eye, so the patient sees double when he looks to the right. The glasses have a lightweight Fresnel prism applied to the outer half of the right lens to compensate for the poor abduction

If a squint is not expected to resolve and cannot be managed successfully by conservative measures such as prisms, then it may be possible to restore binocular vision by surgery. This is often undertaken for:

- longstanding decompensated squints
- sixth nerve palsy
- fourth nerve palsy
- thyroid eye disease.

Third nerve palsy is difficult to treat surgically. In most elderly patients a conservative course is best. Fortunately, most have a total ptosis which relieves the intractable diplopia that would otherwise result.

Patients with chronic progressive external ophthalmoplegia often preserve binocular function despite having a very poor range of eye movement. If diplopia arises it can usually be corrected by prisms, and surgery is not indicated.

Rehabilitative measures for patients with poor vision

Low vision aids

Low vision aids (LVAs) are devices that magnify the image in order to assist resolution of the image in the presence of acuity loss. LVAs may take the form of a hand-held magnifier (with or without built-in illumination), a telescopic magnifier mounted on a spectacle frame, or closed circuit camera systems.

In order to prescribe an appropriate system it is necessary to assess the nature of the patient's visual handicap and to ensure that the system provided is suitable in the light of the patient's lifestyle and other handicaps. It is important that these patients are followed up in order to ensure that they have adapted to using the system; in the absence of follow-up patients easily get discouraged and discard the aid. This task is best handled by an optometric professional specialising in this area.

Hemianopia generates specific rehabilitative problems. Many patients with hemianopia are not conscious of the 'missing' hemifield from minute to minute and are at risk of accident in unfamiliar surroundings and especially when crossing roads. Reading may be impaired, particularly when it is the right hemifield that is lost, because the patient cannot see the next word in the sentence as it is within the blind hemifield. This can be very difficult to rehabilitate. Patients with a left hemifield loss have problems acquiring the next line on the page (as this requires an eye movement into the blind hemifield) but this is more amenable to rehabilitation.

Box 20.4 Emergency referrals in ophthalmology

Same day
- Acute glaucoma
- Macula-on retinal detachment
- Central retinal artery occlusion

Next working day
- 'Wet' ARMD
- Sudden diplopia
- Proliferative diabetic retinopathy
- Macula-off retinal detachment

'Soon'
- Other retinal vascular occlusions
- Diabetic maculopathy
- Cerebral infarction
- Suspected pituitary lesion

Routine
- Cataract
- Posterior capsule thickening
- Lid problems

Bibliography and further reading

Findlay, R. D. & Payne P. A. G. (1998), *The Eye in General Practice*, 10th ed, Butterworth-Heinemann.

Fraser, S., Asaria, R. & Kon. C. (2001), *Eye Know How*, B. M. J. Books.

Khaw, P. T., & Elkington A. R. (1999), *ABC of Books*, 3rd ed, B. M. J. Books.

Parr, J. (1996), *Introduction to Ophthalmology*, University of Otago, N.Z.

Parsons, J. H., Sir (1978), *Parsons' Diseases of the Eye*, 16th ed, Churchill Livingstone, New York

Kanski, J. J. (1999), *Clinical Ophthalmology. A Systematic Approach*, 4th ed, Butterworth-Heinemann.

Chapter 21
Glaucoma

ANDREW BRAGANZA and RAVI THOMAS

Introduction

Glaucoma is not a single disease but refers to a large group of diseases, all of which eventually result in damage to the optic nerve head. The damage is manifest as a characteristic ophthalmoscopic appearance of the optic disc and nerve fibre layer defects, with corresponding defects in the visual field. For a long time it was believed that glaucoma was synonymous with raised intraocular pressure (IOP). Raised IOP is a major risk factor for glaucoma; indeed it is the only known causal risk factor for this disease. However, there are other risk factors and glaucoma can occur in the absence of raised IOP.

The glaucomas are broadly grouped into primary and secondary glaucomas. Primary open angle glaucoma (POAG) is the most common adult onset glaucoma seen in Western populations. In Asian populations, primary angle closure glaucoma (PACG), the other major adult onset primary glaucoma, may be as common as POAG, or even more so.

Secondary glaucomas, with the exception of lens related glaucomas and neovascular glaucoma, are probably relatively unimportant in the geriatric age group. Only a few specific entities will be discussed here. The purpose of this chapter is to emphasise some important concepts in the diagnosis and management of glaucomas that may be required in a geriatric practice.

Table 21.1 outlines the broad classification of glaucoma and mentions a few specific examples in each category. The list is by no means comprehensive. Entities printed in bold typeface are discussed in the text.

Epidemiology

Glaucoma is an important cause of irreversible blindness in adults; in some areas of the world it is the leading cause of blindness in persons over 60 years of age. Using the WHO criteria for blindness (corrected visual acuity < 3/60 in the better eye) it is estimated that there are over 3 million people worldwide who are blind due to glaucoma. This makes it the third most important cause of blindness overall, after cataract and trachoma. Further, it is estimated that there are nearly 65 million individuals affected by glaucoma worldwide, of whom 7 million are expected to go blind. The prevalence of the

Table 21.1 Classification of the glaucomas based on aetiology

Primary glaucomas	Developmental glaucomas	Secondary glaucomas
Primary congenital glaucoma	Hereditary juvenile glaucoma	*Glaucomas associated with corneal endothelial disorders* Irido-corneo-endothelial (ICE) syndrome
Primary open angle glaucoma	*Other developmental glaucomas with associated anomalies* Axenfeld-Rieger syndrome Peter's anomaly	*Glaucoma associated with iris anomalies* Pigmentary glaucoma
Primary angle closure glaucoma		*Glaucomas associated with lens disorders* **Phacomorphic glaucoma** **Phacolytic glaucoma** Ectopia lentis Exfoliation syndrome *Glaucomas associated with posterior segment disorders* **Neovascular glaucoma** Schwartz syndrome *Glaucoma associated with elevated episcleral venous pressure* Thyroid ophthalmopathy Sturge-Weber syndrome *Glaucoma associated with intraocular tumours* Uveal melanomas *Uveitic glaucoma* ***Steroid induced glaucoma*** *Glaucomas associated with intraocular haemorrhage* Hyphaema Ghost cell glaucoma *Traumatic glaucoma* Angle recession glaucoma *Glaucoma following ocular surgery*

primary adult glaucomas and their geographic distribution is shown in Table 21.2. This has been derived and summarised from several population based studies published in the medical literature.

Hospital based studies on white populations in the Western world suggest that POAG is about 5 times as common as PACG. However, there is a strong racial influence on the distribution of the primary glaucomas. For instance, in an urban South Indian population, PACG was 4.5 times more common than POAG in the 30–60 year age group. Hospital based studies in India suggest that PACG is overall at least as common as POAG. This is similar to results from other population based studies in Asia. The large differences in prevalence rates from various sources can be partly explained by differing diagnostic criteria and methods of examination. However, there is little doubt that racial differences in anterior chamber anatomy and angle configurations do exist.

Table 21.2 Prevalence of primary adult glaucomas in the over 40 age group from selected population based studies

Geographic area	Racial group	Prevalence (%)
Baltimore	Whites	1.1
	Blacks	4.7
Singapore	Chinese	3.2
Mongolia	Chinese	2.4
Japan	Japanese	3.1
Barbados	Blacks	5.3
Vellore	Indians	4.7

Source: Acknowledgment to Dr Paul Foster for much of the data.

Pathophysiology

PACG

Aqueous humour is produced by the ciliary epithelium of the ciliary processes in the posterior chamber and, under normal circumstances, flows through the pupil into the anterior chamber of the eye. From here it drains through the trabecular meshwork in the angle into Schlemm's canal and eventually into the aqueous veins. In PACG, the anterior chamber is shallow and configuration of the structures in the anterior segment is such that there is a resistance to the flow of aqueous from anterior to posterior chamber through the pupil. This 'pupillary block' causes an increase in pressure in the posterior chamber, resulting in a forward bowing of the peripheral iris (iris bombé). The peripheral iris can come into contact with and block the outflow channels in the angle. This results in increased pressure in the anterior chamber, increased contact between the lens and the iris, worsening of the pupillary block and a vicious cycle that can result in sudden acute elevation of IOP and an attack of acute angle closure glaucoma (ACG). Alternatively, and more commonly, there is intermittent closure of the angle with gradual permanent adhesions or peripheral anterior synechiae. The peripheral anterior synechiae (PAS) forming between the iris and the trabecular meshwork result in chronically elevated IOP and chronic ACG. Combinations of raised IOP, closed angles on gonioscopy (a clinical method of viewing the anterior chamber angle) usually with PAS, optic disc changes and field defects are diagnostic of chronic ACG. It will be easily understood from Figures 21.1 to 21.3 how pupillary block could cause blockage of the angle and how a peripheral iridotomy (PI) will be curative in the initial stages before PAS formation is extensive. However, all primary angle closure glaucomas are not exclusively due to pupillary block and hence in some cases a PI alone may not be sufficient.

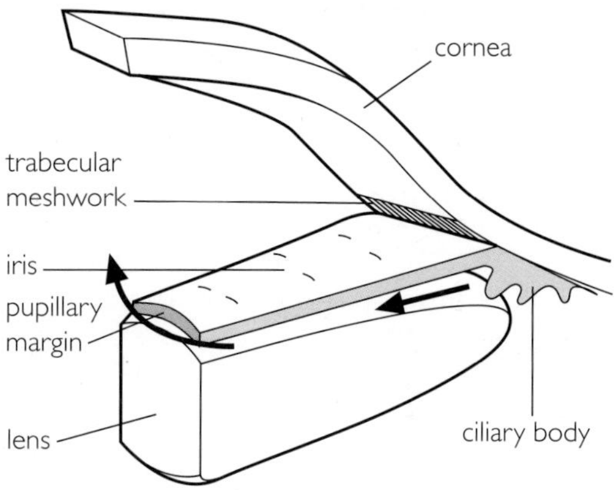

Figure 21.1 Diagram of normal anterior chamber angle. Arrows indicate normal direction of aqueous flow

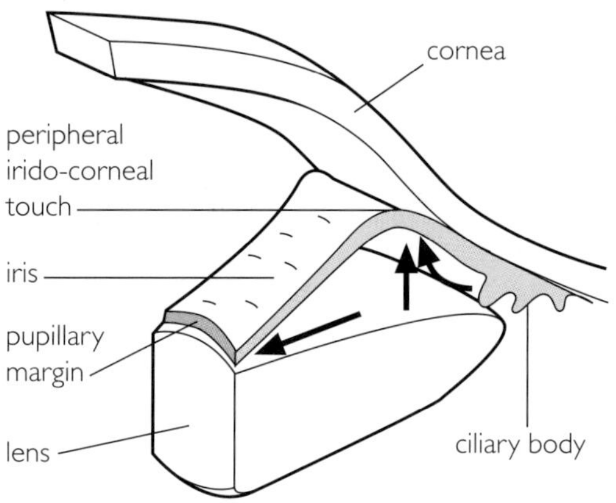

Figure 21.2 Diagram of anterior chamber angle configuration with pupillary block. The increase in pressure in the posterior chamber (see arrows) results in peripheral bowing forward of the iris

POAG

The maximum resistance to the outflow of aqueous occurs in the trabecular meshwork overlying Schlemm's canal. The IOP is essentially a balance

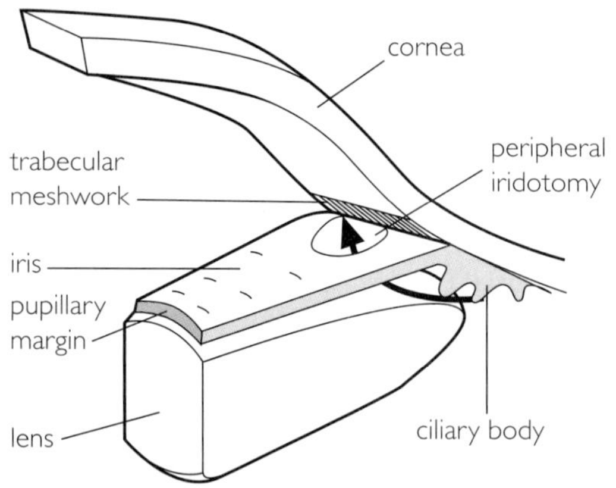

Figure 21.3 Diagram of the anterior chamber angle with a peripheral iridotomy. By providing an alternate route of flow of aqueous from posterior to anterior chamber (see arrow), this relieves pupillary block

between the amount of inflow, governed by various factors operating in the ciliary body, and the facility of outflow. In POAG, changes in the trabecular meshwork result in increased resistance to outflow, thereby raising the IOP. Not all raised IOP results in glaucoma. It must be remembered that, like all biological parameters, 'normal' IOP is simply a statistical definition based on the Gaussian distribution of IOP in a normal population. The mean IOP in a normal population is around 16 mmHg and two standard deviations above this puts the upper limit of 'normal' at 21 mmHg. This simply means that 97.5% of normal individuals will have IOP less than 22 mmHg. This does *not* mean that IOP more than 21 mmHg is abnormal; after all, 2.5% of the normal population will have IOP above the normal range.

POAG is defined on the basis of evidence of disc damage, such as loss of the nerve fibre layer or typical field defects; some discs may be able to withstand higher levels of IOP while others may show glaucomatous changes at 'normal' levels of IOP. Such cases may be thought of as having discs that for some reason are more susceptible to IOP induced damage. POAG is thus characterised by typical disc and field changes with or without IOP elevated beyond the statistical range of normal. Raised IOP is only a risk factor for disc damage; the higher the IOP the greater the risk. It is the only causal risk factor we know of which we can modify therapeutically. However, raised IOP is not mandatory for diagnosis. Other factors that increase susceptibility are yet largely unknown.

Lens induced glaucomas

Phacolytic glaucoma

Cataract is essentially a degenerative change in the lens. Advanced stages of cataract result in a hypermature cataract whose capsule may develop micro leaks, allowing high molecular weight lens proteins into the aqueous. These incite an inflammatory response, causing breakdown of the normal blood–aqueous barrier, with migration of inflammatory cells into the aqueous. Macrophages laden with phagocytosed lens proteins can block the trabecular meshwork. Also, the increased viscosity of the protein rich aqueous makes drainage less efficient. This can result in an acute rise in IOP and a painful red eye typical of phacolytic glaucoma (phacolytic: relating to dissolution of the lens), constituting an ophthalmic emergency. In developing countries this is a significant problem, as patients who have undergone cataract surgery in one eye and are visually rehabilitated tend to ignore the loss in vision in the other eye until a complication such as phacolytic glaucoma ensues. In more developed countries this is a problem of aged, indigent patients who are mostly unattended and may ignore unilateral visual loss until pain sets in.

Phacomorphic glaucoma

The normal human lens slowly increases in size with increasing age as more lens fibres are laid down. Also, with developing cataract, the lens tends to swell with water clefts forming between the degenerating fibres (intumescent cataract). This increase in size has to be accommodated within the normal anterior segment, as the eyeball itself does not grow in size with advancing age. The large lens may cause physical crowding of the angle as well as increase the propensity of the eye to develop pupillary block, resulting in an acute painful red eye with high IOP or phacomorphic glaucoma (phacomorphic: relating to the shape of the lens). Presenting features include severe pain, redness and diminution of vision. Phacomorphic glaucoma is more common in eyes with shallow anterior chambers and a crowded anterior segment. Again, this is more of a problem in developing countries where a cataract may progress to a stage where complications set in. Further, Asian eyes tend to have smaller, more crowded anterior segments and are more prone to developing angle closure glaucoma and possibly phacomorphic glaucoma.

Pseudoexfoliation glaucoma (exfoliation syndrome)

This entity has come to be well recognised over the last half-century as a distinct and fairly common form of secondary open angle glaucoma. Pseudoexfoliation refers to the release of dandruff-like flakes in the anterior segment of the eye, possibly originating from the lens capsule or iris basement membrane. This material, possibly by blocking the trabecular meshwork, causes a rise in IOP in the affected eye and eventually glaucomatous disc damage. All eyes with pseudoexfoliation do not have glaucoma, but as many as 50% may develop a rise of pressure with time. There is a strong geographic and racial predilection for this disease. It was originally described in Scandinavia and persons of Scandinavian origin continue to be at an increased risk. Africans and Asians, especially Indians, also show a high prevalence of this condition with a high incidence of glaucoma. Another important consideration is that pseudoexfoliation becomes more common with advancing age. Once detected, a patient with pseudoexfoliation must be followed up regularly to detect developing glaucoma in the early stages. Pseudoexfoliation glaucoma is more aggressive and rapidly progressive than the primary open angle variety, and hence follow-ups should be more frequent, usually around 3–4 times a year.

Steroid induced glaucoma

It has long been known that some patients develop an ocular hypertensive response to therapeutically administered steroids. This response is believed to have a genetic basis, the magnitude of the response to a standard dose being governed by the homozygous or heterozygous state of the gene. The rise in IOP is usually seen after 2–6 weeks (or more) of topically administered steroids; it may take longer to develop with systemically administered steroids. There is a distinct dose–response relationship to the IOP response. This type of glaucoma is usually managed medically. However, if long-term steroid therapy is needed, argon laser trabeculoplasty or glaucoma surgery (see below) may be indicated.

Neovascular glaucoma (NVG)

Neovascular glaucoma constitutes the most common form of secondary angle closure glaucoma in developed countries. It results from the development of new vessels from the iris and ciliary vasculature in the form of a neovascular membrane that initially obstructs the outflow channels in the angle and eventually contracts to cause permanent peripheral anterior synechiae. The stimulus for neovascularisation is posterior segment pathology. An ischaemic retina produces an angiogenic factor that finds its way into the aqueous and through the pupil and anterior chamber into the trabecular meshwork. This is the reason that new vessels are initially seen at the pupillary margin and then in the angle. In pigmented eyes new vessels at the pupillary margin may be difficult to detect. Hence, a careful gonioscopy in all patients at risk for NVG is mandatory.

The most common cause of NVG is proliferative diabetic retinopathy. The same stimulus that produces fibrovascular proliferation in the posterior segment acts in the anterior segment also. Retinal vein occlusions are another important cause. Carotid artery occlusive disease can cause NVG as well. NVG may be a rare mode of presentation of intraocular malignancies (masquerade syndromes).

Clinical features include a painful red eye, cloudy oedematous cornea and profound visual loss, the latter usually due to the primary underlying condition rather than the NVG itself. In the early stages, however, NVG may be symptomless, and if the retinal pathology has spared the macula, visual acuity may be good as well. Early recognition of the condition is vital in these cases if useful vision is to be preserved.

Treatment is aimed at controlling the underlying disease, causing as much of the neovascular membrane as possible to regress and then addressing the issue of IOP control as with other glaucomas.

Clinical tests

Tonometry

Measurement of IOP is part of the basic ophthalmic examination and is essential for the diagnosis and management of glaucoma. There are two main principles involved in measurement of IOP: indentation and applanation. Indentation tonometers work by displacement of a volume of aqueous and measurement of the force required to achieve the displacement. The well known Schiotz tonometer is one such instrument. Applanation tonometers work by estimating the force needed to flatten a measured area of cornea. These instruments are less affected by the inherent rigidity of the eyeball, which may vary widely in individuals, and are therefore more accurate. In fact, the Goldmann applanation tonometer is considered the gold standard in tonometry. Tonometers such as the non-contact tonometer, which uses an air puff to achieve applanation and measures the applanated area optically, or the Tono-pen™, which is a small electronic device working on an applanating principle, are also acceptable alternatives. The non-contact tonometer is, however, expensive and offers no real advantage over the Goldmann applanation tonometer. Also, abnormal readings of IOP on non-contact tonometry usually need confirmation by Goldmann applanation tonometry. The Tono-pen™ on the other hand, although expensive, is small, portable and can be used with the patient in any position. It has the advantage of applanating a very small area, making it accurate in scarred or irregular corneas.

Gonioscopy

A gonioscope is a device used to view the angle of the anterior chamber. The angle is not normally visible as total internal reflection at the cornea prevents reflected light from the angle escaping the eye. The details and principles of gonioscopy are not pertinent to the present discussion. Suffice it to say that the distinction between the two main types of primary glaucomas, POAG and PACG, depends on a gonioscopic assessment of whether the angle is open or not. Further, the diagnosis of many secondary glaucomas will depend on gonioscopic findings. Thus an ophthalmologist attempting to make a diagnosis of glaucoma must be skilled in performing this essential clinical examination.

Optic disc examination

The optic nerve head is the end organ that suffers damage in glaucoma. Much thought and effort have gone into determining how the nerve is damaged in glaucoma. Debate is still active between proponents of the mechanical theory, who believe damage occurs as a direct result of pressure on the nerve fibres, and those supporting the vascular theory, that the pathology lies in pressure induced effects on the blood supply of the optic nerve head. The truth probably lies somewhere in between but, regardless of the mechanism, optic nerve head damage in glaucoma has a very characteristic appearance and must be looked for and recognised by the ophthalmologist.

Classical teaching was that cupping of the optic disc was a major characteristic of glaucomatous damage. A cup–disc ratio of over 0.3 was considered highly suspicious. With the current recognition that the optic disc can vary in size from about 0.9 mm to almost 3.0 mm, the finding of an enlarged cup has to be interpreted in the light of the actual disc size. As the number of nerve fibres in the disc is more or less constant, the neuroretinal rim (formed by the actual axons) will occupy less space in a large disc than in a small one; the cup is simply the area of the disc not occupied by nerve fibres. More important and specific is a difference of 0.2 or more in cup–disc ratio between the two eyes, but this also has to be interpreted in the context of disc size. One disc may be larger than its fellow and, by the above reasoning, will be expected to have a larger cup. Notching of the rim (extension of the cup to the edge of the disc), nasal shift of vessels, splinter haemorrhages and wedge defects in the nerve fibre layer are also significant signs of glaucomatous damage. Recent understanding of the normal morphology of the neuroretinal rim has led to the observation that the normal rim is thickest **i**nferiorly, then **s**uperiorly, **n**asally and **t**emporally —the 'ISNT' rule. This morphology is altered early with glaucomatous damage and is a sensitive and fairly specific indicator for glaucomatous disc damage. Assessing an optic disc for glaucoma should be done by a specialist. It necessitates a stereoscopic magnified view obtained on slit-lamp indirect ophthalmoscopy with a 60D or 78D lens. Imaging techniques designed to view the optic nerve head and detect early glaucomatous change are also available. The Heidelberg Retinal Tomogram™, the GDX™ system and systems based on optical coherence tomography are slowly moving out of research establishments and are acquiring clinical applicability. From the point of view of the medical practitioner screening patients with a direct ophthalmoscope, it is probably warranted to refer a patient with a cup–disc ratio > 0.5 or asymmetry of 0.2 or more in the cup–disc ratio for a detailed glaucoma assessment. With the acquisition of a little more skill in assessing a disc, the significant alteration of the ISNT rule is a good sign to look for and to refer patients with. The screening for glaucoma will be discussed subsequently in the text. Figures 21.4 and 21.5 show a normal disc and one with a significant notch, respectively. Figure 21.6 shows a disc with advanced glaucoma and total glaucomatous optic atrophy.

Visual field testing

It was stressed earlier that the optic nerve head and the nerve fibre layer are the target tissues that are damaged in glaucoma. It is important, therefore, to try and identify the compromise in function caused by this damage and to quantify it. This is what visual field testing or perimetry attempts to do.

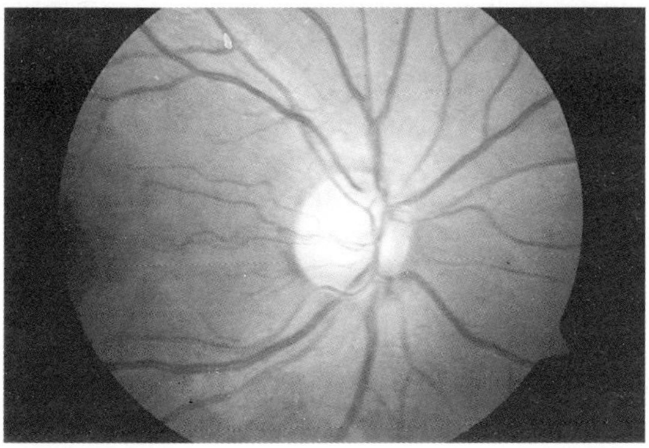

Figure 21.4 Photograph of a normal optic disc. Note the thickness of the neuroretinal rim following the 'ISNT' rule

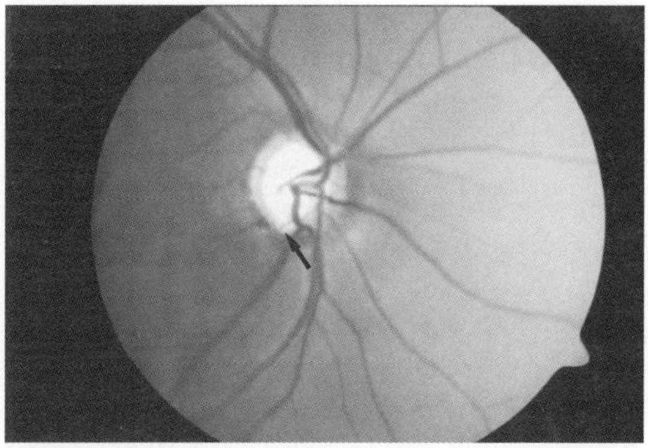

Figure 21.5 Photograph of an optic disc with glaucomatous changes. The arrow indicates an inferior notch in the neuroretinal rim

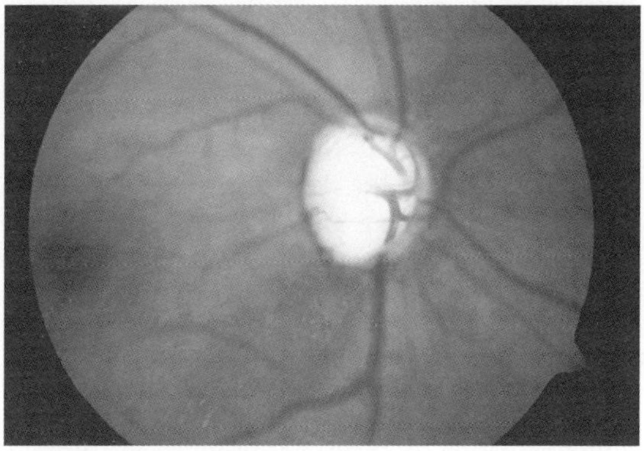

Figure 21.6 Photograph of an optic disc showing near total glaucomatous optic atrophy

The current gold standard in perimetry is an automated computerised perimeter performing full-threshold static testing, with a database of normative data, and statistical functions available to make quantitative assessments and comparisons. It is important that the demonstration of a typical field defect correlating with the disc findings is mandatory for the diagnosis of POAG. It is only on demonstration of a field defect that treatment is indicated and certainly surgical treatment should be considered in POAG only when a significant field defect is present. In secondary glaucomas, on the other hand, the diagnosis is based only on the level of IOP and the associated clinical findings—for example, neovascularisation of the iris or pseudoexfoliation of the lens capsule. Here perimetry may have a role in follow-up (assuming that media opacities and other problems do not interfere with testing and interpretation) and in prognostication but is not essential for diagnosis.

The follow-up of any glaucoma, however, relies heavily on perimetry. All modalities of treatment eventually are aimed at stopping or slowing down the progressive loss of ganglion cells and thus loss of the nerve fibre layer. Perimetry is a qualitative and quantitative test of visual function of the peripheral retina, and will show up progressive damage as an enlarging field defect. Thus most glaucoma specialists will follow their patients with repeated field assessments, probably every 4–6 months, or more often, depending on the clinical situation.

While technology has made field testing faster, more accurate and easier on the subject, it is still a tedious exercise and requires a considerable amount of co-operation from the patient. Interpretation of the result is not always easy and must be made in the context of the overall clinical picture. Figure 21.7 shows the field of the patient whose disc is shown in Figure 21.5. There is a typical superior arcuate defect in the field corresponding to the inferior notch seen in the optic disc.

A newer means of testing the visual field using the physiological phenomenon of frequency doubling has recently become available. Frequency doubling perimetry (FDP) has promise as a simple, fast and sensitive means of testing the visual field to detect glaucomatous field defects. The machine is portable and testing does not require a skilled technician. This test may make screening for glaucomatous field defects possible. It may also be of some use in the detection of neurological field defects. However, glaucomas detected by FDP will still need confirmation and follow-up with conventional automated perimetry.

Diagnosis

PACG

A combination of elevated IOP, angles closed on gonioscopy either with PAS or simply appositionally closed, and characteristic disc and field changes serves to identify the patient with chronic PACG. Secondary causes of angle closure (e.g. neovascularisation) must be ruled out. It is not mandatory for disc changes to be present; raised IOP with PAS or appositional closure is sufficient to diagnose chronic PACG. Conversely, IOP within the normal range but with evidence of closure (PAS or appositional closure on gonioscopy) and disc and field changes also gives us a positive diagnosis of chronic PACG. Acute angle closure glaucoma is easier to diagnose and more dramatic in presentation, as described earlier.

POAG

Open angles on gonioscopy with normal or elevated IOP with typical disc and field changes give us a diagnosis of POAG. The disc and field changes are mandatory for diagnosis. Often a situation arises where IOP is elevated (or normal) and discs may show evidence of typical glaucomatous damage but the fields are normal. Such cases are usually categorised as POAG suspects or even 'pre-perimetric glaucoma' and need a close lifelong follow-up. They have a high chance of developing field defects and clinching the diagnosis of POAG. Other patients may have elevated IOP alone with no disc or field evidence to suggest glaucoma. These used to be referred to as 'ocular hypertensives', but are better termed 'glaucoma suspects' and followed up as such. A significant percentage will show evidence of progressive glaucomatous disc damage with time, necessitating treatment. The decision to treat raised IOP alone with no evidence of target organ damage in the form of field defects is a difficult one. In general, experience has shown that an IOP greater than 30 mmHg considerably increases the risk of developing field defects compared to an IOP less than 30 mmHg. Other risk factors—such as a positive family history of POAG, myopia and diabetes—which may increase the risk of development of field defects are also taken into account in this decision.

Screening for glaucoma

To be eligible for an effective screening program, a disease must have characteristic and unique identifying features and a sensitive and specific test or combination of tests to identify it. The tests must be relatively inexpensive and easy to administer.

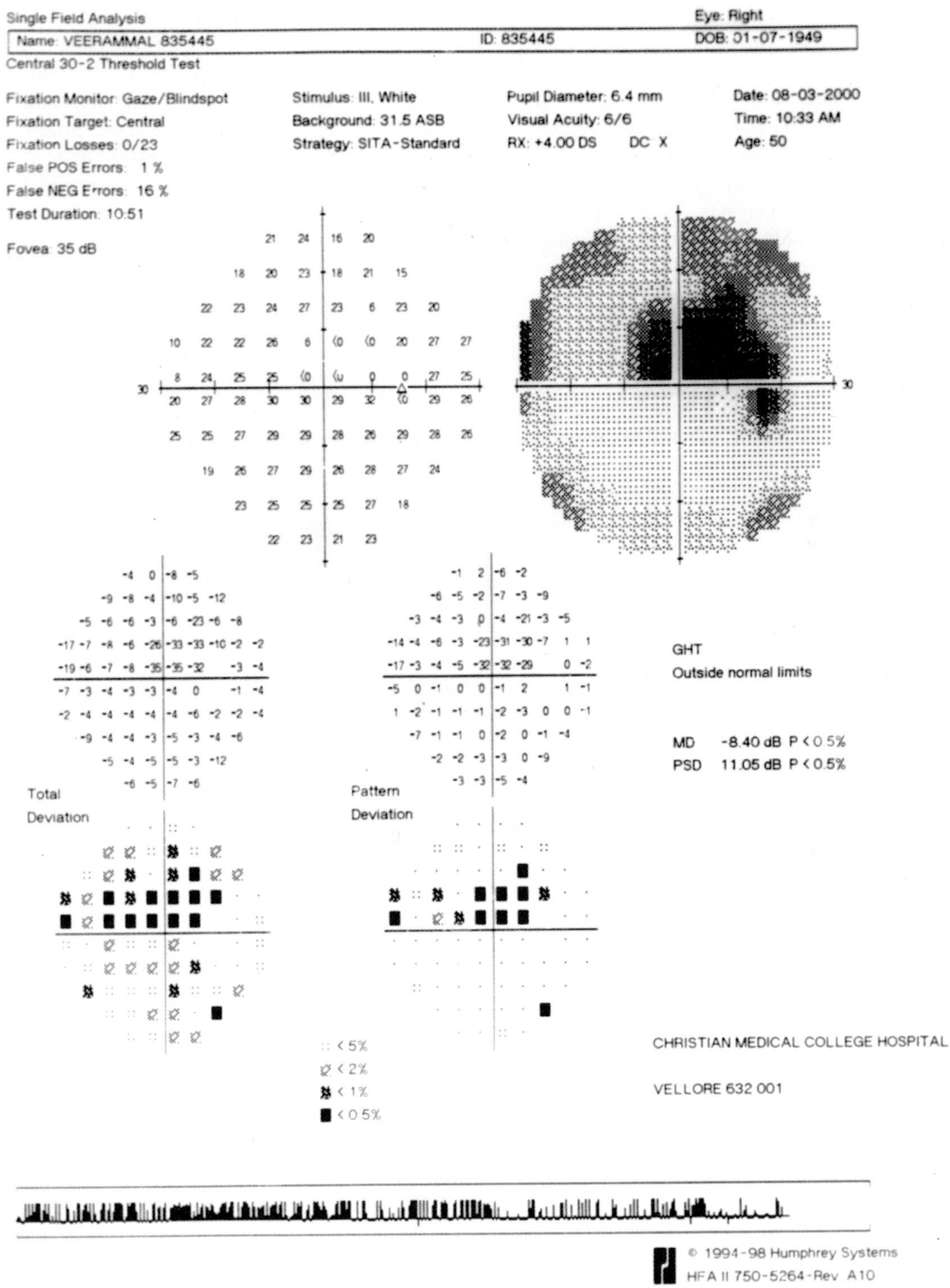

Figure 21.7 Automated perimetry printout (Humphrey's Field Analyzer) of the eye shown in Figure 21.5. Note the superior arcuate field defect corresponding to the inferior notch in the neuroretinal rim

Further, the screening program must have a definite goal for which to aim once the disease is detected—that is, an effective treatment must be available. POAG does fit these requirements fairly well. It has characteristic features and effective treatment is available. The screening tests could be IOP, disc examination or visual field testing or a combination of any of these. IOP alone has a poor sensitivity and specificity at a cut-off of 21 mmHg. Increasing the cut-off to 24 mmHg or even more makes it more specific, but very much less sensitive; this means most of those picked up on screening would have glaucoma but many patients with glaucoma would be excluded.

Disc examination is more sensitive and specific but it requires a skilled examiner. A combination of IOP and disc examination is a good screening tool. Field testing combined with either IOP or disc examination has the best sensitivity and specificity, but the machine is expensive and the test time-consuming.

The best measure of the effectiveness of a screening test is the positive predictive value of the test (PPV: likelihood of a subject testing positive actually having the disease). The PPV of a test is dependent on the actual prevalence of the disease in the population being screened. A rare disease of low prevalence will result in a good test having a poor PPV, while a common disease, even when screened for with a test of poor sensitivity and specificity, will demonstrate a good PPV for the test. Thus, a disease with low prevalence is very hard to screen for, even with a highly sensitive and specific test. Glaucoma, with a prevalence of around 2–5%, gives a poor PPV. On the other hand, if a disease is common, with a prevalence of, say, 20–50%, almost any test would give an excellent PPV. We can artificially increase the prevalence of glaucoma in the population we screen (the pretest probability) by screening only the age groups and persons with risk factors for the disease. In fact, this is what ophthalmologists are routinely doing in their daily practice. This selective screening or case detection could even take place in a general practitioner's clinic to test the over 40 age group. IOP could be measured using the electronic Tono-pen™ described earlier, which needs no skill to operate, unlike the Goldmann or Perkins tonometers. This, combined with a direct ophthalmoscopic view of the disc, could form a good screening tool.

The recently developed Frequency Doubling Perimeter (FDP) is a small, compact, easy-to-operate device and seems the most promising screening tool currently available (see Figure 21.8). Preliminary data shows excellent sensitivity and reasonable specificity for POAG. Abnormal readings may occur due to cataract and neurological lesions which affect the visual field, but it could be argued that all these would anyway need referral to an ophthalmologist. It is distinctly possible that the FDP may be used as a screening device for general ophthalmic pathology in a general clinic, or even become the basis for a community screening program for glaucoma, which has not been possible till now.

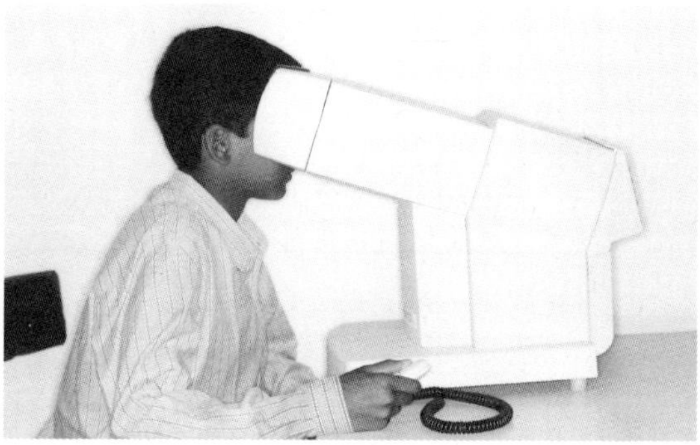

Figure 21.8 Patient undergoing a test with the Frequency Doubling Perimeter

Treatment

For specific glaucoma entities where the pathogenic mechanism is known and can be treated, specific treatment is first performed. For example, pupillary block is treated with a laser peripheral iridotomy to open the angles, or neovascular glaucoma in a diabetic with proliferative retinopathy is treated with pan retinal photocoagulation initially. Once the specific mechanism is addressed, the IOP has to be then brought under control if this has not been achieved. In POAG, the only treatment possible currently is the lowering of IOP.

The goal of treatment in glaucoma is the prevention of blindness. Thus the ophthalmologist's efforts are directed towards preserving the patient's vision so that it lasts the patient's lifetime. This mandates an individual approach to each patient, as the risk–benefit ratio of each treatment modality may vary between patients. Treatment for POAG is traditionally begun in a stepwise manner, starting with topical medical treatment with one or more drugs, adding on a laser procedure and finally considering a surgical option if the earlier treatment becomes ineffective. This approach need not always be followed; some ophthalmologists prefer to utilise a laser procedure first while others may opt for primary surgery. There are valid arguments for each of these philosophies. Essentially, if the patient lives long enough, almost any mode of therapy will eventually fail. The goal is literally to make vision outlast the patient; the purpose of treatment is to buy time. If one is successful in this, the goal of preventing blindness through the patient's lifetime is achieved.

Repeated checks of IOP, review of the disc appearance (ideally documented by disc photographs) and visual field testing monitor the effectiveness of therapy.

Medical therapy

There are several classes of drugs used in treating glaucoma. Most drugs are delivered by the topical route where they enter the eye through the cornea after being instilled in the conjunctival sac. Some drugs, such as acetazolamide, are administered orally and others, such as mannitol, parenterally. Topical therapy is the preferred route as this minimises the systemic side effects of the very potent agents used. However, it is a fact little appreciated among non-ophthalmologists that significant quantities of topically administered medications in the eye find their way into the circulation via the nasolacrimal duct and the nasal mucosa. Thus topically administered β-blockers can precipitate status asthmaticus in susceptible patients. Add to this the fact that most patients with glaucoma are elderly and already on several systemic drugs whose effects can be potentiated or interact with the topical therapy, and a potentially dangerous situation is created if the treating physician and ophthalmologist are not aware of the possible problems. In addition, there is considerable variation in the individual response to a topically applied drug. It makes therapeutic sense for glaucoma specialists to conduct a uniocular trial of a medication to establish that it is indeed effective in the individual patient before committing that patient to lifelong use of the drug.

Medical therapy controls IOP by one of two strategies: on the one hand drugs are used to reduce the production of aqueous; on the other, drugs which improve the facility of outflow are also used. There is a complicated control mechanism involving the sympathetic and parasympathetic nervous systems, which control the production and egress of aqueous. Hence β-blockers, α-adrenergic agents and cholinergic agents may all be employed. In addition, carbonic anhydrase inhibitors are potent in retarding aqueous production as they inhibit the active secretory component of production in the ciliary processes. Recently drugs that can act on a non-conventional outflow of aqueous via what is termed the 'uveo-scleral outflow pathway' have been recognised. This is not normally significant, being responsible for only 5% or less of the total outflow, but under some conditions this can increase considerably. Latanoprost is an example of this class of drug.

β-blockers

These have long been the mainstay of medical treatment in glaucoma. The mechanism of action is by reduction of aqueous production. The drugs include non-selective blockers such as timolol, carteolol and levobunolol, or cardioselective drugs such as betaxolol. β-blockers are contraindicated in patients with bronchial asthma or other respiratory illnesses. Patients on systemic β-blockers may find that the hypotensive effect of the systemic drug is potentiated by the topical preparation. There is consistent lowering of heart rate, and bradyarrhythmias may be seen. Worsening of congestive heart failure has been reported. CNS side effects such as fatigue, emotional lability, anxiety and depression with memory impairment and disorientation have been reported.

Adrenergic agents

Epinephrine and similar compounds which have equal α and β-stimulating properties lower intraocular pressure by increasing the outflow. This action is only slightly offset by the small increase in aqueous production they cause. Drugs commonly used are epinephrine and dipivefrin. The former has fallen out of favour owing to the local and systemic side effects. Dipivefrin is a pro-drug form of epinephrine, which is easily absorbed into the eye and converted to the active compound. It has the advantage of delivering the active agent safely and with minimal side effects. Adverse reactions to this class of drugs include allergy, irritation, madarosis and local pigmentation. Dipivefrin has been known to cause giant papillary conjunctivitis, which may cause discomfort to contact lens wearers. Increase in heart rate and blood pressure is rare with dipivefrin but can occur.

Brimonidine is a recent addition to the therapeutic armamentarium. It is a selective α_2 agonist and acts by reduction of aqueous secretion as well as by some action on the uveoscleral outflow. There is also some experimental evidence to suggest that the drug may have a neuroprotective effect as well; this needs confirmation. The drug has some depressive action on blood pressure and heart rate. Its main side effect is drowsiness and sedation. It is relatively contraindicated in combination with systemic β-blockers and should be used with caution in patients on tricyclic antidepressants and monoamine oxidase inhibitors. The CNS depressant action can worsen the effects of alcohol, so patients on this drug should be warned not to drive after consuming even small amounts of alcohol.

Miotics

Pilocarpine is the prototype of this class of drug and acts by direct cholinergic stimulation of the sphincter pupillae and ciliary muscle. This serves to open the trabecular meshwork and reduce the resistance to aqueous outflow. The pupillary constriction can reduce vision in patients with cataracts. Ciliary body spasm leading to spasm of accommodation and consequent myopia can be frustrating for some patients, especially as the drug is very short-acting and results in cyclic changes in the refractive state through the day. Headache, browache, burning, conjunctival congestion and occasional eyelid twitching are local side effects. Systemic side effects can occur with overdosage and manifest as diarrhoea, nausea, vomiting, abdominal cramps, salivation, bradycardia and muscle weakness. Pilocarpine is often prescribed with a β-blocker and the additive cardiopulmonary side effects can be dangerous.

Pilocarpine is the prototype short-acting miotic. Long-acting potent miotic compounds, notably organophosphorus compounds such as echothiophate, are also used in glaucoma. These agents have essentially the same action as the shorter-acting variety, but tend to produce a much more profound pressure lowering effect. However, this is balanced by the increased rate of side effects. Echothiophate in particular has been shown to cause cataracts (mechanism unknown) and is thus reserved for glaucomas in aphakic or pseudophakic patients. All miotics are associated with an increase in the rate of rhegmatogenous retinal detachments, presumably due to the peripheral tug on the vitreous base created by the ciliary body contraction. This complication is more often seen with long-acting miotics. Because of their destabilising effect on the blood–aqueous barrier, miotics produce a severe fibrinous reaction postoperatively in eyes that undergo intraocular surgery. Hence these agents are usually discontinued a few weeks before surgery is scheduled. The long-acting miotics are no longer used; pilocarpine is the only miotic that continues to find a place in therapy.

Prostaglandins

Latanoprost, a synthetic prostaglandin, has recently become available for use as a topical preparation. It acts principally by increasing the uveoscleral outflow by mechanisms that are still not fully understood. Side effects may include a dramatic change in iris pigmentation seen in light-coloured irides. This change has been shown to be due to increase in the melanin content of melanocytes and not due to melanocytic proliferation. As prostaglandins are mediators of inflammation, this drug is contraindicated in patients with uveitis and immediately following intraocular surgery. There have been reports of cystoid macular oedema in pseudophakic eyes. The drug is used in extremely minute concentrations (0.005%) and in a once daily dosage, so the theoretical side effects of systemic actions of a prostaglandin are not usually seen.

However, some cases of derangement of liver function have been reported. Reactivation of healed herpetic keratitis has been reported with latanoprost. As this drug has only recently been introduced, time is likely to reveal other side effects.

Carbonic anhydrase inhibitors (CAIs)

Acetazolamide given orally is a potent inhibitor of aqueous formation. Unfortunately, side effects are common and usually necessitate discontinuance of therapy. The side effects include paresthesias of fingers, toes and the perioral area and increased frequency of micturition due to the diuretic effect of the drug. These are seen in a large majority of patients, are usually transient and do not necessitate stoppage of treatment. Serum electrolyte imbalances, potassium depletion and metabolic acidosis are more serious and occur with high doses and long duration of treatment. Malaise, weight loss, fatigue, anorexia, depression and decreased libido are correlated with the degree of metabolic acidosis and provide a clinical warning signal of the condition. Gastrointestinal symptoms—including nausea, metallic taste and diarrhoea—are common and may be reduced by taking the medication with meals. It is important to realise that the CAIs are sulfonamides and all the side effects of this group of drugs may be seen with their use. Methazolamide is a more potent longer-acting CAI than acetazolamide and may be tolerated better by some patients. Recently, topical CAIs—notably dorzolamide, which is used in a 3 times daily regimen—have become available. However, it is not free of side effects, although these may be rarer than those seen with the oral preparations.

Hyperosmotic agents

Oral hyperosmotic agents, such as glycerol and isosorbide, or intravenously administered drugs, like mannitol and urea, act to reduce intraocular pressure by their osmotic effect in creating a gradient between the blood and the ocular tissues, thereby drawing fluid out of the eye. The reduction in intraocular fluid volume (around 4–5%) is sufficient to reduce IOP rapidly; these agents are thus used mainly in emergency situations. Side effects include diuresis and circulatory overload.

Neuroprotection

It has been stressed that, until now, IOP lowering has been the only method of controlling glaucomatous damage to the disc. As pathogenic mechanisms of disc damage are better understood, it has become theoretically possible to therapeutically modify them. Some drugs claiming neuroprotective effects are already on the market, while others are in a developmental stage. Drugs that modify the perfusion of the optic nerve head, such as calcium channel blockers (nifedipine, nimodipine), serotonin antagonists (naftidofudryl) and even some classes of steroids, are under investigation. The next few years are likely to see a number of newer therapeutic options available.

Laser treatment

The Nd: YAG laser is used in angle closure glaucoma to create a peripheral iridotomy, thereby relieving pupillary block and establishing free communication between the anterior and posterior chambers. It is used instead of a surgical iridectomy and has the advantage of being a non-invasive outpatient procedure.

Argon laser trabeculoplasty is used as an adjunct to medical treatment in open-angle varieties of glaucoma and works by increasing aqueous outflow. Many surgeons prefer this as a primary procedure before starting drug therapy.

Laser goniotomy and sclerostomy are used as an alternative to filtration surgery (see below), but have not yet found wide acceptance.

Surgical treatment

Filtration surgery is the mainstay of surgical therapy in glaucoma. The principle is to create a guarded fistula between the anterior chamber and the subconjunctival space, thus providing an alternative outflow channel for aqueous which is then absorbed by the conjunctival and scleral vessels. Many surgical techniques are described and used, but the classic trabeculectomy is still the most commonly performed procedure. The overall success of filtration surgery is 75–80% at 5 years and diminishes somewhat thereafter. Techniques of filtration surgery continue to evolve. This is typified by the 'non-penetrating' surgery that is popular with some glaucoma specialists.

Artificial drainage devices are another mode of surgical therapy usually employed when one or more filtering surgeries have failed. These consist of a tube which is implanted into the anterior chamber and connects to a plate that is sutured to the sclera in the sub-Tenon's space near the equator of the eyeball. Aqueous drains into this space which is kept open by the presence of the plate. Various devices are in use of which the Molteno implant, the Baerveldt implant and the American glaucoma valve are some of the better known.

Cyclodestructive procedures are the last surgical resort in glaucoma and are generally reserved for eyes with little or no useful vision. The destruction of the ciliary body may be achieved by external cryotherapy or laser application to the ciliary body. Laser cyclophotocoagulation is done either transsclerally or through the pupil. The main problem with cyclodestruction used to be the unpredictability of results, but newer and more effective laser techniques have made the procedure more acceptable. Laser cyclophotocoagulation is now under evaluation as a primary procedure in seeing eyes.

Prognosis

The goal of prevention of blindness due to glaucoma can be successfully achieved in the majority of cases. As nerve damage due to glaucoma is irreversible, success of treatment depends on how advanced the disease is at diagnosis. A diagnosis of glaucoma mandates a lifelong follow-up for a patient. As we stated earlier, the mode of therapy chosen depends on the individual factors that play a role in each patient. These include the state of the visual fields at presentation, a 'one-eyed' status, tolerance of and compliance with medical treatment, and the assessment of progression of field defects. The latter is the most difficult decision a glaucoma surgeon has to make. Perimetry is a psychophysical test and much depends on the reliability of patient response. As with all psychophysical tests, there is an inherent normal variability, and pathologic change has to be seen to be demonstrably outside the limit of normal variability. If a decision to change a mode of therapy is made on the basis of worsening of field defects, the field tests must be repeated to document consistent change on at least two successive tests. Perimetry is a tedious business for the patient; many will refuse to repeat a recently performed test. The glaucoma surgeon has thus to ride a delicate line between overstressing his patient and obtaining enough information to make a valid and defensible decision. Added to this is the fact that all treatment eventually fails and results in gradual escape of IOP from control. Thus the ophthalmologist, the medical practitioner and the patient must be involved in a three-way relationship that ensures that the patient gets as comfortable a treatment as possible, understands the need for and complies with the schedule of medication and follow-up and lives out her life productively with useful vision.

Bibliography and further reading

Kanski, J. J., McAllister, J. A. & Salmon, J. F. (1996), *Glaucoma. A Colour Manual of Diagnosis and Treatment*, 2nd edn, Butterworth-Heinemann, Oxford.

Ritch, R., Shields, M. B. & Krupin, T. (1996), *The Glaucomas*, 2nd edn, Mosby, St Louis, MO.

Shields, M. B. (1998), *Colour Atlas of Glaucoma*, Williams & Wilkins, Baltimore, MD.

Part VI

Cardiac and pulmonary conditions

Chapter 22

Chest pain and palpitation

VERA CHIAMVIMONVAT

Evaluation of chest pain

The assessment of chest pain is both a common and challenging problem in clinical medicine as chest pain can be due to diverse aetiologies (Table 22.1). Chest pain may indicate a serious disorder, such as ischaemic heart disease, requiring rapid treatment. However, incorrect diagnosis of cardiac disease can result in unnecessary testing and have potential psychological consequences. The initial evaluation of chest pain usually centres on determining whether the pain is due to coronary artery disease or to other conditions that can mimic the symptoms. As well, other potentially life-threatening conditions, including aortic dissection and pulmonary emboli, must be considered.

The history remains the cornerstone of an accurate diagnosis, along with careful physical examination and simple initial laboratory testings. Frequently, after the initial evaluation, myocardial

Table 22.1 Common differential diagnosis of chest pain

Cardiovascular	Gastrointestinal	Pulmonary	Neuromusculo-skeletal	Psychiatric
Ischaemic origin	Oesophageal reflux	Pulmonary embolus	Costochondritis	Anxiety
Coronary artery disease	Oesophageal spasm	Pneumonia	Arthritis	Panic attack
Aortic stenosis or insufficiency	Peptic ulcer disease	Pleuritis	Thoracic outlet syndrome	Depression
Hypertrophic cardiomyopathy		Pneumothorax		
Pulmonary hypertension				
Non-ischaemic origin				
Aortic dissection				
Pericarditis				
Mitral valve prolapse				

ischaemia must be entertained until further clarification is obtained through continued observation, additional testing or response to therapy.

History of chest pain

Chest pain due to myocardial ischaemia

Important features of the history that should be elucidated include the location, radiation and quality of the pain, aggravating and relieving factors, duration of the pain, and other associated symptoms.

Angina pectoris is defined as chest pain of cardiac origin due to myocardial ischaemia with a transient imbalance of myocardial oxygen supply and demand. Ischaemia can occur in settings of decreased myocardial oxygen supply, increased demand or frequently due to a combination of both.

The most distinct characteristics of angina are:

1. the location and quality of pain
2. the precipitating and relieving causes
3. the duration and mode of onset of the symptom.

Typical angina is defined as discomfort that is:

- located in the central chest
- precipitated by exertion
- relieved within 10 minutes by rest or nitroglycerine.

The discomfort is classified as atypical angina if only two of the three features are present, and non-anginal pain if only one feature is present.

Although angina pain can be felt anywhere between the lower jaw and the epigastrium, the most common location is the lower retrosternal area or slightly left of the midline. The pain tends to radiate across the chest into the arms, the left more often than the right. Radiation down the arms to the fingers classically follows the ulnar nerve distribution. The pain also commonly radiates into the shoulders, throat, lower jaws and even into the lower teeth. Less frequent sites of radiation are the armpits, interscapular area and rarely the occiput. At times, angina can be atypical in that it occurs in these locations in the absence of chest pain.

Angina means 'choking' and patients may describe angina not as a pain at all but as an unpleasant sensation in the chest. The quality of angina is commonly described as a band across the chest, tightness, pressure, squeezing, heaviness, weight on the chest, aching, constricting or burning. The pain is usually dull and deep, not sharp and superficial. Angina, like other pain of visceral origin, is poorly localised. Pain that can be well localised to a small area and can be indicated with one or two fingers is less likely to be ischaemic in origin.

Angina due to coronary stenosis usually occurs in situations of increased myocardial oxygen demand, such as increased physical exertion or emotional stress. Typical angina frequently occurs when hurrying or walking up an incline. Angina with exertion is frequently reproducible with a certain of level of activity, although the exact threshold may vary slightly from day to day due to the contribution of dynamic coronary tone. Angina is provoked more easily in the morning, most likely due to higher vasomotor tone. Patients may experience more angina with activity on cold, windy days and after eating a large meal. Activity with arm movement, especially using the arms above the head, which involves more isometric exercise, is more likely to provoke angina than leg exercise, which is more isotonic in nature.

When angina is provoked by exercise, slowing down the pace or resting typically relieves the symptom. Some patients described gradual disappearance of chest pain even with continued exercise, a phenomenon called 'walk-through angina'. This is thought to be due to the opening of functioning coronary collaterals in response to ischaemia.

Chest pain that occurs at rest and is not related to exertion is less likely to be angina. However, in patients with coronary artery disease, angina can also occur at rest. Rest angina is related to a decrease in myocardial supply due to various factors, including thrombosis, changes in coronary tone with coronary vasoconstriction and spasm, intermittent arrhythmia or labile hypertension. The possibility of coronary vasospasm should be considered when typical angina symptoms occur without relation to any activity or occur frequently at rest.

Angina has a gradual onset and resolution. Chest pain of sudden onset that is most severe from the beginning is less likely to be angina. Angina typically lasts 5–15 minutes, although it can be as short as 30 seconds or as long as 1 hour. Any pain that is shooting or fleeting, lasting seconds, is likely to be non-ischaemic in origin and is usually musculoskeletal in nature. On the other hand, usual angina pain should not last for more than 30–60 minutes, as this would imply progression to unstable angina or acute myocardial infarction. Therefore, the description of prolonged and recurrent episodes of chest pain would argue against an ischaemic origin. Other prominent causes of central chest pain not due to cardiac origin are discussed subsequently in this chapter.

The use of nitroglycerine should bring relief promptly within minutes and this can be of diagnostic value, although pain from oesophageal spasm may also improve with nitroglycerine. On the other hand, delayed relief with nitroglycerine is not diagnostic of angina.

The diagnosis of unstable angina or myocardial infarction should be suspected when angina pain is prolonged, severe, radiating more widely or occurring without any precipitating factor.

Angina may be accompanied by other symptoms, including dyspnoea, diaphoresis, presyncope, nausea, vomiting or hiccups. The symptom of dyspnoea may be an 'anginal equivalent' in the absence of chest pain. Dyspnoea can result with severe ischaemia, causing significant myocardial dysfunction and increase in left ventricular end-diastolic pressure.

When assessing whether chest pain is due to ischaemia, it is also important to assess the likelihood of *coronary artery disease* (CAD) based on the risk factor profile and other associated symptoms. These symptoms would indicate other manifestations of vascular disease, such as intermittent claudication, transient ischaemic attack or stroke, which increase the likelihood of co-existing CAD.

Other cardiac disease can also cause angina by the mechanism of increased demand, with or without underlying atherosclerosis. In *aortic stenosis*, *hypertrophic cardiomyopathy* and *systemic hypertension*, myocardial oxygen demand is increased due to an increased wall tension and the presence of left ventricular hypertrophy. In aortic regurgitation, there is increased demand from the increased left ventricular size as well as decreased supply from the reduced diastolic perfusion pressure of the coronary arteries. With pulmonic stenosis, pulmonary hypertension or large pulmonary emboli, angina can occur on the basis of increased right ventricular demand and ischaemia.

Other cardiac causes of chest pain

Aortic dissection is an important and life-threatening cause of chest pain. The chest pain of aortic dissection is usually sudden and severe, with the pain most severe at its onset. The pain tends to have a sharp, tearing quality, commonly starting at the interscapular area, and may radiate or shift to other areas, including the chest, neck, back, abdomen or even the lower extremities depending on the path of the dissection. With the exception of Marfan's syndrome or other connective tissue disease, most patients with aortic dissection have a history of hypertension.

Pericarditis is a relatively common cause of chest pain. The differentiating feature of pericardial pain is its pleuritic quality and the changes in intensity with body position. Sitting up and bending forward often decrease the pain. Occasionally, the pain may worsen by swallowing. The chest pain of pericarditis is typically sharp and can radiate to the shoulders, neck and upper back. The pain is usually constant and prolonged, lasting for several hours, and is not aggravated by physical activity. It must be kept in mind that pericarditis may be a complication of more serious disorders such as post-myocardial infarction or aortic dissection.

Gastrointestinal causes of chest pain

Because the heart and oesophagus share the same spinal sensory innervation, chest pain of oesophageal origin is often indistinguishable from angina. The pain can be restrosternal, burning or squeezing in quality, although radiation to the arms or jaw is less common. A useful feature in the differentiation of an oesophageal cause of chest pain is the association of the pain with eating or after meals and precipitation by certain types of food, such as very hot or cold drinks. The pain may also be precipitated by changes in position, such as bending over or lying down, and can also wake the patient from sleep. Patients with oesophageal pain tend to have accompanying symptoms, such as dysphagia, food regurgitation and acid regurgitation. The pain is usually more prolonged, lasting for hours, and can be relieved by antacid medication. However, some features of oesophageal pain can mimic ischaemic chest pain. *Oesophageal reflux* or *spasm* can be precipitated by exercise or emotional stress. As well, the pain of oesophageal spasm can be relieved by nitroglycerine, which relaxes smooth muscle.

Peptic ulcer disease usually causes epigastric pain that can also be felt in the lower sternal area. The pain is usually prolonged, lasting hours. The relationship to meals and the relief by antacids are useful diagnostic features. Pain of biliary origin is usually epigastric and also tends to be prolonged.

Pulmonary causes of chest pain

Patients with acute massive *pulmonary embolism*, in addition to pleuritic chest pain, may also have ischaemic-like chest pain due to acute right ventricular strain and ischaemia. Pulmonary emboli are usually suggested by the accompanying symptoms of dyspnoea, tachypnoea and cyanosis and may be suspected in patients with risk factors for thromboembolic diseases. Patients with pulmonary hypertension can also have angina-like chest pain, probably due to right ventricular strain and ischaemia.

Other pulmonary causes of chest pain, such as *pneumonia*, *pleuritis* or *pneumothorax*, usually produce sharp, pleuritic pain, along with associated dyspnoea and other pulmonary symptoms.

Neuromusculoskeletal causes of chest pain

Thoracic outlet syndrome can produce pain along the ulnar distribution of the arm, which can be confused with angina. Unlike angina, the pain is usually precipitated by arm movement and not by physical exertion. The pain can also be accompanied by paraesthesias.

Costochondritis can cause acute chest pain that is usually worsened by movement and deep breathing. The pain is localised and reproducible on palpation. Degenerative *arthritis* can produce band-like pain around the chest and back, which can also radiate into the arms. The pain is usually brought on by certain posture or movement, and can be aggravated by coughing or sneezing.

Psychiatric causes of chest pain

Although non-specific chest pain is a common symptom in patients with *anxiety* disorders or *depression*, this should remain a diagnosis of exclusion and other organic causes of chest pain need to be ruled out. Psychogenic chest pain tends to be atypical, usually localised, and sharp or stabbing in quality. The pain usually occurs at rest or with a stressful situation, but uncommonly with activity. The pain can at times be quite prolonged, lasting for hours or days.

Physical examination

In the patient with angina, physical examination may disclose the presence of co-existing vascular disease, such as bruits or decreased peripheral pulses. Signs of hypercholesterolaemia, such as xanthelasma or tuberous xanthoma, increase the likelihood of CAD.

Physical examination can indicate the presence of other diseases that can be associated with angina, including aortic valve disease, hypertrophic cardiomyopathy, and pulmonary hypertension.

In patients with severe chest pain, clues to aortic dissection include absent pulses or unequal blood pressure in the arms or legs, murmur of aortic insufficiency or a pleural effusion. In patients with suspected pericarditis, physical examination would include the presence of pericardial rub, pericardial effusion and evidence of cardiac tamponade with manifestations of cardiac failure and haemodynamic instability.

Physical examination can also point to other causes of chest pain, such as the presence of chest wall tenderness that reproduces the pain, evidence for thoracic outlet syndrome, or signs of arthritis.

Electrocardiogram

An electrocardiogram (ECG) obtained while a patient is experiencing chest pain is helpful in delineating a specific diagnosis. ST segment depression or elevation, T wave inversion and the presence of Q waves suggest ischaemic heart disease. However, a normal ECG during chest pain does not rule out ischaemia. Diffuse ST segment elevation suggests pericarditis. With pulmonary emboli, the ECG may show signs of acute right ventricular strain, with incomplete or complete right bundle branch block, an S wave in lead I and Q wave and T wave inversion in lead III. ECG can also show evidence of underlying structural heart disease with a ventricular hypertrophy pattern.

Emergency evaluation of chest pain

In the assessment of a patient with ongoing chest pain, emphasis is placed on rapid triage to rule out life-threatening aetiologies of pain, such as acute ischaemic syndrome, aortic dissection or pulmonary emboli. This requires a focused assessment, physical examination, ECG, chest X-ray and routine laboratory evaluation. The optimal triage and management of patients who present with acute chest pain is well summarised in several reviews, listed in the Bibliography and Further Reading.

Outpatient evaluation

Commonly, patients present after the chest pain episode has resolved. In this situation, the assessment should focus on whether the presentation suggests unstable coronary disease, in which case hospitalisation should be considered. If the history does not suggest unstable coronary disease, further investigation can proceed on an outpatient basis, usually with initial non-invasive investigations. In patients with recurrent episodes of chest pain, after consideration of other possible diagnoses, non-invasive testing may be indicated to rule out underlying CAD.

The basis of non-invasive testing is the detection of a significant coronary stenosis by provoking ischaemia and/or differential flow under conditions of physiological or pharmacological stress. Ischaemia and/or differential flow can then be detected by the occurrence of any symptoms suggestive of angina, ECG changes, flow differences on myocardial perfusion imaging, or wall motion abnormality detected by echocardiography. The addition of imaging techniques either with myocardial perfusion imaging or echocardiography increases the sensitivity, specificity and accuracy of the test.

Exercise stress test

The exercise stress test is the most widely available and commonly used non-invasive test for CAD. In patients with CAD, exercise using either treadmill or bicycle ergometry provokes ischaemia by increasing the heart rate, blood pressure, contractility and myocardial oxygen demand. Ischaemia is detected by the occurrence of symptoms consistent with angina and positive ECG changes of ≥ 1 mm of ST segment depression or elevation from baseline. The exercise stress test has a reported sensitivity and specificity in the range of 60–70% and 70–80% respectively. The test is useful only if the patient is able to attain an adequate level of stress, usually to a target heart rate based on age. As well, the patient should have a relatively normal resting ECG, since baseline ST segment changes, left bundle branch block and ventricular hypertrophy can make the ECG changes uninterpretable. The exercise stress test also provides important prognostic information. Early positive ECG changes at a low exercise level, marked, diffuse and prolonged ST segment changes, a drop in blood pressure or ventricular arrhythmias indicate significant CAD.

Myocardial perfusion imaging

Myocardial perfusion imaging detects ischaemia and/or differential flow with physiological stress from exercise or pharmacological stress using dipyridamole, adenosine and dobutamine. The radionuclides commonly used for imaging are thallium or technetium-99m based agents.

Myocardial perfusion imaging provides greater diagnostic accuracy for CAD compared to the exercise stress test, with a reported sensitivity and specificity in the range of 80–90% and 70–90% respectively. Patients with an abnormal exercise stress test result can undergo myocardial perfusion imaging to further clarify the diagnosis. Myocardial perfusion imaging is also indicated in patients with an abnormal resting ECG who are likely to have uninterpretable exercise test results.

Pharmacological stress imaging with dipyridamole or adenosine is used for patients who are unable to exercise adequately. These agents are contraindicated for patients with significant bronchospasm. For patients with significant lung disease who are unable to exercise, dobutamine stress with either perfusion imaging or echocardiography can be performed instead.

Special consideration is given to patients with left bundle branch block, where an exercise stress test would be uninterpretable and exercise perfusion imaging can be associated with a false positive abnormality. Dipyridamole or adenosine perfusion imaging provide better accuracy in these patients.

Stress echocardiography

Stress echocardiography detects wall motion abnormality due to ischaemia with physiological stress of exercise or with pharmacological stress, commonly using dobutamine. Overall, stress echocardiography has a similar accuracy to perfusion imaging, with slightly less sensitivity but greater specificity. Indications are similar to those of perfusion imaging. Dobutamine stress echocardiography can be used for patients who are unable to exercise.

Coronary angiography

Coronary angiography is the most accurate test in diagnosing and defining the extent of CAD. Anatomic information from angiography is used to determine the patients' suitability for angioplasty or bypass surgery.

Selection of diagnostic tests for outpatient evaluation of chest pain

The appropriate selection of non-invasive tests depends on the patient's pretest likelihood of CAD as well as the baseline ECG, exercise capacity and the ability to tolerate pharmacological stress agents.

It is useful to consider the age, gender and chest pain quality of the patient to arrive at an estimate of the likelihood of CAD. As previously described, typical angina is defined as discomfort in the central chest, precipitated by exertion and relieved within 10 minutes by rest or nitroglycerine. The discomfort is called atypical angina if only two of the three features are present, and non-anginal pain if only one feature is present. When age and gender is considered along with the chest pain characteristics, an estimation of the probability of CAD is significantly improved. In any given chest pain category, the likelihood of CAD increases with age. However, the likelihood of CAD in a premenopausal woman with any given chest pain category is substantially lower than an age-matched man. After menopause, this probability in women rapidly approaches men of similar age and symptomatology (Table 22.2).

Finally, prediction of the probability of CAD can be further aided by consideration of the patient's risk factor profile, including diabetes, hypertension, smoking, hyperlipidaemia and family history of premature CAD. After consideration of these factors, a patient can be estimated as having low (< 20%), intermediate (20–80%) or high (> 80%) pretest likelihood of CAD. The post-test likelihood of CAD is then determined by the results of the non-invasive tests (Figure 22.1).

Table 22.2 Likelihood (%) of coronary artery disease based on age, sex and chest pain quality

	Non-anginal pain		Atypical angina		Typical angina	
Age (years)	**Men**	**Women**	**Men**	**Women**	**Men**	**Women**
30–39	5.2	0.8	21.8	4.2	69.7	25.8
40–49	14.1	2.8	46.1	13.3	87.3	55.2
50–59	21.5	8.4	58.9	32.4	92.0	79.4
60–69	28.1	18.6	67.1	54.4	94.3	90.6

Source: Adapted from G. Diamond & J. Forrester (1979), 'Analysis of probability as an aid in the clinical diagnosis of coronary artery disease', *New England Journal of Medicine*, 300, pp. 1350–8.

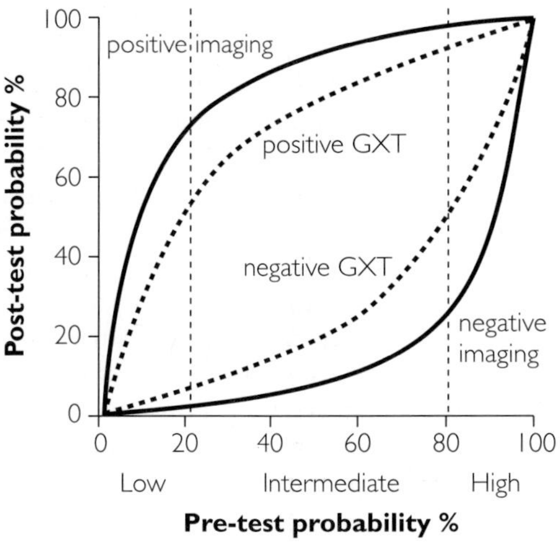

Figure 22.1 Post-test probability of coronary artery disease based on the pretest probability and type of test (exercise ECG stress test and myocardial perfusion imaging or stress echocardiography)

The pretest likelihood of CAD can therefore guide the initial selection of non-invasive testing. For example, young patients with atypical or non-anginal pain and without any risk factors have a low likelihood for CAD (< 20%). The great majority of these patients will therefore have negative ECG stress test results. Such a result effectively rules out any significant CAD and patients can be reassured.

Conversely, older patients with typical angina, especially with one or more risk factors, have a high likelihood for CAD (> 80%). In these patients, the diagnosis of CAD can usually be established on clinical grounds alone. Non-invasive testing is most useful in determining the prognosis and the need for cardiac catheterisation. While both exercise stress testing and stress imaging yield important prognostic markers, imaging studies provide better assessment of the degree of ischaemia and, overall, have superior prognostic value. With perfusion imaging, the number of defects, size and degree of reversibility correlate directly with prognosis. Similarly, with stress echocardiography, the prognosis is correlated to the extent of wall motion abnormality.

Older patients with atypical or non-anginal pain, with, at most, one risk factor, have an intermediate risk for CAD (20–80%). This subgroup presents the greatest diagnostic challenge. The increased diagnostic accuracy by the additional use of imaging, either with perfusion imaging or echocardiography, provides optimal differentiation in such patients. In addition, the results of both the exercise and the imaging components can be combined to provide greater diagnostic and prognostic value. Concordant normal exercise stress test and imaging results indicate a low likelihood for CAD with a good prognosis, while concordant abnormal results confirm the high likelihood for CAD. Discordant test results are seen commonly. Although the likelihood of CAD may not be clarified by such results, there are still prognostic values to the tests. For example, a normal imaging in the setting of an abnormal ECG stress test result has been correlated with an excellent prognosis, regardless of the clinical setting, and may not require further evaluation.

Cardiac catheterisation is indicated in patients with high-risk, non-invasive test results consistent with multivessel disease and in patients whose symptoms are refractory to medical treatment. Cardiac catheterisation may also be indicated for diagnosis in patients whose non-invasive test results are inconclusive, since accurate diagnosis can have a significant impact on quality of life and longevity.

Conclusion

The assessment of chest pain is a common and challenging problem in clinical medicine. Central to the differentiation of ischaemic chest pain from other aetiologies is careful history taking along with consideration of the patient's clinical profile and cardiovascular risk factors. The history and clinical evaluation, along with routine tests, can also screen for potentially life-threatening aetiologies requiring urgent management. In stable patients, further outpatient evaluation is guided by the patient's profile and likelihood for CAD.

Evaluation of palpitation

Palpitation is a frequent but relatively non-specific cardiac symptom and may be described by many terms, including 'skipping', 'stopping', 'fluttering', 'pounding' or 'racing sensation'. Palpitation is defined as an uncomfortable awareness of the heart beat due to a change in cardiac rhythm, rate and/or contractility.

Since palpitation may signify a life-threatening condition, complaints of palpitation usually prompt a search for cardiac arrhythmia. However, the aetiology of palpitation is benign in many cases and the subjective awareness of palpitation is frequently not correlated with the presence of arrhythmias. Nevertheless, palpitation of new onset can be a frightening experience to many patients, often out of keeping with the severity or seriousness of the cause. The resultant anxiety with increased adrenergic drive can lead to increases in heart rate and cardiac contractility and further aggravate the palpitation. Therefore, in many situations, a clear explanation of the aetiology will allay the anxiety and improve the symptom by itself.

Palpitation can occur under normal circumstances when there is an obvious cause, such as exercise or emotional stress, when the normal sinus rhythm is experienced by the patient as a rapid heart rate and/or forceful cardiac contraction. Normal sinus rhythm can also cause palpitation by the same mechanism during pathologic states such as hyperkinetic circulatory states with valvular regurgitation, fever, anaemia or thyrotoxicosis. Palpitations can also occur in association with anxiety, panic attack or depression. Many cases of palpitation are due to intermittent awareness of sinus rhythm.

When palpitation occurs without any obvious cause, it may be due to arrhythmia with changes in cardiac rhythm or rate, including tachyarrhythmia, bradyarrhythmia and extrasystoles (Table 22.3).

Table 22.3 Common causes of palpitation

Change in cardiac rhythm	Increase in heart rate and/or contractility
Tachyarrhythmia	Physiological states
Supraventricular	Exercise
Ventricular	Emotional stress
Bradyarrhythmia	Pathologic states
Sinus pauses	Valvular regurgitation
Atrioventricular block	Fever
Extrasystoles	Anaemia
Atrial premature beats	Thyrotoxicosis
Ventricular premature beats	

The sensitivity to changes in cardiac rhythm and rate varies quite widely between individuals. Some patients with frequent and significant arrhythmia are asymptomatic, whereas others are able to sense every extrasystole. In general, the perception of the heart beat is keener at night, especially when patients first lie down to sleep, when they lie on their left side, or in quiet moments. Patients with normal cardiac contractility tend to be more aware of arrhythmia, whereas patients with organic heart disease and poor contractility may not feel any palpitation at all even with serious arrhythmia. Generally, the awareness of palpitation decreases as the arrhythmia becomes chronic.

History of palpitation

History taking is an important diagnostic tool since most patients are seen between their attacks. Although a precise diagnosis can only be made if the rhythm is recorded during the episode, consideration of history, physical findings, ECG and other associated cardiac investigations can give clues to the diagnosis and, more importantly, the prognosis of the palpitation.

Characteristics of palpitation

When asking patients to describe their symptoms, it is important to keep in mind the different kinds of arrhythmia. The patients should be asked to tap out exactly what they feel. It may be helpful for the physician to tap and demonstrate different kinds of rhythm, including premature beats, slow and rapid rhythm, and regular and irregular rhythm, to assist the patients in their description.

For example, with extrasystoles, the patients may sense the premature contraction and/or the post-premature beat as a brief sensation of 'skipping', 'flip-flopping', 'fluttering' or as the heart 'turning over'. Patients may sense the pause following the premature beat as a feeling that the heart has 'stopped', and this has been shown to have a good correlation, especially with ventricular premature contraction. The post-premature beat has increased contractility and can be sensed as a 'pounding' or 'thudding'. When patients describe such brief, isolated symptoms, extrasystoles are the most likely cause. However, if extrasystoles are very frequent, such as in bigeminal or trigeminal patterns, patients may feel continuous regular or irregular palpitation. This pattern may be difficult to differentiate from other arrhythmias, although extrasystoles should not feel rapid.

A description of rapid palpitation would be consistent with tachyarrhythmia. Rapid, chaotic and irregular palpitation can suggest atrial fibrillation, atrial flutter with variable block or multifocal atrial tachycardia. However, in the case of atrial fibrillation with rapid ventricular response, patients may have difficulty feeling the irregularity and may describe a more rapid regular palpitation. More commonly, rapid regular palpitation is consistent with atrioventricular (AV) node-dependent supraventricular tachycardia, atrial flutter with constant block or ventricular tachycardia.

One differentiating feature is the presence of associated rapid regular neck palpitation, which is suggestive of AV nodal re-entry tachycardia. Neck pounding is due to simultaneous contraction of the atria and ventricles, causing contraction of the right atrium against a closed tricuspid valve with reflux of blood back into the superior vena cava. In ventricular tachycardia, neck palpitation can also occur but in a slower irregular fashion due to complete AV dissociation and intermittent contraction of the right atrium against a closed tricuspid valve. Intermittent neck pounding can also occur with premature ventricular beats and this can also cause transient dyspnoea.

Slow palpitation suggests sinus bradycardia, junctional rhythm or complete heart block.

Mode of onset and termination

Abrupt onset and termination of rapid palpitation suggests a tachyarrhythmia and patients liken the sensation to a switch inside 'being turned on and off'. On the other hand, gradual onset and termination of rapid palpitation suggest sinus tachycardia. However, because of high adrenergic tone during tachyarrhythmia due to the discomfort, anxiety or a drop in blood pressure, patients frequently have sinus tachycardia at the termination of their tachyarrhythmia, which then gradually slows down. They may, therefore, describe the termination as being of more gradual offset. Conversely, patients with sinus tachycardia can also feel abrupt onset and offset of their symptoms.

Patients with AV nodal re-entry tachycardia may describe the tachycardia as starting when they stand up after bending over. These patients may learn by trial and error to terminate their arrhythmia by vagal manoeuvres, such as breath holding, induced gagging, vomiting, lying down, taking a cold shower or even performing carotid sinus massage.

Associated symptoms

Associated symptoms of haemodynamic compromise, including presyncope, syncope, angina or congestive heart failure, strongly suggest ventricular tachycardia as the aetiology of the palpitation. In some patients with ventricular tachycardia and severe heart disease, these symptoms can occur without any awareness of palpitation.

Syncope can occur in patients with supraventricular tachycardia, even in those without heart disease, and can be due to either a vasovagal-like response to the discomfort of the palpitation or to the extremely rapid rate with low cardiac output. Syncope occurring after the termination of rapid palpitation suggests the presence of tachycardia–bradycardia syndrome with a pause following the tachycardia.

Non-specific chest pain or chest pain suggestive of angina can also occur with tachycardia even in healthy patients.

Associated anxiety, the sensation of a lump in the throat, dizziness and tingling in the hands and feet suggest that the palpitation is due to sinus tachycardia occurring with an anxiety state and hyperventilation.

Precipitating factors

The circumstances in which palpitation occurs are also helpful in the diagnosis. Idiopathic ventricular tachycardia, especially that originating from the right ventricular outflow tract, and ventricular tachycardia due to the long-QT syndrome, can be precipitated by increased catecholamine states, such as exercise, emotional stress or acute awakening.

Supraventricular tachycardia, particularly atrial fibrillation, can also be precipitated during exercise or immediately post-exercise due to the withdrawal of sympathetic tone and the acute increase in vagal tone. This is described particularly in athletic men in their 30s to 60s.

Palpitation that is felt more at night or only during quiet periods suggests a more benign aetiology, such that daytime distractions are masking the symptoms. Patients with serious arrhythmia would be expected to have symptoms regardless of any distracting factors.

Age of onset

Palpitations that began in childhood suggest AV node-dependent tachycardia. Idiopathic ventricular tachycardia and long-QT syndrome ventricular tachycardia can begin in adolescence or in the 20s.

General medical history

The medical assessment should include a thorough cardiac history and cardiac symptoms. A family history of syncope or sudden death suggests inherited disorders such as cardiomyopathy or long-QT syndrome. In addition, questions should also be asked about general medical conditions that can be associated with palpitation, such as thyroid disease, anaemia, hypoglycaemia and pheochromocytoma. A review of systems should include questions regarding use of alcohol, tobacco, caffeine, illicit drugs, drugs with sympathomimetic or anticholinergic effects, thyroid supplement, psychoactive drugs and theophylline. In patients who are taking vasodilator medication, such as for hypertension, palpitation can occur due to reflex tachycardia secondary to an orthostatic drop in blood pressure. Palpitation can occur with menopausal symptoms of hot flushes and sweating.

Psychiatric disorders, including panic or anxiety disorders, are a common cause of palpitation, although cardiac arrhythmia must first be excluded. Studies have shown that some patients with palpitation due to supraventricular tachycardia, especially women, were initially diagnosed with panic disorder. In many patients, the two diagnoses can co-exist.

Physical examination

The physical examination should focus on uncovering stigmata of underlying structural heart disease. Physical findings of systemic conditions that can be associated with palpitation as discussed above should be carefully looked for.

Electrocardiogram

An ECG even between episodes may provide useful clues to the underlying aetiology. A long QT interval would suggest ventricular tachycardia. Pre-excitation with a short PR interval and delta waves predispose to either AV re-entry tachycardia or atrial fibrillation. Bradyarrhythmia may be suggested by the presence of a conduction defect or AV block. Atrial or ventricular ectopy may be seen. Evidence of previous myocardial infarction or myocardial ischaemia increases the likelihood of ventricular tachycardia. Left ventricular hypertrophy can be associated with atrial fibrillation or can be a clue to cardiomyopathy, such as hypertrophic or dilated cardiomyopathy, which predispose to ventricular tachycardia. Ventricular tachycardia due to the presence of arrhythmogenic right ventricular dysplasia is suggested by the presence of a late right ventricular activation wave, called an epsilon wave in ECG leads V1 and V2, and an accompanying inverted T wave.

Risk stratification

Risk stratification of the seriousness of the palpitation is an important part of the assessment, since in many patients whose palpitations are infrequent, the definitive diagnosis may not be established immediately. In patients at high risk for significant or life-threatening arrhythmia, more aggressive or even invasive investigations may be required urgently. Patients with underlying structural heart disease or severe associated symptoms of haemodynamic compromise are at risk of serious arrhythmia, particularly ventricular tachycardia, and require further investigation (Table 22.4).

On the other hand, in patients without high-risk markers who are likely to have more benign

Table 22.4 Selected diagnostic tests for palpitation

Test	Indication
Non-invasive	
Electrocardiogram	Screening test for all patients
Ambulatory ECG monitoring	Patients with frequent symptoms
Ambulatory event recorder	Patients with infrequent symptoms where significant arrhythmia is suspected
Exercise stress testing	Patients with exercise-related symptoms Screening test for ischaemic heart disease
Echocardiogram	Assessment of underlying structural heart disease
Stress nuclear imaging	Assessment of ischaemic heart disease
Stress echocardiogram	Assessment of ischaemic heart disease
Head-up tilt testing	Assessment for vasovagal aetiology
Invasive	
Electrophysiologic study	Diagnosis of suspected significant arrhythmia Therapeutic ablation of certain types of arrhythmia

arrhythmia, a few screening tests may suffice and further investigation is pursued as dictated by symptoms.

Further investigation

Further investigation is usually indicated in two groups of patients: those who are at high risk of serious arrhythmia and those whose symptoms and initial investigation suggest an arrhythmic aetiology. Further investigation may also be justified in patients who are anxious about their conditions and require definitive diagnosis for reassurance.

Ambulatory ECG Holter monitoring is useful in patients with frequent symptoms, occurring daily or almost daily. On the other hand, in patients with sporadic episodes, ambulatory monitoring has very low diagnostic value. Correlation of symptoms with rhythm finding is essential as many arrhythmias can be seen normally and may not necessarily be the cause of the palpitation. Frequently, the lack of arrhythmia in the presence of symptoms can be used to reassure patients.

In patients with infrequent palpitation, a continuous loop event recorder may provide greater diagnostic yield. The loop recorder monitors the rhythm continuously but records the data only when manually activated by the patient. When the monitor is activated with an event, the rhythm from the preceding few minutes before and after is saved as preprogrammed. The loop recorder can be worn for a longer period than the Holter monitor and two weeks of monitoring are usually enough to make the diagnosis in the majority of patients.

Electrophysiological investigation can be a cost-effective way of diagnosing palpitation. In patients at high risk of life-threatening arrhythmia and those in whom definite arrhythmia is suggested on screening tests, early electrophysiological study for both diagnosis and treatment may be indicated.

Other cardiac investigations may also be indicated if there is a suspicion of underlying heart disease. These may include assessment for myocardial function, valvular disease and ischaemic heart disease (Table 22.5).

Conclusion

Palpitation is a frequent but relatively non-specific cardiac symptom. The evaluation usually centres on the differentiation of potentially life-threatening causes of palpitation from more benign aetiologies, based on the patient's clinical profile, features of palpitation and associated symptomatology. Test selection is based on the likely aetiology, frequency of symptoms and suspicion of other underlying cardiac disease. The treatments of specific arrhythmias are well summarised in several reviews.

Table 22.5 Risk stratification for significant or life-threatening arrhythmia

Low risk	High risk
No history of associated haemodynamic compromise or severe symptoms with the palpitation: • No syncope or presyncope • No angina or congestive heart failure	History of associated haemodynamic compromise or severe symptoms with the palpitation: • Syncope or presyncope • Angina or congestive heart failure
No underlying structural heart disease or ischaemic heart disease	Underlying structural heart disease: • Left ventricular dysfunction • Ischaemic heart disease • Cardiomyopathy • Significant valvular disease • Conduction system disease • Pre-excitation • Long-QT syndrome
No family history of syncope or sudden cardiac death	Family history of syncope or sudden cardiac death

Bibliography and further reading

A report of the American College of Cardiology/American Heart Association Task Force on Practice Guidelines (1995), 'ACC/AHA guidelines for clinical intracardiac electrophysiological and catheter ablation procedures', *Circulation*, 92, pp. 673–91.

Barsky, A., Cleary, P., Barnett, M., et al. (1994), 'The accuracy of symptom reporting by patients complaining of palpitations', *American Journal of Medicine*, 97, pp. 214–21.

Brugada, P., Gursoy, S., Brugada, J. & Andries, E. (1993), 'Investigation of palpitations', *Lancet*, 341, pp. 1254–8.

Chen, P. S., Athill, C. A., Wu, T. J., Ikeda, T., Ong, J. J. & Karagueuzian, H. S. (1999), 'Mechanisms of atrial fibrillation and flutter and implications for management', *American Journal of Cardiology*, 84, pp. 125R–130R.

Christie, L. G. & Conti, C. R. (1981), 'Systematic approach to the evaluation of angina-like chest pain', *American Heart Journal*, 102, pp. 897–903.

Constant, J. (1983), 'The clinical diagnosis of nonanginal chest pain: the differentiation of angina from nonanginal chest pain by history', *Clinical Cardiology*, 6, pp. 11–20.

Diamond, G. A. & Forrester, J. S. (1979), 'Analysis of probability as an aid in the clinical diagnosis of coronary artery disease', *New England Journal of Medicine*, 300, pp. 1350–8.

Douglas, P. S. & Ginsberg, G. S. (1996), 'The evaluation of chest pain in women', *New England Journal of Medicine*, 334, pp. 1311–15.

Fleet, R. P. & Beitman, B. D. (1997), 'Unexplained chest pain: when is it panic disorder?', *Clinical Cardiology*, 20, pp. 187–94.

Ganz, L. I. & Friedman, P. L. (1995), 'Supraventricular tachycardia', *New England Journal of Medicine*, 332, pp. 162–73.

Gerson, M. C. (1997), 'Test accuracy, test selection and test result interpretation in chronic coronary artery disease,' in Gerson, M. C. (ed.), *Cardiac Nuclear Medicine*, McGraw-Hill, New York, pp. 527–80.

Gibbons, R. J. (2000), 'Myocardial perfusion imaging', *Heart*, 83, pp. 355–60.

Graboys, T. (1992), 'Appropriate indications for ambulatory electrocardiographic monitoring', *Cardiology Clinics*, 10, pp. 551–4.

Gregoratos, G., Cheitlin, M. D., Conill, A., Epstein, A. E., Fellows, C., Ferguson, T. B. Jr, Freedman, R. A., Hlatky, M. A., Naccarelli, G. V., Saksena, S., Schlant, R. C. & Silka, M. J. (1998), 'ACC/AHA guidelines for implantation of cardiac pacemakers and antiarrhythmia devices: a report of the American College of Cardiology/American Heart Association Task Force on Practice Guidelines (Committee on Pacemaker Implantation)', *Journal of the American College of Cardiology*, 31, pp. 1175–209.

Lee, T. H. & Goldman, L. (2000), 'Evaluation of the patient with acute chest pain', *New England Journal of Medicine*, 342, pp. 1187–95.

Lessmeier, T. J., Gamperling, D., Johnson-Liddon, V., et al. (1997), 'Unrecognized paroxysmal supraventricular tachycardia. Potential for misdiagnosis as panic disorder', *Archives of Internal Medicine*, 157, pp. 537–43.

Levine, H. J. (1980), 'Difficult problem in the diagnosis of chest pain', *American Heart Journal*, 100, pp. 108–18.

Mangrum, J. M. & DiMarco, J. P. (2000), 'The evaluation

and management of bradycardia', in *New England Journal of Medicine*, 342, pp. 703–9.

Pellikka, P. A. (1997), 'Stress echocardiography in the evaluation of chest pain and accuracy in the diagnosis of coronary artery disease', *Progressive Cardiovascular Disease*, 39, pp. 523–32.

Prystowsky, E. N., Benson, D. W., Fuster, V., et al. (1996), 'Management of patients with atrial fibrillation: a statement for healthcare professionals from the subcommittee on electrocardiography and electrophysiology', *Circulation*, 93, pp. 1262–77.

Prystowsky, E. N. (1997), 'Atrioventricular node reentry: physiology and radiofrequency ablation', *PACE*, 20, pp. 552–71.

Richter, J. E. (1996), 'Typical and atypical presentations of gastroesophageal reflux disease. The role of oesophageal testing in the diagnosis and management', *Gastroenterology Clinics of North America*, 25, pp. 75–101.

Simons, G. R., Klein, G. J., Natale, A. (1997), 'Ventricular tachycardia: pathophysiology and radiofrequency catheter ablation', *PACE*, 20, pp. 534–51.

Chapter 23
Hypertension

JUDITH A. WHITWORTH

Introduction

Hypertension is a major global health problem, affecting over 600 million people worldwide, in both developed and developing countries. Although mortality from cardiovascular disease has decreased substantially over the last few decades in Australia, it remains the major cause of death, and with ageing of the population contributes to a significant disease burden. At the same time, a so-called second wave of cardiovascular disease is occurring in both the former socialist republics and developing countries.

Most hypertension worldwide is undiagnosed, let alone adequately treated, and before 2020 cardiovascular disease, for which hypertension is the major risk factor, will be the world's biggest killer. Further, the morbidity and mortality attributable to hypertension is not confined to heart attack and stroke. Hypertension is a major cause of heart failure, an increasing problem in Western societies; and a major determinant of progression of diabetic and non-diabetic renal failure, of other diabetic complications including blindness, and of dementia. Much of the burden of disease caused by hypertension is borne by the elderly, and the number of elderly people is increasing in our community and globally.

Hypertension in the elderly has been undertreated in the past because of uncertainty of treatment benefits, and concern about treatment side effects. This is now changing as treatment trials in the elderly have shown evidence of unequivocal benefit.

Aetiology

The causes of hypertension are well covered in standard texts, and a discussion of the possible aetiologies of essential hypertension is beyond the scope of this chapter.

In population studies approximately 5% of hypertension is secondary. About 3% is attributable to renal disease and around 1% to renal artery disease. Both are important causes of hypertension in the elderly (in whom secondary hypertension is more common than in younger patients) and will be considered further, as will iatrogenic hypertension.

Other important causes of secondary hypertension such as phaeochromocytoma, Cushing's syndrome and Conn's syndrome will not be discussed, although it is important to realise that the latter condition appears to be much more common than previously thought and most cases have normal, as opposed to low, serum potassium.

Hypertension and renal disease

Renovascular disease

Atheromatous renal disease should be considered in elderly patients when there are characteristic clinical findings (particularly in smokers with a renal artery bruit), severe refractory difficult to control hypertension, recent onset hypertension, evidence of associated atheromatous disease or renal impairment either pre-existing or following use of angiotensin-converting enzyme (ACE) inhibitors. Atheromatous renal disease, usually bilateral, is a major cause of progressive renal failure in the elderly, as is cholesterol embolisation from aorto-renal atheroma.

Atherosclerotic renal vascular disease is accompanied by hypertension in only around half the cases. The diagnosis is most important as mortality is high when untreated, whereas surgery or angioplasty/stenting can preserve or improve renal function.

Diagnosis depends on demonstration of abnormal renal artery anatomy (> 80% stenosis), and angiography remains the definitive investigation. Non-invasive methods, such as duplex ultrasound scanning and radionuclide scanning, are particularly valuable in following lesion progression.

Risks of angiography include contrast induced acute renal failure and cholesterol embolisation, but angiography has the great advantage of allowing immediate percutaneous transluminal renal angioplasty or stenting. In older patients it is unusual for hypertension to be cured, although blood pressure control may become easier—the major advantage of the procedure is preservation of renal function. Thus investigation is only indicated where intervention would follow.

Renal parenchymal disease

Hypertension is an important manifestation of renal parenchymal disease and the hypertension in turn is a major determinant of progression of renal failure.

Renal parenchymal disease should always be suspected in the hypertensive patient with renal impairment, as in the absence of malignant phase hypertension or atheromatous renal disease there is little evidence that essential hypertension can cause progressive renal impairment in Caucasian populations. Renal parenchymal disease should also be suspected when the urine contains blood or protein, even when renal function is apparently normal.

Glomerulonephritis (primary and secondary) and diabetic nephropathy are common causes of renal failure in elderly people, in whom other conditions to consider include obstruction, particularly secondary to benign prostate hypertrophy, or malignancy, amyloidosis and multiple myeloma. Investigation will include definition of renal and urinary tract anatomy and possibly renal biopsy.

Management will be guided by the nature of the underlying renal disease but aggressive control of blood pressure is particularly important and ACE inhibitors may have additional benefits in preserving renal function over and above their blood pressure lowering effects.

Iatrogenic hypertension

Iatrogenic hypertension secondary to drug therapy is a particular problem in older patients who frequently have associated medical conditions for which they are taking prescribed or over-the-counter medications.

Non-steroidal anti-inflammatory drugs are very commonly used in older patients, and can cause increases in blood pressure and interfere with antihypertensive medication. These drugs tend to be overprescribed. In many patients with osteoarthritis, for example, other treatment, such as weight reduction and simple analgesia, will allow NSAID withdrawal.

Sympathomimetic agents are important causes of iatrogenic hypertension and nasal decongestants are not infrequently used in the older age group. Monoamine oxidase inhibitors can precipitate severe hypertension in patients if they eat foodstuffs containing tyramine (e.g. cheese, pickles). Clonidine withdrawal can also cause profound blood pressure rises.

Corticosteroid therapy contributes significantly to elevation of blood pressure and cardiovascular risk, and it is important that steroids (whether given orally, locally or topically) are given in the minimum dose for disease control. Cyclosporin also has substantial effects on blood pressure and hypertension is a common side effect. This is also a problem when erythropoietin is given to patients with renal failure.

Non-prescription drugs should also be considered: certain types of ginseng can elevate blood pressure, as can liquorice taken as confectionery. Alcohol also has a significant pressor effect.

Epidemiology

Hypertension and cardiovascular risk

Both systolic and diastolic blood pressure relate positively and continuously to risk of stroke. Although the early studies which showed a benefit of treatment of hypertension were based on diastolic pressures, it is now recognised that systolic pressure is a more reliable predictor of cardiovascular events. This is particularly relevant to elderly subjects. In elderly populations some two-thirds of hypertensives have isolated systolic hypertension (ISH). Over 20% of people over 80 years have ISH in Western populations.

The slope of association appears to decline with increasing age, but age itself is such a major risk factor for cardiovascular disease that most strokes affect elderly people. A similar although less marked relationship exists for hypertension and coronary heart disease. There is no good evidence for the existence of a 'J-curve', and the relationship between risk and pressure appears to be linear.

Hypertension is associated with a sixfold greater risk of heart failure and in patients with pre-existing disease is a major determinant of progression to renal failure. Both conditions are particularly prevalent in older people.

Table 23.1 Factors influencing prognosis, from 1999 WHO-ISH Guidelines for Management of Hypertension

Risk factors for cardiovascular diseases	Target organ damage[(a)]	Associated clinical conditions[(b)]
1. *Used for risk stratification* • Levels of systolic and diastolic blood pressure (grades 1–3) • Men > 55 years • Women > 65 years • Smoking • Total cholesterol > 6.5 mmol/L (250 mg/dL) • Diabetes • Family history of premature cardiovascular disease 2. *Other factors adversely influencing prognosis* • Reduced HDL cholesterol • Raised LDL cholesterol • Microalbuminuria in diabetes • Impaired glucose tolerance • Obesity • Sedentary lifestyle • Raised fibrinogen • High-risk socioeconomic group • High-risk ethnic group • High-risk geographic region	• Left ventricular hypertrophy (electrocardiogram, echocardiogram or radiogram) • Proteinuria and/or slight elevation of plasma creatinine concentration (1.2–2.0 mg/dL) • Ultrasound or radiological evidence of atherosclerotic plaque (carotid, iliac and femoral arteries, aorta) • Generalised or focal narrowing of the retinal arteries	*Cerebrovascular disease* • Ischaemic stroke • Cerebral haemorrhage • Transient ischaemic attack *Heart disease* • Myocardial infarction • Angina • Coronary revascularisation • Congestive heart failure *Renal disease* • Diabetic nephropathy • Renal failure (plasma creatinine concentration > 2.0 mg/dL) *Vascular disease* • Dissecting aneurysm • Symptomatic arterial disease *Advanced hypertensive retinopathy* • Haemorrhages or exudates • Papilloedema

(*a*) 'Target organ damage' corresponds to previous WHO stage 2 hypertension.

(*b*) 'Associated clinical conditions' corresponds to previous WHO stage 3 hypertension.

Age, gender and cardiovascular risk

Risks of cardiovascular disease rise steeply with age. The greater risk observed in men compared with women declines with age, and is less evident for stroke than coronary heart disease. At any age a history of cardiovascular disease, diabetes or renal disease is an important predictor of future events. A 65-year-old man with a blood pressure of 145/90 mmHg who has diabetes and a history of transient ischaemic attacks has an annual risk of a major cardiovascular event more than 20 times that of a 40-year-old man with the same blood pressure and no history of diabetes or transient ischaemia.

Other risk factors

Smoking increases cardiovascular risk throughout life, but the magnitude of the cardiovascular risk (as opposed to lung pathology) appears lower in elderly than younger people. Similarly, relative risks due to an increase in both total and low-density lipoprotein (LDL) cholesterol decline with age, although absolute risks increase. Conversely, the beneficial effect of high-density lipoprotein (HDL) cholesterol on cardiovascular risk does not appear to be age related. The risks of obesity appear to decline with age.

Other risk factors for cardiovascular disease include fibrinogen, alcohol (protective at low consumption, deleterious with high consumption and binge drinking), physical inactivity, lower socioeconomic status and ethnicity.

Evidence from major clinical trials in the elderly

Evidence from clinical trials shows that much of the benefit of blood pressure lowering anticipated from epidemiological studies is achieved by treatment, with proportional reduction being similar across different age groups. Because older people have a greater absolute risk, they have a greater absolute benefit. Trials in the elderly have shown a 34% reduction in risk, with 5 strokes prevented for every 1000 patients. For coronary heart disease, there was a 19% reduction in relative risk, which translated to 3 fewer events in every 1000 patients. Although early trials looked predominantly at diastolic blood pressure, both the Systolic Hypertension in the Elderly Program (SHEP) and the Systolic Hypertension in Europe (Syst-Eur) trials have shown that reduction of systolic pressure in the elderly reduces morbidity and mortality.

It is important to recognise that these randomised controlled trials will underestimate the effects of blood pressure lowering in practice, because of cross-over between treatment groups (where control patients begin and treated patients stop therapy), limited duration of the trials, and exclusion of high risk patients (who are most likely to benefit).

Trials in the elderly have suggested greater reduction in risk for diuretic based therapy rather than β-blocker based therapy but direct comparisons have not had sufficient power to confirm this.

More recent trials have examined a variety of new antihypertensive agents. In the Syst-Eur study, calcium channel blocker based therapy with nitrendipine produced a 42% reduction in stroke. Because of the low rate of coronary events, no firm conclusion could be reached on the effects of calcium antagonists on coronary heart disease risk. The Captopril Prevention Project (CAPPP) study compared a captopril based regimen with other treatment. There was no evidence of advantage for captopril, but the study should be interpreted with caution because the captopril treated group had higher entry blood pressure.

It is important to remember that hypertension, albeit a very important risk factor for cardiovascular disease, is one of a range of risk factors and treatment should include attention to all relevant factors (see 'Treatment').

Randomised trials have shown the benefits and safety of antihypertensive treatment in patients up to 80 years. Absolute effects are greater in older individuals because of their higher risk. Benefits of treatment have been demonstrated among older patients with both classical hypertension and isolated systolic hypertension.

Few studies have included the very elderly and there is uncertainty about the value of antihypertensive treatment for patients over the age of 80 years. The Hypertension in the Very Old Trial (HYVET) is recruiting hypertensive patients aged over 80 years and results are awaited with interest.

The very elderly are the fastest growing part of many populations, and they may be different from the 'younger' elderly in that they have been 'selected' for longevity.

Diastolic blood pressure usually rises with age until the mid-50s, then declines, whereas systolic blood pressure continues to rise until at least 80. But this rise does not seem to continue into very old age and very old people frequently have blood pressures regarded as normal in young people. In very old people positive associations with blood pressure and survival have been observed. This could relate to confounding by underlying illness leading to lower blood pressure, but data are somewhat conflicting, and hence the results of the HYVET study will be most valuable in determining how to manage the very old hypertensive.

A subgroup meta-analysis of antihypertensive drugs in very old people (> 80 years) suggested treatment decreased stroke, major cardiovascular events and heart failure, but had no benefit on cardiovascular or all cause death.

Hypertension is a recognised risk factor for dementia. The Syst-Eur trial suggested that antihypertensive treatment may reduce the risk of dementia, but the number of affected patients was small. The hypothesis that blood pressure lowering might reduce the incidence of dementia is being investigated in patients with cerebrovascular disease by a large Australasian initiated multinational study called PROGRESS (Perindopril Protection Against Recurrent Stroke Study) and in the multinational Study on Cognition and Prognosis in the Elderly (SCOPE) trial.

Pathophysiology

Essential hypertension is characterised by normal cardiac output and an elevated total peripheral vascular resistance.

Diastolic blood pressure rises into the 50s in Western populations then tends to fall, whereas systolic blood pressure continues to increase at least to the 80s, with increased stiffness of large arteries and increased pulse pressure. Renal blood flow is reduced and renal vascular resistance increased, but glomerular filtration rate is usually normal or only slightly decreased, so that filtration fraction is increased. Renal structural changes include medial hypertrophy of intrarenal arteries and arterioles with segmental hyalinosis and increased wall–lumen ratio. There may be ischaemic changes in the glomerular tuft. These occur on a background of age-related decline in renal size and function.

These changes are relevant clinically. Because of reduced muscle mass, serum creatinine concentration may be normal in older people even though renal function is substantially reduced, and age related changes in renal function may necessitate dose reduction in renally excreted drugs. Salt sensitivity increases with age, presumably due to diminution of renal excretory capacity.

With advancing age there is a decrease in cardiac output predominantly reflecting a fall in stroke volume. Arteries show thinning and fragmentation of elastic fibres predominantly in the media, with calcification in areas of degeneration leading to stiffer arteries, particularly in central vessels, whereas hyaline thickening increases wall–lumen ratio in small arteries and arterioles and reduction in the size of the peripheral vascular bed. Thus decreased arterial compliance is common in older subjects.

Baroreceptor function decreases, so that postural hypotension may occur, and this is exacerbated by decreased cardiovascular sensitivity to catecholamines and reduced activity of the renin-angiotensin-aldosterone system. Post-prandial hypotension can also be a problem in the elderly.

Other physiological consequences of ageing include reduction in hepatic blood flow with consequent decreased metabolism of some drugs, and altered intestinal absorption. Volume of distribution of water soluble drugs is decreased but lipid soluble drugs have a greater volume of distribution consequent on decrease in lean body mass and increase in body fat.

Clinical tests

Evaluation of the hypertensive patient aims to confirm the diagnosis (see below) and determine the level of blood pressure elevation, to identify any secondary cause of hypertension, to evaluate associated target organ damage and to assess associated cardiovascular risk factors and other conditions that may modify treatment.

The history should include: family history of hypertension, coronary heart disease, diabetes mellitus, dyslipidaemia, stroke or renal disease; duration and levels of hypertension and details of previous antihypertensive drug treatment; history of coronary heart disease and heart failure, cerebrovascular disease, peripheral vascular disease, diabetes mellitus, gout, dyslipidaemia, bronchospasm, sexual dysfunction, renal disease or other illness; any symptoms suggestive of secondary causes of hypertension; assessment of diet, sodium and alcohol intake, smoking, physical activity and weight; drugs that can raise blood pressure, including non-steroidal anti-inflammatory drugs, liquorice, erythropoietin, cyclosporin or steroids; and other personal, psychosocial and environmental factors.

Physical examination should include weight; heart size; evidence of heart failure and arterial disease in the carotid, renal and peripheral arteries; abdominal examination for renal bruits or renal enlargement; and examination of the optic fundi to assess retinal vessels and evidence of accelerated hypertension (haemorrhages and exudates).

Routine investigations should include urinalysis for blood, protein and glucose; microscopic examination of urine; and estimation of serum potassium, creatinine, fasting glucose and total cholesterol concentrations. An electrocardiogram should also be performed.

Optional investigations will be guided by the findings from the history, examination and routine investigations. They are indicated if they carry implications for management.

Diagnosis

Measurement of blood pressure

The diagnosis of hypertension should be based on multiple blood pressure measurements, on several separate occasions.

Blood pressure should be measured with the patient sitting, after several minutes in a quiet room, using a mercury sphygmomanometer or other non-invasive device. Blood pressure should also be measured standing in elderly subjects, in whom orthostatic hypotension is common.

The cuff should be at heart level. The size of the cuff is important. The standard cuff has a bladder that is 12–13 cm × 35 cm, but a larger bladder is needed for fat arms. Phase 5 Korotkoff sounds (disappearance) should be used to measure the diastolic pressure.

Non-invasive semi-automatic and automatic devices are available for blood pressure measurement at home and for ambulatory blood pressure monitoring over longer periods. Both of these approaches provide useful additional clinical information. Home blood pressure measurement can provide values on different days in daily life conditions. Self-blood pressure measurement has been shown to be acceptable in older patients. Ambulatory blood pressure monitoring should be considered when there is unusual variability of blood pressure; hypertension in subjects with low cardiovascular risk; symptoms suggesting hypotensive episodes; and hypertension resistant to drug treatment.

In some older patients it is difficult to compress the arterial wall, resulting in a falsely high reading —Osler's sign, so-called pseudohypertension. If this is the case, despite brachial occlusion the pulseless radial artery will be palpable.

Definition of hypertension

The 1999 WHO-ISH Guidelines for Management of Hypertension define the lower limits of hypertension as 140 mmHg systolic and 90 mmHg diastolic. The Guidelines emphasise that the decision to lower blood pressure in an individual patient is not based on the level of blood pressure alone but also on assessment of that patient's total cardiovascular risk (see Table 23.2).

Treatment

Risk factor reduction

Smoking cessation reduces the risk of many diseases, including heart attack and stroke. Although the benefits of smoking cessation on cardiovascular disease are not as great in the elderly as in younger people, they remain significant and the associated

Table 23.2 Definition and classification of blood pressure levels, from 1999 WHO-ISH Guidelines for Management of Hypertension

Category	Systolic (mmHg)	Diastolic (mmHg)
Optimal	< 120	< 80
Normal	< 130	< 85
High-normal	130–139	85–89
Grade 1 hypertension ('mild')	140–159	90–99
Subgroup: borderline	140–149	90–94
Grade 2 hypertension ('moderate')	160–179	100–109
Grade 3 hypertension ('severe')	⩾ 180	⩾110
Isolated systolic hypertension	⩾ 140	< 90
Subgroup: borderline	140–149	< 90

Note: When a patient's systolic and diastolic blood pressure falls into different categories, the higher category should apply.

benefits (e.g. prevention of malignancy disease) are real.

Cholesterol lowering reduces coronary heart disease events in patients with a history of coronary heart disease and those with high cholesterol concentrations. Reductions in risk of stroke have been observed in trials of 3-hydroxy-3-methylglutaryl-coenzyme A (HMG-co A) reductase inhibitors.

In patients with a history of cardiovascular disease, aspirin reduces risks of cardiovascular events and death. In those with no such history, coronary disease events are also reduced. In the Hypertension Optimal Treatment (HOT) study aspirin produced a one-third reduction in coronary events, but increased risk of bleeding twofold, although in these subjects with well controlled blood pressure there was no increase in cerebral haemorrhage. Aspirin should not be used in patients with poorly controlled hypertension.

Who to treat? Stratification by absolute cardiovascular risk

Decisions about management should not be based simply on the blood pressure but also on the presence of other risk factors, concomitant diseases, target organ damage and other aspects of the patient's situation.

The 1999 WHO-ISH Guidelines (see Table 23.3) define four categories of risk (low, medium, high and very high risk). Within each, the risk of any individual will be determined by the severity and number of risk factors present. By definition, elderly patients, all of whom have age as a risk, are not in the low risk group.

The medium risk group includes patients with a wide range of blood pressures and risk factors. Some have lower blood pressures and multiple risk factors, whereas others have higher blood pressure and no or few other risk factors.

The high risk group includes patients with grade 1 or grade 2 hypertension who have three or more risk factors, diabetes or target organ damage, and patients with grade 3 ('severe') hypertension without other risk factors. Risk of a major cardiovascular event in the following 10 years is typically about 20–30%.

The very high risk group includes patients with grade 3 hypertension and one or more risk factors and all patients with clinical cardiovascular disease or renal disease and a risk of cardiovascular events of the order of 30% or more over 10 years.

Treatment goals

Treatment goals in the elderly should be to achieve at least high normal blood pressures, below 140/90 mmHg. In patients with diabetes or renal disease even lower target pressures should be sought.

Management

In the older hypertensive, the options are to institute immediate drug treatment for the hypertension and other risk factors or conditions present (high and very high risk groups) or to monitor blood pressure and other risk factors over weeks before deciding whether to institute drug treatment (medium risk group).

The individual treatment plan will involve monitoring of blood pressure and other risk factors, lifestyle measures and drug treatment.

Table 23.3 Stratification of risk to quantify prognosis, from 1999 WHO-ISH Guidelines for Management of Hypertension

	Blood pressure (mmHg)		
Other risk factors and disease history	**Grade 1 Mild hypertension (SBP 140–159 or DBP 90–99)**	**Grade 2 Moderate hypertension (SBP 160–179 or DBP 100–109)**	**Grade 3 Severe hypertension (SBP ≥ 180 or DBP ≥ 110)**
I. No other risk factors	Low risk	Medium risk	High risk
II. 1–2 risk factors	Medium risk	Medium risk	Very high risk
III. 3 or more risk factors or TOD[(a)] or diabetes	High risk	High risk	Very high risk
IV. ACC[(b)]	Very high risk	Very high risk	Very high risk

(*a*) TOD—Target organ damage (see Table 23.1).
(*b*) ACC—Associated clinical conditions, including clinical cardiovascular disease or renal disease (see Table 23.1).
Note: Risk strata (typical 10 year risk of stroke or myocardial infarction):
Low risk = less than 15%
Medium risk = about 15–20%
High risk = about 20–30%
Very high risk = 30% or more

Lifestyle measures should be instituted wherever appropriate in all patients, including those who require drug treatment.

Lifestyle measures

Although it has been claimed that elderly patients will not follow lifestyle measures, the TONE study (Trial of Nonpharmacologic Interventions in the Elderly) showed that modification was possible in this group.

All hypertensive patients who smoke should receive appropriate counselling for smoking cessation, and nicotine replacement therapy should also be considered.

Weight reduction of as little as 5 kg reduces blood pressure in overweight hypertensive individuals and has a beneficial effect on insulin resistance, diabetes, hyperlipidaemia and left ventricular hypertrophy. The blood pressure lowering effects of weight reduction may be enhanced by physical exercise, alcohol moderation in overweight drinkers and, most particularly in the elderly, by reduction of sodium intake.

Hypertensive patients should be advised to limit their consumption to under 20–30 g of alcohol per day for men, and 10–20 g per day for women. They should be warned against the risks of stroke associated with binge drinking.

Individuals vary considerably in their responses to changes in dietary salt, with obese and elderly subjects being the most sensitive. The aim of dietary sodium reduction is to achieve an intake of less than 100 mmol (5.8 g) per day of sodium or less than 6 g per day of sodium chloride. Patients should be advised to avoid added salt, obviously salted foods, particularly processed foods, and to eat more meals cooked directly from natural ingredients.

Other dietary factors are also important in blood pressure lowering and older patients should be advised to increase fruit and vegetable consumption, reduce fat intake and to eat more fish.

Sedentary patients should be advised to take up modest levels of aerobic exercise on a regular basis, such as a brisk walk or a swim for 30–45 minutes, 3–4 times a week.

Drug treatment

The six main drug classes used for blood pressure lowering treatment are: diuretics, β-blockers, calcium antagonists, ACE inhibitors, angiotensin II receptor antagonists and α-adrenergic blockers.

There is no consistent difference between drug classes in their effects on blood pressure, but there are differences in the side effect profiles of each class. While there is much data demonstrating the benefits of diuretics and β-blockers, there are fewer data available for newer drugs.

Principles of treatment include the use of the lowest doses of drugs to initiate therapy; the use of drug combinations to maximise efficacy while minimising side effects; changing to a different drug class if there is poor response or tolerability to the first drug used; and the use of long-acting drugs once daily to improve adherence to therapy and minimise blood pressure variability.

For patients in the high and very high risk groups, drug treatment should be instituted within a few days as soon as repeated measurements have confirmed the high blood pressure.

For patients in the medium risk group it is desirable to continue with lifestyle measures for at least 3 months before considering drug treatment. If goal blood pressures are not attained within 6 months, drug treatment should be initiated.

Patients with high-normal blood pressure who also have diabetes mellitus and/or renal insufficiency should receive early and active drug treatment. The choice of drugs will be influenced by cardiovascular risk factor profile and the presence

Table 23.4 Guidelines for selection of drug treatment of hypertension in elderly patients, from 1999 WHO-ISH Guidelines for Management of Hypertension

Class of drug	Compelling indications	Possible indications	Compelling contraindications	Possible contraindications
Diuretics	Heart failure Elderly patients Systolic hypertension	Diabetes mellitus	Gout	Dyslipidaemia Sexually active males
β-blockers	Angina After myocardial infarct Tachyarrhythmias	Heart failure Diabetes mellitus	Asthma and chronic lung disease Heart block[(a)]	Dyslipidaemia Peripheral vascular disease
ACE inhibitors	Heart failure Left ventricular dysfunction After myocardial infarct Diabetic nephropathy		Hyperkalaemia Bilateral renal artery stenosis	
Calcium antagonists	Angina Elderly patients Systolic hypertension	Peripheral vascular disease	Heart block[(b)]	Congestive heart failure[(c)]
α-blockers	Prostatic hypertrophy	Glucose intolerance Dyslipidaemia		Orthostatic hypotension
Angiotensin II-receptor antagonists	ACE inhibitor cough	Heart failure	Bilateral renal artery stenosis Hyperkalaemia	

(a) Grade 2 or 3 atrioventricular block.
(b) Grade 2 or 3 atrioventricular block with verapamil or diltiazem.
(c) Verapamil or diltiazem. ACE, angtiotensin-converting enzyme.

of target organ damage or cardiovascular or renal disease, and diabetes.

Diuretics are cheap, effective and well tolerated. Diuretic based treatment regimens have been shown to prevent stroke and coronary heart disease. Many of their side effects (e.g. potassium depletion, reduced glucose tolerance, ventricular ectopic beats and impotence) were associated with inappropriately high doses. Diuretics should be used in low doses (e.g. 12.5 mg daily of hydrochlorothiazide) and are particularly recommended for elderly patients. Serum potassium concentrations should be maintained in the normal range, as there is some evidence that the benefits of treatment are not seen in the presence of hypokalaemia. It should be recognised that elderly patients are particularly susceptible to volume depletion and hence dehydration, uraemia, postural hypotension and hyponatraemia with excess diuretic therapy are all more common in older patients.

β-adrenoceptor blocking drugs are safe, cheap and effective as monotherapy in the general hypertensive population or in combination with diuretics, dihydropyridine calcium antagonists or α-blockers. They are used particularly in patients with coronary artery disease. β-blockers should be avoided in patients with obstructive airways disease and peripheral vascular disease, and may be associated with depression, another common problem in the elderly. Trial evidence for reduction of morbidity in cardiovascular events in the elderly is less compelling than for diuretic or calcium channel blocker therapy, but comparisons have not had sufficient power to reliably indicate advantages for one class compared with another.

ACE inhibitors are safe and effective in lowering blood pressure and in reducing morbidity and mortality in heart failure and in retarding the progression of renal disease. Dry cough is common. In elderly patients—particularly those with cardiac failure, renal impairment or dehydration—they can cause reversible renal impairment.

Calcium antagonists are effective and well tolerated and have been shown to prevent stroke in elderly patients with systolic hypertension. Long-acting calcium antagonists are preferred and rapid onset, short-acting calcium antagonists should be avoided. Adverse effects include tachycardia, flushing, ankle oedema and constipation with verapamil. The latter can be particularly troubling in older patients.

Angiotensin II-receptor antagonists have many features in common with ACE inhibitors, but less cough.

α-blockers are effective in lowering pressure but in the Antihypertensive and Lipid Lowering Heart Attack Treatment (ALLHAT) study doxazosin was associated with a higher incidence of congestive heart failure than chlorthalidone. They are often used in older men with prostatism, as they improve symptoms in this condition. Because of the increased risks of orthostatic hypotension it is imperative that therapy should be initiated at the lowest dose at bedtime.

Effective drug combinations utilise drugs from different classes in order to obtain additive hypotensive effect, while minimising side effects. They include diuretic and β-blocker; diuretic and ACE inhibitor (or A II-receptor antagonist); calcium antagonist (dihydropyridine) and β-blocker; calcium antagonist and ACE inhibitor; α-blocker and β-blocker.

Patient education and the patient–doctor relationship are key to compliance with therapy. Failure to respond to treatment (refractory hypertension) may be apparent (white coat hypertension, inappropriate cuff size) or real, due to unsuspected secondary hypertension, particularly renovascular disease, poor compliance, interfering drugs (e.g. NSAIDs), weight gain, heavy alcohol intake or volume overload due to inadequate diuretic therapy, renal insufficiency or high sodium intake.

Provided antihypertensive medication is prescribed appropriately, side effects are not a greater problem in older people. Care should be taken to avoid postural (and post-prandial) hypotension and practitioners should be sensitive to possible effects on sexual function which older patients may not volunteer. Concomitant disease may restrict drug choice.

Whatever drugs are used, the regimen should be as simple as possible, and this is particularly true for older patients with cognitive impairment. Polypharmacy is a common problem, as older patients frequently have associated disease requiring medication which may interact with antihypertensive medication (e.g. NSAIDs, antidepressants).

Cost effectiveness of treatment of hypertension in the elderly

Because absolute risk is greater in older patients, treatment of older people is more cost effective in terms of events prevented than in younger people. It has been claimed that treatment of hypertension in women over 70 may provide overall cost savings.

Prognosis

The prognosis of hypertension in the elderly, untreated, has been discussed under the heading of 'Epidemiology'. Depending on other risk factors, there are substantial risks of heart attack and stroke, dementia and renal failure. Age is of itself a risk factor for cardiovascular disease.

Treatment of hypertension in the elderly, as discussed above, significantly reduces the risks of cardiovascular events, and the absolute benefit of treatment in an individual patient will depend on a range of factors, including the level of absolute risk, the successes or otherwise in modifying concomitant risk factors, compliance with therapy and the levels of blood pressure achieved.

The days of therapeutic nihilism in hypertension in the elderly are long gone. Individual patients should profit from the increasing body of evidence of the value of blood pressure lowering in the elderly.

Acknowledgment

Ms Laura Vitler assisted in the preparation of the manuscript.

Bibliography and further reading

ALLHAT Collaborative Research Group (2000), 'Major cardiovascular events in hypertensive patients randomised to doxazosin vs chlorthalidone: The antihypertensive and lipid-lowering treatment to prevent heart attack (ALLHAT)', *Journal of the American Medical Association*, 283, pp. 1967–75.

Dahlof, B., Lindholm, L., Hansson, L., Schersten, B., Ekbom, T. & Wester, P.-O. (1991), 'Morbidity and mortality in the Swedish Trial in Old Patients with Hypertension (STOP—Hypertension)', *Lancet*, 338, pp. 1281–5.

Flack, J. M., McVeigh, G. & Grimm, R. H. (1993), 'Hypertension therapy in the elderly', *Current Opinion in Nephrology and Hypertension*, 2, pp. 386–94.

Forette, B. (1999), 'Hypertension in very old subjects', *Clinical and Experimental Hypertension*, 21, pp. 917–25.

Gueyffier, F., Bulpitt, C., Boissel, J. P., INDANA Group et al. (1999), 'Antihypertensive drugs in very old people: A sub-group meta-analysis of randomised controlled trials', *Lancet*, 353, pp. 793–6.

Hansson, L., Zanchetti, A., Carruthers, S. G. et al. for the HOT Study Group (1998), 'Effects of intensive blood pressure lowering and low dose aspirin in patients with hypertension: Principal results of the Hypertension Optimal Treatment (HOT) randomised trial', *Lancet*, 351, pp. 1755–62.

Meyrier, A. (1996), 'Renal vascular lesions in the elderly: Nephrosclerosis or atheromatous renal disease?', *Nephrology Dialysis Transplantation*, 11(Suppl. 9), pp. 45–52.

(1992), 'MRC Working Party Medical Research Council trial of treatment of hypertension in older adults: Principal results', *British Medical Journal*, 304, pp. 405–12.

Prisant, L. M. & Moser, M. (2000), 'Hypertension in the elderly: Can we improve results of therapy?', *Archives of Internal Medicine*, 160, pp. 283–9.

SHEP Co-operative Research Group (1991), 'Prevention of stroke by anti-hypertensive drug treatment in older persons with isolated systolic hypertension: Final results of the Systolic Hypertension in the Elderly Program (SHEP)', *Journal of the Amercian Medical Association*, 265, pp. 3255–64.

Starr, J. (1999), 'Blood pressure and cognitive decline in the elderly', *Current Opinion in Nephrology and Hypertension*, 8, pp. 347–51.

WHO (1999), 'WHO-ISH Guidelines for Management of Hypertension', *Journal of Hypertension*, 17, pp. 151–83.

Chapter 24
Cardiac failure

A. PETER PASSMORE

Introduction

Cardiac failure is a common condition which usually results from coronary heart disease but is in effect the final stage of any disease of the heart. Although a variety of definitions exist, mostly based on pathophysiology, for clinicians the clinical syndrome is most meaningful and includes dyspnoea, fatigue and oedema.

Cardiac failure is more common in older people and accounts for a significant percentage of hospital admissions. The incidence is likely to increase in the future because of population demographics and improvements in the management of contributory causes. Although hypertension was usually cited as the most common cause, coronary heart disease is now said to be the main factor in Western societies, with valvular heart disease and arrhythmias accounting for a smaller proportion. Cardiac failure may also be precipitated by conditions such as anaemia, pneumonia, pulmonary embolism, non-steroidal anti-inflammatory drugs and negative inotropes.

The diagnosis of cardiac failure is a clinical one where symptoms may include reduced exercise tolerance, fatigue and orthopnoea or dyspnoea, and examination may reveal raised jugular venous pressure, third heart sound, lung crepitations and peripheral oedema. However, diagnosis can be difficult, especially in the early stages where there may be few clinical features and specific investigations are often indicated. This is often the case in older patients where the diagnosis presents even more difficulty.

The best form of treatment of cardiac failure is prevention through the aggressive management of coronary disease, hypertension and other predisposing conditions. It is important to make an accurate diagnosis and identify the underlying cause where possible. Any precipitating factors should be managed. The aims of treatment are to improve symptoms and prognosis. Although treatment of cardiac failure usually involves the early use of medication, non-pharmacological measures are important. These may involve bed rest, oxygen and fluid or salt restriction. For mild heart failure exercise is important. It is also important to educate the patient about her condition.

Diuretics are an integral part of management. Where left ventricular dysfunction is diagnosed, ACE inhibitors should be used early. These drugs have been shown to improve symptoms and prognosis in all stages of heart failure and to reduce hospitalisation. β-adrenoceptor blocking drugs have recently been shown to be beneficial in certain groups of patients with heart failure and the use of spironolactone in small doses has been shown to reduce mortality. Digoxin is also useful and nitrates are often indicated. Depending on the cause, surgical intervention, pacemakers and ventricular assist devices may be indicated.

Aetiology and epidemiology

Cardiac failure can be considered as acute or chronic and where left ventricular systolic function is reduced or normal. There have been a number of studies on the epidemiology of cardiac failure. Any discrepancy between the reported incidence and prevalence relates to different definitions employed. The Task Force of the European Society of Cardiology has published guidelines on diagnosis, citing 'symptoms of heart failure, objective evidence of cardiac dysfunction and response to treatment directed towards heart failure'. The increasing use of echocardiography in the assessment of cardiac function in recent studies has helped produce some consensus.

Incidence, prevalence and aetiology

The most important source of information relating to the epidemiology of heart failure has come from the Framingham heart study. The age adjusted prevalence was similar in men and women and approximately doubled with each decade of ageing. Prevalence ranged from 8 per 1000 population aged 50–59 years to 72 per 1000 population aged 80–89. The annual incidence showed a rise of 3 per 1000 population aged 50–59, to 24 per 1000 aged 80–89. An echocardiographic study in Glasgow of the prevalence of significantly impaired left ventricular contraction (ejection fraction < 30%) showed rates increased with increasing age, ranging from 1.4% (45–54 years) to 3.2% (65–74 years) in men, with similar rates in women, for symptomatic cases, while prevalence of asymptomatic cases were seen in 3.2–4.4% of men with little apparent relation to age.

In a population study of 151 000 people in Hillingdon, West London, England, the overall incidence of cardiac failure was 1.3 cases per 1000 population per year for those aged over 25 years, with an incidence rate of 11.6 per 1000 per year for those aged 85 years and over. The incidence was higher in males than females and the median age at presentation was 76 years. Overall the primary aetiologies were coronary heart disease (36%), unknown (34%), hypertension (14%), valve disease (7%), atrial fibrillation alone (5%) and other (5%). Coronary heart disease frequently coexisted with a history of hypertension (51% cases), while 44% of all cases had a history of hypertension although this was considered to be the primary aetiology in only 31% of these cases, giving the 14% overall figure for hypertension. Causes of heart failure are listed in Box 24.1.

Box 24.1 Causes of heart failure

- Coronary heart disease
- Hypertension
- Cardiomyopathy
- Valvular and congenital heart disease
- Arrhythmias
- High output failure
- Pericardial disease
- Primary right heart failure

Quite often echocardiographic studies in older people with cardiac failure show preserved left ventricular function. As many as 30–40% of patients with cardiac failure may have normal systolic contraction. These individuals can be considered as having diastolic dysfunction which results from impaired myocardial relaxation, with increased stiffness in the ventricular wall and reduced left ventricular compliance leading to impairment of diastolic ventricular filling. Diastolic dysfunction can result from hypertension, particularly when left ventricular hypertrophy is present, and from coronary heart disease. Ventricular compliance is also reduced with ageing due to an accumulation of fat, fibrous tissue, lipofuscin and amyloid. Diastolic dysfunction can be assessed using echocardiography or cardiac catheterisation techniques but there is no consensus on the most accurate index. In most patients with cardiac failure both systolic and diastolic dysfunction can be present. Most studies in heart failure have used indices of systolic dysfunction as primary entry criteria and give clear guidelines on management of heart failure in this situation, whereas there are few, if any, studies of heart failure with normal systolic function—a very common manifestation in older people.

Precipitants

In older patients there is often significant co-morbidity and concomitant medication. Even in older people without cardiac dysfunction, some concurrent conditions and treatments can precipitate heart failure. Arrhythmia, particularly atrial fibrillation, is a common precipitant, especially where there is diastolic filling impairment and a contribution is needed from atrial contraction. Any bradyarrhythmia may cause or exacerbate cardiac failure. Hyperdynamic circulation such as that found in hyperthyroid states, anaemia or fever will exacerbate cardiac failure. Older people are often on a variety of medications and very often these are the cause of cardiac failure or worsening cardiac decompensation. These causes are listed in Box 24.2.

Box 24.2 Precipitants of heart failure

- Angina pectoris
- Acute myocardial infarction (may be silent in older people)
- Arrhythmias, particularly atrial fibrillation
- Infections, particularly chest infections
- Thyroid disorders (thyrotoxicosis and hypothyroid disease)
- Anaemia
- Pulmonary embolism
- Iatrogenic
  - Fluid replacement
  - Corticosteroids
  - Mineralocorticoids
  - Non-steroidal anti-inflammatory drugs
  - Anti-arrhythmics
  - β-blockers
  - Calcium channel blockers

Drugs which exert a negative chronotropic or inotropic effect such as β-blockers, some calcium channel blockers or anti-arrhythmics are often implicated. The other medications that are often to blame are drugs—such as non-steroidal anti-inflammatory drugs, corticosteroids or mineralocorticoids—which cause retention of sodium and water.

There are ethnic and societal variations in the epidemiology of cardiac failure. In Western countries, coronary heart disease and hypertension are common causes, while in the developing world, valvular heart disease and nutritional cardiac disease are more common. In a UK study the most common aetiological factor for black Afro-Caribbean patients was hypertension, for Indo-Asians coronary heart disease and diabetes, and for whites coronary heart disease.

Pathophysiology

Age related changes

It is important to consider the effects of physiological changes with ageing upon the cardiovascular system. The ability to increase heart rate during exercise is attenuated. Ventricular mass increases without coronary artery disease or hypertension, not because of hyperplasia but due to increased myocyte size. An increased myocardial collagen is also seen. As a result, ventricular compliance is decreased and both systolic and diastolic function are affected, although the latter predominates. Impaired diastolic function leads to left ventricular underfilling and a fall in cardiac output. This is compensated for by an overall reduction in myocardial oxygen demand due to a reduction in lean body mass.

Overview

Although cardiac failure implies the problem lies only in the heart, the syndrome must be considered a multisystem disorder, characterised by stimulation of the sympathetic nervous system, a complex pattern of neurohormonal changes, and abnormalities of renal and peripheral vascular function, skeletal muscle physiology and pulmonary dynamics. Although heart failure can resolve after definitive treatment of its cause—for example, surgery for valve lesions—the syndrome is usually a progressive process. Initial responses include dilatation and hypertrophy leading to cardiac remodelling. A fall in cardiac output results in activation of several neurohormonal compensatory mechanisms. Under normal physiological circumstances these mechanisms provide support for the heart, but in cardiac failure their activation can play an important part in cardiac remodelling and in the progression of cardiac failure.

Neurohormonal systems

Early neurohormonal changes involve changes in the sympathetic nervous system and atrial natriuretic peptide. An increase in ventricular diastolic volume increases the force of contraction through the Frank-Starling principle. Sympathetic activation occurs as a result of low and high pressure baroreceptor stimulation and increases both force and frequency of contraction through stimulation of ventricular β-adrenoceptors, leading to preservation of cardiac output. An increase in atrial stretch leads to a release of atrial natriuretic peptide which has both natriuretic and vasodilatory effects.

Chronic activation of these mechanisms may have deleterious effects and lead to further deterioration in cardiac function. Continued atrial distension leads to depletion of natriuretic peptides. Sustained sympathetic stimulation further activates the renin angiotensin aldosterone system, resulting in increased concentrations of renin, angiotensin II and aldosterone. Angiotensin II is a potent vasoconstrictor of renal efferent and peripheral arterioles, and stimulates noradrenaline release from sympathetic nerve terminals, inhibits vagal tone and promotes release of aldosterone. This in turn causes sodium and water retention and potassium excretion. The increased renin angiotensin activation and sympathetic stimulation results in increased arterial and venous tone, an increase in plasma noradrenaline concentrations and further retention of sodium and water with resultant development of oedema. Both noradrenaline and angiotensin II can exert toxic effects on myocardial cells, causing cardiac myocyte apoptosis, hypertrophy and focal myocardial necrosis. In the long term this high level of catecholamines causes a down regulation of cardiac β-receptors and a resultant attenuated myocardial response.

In addition to atrial natriuretic peptide (ANP), brain natriuretic peptide (BNP) is released from ventricles in response to volume expansion and pressure overload and, by causing natriuresis and vasodilatation, acts in opposition to angiotensin II.

Antidiuretic hormone concentrations are increased in chronic severe cardiac failure, particularly in patients receiving diuretics, and this may contribute to development of hyponatraemia. Endothelin is a potent vasoconstrictor peptide secreted by vascular endothelial cells; it has pronounced effects on the renal vasculature promoting sodium retention. Higher levels of endothelin are seen in cardiac failure.

Peripheral vasculature

There is an increased vascular resistance and decreased distal arterial compliance which occurs as a result of increased sympathetic tone, activation of the renin-angiotensin-aldosterone system, increased endothelin release and impaired release of endothelium derived relaxing factor. Mechanical changes contributing to increased vascular impedance in cardiac failure include sodium and water retention within vessel walls and in the interstitium and structural changes in vessel walls.

Skeletal muscle

In the context of older people, abnormalities in the structure and function of the peripheral skeletal musculature are particularly important in the pathogenesis of reduced exercise tolerance in cardiac failure. There are reductions in muscle mass and abnormalities in muscle structure metabolism and function. Some of these changes are due to vasoconstriction produced as a result of neurohormonal activation. Peripheral vasoconstriction results in reduced blood flow to active skeletal muscle. These changes, including those in respiratory muscles, contribute to fatigue and lethargy. Raised pulmonary capillary pressure and abnormalities of pulmonary perfusion also contribute to fatigue, dyspnoea and reduced exercise capacity.

Clinical assessment

Heart failure is a clinical syndrome and in assessment of patients it is important to establish the diagnosis, to characterise the nature and extent of the functional limitation (symptoms), to assess the presence and severity of fluid retention (physical signs) and to identify the nature and severity of the cardiac abnormality or any predisposing factors (symptoms, physical signs and investigations).

Clinical features

Cardiac failure is associated with a number of classical symptoms and signs, many of which are non-specific, particularly in an older population. This is complicated by the fact that cardiac failure develops gradually in most patients and the interpretation of symptoms and signs may be complicated by the presence of non-cardiac disease. This often means that investigations are relied upon to confirm the diagnosis that is suspected clinically. The common symptoms of cardiac failure include dyspnoea, fatigue, exercise intolerance and swollen ankles. In older people, history taking is often not straightforward due to the co-existence of deafness or even mild cognitive impairment. The history from relatives or those close to the patient is often valuable.

Symptoms

Dyspnoea

The initial manifestation of cardiac failure is dyspnoea on exertion. This can also be due to lack of fitness in older people or to anaemia, pulmonary disease or renal disease. Renal disease can produce dyspnoea because of oedema, uraemia or acidosis. It is important to clarify the extent of exertional dyspnoea and to ascertain whether exercise is limited by symptoms of cardiac failure or by other disorders that may affect effort tolerance (e.g. angina, musculoskeletal disorders or intermittent claudication). If exercise is limited by dyspnoea or fatigue, it is important to determine whether the principal cause is heart failure, pulmonary disease or some other abnormality. Sometimes these disorders co-exist in the same patient. Orthopnoea is said to be a more specific symptom but may not be that sensitive. Paroxysmal nocturnal dyspnoea results from increased left ventricular filling pressures and has a better sensitivity and specificity. It does need to be differentiated from nocturnal dyspnoea associated with pulmonary disease.

Fatigue and lethargy

These can be common symptoms in older people and may as such be quite non-specific. However, older people with low cardiac output complain of tiredness and may sleep more and even spend much of their time in bed. Fatigue and lethargy relate not only to the low output but also to abnormalities in skeletal muscle. Here there may be premature muscle lactate release, impaired muscle blood flow, deficient endothelial function and abnormalities in skeletal muscle structure and function. A reduction in cerebral blood flow may contribute to somnolence and confusion in older people.

Oedema

This is a common presenting feature of cardiac failure, although in older people there may be a tendency to label all ankle oedema as cardiac failure whereas there may be a number of other causes. This is particularly so where there is chronic neurological or joint disease or venous insufficiency, or in frail people where albumin levels may be low. This gravitational oedema is often due to immobility associated with these states. Quite often where old people have cardiac failure and are more immobile or staying longer in bed, the oedema is seen at the sacrum, assuming more significance and being more helpful in diagnoisis. In severe cardiac failure oedema may extend to ascites.

In older people particularly it is important to assess the type, severity and duration of the symptoms discussed above in order to obtain an idea of the patient's functional capability. In clinical practice the severity of symptoms is gauged by a subjective scale first introduced by the New York Heart Association (NYHA). This scale is still widely used (see Table 24.1).

Physical signs

In the early stages of heart failure, examination is likely to be unrewarding. Peripheral oedema,

Table 24.1 NYHA Classification of Heart Failure

Class I	No limitation of physical activity	No symptoms on ordinary activity
Class II	Slight limitation of physical activity	Symptoms on ordinary activity
Class III	Marked limitation of physical activity	Symptoms on less than ordinary activity
Class IV	Any physical activity causes discomfort	Symptoms at rest

hepatomegaly and raised venous pressure are the classical signs of congestion in systemic veins. The most specific signs in descending order are tachycardia, neck vein distension, gallop rhythm, oedema and crepitations. Raised jugular venous pressure and positive hepatojugular reflex are quite specific, although these signs may be absent, even in severe heart failure, and interrater reliability is poor. A third heart sound is common in severe heart failure and is quite specific but, again, interobserver variability is unreliable. Pulmonary crepitations in older people are quite common and may be a chronic finding or represent infection or pulmonary fibrosis. It is important on examination to look for other clinical features which may indicate an underlying cause or precipitant of cardiac failure. Thus anaemia, infection, thyroid status, arrhythmias, the presence of hypertension, heart murmurs and respiratory examination are all important.

Diagnosis

The guidelines for diagnosis of cardiac failure published by the European Society of Cardiology are quite useful and pragmatic (see Box 24.3). In the preceding section it is clear that symptomatology and physical examination may be imprecise, particularly in older people. It is therefore important to have objective measures of cardiac function and this is a stipulation of the European guidelines. However, it can be seen from Box 24.3 that essential features include both symptoms and objective evidence. Hence clinical assessment is mandatory prior to performance of detailed investigations. The most useful test is the two-dimensional echocardiogram which is increasingly accessible on an 'open access basis' but investigations which should be performed before referral include haematological and biochemical testing, 12-lead electrocardiography and chest x-ray.

Box 24.3 European Society of Cardiology Guidelines for Diagnosis of Heart Failure

Essential features

- symptoms of heart failure (e.g. breathlessness, fatigue, ankle swelling) and
- objective evidence of cardiac dysfunction at rest

Non-essential features

- response to treatment directed towards heart failure (in cases where diagnosis is in doubt)

Haematology and biochemistry

Anaemia can cause a high output cardiac failure or may exacerbate existing cardiac failure in older patients. This is usually easy to correct and it is important not only to detect and quantify but also to identify and treat any underlying cause.

The electrolytes and renal function must be measured. Although in mild cardiac failure these are usually normal, it is important to obtain a baseline measure prior to initiation of treatment. Hyponatraemia may indicate a dilutional effect due to inability to excrete water. Elevations of serum creatinine may indicate pre-existing renal damage (e.g. due to longstanding hypertension or an effect of the cardiac failure on glomerular filtration rate and renal blood flow). Potassium levels are also important. In untreated mild cardiac failure these should be unchanged, but where treatment is already incorporated hyperkalaemia or hypokalaemia may develop, with potential effects on cardiac arrhythmias or drug interaction. Liver function tests are often an indication of the degree of hepatic congestion. In an older population the presentation of thyroid disease is often atypical. For example, thyrotoxicosis often presents as atrial fibrillation and cardiac failure while hypothyroidism can also manifest in this fashion. In older people generally there is a good rationale for having thyroid function as a screening blood test. This is particularly the case in older people with cardiac failure.

12-lead electrocardiography

Most general practitioners should have access to 12-lead electrocardiography. This would be useful for establishing the diagnosis of cardiac failure and for assessing aetiology and arrhythmias. In most cases of cardiac failure the ECG is abnormal. A normal ECG makes it unlikely that the patient has cardiac failure secondary to left ventricular dysfunction since this test has a high sensitivity and a negative predictive value. The ECG should be examined for arrhythmia, the presence of Q waves indicating previous myocardial infarction, T wave abnormalities or ST segment changes indicative of ischaemic heart disease and left ventricular hypertrophy or bundle branch block. If the patient complains of palpitations or dizziness, Holter monitoring or use of a Loop recorder (a device which can be carried by the patient and which may be activated when palpitations or dizziness appears, resulting in a cardiac recording which can assist in diagnosis) may detect paroxysmal arrhythmias. However, the ECG alone will not diagnose cardiac failure.

Chest x-ray

A chest x-ray is also an important investigation in general practice prior to further investigations or specialist referral. This is for detecting cardiac enlargement, pulmonary congestion or pulmonary disease. A good quality postero-anterior film is essential. While a cardiothoracic ratio of over 50% may be helpful, cardiomegaly is dependent upon the severity of haemodynamic disturbance and its duration. An increased cardiothoracic ratio may be due to left ventricular hypertrophy, dilatation of either ventricle or, more rarely, pericardial effusion (pear-shaped heart). Cardiomegaly may be absent in acute left ventricular failure or acute valvular regurgitation.

The presence of pulmonary congestion and cardiomegaly provides useful support for the diagnosis of cardiac failure. There are varying degrees of pulmonary venous congestion. In left ventricular failure, pulmonary venous congestion occurs initially in the upper zones. Further increases in pulmonary venous pressure may result in appearance of fluid in the horizontal fissure and costophrenic angles (Kerley B lines). At higher levels of pulmonary venous pressure, there is an appearance of pulmonary oedema where the lungs are said to have a 'bats wing' appearance. The chest x-ray will often reveal pleural effusions in this situation. These may be bilateral, but if unilateral the right side is more commonly affected. Pulmonary congestion on chest x-ray may be indicative of other disease processes, such as renal impairment, and should not be used in isolation without taking account of the features on history and examination. In older people the chest x-ray often shows unfolding of the aorta and calcification in the aortic wall. Occasionally there may be the appearances of a thoracic aortic aneurysm, valve calcification or a suggestion of left ventricular aneurysm.

Echocardiography is usually necessary for determining the cause of cardiomegaly and for clarifying some of the findings seen on chest x-ray.

Echocardiography

Echocardiography is important for the accurate diagnosis of cardiac failure and should be performed in all patients with suspected heart failure. This is especially true in older people where symptoms and signs may be conflicting. The benefits in older patients are the non-invasive nature of the test which causes minimal distress and results in fewer refusals to have the test performed. While clinical evidence—together with initial screening blood tests, electrocardiography and chest x-ray—provide a major platform for diagnosis of cardiac failure, there is a requirement to furnish objective evidence. The echocardiogram provides the necessary objective assessment of cardiac structure and function. The two-dimensional echocardiogram, coupled with Doppler flow studies, shows whether the primary abnormality is pericardial, myocardial or endocardial and, if myocardial, whether the dysfunction is primarily systolic or diastolic. The echocardiogram allows the quantitative assessment of the dimensions, geometry, thickness and regional motion of the right and left ventricles as well as the qualitative evaluation of pericardial, valvular and vascular structures. This is useful since patients with cardiac failure, particularly older patients, may have more than one cardiac abnormality.

The primary information gained from the echocardiogram is measurement of left ventricular ejection fraction. This is the stroke volume—that is, the difference between end diastolic and end systolic volumes, expressed as a percentage of the left ventricular end diastolic volume. Measurements are less reliable in patients with atrial fibrillation or regional abnormalities in wall motion. Patients with ejection fraction of less than or equal to 40% are generally considered to have systolic dysfunction. The left ventricular ejection fraction is important because of the correlation with outcome and survival in cardiac failure. Lower levels of left ventricular systolic function are associated with reduced survival. The detection of left ventricular systolic dysfunction with echocardiography is important since it may precede clinical or radiological signs.

As previously stated, older patients with cardiac failure may have more than one underlying aetiology or precipitating factor. Echocardiography may also show pericardial or valvular disease and other problems, such as left ventricular aneurysm or intracardiac thrombus. In older patients valvular abnormalities are commonly found. Ejection systolic murmurs are commonly heard and the only way to clearly identify these is by echocardiography. Quite often the cause is found to be calcific aortic sclerosis but aortic stenosis is an important finding because of implications for management or specific pharmacological treatment. Mitral incompetence is commonly seen at echocardiography in cardiac failure patients. This can be either due to intrinsic mitral valve disease or secondary to ventricular dilatation. Two-dimensional echocardiography allows assessment of valvular structure, while Doppler echocardiography permits quantitative assessment of flow across valves and identification of valve stenosis, as well as assessment of right ventricular pressures and presence of pulmonary hypertension. The prevalence of diastolic dysfunction is said to be common in older people. However, while Doppler studies have been used in the measurement of diastolic dysfunction, there is no single reliable echocardiographic measure of diastolic dysfunction.

Colour flow Doppler techniques are sensitive in detecting the direction of blood flow and the presence of valvular incompetence. Access to transoesophageal echocardiography can be helpful. This technique allows detailed assessment of the atria, valves, pulmonary veins and cardiac masses, including valvular vegetations and thrombi. Infective endocarditis does present problems in diagnosis in older people and transoesophageal echocardiography has made a significant difference to diagnosis of this condition. It is slightly more invasive but seems to be acceptable and well tolerated by older patients.

It is clear from the above that echocardiography is the 'gold standard' in diagnosis of cardiac failure in terms of providing the objective evidence required. Ideally this should be available for every patient in whom heart failure is suspected clinically. Clearly many of these patients are older and there will be increasing demand, not least because of demographic predictions. There is clear evidence that intervention strategies in heart failure produce reductions in morbidity, hospitalisations and mortality and are cost effective. There is therefore a need for agreement about the assessment and definitive diagnosis of patients with heart failure, particularly in relation to the role of echocardiography and the availability of this technique to general practitioners.

Other investigations

There are a number of other investigations providing information about the nature and severity of the cardiac abnormality which may be indicated. These are performed more commonly in younger people where the main indications would include where the cause of cardiac failure is unclear.

Radionuclide ventriculograms allow the assessment of the global left and right ventricular function and are useful where echocardiography is not possible or technically difficult. Measurements of ejection fraction, systolic filling rate, diastolic emptying rate and wall motion abnormalities are possible. These studies can also assess myocardial perfusion and the presence or extent of coronary ischaemia.

Where the cause of cardiac failure remains unclear, further testing may be indicated, including exercise tolerance testing, stress studies, ventilation perfusion lung scanning, cardiac catheterisation and coronary angiography. Exercise tolerance testing may include a treadmill test, cycle ergometry or a 6 minute walking test. This is a simple objective measure of functional exercise capacity. Subjects are asked to walk as far as they can over a measured course in a 6 minute period. Respiratory physiological measurements made during exercise are useful and measurement of the upper limit of aerobic exercise tolerance using maximum oxygen consumption is a useful indicator of the severity and prognosis in heart failure. Stress studies employ graded physical exercise or pharmacological stress with agents such as adenosine, dipyridamole or dobutamine. Stress echocardiography is emerging as a useful technique for assessing myocardial reversibility in patients with coronary heart disease. Angiography should be considered in patients with recurrent ischaemic chest pain associated with cardiac failure and in those with evidence of severe reversible ischaemia or hibernating myocardium. Left ventricular angiography can show impairment of function and assess end diastolic pressures while right-sided catheterisation allows assessment of pressures in the right atrium, right ventricle and pulmonary arteries along with pulmonary artery capillary wedge pressure in addition to oxygen saturations.

For older people exercise testing with respiratory physiology can be easily performed and stress tests can also be useful. Angiography and cardiac catheterisation are not performed very often in older patients and particularly not in very old patients.

Management

The therapeutic approach to cardiac failure has undergone considerable change over the past 10 years. For many years management of cardiac failure meant the use of pharmacological and non-pharmacological approaches to relieve symptoms. Nowadays there is focus on prevention of occurrence and progression of cardiac failure, modulation of the progression of asymptomatic left ventricular dysfunction to symptomatic heart failure and a reduction in mortality (Box 24.4). The neurohormonal response to cardiac failure, cytokine responses, renal and peripheral vascular changes, skeletal muscle and lung function changes and retention of sodium and water are all important. In particular the neurohormonal and cytokine activation are linked to the occurrence of cardiac failure, clinical expression and prognosis. Limitation of this activation and reversal of the extracardiac abnormalities are major treatment objectives.

Box 24.4 Aims of treatment

1. **Prevention**
   (a) prevention of disease leading to cardiac dysfunction and heart failure
   (b) prevention of progression to heart failure once cardiac dysfunction is established
2. **Morbidity**
   Maintenance or improvement in quality of life
   (a) Diuretics
   (b) Digoxin
   (c) ACE inhibitors
3. **Mortality**
   Increased duration of life
   (a) ACE inhibitors
   (b) β-blockers
   (c) Oral nitrates + hydralazine
   (d) Spironolactone

Prevention

The primary prevention of disease which leads to cardiac dysfunction and heart failure is a very important issue but is not one which can be addressed in sufficient detail in this chapter. The prevention of cardiac failure must always be a prime objective. It is important where possible to treat potential causes of myocardial damage and reduce the extent of myocardial damage. This is particularly important in the treatment of acute myocardial infarction and hypertension, prevention of reinfarction and modulation of risk factors for coronary heart disease.

When myocardial dysfunction is already present, the first objective is to remove the underlying cause of ventricular dysfunction, if possible. The second objective of modern therapy is to modulate the progression from asymptomatic left ventricular dysfunction to cardiac failure. This is described below.

Non-pharmacological management

See Table 24.2.

Table 24.2 Treatment options

1. General advice	Counselling: symptoms, monitoring of body weight
	Social activity
	Travel
	Vaccination
2. General measures	Diet: obesity, salt, fluid intake
	Smoking
	Alcohol
	Exercise (including training programs)
	Rest (acute heart failure or exacerbations of chronic heart failure)

Education and counselling

Education and counselling are effective, even in older people. Written information should accompany verbal advice. The written information should be in simple straightforward language that is easily understood. There should be a clear explanation about the condition, including exacerbating factors and predisposing conditions, details about symptoms and signs and non-pharmacological as well as pharmacological strategies. It is often very useful to involve relatives or carers in this educative process. Patients should be informed about the importance of drug compliance and it can be very useful to instruct the patient about the value of sudden weight increases and how additional medication can be self-administered to avoid deterioration if this develops. This should also alert the patient to seek advice.

Lifestyle

It is important that patients modify their lifestyle, although social activities should be encouraged so that mental and social isolation are avoided.

Travel

While one does not associate older people with significant amounts of travel, it is clear that greater potential exists for travelling by air and to areas where high temperatures and humidity occur. Long flights may cause problems such as dehydration, leg oedema and risk of thrombosis in severe heart failure. If air travel of this type is necessary, the patient should be advised about fluid intake, use of diuretics and mobility during travel. It is important to warn about the possibility of gastrointestinal upset and the effects of high temperature and humidity on fluid balance and diuretic use.

Immunisation and antibiotic prophylaxis

As well as predisposing to pulmonary infection, cardiac failure can also be exacerbated by this condition. Vaccinations for influenza and pneumococcal disease should be considered in all patients with cardiac failure. Similarly, it may be advisable to treat early with antibiotics where there is any clinical suspicion of pulmonary infection in patients with cardiac failure. Antibiotic prophylaxis for dental and other surgical procedures is mandatory in patients with primary valve disease and prosthetic heart valves.

Obesity

Since excess body mass increases cardiac workload during exercise, weight loss in obese patients should be encouraged. This means encouraging weight reduction to within 10% of optimal body weight.

Nutrition

Patients with cardiac failure are at increased risk from malnutrition as a result of anorexia which may be related to therapy, hepatic congestion or metabolic disturbance. Malabsorption may occur in severe cardiac failure and there may be increased nutritional requirements due to an increase in basal metabolic rate which can rise up to 20%. These can result in a catabolic state where lean muscle mass is reduced, leading to an increase in symptoms and reduced exercise capacity. Cardiac cachexia is a serious development since it is an independent risk factor for mortality. Combined management by a physician and dietician is important.

Salt

While there are no good studies of salt restriction in cardiac failure, it seems that avoidance of a high sodium intake is advisable. Patients should be educated about foods that are high in sodium (see Box 24.5) and cautioned about adding salt to food at the table.

Box 24.5 Foods with a high sodium content

- Bread and biscuits
- Butter and cheese
- Tinned foods
- Ham, bacon, sausages
- Chocolate
- Crisps and salted peanuts

Fluid intake

High fluid intake negates the positive effects of diuretics and can induce hyponatraemia. Generally, it is difficult to be proscriptive about fluid intake in milder degrees of cardiac failure, but in more severe cardiac failure where higher doses of diuretics are needed, fluid restriction of 1.5–2 L daily should be considered; however, in warmer climates this should be assessed.

Exercise training

Exercise training has been shown to benefit patients with cardiac failure. There may be improvement in symptoms, exercise capacity and quality of life. The effects on prognosis are unknown. Patients with stable cardiac failure should be encouraged to participate in a simple exercise program. Specific exercise training needs to be tailored to the appropriate level of the patient's disease and should always be performed under medical guidance. For older people specifically, a low level of endurance activity (such as walking) should be encouraged. However, even in older people an exercise routine that includes walking, cycling or swimming may be appropriate, although patients should be aware of their own limitations. These measures will ensure that physical deconditioning is avoided, with the resultant avoidance of peripheral and central abnormalities and skeletal muscle changes. In patients with acute heart failure or those with exacerbations of chronic heart failure, rest is advisable.

Drug treatment

The management of cardiac failure is aimed at improving quality of life and survival. Some drugs only improve symptoms, while others improve both symptoms and survival. Diuretics and digoxin have been central to the management of cardiac failure for many years. More recently, angiotensin-converting enzyme inhibitors have become an integral part of management because of evidence showing improvements in mortality as well as symptoms. Spironolactone has now been shown to be beneficial in stable cardiac failure, while there has also been an emerging literature about the potential benefits of β-adrenoceptor blockers.

Diuretics

Diuretics are the most effective symptomatic treatment for cardiac failure. They alleviate the sodium retention characteristic of cardiac failure, thereby lowering ventricular filling pressure and improving symptoms of oedema and dyspnoea. Treatment with loop diuretics is usually required, although some patients with very mild heart failure and no renal impairment may be adequately controlled with thiazide diuretics.

The diuretics of choice are loop diuretics, which act on the ascending limb of the loop of Henle and have a rapid onset of action. They are used intravenously in acute cardiac failure (onset 5 minutes) and when used orally will act within 1–2 hours with a duration of effect of 4–6 hours. Loop diuretics often have to be given intravenously in congestive heart failure where there is considerable oedema and problems with absorption. This particularly applies to frusemide, while in the case of bumetanide the pharmacokinetics may allow improved bioavailability. Loop diuretics should be used in moderate doses with careful monitoring of symptoms, body weight and blood chemistry. It is important to monitor for hypokalaemia and potassium supplementation, or potassium-sparing diuretics should be used unless there is renal dysfunction. The potassium-sparing diuretic of choice today should probably be spironolactone. Since all patients with cardiac failure on diuretics are likely to be on an ACE inhibitor, the spironolactone should be added in low dose to this combination and electrolytes monitored (see later).

The use of spironolactone in cardiac failure has recently been highlighted. The importance of aldosterone in heart failure has been overlooked in recent years because angiotensin-converting enzyme (ACE) inhibitor related reductions in angiotensin were thought to eliminate aldosterone production. However, suppression of aldosterone is brief and incomplete, other mechanisms stimulate aldosterone and there is reduced clearance due to liver congestion. In a recently published comparison of spironolactone and placebo added to diuretic and ACE inhibitor in patients with severe heart failure and left ventricular dysfunction, spironolactone improved mortality by 30%, reduced hospitalisation by 35% and improved functional status. This study suggests that spironolactone confers additional benefits to diuretic and ACE inhibitor therapy in patients with severe heart failure when used at doses of 25 mg and does not cause major problems with hyperkalaemia when patients have a serum creatinine of less than 221 mmol/L and potassium less than 5 mmol/L.

Thiazide diuretics act on the cortical-diluting segment of the nephron and are not effective when used alone if glomerular filtration rate is markedly reduced. Where severe chronic congestive cardiac failure is refractory to loop diuretics, thiazide or thiazide-like diuretics (metolazone) can be added. This provides sequential nephron blockade and can promote diuresis. These combinations can produce marked diuresis with associated electrolyte abnormalities and the effects should be carefully monitored. This is easily performed in a hospital setting where the combination may be used every day, but often after satisfactory diuresis and symptom relief has been achieved the doses are reduced and metolazone may be needed only 2 or 3 times weekly. In general practice the use of metolazone should be gradual, starting with low doses and slowly building up dosage and frequency of administration, in keeping with the ability to monitor clinical state and electrolytes in the patient. It has also been shown that the ability to respond to the addition of metolazone is a positive prognostic sign.

ACE inhibitors

Large randomised placebo controlled studies have established that ACE inhibitors prolong survival and reduce progression of cardiac failure in patients with left ventricular dysfunction, in all grades of severity, and also in patients with asymptomatic left ventricular dysfunction. ACE inhibitors have also been shown to be beneficial in patients after myocardial infarction.

ACE inhibitors work by inhibiting production of angiotensin II, a potent vasoconstrictor, and by increasing concentrations of bradykinin by inhibiting its degradation by kininase. Bradykinin may be responsible for ACE induced cough. ACE inhibitors also reduce activity of the sympathetic nervous system. These drugs are effective in all grades of systolic heart failure. This was first shown to be effective for severe heart failure (CONSENSUS I), then mild to moderate heart failure (SOLVD-T, V-HeFT, Munich Study) and finally in asymptomatic left ventricular dysfunction (SOLVD-P). Several studies have shown the benefits of ACE inhibitors after myocardial infarction where mortality is improved in those with impaired systolic function.

It is important to note that the majority of cardiac failure patients are older, a significant percentage have preserved systolic function and that the full age and disease spectrum has probably not been represented in the trials conducted to date. However, from the data available, the older people in the studies seem to have derived the same benefits as those at the younger end of the age spectrum. Studies of older patients with heart failure and preserved systolic function are now starting.

ACE inhibitors are effective and well tolerated in older patients, although care may be needed in initiation and titration. Some patients are at high risk of adverse events (Box 24.6) and treatment under supervision may need to be introduced. In practice this need not mean hospitalisation since supervision can take place in a daycare setting. In general, ACE inhibitors should be introduced at very low doses, followed by a gradual dose escalation to the maximum tolerated maintenance level. Often patients are started on ACE inhibitor therapy and remain on low doses. Based upon trial evidence, this is not appropriate, and patients should have doses increased to the levels shown in clinical trials to reduce morbidity and mortality (e.g. for enalapril 20 mg daily). It is important to measure renal function before and after initiation of treatment. Electrolytes and creatinine should be monitored 1–2 weeks after the start of treatment and at periodic intervals thereafter. The adverse effects of ACE inhibitor therapy include cough, dizziness and deterioration in renal function. Cough is said to be more common in females and older patients with an incidence of 5–15%. It occurs early in therapy, disappears within 1–2 weeks of discontinuing treatment and recurs within days of rechallenge. Older patients with cardiac failure may cough for other reasons. The decision to discontinue therapy should be based upon the severity of the cough and after the benefits of therapy have been adequately explained to the patient.

Box 24.6 Initiation of ACE inhibitors—high-risk patients

- Severe heart failure (NHYA class IV) or decompensated heart failure
- Low systolic blood pressure (< 100 mmHg)
- Resting tachycardia > 100 beats per minute
- Low serum sodium concentration (< 130 mmol/L)
- Other vasodilator treatment
- Severe chronic obstructive airways disease and pulmonary heart disease (cor pulmonale)

Angiotensin receptor antagonists

Angiotensin II type 1 receptor antagonists (AIIRAs) are a recent development in blockade of the renin angiotensin system. These drugs resemble ACE inhibitors in effects but do not produce the cough. An initial comparison of losartan and captopril in older patients with mild to severe cardiac failure (ELITE 1) suggested that losartan had significant benefits in reducing mortality. A follow-up study (ELITE II) did not confirm these findings. AIIRAs should be reserved for use in patients with cardiac failure who cannot tolerate ACE inhibitors.

Hydralazine and oral nitrates

The combination of venous (nitrates) and arterial (hydralazine) dilators was considered useful since venous capacitance and arterial resistance are important determinants of cardiac performance. The combination has been studied in two large-scale trials. In V-HeFt I hydralazine and isosorbide dinitrate decreased mortality by 25–30% compared to prazosin and placebo when each treatment was added to diuretic and digoxin therapy. However, by the end of 6 months only half were taking the full doses of both drugs. In the V-HeFT II trial patients with mild to moderate heart failure were randomised to a combination of hydralazine plus isosorbide dinitrate or enalapril which were added to therapy with digoxin and diuretics. Treatment with enalapril was associated with a 28% lower risk of death at two years compared to the vasodilator combination. However, the vasodilator combination had more favourable effects on exercise tolerance and ejection fraction than the ACE inhibitor. The consensus is that this vasodilator combination should be considered only in those who cannot tolerate an ACE inhibitor.

Calcium antagonists

Quite often patients with cardiac failure suffer from angina and the issue of therapy with calcium antagonists arises. The calcium antagonists have different properties. There is evidence that amlodipine and felodipine are neutral in cardiac failure, or that they may be beneficial in non-ischaemic dilated cardiomyopathy. On the other hand, diltiazem and verapamil have negatively inotropic and chronotropic properties and thus have a potential to exacerbate cardiac failure. In any setting where the patient has decompensated heart failure, calcium antagonists of any type are better withdrawn as the acute situation is treated.

Digoxin

Digoxin usage for heart failure varies internationally. Digoxin has positive inotropic effects but also may decrease central sympathetic outflow and suppress renin secretion from the kidneys. Several small trials have shown that, when administered over 1–3 months, digoxin can improve symptoms, quality of life, functional capacity and exercise tolerance in patients with mild to moderate heart failure. The RADIANCE and PROVED trials showed that withdrawal of digoxin in patients with chronic heart failure was associated with worsening heart failure and increased hospital admission rates. The long-term effects of digoxin were studied in the DIG trial, where patients with mild to moderate heart failure were randomised to placebo or digoxin, which were given in addition to diuretics and an ACE inhibitor for 28–58 months (mean 37 months). Treatment with digoxin did not affect survival but reduced hospitalisation for heart failure by 28%.

Digoxin is invaluable in patients with atrial fibrillation and co-existent heart failure. Digoxin is also useful in patients with chronic heart failure secondary to left ventricular systolic impairment, in sinus rhythm, who remain symptomatic despite optimal doses of diuretics and ACE inhibitors. Particular thought should be given to the initiation of treatment with digoxin in older people. The dosage may need to be reduced, particularly where there is renal dysfunction. Consideration must also be given in the setting of some concomitant therapy where interaction may occur. In general 125 μg is the usual maintenance dose, except where there is impaired renal function, in which case 62.5 μg should be used. Electrolytes should be monitored and serum levels may also be required, particularly where the patient becomes unwell for any reason. Digoxin toxicity is often difficult to diagnose in older people and a high index of suspicion is needed. Often digoxin should be stopped while the clinical situation is evaluated.

The study of alternative inotropes in heart failure has been consistently met with disappointing results when these drugs are used over the long term.

β-adrenoceptor blocking drugs

The traditional teaching about β-blockers has been that they should be avoided in heart failure. In recent times, however, that attitude has been changed as a result of a number of trials. There is a body of evidence which suggests that β-blocking drugs are useful in patients with chronic stable heart failure resulting from left ventricular systolic dysfunction. These studies have shown that β-blocker therapy is well tolerated, has improved mortality and is associated with improved morbidity in terms of progressive heart failure and numbers of hospitalisations.

Each of the recently reported studies of β-blockade in chronic heart failure is characterised by:

1. inclusion of patients with primarily mild to moderate heart failure;
2. inclusion of patients with stable heart failure; and
3. a slow dose titration procedure.

The studies did not include significant numbers of older patients which is a major weakness. It is also important to note that β-blocker therapy was added to ACE inhibitor and diuretic therapy. The drugs studied were bisoprolol, metoprolol and carvedilol. In all studies therapy was initiated at low dose with subsequent slow dose titration over a 2–3 month period. These regimens have implications for clinical practice. Patients should be reviewed at regular intervals over a short period of time. Problems arise if there is cardiac decompensation during this period. It is suggested that β-blockade should be initiated under the care of individual physicians with an interest in heart failure and experience in the use of β-adrenoceptor blockers in this situation. For now, it is not recommended that β-blockade is initiated in primary care.

Anti-arrhythmic treatment

For patients with atrial fibrillation, restoration and long-term maintenance of sinus rhythm is an important objective. Digoxin has been discussed and will control ventricular rate in patients with chronic atrial fibrillation. Amiodarone can be added in resistant cases. Where there has been recent onset of atrial fibrillation, treatment with amiodarone increases the long-term success of cardioversion.

Ventricular arrhythmias are a common cause of death in severe heart failure. Patients should be monitored carefully for electrolyte disturbance, digoxin toxicity, drugs causing electrical instability (antidepressants, anti-arrhythmics) and recurrent myocardial ischaemia. Amiodarone is effective for the symptomatic control of ventricular arrhythmias in chronic heart failure and should probably be reserved for patients who also have symptomatic ventricular arrhythmias. Studies are ongoing in relation to the role of implantable defibrillators.

A summary of drug management in chronic heart failure is given in Table 24.3.

Antithrombotic treatment

The incidence of thromboembolism and stroke is higher in patients with heart failure where there is atrial and left ventricular dilatation and severe left ventricular dysfunction. Although studies are in progress, anticoagulation should be considered where there is atrial fibrillation, mobile ventricular thrombus and severe cardiac impairment. Heart failure in association with atrial fibrillation gives a high risk of thromboembolism, which is reduced by long-term warfarin treatment.

Hospital referral

There are two main roles for hospitals in management of chronic heart failure: first, to help make a correct diagnosis and, second, to initiate and change therapy, some of which may not be available to or appropriate for the general practitioner. The selection of patients who should be referred to hospital is dependent to a degree upon the facilities available in the general practice and the range of investigations to which the GP has open access. The majority of patients can probably be seen by a general physician, although certain patients may benefit from direct referral to a cardiologist. A guide on consideration for specialist referral is shown in Box 24.7.

Prognosis

The prognosis of heart failure, particularly in its most severe form, compares unfavourably with many forms of cancer, and there is considerable morbidity associated with the syndrome. Follow-up data from Framingham (16 years) shows that within 2 years of diagnosis 37% of men and 38% of women had died, with the corresponding figures at 6 years

Table 24.3 Summary of drug management in chronic heart failure

Drug class	Potential therapeutic role
Diuretics	Improves congestive symptoms Spironolactone improves survival in severe (NYHA class IV) heart failure
ACE inhibitors	Improves symptoms, exercise capacity and survival in patients with asymptomatic and symptomatic systolic dysfunction
Digoxin	Improves symptoms and exercise capacity and reduces hospital admissions
AIIRAs	Useful in treatment of symptomatic heart failure in patients intolerant of ACE inhibitors
Nitrates and hydralazine	Improves survival in symptomatic patients intolerant of ACE inhibitors or AIIRAs
β-blockers	Improves symptoms and survival in stable patients already receiving ACE inhibitors
Amiodarone	Prevents arrhythmias in patients with symptomatic ventricular arrhythmias

Box 24.7 Considerations for referral to hospital specialist

- Patients in whom the diagnosis is in doubt, or when the aetiology of heart failure is not known
- Patients with severe uncontrolled heart failure, or when the condition is rapidly progressive
- Patients with a potentially reversible condition (e.g. valvular heart disease)
- All young patients with chronic heart failure

being 82% and 67%, respectively. The prognosis of the various grades of heart failure is shown in Table 24.4. The mortality in the placebo group of the CONSENSUS study was 44% at 6 months. Approximately half the patients who die of heart failure die suddenly, with many of the remaining dying because of progression of the heart failure. The reasons for sudden cardiac deaths are not clear, although it is recognised that the disturbance of electrolyte levels and high levels of neurohormones found in heart failure may predispose to malignant arrhythmias. It is therefore important to intervene in patients to reduce these statistics. The therapies which can have an impact are detailed above. The evidence on interventions that reduce morbidity and mortality is clear. This must be applied to patients diagnosed with heart failure.

Table 24.4 Prognosis related to severity of heart failure

NYHA grade	Mortality at 5 years (%)
I	10
II	10–20
III	60–70
IV	70–90

Bibliography and further reading

Cohn, J. N., Archibald, D. G., Ziesche, S., Franciosa, J. A., Harston, W. E., Tristani, F. E. et al. (1986), 'Effect of vasodilator therapy on mortality in chronic congestive heart failure: Results of the Veterans Administration Cooperative Study', *The New England Journal of Medicine*, 314, pp. 1547–52.

Cohn, J. N., Johnson, G., Ziesche, S., Cobb, F., Francis, G., Tristani, F. et al. (1991), 'A comparison of enalapril with hydralazine-isosorbide dinitrate in the treatment of chronic congestive heart failure', *The New England Journal of Medicine*, 325, pp. 303–10.

Cohn, J. N., Ziesche, S., Smith, R., Anand, I., Dunkman, W. B., Loeb, H. et al. (1997), 'Effect of the calcium antagonist felodipine as supplementary vasodilator therapy in patients with chronic heart failure treated with enalapril. V-HeFT III', *Circulation*, 96, pp. 856–63.

'Consensus recommendations for the management of chronic heart failure' (1999), *American Journal of Cardiology*, 83(2A), pp. 1A–38.

CONSENSUS Trial Study Group (1987), 'Effects of enalapril on mortality in severe congestive heart failure. Results of the North Scandinavian enalapril survival study', *The New England Journal of Medicine*, 316, pp. 1429–35.

Digitalis Investigation Group (1997), 'The effect of digoxin on mortality and morbidity in patients with heart failure', *The New England Journal of Medicine*, 336, pp. 525–33.

Ho, K. K., Pinsky, J. L., Kannel, W. B. & Levy, D. (1993), 'The epidemiology of heart failure: The Framingham study', *Journal of American College of Cardiology*, 22, pp. 6–13A.

Kleber, F. X., Niemoller, L. & Doering, W. (1992), 'Impact of converting enzyme inhibition on progression of chronic heart failure: Results of the Munich Mild Heart Failure Trial', *British Heart Journal*, 67, pp. 289–96.

Packer, M. (1992), 'The neurohormonal hypothesis: A theory to explain the mechanisms of disease progression in heart failure', *Journal of American College of Cardiology*, 20, pp. 248–54.

Packer, M., Georghiade, M., Young, J. B., Costantini, P. J., Adams, K. F., Cody, R. J. et al. (1993), 'Withdrawal of digoxin from patients with chronic heart failure treated with angiotensin converting enzyme inhibitors', *The New England Journal of Medicine*, 329, pp. 1–7.

Packer, M., O'Connor, C. M., Ghali, J. K., Pressler, M. L., Carson, P. E., Belkin, R. L. et al. (1996), 'Effect of amlodipine on morbidity and mortality in severe chronic heart failure', *The New England Journal of Medicine*, 335, pp. 1107–14.

Pitt, B., Segal, R., Martinez, F. A., Meurers, G., Cowley, A. J., Thomas, I. et al. (1997), 'Randomised trial of losartan versus captopril in patients over 65 with heart failure', *Lancet*, 349, pp. 747–52.

Pitt, B., Zannad, F., Remme, W. J., Cody, R., Castaigne, A., Perez, A. et al. (1999), 'The effect of spironolactone on morbidity and mortality in patients with severe heart failure', *The New England Journal of Medicine*, 341, pp. 709–17.

The SOLVD Investigators (1991), 'Effects of enalapril on survival in patients with reduced left ventricular ejection fractions and congestive heart failure', *The New England Journal of Medicine*, 325, pp. 293–302.

The SOLVD Investigators (1992), 'Effects of enalapril on mortality and the development of heart failure in asymptomatic patients with reduced left ventricular ejection fractions', *The New England Journal of Medicine*, 327, pp. 685–91.

Squire, I. B. & Barnett, D. B. (2000), 'The rational use of β-adrenoceptor blockers in the treatment of heart failure. The changing face of an old therapy', *British Journal of Clinical Pharmacology*, 49, pp. 1–10.

The Task Force on Heart Failure of the European Society of Cardiology (1995), 'Guidelines for the diagnosis of heart failure', *European Heart Journal*, 16, pp. 741–51.

The Task Force of the Working Group on Heart Failure of the European Society of Cardiology (1997), 'The treatment of heart failure', *European Heart Journal*, 18, pp. 736–53.

Uretsky, B. F., Young, J. B., Shahidi, F. E., Yellen, L. G., Harrison, M. C., Jolly, M. K. et al. (1993), 'Randomized study assessing the effect of digoxin withdrawal in patients with mild to moderate chronic congestive heart failure: Results of the PROVED trial', *Journal of American College of Cardiology*, 22, pp. 955–62.

Chapter 25
Cardiac arrhythmias

EHUD I. GOLDHAMMER

Basic guidelines for rhythm analysis

A systematic approach to the analysis of abnormal cardiac rhythms will assist in their identification and management. However, prior to any rhythm analysis one should be acquainted with the basic electrocardiogram (ECG) features and these basic features should be analysed systematically as well.

P wave morphology

- The P wave contour is usually smooth, positive and monophasic. There are two exceptions: in lead V1 it is usually biphasic and in lead aVR it is negative.
- Its duration is normally less than 0.12 sec.
- Its amplitude is normally less than 0.25 mV in all leads.
- The P wave reflects atrial activation.

The PR interval

- This interval measures the time required for the depolarisation wave to be propagated and conducted from the atria through the atrioventricular (AV) node to the ventricular myocardium adjacent to the fibres of the Purkinje network.
- The normal PR duration is 0.10–0.20 sec. In childhood it is somewhat shorter (0.10–0.12 sec), somewhat longer in adolescence (0.12–0.16 sec), and in the elderly, 0.14–0.20 sec.
- The PR interval varies with the heart rate, being shorter at faster rates and longer with slower rates according to sympathetic/parasympathetic dominance.

QRS complex

- The QRS complex reflects the depolarisation of the right and left ventricular myocardium.
- The initial small negative deflection of the QRS complex is the Q wave that reflects the initial depolarisation wave of the interventricular septum from left to right. In all the 'left' leads—I, aVL, V5 and V6—these small negative deflections are easily detected, while in the right precordial lead V1, a small R wave is the equivalent of this normal septal Q wave.
- Q wave duration is normally less than 0.03 sec. It may be enlarged following myocardial infarction, in ventricular hypertrophy or in dilatation.

- The R and S waves reflect the electrical activity progressing to both ventricles, from the thinner right ventricle to the thicker left ventricle. The positive R wave normally increases in amplitude from leads V1 to V4.
- The duration of the QRS complex (= QRS interval) is 0.08–0.10 sec (= 2–2.5 small squares of the ECG tracing). The amplitude has wide normal limits. Amplitudes as much as 30 mm or more, or less than 5 mm (0.5 mV) in any of the limb leads, and no more than 10 mm (1.0 mV) in any of the precordial leads are considered abnormal.

The T wave and the QT interval

- The T wave reflects normal repolarisation of the ventricles. Its duration is not usually measured, but is instead included in the QT interval. T waves do not normally exceed 5 mm in any limb lead, or 10 mm in any precordial lead.
- The QT interval (Q wave to the end of the T wave) varies with the heart rate, gender and even time of day. There are several methods of correcting for heart rate; the simplest is by Bazett's formula, in which QT_c is the corrected length of the QT interval:

$$QT_c = \frac{QT}{\sqrt{R\text{–}R\ interval}}$$

- The normal QT interval is 350–430 msec, and whatever the rate, a QT interval of greater than 440 is probably pathological.

Systematic approach

Following the general analysis of the basic ECG features, the next step is a simple systematic approach to rhythm analysis (Box 25.1).

Box 25.1 A systematic approach to rhythm analysis

The P wave

- Are P waves present?
- What is the P wave rate?
- Are they normal P waves?
- If atrial activity is present but P waves are of different morphology, are they ectopic P waves?
- Is there evidence of retrograde conduction to the atria; that is, negative P waves in leads II, III and aVF?
- Is there atrial flutter ('saw-toothed line') or fibrillation?

QRS complex

- Is the QRS rhythm regular?
- What is the QRS rate?
- Is the QRS complex narrow (< 0.12 sec) or wide (> 0.12 sec)? A narrow QRS practically guarantees a supraventricular origin.

The P–QRS relationship

- Is the P wave related to the QRS?
- Is each P wave followed by a QRS?
- Is the PR interval normal and constant?

Intervals

- Is the PR interval within normal limits?
- Is the PR interval variable?
- Are the PP and RR intervals variable?
- Is the QT interval, corrected for heart rate, within normal limits?
- Is it variable?

Rate, regularity and rhythm

Sinus rhythm is the only normal sustained rhythm of the heart and has a regular rate of 60–100 beats per minute. It may be slightly irregular with variable RR intervals. The variability in heart rate is due to changes in autonomic balance: when parasympathetic tone dominates, variability is pronounced, and when sympathetic tone prevails, variability is reduced. Minor variations in the autonomic balance are produced by the phases of the respiratory cycle; the sinus rate accelerates with inspiration and slows with expiration. The term 'sinus arrhythmia' or 'respiratory arrhythmia' is used to describe this normal variation in heart rate.

It is a common normal finding in children, young adults and athletes, and becomes less evident with increasing age. It is lost in conditions such as diabetic neuropathy, congestive heart failure and in post-extensive myocardial infarction patients.

The normal rhythm is called 'sinus rhythm' to indicate that the site of formation of the initial electrical impulses, the depolarisation wave, is the sinoatrial (SA) node. Below 60 beats/min the rhythm is called 'sinus bradycardia', and above 100 beats/min 'sinus tachycardia'.

Determination of cardiac rate and regularity requires understanding of the grid markings of the ECG paper. There are thin vertical lines every 1 mm and thick lines every 5 mm. At the usual ECG recording speed of 25 mm/sec, the thin lines are at 0.04 sec (40 msec) intervals, and the thick lines at 0.2 sec (200 msec or 1/5 sec). At the usual calibration of 10 mm/mV, the thin line indicates 0.1 mV increments and the thick lines 0.5 mV increments. It is most convenient to select the most prominent ECG waveform, generally the R wave that begins on a thick line, and then count the number of large squares before the same waveform of the next following cycle recurs. Thus, if 2 consecutive QRS complexes are separated by 2 thick lines (= 1 large square, 0.2 sec), then the cardiac rate is 60/0.2 = 300 beats/min; if they are separated by 3 thick lines (2 large squares, 0.4 sec), then the rate is 60/0.4 = 150 beats/min and, similarly, being separated by 4 thick lines (3 large squares, 0.6 sec), then the rate is 60/0.6 = 100 beats/min, by 5 thick lines (four large squares, 0.8 sec), the rate is 60/0.8 = 75 beats/min, and so on.

Sinus bradycardia

Sinus bradycardia is a regular sinus rhythm with a P wave rate below 60 beats/min. The P wave maintains its normal configuration. Sinus bradycardia ranges from a benign asymptomatic physiological adjustment in heart rate to pathological symptomatic expression of sinus node dysfunction.

The physiological form refers in general to exercise training effect or sleep, and the pathological form refers to hypothyroidism, hypothermia, jaundice, raised intracranial pressure, acute inferior myocardial infarction and drug effects (e.g. digitalis, amiodarone, verapamil, diltiazem, β-blockers).

Sinus tachycardia

Sinus tachycardia is a regular sinus rhythm at a P wave rate above 100 beats/min. Sinus tachycardia is the appropriate response of the circulatory system to exercise, excitement, fright, anaemia, pregnancy, hypotension and loss of circulatory volume. It may also be a compensatory mechanism to reduce cardiac stroke volume in congestive heart failure. It is a common, albeit not specific, clinical sign of, for example, phaeochromocytoma or pulmonary embolism.

Sinus tachycardia is often symptomatic, and 'palpitation' is the common complaint attributed to it. Usually the relationship of such palpitations to a precipitating cause is obvious, and the individual, unless he is concerned about the problem, does not feel the need to seek medical advice.

Maximal sympathetic stimulation can increase sinus rate to 200 beats/min and, rarely, to 220 beats/min in younger individuals. The rate rarely exceeds 160 beats/min in non-exercising adults and 140 beats/min in the elderly. The PR interval is shorter in sinus tachycardia than during normal sinus rhythm.

Ectopic beats

An impulse arising outside the sinus node (in the atria, atrioventricular junction or ventricles) which is premature in the cardiac cycle is defined as an ectopic beat or extrasystole or premature contraction.

The interval between the ectopic beat and the preceding beats is defined as the 'coupling interval'. An ectopic beat is premature by definition, so the coupling interval is shorter than the RR interval (cycle length) of the basic rhythm.

If the premature beat does not disturb the sinus rhythm but merely takes the place of a conducted beat, then the interval from the conducted beat prior to the premature beat to the following conducted beat will be equal to 2 sinus cycles. This interval is termed a 'compensatory pause' because the cycle following the premature beat compensates for its prematurity, and the sinus rhythm resumes on schedule. A complete compensatory pause is present when the sum of the coupling interval and the compensatory pause is equal to twice the basic sinus cycle length; it is characteristic of a ventricular ectopic beat that fails to conduct retrogradely to the atria, thus leaving the sinus node undisturbed. An incomplete compensatory pause occurs when the sinus node is discharged early by an ectopic beat or by a retrogradely conducted ventricular ectopic beat.

Atrial premature beats

The usual atrial premature beat (APB) or atrial premature contraction (APC) has three basic features (see Figure 25.1):

1. There is a premature P wave with abnormal morphology (labelled 'P').
2. The QRS complex of the premature beat is similar to that of the conducted sinus beats.
3. It has a following cycle that is less than compensatory.

It should be noted that atrial ectopies arising early in the cardiac cycle may find part of the conduction system still partially or completely refractory. If the atrioventricular node is completely refractory, then the ectopic P is not followed by a QRS complex. The 'blocked APB' is the most common cause of a pause interrupting regular sinus rhythm encountered in clinical settings. If a bundle branch, usually the right, is refractory, then a phasic aberrant ventricular conduction occurs. The QRS complex following the ectopic P wave shows a wide, bundle branch block pattern, simulating a ventricular premature beat (see Figure 25.2).

The duration of the refractory period of the bundle branches is proportional to the duration of the preceding RR interval. Aberration may occur when a short RR interval follows a long RR interval. This is termed 'Ashman's phenomenon' and is frequently observed in atrial fibrillation.

Premature beats, either atrial or ventricular, can appear singly or in pairs (couplets) (see Figure 25.3); 3 or more ectopic complexes in rapid succession over 100/min is, by definition, tachycardia. The ectopic beat may come and go randomly, or can constantly or episodically appear as bigeminy, trigeminy or quadrigeminy, so that every second, third, or fourth complex, respectively, is a premature beat (see Figure 25.4).

The clinical significance and management of APBs

APBs occur frequently in normal individuals and usually do not require treatment. They are frequent in thyrotoxicosis and accompany the usual drug treatment of hypothyroidism, in patients with mitral valve prolapse, in pericarditis, in all cardiac conditions associated with atrial distension, elevated ventricular filling pressures, and congestive heart failure.

In normal individuals removal of the inciting factors, such as coffee, cigarettes, alcohol and mental stress, is generally sufficient. In cardiac

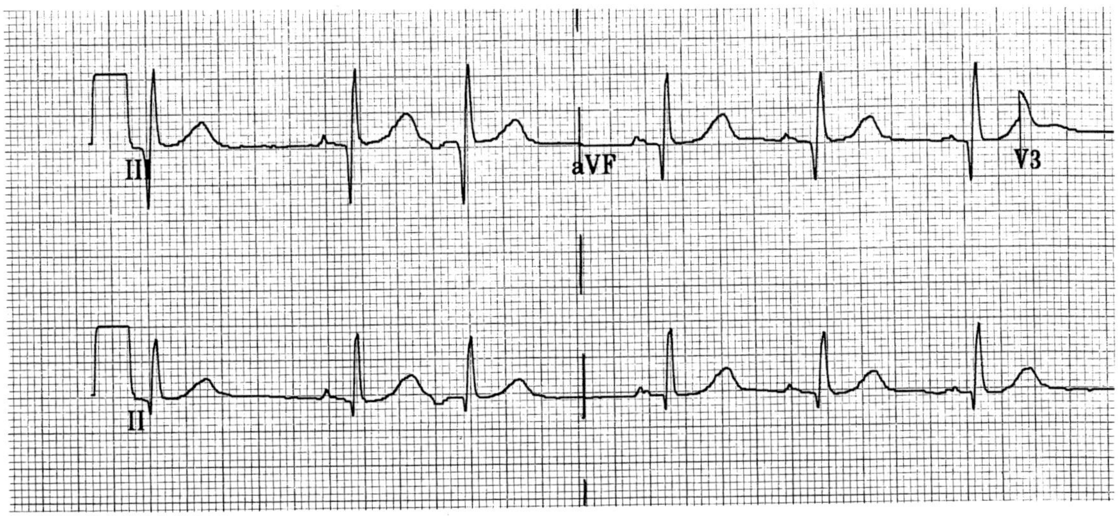

Figure 25.1 An atrial premature beat. The third QRS complex is premature and is preceded by a P wave of different morphology. The QRS morphology and vector are identical to the normal sinus beats

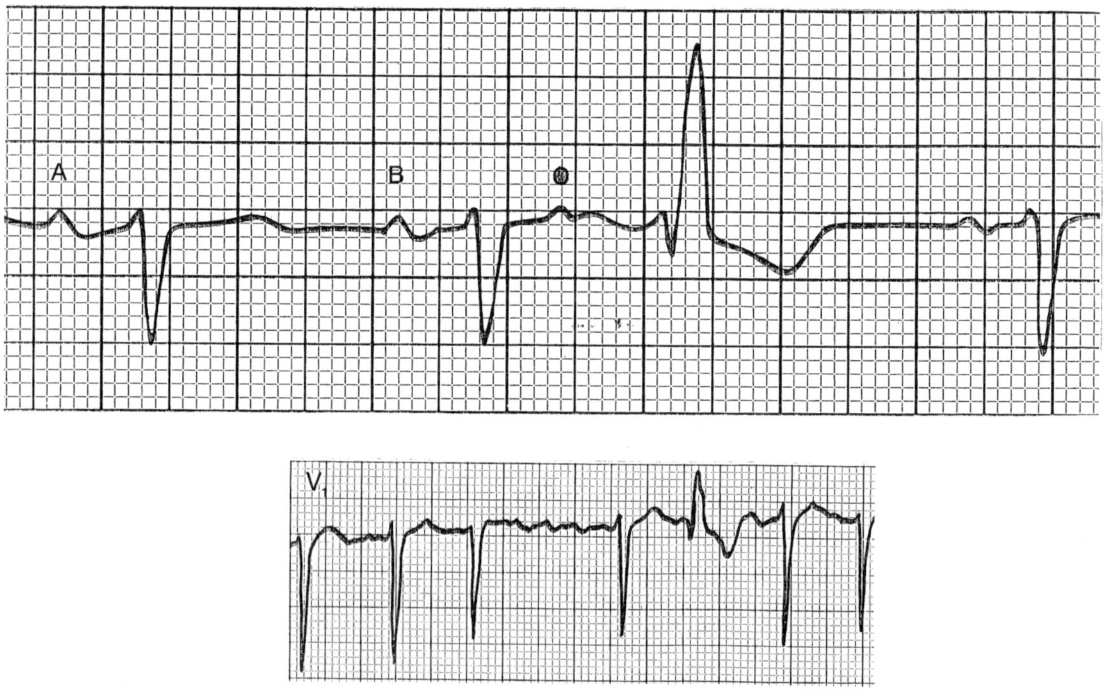

Figure 25.2 Aberrant conduction of an atrial premature beat with RBBB pattern (marked with a dot), and aberrant conduction in the settings of atrial fibrillation (Ashman's phenomenon)

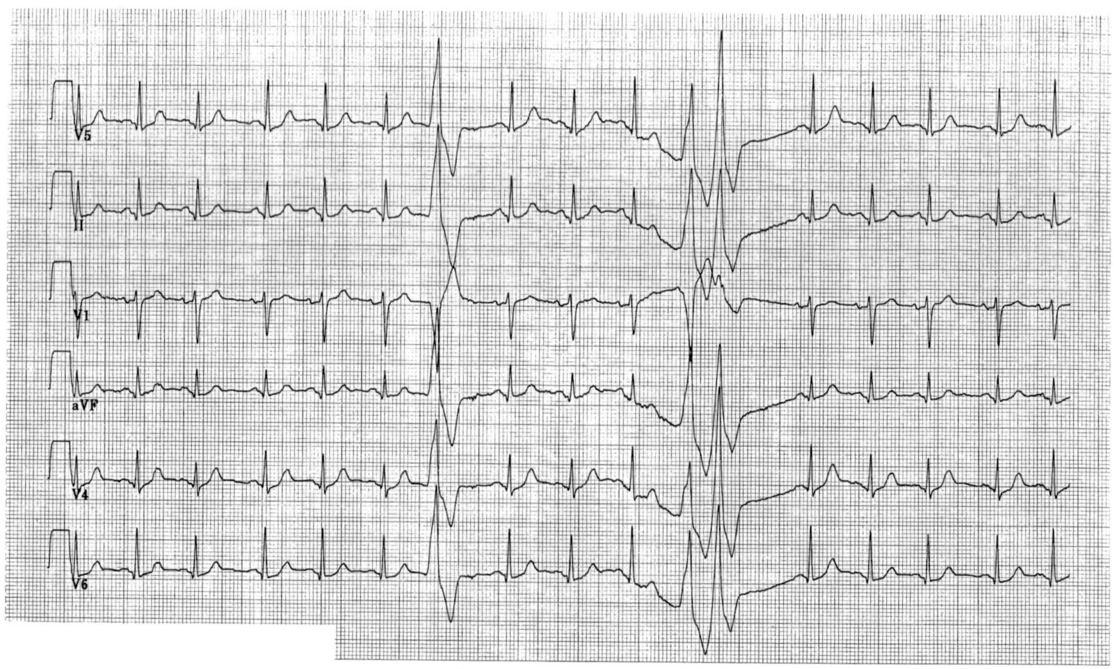

Figure 25.3 A single ventricular premature beat and a couplet of VPBs

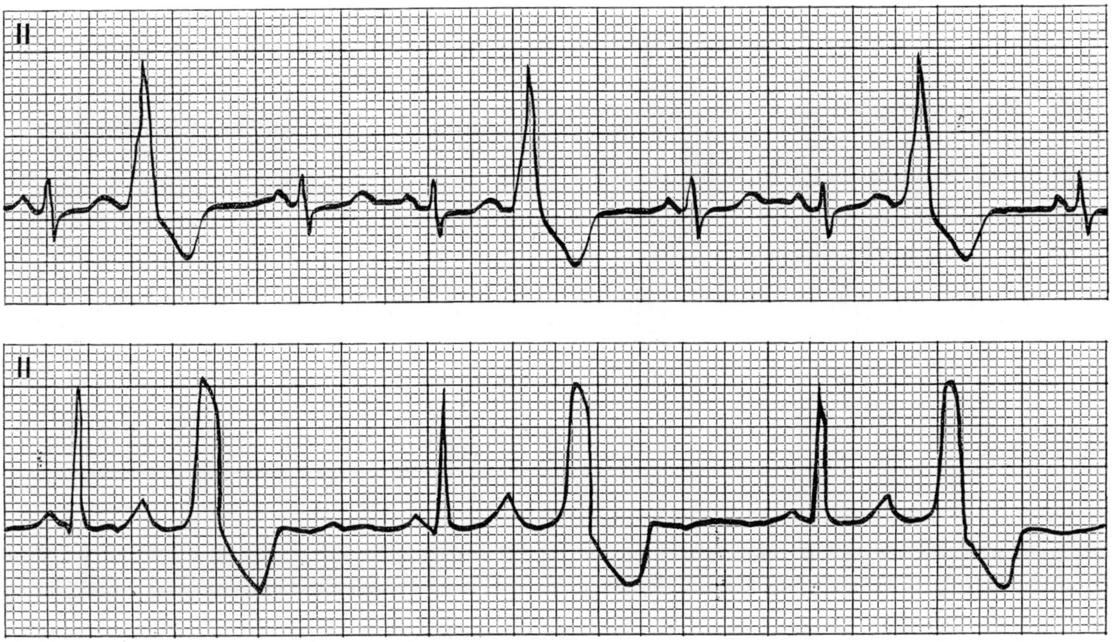

Figure 25.4 Ventricular bigeminy and trigeminy

patients an adequate treatment of the underlying disease is required for the eradication of the ectopic beats. By improving the underlying disease, diuretics, ACE-inhibitors, β-blockers and digoxin lead to the diminution and disappearance of APBs. Conventional antiarrhythmic drugs (except for the β-blockers), even though they are potentially effective, are not indicated or recommended. The only exclusion is in patients with the Wolf-Parkinson-White (WPW) syndrome in whom APBs may induce supraventricular tachycardia and atrial fibrillation, which may in turn induce ventricular fibrillation! The drug of choice in these patients is amiodarone.

Supraventricular tachyarrhythmias

Supraventricular tachycardias (SVTs) include all tachyarrhythmias that originate above the bifurcation of the bundle of His.

Any type of tachyarrhythmia, whether supraventricular or ventricular, is initiated and sustained by one or two mechanisms:

1. re-entry circuit
2. enhanced automaticity.

For re-entry to occur, several conditions must be met. Firstly, there must exist an anatomical substrate of cardiac tissue with certain electrical properties in which re-entry may occur. Secondly, the loop of re-entry (re-entrant loop) should comprise 2 limbs of excitable tissue with electrical continuity but with different conduction velocities and refractoriness.

One limb should have a slow conduction velocity and a short refractory period, and the other limb a fast conduction velocity with a long refractory period. The longitudinal dissociation formed by the different electrophysiological properties leads to a unidirectional block that the excitation wave front must encounter (see Figure 25.5). Thirdly, the excitation wave front must be able to circulate around the central area, focus, of the block.

Let us assume that the re-entry loop is entirely within the AV node; normally the conduction is anterograde (forward) in both limbs of such a pathway, but an anterograde impulse may pass normally down one and be blocked in the other (due to a longer refractory period). From the point

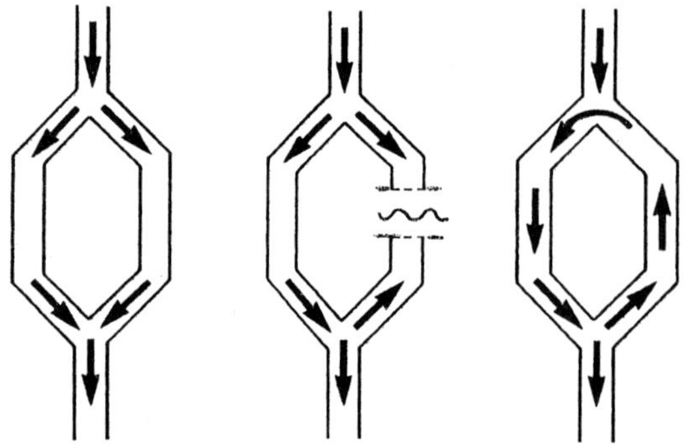

Figure 25.5 Re-entry loop

at which the pathways rejoin, the depolarisation wave can spread retrogradely (backwards) up the abnormal branch. If it arrives when that pathway is no more refractory to conduction, it can then pass right around the circuit and reactivate it. Thus, a circular re-entry pathway is set, around which depolarisation reverberates, causing a tachycardia.

The re-entry loop may be in the SA node itself, in the atria, in the AV node and in the AV node plus an atrioventricular bypass tract (Kent bundle in WPW syndrome). Depending on the loop's size, there may be micro and macro re-entry loops.

Enhanced automaticity occurs whenever an atrial or ventricular focus gains the ability that is normally reserved only for the specialised cardiac cells to achieve spontaneous depolarisation. Such a focus functions then as a 'pacemaker', which may fire at high rates.

How can one distinguish between re-entrant and enhanced automaticity supraventricular tachycardia? Table 25.1 lists the distinguishing features of each.

SVTs are categorised into three groups, based on duration: paroxysmal (PSVT), persistent and chronic. Arrhythmias that are paroxysmal in onset and offset tend to be recurrent and of short duration (seconds to hours). Those that are persistent are paroxysmal as well but last for longer periods of time (days or weeks) and tend to be recurrent. Usually they are associated with drug toxicity (digitalis), electrolyte disturbances and chronic obstructive pulmonary disease (COPD). Chronic SVTs do not revert spontaneously and often fail to revert with attempted medical and electrical cardioversion.

Table 25.1 Distinguishing features of re-entry and enhanced automaticity supraventricular tachycardia

Re-entry	Enhanced automaticity
Common	Less common
Paroxysmal	'Non-paroxysmal', sustained
Initiated by an ectopic beat	Warm-up phenomenon (gradual increase to the maximal rate)
Sudden onset and sudden cessation	
Relatively higher atrial rates	Relatively lower atrial rate

PSVT due to AV nodal re-entry

PSVT due to AV nodal re-entry (see Figure 25.6(a) and (b)) is characterised by an abrupt onset and offset, and usually has a narrow QRS complex without clearly discernible P waves. The rate is usually in the range of 160–190/min. When a pre-existing bundle branch block is present, the tachycardia will reflect the pre-existing pattern; however, a functional rate dependent BBB pattern (LBBB or RBBB) may also occur.

PSVT due to AV nodal re-entry is well tolerated by normal, healthy individuals. Usually the only complaints are palpitations, 'heart is running away' and polyuria following termination of the tachycardia. Polyuria is due to a significant increase in cardiac output secondary to an increase in heart rate in an individual with normal systolic myocardial function. Rest and sedation vagotonic manoeuvres (e.g. carotid sinus massage) are simple ways of reverting acute episodes. However, when ischaemic heart disease, hypertrophic obstructive cardiomyopathy (HOCM; idiopathic hypertrophic subaortic stenosis) or mitral stenosis co-exist, then it may be poorly tolerated and requires prompt intervention. Intravenous adenosine, verapamil, digoxin or β-blockers are equally effective. Adenosine, 6 mg IV, followed by one or two 12 mg boluses if

(a)

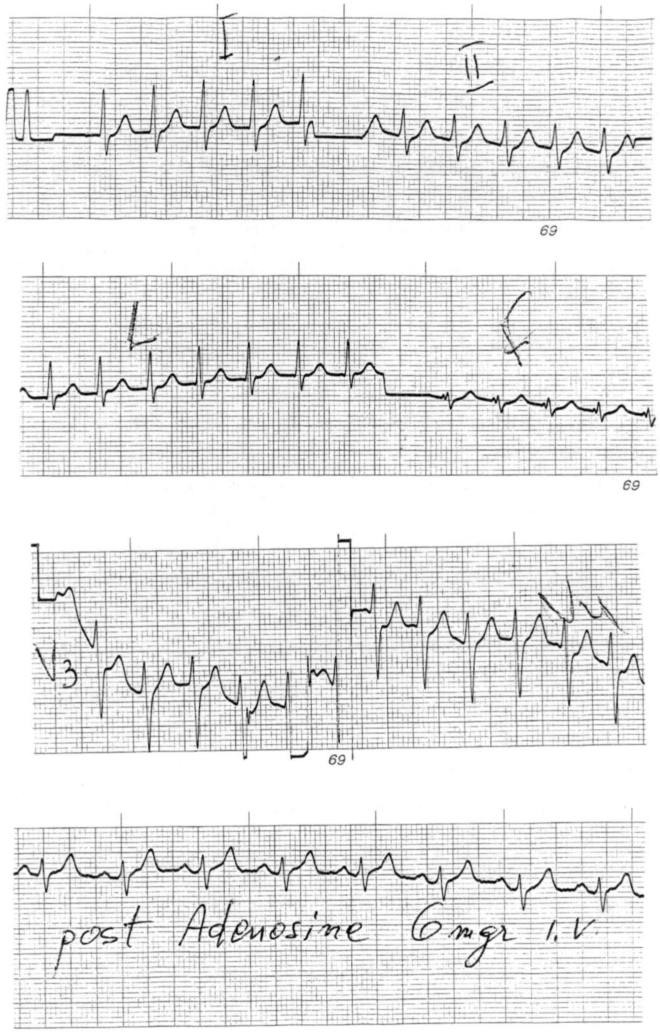

(b)

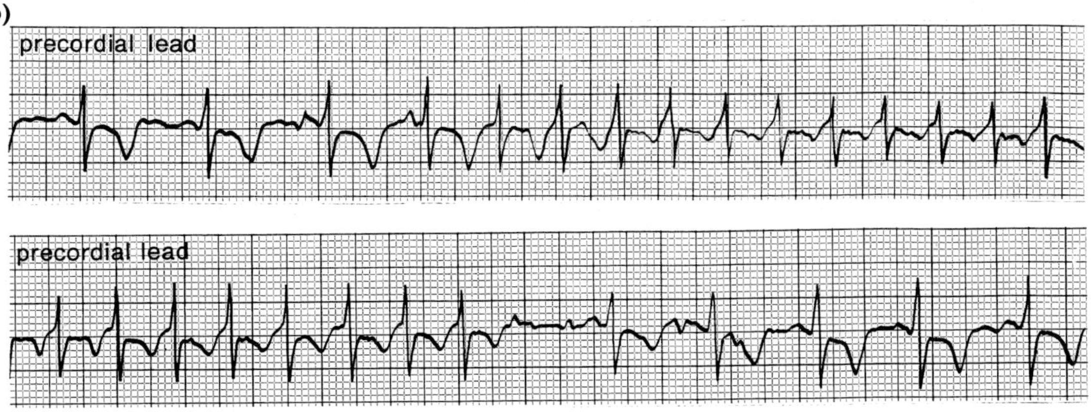

Figure 25.6 (a) and (b) Two examples of PSVT

necessary, is an effective and safe approach, and due to its very short duration of action and lack of negative inotropic effect, it is considered the preferred approach for treatment. If long-term control of recurrent PSVT due to AV nodal re-entry with pharmacological therapy fails, then catheter ablation, radiofrequency ablation (RFA), surgical techniques or electronic antitachycardia pacing devices are used.

PSVT due to WPW syndrome

In PSVT due to WPW syndrome, the re-entry pathway consists of the AV node and an accessory extranodal bypass tract (Kent bundle).

It may occur in a concealed form, in which the standard ECG is normal during sinus rhythm because of the inability of the bypass tract to conduct in the antegrade direction. It can conduct only in a retrograde direction (ventricle to atria), so ventricular pre-excitation cannot occur. It may be an overt, not concealed or 'revealed' form; in such a case it is capable of bidirectional conduction. Antegrade 1:1 conduction through the bypass tract facilitates very rapid ventricular rates that may exceed 300 beats/min in atrial fibrillation, with possible degeneration to ventricular fibrillation.

A premature atrial beat may be blocked at the accessory tract and conduct antegradely down the normal pathway, ultimately entering the accessory tract in the retrograde direction, re-entering the atrium to establish a circus movement; the re-entrant tachycardia is termed 'orthodromic'. In this case, due to the use of the normal pathway for ventricular activation, the typical delta wave of WPW is lost and the QRS complex is normal and narrow.

A shorter refractory period in the accessory tract leads to a block of the initiating atrial premature beat in the normal pathway, with antegrade conduction down the accessory tract and then retrograde conduction to the normal AV nodal pathway to initiate an antidromic tachycardia. The QRS complex is wide, having the characteristics of a ventricular complex originating near the insertion site of the accessory bypass tract. There is an LBBB pattern when the tract is right-sided and a RBBB pattern when it is left-sided.

Procainamide, disopyramide, quinidine, amiodarone and β-blockers may be used to convert re-entrant PSVT due to WPW. Verapamil and digoxin can shorten the refractory period of the accessory pathway, accelerating the ventricular rate and thereby placing the WPW patient with atrial fibrillation at increased risk for ventricular fibrillation. Successful surgical or radiofrequency ablation can be achieved in most patients.

Atrial tachycardia due to enhanced automaticity

The two most common forms of atrial tachycardia due to enhanced automaticity are:

1. paroxysmal atrial tachycardia (PAT) with block
2. multifocal atrial tachycardia (MAT) (see Figure 25.7).

PAT with AVB is typically associated with digitalis toxicity. Digitalis has a parasympathetic effect on the SA and AV nodes, resulting in AVB whenever the ectopic focus fires at a high rate.

Acute or chronic severe pulmonary disease with acute exacerbation is the most common cause for

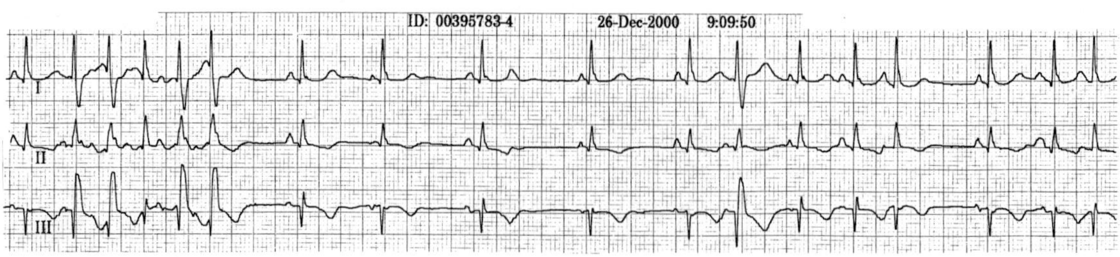

Figure 25.7 ECG features of MAT, showing the different P wave morphology and variable P wave amplitude, with short bouts of SVT

bouts of an irregular atrial tachycardia with multiple P waves of different morphology appearing. Therefore it is considered a transitional form of arrhythmia between frequent APBs and atrial fibrillation (Figure 25.7).

Treatment of PAT with block consists of reducing or withholding digoxin and potassium supplement. Antiarrhythmic treatment of MAT usually fails and this peculiar arrhythmia regresses only when the underlying pulmonary disease improves.

Atrial flutter

Atrial flutter is a rapid, regular re-entrant tachyarrhythmia that occurs most often in patients with organic heart disease—especially with underlying atrial abnormalities such as congenital heart disease, mitral valve disease and cardiomyopathies—and frequently post-cardiac surgery (see Figure 25.8(a) and (b)).

(a)

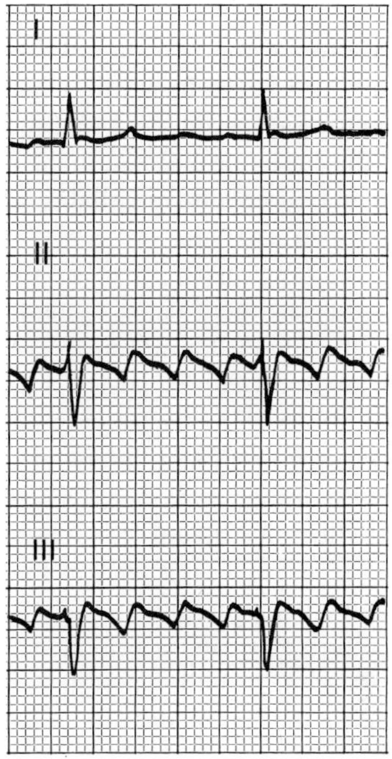

(b)

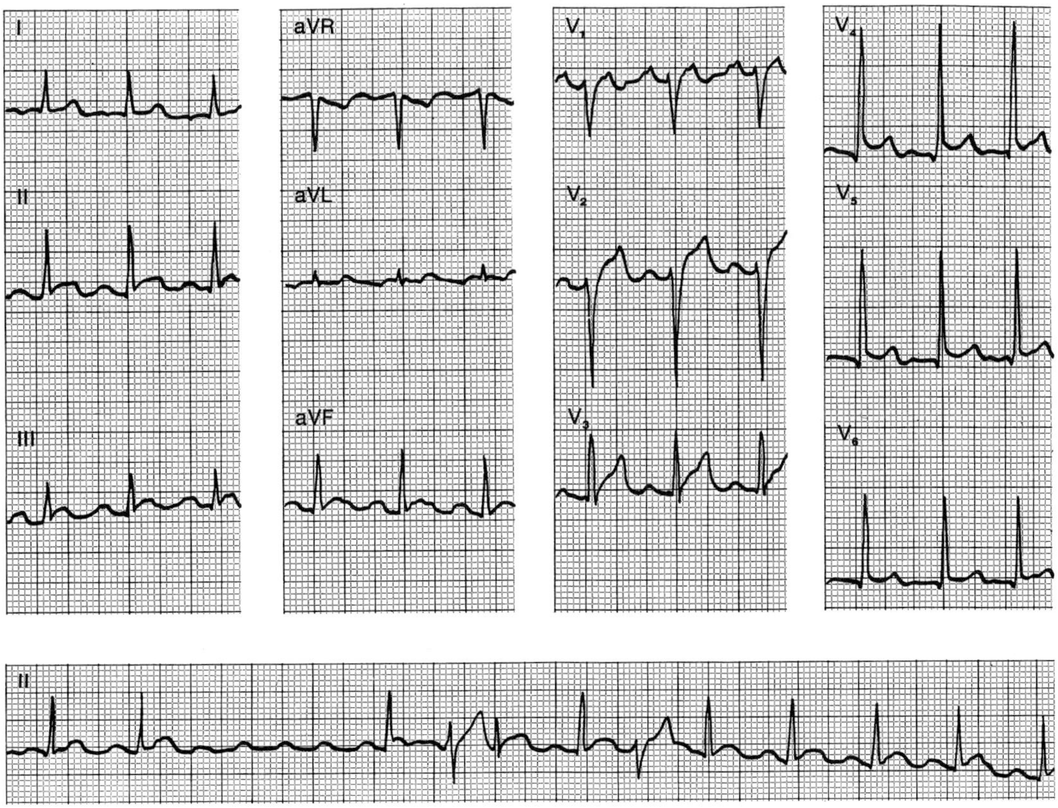

Figure 25.8 Atrial flutter. In **(b)** flutter waves can be detected only in lead II

There are two types of atrial flutter—type 1 and type 2—distinguished by the atrial rate. In type 1, the rate is usually 280–320/min with 2:1 conduction, thus the ventricular response is 140–160/min. In type 2 flutter the atrial rate is faster, in the range of 350–450/min and 4:1 conduction; that is, a ventricular response of 90–110/min.

Atrial flutter has a typical pattern of atrial activity in the ECG—the saw-tooth pattern identifiable easily in leads II, III and aVF. Carotid sinus massage enables us to make the correct diagnosis if a narrow QRS tachycardia at a rate of 140–160/min occurs. Carotid sinus massage will not interrupt atrial flutter, but because of the parasympathetic stimulation it will reduce AV nodal conduction to 70–80/min, thus revealing occult, typical flutter F waves—the saw-tooth appearance.

When the ventricular rate is tolerated, drug treatment is indicated, to either revert to sinus rhythm or to control the ventricular rate. Ventricular rate should be slowed with digitalis or verapamil, and the conventional antiarrhythmic drugs may be used to convert flutter to sinus rhythm. Quinidine and other class 1A agents as well as class 1C, propafenone, or class III, amiodarone, are equally effective. However, if the flutter rate is poorly tolerated as expected in patients with ischaemic and congestive heart failure, then electrical cardioversion is preferred. Energies as low as 15–25 J are usually effective.

Atrial fibrillation

Atrial fibrillation (AF) is the most common sustained arrhythmia encountered in primary care practice. According to the Framingham Heart Study, AF has a prevalence of 4% in the adult population. As the patient population continues to age, the prevalence of this arrhythmia rises as well, from < 0.5% in patients 25–35 years of age to > 5% in patients > 69 years of age. The incidence of AF increases with age and is related to left atrial size.

AF may be seen in normal individuals, especially during emotional stress, after exercise, surgery or acute alcoholic intoxication. The five most common conditions that produce atrial fibrillation are:

1. rheumatic heart disease
2. ischaemic heart disease
3. heart failure of any aetiology
4. hypertensive heart disease
5. thyrotoxicosis.

AF is associated with significant morbidity, including an increased susceptibility to embolic stroke. It is estimated that the annual risk of stroke in patients with AF is as high as 4.5%. It can also decrease exercise tolerance due to the loss of atrial contribution to left ventricular diastolic filling that may contribute up to 20% of the cardiac output. Clinical presentation ranges from minimal symptoms to acute pulmonary oedema in patients with significant mitral or aortic stenosis.

ECG features

AF is characterised by an irregular, disorganised atrial activity in the form of an irregular undulation of the baseline with an irregular ventricular response. Atrial fibrillatory waves (F waves) are best seen in standard lead V1 and are usually also evident in II, III and aVF as well (see Figure 25.9). The F waves may be quite large and coarse or almost imperceptible; however, there is no correlation between the F waves' size and atrial size or the type of heart disease.

A common phenomenon associated with AF is aberrant conduction. This occurs when a long ventricular cycle is followed by a short cycle. The long–short cycle sequence terminated by an aberrantly conducted beat is termed 'Ashman's phenomenon'. The aberrant beat usually shows the right bundle branch block pattern (Figure 25.2).

AF may be divided into acute and chronic forms:

- Paroxysmal AF is defined as recurrent episodes of spontaneously terminating AF.
- Persistent AF is defined by persistence of the arrhythmia for over 48 hours or until cardioversion is performed.
- Permanent AF is refractory to attempts at cardioversion. Thus, cardioversion is used only in cases of acute and chronic persistent AF and not in cases previously demonstrated to be refractory.

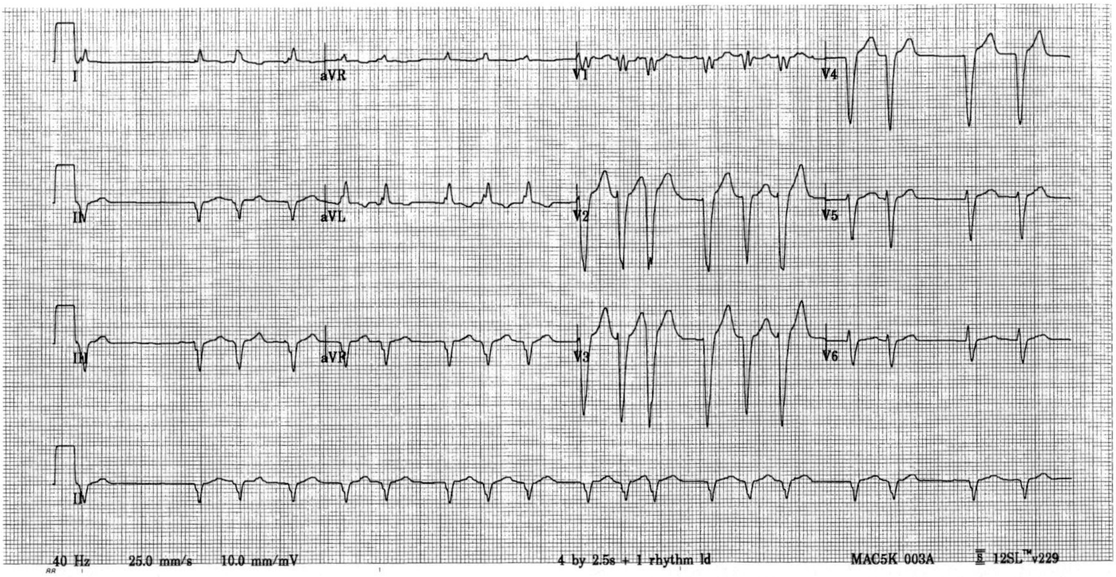

Figure 25.9 Atrial fibrillation

Therapy

The major goals of therapy include prevention of stroke, reduction of symptoms, and overall improvement in survival. Management strategies include rate control, rhythm control, anticoagulation therapy, or a combination of these strategies.

For patients with a rapid ventricular response, intravenous verapamil with an initial bolus of 0.1 mg/kg (5–10 mg) is highly effective and tends to slow the ventricular response by about 30%. Intravenous esmolol, an ultra-short-acting β-blocker, is also useful in controlling ventricular response within a few minutes. Other β-blockers, such as class IV agents, metoprolol or propranolol, can also be used.

Intravenous ibutilide, a new class III agent, is effective in terminating AF within 1 hour in approximately 35% of cases. Intravenous procainamide, given at a dose of 15 mg/kg over 0.5 hour is an acceptable approach. Oral quinidine, or a bolus dose of propafenone (600 mg) or oral flecainide (300 mg) are all effective in facilitating conversion of AF to sinus rhythm.

Acute termination, including spontaneous reversion, occurs in 60% of patients within 48 hours following rate control.

Electrical cardioversion, effective in about 85% of cases, is the most effective means of terminating AF. In a patient with AF and overt pre-excitation, direct circuit (DC) cardioversion is the therapy of choice. Non-pharmacological therapies, including pacing techniques, ablation of the atrioventricular (AV) node ('ablate and pace'), AV node modification, implantable atrial defibrillators, operative therapy and direct ablation of AF are reserved for patients who continue to be significantly disabled either from the arrhythmia per se or from the drugs used for treatment of AF. In patients with persistent AF resistant to treatment, management consists of rate control and lifelong anticoagulation therapy with warfarin.

Ventricular arrhythmias

Ventricular premature beats

The usual ventricular premature beat (VPB) has several typical ECG characteristics (Figures 25.3 and 25.4):

- Premature, wide QRS complex (> 120 msec) ectopic beats originating in the right ventricle have an LBBB morphology and those with left ventricular origin have an RBBB pattern.
- It is not preceded by a P wave. The P wave of the next normal sinus beat is normal in timing

and may distort the QRS complex, the ST segment or the T wave of the ectopic beat.

- It has an abnormal ST segment and T wave (usually opposite in polarity to the QRS complex due to the abnormal pattern of repolarisation).
- It has a full compensatory pause (unless the ectopic beat conducts retrogradely and resets the sinus node).

Common forms of VPBs are coupled to the preceding sinus beat by a fixed coupling interval. This is usually the rule when the VPBs are unifocal; however, because VPBs have different QRS morphologies they may have different coupling intervals.

Parasystolic rhythm refers to an independent, automatic ectopic rhythm, with the site of origin being protected by an 'entrance block'. Such a protective block means that the normal progressing sinus impulse cannot enter and reset the parasystolic focus but can create an area of refractoriness around this focus, limiting the rate and timing of it.

The VPB may be interpolated between 2 consecutive sinus beats. When a VPB is extremely premature, it cannot be conducted retrogradely because the AV node is still refractory from the last sinus beat. However, the following sinus beat can then be conducted to the ventricles. The result is a VPB interpolated between 2 sinus beats. The PR interval of the beat following the interpolated VPB is usually prolonged due to the fact that the conduction system is partially refractory from the retrograde conduction of the premature beat (see Figure 25.10).

A VPB may occur and vanish randomly, or constantly or episodically appear as bigeminy, trigeminy or quadrigeminy, so that every second, third or fourth complex, respectively, is an ectopic beat (Figure 25.4).

Lengthening of the cardiac cycle favours the generation of ventricular premature beats; the long compensatory pause following a VPB lengthens the heart rate and therefore the ventricular recovery—refractory time—measured by the QT interval which varies with rate (QT_c). Longer refractory time creates the potential for re-entry, facilitating the development of another ectopic beat. Thus, once started, the VPB has an inherent tendency to be self-perpetuating as ventricular bigeminy, a phenomenon often termed the 'rule of bigeminy'.

VPBs may be 'benign' unifocal, 'malignant' multiform or multifocal. Multifocal VPBs require attention and prompt treatment because they may precipitate life-threatening arrhythmias (ventricular tachycardia and fibrillation). Similarly, VPBs occurring very early in the cardiac cycle, during the early phase of recovery—'R-on-T VPBs'—are considered capable of inducing ventricular fibrillation, especially during the early phases of myocardial infarction.

Management of VPBs

VPBs occur frequently in healthy individuals and generally do not require any treatment. Furthermore, the risk–benefit ratio of antiarrhythmic drugs does not support treatment. Treatment with β-blockers may be required in patients with mitral valve prolapse with exercise-induced arrhythmias.

VPBs in acute coronary syndromes

Clinical settings characterised by myocardial reperfusion, such as thrombolysis in acute myocardial infarction, coronary angioplasty and stenting, are

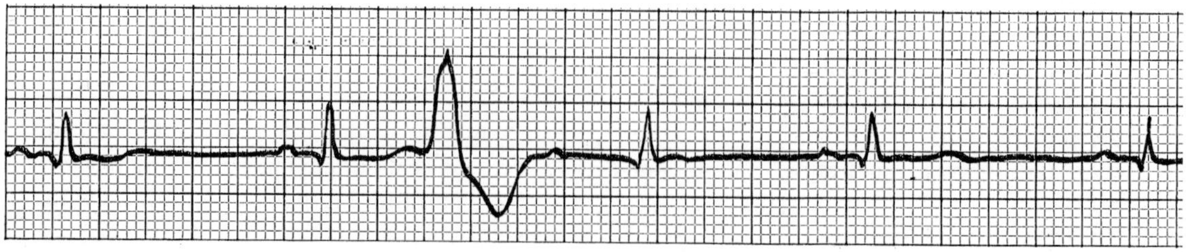

Figure 25.10 Interpolated VPB. The PR interval following the premature ventricular beat is prolonged due to partial refractoriness of the conduction system

frequently accompanied by reperfusion arrhythmias. These arrhythmias are usually transient and self-limiting and therefore do not require treatment unless they evolve to ventricular tachycardia or fibrillation.

The treatment of choice in acute myocardial infarction settings is still intravenous lidocaine (50–100 mg bolus followed by continuous infusion of 2–4 mg/min).

Treatment of patients with chronic ischaemic heart disease, hypertensive heart disease and cardiomyopathies has changed dramatically in the last 2 decades. The main reasons for change were the results of the CAST (Cardiac Arrhythmia Suppression Trial) study, which clearly demonstrated a significant excess risk of sudden cardiac death and total cardiovascular mortality in patients receiving class IC agents, such as flecainide.

β-blockers are the drugs of choice in post-myocardial infarction patients with asymptomatic or mildly symptomatic VPBs. In patients with symptomatic repetitive forms of VPBs, amiodarone is usually recommended (loading dose of 2.5–3 g within 2–4 days, then 20–400 mg daily).

Amiodarone and class IA drugs (e.g. procainamide) are the preferred drugs for suppression of VPBs in hypertrophic cardiomyopathy (obstructive and non-obstructive).

Non-sustained ventricular tachycardia

This term refers to a run of 6 or more consecutive VPBs lasting up to 30 seconds. Runs of 3–5 consecutive VPBs are termed 'non-sustained runs' of ventricular tachycardia (see Figure 25.11). Treatment is generally similar to that for symptomatic, multiform VPBs.

Sustained ventricular tachycardia

Ventricular tachycardia (VT), by definition, occurs at a rate of 100/min or more and lasts for 30 sec or more; most commonly the rate is in the range of 140–200/min. It is due to a local re-entry mechanism distal to the bundle of His. As in supraventricular re-entry tachycardias, it is initiated by an appropriately timed ventricular ectopic beat.

ECG recognition

ECG recognition of VT includes the following:

- The presence of ventricular/atrial dissociation, with clearly discernible P waves, independent of a regular wide QRS rhythm, is strongly suggestive of VT (see Figure 25.12).
- If P waves cannot be seen during the tachycardia, then indirect evidence of independent atrial activity is provided by capture beats. A capture beat occurs when a normal sinus beat is so timed that it is conducted to the ventricles, arriving before the next expected beat of the VT. If this atrial beat penetrates the ventricles a little later, it may fuse with the next expected beat of the VT, resulting in a fusion beat.
- The QRS complex is always wide, greater than 120 msec. A QRS duration above 160 msec is virtually diagnostic for VT (except for antidromic SVT in WPW syndrome in which QRS duration in excess of 240 msec is common). A QRS duration above 140 msec favours diagnosis of VT but does not rule out SVT with aberration or with pre-existing BBB.
- Left axis, −30° or beyond in frontal plane indicates VT over aberration.

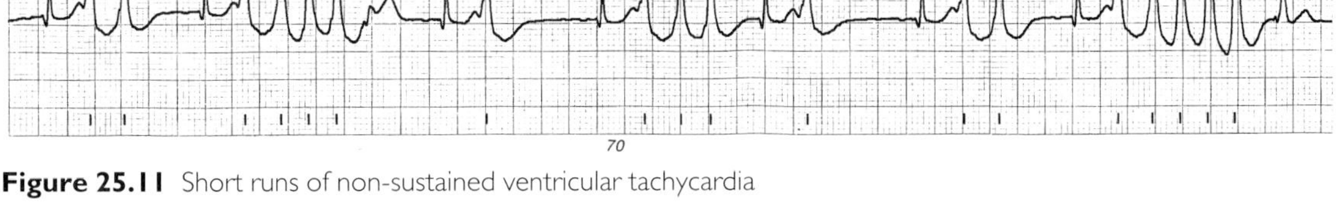

Figure 25.11 Short runs of non-sustained ventricular tachycardia

- Concordantly, positive or negative QRS complexes across the precordium from leads V1 to V6 are highly suggestive of VT.
- In lead V1, a RBBB pattern that is monophasic (R) or biphasic (qR) suggests VT, while a triphasic rSR' pattern indicates SVT with aberration.
- R wave amplitude in lead V1 during tachycardia exceeding that during sinus rhythm suggests VT.
- Sustained monomorphic VT commonly occurs at rates of 150–180/min, while polymorphic VT is more rapid, and rates may be in excess of 250/min.

Monomorphic VT (Figure 25.12) is a re-entrant tachycardia, and is more frequent in acute or chronic heart disease syndromes and in idiopathic dilated or hypertrophic cardiomyopathy. Polymorphic VT (see Figure 25.13) is encountered more often in patients with transient myocardial ischaemia. The mechanism may be either re-entrant or automatic. Greater cycle length variability, greater regional dispersion of ventricular repolarisation time and heterogeneity of ventricular repolarisation play a major role in the genesis of polymorphic VT.

Treatment

In acute myocardial infarction settings, if the patient is stable, a bolus of 75–100 mg IV lignocaine followed by continuous drip of 2–4 mg/min should be

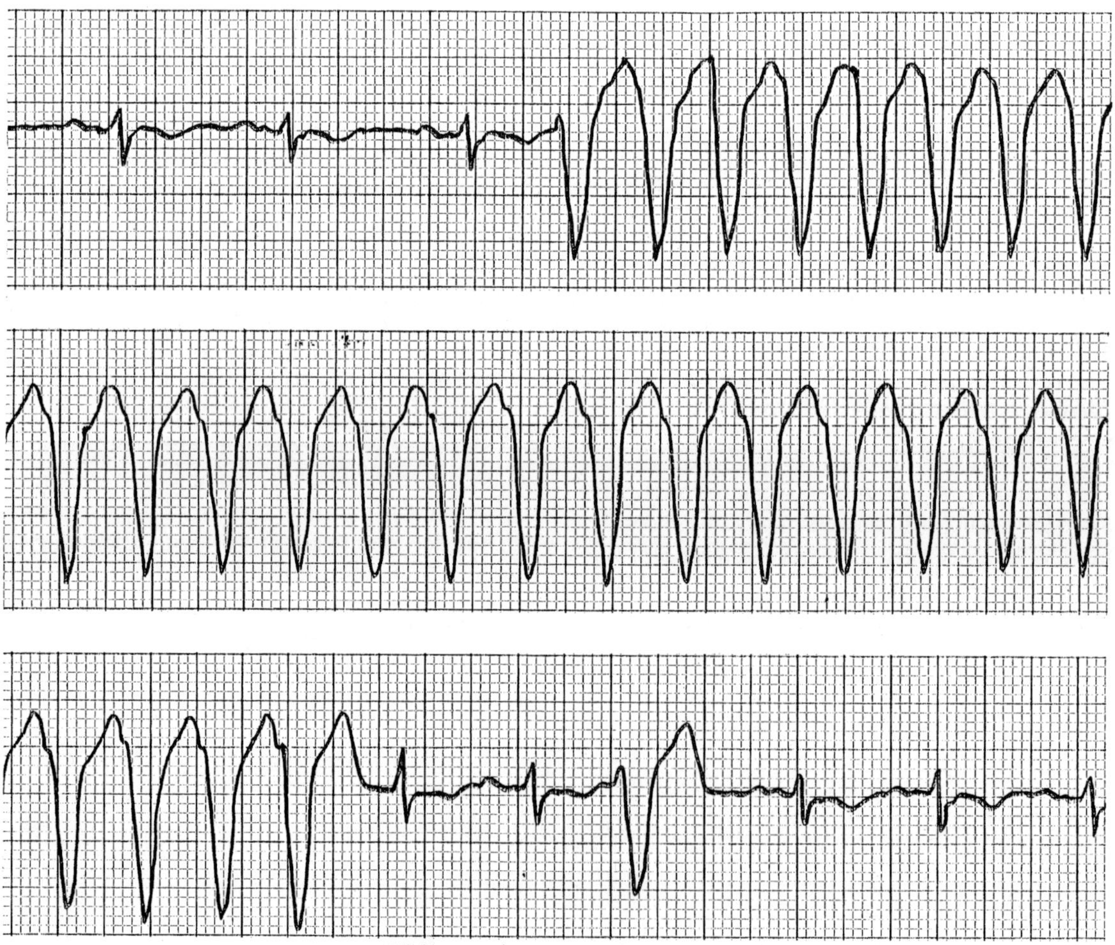

Figure 25.12 Ventricular tachycardia

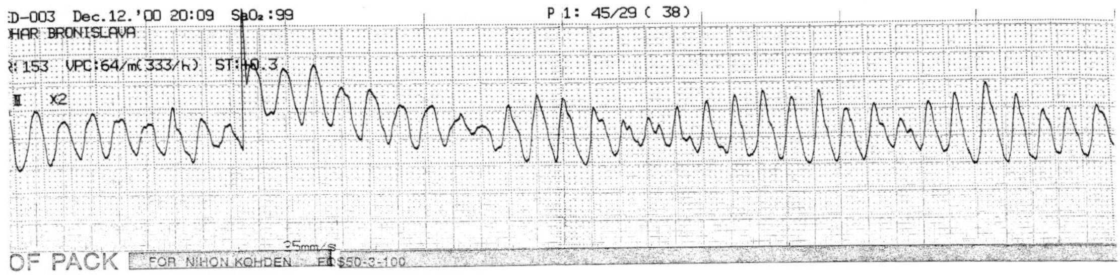

Figure 25.13 Polymorphic VT

tried. If the VT does not revert or if the patient is hypotensive, immediate electrical cardioversion is required. If VT recurs, lignocaine should be tried again and then 100 mg boluses of procainamide are administered at 5 minute intervals to a total loading dose of 500–1000 mg. Refractory VT should be treated with amiodarone, 300 mg bolus followed by continuous drip of 1200–2000 mg/24 hours for 2–3 days and by oral amiodarone.

Automatic implantable defibrillation is recommended for patients with recurrent sustained VT and a moderate to severe reduction in left ventricular systolic function (LVEF% = 25–35).

Torsade de pointes

Torsade de pointes is a peculiar variant of polymorphic VT that is characterised by QRS peaks that seem to twist around the baseline and are fusiform in appearance, with 'twisting of the points' (see Figure 25.14). There are undulations of varying amplitude which alternate above and below the baseline. Usually it is considered part of a syndrome that includes a prolonged QT interval and a precipitating factor. The precipitating factor may be the proarrhythmic effect of drugs that prolong ventricular recovery time, including quinidine, procainamide, disopyramide, amiodarone, sotalol, phenothiazine and tricyclic antidepressants. It often occurs with hypokalaemia and hypomagnesaemia, subarachnoid haemorrhage, bradyarrhythmias and congenital long QT syndromes.

Management

Intravenous magnesium sulphate is often effective, especially when the torsade is due to quinidine. It should be administered in a dose of 1.5–2 g within 2 minutes, followed by an infusion of 2–20 mg/min.

Administration of isoproterenol will shorten the prolonged QT interval; however, the unavoidable acceleration of heart rate limits its use in patients with symptomatic ischaemic heart disease. Lidocaine and mexiletine may be beneficial, while class IA (e.g. quinidine, procainamide) and class III (e.g. amiodarone, bretilium and sotalol) antiarrhythmic drugs should be avoided.

Although electrical cardioversion may interrupt torsade de pointes, it frequently recurs.

Bidirectional VT

When the polymorphic VT is regular and there are two alternating QRS morphologies with opposite

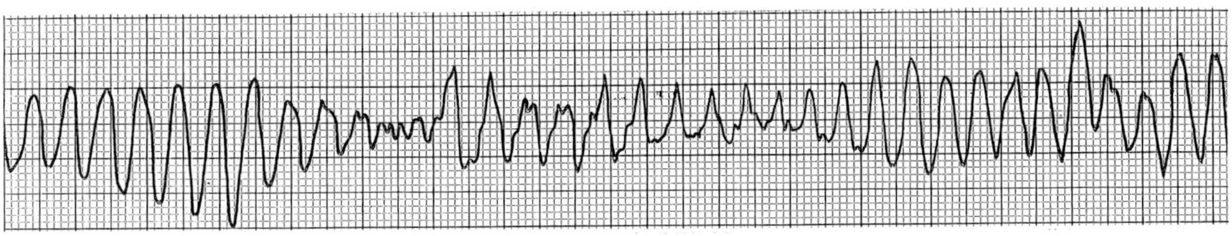

Figure 25.14 Torsade de pointes: QRS undulations of varying amplitude above and below the baseline

polarity, the term 'bidirectional tachycardia' is applied. It is usually a manifestation of digitalis intoxication.

Ventricular fibrillation

Ventricular fibrillation (VF) (see Figure 25.15) is a rapid, irregular chaotic rhythm regarded as a potentially lethal, terminal arrhythmia. Since co-ordinated contraction of the ventricular myocardium is impossible, there is a circulatory arrest and loss of consciousness requiring prompt defibrillation and cardiopulmonary resuscitation.

It is often precipitated by a VPB with a very short coupling interval, falling in the vulnerable period of the preceding T wave ('R-on-T' phenomenon).

VF occurs most commonly in the setting of acute ischaemic events, in acute myocardial infarction (AMI) in particular. Primary VF occurs during the first 4–6 hours of AMI, and the incidence is highest in the first hour, decreasing dramatically thereafter. The overall incidence in AMI patients is 2–4%. Defibrillation is usually successful and the prognosis is good. Secondary VF complicating cardiogenic shock or cardiac failure is less successful and implies a poor subsequent prognosis.

VF is the mode of death in 25–50% of fatalities among patients with cardiomyopathies. Amiodarone (with or without β-blockers) and the implantable cardioverter-defibrillator (ICD) are considered the two major therapeutic tools for preventing sudden arrhythmic death in patients with organic heart disease and poor left ventricular function.

Ventricular flutter

Ventricular flutter is characterised by a sine wave configuration with a cycle length of 200–240 msec (see Figure 25.16). Management is identical to that of VF.

As patients with ventricular flutter may remain apparently stable for several seconds and the morphological ECG pattern mimics an external electrical artefact, initiation of emergency therapy is usually delayed until the patient loses consciousness.

Accelerated junctional and ventricular rhythms

Accelerated rhythms derive from subordinate pacemakers and foci in the conduction system whenever the sinus rate is less than the rate of the normally suppressed 'lower' subordinate focus. Such a rhythm typically represents the enhanced automaticity mechanism.

Inferior wall myocardial infarction, hypokalaemia, hypoxaemia and digitalis intoxication are

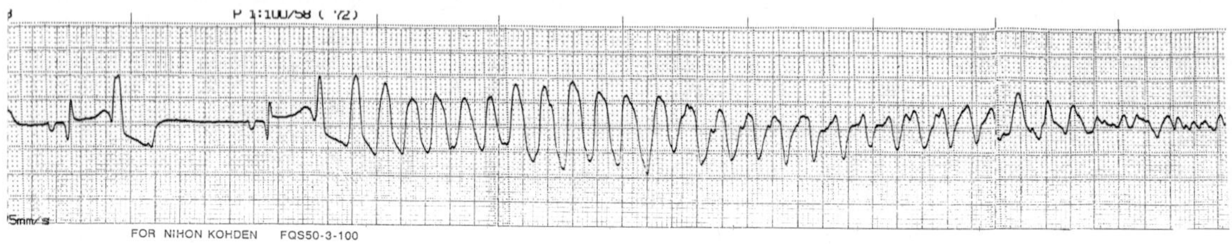

Figure 25.15 VT degenerating to ventricular fibrillation

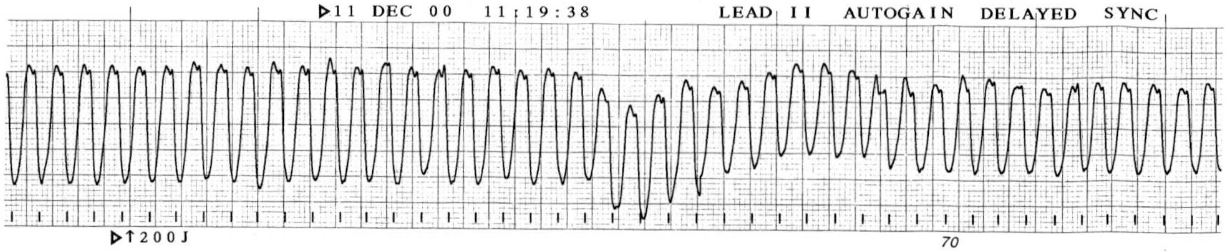

Figure 25.16 Ventricular flutter

usually the clinical settings in which the accelerated idioventricular rhythm (AIVR) and accelerated idionodal rhythm (AINR) occur (see Figures 25.17 and 25.18).

Sinoatrial block

SA block refers to the failure of an impulse formed in the SA node to conduct normally to the adjacent

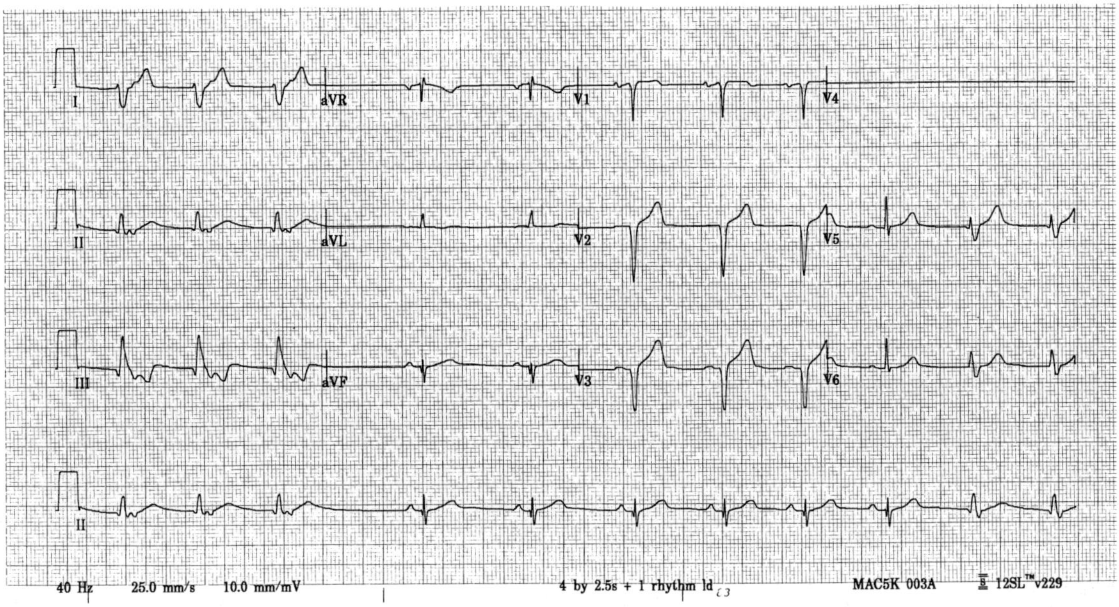

Figure 25.17 Idionodal rhythm: alternating normal sinus rhythm originating in the SA node and AV nodal rhythm (low nodal, retrograde P waves, first 3 beats), and AV nodal rhythm originating higher in the AV node (P waves indiscernible, last 2 beats)

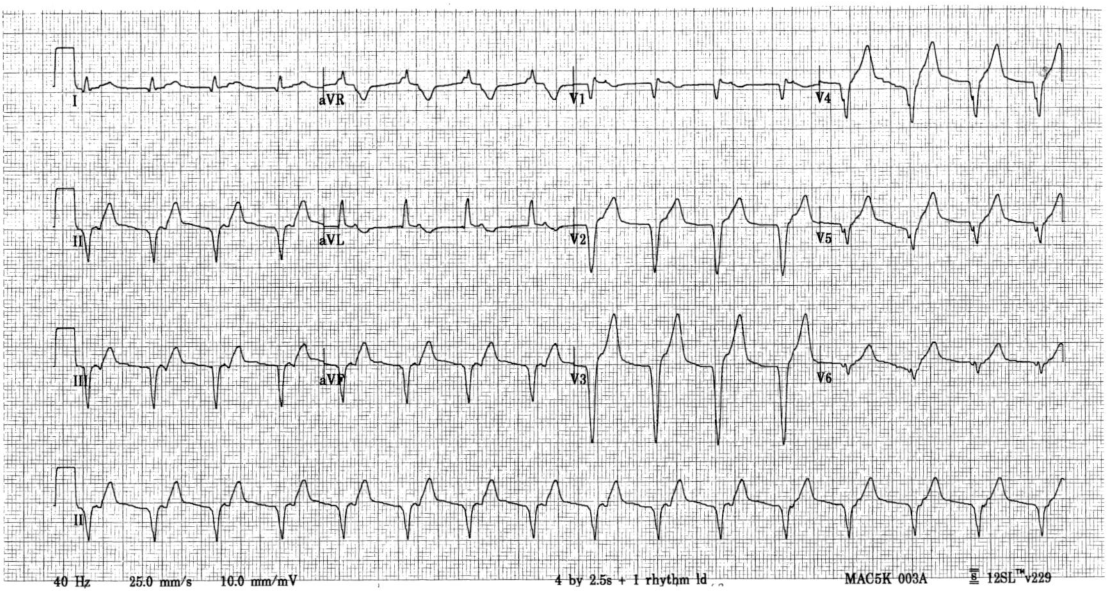

Figure 25.18 Idionodal rhythm

atrial muscle. In this case the PP intervals are multiples of the preceding sinus cycle length. SA block can be classified as first, second or third degree block. First and third degree blocks cannot be recognised on the standard ECG. Only the second degree SA block can be recognised because of its intermittent pattern (see Figure 25.19).

Atrioventricular block (AVB)

The normal PR interval measures 0.12–0.20 sec.

First degree AVB

In first degree AVB, the PR interval is prolonged, > 0.2 sec, indicating prolongation of AV conduction time. Each P wave is followed by a QRS complex (see Figure 25.20). Isolated first degree AVB is never symptomatic and does not require pacing. The only exception refers to patients with chronic advanced bundle branch block, for example, chronic RBBB and LAHB, chronic RBBB and LPHB, or chronic LBBB in whom an occasional 'pseudonormalisation' of the QRS complex occurs, where a narrow QRS complex is preceded by a long PR interval. This refers to a bilateral bundle branch block; both ventricles are depolarised slowly due to conduction delay in both bundles, but arriving simultaneously at both ventricles with a resultant prolonged PR interval and a narrow QRS (concealed bilateral BBB).

Second degree AVB

Second degree AVB is the intermittent failure of AV conduction of a P wave with a drop-out of a QRS complex. The drop-out pattern is often repetitive, that is, normal AV conduction of 1 out of 2 P waves, 2 out of 3 or 3 out of 4 P waves, resulting in a conduction ratio of 2:1, 3:2, 4:3, and so on.

Second degree AVB is subdivided into Mobitz type I (Wenkebach) and Mobitz II block. Second degree AVB usually occurs in the AV node. Mobitz I is commonly associated with acute inferior wall myocardial infarction, while Mobitz II is associated with digitalis toxicity, β-blockers and calcium channel blockers. The block is usually transient and reversible; however, chronic second degree AVB may occasionally occur in aortic valve disease and amyloidosis.

Mobitz I (Wenkebach) (see Figure 25.21) is characterised by a progressive lengthening of the PR interval over a successive number of P–QRS cycles, usually 3 or 4, until a QRS complex drops out. The subsequent pause enables the conduction pathways to recover so the PR interval of the next following P–QRS cycle is shortened. In the typical Mobitz I block, along with the progressive PR interval prolongation, a progressive shortening of RR interval is noticed. Even though the absolute PR interval is longer, the change in PR is less in the subsequent PR intervals, with resultant progressive

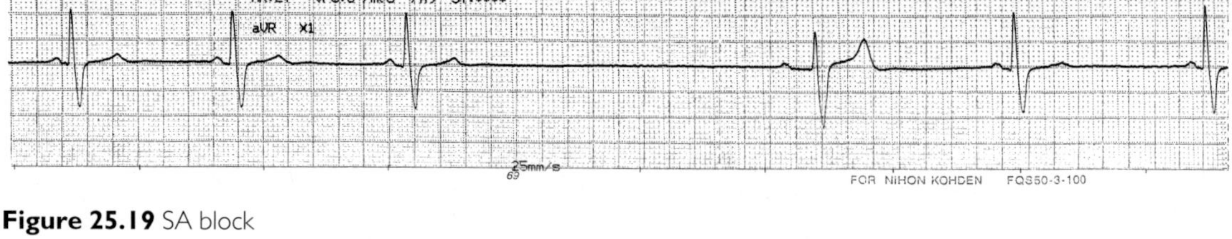

Figure 25.19 SA block

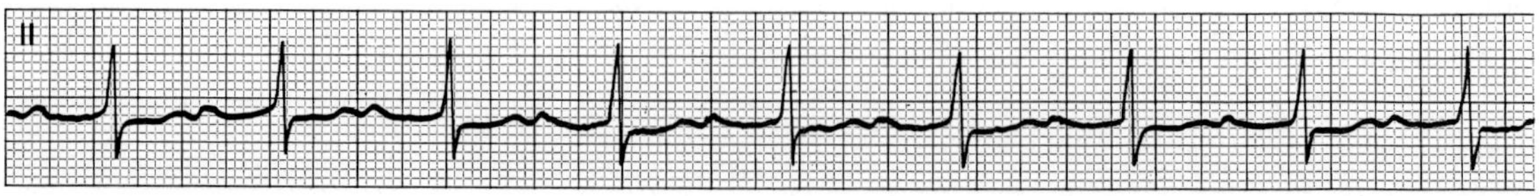

Figure 25.20 First degree AVB

shortening of RR intervals before the pause caused by the dropped beat.

The site of the block is above or within the AV node. In Mobitz type II block, an appropriately timed P wave fails to conduct, but the PR interval is not characterised by progressive PR lengthening (see Figure 25.22). The site of the block is infra-nodal as a rule.

Third degree AVB

Third degree AVB (complete AVB) is characterised by a complete cessation of AV conduction (see Figure 25.23).

The criteria for third degree AVB are:

1. evidence of atrial activity, usually in the form of sinus P waves, less common atrial tachycardia, atrial fibrillation or flutter
2. AV dissociation with independent atrial and ventricular activation
3. escape rhythm, AV junctional or ventricular. Automaticity is enhanced by the slow rhythm, thus when the escape is junctional, QRS complex may be narrow, and when the escape rhythm is ventricular, then QRS is wide.

Complete AVB can be symptomatic and may cause lightheadedness, worsen or precipitate heart failure. If ventricular rate falls below a critical level, the patient may lose consciousness in a Stokes-Adams attack.

Permanent pacing (either ventricular or physiological dual chamber pacing) is required unless those factors responsible for the block can be removed (e.g. digoxin, calcium channel blockers, β-blockers) or when the block complicates an acute inferior wall myocardial infarction.

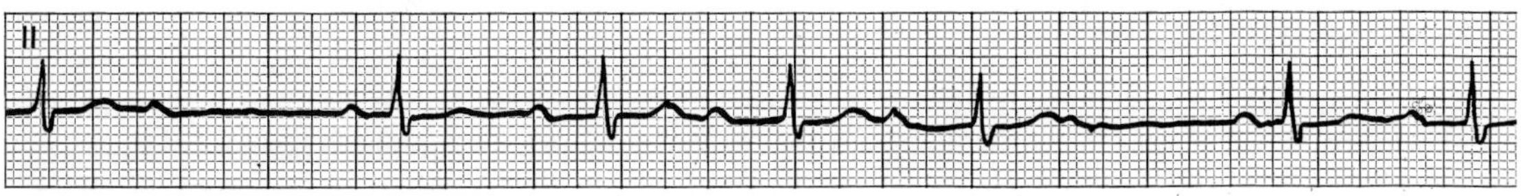

Figure 25.21 Second degree AVB, Mobitz I

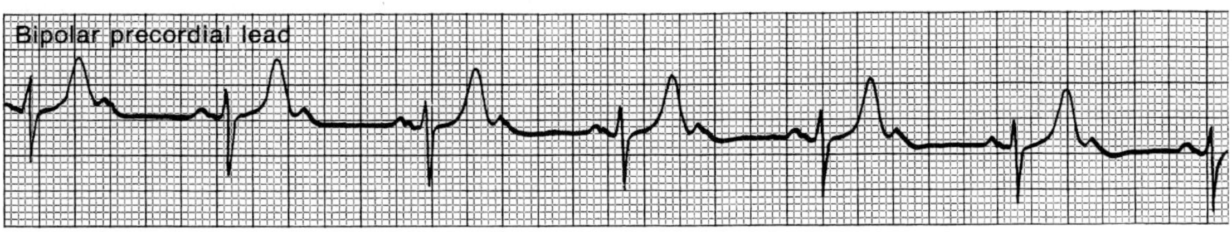

Figure 25.22 Second degree AVB, Mobitz II

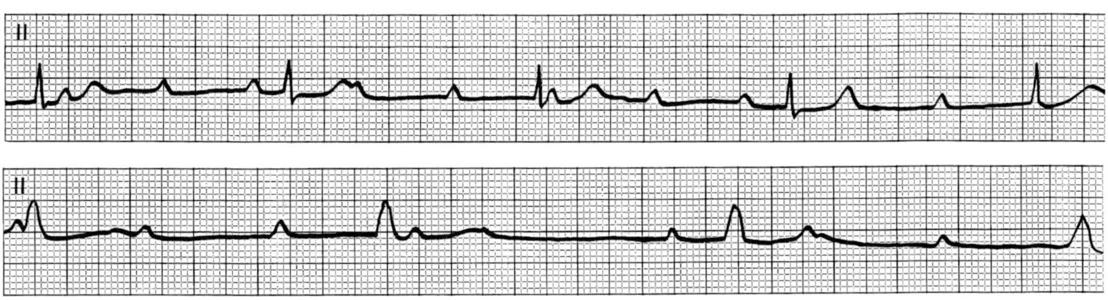

Figure 25.23 Third degree AVB: complete AVB with AV dissocation

Sick sinus syndrome

Sick sinus syndrome (SSS) is a clinical entity based on abnormal sinus node impulse formation with or without abnormal intra-atrial and AV conduction. Rhythm disturbances encountered in SSS are various and may be manifested as persistent, inappropriate sinus bradycardia even on exercise (chronotropic incompetence), sinus arrest, sinoatrial block or combinations of alternating supraventricular tachyarrhythmias with bradyarrhythmias ('brady-tachycardia syndrome').

Negative inotropic agents, such as β-blockers, digitalis and calcium channel blockers, should be avoided or discontinued. Oral anticoagulation and dual chamber (DDD) and physiological pacing are usually required. The dual chamber (atrioventricular) pacemaker is superior to the simple, single chamber (VVI) pacemaker because of the lower associated incidence rate of atrial fibrillation.

Pacemaker signals

All current artificial pacemakers have a built-in standby or 'demand' mode, because rhythm and conduction abnormalities that require their implantation may occur intermittently. Figure 25.24 illustrates a typical example of a normally functioning demand pacemaker. In this mode, whenever the device senses a ventricular R wave, it does not generate an artificial impulse, but when the R wave fails to occur within a certain time interval that corresponds to a predetermined cycle length (i.e. predetermined heart rate), it then generates an appropriate artificial stimulus.

The pacemaker signal, the 'spike', may initiate the P wave or the QRS complex or both, depending on the type of pacing system. If the pacing mode is AAI (atrial pacing, atrial sensing and atrial inhibition), the 'spike' will initiate the P wave (see Figure 25.25); if the pacing mode is VVI (ventricular pacing, ventricular sensing and ventricular inhibition), then the 'spike' initiates the QRS complex (Figure 25.24). With DDD or DVI pacing these signals may initiate the P wave or QRS complex, or both (see Figure 25.26). In this mode, both chambers are paced but only the ventricle is capable of sensing, responding in both a ventricular and atrial inhibited fashion (atrial and ventricular rates are identical and separated by a fixed AV delay).

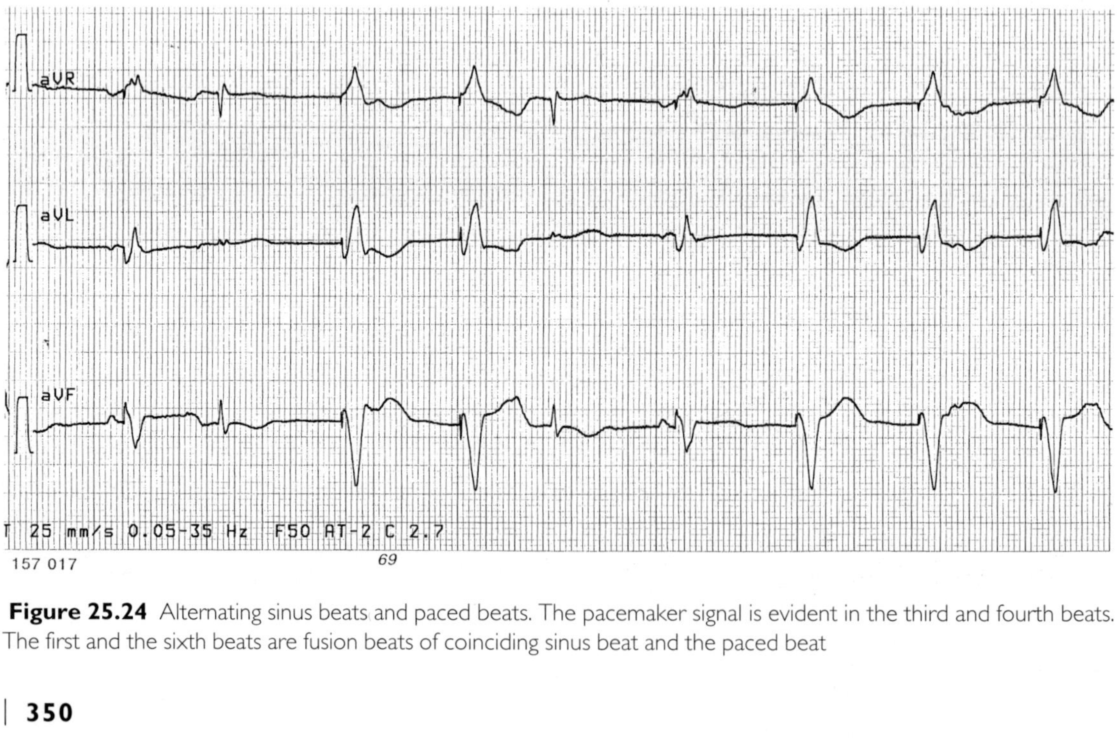

Figure 25.24 Alternating sinus beats and paced beats. The pacemaker signal is evident in the third and fourth beats. The first and the sixth beats are fusion beats of coinciding sinus beat and the paced beat

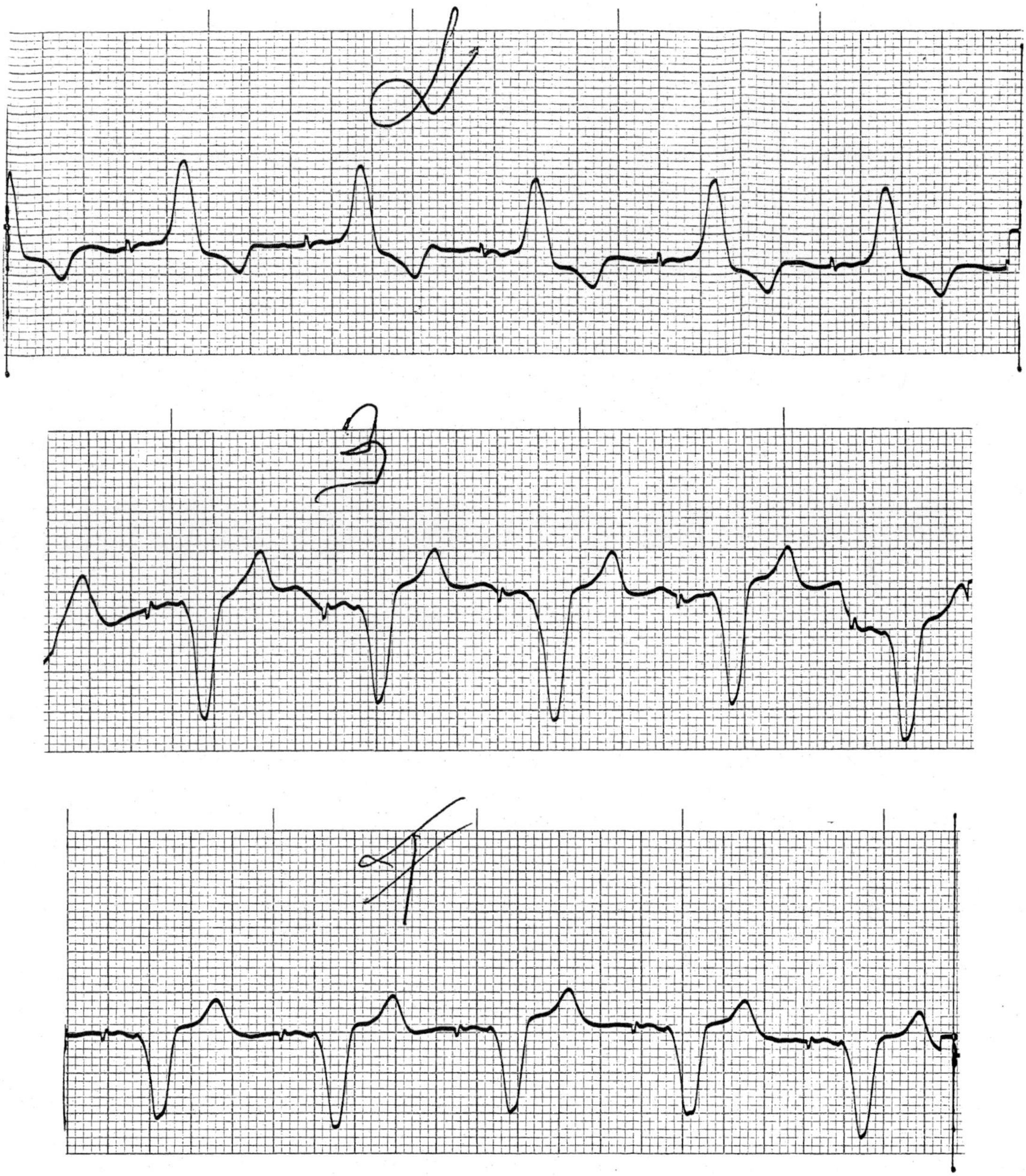

Figure 25.25 Atrial pacing. A pacemaker signal precedes every P wave

Pacemaker failure to sense or to pace is easily recognised; if the pacemaker 'spike' occurs prematurely, resembling an ectopic premature beat, then a pacemaker-sensing failure is diagnosed. If no 'spike' appears following a pause that is longer then the preset pacemaker cycle length (i.e. pacemaker rate), a sensing failure may be the case as well due to faulty interpretation of a small voltage P wave as

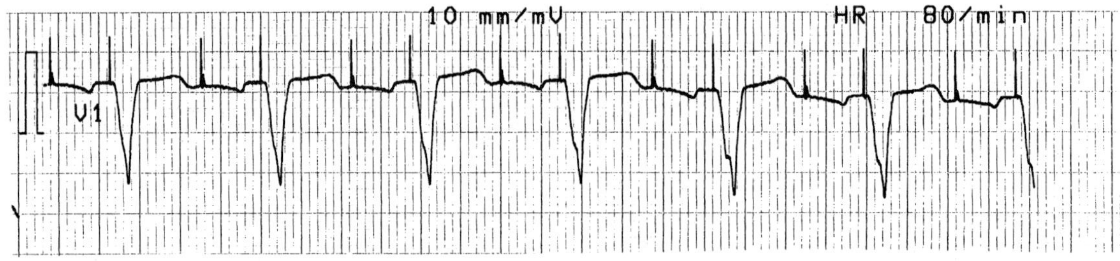

Figure 25.26 Dual chamber pacing (DDD). Each P wave and QRS complex are initiated by an artificial pacemaker signal. In this patient the PR interval was set at 0.242 msec

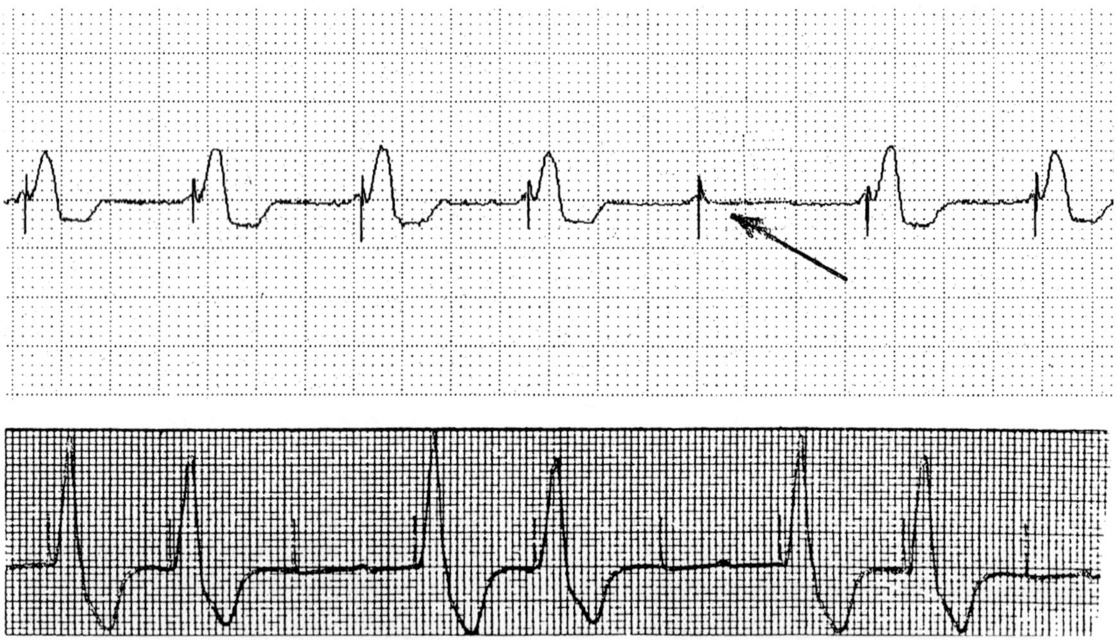

Figure 25.27 Pacing failure is diagnosed by the intermittent absence of pacemaker stimulus ('spike')

a normal ventricular R wave. In such a case, the pacemaker is expected to remain inactive. In Figure 25.27, two different examples of pacing failure are shown; ventricular depolarisation does not follow a pacemaker's 'spike'.

Bibliography and further reading

Blake, T. M. (ed.) (1999), *Annotated Atlas of Electrocardiography: A Guide to Confident Interpretation, Contemporary Cardiology*, Vol. 3, Humana Press, Totowa, NJ.

Cavallaro, D., Grauer, K. M. D. & Cavallaro, D. (1997), *Arrhythmia Interpretation: ACLS Preparation and Clinical Approach*, 1st edn, Mosby-Year Book, St Louis, MO.

Fuster, V. (ed.) (2000), *Hurst's The Heart*, 10th edn, McGraw-Hill, New York.

Hampton, J. R. (ed.) (1997), *The ECG in Practice*, 3rd edn, Churchill Livingstone Publishing, Philadelphia.

Hohnloser, S. H. (1999), 'Implantable devices versus antiarrhythmic drug therapy in recurrent ventricular tachycardia and fibrillation', *American Journal of Cardiology*, 84(9A), pp. 56R–62R.

Jalife, J., Delmar, M. & Davidenko, J. M. (eds) (1998),

Basic Cardiac Electrocardiography, Futura Publishing, Armonk, NY.

Lampert, R. & Ezekowitz, M. D. (2000), 'Management of arrhythmias', *Clinics in Geriatric Medicine*, 3, pp. 593–8.

Naccarela, F., Lepera, G. & Rolli, A. (2000), 'Arrhythmic risk stratification of post-myocardial infarction', *Current Opinions in Cardiology*, 1, pp. 1–6.

Schamroth, L. & Schamroth, C. (1990), *Introduction to Electrocardiography*, 7th edn, Blackwell Science Publishing, Boston.

Wagner, G. S. (ed.) (1994), *Marriott's Practical Electrocardiography*, 9th edn, Lippincott, Williams & Wilkins, Philadelphia.

Yap, Y. P. & Camm, A. J. (1999), 'Lessons from antiarrhythmic trials involving Class III antiarrhythmic drugs', *American Journal of Cardiology*, 84, pp. 9A, 83R–9R.

Chapter 26
Pulmonary embolism

D. J. CHRISTOPHER and RICHARD E. RUFFIN

Introduction

Pulmonary embolism (PE) is a disorder that holds the interest of a wide variety of practitioners, namely general practitioners, pulmonologists, cardiologists, general physicians, surgeons, obstetricians, radiologists, nuclear physicians, pathologists and others. Despite an improved understanding of the pathogenesis and consequently the use of preventive measures, PE remains a major cause of morbidity and mortality. Furthermore, deaths from pulmonary embolism are often sudden and unexpected. Although there have been technological advances in management, for many clinicians the only confirmative test available is ventilation-perfusion lung scanning. In actual practice, treatment is often offered on the basis of a subjective diagnosis based on clinical features. In this chapter, we provide an overview of PE with a focus on the diagnostic approach and the management of this problem.

Epidemiology

It has been estimated that a district hospital with a catchment population of 200 000 is likely to diagnose 50 cases of pulmonary embolism annually. Two population-based studies from America suggest that the overall incidence of this problem is 1 in 1000 per year. The risk increased with age, doubling with every 10 year increase, and there was a male preponderance. Pulmonary embolism has been shown by autopsy studies to be the cause of mortality in 10% of all hospital deaths and contributing to mortality in a further 10%; 60–80% of the fatal PE cases are clinically unsuspected and undiagnosed.

Pathophysiology

Pulmonary embolism and deep venous thrombosis should be considered part of the same pathological process; together they are often referred to as 'venous thromboembolism'. Current evidence confirms that the triad of factors related to clot formation (Virchow's triad) are venous stasis, increased blood coagulability and injury to the vein wall. The most common source of PE is thrombosis in the deep veins of the lower limbs, particularly between the knee and the inguinal ligament. Pulmonary embolism is infrequently due to thrombosis of the pelvic veins, veins of the upper extremities or other organ systems (e.g. hepatic and renal veins). The thrombus dislodges and travels through the venous circulation and lodges in one of the pulmonary arteries. The embolism results initially in an area of the lung that is ventilated but underperfused, resulting in an alveolar dead space. Release of vasoactive substances like serotonin from the platelets and the blockade of the pulmonary artery by the clot cause a rise of pulmonary vascular resistance. This results in an increase in right ventricular work load, leading to a redistribution of blood flow and increase in right ventricular work load, which if excessive may result in right ventricular failure. Once this occurs there is a fall in the pulmonary blood flow and reduction of left ventricular filling, causing systemic hypotension.

Airway obstruction resulting from the reflex bronchoconstriction further contributes to the ventilation-perfusion (V/Q) mismatch. After about 24 hours, there is depletion of surfactant and this may result in atelectasis and oedema in the affected area. Pulmonary infarction itself is an uncommon consequence of pulmonary embolism, because the pulmonary parenchyma has three potential sources of oxygen, namely the pulmonary arteries, the bronchial arteries and the alveoli. Generally, two of these sources need to be compromised before infarction develops and this usually happens only in patients with coexisting cardiopulmonary disease. Also, complete occlusion of the pulmonary artery is infrequent.

Although the site of the clot and the extent of obstruction determine the severity of the disease and the outcome, in the presence of pre-existing cardiopulmonary disease, a small embolic event in the pulmonary artery may result in serious consequences. Conversely, a major occlusion in one of the main pulmonary arteries may have lesser consequences in a person with a normal pre-existing cardiopulmonary status.

Risk factors

Although venous thromboembolism can occur *de novo* without any identifiable risk factors, in the vast majority of the patients, one or more risk factors are identified (Table 26.1). In a published series, 96.3% of the patients had at least 1 risk factor, 76% had at least 2 risk factors and 39% had at least 3 risk factors. The chance of having the disease increases proportionately with the increase in the number of risk factors. Therefore, it is important to be aware of the known risk factors, to make a clinical diagnosis and select the patients requiring further investigations. Age is an important risk factor; in one series, 88.5% of the patients diagnosed with PE were aged 40 years or more. The other major risk factors are as follows.

Immobilisation

Immobilisation for more than a week is an important risk factor. Diminished muscle activity in the lower limbs reduces venous return, facilitating accumulation of activated clotting factors.

Surgery and fractures

Recent surgery and fractures, particularly of the femur and tibia, pose an increased risk. In surgical patients, the high risk groups are those that have major high-risk operations performed for abdominal or pelvic malignancy and major orthopaedic surgery, or any surgery requiring intensive care. The likely causative factors are immobility and liberation of clotting factors.

Cardiorespiratory disorders

The source of the emboli in these diseases is also the veins of the lower limbs, rather than the heart itself. In these situations, the risk of clot formation in the leg veins is probably enhanced by the reduction in the peripheral blood flow. Venous thromboembolism has been reported to be over 3 times more common in patients with heart disease (aged 30 years or more) than in age-matched controls.

Malignancy

Although the exact mechanism for this is unknown, abnormalities of haemostasis occur in patients with neoplastic disease. A well known example of this is the association of thrombophlebitis migrans with gastrointestinal tract malignant disease. The association of venous

Table 26.1 Risk factors for pulmonary embolism

Category	Risk factors
Surgery and fractures	Major surgery Surgery requiring intensive care Lower limb surgery Bone fractures, especially of tibia and femur
Immobilisation (especially lower limb)	Plaster of Paris cast Paralysis
Malignancies	Pancreatic Bronchial Genitourinary Stomach and colon Breast
Cardiorespiratory	Myocardial infarction Chronic congestive cardiac failure Congenital heart disease Chronic obstructive airways disease
Obstetric	Pregnancy and puerperium
Miscellaneous	Increasing age Obesity Previous proven PE or DVT Primary hypercoagulable states (e.g. antithrombin III, protein C and protein S deficiency)

thromboembolism is seen most often with pancreatic cancer, followed in the order of frequency by carcinomas of the bronchial tree, genitourinary tract, colon, stomach and breast. In one series, cancer was found to be a risk factor in 22.3% of the patients with venous thromboembolism.

Pregnancy and puerperium

In pregnancy and puerperium, the clot formation is probably due to venous stasis in the lower limbs resulting from decreased venous return due to direct pressure from the enlarged uterus. Increased levels of some of the clotting factors and possible reduction in fibrinolytic activity may also contribute. In women during pregnancy and puerperium, the reported incidence varies from 1 in 200 to 1 in 1600.

Obesity

In postoperative patients 40 years of age or older, one study reported the incidence of deep venous thrombosis (DVT) to be significantly higher in obese patients when compared to non-obese patients (47.9% versus 24.5%). This finding has not been replicated by investigators who controlled for other risk factors. Thus obesity cannot be considered an independent risk factor, but it may have an additive effect in combination with other risk factors.

Oral contraceptives (OCP)

Earlier reports suggested an increase in venous thromboembolism with the use of OCPs. This risk has currently declined drastically with the availability of low dose formulations.

Clinical features

Data from post-mortem studies suggest that many patients with PE are undiagnosed and unrecognised (see Figure 26.1). Therefore, a substantial number of asymptomatic PE may exist. Furthermore, only in a third of the patients suspected of having PE is the disease subsequently confirmed.

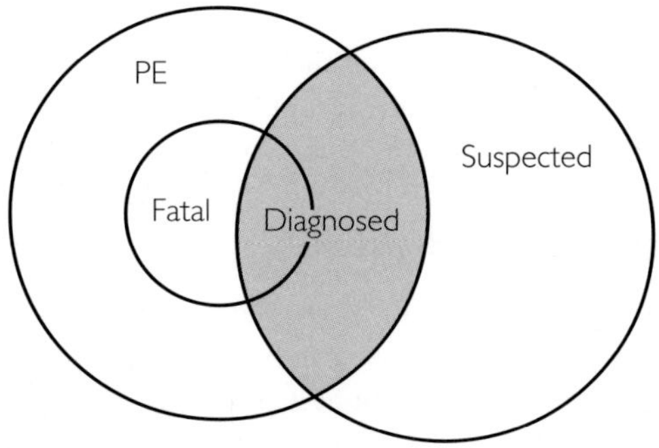

Figure 26.1 Relationship between suspected and diagnosed PE

The data on the clinical features is from studies where the diagnosis has been confirmed by specific tests. Dyspnoea, pleuritic chest pain, apprehension and cough are the most important symptoms. Dyspnoea is the most common presenting symptom of PE and it is classically sudden in onset, although it may set in more insidiously in some. Haemoptysis is neither common nor frequent. The common presenting symptoms and their frequencies are summarised in Table 26.2.

The symptoms with high sensitivity have low specificity and those with high specificity have low sensitivity. Therefore, on the basis of individual symptoms, it is not possible to exclude or confirm PE and so some authors have attempted to use a combination of clinical features.

The initial presentation usually falls into one of the three following types:

1. *Pulmonary infarction syndrome.* The patients who fall in this category present with dyspnoea and pleuritic chest pain. The severity of PE in these patients is deemed to be mild. This is the most common mode of initial presentation; in one study, three-quarters of the patients presented in this fashion.
2. *Isolated dyspnoea.* In these patients, the only symptom is acute shortness of breath. These patients are often hypoxic, and PE in these patients is deemed to be moderate. This presentation probably is encountered in roughly one-fifth of the patients.
3. *Circulatory collapse.* Patients in this category present with circulatory collapse, characterised by shock or syncope. PE in these people is deemed to be severe.

Table 26.2 Common presenting symptoms and signs

Symptoms	%	Signs	%
Dyspnoea	73	Tachypnea (RR ≥ 20/min)	70
Pleuritic pain	66	Rales	51
Cough	37	Tachycardia (HR > 100/min)	30
Leg pain	26	Fourth heart sound	24
Haemoptysis	13	Loud S_2P	23
		Deep vein thrombosis	11

Source: Data derived from P. D. Stein et al. (1991), 'Clinical, laboratory, roentgenographic, and electrocardiographic findings in patients with acute pulmonary embolism and no pre-existing cardiac or pulmonary disease', *Chest*, 100(3), pp. 598–603.

The physical signs that are commonly encountered in PE are tachypnea, crackles and tachycardia. These findings are common to several cardiopulmonary disorders and so have a low specificity. Other signs include fever, diaphoresis, cyanosis, parasternal heave, loud pulmonary component of the second heart sound, a third or fourth heart sound, wheezes, pleural friction rub, hepatomegaly and hepatojuglar reflux.

Since lower limb DVT is the cause of PE in the majority of cases, it is prudent to look for features of DVT, namely local swelling, pain and tenderness, redness and warmth. Unfortunately, these signs are also non-specific and may even be misleading at times.

Investigation

All patients suspected of PE should undergo the basic tests discussed below. Although they seldom provide confirmation of the diagnosis, they are helpful in ruling out alternate diagnoses.

Chest radiography

A chest radiograph is usually the first test ordered for patients when they present with symptoms of PE. It is of limited value in the diagnosis of PE, falling short in both sensitivity and specificity. It is invaluable in ruling out conditions like cardiac failure, pneumonia, lung cancer and pneumothorax that present with similar clinical features. Furthermore, when the chest radiograph is normal in a breathless patient with hypoxia, the probability of having a diagnosis of PE increases. The Prospective Investigation of Pulmonary Embolism Diagnosis (PIOPED) study data suggests that perhaps 12% of the patients with PE had normal chest radiographs. The most common radiographic feature in patients with proven PE was atelectasis. The other common radiologic findings are focal infiltrate, raised hemidiaphragm and small pleural effusion. A wedge-shaped pleural based density, often sought by clinicians, is very uncommon and is also a non-specific radiologic finding.

The radiologic signs are listed in Box 26.1.

Box 26.1 Radiologic signs of PE

Common

- Atelectasis
- Raised hemidiaphragm
- Focal infiltrate
- Small pleural effusion

Rare

- Focal oligaemia (Westermark's sign)
- Wedge shaped density above the diaphragm (Hampton's sign)
- Enlarged right descending pulmonary artery (Palla's sign)
- Cardiomegaly

Electrocardiography

Non-specific changes in the ST segment and/or T wave are often seen in the electrocardiogram (ECG) of patients with PE. Features of right heart strain are common with massive emboli. The most common abnormality seen is T wave inversion in the anterior leads, especially V1–V4. Occasionally, the much talked about pattern S1Q3T3 may be seen. Admission ECG in 76% of the patients with PE in a series had at least 3 out of 7 predefined features of right heart strain or ischaemia. Sinus tachycardia is common but the other rhythm abnormalities, including new onset right bundle branch block and atrial fibrillation, are uncommon. ECG also has an important role in ruling out acute myocardial infarction and pericardial disease. It should be borne in mind that the presence of ECG features of acute myocardial infarction do not always rule out PE, since the two conditions can co-exist.

Arterial blood gases

Typical abnormalities of arterial blood gases in PE are hypoxaemia, hypocarbia and a high alveolar-arterial oxygen gradient as a consequence of ventilation-perfusion (V/Q) mismatch and hyperventilation. The hypoxaemia is proportionate to the degree of embolism. Normal PaO_2 and $PaCO_2$ may be encountered, particularly if the embolism is minor. It is not possible to confirm or rule out the diagnosis on the basis of the arterial blood gas abnormalities. In patients recruited for the PIOPED study, 38% of the patients without and 14% of patients with pre-existing cardiopulmonary disease had PE despite having normal arterial blood gas results.

Specific tests for PE

Radioisotope ventilation-perfusion lung scanning (V/Q scan)

This is the most commonly used specific test for PE and is invariably performed before any other. It has the advantage of being non-invasive and it is available in most acute care hospitals.

Xenon-133 (^{133}Xe) is the most frequently used agent for performing ventilation scans. Krypton-81 (^{81m}Kr), technegas and Tc-DPTA aerosol are other substances used. Perfusion scans are performed using ^{99m}Tc-labelled macroaggregates of albumin or human albumin microspheres. The mandatory views obtained are anterior, posterior, right and left posterior oblique. Lateral views could also be obtained. The reporting is based on the principle that the vascular obstruction should give rise to perfusion defects in areas with normal ventilation. A good quality chest radiograph is required for correlation, and liaison with the clinician is invaluable in improving the quality of the result.

The scan is reported as low, intermediate or high probability for PE, or normal, using the modified PIOPED criteria (Box 26.2). A normal scan rules out pulmonary embolism. Generally in patients suspected of PE, a high probability scan report is

Box 26.2 Amended PIOPED criteria for interpreting V/Q scans

High probability for PE

- ≥ 2 large[a] segmental V/Q[d] mismatched defects without corresponding chest radiographic abnormalities
- 1 large and > 2 moderate[b] segmental V/Q[d] mismatched defects without corresponding chest radiographic abnormalities
- ≥ 4 moderate[b] segmental V/Q[d] mismatched defects without corresponding chest radiographic abnormalities

Intermediate probability for PE

- 1 moderate[b] or < 2 large[a] segmental V/Q[d] mismatched defects without corresponding chest radiographic abnormalities
- Matched V/Q[d] defects and corresponding abnormalities in the lower lung zone
- Single moderate[b] matched V/Q[d] defects without corresponding chest radiographic abnormalities
- Matched V/Q[d] defects with a small pleural effusion on chest radiograph
- Difficulty in categorising scan as normal, low or high probability of PE

Low probability for PE

- Multiple matched V/Q[d] defects, regardless of size, without corresponding chest radiographic abnormalities
- Matched V/Q[d] defects in the upper and middle zones with corresponding chest radiographic abnormalities
- Matched V/Q[d] defects and a large pleural effusion on chest radiography
- Any perfusion defects with substantially larger abnormality on chest radiography
- Perfusion defects surrounded by normally perfused lung (stripe sign)
- > 3 small[c] segmental perfusion defects without abnormalities on chest radiography
- Non-segmental perfusion defects (cardiomegaly, aortic impression, enlarged hila)

Very low probability of PE

- ≤ 3 small[c] segmental perfusion defects without abnormalities on chest radiography

Normal findings

- No perfusion defects, perfusion outlining the shape of the lung in a chest radiograph

(*a*) > 75% of a segment.
(*b*) 25–75% of a segment.
(*c*) < 25% of a segment.
(*d*) Ventilation-perfusion.

Source: Data from D. F. Worsley & A. Alavi (1995), 'A comprehensive analysis of the results of the PIOPED study', *Journal of Nuclear Medicine*, 36, pp. 2380–7.

accurate in confirming the diagnosis in nearly 90%, and low probability and normal scans in ruling out the diagnosis in about 86% and 96% of the patients, respectively.

Analysis of the PIOPED study data suggested that the scans with the most diagnostic value are those that have a very low, low or high probability of PE in patients with concordant clinical features. However, the very low or low scan results in patients with certain risk factors—prolonged immobilisation, lower limb trauma, recent surgery or central venous instrumentation—was associated with a fourfold increase in the incidence of PE compared with the patients without these risk factors. Thus for these patients, and for those who have had an intermediate probability scan, or whose clinical condition does not correlate with the scan result, further investigation is necessary.

The following clinical situations may render the interpretation of lung scans difficult or misleading: COPD, left heart failure, previous PE (unless a follow-up scan has demonstrated resolution of the thrombus), pulmonary fibrosis, and lung cancer causing vascular occlusion. Age by itself does not affect the interpretation of the test.

More recently there is evidence that the ventilation scans add very little to the information provided by the perfusion scans. One group (PISA-PED) has obtained comparable results using perfusion scans alone and their 4 category grading is very simple to use (see Box 26.3). It is likely that perfusion scans alone may come into vogue, and render performing additional ventilation scans redundant.

Box 26.3 PISA-PED criteria for the interpretation of perfusion scans

Normal

No perfusion defects of any kind

Near normal

Perfusion defects smaller or equal in size and shape to the following roentgenographic abnormalities: cardiomegaly; enlarged aorta, hila and mediastinum; elevated diaphragm; blunting of the costophrenic angle; pleural thickening; intrafissural collection of liquid

Abnormal (PE+)

Single or multiple wedge-shaped perfusion defects with or without matching chest-roentgenographic abnormalities. Wedge-shaped areas of overperfusion usually coexist

Abnormal (PE–)

Single or multiple perfusion defects other than wedge-shaped, with or without matching chest-roentgenographic abnormalities. Wedge-shaped areas of overperfusion are usually not seen

Source: Data from M. Miniati, M. Pistolesi, C. Marini, G. Di Ricco, B. Formichi, R. Prediletto et al. (The PISA-PED investigators) (1996), 'Value of perfusion lung scan in the diagnosis of pulmonary embolism: Results of the prospective investigative study of acute pulmonary embolism diagnosis (PISA-PED)', *American Journal of Respiratory and Critical Care Medicine*, 154, pp. 1387–93.

Spiral computerised tomography and magnetic resonance imaging

Spiral CT (single-slice helical CT or SSHCT) of the chest with contrast medium is a very promising diagnostic modality. An added advantage is its ability to evaluate the entire thorax and detect, for example, lymphadenopathy, lung tumours, pneumonia, emphysema, pleural and pericardial disease, aortic dissection and some oesophageal disease. It is most effective in diagnosing PE in the main, lobar and segmental arteries, but has only limited ability to detect disease in the subsegmental branches. The reliability of spiral CT in the diagnosis of PE has been demonstrated and is more sensitive than the V/Q scan. It has a sensitivity of 94% and specificity of 96%, compared with pulmonary angiography. Its accuracy as the initially performed specific test has been compared with the V/Q scan. Although the detection rate was similar, a confident diagnosis was possible in more patients when spiral CT was performed first. This and its greater out-of-hours availability may result in spiral CT replacing V/Q scan as the most frequently performed confirmatory test for PE.

Multi-slice helical CT (MSHCT) is 8 times faster than most SSHCT systems. The increased speed results in rapid scanning with fewer motion artefacts and the need for only a shorter breath hold. The thinner slices have an improved spatial resolution and thus increase diagnostic accuracy. Quicker scan time requires a faster administration of the intravenous contrast and this renders the arteries, veins and pathological conditions more conspicuous. However, the efficacy of this procedure is unknown and awaits results of clinical trials.

MRI may prove to be a valuable tool for the assessment of PE but its role has not yet been adequately assessed. It provides the opportunity to simultaneously assess the lower limb for DVT.

Gadoline-enhanced magnetic resonance pulmonary angiography seems to be a promising new technique.

Pulmonary angiography

Pulmonary angiogram continues to be the gold standard for the diagnosis of PE. It is believed that at least a third of the patients require this test for confirmation of diagnosis. It is an invasive procedure with potential risks and is therefore performed very infrequently. Only 15% of the radiology departments in British hospitals offer this service. It is indicated when cardiovascular collapse and hypotension are present and when other investigations are inconclusive. The dye is injected into the pulmonary artery via a catheter inserted through the femoral, internal jugular or the subclavian vein. The features indicating the presence of an embolus include intraluminal filling defect and abrupt vascular cut-off in pulmonary arteries.

Fatal complications occur in 0.5–1.3% of the procedures and minor complications in 2%. There is correlation between the presence of pulmonary hypertension and the development of major complications. The complication rate is reduced if the patients are carefully selected and if the procedure is withheld from patients with renal failure, cardiac failure and pulmonary hypertension. The introduction of low osmolar non-ionic contrast media reduces complications.

Interpretations of pulmonary angiograms using digital subtraction angiography (DSA) techniques have a lower interobserver variability. Additional benefits of DSA pulmonary arteriography over conventional angiography are the requirement of less contrast material and eliminating the need for immediate film processing, thus substantially decreasing procedural time. These factors potentially improve the safety of the procedure. The disadvantages of DSA are that it:

1. is not widely available
2. requires highly skilled operators
3. is invasive
4. is expensive.

Intravenous DSA does not require pulmonary catheterisation, but is neither as sensitive nor as specific as pulmonary angiography.

Leg imaging

Since lower limb deep vein thrombosis is the cause of the majority of PE, clots may be demonstrated even in the absence of clinical evidence of DVT. If clots are present, that in itself is an indication for treatment. Leg vein imaging is indicated as the first performed specific test in those with clinical evidence of DVT, in patients with chronic cardiorespiratory disease and in situations of an indeterminate V/Q scan. The test should be performed within 24 hours.

Leg vein imaging is usually performed by ascending contrast venography or ultrasound techniques. Ultrasonographic techniques are now established as first-line imaging modalities. Among these, colour Doppler ultrasonography, which has a sensitivity of 95% and a specificity of 98% for the diagnosis of femoral and popliteal vein thrombosis, has reached a position of pre-eminence. Impedance plethysmography and radioisotope techniques have limitations and are therefore not widely used in clinical practice. Venography is the gold standard for the diagnosis of DVT, but it is invasive and may be technically inadequate in up to 20% of the cases.

If the test is negative, in patients with inadequate cardiopulmonary reserve a pulmonary angiogram should be considered. In those with adequate cardiopulmonary reserve, a repeat scan in 3–7 days will be the preferred option.

Echocardiography

Doppler or two-dimensional echocardiography via transthoracic or transoesophageal route may provide evidence of PE by demonstrating either signs of right ventricular dysfunction or intracardiac clots. It may also exclude other diseases, such as myocardial infarction, aortic dissection and pericardial tamponade, which mimic PE. The presence of right heart stress indicates a poor outcome and clots observable on echocardiography are frequently associated with a fatality. The test has been recommended in all cases of suspected PE in order to effect early operative or thrombolytic intervention. However, its yield is highest in the presence of systemic hypotension and so, in practice, the testing is often confined to this category of patients.

Plasma D-dimer

The concentration of D-dimer, a fibrin degradation product, rises with intravascular coagulation and has been investigated as a potential marker for PE. A recent meta-analysis reviewed 29 studies that have compared D-dimer results with other confirmatory tests for DVT or PE and reported a sensitivity of 48–96% and a specificity of 21–100% for the latex agglutination test, and a sensitivity of 88–100% and a specificity of 10–68% for enzyme linked immunosorbent assay (ELISA). A raised D-dimer level is a common finding in hospitalised patients. Also, a normal value is rare in patients with venous thromboembolism. Therefore the test may be reliable in excluding venous thromboembolism and thus reduce the need for further investigation. It is not useful for confirmation of the diagnosis in patients with clinical suspicion. Further studies will be required before ascertaining the role of this test in the diagnostic algorithm of PE.

Approach to diagnosis

Since the clinical features of PE are non-specific, a wide spectrum of disorders figure in the differential diagnosis (Box 26.4).

Clinical suspicion is crucial and the aim is to identify all patients with suggestive clinical features with a view to subjecting them to further appropriate investigations. Since 97% of patients have dyspnoea, tachypnoea or chest pain and the rest either have chest radiographic changes or a low $P\hat{a}O_2$, the absence of these features virtually excludes PE. It is important to develop an algorithm for the diagnostic analysis and treatment of patients with PE, keeping in mind the resource constraints of the hospital. One such algorithm compiled by the British Thoracic Society (BTS) Standards of Care Committee for patient assessment (see Chart 1 of 'Appendix 26.1') and management (see Chart 2 and Notes of 'Appendix 26.1') has been included.

Box 26.4 Differential diagnosis of PE

- Pneumonia
- Pneumothorax
- Acute asthma
- Acute exacerbation of chronic obstructive airways disease
- Pulmonary oedema
- Pericardial tamponade
- Myocardial infarction
- Aortic dissection
- Pleurisy
- Lung cancer
- Rib fracture
- Costochondritis

Treatment

The choice of primary therapy depends on the size of the embolus and the severity of the patient's condition. Unless specific contraindications exist, all haemodynamically stable patients with PE are anticoagulated. In patients with an intermediate or high suspicion of PE, anticoagulation should be started before completion of investigations as the risk of recurrent PE outweighs the risk of complications secondary to anticoagulation. A case can be made for offering thrombolytic treatment for those who are haemodynamically unstable from massive PE, and if this fails, for surgical embolectomy when the expertise to perform this is available. (Refer to Chart 2 of 'Appendix 26.1' for an algorithm for management, Chart 3 for the drug regimens and Chart 4 for the discharge check list.)

Anticoagulation

Heparin

Anticoagulation with heparin remains the mainstay of treatment of PE and reduces the incidence of fatal recurrent embolism. This prevents further clot formation while allowing endogenous fibrinolysis to proceed. It is unlikely that heparin itself has any direct role in fibrinolysis. If contraindications do not exist, heparin should be administered when a high or intermediate clinical suspicion is present pending the results of investigations. A loading dose of 5000–10 000 units should be given followed by 18 IU/kg/hr daily as a continuous infusion. Dose adjustments should be made to maintain the activated partial thromboplastin time (APTT) at 1.5–2.5 times the control values. The first measurement of APTT should be performed 4–6 hours after starting treatment to ensure adequate anticoagulation and repeated 6–10 hours after every change of dose and subsequently at least daily. Dosing based on patient's body weight is preferable to a standard regimen, since it causes fewer fluctuations in APTT and achieves a therapeutic level more quickly with a shorter warfarin overlap. Heparin should be continued until adequate maintenance anticoagulation with warfarin is achieved. A 5-day course appears to be as good as a 7–10 day course. If continued beyond 5 days, the platelet count must be monitored because of the risk of heparin induced thrombocytopenia with thrombosis.

In some patients with venous thrombosis associated with metastatic malignancy, heparin is used as short-term and long-term treatment, because oral anticoagulation often fails to prevent recurrent venous thrombosis.

Low molecular weight heparin (LMWH)

Trials have confirmed the efficacy of LMWH administered subcutaneously and it has been advocated as an alternative to intravenous unfractionated heparin in haemodynamically stable PE and DVT. It has the advantages of a simple subcutaneous administration, and does not require laboratory monitoring. Recent reports have suggested that it may be as efficacious as unfractionated heparin in non-life-threatening PE.

Several meta-analyses have shown that treatment with LMWH results in fewer episodes of recurrence and bleeding than unfractionated heparin and it might provide a small survival benefit for patients with malignancy and venous thromboembolism. It also opens up the possibility of treating selected patients with PE in an outpatient setting. The available evidence seems to suggest that subcutaneously administered LMWH may replace IV unfractionated heparin in the initial treatment of venous thromboembolism.

Warfarin

Warfarin may be started as soon as the diagnosis is confirmed. A delayed start is associated with increased hospital stay and higher recurrence. Paradoxically, the first 24 hours of warfarin treatment is associated with a transient hypercoagulable state and heparin should not be stopped until the international normalised ratio (INR) reaches therapeutic range 2.0–3.0 and remains so for at least 2–3 days.

Duration of anticoagulation

Most studies on the duration of anticoagulation suggest that treatment for 6 weeks to 3 months is adequate for venous thromboembolism. When there are temporary risk factors for venous thromboembolism, such as the postoperative period, recurrence during and after treatment is unusual. Recurrent embolism in the absence of a recurrent or new risk factor should be treated with long-term anticoagulation. In patients with persisting underlying risk factors, such as deficiency of antithrombin III, protein C or protein S, the anticoagulation is usually prolonged to several years, possibly lifelong.

General supportive measures

Analgesia should be given to patients with severe pleuritic pain, but opiates should be avoided in patients with incipient cardiovascular collapse since they cause vasodilatation. Hypoxaemia should be treated with a high percentage inspired oxygen, and severe hypoxia may require ventilation. In hypotensive patients colloid should be administered while monitoring central venous pressure and the right atrial pressure should be maintained high (15–20 mmHg) to ensure maximal right ventricular filling. Use of inotropic agents may be required to provide circulatory support. Diuretics and vasodilators are not indicated.

Thrombolytic treatment

Heparin reduces the incidence of recurrent PE, but clot lysis is effected only by endogenous fibrinolysis. This occurs over a variable period of time ranging from a week to several months. Organisation of the thromboemboli may occur when there is incomplete resolution, leading to chronic narrowing or obliteration of the pulmonary vascular bed. Thrombolytic therapy could therefore potentially have several advantages by actually dissolving thromboemboli. Streptokinase, urokinase and recombinant tissue plasminogen activator (rtPA) are the agents now used. They have comparable efficacy and safety when equivalent doses are delivered at the same rate over a short period of time. Some regimens are outlined in Chart 3 of 'Appendix 26.1'.

Thrombolytic therapy is equally effective via a peripheral vein or a pulmonary artery catheter. Thrombolysis is indicated primarily in patients who are haemodynamically unstable, particularly in the presence of systemic hypotension or shock. It has no role in the management of haemodynamically stable patients, except perhaps in the subgroup of patients with right ventricular dysfunction but normal systemic arterial pressure, where there is some evidence for its efficacy. Thrombolytic treatment is most effective when administered soon after PE, but benefit may extend for up to 14 days from the onset of symptoms.

Bleeding complication from treatment of PE

Anticoagulation could be complicated by bleeding. The risk of bleeding is higher when a thrombolytic agent is added. The risk of bleeding is 1% in low-risk patients but is substantially higher (10%) in high-risk patients. High-risk patients include those who have had recent surgery, obstetric delivery or invasive vascular studies and those with history of peptic ulcer disease, gastrointestinal or urinary tract bleeding, bleeding disorders, or a platelet count less than 150×10^9/L. Absolute contraindications to anticoagulation and thrombolytic treatment are recent haemorrhage, stroke and current gastrointestinal haemorrhage.

Surgical embolectomy

Most of the data on surgical embolectomy precedes the advent of thrombolytic treatment. Given the efficacy of thrombolytic treatment in clot lysis, the role of surgical embolectomy is not clear and there is paucity of data comparing the two treatments. Surgery should be considered in patients with a massive PE who fail to respond to thrombolytic therapy in the first hour and when thrombolytic treatment is contraindicated. Embolectomy is performed either by percutaneous catheter techniques or open operation.

Inferior venacaval (IVC) filters

IVC filter devices placed in the inferior vena cava protect the pulmonary circulation from emboli. Their role in the primary prophylaxis is controversial. The two main indications are: contraindication of anticoagulation, and recurrent embolism despite anticoagulation. Several filters have been evaluated, but their comparative efficacy is unknown. Filter insertion should be carried out by an experienced interventional radiologist.

Prevention

The adage 'prevention is better than cure' is very true for PE, since it is difficult to detect and treatment is not always successful. All hospitalised patients should be stratified according to their risk for PE and appropriate prophylaxis should be instituted.

Mechanical approaches to prevention include the use of graduated-compression stockings, devices that provide intermittent pneumatic compression, and IVC filters alone or in combination. Intermittent pneumatic compression increases venous blood flow to the legs and also promotes endogenous fibrinolysis by stimulating the vascular endothelial wall. Although compliance for this treatment among patients in an intensive care unit is reasonable, it is not so among less critically ill patients. Foot pumps, which compress the plantar venous plexus, have been used, but they have not yet been adequately investigated.

Low dose subcutaneous heparin (5000 units 2–3 times daily) has been used without laboratory monitoring for peri-operative prophylaxis and this strategy reduces the rate of fatal pulmonary embolism by two-thirds. The first dose is administered 2 hours before surgery and the treatment is continued until the patient is discharged and fully ambulatory. Low molecular weight heparin has increasingly replaced unfractionated heparin because of its superior bioavailability and absorption, the need for less frequent doses, and lower rates of heparin induced thrombocytopenia. However, it is more expensive. The efficacy of aspirin is inadequate for use as a single agent for prophylaxis for PE. There is lack of consensus regarding several aspects of the prevention of pulmonary embolism, including the optimal timing and the duration of prophylaxis in various clinical settings.

Acknowledgment

The authors wish to thank Dr Mark L. H. Tie FRANZCR, consultant radiologist, for reading through the section of the manuscript on imaging and forwarding his valuable comments.

Bibliography and further reading

Anderson, F. A. & Wheeler, H. B. (1995), 'Venous thromboembolism risk factors and prophylaxis', *Clinics in Chest Medicine*, 16, pp. 235–51.

Arcasoy, S. M. & Kreit, J. W. (1999), 'Thrombolytic therapy of pulmonary embolism: a comprehensive review of current evidence', *Chest*, 115(6), pp. 1695–707.

British Thoracic Society Standards of Care Committee (1997), 'Suspected acute pulmonary embolism: a practical approach', *Thorax*, 52(Suppl. 4), pp. S1–24.

Fennerty, T. (1997), 'Fortnightly review: the diagnosis of pulmonary embolism', *British Medical Journal*, 314(7078), pp. 425–9.

Goldhaber, S. Z. (1998), 'Medical progress: pulmonary embolism', *New England Journal of Medicine*, 339(2), pp. 93–104.

Hyers, T. M., Hull, R. D., Morris, T. A., Tapson, V. & Weg, J. G. (2001), 'Antithrombotic therapy for venous thromboembolic disease (Sixth ACCP Consensus Conference on Antithrombotic Therapy)', *Chest*, 119, pp. 1765–935.

Ryu, J. H., Olson, E. J., Pellikka, P. A. & Patricia, A. (1998), 'Clinical recognition of pulmonary embolism: problem of unrecognised and asymptomatic cases', *Mayo Clinic Proceedings*, 73(9), pp. 873–9.

Stein, P. D., Terrin, M. L., Hales, C. A., Palevsky, H. I., Saltzman, H. A., Thompson, B. T., Tai, N. R., Atwal, A. S. & Hamilton, G. (1991), 'Modern management of pulmonary embolism', *The British Journal of Surgery*, 86(7), pp. 853–68.

Weg, J. G. (1991), 'Clinical, laboratory, roentgenographic, and electrographic findings in patients with acute pulmonary embolism and no pre-existing cardiac or pulmonary disease', *Chest*, 100(3), pp. 598–603.

Appendix 26.1

The following charts were prepared by the Standard of Care Committee of the British Thoracic Society (British Thoracic Society Standards of Care Committee (1997), 'Suspected acute pulmonary embolism: A practical approach', *Thorax*, 52(Suppl. 4), pp. S1–24), set up to review available literature and recommend a strategy for the diagnosis and management of suspected acute pulmonary embolism. We have modified it in keeping with current understanding. These are simple and practical and so they could be incorporated into junior doctors' handbooks as such or after modification, depending on the local resource constraints.

Chart 1 Initial assessment and action

STEP 1—Assess probability of pulmonary embolism

Clinical patterns of PE include:
(a) sudden collapse with raised jugular venous pressure (faintness and/or hypotension)
(b) pulmonary haemorrhage syndrome (pleuritic pain and/or haemoptysis)
(c) isolated dyspnoea (i.e. no cough/ sputum/chest pain)

PE is easily missed:
(a) in severe cardiorespiratory disease
(b) in elderly patients
(c) if only symptom is breathlessness 'isolated dyspnoea')

- Most are breathless and/or tachypnoeic (rate > 20/min).
- PE is rare if age < 40 with no risk factors.
- Oestrogens are only a minor risk factor.

If PE is suspected, ask the following questions:

1. Are other diagnoses unlikely?
- on clinical grounds
- after basic investigations:
  - white cell count
  - chest radiography
  - ECG
  - spirometry or peak flow
  - blood analysis

If YES, score + 1

2. Is a major risk factor present?
- recent immobilisation or major surgery
- recent lower limb trauma and/or surgery
- clinical deep vein thrombosis
- previous proven DVT or PE
- pregnancy or post-partum major medical illness

If YES, score + 1

STEP 2—Take action according to score

Action	**Score Probability**	**2 High**	**1 Intermediate**	**0 Low**
Heparinise?		Yes[(a)]	Yes[(a)]	Wait
Tests for PE?		Urgent[(b)]	Early[(b)]	Consider
Another diagnosis?		Consider	Seek	Seek

(*a*) Unless contraindicated.
(*b*) See chart 2.

Chart 2 Investigations and action

This diagram is a template that can be modified according to local facilities and expertise.

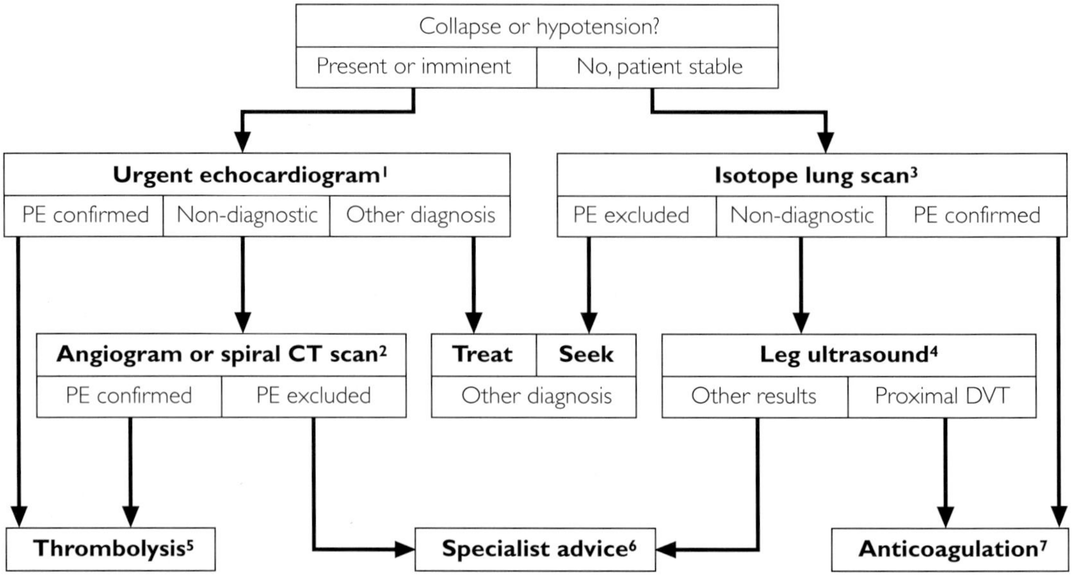

Notes (Chart 2)

1. Contact senior staff urgently (a) because of severity of illness, (b) to expedite investigations. If massive PE obvious clinically (a) start heparin, (b) arrange angiography or spiral CT immediately. 'Other diagnoses' mimicking massive PE include aortic dissection, pericardial tamponade, acute myocardial infarction. 'Non-diagnostic', start heparin (unless active gastrointestinal bleeding, cerebral haemorrhage).
2. Whichever can be arranged more quickly, as far as possible within 1 hour. Perfusion (without ventilation) lung scan is an alternative urgent investigation. Spiral CT scanning may miss a small PE, but this rarely causes cardiovascular collapse.
3. Start heparin unless (a) contraindicated or (b) low clinical probability. Preferably request leg imaging at the same time; it can be cancelled if lung scan is diagnostic. Consider leg imaging instead if (a) previous proven PE, (b) in pregnancy or (c) poor cardiorespiratory reserve. 'PE excluded' by lung scan either if normal, or if low probability plus low clinical probability. 'PE confirmed' if lung scan high probability plus high clinical probability.
4. Compression ultrasound, preferably with colour Doppler imaging. 'Other' includes (i) calf vein DVT, (ii) poorly visualised veins, (iii) normal study. Specialist will advise either:
   (a) treat as possible PE, especially if either (i) or (ii) in those with poor cardiorespiratory reserve
   (b) that PE has been excluded, especially if (iii) and low clinical probability
   (c) further imaging—either pulmonary angiography or repeat ultrasound at 3–7 days.
5. Surgical or catheter embolectomy is an alternative, especially if medical treatment is contraindicated. Thrombolysis is followed by anticoagulation.
6. Advice from a senior chest physician or cardiologist should be sought if:
   (a) there is undue delay in arranging investigations
   (b) diagnostic uncertainty remains after both lung scanning and leg imaging
   (c) PE has been excluded but the correct diagnosis remains elusive.

7. IVC filter should be considered if anticoagulation is contraindicated. For anticoagulation with heparin + warfarin, see Treatment section.

Pulmonary angiography, where readily available, may be chosen as the initial imaging modality.

Close co-operation with imaging departments is essential.

Chart 3 Anticoagulant drug regimens

Intravenous thrombolysis		
	Initial treatment	**Further treatment**
rtPA	100 mg in 2 hours	
Streptokinase[(a)]	250 000 units in 20 minutes	100 000 units/hour for 24 hours
Urokinase	4400 IU/kg in 10 minutes	4400 IU/kg/hour for 12 hours
Before treatment, stop heparin; after treatment, use maintenance dose as below (*a*) Plus hydrocortisone to prevent further circulatory instability		

Intravenous heparin		
	Initial dose	**Maintenance dose**
Standard	5000–10 000 IU	1300 IU/hour
Weight adjusted	80 IU/kg	18 IU/kg/hour
Adjust infusion rate until APTT = 1.5–2.5 times control (45–75 seconds)		
APTT monitoring	After initial bolus	4–6 hours later
	After any dose change	6–10 hours later
	APTT in therapeutic range	Daily
Discontinue heparin 5 days after starting warfarin if INR at least 2.0		

Low molecular weight heparins		
	Dosage to be administered subcutaneously	**Maximum strength of single dose**
Dalteparin sodium	200 anti-Coagulant IU/kg/day	18 000 IU
Enoxaparin sodium	1 mg/kg Coagulant every 12 hours or 1.5 mg/kg per day	180 mg
Nadroparin calcium	86 anti-Coagulant IU/kg every 12 hours or 171 anti-Coagulant IU/kg per day	17 000 IU
Tinzaparin sodium	175 anti-Coagulant IU/kg per day	
• Check platelet count between 3 to 5 days • Stop LMWH therapy after at least 4–5 days of combined therapy with warfarin when INR > 2		

Warfarin	
Initial doses	5–10 mg daily for 2 days
Subsequent treatment	1–10 mg
Adjust dose to INR = 2–3 times control, initially measured every 1–2 days	

Chart 4 Discharge check list

1. The international normalised ratio (INR) is between 2.0 and 3.0.
2. The general practitioner:
   - is aware the patient is on anticoagulant, and
   - has been informed of the proposed duration of treatment, and
   - has a discharge summary stating diagnosis as either PE suspected or PE confirmed.
3. The patient:
   - is aware of side effects of anticoagulants and interactions with other drugs, and
   - has written information on warfarin therapy and
   - has an appointment for anticoagulant supervision.
4. Follow-up review at 6–12 weeks has been arranged. At that time, if:
   - first episode and temporary risk factors, anticoagulation may be discontinued;
   - idiopathic or recurrent episode, consider (a) thrombophilic disorder, (b) occult cancer.
5. Specialist advice has been sought for female patients on oral contraception.

Abbreviations

APTT activated partial thromboplastin time
CT computerised tomography with contrast
DVT deep vein thrombosis
ECG electrocardiogram
INR international normalised ratio
IU international units
IVC inferior vena cava
PE pulmonary embolism
rtPA recombinant tissue plasminogen activator

Chapter 27

Cough, dyspnoea and haemoptysis

MARY IP

Introduction

Respiratory symptoms are very common in the general population, and due to the overall decline in health with ageing, symptoms such as cough and dyspnoea are highly prevalent even in the ambulatory elderly cohorts. Epidemiological studies indicate that various respiratory symptoms singly or in combination may affect over half of elderly community cohorts in various countries. These symptoms reflect diverse underlying diseases, which account for significant disability, morbidity and ultimate mortality in the geriatric age group.

Cough, dyspnoea or haemoptysis are usually indicative of pathologies in the respiratory system, although they are also often due to cardiac diseases. This chapter provides a comprehensive framework of approach to the elderly who present with symptoms of cough, dyspnoea and haemoptysis to the general practitioners, the primary doctors looking after the ageing population.

Cough

Cough is a body reflex that occurs when irritant receptors in the respiratory system are stimulated. There is evidence to suggest that the cough centre is diffusely located in the medulla, and cough is effected by an increased expiratory effort from increased intrathoracic pressure and high gas flows which result from increased respiratory muscle contraction in the face of a transiently closed glottis.

Cough has diverse roles. Cough is primarily an important defence mechanism of the airways to clear excessive secretions and foreign materials, most of which are obnoxious to the body. Cough may be a manifestation of underlying pathology due to either disease of the lung parenchyma, the airways or the pulmonary vasculature and, occasionally, of a more systemic nature beyond the chest itself. Inadvertently, cough is also an important factor that leads to the spread of airborne infections, especially in confined environments.

Hence cough as a body reaction may occur during both 'health' and disease states of an individual and it is therefore a very common symptom for which medical attention may be sought. When either the afferent pathway or the effector mechanisms are blunted by any physiological, pathological or pharmacological process, a phenomenon not uncommon in the elderly population, the cough reflex becomes diminished or the cough effort is ineffective. This compromises the important functions of cough as a body defence mechanism in the elderly.

Chronic cough is a common symptom in the elderly and has been reported to occur at a prevalence rate of 10% to over 50% in studies of European or Asian populations. The most important determinant has been reported to be smoking, although there are many other causes of chronic cough as discussed below.

Evaluation of cough

The common causes of acute cough (arbitrarily defined as less than 3 weeks) and chronic cough are different (see Table 27.1), although there is overlap because acute cough may persist while chronic cough may have acute exacerbations. There may also be multiple aetiologies of cough in one person.

Table 27.1 Causes of cough in the elderly

Duration of cough	Cause
Acute cough (cough lasting for less than 3 weeks)	Respiratory infections—common cold, acute tracheobronchitis, pneumonia Pulmonary oedema Exacerbation of chronic bronchitis and emphysema Exacerbation of chronic asthma Aspiration Pulmonary embolism
Chronic cough (cough lasting at least 3–8 weeks)	Chronic bronchitis Asthma Bronchiectasis Gastroesophageal reflux 'Silent' aspiration Tuberculosis Post-infectious cough Post-nasal drip Interstitial lung disease Drugs

Several prospective studies have investigated the aetiologies of chronic cough in adults. Asthma, post-nasal drip and gastroesophageal reflux disease (GORD) are the most common causes of cough, either singly or as a triad. However, the studies involved patients referred for cough; smokers with chronic bronchitis were probably screened out already. Furthermore, the mean ages in those studies were less than 60 years old, and the findings may not be directly applicable to the geriatric population, but they can certainly be adapted for use in the diagnostic approach to elderly subjects presenting with chronic cough.

History

Bearing the possible aetiologies of cough in mind, the history should focus on the following features:

- onset and duration of cough
- history of smoking and other known respiratory or cardiac conditions
- precipitating factors
- concomitant symptoms, such as production of phlegm
- haemoptysis and dyspnoea
- rhinitis
- gastroesophageal reflux
- recently introduced medications for any illness
- previous or current occupation
- exposure to inhaled irritants
- systemic symptoms.

The importance of considering the total picture with the combination of symptoms and any background illness cannot be overemphasised. The history taking in chronic cough should not only focus on the underlying diagnosis, but also on the impact of cough and its complications on the patient's daily functions.

Physical examination

General physical signs that may be related to underlying problems causing cough are fever, clubbing of fingers, lymphadenopathy and ankle oedema. Particular attention should be given to the respiratory and cardiac systems. In acute cough with symptoms compatible with acute respiratory tract infection, examination of the throat may find evidence of upper respiratory tract infection, such as post-nasal drip in the pharynx or congestion. Elderly patients with signs of lower respiratory tract infection, such as crackles, rhonchi or bronchial breathing on auscultation, are at risk of a more adverse outcome and need more monitoring. If acute pulmonary oedema is suspected, the signs of tachycardia, lung crackles with or without elevated jugular venous pressure (JVP) and ankle oedema should be sought. Subjects with cough as part of chronic obstructive pulmonary disease (COPD) or asthma usually have wheezing during acute exacerbations, but wheezing may not be present in the chronic phase or in cough variant asthma.

The appropriate sequence and extent of investigations depend on the priority ranking of the differential diagnosis after history and physical examination. The salient diagnostic tests for each of the differential diagnoses are outlined in Table 27.2.

Table 27.2 Selected diagnostic tests in chronic cough

Cause of cough	Diagnostic test
Chronic bronchitis	Spirometry Carbon monoxide diffusing capacity
Asthma	Spirometry Bronchodilator reversibility
Post-nasal drip	X-ray sinus in selected cases
Gastroesophageal reflux disease	24 hours oesophageal pH monitoring
Bronchiectasis	HRCT[a] of thorax Sputum microbiology
Interstitial lung disease	HRCT thorax Lung biopsy
Bronchogenic carcinoma	CT thorax Fibreoptic bronchoscopy
Foreign body	Fibreoptic bronchoscopy
Tuberculosis	Sputum microbiology

(*a*) HRCT = High-resolution computerised tomography.

Common differential diagnoses

Chronic bronchitis

Chronic bronchitis is clinically defined as productive cough for at least 3 months a year for 2 consecutive years, with no other specific cause for cough being identified. Hence, the diagnosis of chronic bronchitis is based on the exclusion of other diseases leading to the symptom. The majority of chronic bronchitis is related to smoking; less commonly it is due to chronic exposure to gaseous irritants in the environment at work or at home. Cough and phlegm usually improve but may not always completely resolve with cessation of smoking. Smokers tend to accept a minor degree of cough and phlegm due to smoking, and may not seek medical attention unless there are additional symptoms, such as exertional dyspnoea from airflow obstruction or other new complications. It is therefore imperative to ask about other respiratory symptoms. If the subject is a non-smoker with no predisposing irritant exposure history, other causes of cough as outlined below should be considered.

Asthma

Asthma is a common disease and may present for the first time in old age, although its diagnosis tends to be overlooked in this age group. Its prevalence is difficult to ascertain due to diagnostic confusion with smoking-related COPD (Chapter 28) or even heart failure (Chapter 24), which may have similar symptoms. Presentation of asthma in the elderly is similar to that in the young with cough, chest tightness and wheeze, but symptoms may be less well perceived. Cough may be the sole or dominating symptom for weeks or months before other symptoms such as wheeze, dyspnoea or chest tightness become manifest. Cough may also be the only symptom without any evidence of airflow obstruction in cough variant asthma, the diagnosis of which is often one of exclusion of other causes of cough, supported by evidence of bronchial hyperreactivity, and response to therapeutic trial of anti-asthma medications. The prevalence of cough variant asthma in the elderly is not known, and population studies of asthma in the elderly suggest that they tend to have more persistent airflow obstruction which may be 'fixed', even in non-smokers.

Gastroesophageal reflux disease (GORD)

Gastroesophageal reflux is a common disorder in which gastric acid refluxes back into the oesophagus and is then aspirated into the respiratory tract. Hence GORD is associated with many respiratory symptoms from the larynx to the lower respiratory tract. In one series, it has been found to be the sole cause of the symptom in about 1 in 10 adults with chronic cough. The classical symptoms of GORD are waterbrash, heartburn and retrosternal discomfort. However, GORD may lead to chronic cough without marked gastrointestinal symptoms, thus making the diagnosis difficult. GORD may also be one of the triad together with asthma and post-nasal drip in causing cough in the same individual.

Bronchiectasis

Patients with bronchiectasis due to cystic fibrosis (CF) are not a geriatric problem, and are not considered further here. Non-CF bronchiectasis is common in adult populations in some localities in Asia, but reported to be uncommon in countries such as the US, although two series on chronic cough detected bronchiectasis as the cause in 4% and 17% of subjects, respectively. In geriatric subjects presenting with chronic cough due to bronchiectasis, the aetiology is either idiopathic or post-infectious, and occasionally due to repeated minor aspirations or post-obstruction from an aspirated object. Cough in bronchiectasis is usually accompanied by production of sputum, although occasional cases have non-productive cough. Subjects are also prone to intermittent exacerbations with increased infective symptoms and even haemoptysis.

Post-nasal drip

In adults, post-nasal drip induced cough has been reported to be the most common aetiology of chronic cough. Although there has been no study specifically on cough among the elderly, clinical experience and epidemiological studies in the elderly suggest that chronic cough is due to causes other than post-nasal drip. Post-nasal drip as a cause for cough is diagnosed by the history of nasal/sinus symptoms with no evidence of other causes of cough, and the diagnosis needs to be confirmed by prompt resolution of cough to specific therapy for post-nasal drip.

Bronchogenic carcinoma or lung metastasis

Cough is a common symptom associated with bronchogenic carcinomas, although it accounts for only a small percentage of subjects presenting with cough. It has been reported in various series on chronic cough as the cause in 0–2% of adult subjects, but the index of suspicion for a malignant cause should be greater in the elderly due to the increased incidence of malignancies, both primarily of lung origin or metastatic. Cough presents earlier if the tumour is endobronchially situated, and such tumours are mostly of squamous and small cell type, related to smoking. Cough in a smoker tends to be attributed to chronic bronchitis and therefore ignored by the patient and overlooked by the physician. Adenocarcinoma is rising in incidence worldwide and more often occurs in non-smokers. Age alone does not prohibit surgery, and therefore referral for further assessment should be made if the patient is deemed fit and the tumour operable. Lung metastasis tends to give rise to cough only late in the course of lung involvement.

Aspiration

Gag reflex may be diminished even in the healthy elderly, and further compromised in the presence of co-morbid illnesses. Hence, apart from GORD which predisposes to aspiration of gastric acid and hence cough, the ill elderly are prone to more severe forms of aspiration. Significant aspiration of food particles or tablets results in choking and acute cough. This may subside after the acute event without the aspirated object being expelled and the patient subsequently presenting with cough or even haemoptysis. In the elderly with multiple morbidities, especially those with impaired neurological functions, relatively silent aspiration of oropharyngeal contents or even gastroesophageal contents with resultant chronic cough and episodic pneumonia is a definite possibility.

Respiratory infections

Acute cough is frequently due to the common cold. Usually this resolves within a few weeks, but may sometimes persist as post-infectious cough for 8–12 weeks before spontaneously resolving. Symptoms of infection in the elderly may be non-specific and non-localising, probably due to decreased cough reflex. The subject may merely present with overall deterioration and subtle symptoms of cough. It is important to be vigilant for subsequent lower respiratory tract infection, as pneumonia can cause serious morbidity and mortality in the elderly.

More insidious infections such as tuberculosis should be considered in subjects with prolonged cough with or without constitutional symptoms. In localities where the condition is common, the prevalence of tuberculosis and mortality is highest in the elderly, and the majority is due to reactivation. In developed countries, tuberculosis may not be common but its prevalence is increasing, with a disproportionate increase in the elderly. The preponderance in the elderly may be partly due to decreased immunity and partly the ease of transmission among institutionalised elderly subjects. There is an increased risk of tuberculosis in nursing homes and residential homes since spread of the infection can have implications beyond the individual patient.

Drugs

Notably, angiotensin-converting enzyme inhibitor (ACEI), given for hypertension or heart failure, leads to cough in about 1% of subjects. Cough may appear within a few hours to months after initiation of ACEI, therefore the diagnosis should be considered in a patient who develops cough while taking ACEI. Usually, the cough disappears or improves substantially within 4 weeks of discontinuation of the medication.

Drugs may also lead to cough by causing interstitial lung disease. The list of drugs with this potential side effect is long, and the more commonly implicated are amiodarone, gold, penicillamine, nitrofurantoin, sulphasalazine and bisulphan.

Drugs such as propranolol may also aggravate cough and airflow obstruction in those with asthma.

Psychogenic/habit cough

This is a diagnosis of exclusion. It has been said to be more common in children and the prevalence in the elderly is not known. The throat-clearing habit probably reflects a withdrawn or self-conscious personality. It is important to consider post-nasal drip that may result in a similar type of cough.

Investigations

Bearing the common causes in mind, the history and physical examination should prioritise some of the major causes, to proceed with further investigations if necessary. Acute cough caused by acute respiratory tract infection requires investigation but may be necessary if constitutional upset occurs. If lower respiratory tract infection is suspected, a chest X-ray is needed. The management of respiratory tract infection is discussed elsewhere (Chapter 51). If pulmonary embolism is suspected, chest X-ray and other appropriate management steps are necessary.

Algorithms for the management of chronic cough have been proposed and such algorithms can be adapted for elderly patients. In those patients in whom cough is attributed to ACEI, stopping the drug to see if cough resolves, usually within 4 weeks, is the first step. If there are symptoms suggestive of post-nasal drip, a trial of decongestants/antihistamines can be given before further more extensive investigations, although sinus films may be needed when the patient cannot give a clear history of nasal symptoms.

For all other patients with chronic cough, a chest radiograph is indicated and if this is not immediately informative, a spirometry with bronchodilator test for reversible airflow obstruction should be done. The differential diagnosis can then be reprioritised according to the history, physical signs and the findings of chest radiograph (chest X-ray) and spirometry. Depending on which diagnosis is the most likely, further investigations can be requested according to the availability of facilities as well as the overall condition of the patient (see Table 27.2). In most cases, at this stage, there would be clues for causes such as chronic bronchitis, asthma, lung tumours, tuberculosis, bronchiectasis and interstitial lung disease.

If the history and physical signs are not directive, and chest X-ray and spirometry do not show significant lung abnormality, conditions such as cough variant asthma or GORD should be considered. For cough variant asthma, if a patient is generally fit and facilities available, bronchial challenge should be considered. If not, a therapeutic trial of anti-asthma medications is practical. In GORD, presence of hiatus hernia on chest X-ray should raise this suspicion, although usually chest X-ray is non-revealing. A 24 hours pH monitoring for a definitive diagnosis is highly desirable since effective treatment may entail a long course of proton-pump inhibitors and motility drugs. If the test is indeed not available or not feasible, and the diagnosis is highly suspected, a trial of antireflux therapy may be given. If cough persists despite the above measures, it would be necessary to repeat the chest radiograph as evolutionary changes may have occurred and one should also consider multiple aetiologies of cough in one subject. If the chest radiograph remains normal or non-specific, and the symptom is significant, one should consider CT thorax and/or fibreoptic bronchoscopy.

If cough is productive of phlegm with constant or frequent infective characteristics, and chest crackles are present, bronchiectasis should be considered even if chest X-ray is not revealing, as chest radiographs are not sensitive or specific for bronchiectasis. A high resolution CT thorax is indicated for the diagnosis. Sputum bacterial culture further aids subsequent treatment. If the cough is dry or scantily productive and there is also dyspnoea with fine crackles in the chest, it is important to re-examine the chest X-ray and spirometry for subtle features of reticulonodular shadows and restrictive pattern, respectively. If indicated, CT thorax and full lung function tests with lung volumes and carbon monoxide diffusing capacity would be very informative.

If the chest X-ray shows an abnormality that suggests a diagnosis such as lung tumour or tuberculosis, relevant investigations such as sputum analysis, computerised tomography of chest and referrals for invasive tests such as fibreoptic bronchoscopy would be indicated.

In patients who have one cause of cough identified and are treated adequately without satisfactory resolution of cough, multiple aetiologies should be considered.

Complications of cough

Apart from the underlying process that the cough indicates, it is important to remember that cough as a symptom can lead to undesirable consequences, some of which the elderly are particularly prone to. Some of these complications can be dangerous or, although not directly life-threatening, detrimental to overall quality of life. Common complications of cough in geriatric practice are listed in Box 27.1.

Treatment of cough

Box 27.1 Common complications of cough

- Urinary incontinence
- Uterine prolapse (especially in multiparous females)
- Musculoskeletal pain and rib fractures (cough fractures)
- Cough syncope
- Arrhythmias
- Gastroesophageal reflux
- Aggravation of hernias
- Exhaustion and sleep deprivation
- Decreased quality of life

Depending on the cause of the cough, treatment is best directed specifically to the underlying disease. Sometimes the underlying disease/mechanism has no effective specific therapy (e.g. common cold) or the disease process cannot be adequately controlled (e.g. carcinoma of lung), and symptomatic treatment is indicated for alleviation of cough. However, although the use of such symptomatic therapies is a common practice, either prescribed by the physician or by self-prescription with over-the-counter medications, it has a limited role due to the lack of consistently effective agents or side effects. The therapy is generally aimed at either suppression of cough (antitussive) or induction of cough and its related clearance of phlegm (protussive).

Antitussives

Excessive cough should be suppressed when it does not serve any useful function because it is an uncomfortable symptom that may lead to the complications described above. Unfortunately, many medications currently prescribed have no demonstrable efficacy in rigorous trials, while some medications are only shown to be useful for cough reduction in specific conditions or have limited efficacy. The conditions in which medications have been shown to decrease cough in randomised, double-blind, placebo controlled trials include:

- common colds—dexbrompheniramine and pseudoephedrine combination
- bronchitis—ipratropium bromide, guaimesal, diphenhydramine, codeine, dextromethorphan
- carcinoma, tuberculosis, pulmonary fibrosis and bronchitis—codeine, dextromethorphan.

Special caution is needed in the use of antitussives in the elderly. Dextromethorphan or codeine gives rise to dizziness and drowsiness, especially on initial introduction, and almost invariably leads to constipation with prolonged use. Naproxen, although shown to be effective in decreasing cough in a study in rhinovirus colds, has limited applicability for such indications in the elderly due to its potential gastric and renal side effects.

Protussives

Protussive therapy is indicated when cough as a mechanism to clear secretions is desired (e.g. in bronchiectasis) and the patient's own cough is considered inadequate for the purpose. These agents aim at improving cough clearance with or without increasing cough frequency. They may do so by either stimulating cough and/or changing the viscosity of the sputum, which may facilitate mucus clearance by cough (mucolytics). However, only a few agents have been shown to be effective in specific conditions:

- bronchitis—hypertonic saline inhalation
- bronchiectasis—terbutaline inhalation with chest physiotherapy.

Hypertonic saline should be used with caution as it may itself result in very severe cough and it is contraindicated in subjects with asthma as it may precipitate bronchoconstriction. Chest physiotherapy should always be considered if cough clearance is desired.

Cough mixtures or elixirs usually contain a combination of agents, such as an antitussive with an antihistamine for use in common colds, or a protussive with mucolytics for sputum clearance. The habitual use of cough elixirs in chronic cough without determining the cause is not recommended. The aim should always be to determine the aetiology and give specific treatment that would usually abolish or improve the cough. An example is the need for and efficacy of specific anti-asthma medications for increased cough and sputum in asthma exacerbation rather than the use of cough suppressants or mucolytics.

Dyspnoea

Dyspnoea is the subjective awareness of the effort of breathing and it is usually an unpleasant sensation. Elderly subjects, despite a decreased capacity for sensing dyspnoea compared to younger adults, experience more dyspnoea because of age-related decline in lung function and co-morbidities of cardiorespiratory illnesses as well as systemic health problems. In general, the elderly accept a decline in their overall 'fitness' and gradually adjust the level of their daily activities with increasing age. Hence they would only present to health care personnel when the dyspnoea poses a limitation to their daily function, and this may cause a delay in recognition of any underlying pathologic issues.

The assessment of dyspnoea has twofold implications. First, as a presenting symptom, it would lead to the diagnosis and treatment of the underlying disease and, second, dyspnoea itself requires relief since the symptom per se impairs the quality of life.

Mechanisms of dyspnoea

Dyspnoea is a complex symptom that in one or more different diseases may have a different pathophysiological basis. The mechanisms of dyspnoea are not yet fully understood. The sensation of dyspnoea is brought about by a biological loop. Sensory receptors involved with respiration are stimulated by diverse signals—chemical (e.g. hypoxia and hypercapnia acting via chemoreceptors) or mechanical (e.g. stretch receptors in the lungs)—and these signals are sent to the higher brain centres in the central nervous system. Signals are processed and result in, first, a sensation of dyspnoea and, second, subject to modification by the individual's behavioural style and emotional state, efferent responses of the body (also known as the perception of dyspnoea), which would include changes in the breathing pattern. Such changes may themselves modify the sensation of dyspnoea as the mechanical receptors in the respiratory system would be stimulated by the altered pattern of breathing and send further afferent messages to the central nervous system to be interpreted and perceived.

The major mechanisms modifying sensation and perception of dyspnoea may be broadly classified under:

1. increased ventilatory demand due to increased ventilatory drive from metabolic or mechanical stimulus
2. increased ventilatory load, such as airflow obstruction
3. inadequate respiratory muscle function
4. previous experience as stored in the 'central memory' of the individual.

Lung function values and respiratory muscle strength decline as part of ageing. There is also evidence of decreased responsiveness to increased resistive loads and chemical stimuli of hypoxia and hypercapnia in the elderly, suggesting a decreased propensity to feel dyspnoeic. On the other hand, enhanced ventilatory response to exercise has been reported which may contribute to the sensation of dyspnoea on exertion. An important undesirable effect of exertional dyspnoea is the voluntary inhibition of activity in the individual to decrease the work of breathing and hence limit the uncomfortable sensation. This would gradually result in deconditioning of both respiratory muscles as well as other body systems that push the individual to go into a vicious cycle of further dyspnoea and further deconditioning.

Evaluation of dyspnoea

Dyspnoea is a subjective sensation which may vary widely in terms of quality in various individuals and the severity of dyspnoea may not entirely correlate with the underlying physiological severity. The evaluation of dyspnoea focuses on making a diagnosis of the underlying cause, assessing the severity of dyspnoea and evaluating other aspects of the underlying disease. Understanding the mechanisms of dyspnoea operating in the individual is useful as it helps to plan the strategy for relief of dyspnoea. Points of note would therefore include:

- onset and quality of dyspnoea
- precipitating or relieving factors of dyspnoea
- accompanying symptoms and concomitant diseases
- degree of functional impairment from dyspnoea;
- investigations to assist in confirmation and assessment of underlying disease and
- planning of treatment for underlying disease and symptomatic control of dyspnoea in those in whom the underlying disease is not completely reversible.

History

Being a sensation, the description of the uncomfortable awareness of breathing may present as different terminologies in different individuals. Terms such as 'short of air/breath', 'not enough air', 'tight sensation in the chest', 'breathing requires more effort/work', 'rapid breathing', 'suffocating' may be the descriptors used by patients. Studies have shown that certain descriptors are used more frequently in certain conditions: dyspnoea in asthma is often qualified as 'chest tightness', dyspnoea in heart failure is described as 'suffocating' or 'air hunger', while that in COPD or neuromuscular weakness is perceived as increased effort of breathing.

It is useful to note the aggravating factors of dyspnoea, including the body position. Orthopnea is characteristically suggestive of pulmonary congestion.

Since the most common causes of both acute and chronic dyspnoea are cardiopulmonary diseases, followed by neuromuscular disorders (see Table 27.3), questions should focus on features relating to these common conditions. For acute dyspnoea, the most common causes are exacerbations of congestive heart failure, COPD and asthma. Thus, for subjects with these chronic diseases, an increase or acute onset of dyspnoea often reflects an acute exacerbation or complications such as pneumothorax in COPD. Patients with asthma may have chronic cough in the background and present acutely with dyspnoea and wheezing. Elderly subjects who are immobile or bed-ridden are prone to pulmonary embolism that may present with acute dyspnoea, cough, haemoptysis and pleuritic pain.

Table 27.3 Causes of dyspnoea

Duration of dyspnoea	Cause
Acute dyspnoea	Exacerbation of COPD or asthma Congestive heart failure/pulmonary oedema Pulmonary embolism Pneumothorax Respiratory infections Metabolic acidosis (e.g. diabetic ketoacidosis) Upper airway obstruction—tumour, infection, foreign body
Chronic dyspnoea	COPD Congestive heart failure Chronic asthma Pulmonary fibrosis/interstitial lung disease Valvular heart disease Kyphoscoliosis Exudative pleural effusion from malignancies or chronic infections (e.g. tuberculosis) Neuromuscular disease Chronic pulmonary thromboembolism Systemic illnesses (e.g. anaemia) Deconditioning (due to any chronic debilitating illnesses, especially cardiorespiratory diseases)

For chronic dyspnoea, the most common causes are also cardiorespiratory in origin. A long history of smoking with exertional dyspnoea suggests emphysema, and the presence of angina would also suggest ischaemic heart disease causing heart failure as another possibility.

It is important to recognise deconditioning as a cause of dyspnoea, either solely or as an aggravating factor. Usually a careful history of the background wellbeing of the patient would give some clues to the preceding event/events which have led to physical inactivity. Initial resumption of activity is then marked by the sensation of dyspnoea, followed by anxiety/panic or simple voluntary limitation of exertion to reduce the symptom. Deconditioning is not uncommonly an aggravating factor of the symptom in chronic conditions which themselves cause dyspnoea, and some therapeutic strategies may help to alleviate the symptom and improve functional capacity and quality of life even when the underlying disease is not altered. The major components of reconditioning strategy are exercise training, energy conservation training, nutritional manipulation and cognitive-behavioural modulation, which are discussed later in the chapter.

Physical examination

Physical examination should first evaluate the general condition of the patient and the breathing pattern at rest and on exertion. The presence of cyanosis would indicate significant hypoxaemia. Pursed lip breathing is often seen in patients with chronic airflow obstruction, while rapid shallow breathing occurs in pulmonary congestion or lung parenchymal disease. The use of accessory muscles of respiration indicates excessive work of breathing. Other important features are pallor indicating anaemia, cachexia suggestive of COPD, malignancy or deconditioning, stridor in upper airway obstruction, supraclavicular/neck lymph nodes in 'occult' malignancy, unilateral leg swelling suggestive of deep vein thrombosis, or bilateral ankle oedema caused by congestive heart failure.

The presence of wheeze on auscultation is indicative although not specific for airflow obstruction in asthma, COPD or heart failure. On the other hand, the absence of wheeze does not rule out chronic asthma or stable COPD.

The presence of elevated jugular venous pressure (JVP), ankle oedema, a gallop rhythm and bilateral crackles are diagnostic of congestive heart failure, although acute pulmonary oedema may present without ankle oedema or elevated JVP. Rheumatic valvular heart lesions need to be borne in mind, especially in localities where chronic rheumatic heart diseases are not uncommon.

Investigations

Investigations are targeted at diagnosis and assessment of the degree of incapacitation caused by dyspnoea so that treatment strategies may be designed.

Investigations to assist in confirmation or exclusion of specific conditions are always guided by the working diagnosis obtained at history and physical examination. For acute dyspnoea, a chest radiograph is very useful. It would help to provide evidence of pulmonary congestion, infections, pneumothorax or hyperinflation. Bedside oximetry gives a quick idea of the degree of hypoxaemia and the oximeter is now readily available in outpatient clinics or hospital wards. Arterial blood gases may be indicated, depending on the severity of the condition. Other investigations would depend on the clinical picture and the working diagnosis. If pulmonary oedema or heart failure is suspected, an ECG for ischaemia or evidence of myocardial infarction is necessary. If pulmonary embolism is suspected, ECG would provide adjunctive evidence but diagnosis will depend heavily on demonstration of deep vein thrombosis or, better still, pulmonary embolism with ventilation-perfusion (V/Q) scan or spiral high-resolution CT with contrast, which are sensitive and specific yet less invasive than pulmonary arteriography. Dyspnoea in the face of normal oxygenation should raise the suspicion of metabolic acidosis and hyperventilation, and arterial blood pH analysis would provide evidence for the metabolic acidosis.

For chronic dyspnoea, the basic investigations would include a chest radiograph, spirometry and at least oxygen saturation by oximetry if not an arterial blood gas. These tests would suggest or definitively diagnose conditions such COPD, asthma, chronic heart failure and interstitial lung disease. Further selected investigations may be indicated to confirm or evaluate the specific condition (see Table 27.4). ECG and echocardiogram are useful for assessing heart function in chronic heart failure. Measurements of static lung volumes would further assess hyperinflation or restriction. Carbon monoxide diffusing capacity (DLCO) helps to distinguish between persistent asthma with 'fixed' airflow obstruction and emphysema, and CT scan thorax confirms and evaluates bronchiectasis and interstitial lung diseases.

The degree of dyspnoea may or may not concur with the degree of physiological impairment caused by the disease itself. In the strategic management of chronic dyspnoea, the formal evaluation of the severity of dyspnoea and its response to therapy is desirable. This may be done using Borg's scale. It is more practical to assess the degree of functional impairment in relation to the dyspnoea and commonly used scales are the Dyspnoea Rating Scale of Medical Research Council, UK, or the New York Heart Association Functional Scale. Further objective evaluation can be done with a treadmill or cycle exercise test, although in the elderly, a more practical test is the 6-minute walking test to document the distance and oxygen saturation during level ground walking within 6 minutes. This type of assessment is particularly important when it comes to holistic management of the patient as the disease itself may not be entirely reversible with medical treatment, and symptomatic improvement is an important target in management.

Table 27.4 Diagnostic investigations in dyspnoea

Cause of dyspnoea	Diagnostic test
COPD	Spirometry, lung volumes, DLCO
Asthma	Spirometry with bronchodilator test
Interstitial lung disease	HRCT, lung volumes, DLCO, lung biopsy
Congestive heart failure	ECG, echocardiogram
Extensive pneumonia/ effusion	Microbiology, fluid analysis
Pulmonary embolism	V/Q scan or spiral CT with contrast, Doppler scan of legs for deep venous thrombosis
Neuromuscular weakness	Mouth pressures
Upper airway obstruction	Flow volume loop Fibreoptic bronchoscopy
Kyphoscoliosis	Lung volumes
Anaemia	Haemoglobin

Treatment strategies

Symptomatic relief is very important because dyspnoea is a distressing symptom that disrupts normal daily activities, impairs quality of life and may lead to a downward spiral of physical incapacitation. Specific treatment targeted to relieve the underlying condition may be completely or partially effective in resolving the dyspnoea. For instance, drainage of a pneumothorax or bronchodilators for acute asthma addresses the symptom of dyspnoea and also the underlying pathological process. However, the disease process that is the primary cause of the dyspnoea may not be completely reversible in many circumstances.

The various types of treatment set out below may target more than one pathophysiological mechanism of dyspnoea. Only those methods relevant to the non-ventilator dependent subject are discussed here. Many of the measures for alleviation of dyspnoea described below are included in comprehensive pulmonary rehabilitation programs. These programs utilise a multidisciplinary approach for the provision of care to restore a patient to the highest functional capacity allowed by their disease condition and overall life situation. Pulmonary rehabilitation programs cater for patients with chronic respiratory disease, and usually comprise exercise training, physical therapy, patient education regarding use of medications and oxygen, self-management of panic/anxiety reactions, nutritional manipulation, and energy conservation measures. Other rehabilitation programs cater for cardiac patients or stroke patients with special relevance to their disability, but may also have some components that help to manage the dyspnoea which occurs in those diseases. Where rehabilitation programs are not available or not applicable to the individual patient, the following measures may be adopted selectively as appropriate to the patient.

Oxygen therapy

Most conditions with dyspnoea have a variable degree of hypoxaemia. Hypoxaemia may lead to dyspnoea because:

1. it acts as a chemical stimulus to the peripheral chemoreceptors, increasing ventilation
2. it may increase pulmonary arterial pressure, which stimulates ventilation;and
3. it may impair respiratory muscle function.

Supplemental oxygen in hypoxaemic lung conditions decreases ventilation both at rest and during exertion, with a resultant decrease in dyspnoea. A large, multicentre study has shown that supplemental oxygen during physical activity may decrease breathlessness in COPD patients with mild hypoxaemia who did not fulfil the established criteria of long-term oxygen. While supplemental oxygen may reduce exertional dyspnoea, its effects do not directly correlate to the degree of hypoxaemia and the response is not predictable in individuals. Supplemental oxygen should be considered for relief of dyspnoea in those who respond.

The logistics of providing supplemental oxygen may be a disincentive for its use. For relief of exertional dyspnoea, it has to be given during ambulation. Within the house, it can be given through long extension tubing connected to oxygen concentrators, and for outdoor activities, through a portable oxygen source (either liquid oxygen or compressed gas). The delivery through the transtracheal route gives greater relief for the same degree of oxygen supplement, but is an invasive route with its own complications. The development of oxygen-conserving devices has enhanced the utility of portable oxygen as it can prolong the hours of use of one portable cylinder of oxygen.

Physical therapy

Breathing and coughing exercises and postural drainage may help to promote sputum clearance and improve dyspnoea in those with significant phlegm production. An altered pattern of breathing may cause dyspnoea due to altered lung mechanics. Breathing retraining, including diaphragmatic retraining and pursed lip breathing, has been advocated to relieve dyspnoea in obstructive airways disease, but the efficacy of these techniques is highly variable.

Reconditioning

Rehabilitation programs in various disciplines (pulmonary, cardiac, neuromuscular) may all have components that improve dyspnoea since they improve the individual's exercise tolerance and functional capacity which may be limited by deconditioning after a serious illness in that organ/system. The major components of reconditioning are exercise training, energy conservation training by work simplification and modification of living environment, dietary manipulation and cognitive-behavioural modulation. For patients with chronic respiratory disease leading to dyspnoea, exercise training aims to train the lower as well as upper limbs for strength and endurance, which would in turn alleviate the sensation of exertional dyspnoea and improve exercise tolerance. Exercise intensity is increased gradually. The common types of lower limb exercise include treadmill and ergometer cycling. The evidence for a beneficial effect from specific training of inspiratory muscles is controversial and therefore it is only applied in selected patients.

Cognitive-behavioural approach

Patient education about the disease and self-management measures helps to improve self-confidence, reduce stress and modulate anxiety/panic reactions. This has been shown to decrease dyspnoea in asthma, although less clearly so in COPD. This is because such patient education is usually provided as part of a multifaceted pulmonary rehabilitation program for COPD patients and the effects are difficult to distinguish from other components of the program.

Pharmacological/mechanical/surgical therapy

Pharmacological treatment may be specific for the underlying disease process or non-specific for symptom relief.

Specific treatment

- *Drug treatment of airway obstruction* Reducing airflow resistance in conditions with airflow obstruction such as COPD or asthma with bronchodilators will improve dyspnoea. Inhaled β-agonists, ipratropium bromide and oral sustained release bronchodilators have all been shown to improve dyspnoea. The newer longer-acting β-agonists (that can be given once or twice daily) also improve dyspnoea. The degree of improvement seen on spirometry does not predict the degree of relief of dyspnoea. The use of inhaled steroids in asthma is important for controlling airway inflammation and therefore indirectly reduces airflow obstruction. Their overall efficacy in smoking related chronic airflow obstruction is more controversial, and specific beneficial effects on dyspnoea have not been demonstrated.
- *Anti-heart failure regimen* Dyspnoea in heart failure is partly related to pulmonary congestion and partly to decreased cardiac output. Hence specific treatment directed to the removal of pulmonary oedema fluid (e.g. use of diuretics) and measures to enhance cardiac function (e.g. use of ACEI, coronary angioplasty) may help to improve dyspnoea caused by congestive heart failure.
- *Surgical procedures to reduce lung hyperinflation* This includes bullectomy for large space-occupying lung bullae or volume reduction surgery in emphysema. With the alleviation of lung hyperinflation, the mechanics of respiration improve and so does dyspnoea. The identification of candidates who would benefit from such surgery requires rigorous assessment by the relevant pulmonary teams.
- *Positive pressure support* The use of nocturnal positive pressure support ventilation through non-invasive means during sleep is subject to clinical trials in COPD. It is postulated that this would improve respiratory muscle function and lead to daytime improvement in blood gaseous exchange, dyspnoea and exercise capacity. However, the evidence so far is inconclusive and its use is not yet established.

Non-specific treatment

Non-specific pharmacological treatment of dyspnoea has not been very successful because of the limited efficacy and the almost inseparable side effects. The two major groups of drugs that have been tried are opiates and anxiolytics.

- *Opiates* Opiates relieve dyspnoea via the suppression of respiration and blunting of the perceptual responses to any given stimulus, thus decreasing the uncomfortable sensation of dyspnoea. However, side effects of opiates are substantial, including respiratory depression, dizziness, nausea and constipation if used long term. These side effects are more prominent in the elderly. Although opiates have been shown to be effective in acute modulation of dyspnoea in COPD or bronchoconstriction, enabling a greater degree of exertion, there is insufficient evidence to advocate their use in these conditions. They are mainly restricted to improving the breathing discomfort during the dying process of end-stage respiratory failure from diverse causes. To avoid side effects, the drug should be introduced gradually. The dose often needs to be increased due to tolerance.

- *Anxiolytics* Theoretically, anxiolytics such as benzodiazepines can relieve dyspnoea through relief of anxiety as well as suppression of ventilatory drive from hypoxic or hypercapnic stimuli. However, results of clinical trials have not been consistent and, as with opiates, these drugs carry a substantial risk of side effects, especially of respiratory depression in patients with marginal respiratory reserve. They are indicated only in patients who are very anxious and in whom the anxiety is judged to contribute significantly to the sensation of dyspnoea. As with opiates, anxiolytics should be started in low dosage with monitoring for symptomatic response and adverse effects.

Pulmonary rehabilitation programs offer comprehensive evaluation and management of chronic lung disease, mostly COPD. These programs, incorporating many of the therapeutic strategies listed above, have been shown to be effective in decreasing dyspnoea.

Haemoptysis

The expectoration of blood from the airways is usually an alarming symptom and warrants thorough investigation. Clinically, the definition of haemoptysis includes both blood streaked sputum and gross haemoptysis. Before embarking on extensive diagnostic work-up for haemoptysis, it is important to ascertain that the blood is indeed coming from the respiratory tract and not other sites, such as the gastrointestinal tract (haematemesis) or the oral cavity. In haemoptysis, the prodrome is usually a tingling sensation at the throat and blood is then coughed up (not regurgitated or vomited). Blood is usually bright red and frothy or mixed with sputum.

Approach to haemoptysis

Apart from cases where gross life-threatening haemoptysis requires immediate intubation for airway protection, the approach for haemoptysis would follow the usual lines of history taking, physical examination and appropriate investigations.

History

History should focus on information including the onset and amount of haemoptysis (blood streaked sputum versus gross haemoptysis); previous history of haemoptysis; other features, such as fever; quality and quantity of sputum; pleuritic pain; and recent weight loss. Other points of note are history of chronic disease, predisposing factors for deep vein thrombosis and use of medications, especially anticoagulants or antiplatelet agents.

Bearing the common causes of haemoptysis in mind (see Box 27.2), history taking should enable one to form a priority list of differential diagnosis in the individual patient. In those who are acutely unwell with fever, pleuritic pain, cough and purulent sputum, haemoptysis is likely to be part of an acute pneumonia or even lung abscess. In pneumococcal pneumonia, haemoptysis should not be gross, and is usually mixed in sputum as blood streaks or rusty sputum. With necrotising or cavitating pneumonia due to *Staphylococcus*, *Klebsiella* or anaerobes, haemoptysis can be more significant. The elderly are more prone to aspiration because of co-morbid illness or poor dental hygiene, and it is important to think of aspiration pneumonia which can cause necrotising pneumonia or lung abscesses of polymicrobial aetiology, including anaerobes. Underlying bronchial obstruction by malignancy or foreign body may also be the cause of haemoptysis.

Pulmonary oedema may lead to haemoptysis as pink frothy sputum and dyspnoea is usually dominant. In those with mitral stenosis, there may be fresh haemoptysis due to high pulmonary venous pressure, even without pulmonary oedema.

Box 27.2 Causes of haemoptysis

- Pneumonia
- Pulmonary oedema
- Lung cancer
- Tuberculosis
- Bronchiectasis
- Mycetoma
- Lung abscess/cavity
- Mitral stenosis
- Foreign body
- Autoimmune alveolar haemorrhage
- Acute bronchitis

In those with predisposing factors for deep vein thrombosis, such as recent post-operative or bed-bound state, pulmonary embolism may be the cause of haemoptysis. It is usually accompanied by acute pleuritic chest pain, dyspnoea and cough.

A chronic history of purulent sputum or recurrent haemoptysis is very suggestive of bronchiectasis.

In localities where tuberculosis is common, either active tuberculosis or old tuberculosis giving rise to bronchiectasis, destroyed lung or mycetomas must be considered. It has been reported that active tuberculosis in the elderly is less often a cause of haemoptysis compared to infection in the young. On the other hand, bronchiectasis, cavities or mycetoma as sequelae of tuberculosis can give rise to gross haemoptysis. The history taking should look for recent contact with cases of active tuberculosis (in institutions, recently diagnosed cases of tuberculosis in the inmates is an important point to rule out), previous history of tuberculosis and other symptoms, such as cough, or subtle features of constitutional upset, such as weight loss or loss of appetite.

Haemoptysis may be the first presenting symptom of lung malignancy. A careful history may reveal other symptoms of prolonged cough and weight loss. Smoking is an important predisposing factor to squamous or small cell lung cancers which are often endobronchial and more likely to cause haemoptysis. Metastatic malignancies to the lung less commonly present with haemoptysis.

An uncommon cause of haemoptysis in the elderly is pulmonary vasculitis. Autoimmune conditions may lead to alveolar haemorrhage, which is usually part of an autoimmune disease or pulmonary–renal syndrome.

Acute bronchitis or acute on chronic bronchitis is often the final diagnostic label given as the cause of haemoptysis. However, this is a diagnosis of exclusion after appropriate investigations for other causes.

Physical examination

In massive haemoptysis, the first priority is to assess the patient's risk of suffocation from excessive blood in the airways. Symptoms of massive haemoptysis with respiratory distress, stridorous breathing and cyanosis would suggest that urgent action is required to maintain the airway and stabilise the circulation.

General examination should seek clubbing which occurs in lung cancers and bronchiectasis, lymphadenopathy in lung cancer, unilateral swelling suggesting deep vein thrombosis, and bilateral leg swelling suggesting congestive heart failure.

Chest crackles on auscultation may be due to underlying lung pathology such as bronchiectasis or pulmonary congestion, but it may also be due to aspirated blood if haemoptysis is significant. Bronchial breathing of lobar consolidation would indicate pneumonia, while signs of lung collapse may indicate endobronchial obstruction by a tumour, endobronchial tuberculosis or blood clot. Pleural rub may be heard in pulmonary embolism.

Examination of the cardiovascular system should seek signs of pulmonary oedema, mitral stenosis, pulmonary hypertension and/or hypotension in massive pulmonary embolism.

Investigations and management

The extent of investigation required to establish a diagnosis will depend not only on the amount of haemoptysis, but also particularly on the suspected underlying diagnosis. In instances where haemoptysis is consistent with a disease already diagnosed, further extensive or invasive intervention for establishing the cause of haemoptysis is not warranted. In new occurrences of haemoptysis, and if haemoptysis is recurrent, a chest radiograph is mandatory. The chest radiograph may provide evidence to account for the haemoptysis—for example, pneumonia, tuberculosis, a mass lesion, mitral stenosis, pulmonary oedema, or mycetomas; or non-specific conditions such as bronchiectasis (except cystic bronchiectasis where there are specific diagnostic findings) and pulmonary embolism. In cases of infective aetiology, microbiological tests of sputum for pyogenic bacteria or acid-fast bacilli are indicated. Fungal infections should be considered in patients who are immunocompromised by disease or treatment. If primary lung malignancy is suspected, sputum cytology (and, if necessary, bronchoscopy) would confirm the diagnosis. Age alone does not preclude surgery for an operable lung malignancy. Thus specific treatment for the above diseases would usually control haemoptysis.

The chest radiograph in alveolar haemorrhage shows diffuse alveolar shadows similar to pulmonary oedema, and a drop in haemoglobin coincides with haemoptysis. Renal manifestations would occur in patients with Goodpasture's syndrome and Wegener's granulomatosis.

When chest X-ray findings are negative, non-specific or require further delineation, computerised tomography of the chest is often the next step when lung pathology is suspected. High-resolution CT is both sensitive and specific for bronchiectasis. Ventilation-perfusion scans and spiral CT with contrast are indicated for suspected pulmonary embolism. If these investigations are negative, fibreoptic bronchoscopy is indicated. If a primary cardiac cause could be responsible for haemoptysis, then investigations such as ECG and echocardiography would be more appropriate.

If haemoptysis is massive, even if the cause is known, as in bronchiectasis, fibreoptic bronchoscopy may be required to localise the site of bleeding in preparation for therapeutic measures such as bronchial artery embolisation.

In up to 50% of patients with one episode of haemoptysis, no cause can be identified following investigations for the common causes of haemoptysis. The need to pursue further investigations such as a bronchial arteriogram will depend upon the amount of haemoptysis, whether the haemoptysis recurs, and the premorbid state of the patient. If the haemoptysis is not severe, and no diagnosis is forthcoming after the approach as outlined above, it is reasonable to follow up the patient, and if haemoptysis recurs, to review the case again for new clues that may emerge with the course of time.

Bibliography and further reading

The American College of Chest Physicians (1998), 'Managing cough as a defence mechanism and as a symptom—clinical consensus statement', *Chest*, 114, pp. 133S–181S.

American Thoracic Society (1999), 'Dyspnoea: Mechanisms, assessment and management: A consensus statement', *American Journal of Respiratory and Critical Care Medicine*, 159, pp. 321–40.

Bestall, J. C. et al. (1999), 'Usefulness of the Medical Research Council (MRC) dyspnoea scale as a measure of disability in patients with chronic obstructive pulmonary disease', *Thorax*, 54, pp. 581–6.

Braman, S. S., Kaemmerlen, J. T. & Davis, S. M. (1991), 'Asthma in the elderly. A comparison between patients with recently acquired and long-standing disease', *The American Review of Respiratory Disease*, 143, pp. 336–40.

Crystal, R. G., Bitterman, P. B., Rennard, S. I. et al. (1984), 'Interstitial lung disease of unknown cause. Disorders characterised by chronic inflammation of the lower respiratory tract', *The New England Journal of Medicine*, 310, pp. 154–66.

DePaso, W. J., Winterbauer, R. H., Lusk, J. A., Dreis, D. F. & Springmeyer, S. C. (1991), 'Chronic dyspnea unexplained by history, physical examination, chest roentgenogram, and spirometry. Analysis of a seven-year experience', *Chest*, 100, pp. 1293–9.

Dow, L., Coggan, D., Osmond, C. & Holgate, S. T. (1991), 'A population survey of respiratory symptoms in the elderly', *The European Respiratory Journal*, 4, pp. 267–72.

Enright, P. L., Kronmal, R. A., Higgins, M. W., Schenker, M. B. & Haponik, E. F. (1994), 'Prevalence and correlates of respiratory symptoms and disease in the elderly', *Chest*, 106, pp. 827–34.

Haponik, E. & Chin, R. (1990), 'Haemoptysis: Clinicians' perspectives', *Chest*, 97, pp. 469–75.

Haponik, E. F. et al. (1987), 'Computed chest tomography in the evaluation of haemoptysis: Impact on diagnosis and treatment', *Chest*, 91, pp. 80–5.

Irwin, R. S., Curley, F. J. & French, C. L. (1990), 'Chronic cough: The spectrum and frequency of causes, key components of the diagnostic evaluation, and outcome of specific therapy', *The American Review of Respiratory Disease*, 141, pp. 640–7.

Lis, R. J. & Kvetan, V. (1995), 'Evaluation of non-massive haemoptysis', *Pulmonary & Critical Care Update*, 10(16), pp. 1–9.

Mahler, D. A. & Horowitz, M. B. (1994), 'Clinical evaluation of exertional dyspnea', *Clinics in Chest Medicine*, 15(2), pp. 259–69.

Mane, J. M., Estape, J., Sanchez-Lloret, J. et al. (1994), 'Age and clinical characteristics of 1433 patients with lung cancer', *Age and Ageing*, 23, pp. 28–31.

Pratter, M. R., Bartter, T., Akers, S. & Dubois, J. (1993), 'An algorithmic approach to chronic cough', *Annals of Internal Medicine*, 119, pp. 977–83.

Shirakusa, T., Tsutsui, M., Iriki, N. et al. (1989), 'Results of resection for bronchogenic carcinoma in patients over the age of 80', *Thorax*, 44, pp. 189–91.

Silvestri, G. A. & Mahler, D. A. (1993), 'Evaluation of dyspnea in the elderly patient', *Clinics in Chest Medicine*, 14(3), pp. 393–404.

Stein, P. D., Gottschalk, A., Saltzmann, H. A. & Terrin, M. L. (1991), 'Diagnosis of acute pulmonary embolism in the elderly', *Journal of American College of Cardiology*, 18, pp. 1452–7.

Weaver, L. et al. (1979), 'Selection of patients with haemoptysis for fiberoptic bronchoscopy', *Chest*, 76, pp. 7–10.

Chapter 28

Chronic obstructive pulmonary disease

RICHARD E. RUFFIN

Introduction

The term chronic obstructive pulmonary disease (COPD) represents mainly smoking-induced lung disease, but not exclusively so. One of the most recent definitions of COPD by the European Respiratory Society is 'reduced maximum expiratory flow and slow forced emptying of the lungs, which is slowly progressive and mostly irreversible to present medical treatment'. Specific causes of airflow obstruction such as bronchiectasis or cystic fibrosis are excluded. The most common labels of disease existing within the COPD umbrella are emphysema and chronic bronchitis. This definition means that it is mandatory to measure lung function by spirometry or flow volume loops to diagnose COPD.

However, it is not possible to exclude childhood illnesses such as bronchiolitis or bronchopulmonary dysplasia as being subsequent causes of COPD, nor of poorly controlled asthma as also being an underlying cause for some cases of COPD. It is critical to understand that COPD can exist as the only diagnosis in a patient, but can also exist in combination with other specific diseases. For example, COPD can co-exist with asthma. A situation seen in community practice would be a patient with asthma who also smokes. The challenge in managing COPD is to identify the relevant subsets and co-morbidities that can lead to management strategies that improve quality of life.

Aetiology and epidemiology

The reason for considering causative or risk factors of COPD is to provide the reader with information that is useful to include in the history-taking process to enable identification of the underlying causes of COPD and the potential helpful management strategies.

Risk factors for COPD

Each of the risk factors for COPD described below may be operational during each of the four phases of lung development (Table 28.1).

Cigarette smoking

Cigarette smoking is the best-established risk factor for COPD. Cross-sectional surveys have shown a 2.8-fold increased risk of COPD in people who are

Table 28.1 The four phases of lung development

Phase of lung development	Risk factor effect on lung function
In utero	Low initial lung function
Growth (childhood–adolescence)	Low maximum lung function
Plateau (early adult)	Earlier start of decline of lung function
Decline (> 40 years)	More rapid decline of lung function

active smokers compared to non-smokers. Mortality from COPD in smokers of more than 25 cigarettes a day is 20 times greater than that of non-smokers. Smoking is known to accelerate the loss of lung function as measured by forced expired volume in 1 second (FEV_1). In heavy smokers, the average loss in FEV_1 per year has been reported as 33 mL above that due to ageing. Environmental tobacco smoke (passive smoking) is another causative factor in COPD.

Air pollution

The effects of air pollution on COPD are still uncertain in terms of induction of the disease. It appears that living in cities with high pollution or working in areas exposed to organic or coal dust contribute to loss of lung function. One study suggests that a high pollution environment causes lung function loss in the order of heavy smoking. It is clear that particulate pollution, sulphur dioxide and ozone pollution increase COPD exacerbations, hospital admissions and mortality.

Nutrition

It seems plausible that the reduced intake of some dietary factors results in an increased risk of COPD. Antioxidant agents have a role in preventing the damage caused by inhaled free radicals, endogenous oxidants and proteolytic enzymes, which are thought to have a role in the pathogenesis of emphysema. Intake of vitamins C and E, fish oils and magnesium have been reported to have a protective role, or predispose to loss of lung function when deficient. It is uncertain if the above effects are seen in early life only or continue throughout life. Appropriately designed clinical trials are needed to provide absolute evidence on the quantum of effect but the current evidence is enough to support commonsense in advocating a balanced diet for all.

Infection

Infection in childhood is a possible factor in COPD risk. However, the determination of causality is uncertain. That is, it is not clear whether impaired lung function is caused by childhood infection or is itself a pre-existing risk for childhood infection. In adults with COPD, infection is not a cause of accelerated loss of lung function.

Socioeconomic status

Many studies have shown that there is a strong association between COPD mortality and low socioeconomic status. It is a difficult area because of confounding by associated factors of smoking, nutrition, housing and occupation. Some studies, having adjusted for the known risk factors, have claimed the presence of lower lung function in low socioeconomic groups.

Genetic factors

Alpha-1-antitrypsin deficiency is a known risk factor for COPD and basal emphysema. It is very likely that other genes will be discovered that will be shown to predispose to COPD when deficient or altered. The benefit of this knowledge in the future will be to consider targeted preventative strategies or replacement therapy. It is worthwhile asking about a family history of lung disease or COPD in your initial assessment of a patient.

Airway hyper-responsiveness

A number of studies have shown that the presence of airway hyper-responsiveness, as measured by histamine or methacholine inhalation tests, is an independent risk factor for decline in FEV_1 in smokers with COPD. In practice, this becomes an issue in deciding whether your patient has COPD alone or COPD and asthma. Resolution of this problem and having a practical approach is important to providing the best outcomes for individual patients with COPD.

Epidemiology

There are major problems in assessing the prevalence of COPD. Studies reporting only interview data are likely to underestimate vastly the prevalence of COPD and comparisons between countries of COPD mortality and morbidity are unreliable because of misclassification and failure to record COPD as a co-morbidity.

The prevalence of COPD (chronic bronchitis and emphysema) as determined by interview over time in the US is shown in Table 28.2.

Table 28.2 Prevalence of COPD (per 1000) in the US

	1986	1994
Total	56.6	61.8
Males	51.7	54.2
Females	61.2	69.1

This data is surprising when looked at in an age-unadjusted fashion because the higher prevalence of smoking in men would intuitively suggest a higher prevalence of COPD in men. Looking at the prevalence according to age groups shows that the average prevalence climbs steeply with age and in the 65–74 year age group was 136 per 1000 men and 118 per 1000 women. The prevalence rates for men far exceed those for women at ages 75–84 years. In the UK, it has been estimated that COPD is present in 5% of men aged 65–74 years and 20% of men aged over 75 years.

The South Australian adult population experience with self-reported data for the prevalence of COPD has shown an age-unadjusted prevalence of 10.9% (95% CI, 9.8–12.1) in 1998.

In the US in 1996, COPD was the fourth leading cause of death in women and the fifth leading cause of death in men. The age-adjusted death rate for COPD in 1996 was 55 per 100 000 for white men and 135 per 100 000 for white women. At age 70, men had twice the death rate from COPD as women, with a continual widening in the COPD death rate as age increases.

Pathophysiology

The two major components of COPD—chronic bronchitis and emphysema—have quite distinct pathologic appearances and anatomic sites of disease even though cigarette smoke is the main inducer of these diseases.

Chronic bronchitis

Cigarette smoking initially injures the small respiratory bronchioles by inducing inflammation at least partly via the production of reactive oxygen substances.

The pathology of chronic bronchitis is inflammation of the cartilaginous airways (Figure 28.1) and includes mucous gland hyperplasia, smooth muscle hypertrophy and lymphocytic infiltration in the mucosa of the bronchial wall, causing thickening with neutrophilic glandular inflammation.

Chronic bronchitis leads to increased airflow obstruction with a consequent increase in the work of breathing and a ventilation/perfusion (V/Q) mismatch, causing hypoxaemia. The increased airflow obstruction in chronic bronchitis is due to mucus in the airway lumen and thickening of the airway wall (smooth muscle hypertrophy and inflammation of the mucosa) (Figure 28.1).

Emphysema

Reactive oxygen substances resulting from smoking have a role in releasing the proteolytic enzymes in the alveolar regions, which results in the alveolar wall destruction that occurs in emphysema.

Emphysema leads to increased airflow obstruction and increased work of breathing plus hypoxaemia from a V/Q mismatch. The airflow obstruction in emphysema arises from a loss of elastic recoil in the emphysematous lung resulting in a loss of radial traction and expiratory airway narrowing (Figure 28.1).

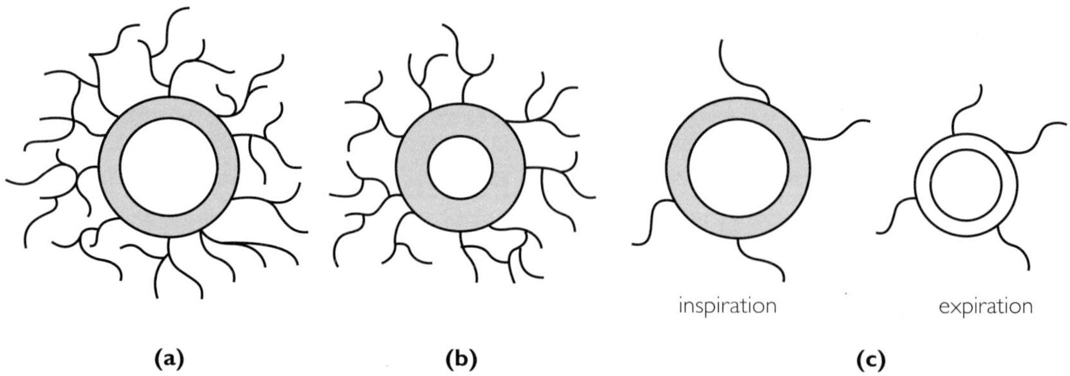

Figure 28.1 Schematic cross-section of an airway: **(a)** normal; **(b)** in chronic bronchitis; **(c)** in emphysema during inspiration and expiration

Airflow obstruction

Airflow obstruction is measured clinically by spirometry or expiratory flow volume loops. The maximum expiratory flow is dependent on the lung volume at which it is measured and also on neuromuscular co-ordination, co-operation with the test, elastic recoil of the lung and airway calibre. Chronic bronchitis directly reduces the airway calibre because the thickened wall encroaches on the airway lumen. Emphysema reduces the elastic recoil of the lung and hence reduces airway calibre during expiration, with airway wall collapse because of loss of support of elastic lung tethering. Often both emphysema and chronic bronchitis are present together in a patient. Airflow obstruction is diagnosed by a reduced ratio of FEV_1/FVC (forced vital capacity) and a lowered FEV_1. An FEV_1/FVC of less than 70% across most age groups is considered to show airflow obstruction. The presence of a more than 200 mL and 12% increase in FEV_1 with inhaled bronchodilator indicates an acutely reversible bronchodilator response, which should make one consider the presence of asthma as well as COPD.

Gas exchange and the work of breathing

In cases of chronic bronchitis and emphysema, hypoxaemia results from a V/Q mismatch. Emphysema results in reduced gas transfer because of the destruction of the alveolar capillary bed. Hypoxaemia induces pulmonary artery constriction, and if present over a lengthy period, causes right ventricular hypertrophy and sometimes cor pulmonale (right heart failure due to underlying lung disease via hypoxaemia). Therefore, in patients where the V/Q mismatch is severe and hypoxaemia is present, it is possible for COPD to result in cor pulmonale. As airflow obstruction increases, there is a balance between the work involved in breathing and the ventilation required to maintain a normal arterial carbon dioxide level (P_aco_2).

The P_aco_2 is inversely related to alveolar ventilation. That is, if alveolar ventilation is halved, the carbon dioxide level doubles, and if alveolar ventilation is doubled, the carbon dioxide level is halved (Table 28.3). A high P_aco_2 level indicates that alveolar ventilation is insufficient to maintain a P_aco_2 in the normal range of 35–45 mmHg. This can result from an acute change in airflow obstruction or can occur chronically where the human body balances a higher P_aco_2 against the cost of increased work of breathing to maintain a normal P_aco_2. This results in a resetting of the P_aco_2 level at which ventilation is increased or a desensitisation to the usual ventilatory drive caused by an elevated P_aco_2. The increased work of breathing occurs because of two factors at least:

- the work done to breathe out (or in, in some cases) against an obstructed airway
- the work done to breathe at higher lung volumes

Table 28.3 Alveolar ventilation and arterial carbon dioxide tension (P_aCO_2)

Situation	Alveolar ventilation (L/min)[a]	P_aCO_2 (mmHg)
Normal	4	40
Hypoventilation	2	80
Hyperventilation	8	20

(a) Alveolar ventilation = respiratory rate × (tidal volume – dead space).

as a result of hyperinflation and an increased function residual capacity.

A consequence of increasing airflow obstruction is a shift to a higher functional residual capacity to maintain airway calibre, which increases the work of breathing. In addition, dynamic hyperinflation results when expiration is prolonged and the patient needs to start the next breath before finishing expiration.

Another consequence of increasing airflow obstruction is a reduction in exercise capacity. This is because the normal response to increasing exercise is an increase in ventilation but COPD limits the ability to achieve this. Hence, exercise capacity is limited by ventilatory capacity ($FEV_1 \times 30$ L per minute) and by physical unfitness in COPD.

We must also consider other co-morbidities that impact on COPD aside from unfitness. Obesity is a problem in that it limits ventilatory capacity but also increases the risk for obstructive sleep apnoea (OSA). The presence of coronary artery disease in this age group can also influence exercise capacity and may be a confounding factor when assessing patients with COPD.

Clinical assessment

The clinical assessment of COPD includes the patient's symptoms, history of exercise ability, previous treatments, hospitalisations, current therapy, occupation, smoking history and evidence of relevant co-morbidity factors (e.g. angina, reflux or OSA). To complete the assessment requires:

- physical examination
- measurement of lung function by spirometry (plus sometimes lung volumes and gas transfer) and radiology
- in special circumstances, arterial blood gas levels, sleep studies, cardiac and pulmonary hypertension assessment and exercise testing may be considered.

Useful markers of the severity of COPD obtained from the history include:

- walking distance (the more the limitation the greater the severity)
- sleep disturbance by dyspnoea (the more the limitation the greater the severity)
- ability to conduct activities of daily living
- hospitalisations
- presence of co-morbidities (e.g. snoring; apnoeic periods and daytime somnolence from OSA; ankle oedema in cor pulmonale).

Useful markers of the severity of COPD obtained by physical examination include:

- cyanosis
- work of breathing:
  - accessory muscle use
  - tachypnoea
  - pulsus parodoxus
  - tachycardia
- intensity of breath sounds
- hyperinflation
- wheeze/crackles
- evidence of pulmonary hypertension.

Cyanosis, increased work of breathing at rest and low intensity of breath sounds are all consistent with severe COPD. Wheeze does not have to be present at rest in a person with severe COPD. Forced expiratory wheeze is a poor discriminatory test of COPD severity. Evidence of pulmonary hypertension (loud pulmonary second sound and right ventricular lift) or cor pulmonale (elevated jugular venous pressure, ankle oedema) make one consider severe COPD causing hypoxaemia or the presence of a co-morbidity such as OSA or, more rarely, heart disease affecting cardiac performance and leading to peripheral oedema.

The presence of early inspiratory crackles may occur in COPD probably due to obstruction of the small airways rather than to cardiac failure, where the crackles are mid to late inspiratory in nature.

Lung function testing

Spirometry or flow volume loops are essential to diagnose COPD: a low FEV_1 and a reduced FEV_1/FVC ratio (< 70%) (Figures 28.2, 28.3). Other patterns, such as a low peak expiratory flow (PEF), may suggest emphysema (Figure 28.4). More formal testing with lung volumes and gas transfer are appropriately done at the time of specialist referral.

Increases in residual volume, function residual capacity and total lung capacity are seen in patients with COPD and are more common in those with emphysema.

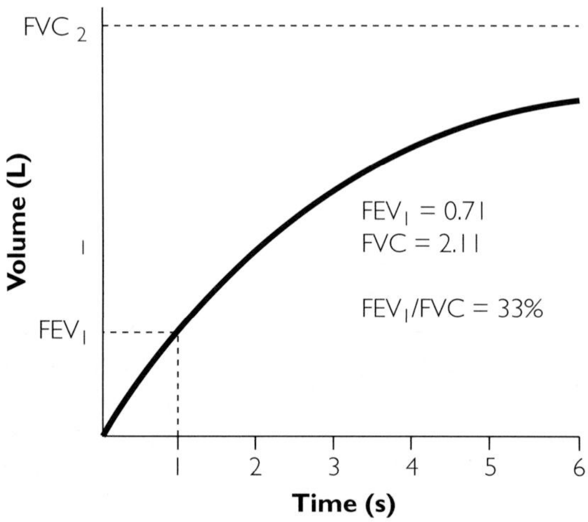

Figure 28.2 Evidence of airway obstruction by spirometry

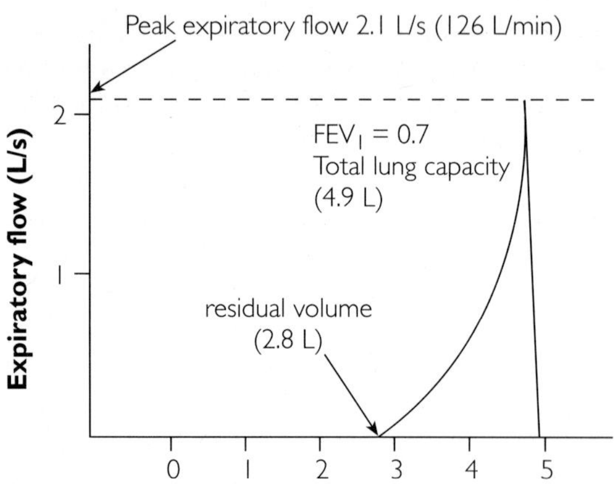

Figure 28.3 Evidence of airway obstruction by flow volume loop

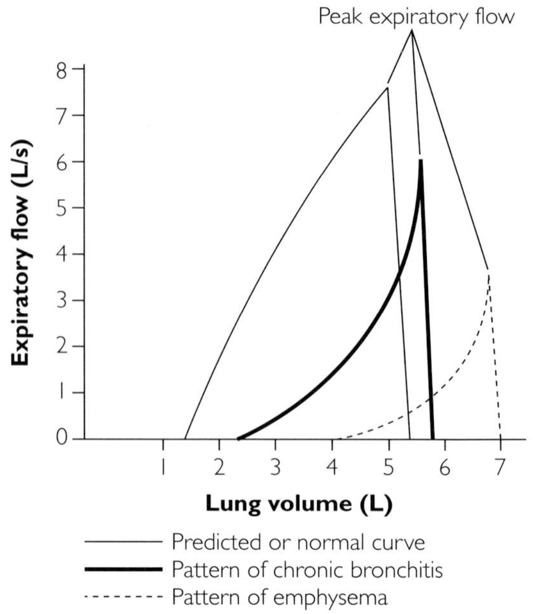

Figure 28.4 Comparison of expiratory flow by flow volume loops for normal patients with those with chronic bronchitis and emphysema

Radiology

A chest X-ray is a standard investigation in patients with COPD to act as a baseline assessment of heart size, to detect hyperinflation and to exclude lung malignancy because of the usual smoking history. The characteristics of a chest X-ray in cases of advanced emphysema are hyperinflation (diaphragm below 11th rib posteriorly on an inspiratory film), flattening of diaphragms, large retrosternal airspace and paucity of vessel marking (Figure 28.5). Computerised tomography (CT) chest scans can be diagnostic for emphysema.

It is likely that, in the near future, guidelines will be altered to recommend spiral CT chest scanning in patients who are at risk of lung cancer by virtue of their smoking history and age (e.g. 1 pack per day for 20 years and over 50 years). This change is due to the increased sensitivity of CT scans in detecting lung masses, and hence the increased cost-effectiveness of detecting stage I lung cancer, which is amenable to curative surgery.

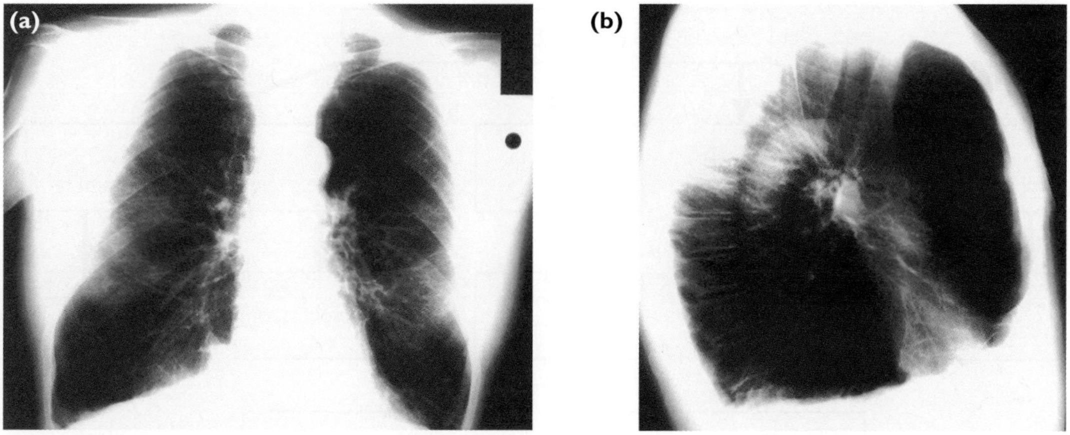

Figure 28.5 **(a)** Posterior-anterior chest X-ray showing posterior rib count of 11 above the diaphragm and a paucity of vascular markings consistent with emphysema. **(b)** Lateral chest X-ray showing flattened diaphragm and a large retrosternal airspace consistent with emphysema

Special tests

Arterial blood gases

The advent of oximetry has simplified the assessment of oxygen saturation (S_aO_2). Oximetry should form part of the initial assessment of COPD. At sea level, an S_aO_2 of 90% corresponds to a P_aO_2 of 60 mmHg and a P_aO_2 of 55 mmHg corresponds to an S_aO_2 of 88%.

Arterial blood gas (ABG) measurement should be done if a stable patient has an S_aO_2 of less than or equal to 90% and during acute exacerbations of COPD. In the former situation, it provides long-term guidance to oxygen therapy (see later). In the latter situation, it provides a means of assessing the severity of the situation and guiding the introduction of ventilation support.

Mystery often surrounds the use and interpretation of ABG measurements. Generally, the use of ABG measurements for COPD management would be at the time of assessment for hospitalisation (and subsequent hospital management), or during an assessment for long-term oxygen therapy, or when determining if a prescription for oxygen therapy should be altered.

Figure 28.6 shows a simple approach to interpreting ABG results. The first issue is that knowledge of the inspired oxygen level is mandatory (e.g. room air = 21% O_2; 2 L per minute O_2 via nasal prongs is approximately 28% O_2). The units used to report the partial pressures or concentrations of gases in blood in Australia are commonly still millimetres of mercury (mmHg) but in the UK and Europe kilopascals (kPa) are used (to convert mmHg to kPa, divide mmHg by 7.5). Then, after noting the inspired oxygen level, look at the pH value. A pH between 7.35 and 7.45 is normal. A value below 7.35 is acidic and above 7.45 is alkalotic. A normal pH does not exclude respiratory disease. If the pH is outside the 7.35–7.45 range, you must ask yourself whether this a respiratory or metabolic cause. The quickest way to ascertain this is to look at the P_aCO_2 value. This value is influenced by a range of factors, but mainly by alveolar ventilation in an inverse relationship (see Table 28.3). The normal range for P_aCO_2 is 35–45 mmHg.

If the pH is less than 7.35 and the P_aCO_2 over 45 mmHg, there is a respiratory or ventilatory component to the picture. The results must be interpreted with the clinical situation. The cause for these values could be suppression of ventilatory drive by narcotics or even excess oxygen, or inadequate ventilation due to severe COPD.

The chronicity of a clinical situation can also be judged by the ABG pattern. If the P_aCO_2 is chronically elevated, the compensatory mechanism of bicarbonate retention occurs. These compensatory mechanisms will not over-compensate. For example, a

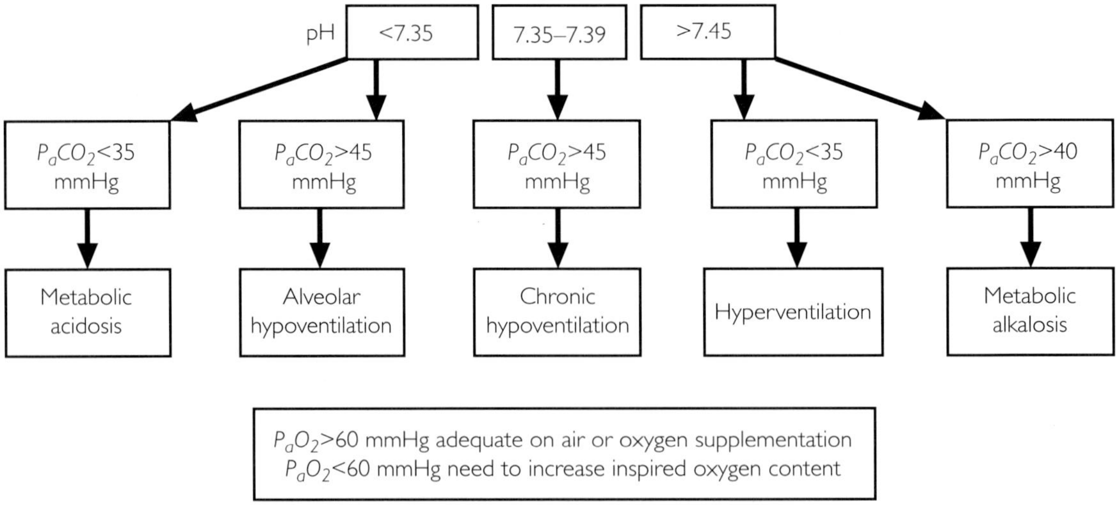

Figure 28.6 Interpretation of arterial blood gas measurements

person with a COPD exacerbation may present with a pH of 7.25 and a P_aCO_2 of 50 mmHg and bicarbonate level of 24 mmol/L. Over several days, the pH increases to 7.38, the P_aCO_2 remains at 50 mmHg and the bicarbonate level increases to 27 mmol/L.

If the pH is less than 7.35 and the P_aCO_2 is less than 40 mmHg, the cause of acidosis is likely to be metabolic. If the pH is above 7.45 and the P_aCO_2 less than 35 mmHg, it is likely that hyperventilation (e.g. psychological or pulmonary embolus) is contributing. If the pH is above 7.45 and the P_aCO_2 over 35 mmHg, the cause is metabolic. As above, a chronic situation could lead to compensation with a pH between 7.40 and 7.45, a low P_aCO_2 and a reduced bicarbonate level.

Finally, look at the P_aO_2 level. The normal P_aO_2 when breathing room air is 80–100 mmHg. As people get older, the alveolar–arterial (A–a) oxygen gradient widens and so a P_aO_2 down to 65–70 mmHg may be normal in the older population.

If the P_aO_2 is less than 60 mmHg (corresponding to an S_aO_2 of 90%), this indicates respiratory failure from respiratory disease, or from breathing in a low oxygen concentration. In most hospital situations, the value of 60 mmHg represents a target for implementing oxygenation. Oximetry can replace arterial blood gases as a guide (i.e. achieve an S_aO_2 > 90%) but does not provide information about the effects of inducing hypoventilation in patients with COPD who are dependent on hypoxic ventilatory drive.

Sleep studies should be considered when there are clinical features of OSA. The features of OSA include snoring, daytime somnolence and episodes of stopping breathing during sleep (apnoeic events).

There is now some evidence published to raise doubts about the usefulness of nocturnal oxygen therapy for overnight hypoxaemia. A respiratory physician should be involved in these tests for diagnosis and treatment.

Cardiac and pulmonary hypertension assessment

If there are symptoms of angina or signs of congestive cardiac failure, then cardiac assessment is required. A minimum investigation is electrocardiography. Findings of 'p pulmonale' or right ventricular hypertrophy are specific for the presence of pulmonary hypertension but not very sensitive.

The decision to investigate cardiac function further with echocardiography or gated blood pool scans, or pulmonary hypertension with Doppler ultrasound or more invasive testing, should be made after an assessment by a respiratory physician.

Exercise testing in patients with COPD would be considered predominantly to see if the exercise capacity of an individual can be improved by oxygen therapy. The decision for oxygen therapy needs to be made by a respiratory physician and the exercise test is undertaken with the patient receiving oxygen or air in a blinded fashion. There is no simpler test to replace this standard approach to determining if oxygen for exercise is indicated.

Treatment

The treatment of COPD consists of:

- general management
- medications for COPD
- possible transplantation or lung volume reduction surgery
- treatment of co-morbidities.

General management

The features of general management are the general principles of smoking cessation, diet, weight control, maintenance of physical fitness and preventive vaccinations against influenza and pneumococcus.

Smoking cessation can be facilitated by the practitioner's advice to stop (5–10% success rate) and further by the use of nicotine replacement therapy (chewing gum and/or patches). These measures with the appropriate advice lift smoking cessation in the medium term to about 25%. The availability of bupropion is a further advance and this tablet will facilitate even higher cessation rates. The emphasis on smoking cessation is the major therapeutic platform for COPD intervention.

Weight control (or reduction in the presence of obesity) is an important principle in the management of COPD and other chronic diseases. Weight gain increases the work of breathing at rest and with exercise, as well as increasing the risk of developing OSA. Balanced diets with appropriate size-related caloric intake are available through dietitians or commercially. Appropriate exercise also facilitates weight control. However, patients with severe COPD who are expending a lot of energy with their breathing require additional caloric intake, which is best achieved through frequent small meals.

Exercise programs have the benefit of assisting weight control but also in maintaining physical fitness. The maintenance of muscle fitness enables more work to be done by a patient with COPD for a given amount of breathing or ventilation. Rehabilitation pulmonary programs may become more widely available in the future.

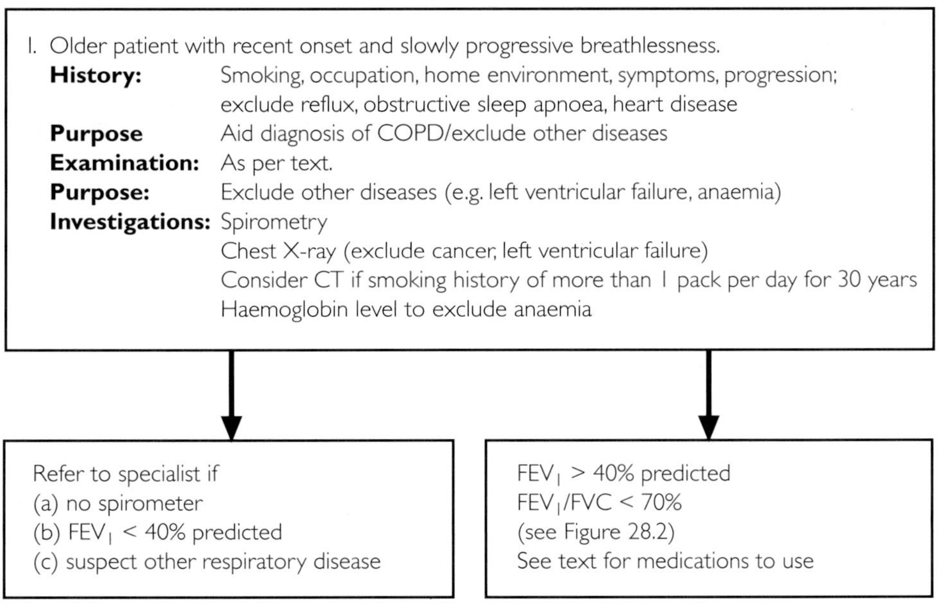

Figure 28.7 Management scenarios for the general practitioner

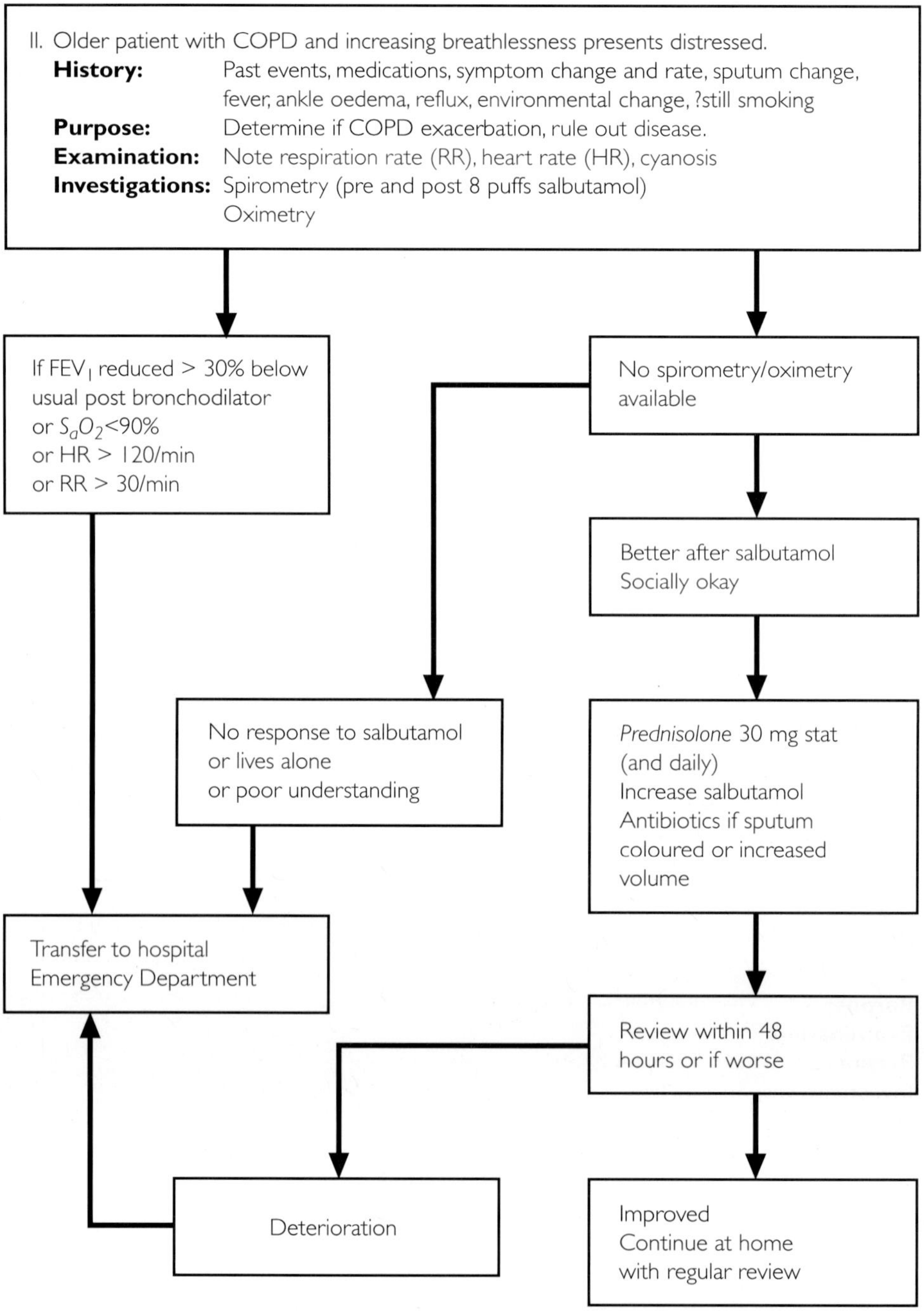

Figure 28.7 Management scenarios for the general practitioner (*continued*)

Frequent, short-distance walking is the easiest way for patients with severe COPD to maintain fitness. However, continuing this type of program can be difficult if the patient is alone and requires the encouragement of the medical practitioner and a support group.

Some hospitals provide rehabilitation programs for patients with COPD and these have been shown to at least improve quality of life for the participants and also reduce breathlessness and improve exercise capacity. Commercial organisations can tailor an exercise program if patients with COPD can afford the cost.

Patients with COPD comprise one of the patient groups in Australia who qualify for subsidised influenza and pneumococcal vaccinations. Maintaining the vaccination status is an important preventive factor against exacerbations and pneumonia.

Medications for COPD

Bronchodilator therapy

Short-acting β_2-agonists

These agents, such as salbutamol or terbutaline, are commonly used as first-line treatment by inhalation. There is good evidence to support the use of metered dose inhalers (MDI) and spacers rather than using nebulising solutions. It has been repeatedly shown that 6–8 puffs of 100 μg/puff salbutamol from an MDI and spacer is at least equivalent to 5 mg salbutamol via a nebuliser. Therefore, even in the situation of a patient with severe COPD, an MDI and spacer should be used with appropriate dosage before nebuliser therapy. The MDI and spacer remain one of the cheapest, quickest and most efficient aerosol delivery systems.

Patients use β_2-agonists to control or reduce symptoms. The subjective benefit of these agents does not correlate with spirometry improvement. These agents can be used frequently and in high doses in severe COPD (e.g. 2 hourly use of 8 puffs salbutamol via spacer to reduce symptoms). The limiting factor is often the side effects of tremor. It is appropriate practice to trial patients on anticholinergic bronchodilators if their subjective response to short-acting β_2-agonists is not optimal or tremor is significant.

Anticholinergic agents

In Australia, ipratropium bromide is currently the only anticholinergic agent available. It has a slower onset of effect than the short-acting β_2-agonists but a longer duration. Although data is not available, it would seem to be commonsense that using an MDI and spacer will be as effective as nebulised delivery providing the MDI dosage is correct. On the basis of the salbutamol data, one would predict that about 80 μg of ipratropium via an MDI and spacer would be equivalent to 500 μg via a nebuliser. The frequency of administration is again related to the patient's symptoms.

Some patients are likely to have greater benefit from ipratropium bromide than salbutamol or terbutaline and vice versa. The only way to identify these benefits is by a trial of treatment.

Combination of β_2-agonists and anticholinergic medications

These can be considered for a trial of treatment when neither β_2-agonists nor anticholinergic agents are providing optimum symptom relief for a patient or as a trial to see if the duration of symptom relief is extended. There is, hence, a degree of reliance on the individual patient's interpretation of her own symptoms, which can be coloured by the thought of a new treatment.

The combination of a short-acting β_2-agonist and anticholinergic agents now exists in one MDI.

Theophylline

Theophylline is not commonly used as an initial treatment because of its side-effect profile and the variation in dose with drug interactions and among patients. However, it can be helpful in some patients where its effect may be more on diaphragm function rather than its bronchodilator effect. An interesting new development that may be of benefit in COPD is that of the new phosphodiesterase inhibitors, which are currently undergoing clinical trials.

Long-acting β_2-agonists

There is still controversy about these agents in COPD management. They are not approved in Australia for use with COPD but there are clinical trials suggesting that the quality of life for patients with COPD can be improved with these agents. This is an area where there may be a change in recommendation and availability in the near future.

Corticosteroids

Inhaled

There is still controversy regarding the use of inhaled corticosteroids in patients with COPD. Large clinical trials have shown them to have no benefit in preventing decline in lung function of patients with COPD. However, one study does suggest that inhaled corticosteroids aid in reducing exacerbations and maintaining quality of life in patients with COPD. Thus, this is another area that may change with further studies.

Oral

Prednisolone is effective in treating exacerbations of COPD (e.g. 30 mg daily for 7 days). Long-term treatment with prednisolone should be avoided because in the elderly the side effects of myopathy, bruising and osteoporosis are major problems with the potential to cause reduction in quality of life. A short (2 week) trial of prednisolone is indicated at the time of diagnosis of COPD to identify any concomitant asthma.

Other medications

The judicious use of additional medications to treat co-morbidities may improve the quality of life of patients with COPD (e.g. antidepressants for depression and diuretics for congestive cardiac failure).

Antibiotics such as amoxycillin or doxycycline have been shown to be helpful in COPD during an exacerbation when there has been an increase in sputum volume or a change in the colour of sputum in association with breathlessness.

Oxygen therapy

Oxygen therapy is commonly an emotive situation to discuss with patients with COPD. However, there are very clear guidelines governing the prescription of long-term oxygen therapy. Under the conditions of the guidelines, evidence has been obtained to show that oxygen therapy for more than 15 hours per day prolongs life for patients with COPD with a low P_aO_2 (see below).

When the decision for long-term oxygen therapy is made, the patient must be in a stable condition (i.e. no recent exacerbations) and have had full medical treatment including a trial of oral prednisolone. The measurement of ABGs should occur on two occasions a month apart. A P_aO_2 below 55 mmHg, or a P_aO_2 below 59 mmHg in the presence of cor pulmonale, indicate the need for long-term oxygen therapy, which is best delivered by an oxygen concentrator. There is currently debate about the value of overnight oximetry indicating the need for long-term oxygen therapy.

Firm guidelines for oxygen for exercise have not been promulgated. The amount of improvement in exercise capacity achieved by oxygen for an individual needs to be assessed carefully to balance nuisance value and embarrassment versus quality of life and improved function before prescribing ambulatory oxygen. In Australia, oxygen therapy is subsidised only when prescribed or approved by a respiratory specialist.

Surgical interventions

Lung transplantation is a possibility for patients with severe COPD and under 60 years of age. An assessment by a respiratory physician and a lung transplant physician is required.

Lung volume reduction surgery is a procedure that may help some patients with severe emphysema with heterogeneous disease and aged under 75 years. This procedure can provide substantial benefit over 3 years but does carry a significant early mortality risk and the procedure is still being evaluated. An assessment by a respiratory physician is mandatory and the presence of significant cardiac disease and pulmonary hypertension are absolute exclusions.

Prognosis of COPD

The poorer prognosis of COPD is seen with:

- lower values of FEV_1
- continued smoking
- hypoxaemia
- increasing age (Table 28.4).

The importance of smoking cessation can be demonstrated by considering the following scenario.

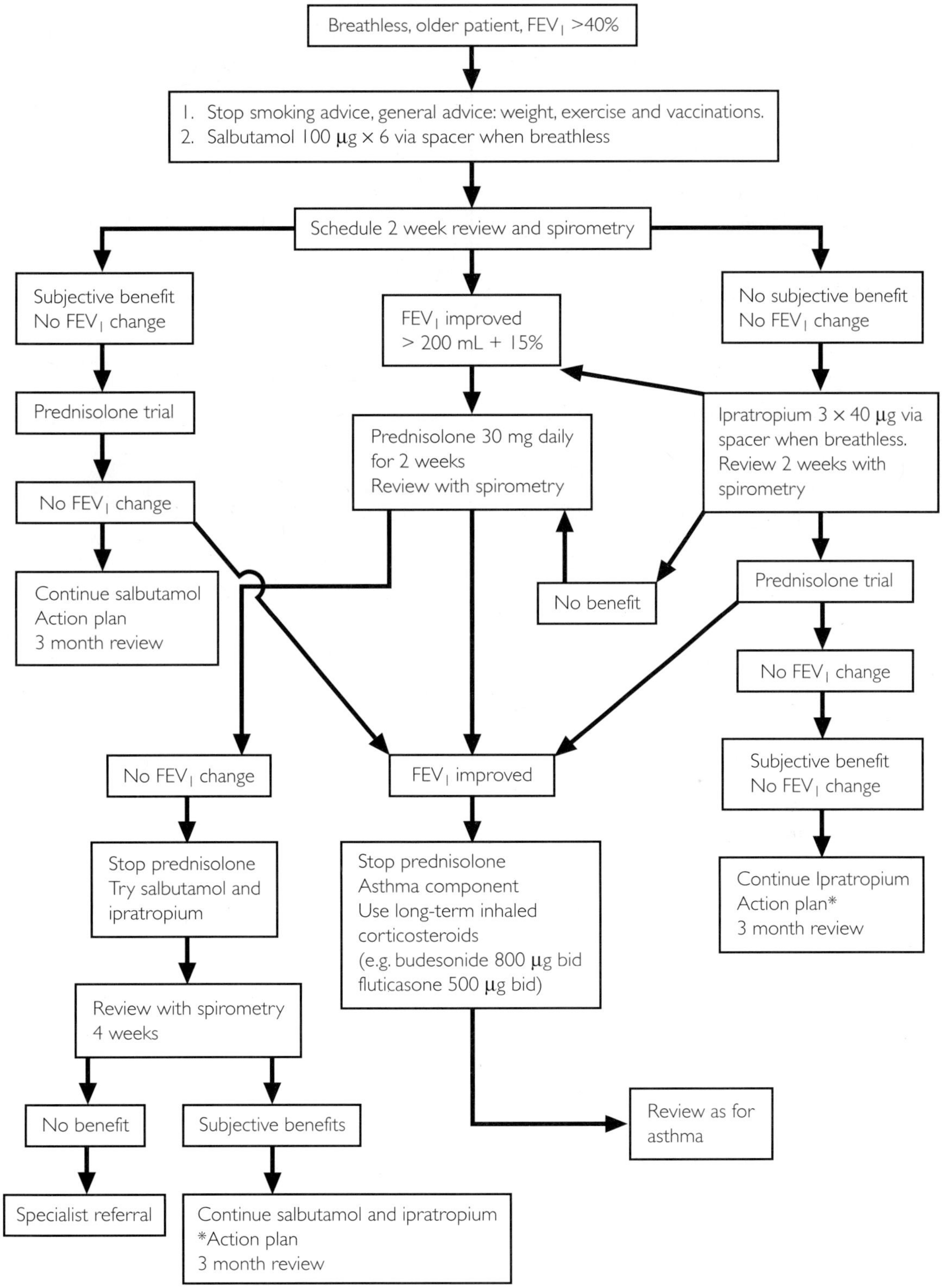

Figure 28.8 Office management of patients with COPD

Regular respiratory medication

1. blue inhaler..........
2. ....
3. ....
4. ....
5. ....

Emergency pack contents

1. Prednisolone 25 mg
2. Antibiotics..........one course

Remember to always have an emergency pack available at home

Date: Signature:

North Western Adelaide Health Service
TQEH
COPD ACTION PLAN

Name:

Doctor: Ph:

Hospital: 8222 6000

Ambulance: 000

ACTION PLAN—Breathing

- If unable to do normal activities due to shortness of breath
- If you wake up more than 2 times overnight with a cough or increased breathlessness
- If you need to use an extra 4 doses of reliever

1. *Commence* prednisolone 1½ × 25 mg for.... days

or *Commence* prednisolone for days
prednisolone for days
prednisolone for days

2. Contact your doctor within 24 hours if not improving

Infection

If your sputum:

- changes colour (especially yellow/green)
- becomes thick or sticky
- coughing up increased amounts

1. Commence antibiotics.....................mg from the emergency pack until completed
2. Contact your doctor within 24–48 hours

Figure 28.9 Sample action plan card for patients with COPD

Table 28.4 Prognosis of COPD

Age (years)	FEV_1 (% predicted)	3-year survival (%)
< 60	> 50	90
> 60	> 50	80
> 60	40–49	75

A 50 year old man of average height smoking 20–30 cigarettes per day has an FEV_1 of 2 L (60% predicted). If he stops smoking, his FEV_1 declines at 25 mL/year. At 70 his FEV_1 is likely to be 1.5 L—a value that should allow a reasonably good quality of life. If he continues smoking, his FEV_1 declines at 60 mL/year, so at 70 his FEV_1 will be 0.8 L—a value that will be likely to cause significant disability.

A recent review at Flinders Medical Centre has looked at the outcomes of patients with COPD who were started on long-term oxygen therapy. There were: 249 males: average age, 69.9 years; FEV_1, 0.86 L; P_aO_2 (air), 52.6 mmHg; 256 females: average age, 71.0 years; FEV_1, 0.65 L; P_aO_2 (air), 50.9 mmHg. The one-year survival rate was 75.2%, the 2-year survival rate was 51.3%, the 5-year survival rate was 18.9% and the 10-year survival rate was 1.1%. These figures emphasise the poor prognosis of severe COPD.

Conclusion

COPD is a common condition causing dyspnoea in the elderly. An accurate diagnosis requires measurement of spirometry, and management is influenced by the presence or absence of co-morbidities such as obesity, OSA, pulmonary hypertension and cor pulmonale.

The most important management factor is smoking cessation. Maintenance of physical fitness and treatment of OSA, cor pulmonale, and hypoxaemia are also critical. The development of appropriate medication plans that minimise side effects and maximise quality of life (without necessarily influencing spirometry) are becoming increasingly evidence-based. Self-management can be promoted for mild-to-moderate exacerbations by the use of personalised action plans. Severe exacerbations warrant hospitalisation and persistent hypoxaemia warrants assessment for oxygen therapy by a respiratory physician.

Bibliography and further reading

Calverley, P. & Bellamy, D. (2000), 'The challenge of providing better care for patients with chronic obstructive pulmonary disease: the poor relation of airways obstruction?', *Thorax*, 55, pp. 78–82.

COPD Guidelines Group of the Standards of Care Committee of the British Thoracic Society (1997), 'BTS guidelines for the management of chronic obstructive pulmonary disease', *Thorax*, 52 (suppl.), pp. S1–S28.

Flaherty, K. R., Kazerooni, E. A. & Martinez, F. J. (2000), 'Differential diagnosis of chronic airflow obstruction', *Journal of Asthma*, 37, pp. 201–24.

Hill, R. D. & Fisher, E. B. Jr (1993), 'Smoking cessation in the older chronic smoker: a review in pulmonary disease in the elderly patient', in Mahler, D. A. (ed.), *Lung Biology in Health and Disease*, vol. 63, Marcel Dekker, New York, pp. 189–218.

McNicholas, W. T. (2000), 'Impact of sleep in COPD', *Chest*, 117, pp. 48S–53S.

Postma, D. S. & Siafakas, N. M. (eds) (1998), 'Management of chronic obstructive pulmonary disease', *European Respiratory Monographs*, 7, pp. 1–302.

Ramsey, S. D. (2000), 'Suboptimal medical therapy in COPD. Exploring the causes and consequences', *Chest*, 117, pp. 335–75.

Siafakas, N. M., Vermeire, P., Pride, N. B., et al. (1995), 'Optimal assessment and management of chronic obstructive pulmonary disease (COPD)', *European Respiratory Journal*, 8, pp. 1398–420.

Part VII

Nutritional status and gastroenterological conditions

Chapter 29
Oral health

RONALD L. ETTINGER

Introduction

Oral health has been defined as: 'A standard of health of the oral and related tissues which enables an individual to eat, speak and socialise without active disease, discomfort or embarrassment, and which contributes to general well being'. Oral health problems have been shown to be among the most prevalent chronic problems with which elderly persons have to deal. In general, physicians are unaware that these problems can lead to impaired nutrition, systemic morbidity, speech problems and decreased satisfaction, resulting in an impaired quality of life. The predominant oral health problems of older adults include tooth loss, dental caries, periodontal disease, xerostomia (dry mouth), tooth wear from various causes, and oral mucosal disease, most significantly oral cancer. Many oral problems can be either prevented or effectively treated if dentists are brought in as part of the health care team.

In most industrialised countries, dental care for many older adults has been an ongoing process in which an older dental practitioner has maintained a heavily restored dentition using conservative, restorative techniques. Preventive regimens have not been a significant component of these dentists' armamentarium. Usually, if a tooth was near the anterior of the mouth, and if the patient could afford it, a fixed partial denture (bridge) was constructed. If the patient could not afford this treatment, a removable partial prosthesis (plate) was offered as an alternative to fill that space. When only a few teeth were left due to a process of progressive tooth loss, the remaining teeth were extracted and a complete denture was constructed. This model of patient–dentist interaction has been quite well documented. However, data from several national and regional studies have shown that over 60% of the elderly population are now retaining some of their natural teeth and the stereotype of the older consumer of health care being toothless and needing complete dentures is outdated.

In the past, when an elderly person was edentulous or had an oral problem, usually he or his caregiver would remove his complete dentures and he would eat mush. This was not good for the quality of life of the patient, but neither was it particularly life-threatening. Now, however, the majority of elderly persons have some natural teeth. As long as such an elderly person remains healthy, few problems occur because he can access a dental office. What happens when a patient of a general dental practice becomes medically compromised, physically disabled or cognitively impaired and so becomes housebound or institutionalised? His oral health care now requires the dentist and physician to work together with the rest of the health care team so that a treatment plan is developed in the best interests of the patient. The following case history illustrates some of the relevant issues.

Case history

A 76-year-old man was referred to the author's unit for treatment by an oral surgeon the man's wife had taken him to. As she explained it, her husband had 'lost anchor teeth for his partials and he could not keep them in'. She went on to say that 'my husband has advanced Alzheimer's and our dentist has retired'. The wife told us that her husband had not been eating well, that he had lost some weight and that he was no longer eating ice cream, which he enjoyed very much.

The patient's medical record, which was supplied by his physician, revealed that the diagnosis of Alzheimer's disease was made 8 years ago. The patient has no history of smoking and denies alcohol or drug abuse. No other family member except his grandfather has developed Alzheimer's disease. The patient has a history of arthritis of the hands and mild hypertension. In the last four years he has progressively lost interest in eating, has had photophobia and visual hallucinations, is disoriented, and sings and taps all the time. He was prescribed Halperidol (Haldol) 0.5 mg for the hallucinations about 4 years ago and Triamterene with hydrochlorothiazide (Dyazide) for the hypertension. He has been taking two 325 mg tablets of acetaminophen (Tylenol) twice a day. The patient is now incontinent but he can walk by himself.

The patient was led into the dental office by his wife. The patient has aphasia and he smiles and hums to himself continuously. If he is disturbed or stressed, his foot tapping increases and the humming gets louder and changes pitch. He is not physically aggressive and can follow simple instructions given to him by his wife. His blood pressure was 112/75, respiration 28.

With some difficulty, and with his wife holding his hands, I was able to get him to open his mouth and could see the following teeth:

- right maxilla—3 molars and a premolar
- left maxilla—premolar and a molar
- left mandible—a canine
- right mandible—no natural teeth.

There was decay in several teeth; especially affected was the premolar and molar of the left maxilla as well as the mandibular canine.

There were no interdigitating pairs of teeth to chew with. His removable partial dentures no longer fitted him. The maxillary denture did not fit at all. The mandibular denture could be stabilised, so with a thermoplastic material I was able to add to the denture and fill the space where natural teeth had been and then make an accurate impression of the soft tissues under the denture. The denture was sent to the laboratory for a reline and the addition of the missing teeth with denture teeth. In the meantime, an appointment was organised to clean his teeth and to restore the decayed teeth. To achieve this required 4 people: his wife to hold his hands, one of us to keep his lips open while another one did the restorative work, and a dental assistant/nurse to handle the instruments and prepare the restorative materials. For the larger restorations, local infiltration with local anaesthetic, Xylocaine with 1:100 000 Epinephrine, was used. We found that if we hummed or sang to him, he calmed down and allowed us to carry out the needed dental care.

At another appointment the relined partial denture was fitted and we taught his wife how to remove it and to place it, and how to brush his teeth without getting accidentally bitten. It was suggested she give him the denture for eating only, as he was likely to take it out and leave it somewhere out of sight. We did not try to make him a new maxillary denture for aesthetics, to replace the missing upper anterior teeth, as we felt that the stress of the appointments was greater than the benefit. This was difficult for his wife, but she accepted the decision, as her husband was no longer concerned about his appearance.

The remaining teeth were treated with a fluoride-containing varnish and the patient was seen a week later. His eating had improved, he was again enjoying his ice-cream and was tolerating the denture. The patient was put on a 3 month recall schedule.

This case history illustrates several significant issues:

1. The majority of older adults are no longer edentulous; most have some natural teeth which require care from a dentist.
2. The difficulty and personnel requirements of treating emergency or restorative dental problems of individuals who are severely cognitively impaired can be problematic.
3. The impact of oral disease on quality of life can be seen here. Poor oral function impairs a person's ability to ingest food or to live without pain or discomfort and is avoidable.
4. If the patient had been referred for dental care by the physician early in the disease, much of the current tooth loss could have been avoided.

Oral disorders in older adults

Tooth loss

Tooth loss can be a very emotionally disabling and handicapping event for some people and can have a profound impact on the quality of their lives. Edentulism or total tooth loss can result in difficulty chewing food. As a group, edentulous persons tend to eliminate certain foods from their diet, such as some fresh fruits, vegetables and nuts. Anything with meat requires an expensive cut or a lot of cooking. Tooth loss is strongly related to age, race, ethnicity and social class. A recent study in Australia reported that, using multivariate analysis, higher rates of edentulism were associated with being older, female, Australian born, having a pensioner health benefit card, having left school early (no high school diploma) and not owning one's own home. A Finnish study found a relationship between edentulousness and a history of bone fracture (odds ratio 2.5) and tobacco smoking (odds ratio 2.42).

A series of recent studies have identified tooth loss as a risk factor associated with morbidity of a number of diseases. For instance, the mean number of missing teeth was significantly higher among those persons who had a history of atherosclerotic vascular disorder, heart failure, ischaemic heart disease and joint disease. Those persons were also more likely to be edentulous than persons who did not have a history of those diseases.

There have been a number of studies that have shown that as a population ages, visits to the physician increase, while visits to the dentist decrease. This finding has been attributed to the increased risk of chronic diseases associated with ageing, the attitude of older people towards disease, the availability of payment for services and the fact that persons who are edentulous often do not perceive a need for regular care. However, data from national surveys in the US, UK and Australia have shown that total tooth loss or edentulousness has declined among elderly people, especially among the new elderly.

In 1979, 60% of elderly Australians were edentulous. By 1989 this figure had decreased to 44%. It has been projected that by the year 2020 only 20% of elderly Australians will be edentulous.

If the majority of older adults are maintaining at least a portion of their natural dentitions, then dentists must be included in multidisciplinary teams. In fact, several studies have shown that older dentate adults are using dental services in a manner similar to younger adults and that the difference in utilisation is not related to age but to the presence of natural teeth.

Caries

Caries is a bacterial infection of teeth that is influenced by the combination of virulence of the acidogenic bacteria in the mouth, the acidogenic potential and pattern of food intake, the ability of the individual to maintain oral hygiene, and the inherent resistance of the teeth to demineralisation. It has been suggested that dental caries is the most costly preventable diet related disease in the industrialised nations and is more costly than coronary heart disease, hypertension or diabetes. There has been a dramatic change in the incidence of caries in these societies, which can be characterised by a decreased caries rate in children and an increasing caries rate in the ageing population. In fact, it has been shown that the incidence of caries in a population aged 65 and older is greater than in a population of 14-year-olds living in a non-fluoridated area.

Several studies of the ageing population have found that untreated caries are most commonly found on the crowns of the tooth (25%), although a substantial number of elderly (18%) also have root caries. A longitudinal study of caries in older adults has found that over 3 years, caries developed on an average of 2.4 coronal surfaces and 1.1 root surfaces per person per year. For persons who are functionally frail and are unable to manage oral hygiene independently, the rates are much higher.

An evaluation of the existing data suggests that caries can be found in more than 95% of the dentate elderly population. Those at highest risk are persons who are physically frail or mentally confused, and the majority of these persons are homebound or institutionalised. A constant problem is whether it is appropriate simply to restore caries in the teeth of older adults without helping them to manage their diet or their personal oral hygiene. It has been shown that topical fluoride can remineralise early carious lesions, that antimicrobials such as chlorhexidine can reduce the number of acidogenic bacteria, and that the use of sugar substitutes reduces the acidogenic environment. The recurring problem is how to educate and motivate the older adult population, and especially significant others or caregivers of frail and functionally dependent older adults, to perform oral hygiene regularly (see Figure 29.1).

The treatment of root surface caries in older adults is often very frustrating. Incipient lesions can be remineralised with topical fluorides, slightly larger lesions can be polished away and the root surface treated with topical fluoride. Larger cavitated lesions will need a restoration but no ideal restorative materials exist. The newer glass ionomer/resin restorative materials are a viable alternative as they can be bonded to dentin and do release fluoride over time, which helps prevent recurrence. However, only a good daily home oral hygiene program is effective. Unfortunately, many older adults have poor vision, poor hand–eye co-ordination and lack motivation to carry out a home care program.

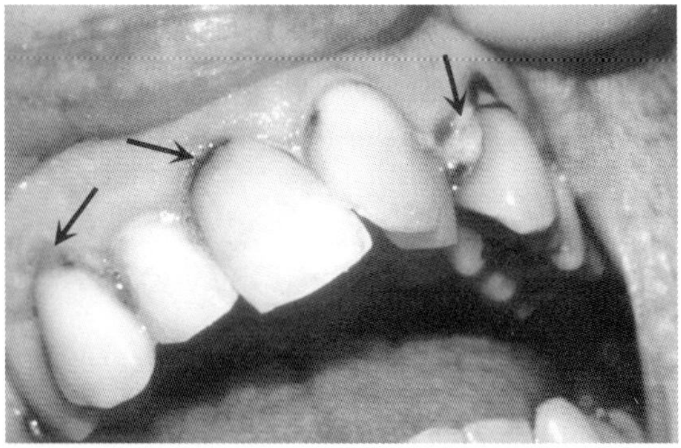

Figure 29.1 This is a picture of the maxillary teeth of a 68-year-old woman who has a history of hypertension for which she is taking a diuretic and β-blocker. The drugs have a xerogenic potential, and when combined with poor plaque control, can cause caries in susceptible persons. The arrows indicate root surface caries along the cemento-enamel junction on the incisors and inter-proximal caries on the canine

Periodontal diseases

The periodontal diseases are a series of plaque induced diseases, which result from the exposure of the teeth to a biofilm, which accumulates on the teeth to form bacterial masses. Dental plaque is very complex—more than 400 species of bacteria have been isolated from the plaque of persons with periodontal diseases. In gingivitis, the infectious, inflammatory and immunological process is limited to the gingival tissues (see Figure 29.2(a)).

Periodontitis is a chronic infectious disease which can result in inflammatory deterioration of the periodontal ligament and alveolar bone. It is characterised clinically by inflammation of the gingival tissues, apical migration of the junctional epithelium of the periodontal tissues, pocket formation and alveolar bone loss (see Figure 29.2(b)).

Early epidemiologic studies of dental patients suggested that gingivitis progressed with time to periodontitis and that once periodontitis was established, tooth loss was inevitable. However, concepts related to the universality of progressive periodontal disease have changed. More recent

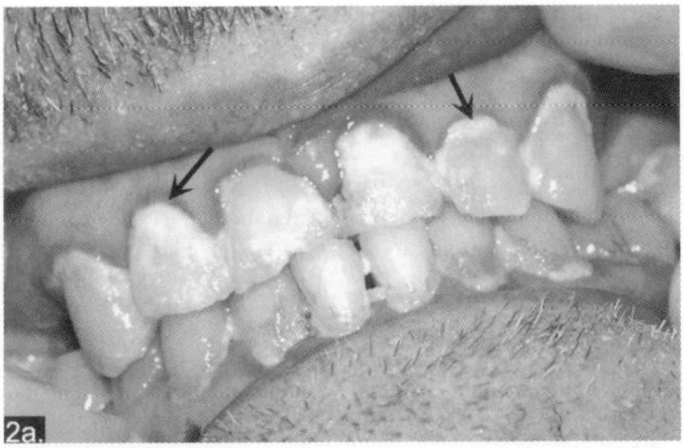

Figure 29.2(a) This is a picture of the dentition of a 72-year-old male with failing eyesight where the marginal gingiva are inflamed due to the heavy deposits of plaque on the teeth (see arrows). This is a reversible condition and the tissues will heal once the plaque with its micro-organisms are removed

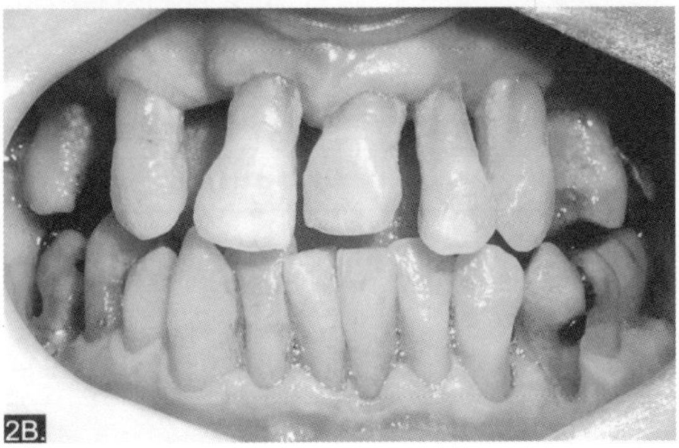

Figure 29.2(b) This is a picture of the dentition of an 82-year-old woman with periodontitis. This is also a plaque induced infectious disease, which results in bone loss, exposure of root surfaces, and mobility of the teeth. The damage created by periodontitis cannot be reversed, but if the soft and hard bacterial deposits are removed and the teeth are kept clean, the disease usually will not progress further

studies have shown that comparatively few older individuals harbour the majority of tooth sites with progressive periodontal disease. These data came from studying untreated patients with pocketing, and showed that progression at any given site occurred infrequently and usually at a slow rate, except in a small group of 'susceptible individuals'. In these susceptible individuals—even those with diagnostic signs and symptoms, such as bleeding on probing, probing depths of 6 mm, and the presence of certain periopathogens—loss has been found to increase only 20–30% during periods varying in length from 1 to 5 years.

It is now accepted that the active phase of periodontal disease is episodic, with bursts of destruction followed by periods of quiescence. These bursts of activity seem to be randomised and their incidence seems to be reduced in persons over the age of 40. Although cross-sectioned epidemiological data suggests that the prevalence and severity of periodontal disease increases with age, longitudinal studies have identified that severe disease only occurs in a small group of at risk patients, as described earlier (see Figures 29.3(a) and 29.3(b)). At this time, because there are no effective tests to identify the high-risk subjects, the dentist needs to follow up older adults carefully to determine who is at risk. Evidence for this concept comes from the more recent longitudinal studies of

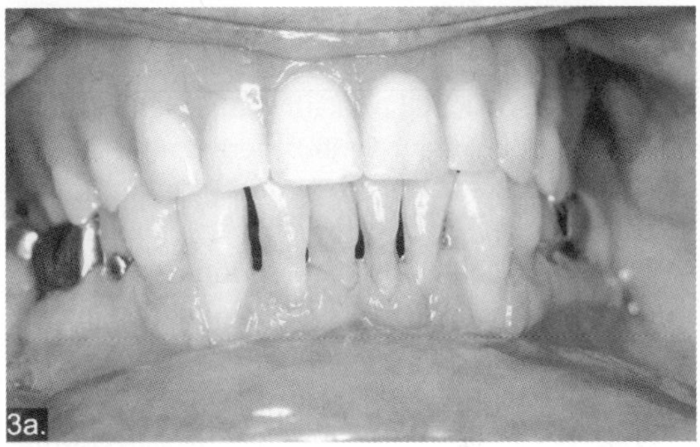

Figure 29.3(a) This is a 66-year-old male who was treated with a complete upper denture and careful scaling and cleaning of the lower teeth

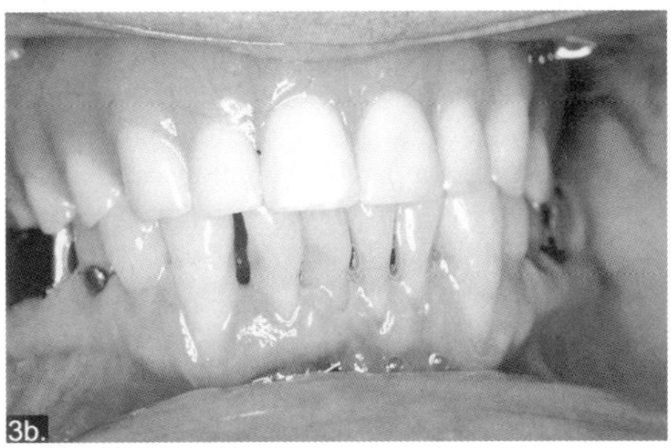

Figure 29.3(b) This is the same patient 15 years later at the age of 81. There has been no recurrence of the disease and no further bone loss due to his good home care and professional cleaning every 4 months

community-dwelling older adults in the US, which showed that all of the population had suffered attachment loss at the beginning of the study. Fifty-five per cent of African-Americans and 27.9% of whites had at least one site with more than 7 mm of attachment loss. Also, 32.7% of African-Americans and 9.9% of whites had at least one tooth with probing depths deeper than 6 mm. After 3 years, 63% of whites and 45% of African-Americans had no loss of attachment. This study concluded that the people who died or became totally edentulous after 3 years had deeper probing depths and more attachment loss at baseline. The authors concluded that this data was 'consistent with an episodic, random hit model of disease, which places overall risk at the patient level with variations at the site level due to site characteristics'. The authors stated categorically that baseline probing depths and attachment level by themselves are not good predictors of future attachment loss.

The clinical implication is that mild forms of gingivitis and periodontal pocketing affect almost all of the ageing population. Serious periodontal disease affects a much smaller proportion of older adults. Therefore, the majority of elderly people need scaling and cleaning as their routine periodontal treatment, which can be carried out by a dental hygienist, while a small minority need complex care, which can only be delivered by a dentist.

The response of the tissues to periodontal therapy can be compromised if patients have insulin dependent diabetes mellitus, are immunocompromised, or have received radiation therapy to the head and neck. The compromised microvasculature and the inability to deal with stress prevent adequate healing of the tissues after periodontal therapy and allow the microflora to overcome the local tissue response. This situation can lead to rapid bone loss and loss of teeth in patients who are not monitored closely to maintain good home oral hygiene habits.

Fibrous hyperplasia of the gingiva can result from many causes. Some causes are idiopathic but the majority are iatrogenic. Until recently, only phenytoin was recognised as causing generalised fibrous gingival hyperplasia. However, more recently cyclosporin A, an immunosuppressant used in organ transplant procedures, and a series of calcium channel blockers (e.g. nifedipine, used for the treatment of vasospastic angina, chronic stable angina and ventricular arrhythmias) have also been implicated (see Table 29.1). The drug induced gingival hyperplasias seem to be similar in epithelial, morphological and inflammatory patterns. It is suggested that the effect is on fibroblasts and that an increase in ground substance causes the hyperplastic response. Poor oral hygiene seems to stimulate the magnitude of the response.

Persons who are functionally dependent because of physical frailty, mental confusion or dementia are at the highest risk for periodontal disease because of their inability to maintain oral hygiene independently. Unless caregivers or significant others are trained and motivated to help these at-risk persons, maintenance of oral health is not possible and periodontal disease with loss of teeth is inevitable.

Table 29.1 Drugs associated with gingival overgrowth

Generic drug	Brand name
Anticonvulsants	
Phenobarbital	Luminal Sodium, Solfoton
Phenytoin	Dilantin, Diphenylan
Valproic acid	Depakene, Depakote
Immunosuppressants	
Cyclosporin A	Sandimmune
Tacrolimust (FK-506)	Prograt
Calcium channel blockers	
Diltiazem	Cardizem, Dilacor XR
Felodipine	Plendil, Renedil
Nifedipine	Procardia, Adalat
Verapamil	Calan, Isoptin

Sources: R. T. Butler, K. L. Kalkwarf & W. B. Kaldahl (1987), 'Drug induced gingival hyperplasia: Phenytoin, Cyclosporine, and Nifedipine', *The Journal of the American Dental Association*, 114, pp. 56–60; L. H. Silverstein, J. T. Garnick, M. Szikman & B. Singh (1997), 'Medication-induced gingival enlargement: A clinical review', *General Dentistry*, 45, pp. 371–80; and S. J. Merow & D. J. Sheridan (1998), 'Medically induced gingival hyperplasia', *Mayo Clinic Proceedings*, 73, pp. 1196–9.

Xerostomia (dry mouth)

Saliva is one of the most important body fluids and serves a series of important physiological functions. Saliva is required to supply lubrication for speech, the formation of the bolus, as well as swallowing, and it protects the teeth and the oral mucosa from infection. This fluid also contains a variety of electrolytes, peptides, lipids and glycoproteins which serve as:

- antimicrobial to kill bacteria and viruses
- protection of the mucosa from trauma and dehydration due to the coating of mucin
- buffers, to maintain pH levels and compensate for the daily ingestion of acidic and basic fluids and foods
- protection of the teeth from demineralisation by adding a super-saturated solution of calcium and phosphates into the oral cavity.

A loss of saliva or even a reduction in flow rates can result in a significantly higher risk of caries, periodontal disease, problems with eating, talking and denture wearing, as well as altered taste sensations (see Figure 29.4). Subjects with dry mouth are also at a higher risk for oral mucosal problems, such as mucositis and candidiasis. The most significant problem for persons with xerostomia is that it results in an overall reduction in the quality of life.

Xerostomia has been defined as the 'subjective feeling of oral dryness' and is due to salivary hypofunction. The prevalence of xerostomia varies from 13% to 28% in older populations and has been reported to be as high as 61% in persons living in long-term care institutions.

The majority of xerostomias are due to drugs and disease. Over 400 drugs have been identified as having a xerostomic potential due to some anticholinergic properties. The most common groups (and some examples) are shown in Table 29.2. The intensity of the effect of a drug will depend upon the dosage of the drug, the duration of administration of the drug, the anticholinergic potential of the drug and the response of the individual. If a dentist notices oral side effects from a drug, she may ask the physician if it is possible to adjust the drug dosages, to modify the drug schedule or to change to a less xerogenic drug, and if that is not possible, to treat the xerostomia jointly.

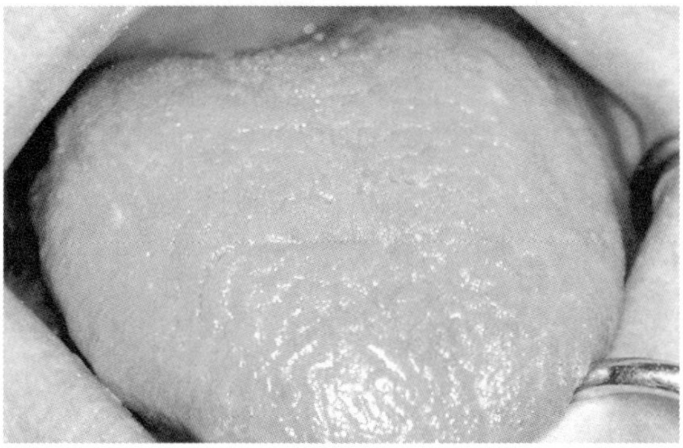

Figure 29.4 Atrophy of the tongue papillae and lobulation in a woman aged 78 years suffering from Sjögren's syndrome which has caused the xerostomia

There is a series of diseases that affect the glands directly. Among them are a group of autoimmune diseases, which include the collagen diseases often associated with rheumatoid arthritis. The most common of these is Sjögren's syndrome. Diseases such as Parkinson's disease, dementia and Alzheimer's disease have also been shown to cause diminished salivary flow rates.

Treatment of xerostomia

The treatment for dry mouth is very frustrating for the patient, as well as for the clinician, because usually the symptoms cannot be eliminated. Relief is usually transient, if there is any at all. If the cause of the xerostomia is dehydration, then fluid replenishment will eliminate the problem. If the cause is a drug, then it may be possible to work with the physician to change the drug, the dosage or the scheduling. If it is not contraindicated and the patient has potentially functioning salivary glands, it may be possible to use cholinergics, such as pilocarpine, to stimulate salivary flow. The patients can sometimes gain relief from chewing sugarless gum or candy. If no salivary gland activity exists, commercial artificial salivas or gels may help to give temporary palliation. In our experience, the most useful moisturising gel is Oral Balance (Laclede, Gardenia, CA, 90048, US). This gel contains lacto-peroxidase and a glucose oxidase inhibitory system. Other systems which give relief contain mucin (Saliva-Orthana, AS-Orthana, Kemisk Fabrick, Denmark, DK-2770). If patients with xerostomia are dentate, they need to use a high concentration fluoride gel (e.g. Prevident-5000) and to be on a professionally designed daily topical fluoride program developed for them by their dentist (see Figures 29.5(a) and 29.5(b)).

Table 29.2 Medications that could cause xerostomia

Generic drug	Brand name	Nursing home (% of pop'n) (*n* = 481)[(a)]	Community dwelling (% of pop'n) (*n* = 3217)[(b)]
Anticholinergics	Bentyl	2.5	0.6
Antidepressants	Elavil	11.7	3.8
Antihypertensives	Inderal	11.0	20.0
Anti-Parkinson's	Cogentin	3.9	0.4
Antipsychotics	Mellaril		
	Thorazine		
	Haldol	16.8	1.1
Diuretics	Lasix		
	Hydrodiuril		
	Dyazide	50.7	39.0
Gastrointestinal	Probanthine	4.0	2.8
Antihistamines/decongestants	Benadryl		
	Actifed		
	Dimetapp	13.1	5.3
Systemic bronchodilators	Theodur		
	Brethine	3.0	2.9

(*a*) Modified from K. A. Baker, S. M. Levy & E. A. Chrischilles (1991), 'Medications with dental significance: Usage in a nursing home population', *Special Care in Dentistry*, 11, pp. 19–25.

(*b*) Modified from S. M. Levy, K. A. Baker & F. J. Kohout (1988), 'Use of medication with dental significance by a non-institutionalized elderly population', *Gerodontics*, 4, pp. 119–25.

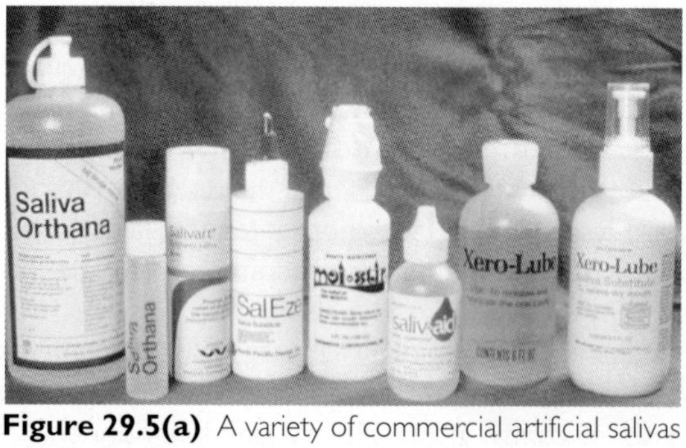

Figure 29.5(a) A variety of commercial artificial salivas which only give very short-term relief. Most are a mix of glycerine and water with carboxymethylcellulose to give them a viscosity similar to saliva, and most contain calcium and phosphate ions. The Orthana product from Denmark is made from bovine mucin and seems to give more effective relief

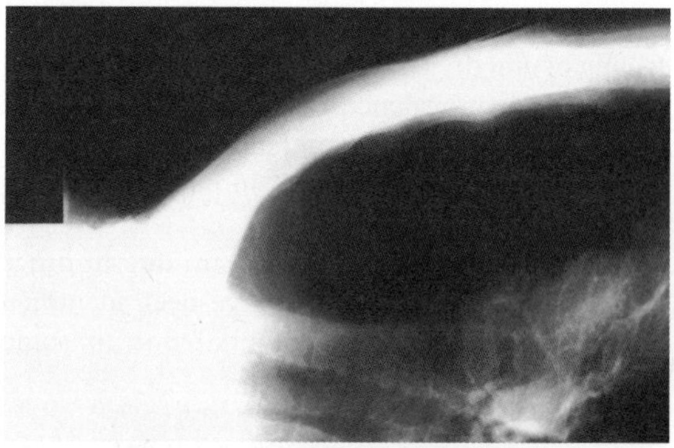

Figure 29.5(b) SALIX is a saliva stimulant containing a buffered citric acid tablet which can be sucked. Karigel-N and Prevident 5000 are topical fluoride gels which are brushed on the teeth. Oral Balance is a topical gel which contains lacto-peroxidase and a glucose oxidase inhibitor system which protects the mucosa

Tooth wear

Dental hard tissues, unlike skin or mucosa, do not have the capacity for repair or replacement. Therefore, over time all persons will show some wear of their dentitions. The rate of tooth wear depends upon a variety of factors which include:

- habits (e.g. biting thread, or chewing a pipe stem)
- diet (e.g. abrasiveness of food)
- stress (e.g. attrition: grinding teeth during sleep (bruxism))

- chemical erosion, e.g.:
  - the diet: sipping carbonated beverages which produce acid
  - the environment: working in a battery factory
  - severe gastroesophageal reflux: acute peptic ulcer, alcoholism, food fads (see Figures 29.6(a) and (b)).

There are very few epidemiological studies of tooth wear. However, Hand et al. investigated the prevalence of occlusal attrition in 520 dentate non-institutionalised older adults living at home. They found that 84.2% of the population had at least one tooth where the enamel was so worn that the dentine showed through, and a further 72.9% had dentinal attrition, when all of the occlusal or incisal enamel was obliterated. Severe attrition was defined when the tooth was worn to the gingival margin and this was found in 3.9% of the population. Most people had some attrition, with about 25% of their teeth affected, and it was more prevalent in the anterior of the mouth. In this same population 56% had some cervical abrasion, and in 30% it was deeper than 1 mm in depth.

The consequences of this tooth wear are significant. Because more older people are keeping more teeth and are reluctant to have these teeth extracted, the dental industry is being asked to develop new materials to restore these dentitions. At this time, the only way to restore many of these patients with extensive wear is through the use of costly porcelain and metal crowns by specialist prosthodontists (see Figures 29.7(a) and (b)). The

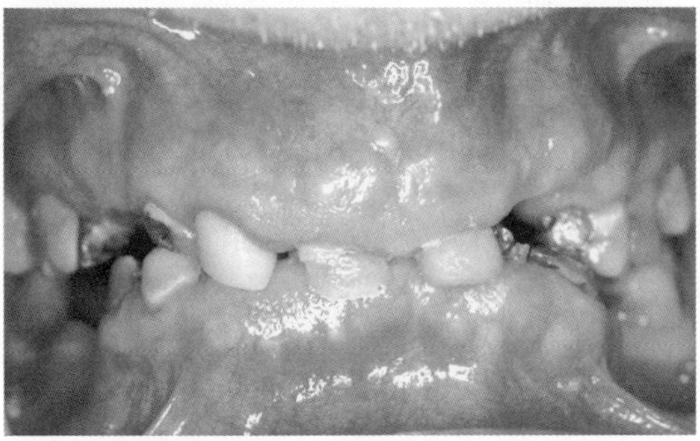

Figure 29.6(a) This is the dentition of a 75-year-old farmer who has lost key posterior teeth and is a bruxer and so has worn down his teeth

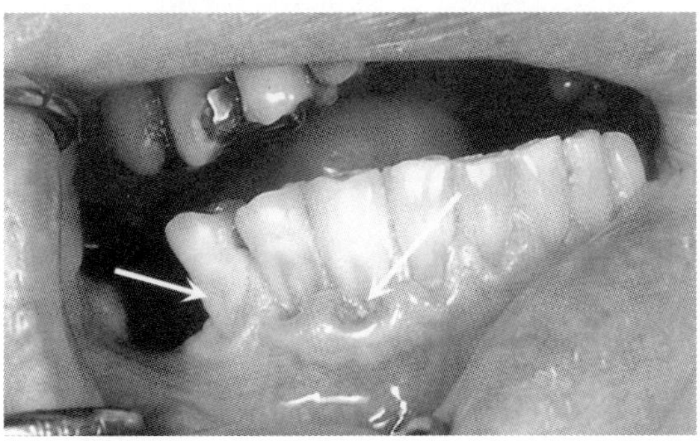

Figure 29.6(b) This is the right side of the dentition of a 69-year-old woman. She is right-handed and has brushed her teeth with a scrubbing action to the point where she has removed all of the enamel and most of the dentine

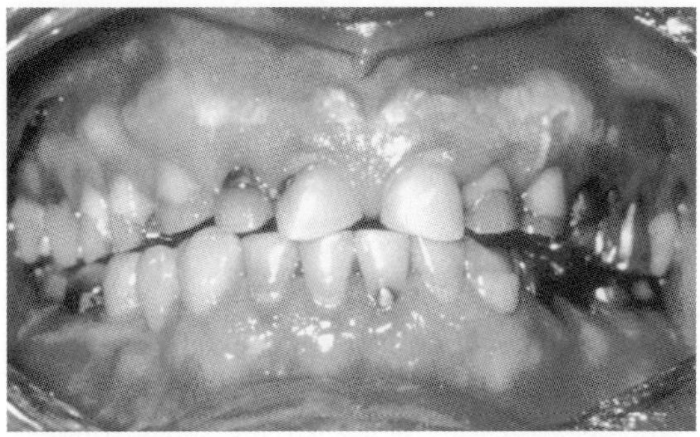

Figure 29.7(a) This is a 66-year-old businessman who had a history of peptic ulcer with reflux oesophagitis which has resulted in significant loss of enamel

PICTURE COURTESY OF DR KEITH THAYER, UNIVERSITY OF IOWA

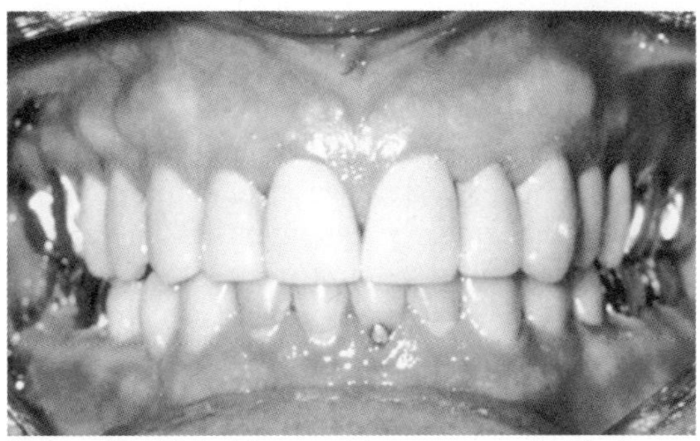

Figure 29.7(b) After receiving treatment for his disease, all the teeth were restored with gold crowns or porcelain fused to gold crowns except the 6 mandibular anteriors. During regurgitation, the tongue protects the mandibular anteriors from the acidic gastric contents

PICTURE COURTESY OF DR KEITH THAYER, UNIVERSITY OF IOWA

other significant problem associated with tooth wear is tooth sensitivity. Although there are fluoride-containing varnishes and resin-bonding agents on the market to desensitise the teeth, they do not solve all patients' problems. There is a group of patients whose sensitivity is so severe that the only solution to maintaining their teeth is endodontics or root canal therapy, which is time-consuming, invasive and costly.

Oral mucosal disease

The health and integrity of the oral cavity depends on an intact mucosa protecting the tissues beneath it from desiccation, infection and chemical, thermal and mechanical injury. The mucosa must be able to impede ingress of noxious or infectious material, to respond to injury, and to mount an effective inflammatory and immune response to deal with any materials or organisms that may try to penetrate the barrier.

Oral mucosal lesions in older adults are associated with a wide variety of causes, such as trauma, infection, immunological based mucosal disease, haematological disorders, oral manifestations of systemic disease, poor nutritional status, pharmacologic side effects and neoplasias. This chapter will focus on only a few of the most common problems.

The loss of teeth and denture wearing are associated with changes in the oral mucosa of elderly persons. Some of the induced changes include mucosal inflammatory changes, such as diffuse and granular denture stomatitis, hyperplastic lesions and atrophic changes. A strong relationship has been shown between the inflammatory changes of stomatitis and the presence of *Candida albicans*. Dentures that are worn continuously and not kept adequately clean develop a plaque that becomes colonised by a variety of organisms, including *C. albicans*. These organisms produce toxins that induce an inflammatory response in the mucosa (diffuse stomatitis), sometimes with an associated hyperplasia which is called granular denture stomatitis or inflammatory papillary hyperplasia. The prevalence of denture stomatitis in older populations varies greatly but has been shown to affect at least 20% of that population wearing dentures. Angular cheilitis is often associated with both the diffuse and the granular forms of denture stomatitis. It does not seem as prevalent as denture stomatitis and has been described as having a multifactorial aetiology (see Figures 29.8(a) and (b)).

If the oral mucosa is stimulated by low-grade chronic irritation, it responds with a hyperplastic reaction. In older adults who wear dentures, there is continuous resorption of the residual ridges beneath dentures, which results in the poor fit of dentures over time and the greater potential for movement and trauma. The most common site for trauma is the periphery of complete dentures, especially in the mandibular arch where support is poor and the rate of resorption is 4 times greater than the maxilla. If the trauma becomes greater, the tissues either ulcerate or they may hyperkeratose to form white patches in the mouth (leucoplakia). These areas of ulceration and hyperkeratosis have the potential to undergo malignant transformation (see Figures 29.9(a) and (b)). The rate of change, with a period prevalence of malignant transformation for leucoplakia, varies from 4% to 6% with follow-up periods of 3–20 years. The transformation of these kinds of denture induced lesions is unknown, however.

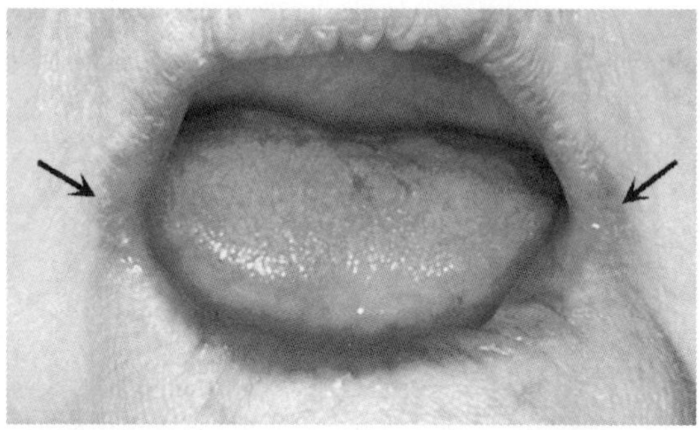

Figure 29.8 This is the mouth of an 82-year-old woman who suffered a stroke 3 years ago. She has been wearing dentures continuously for the last 45 years. She has angular cheilitis and a denture induced stomatitis due to *Candida albicans*. She was advised to remove her dentures when sleeping. The dentures were treated with an antifungal soak (benzylkonium chloride 1:750 dilution). A topical antifungal ointment (Ketaconacole cream 2%) was used on the mucosa and as the dentures were ill-fitting they were stabilised with an interim liner

In Western countries, oral cancer accounts for about 3–5% of all malignant tumours. It has been shown that over 90% of the oral malignant tumours are squamous cell carcinoma. Many oral cancers arise from apparently healthy mucosa but some have been reportedly associated with premalignant lesions. The most common of these premalignant lesions are erythroplakia, speckled leucoplakia and erosive lichen planus. Some other conditions which may predispose to oral carcinoma are syphilitic glossitis, submucous fibrosis and iron deficiency anaemia. Papilloma virus also has been implicated. However, the greatest risk factors are alcohol and the use of tobacco products (see Figures 29.10(a) and (b)).

Oral cancer can be detected by a thorough soft tissue examination and, if found in the early stages, can be readily treated. However, the older adult population tends to see a physician more often than a dentist and very few physicians routinely examine the oral cavity. Thus, the oral cancers have a high morbidity and mortality because they are usually painless, unless the lesion involves a nerve or it becomes secondarily infected. It has been shown that the incidence of oral cancer is higher than for leukaemia and tumours of the brain, liver, ovary, kidney, thyroid, stomach and cervix.

A majority of older persons are likely to have chronic diseases, most of which are age dependent,

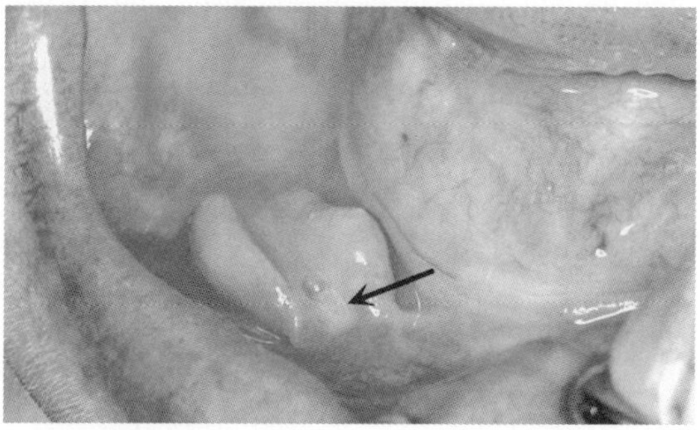

Figure 29.9(a) The arrow is pointing to an ulceration in a fibrous hyperplasia caused by chronic irritation on the mandibular arch of a 77-year-old woman who has worn complete dentures for the last 35 years. She only become aware of the lesion 2 days before because of the ulceration

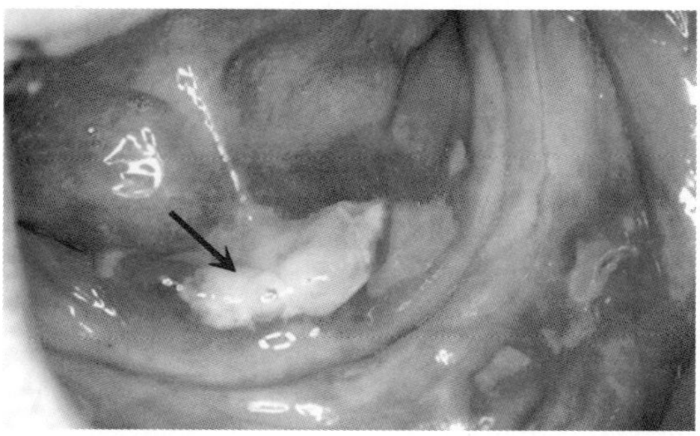

Figure 29.9(b) The arrow is pointing to an area of chronic irritation which has resulted in a white lesion on the floor of the mouth, a leukoplakia. This 67-year-old woman has been wearing an ill-fitting complete lower denture. She is unaware of this lesion which has the potential to undergo malignant transformation

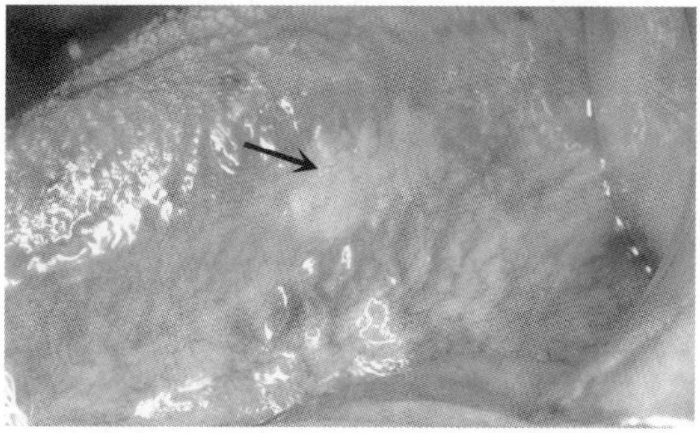

Figure 29.10(a) This is a picture of the lateral border of the tongue of a 94-year-old woman whose chief complaint is that her dentures are loose and uncomfortable when she eats. She is unaware of the white lesion. The patient has a history of hysterectomy (40 years ago); hypertension; cataracts removed 16 years ago; hip fracture 3½ years ago; arthritis of the left arm and shoulder and trigeminal neuralgia for the past 12 years. She has been edentulous for 42 years

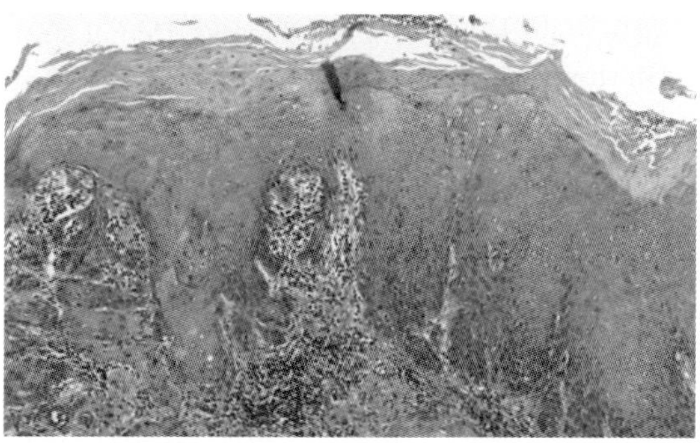

Figure 29.10(b) Excisional biopsy of this lesion which turned out to be a well differentiated squamous cell carcinoma HISTOLOGY COURTESY OF DR STEVEN VINCENT, UNIVERSITY OF IOWA

and so the prevalence of drug treatment increases in complexity with advancing years. Many of these medications may have a direct effect on the oral mucosa by causing hyposalivation or xerostomia, which has been discussed earlier, bleeding disorders of the tissues, lichenoid reactions, tissue overgrowth and hypersensitivity reactions. Therefore, it seems prudent for every older adult to have their oral soft and hard tissue examined at least yearly as a routine preventive measure.

Patient management

Premedication and prevention of medical emergencies

Good communication is required between the physician and the dentist if the oral health needs of their elderly patients are to be safely served. What should the physician know about the medical problems facing the dental team? The first of these is premedication, which may take several forms and include sedation or restraint, antibiotic prophylaxis and complications stemming from underlying disease or medications used to treat those diseases.

Premedication with sedation

Behaviour management is required for a number of older patients who are cognitively impaired. The majority of these patients are functionally dependent older adults suffering from a variety of dementias, psychiatric disturbances or any of the choreas which produce degenerative illnesses. Dental treatment should be scheduled for short appointments at mid-morning or early afternoon and should be accompanied by stress and anxiety reduction techniques. To manage these individuals, the dentist should consult the physician for recommendations if chemical restraint (sedation) is to be used. The physician should help the dentist evaluate whether using chemical restraint is appropriate for a particular patient, because it must be determined if the patient's resistance is due to their cognitive impairment or is a valid desire to refuse dental treatment.

If the patient's resistance or combativeness is a problem, then premedication should be used only if all other behaviour modification techniques have been tried. These can be hand-holding, distraction of the hands with soft squeezable toys or towels, reducing background noise and visual noise, or the presence of familiar people, either family or caretakers, in the dental surgery/operatory. For homebound or institutionalised persons, equipment and treatment at the site of habitat may be necessary. If sedatives are necessary, our preference has been short-acting second-generation benzodiazepines, such as lorezepam or oxazepam. The usual dosage we have used is 10–15 mg of oxazepam or 1–2 mg of lorezepam half an hour before treatment. If the patient is not treatable under these conditions and has significant needs, such as an abscessed tooth, then he will need to be hospitalised and treated under conscious sedation or general anaesthesia. This risk assessment requires extensive communication between the family, the dentist and the physician.

Premedication and antibiotics

There is a group of patients who have a need to be protected from bacteraemias induced by specific dental procedures, such as deep scaling or minor oral surgery. The dental procedures which require prophylaxis are shown in Table 29.3. These at-risk persons include brittle diabetics, immunosuppressant patients, persons at risk for infective endocarditis, and persons who have had a major joint replaced with an artificial substitute. It also includes persons with prosthetic cardiac valves, a previous history of bacterial endocarditis, most congenital cardiac malformations, rheumatic and other acquired valvular regurgitation. The degree of risk associated with these conditions is shown in Table 29.4. Persons who are receiving chemotherapeutic agents, immunosuppressive agents, radiation therapy or long-term steroid therapy usually have an increased susceptibility to infection and should also be given antibiotic coverage. A sometimes forgotten group are patients who have had arterial grafts to replace segments of large arteries which have developed an aneurysm. Because the material used for the graft is dacron, it may take up to a year for epithelisation of the graft. It seems appropriate to cover these patients at appropriate

Table 29.3 Stratification of dental procedures that can cause bacteraemia

Prophylaxis recommended	**Prophylaxis *not* recommended**
Dental extractions	Restorative dentistry with or without retraction cord
Periodontal procedures, including surgery, scaling and root planing, probing and recall maintenance	Local anaesthetic injections (non-intraligamentary)
Dental implant placement and reimplantation of avulsed teeth	Intracanal endodontic treatment; post-placement and build-up
Endodontic (root canal) instrumentation or surgery only beyond the apex	Placement of rubber dams
Subgingival placement of antibiotic fibres or strips	Post-operative suture removal
Initial placement of orthodontic bands but not brackets	Placement of removable prosthodontic or orthodontic appliances
Intraligamentary local anaesthetic injections	Taking of oral radiographs
Prophylactic cleaning of teeth or implants where bleeding is anticipated	Orthodontic appliance adjustment
	Shedding of primary teeth

Source: Modified from A. S. Dajani, K. A. Taubert, W. Wilson et al. (1997), 'Prevention of bacterial endocarditis: Recommendations by the American Heart Association. From the Committee on Rheumatic Fever, Endocarditis and Kawasaki Disease, Council on Cardiovascular Disease in the Young', *The Journal of the American Medical Association*, 277, pp. 1794–801.

times with antibiotics for at least up to 1 year after surgery. If complex dental procedures are planned where multiple appointments are required, it is advisable that at least 10 days be allowed to elapse between appointments to prevent resistant organisms from developing by too frequent exposures to antibiotics.

The universal need for prophylactic antibiotic coverage before dental treatment, in persons who have had a large joint replaced with an artificial substitute, has not been established. Nevertheless, in 1996, a working group drawn from orthopaedics and dentistry in the US recommended prophylaxis. Persons who have been identified as being in the high-risk group for late prosthetic joint infection (Box 29.1), and who must be covered with antibiotics, include insulin dependent diabetics, persons who have had a previous infection in the joint or have lost a previous prosthesis due to infection, those with a history of rheumatoid arthritis, and those who are taking steroids. A patient who has had a joint in place without incident for 2 years is no longer recommended for antibiotic prophylaxis. To reduce bacteraemias, the same protocol is used for the joint as we suggested for prevention of endocarditis.

Box 29.1 Persons at increased risk for blood borne joint infection

Use antibiotics for:

- first 2 years following joint placement
- insulin dependent (type 1) diabetes
- previous joint infection
- haemophilia
- chronic joint dislocation
- rheumatoid arthritis
- systemic lupus erythematosus
- immunosuppression (drugs or radiation)

Source: Modified from (1997), 'Antibiotic prophylaxis for dental patients with total joint replacements', American Dental Association; American Academy of Orthopaedic Surgeons, *The Journal of the American Dental Association*, 128, pp. 1004–8.

Table 29.4 Degree of risk for subacute bacterial endocarditis posed by various cardiac or vascular lesions

High degree of risk	High to moderate	Moderate	Low to negligible[b]
Prosthetic valves	Arteriovenous fistulae	MVP[a] w/regurgitation	Arteriosclerotic plaques
Previous infective endocarditis	Patent ductus arteriosus	tricuspid or pulmonary valve disease	Coronary sclerosis
Recent surgical repair of cardiac valve defect	Ventricular septal defect	Pure mitral stenosis	Small atrial septal defect
	Aortic valve disease	Idiopathic hypertrophic subaortic stenosis	Cardiac pacemaker
	IV catheter (ventriculo-jugular shunt)	Large atrial septal defect	Syphilitic aortitis
	Coarctation of aorta	Cardiomyopathy	Surgically corrected cardiovascular lesion with no prosthetic implant (greater than 6 months post-op.)
	Tetraology of Fallot	Surgically corrected cardiovascular lesion with synthetic prosthetic implant (> 6 months post-op.)	Previous rheumatic fever with no valve dysfunction Coronary artery bypass
	Marfan's syndrome		
	Mitral insufficiency		
	Asplenic patients		

(*a*) MVP = mitral valve prolapse.

(*b*) No premedication required.

Source: Modified from A. S. Dajani, K. A. Taubert, W. Wilson et al. (1997), 'Prevention of bacterial endocarditis: Recommendations by the American Heart Association', *The Journal of the American Dental Association*, 128, pp. 1142–51.

The prevention of medical emergencies in dental offices

In the US it has become accepted procedure for dentists who care for elderly patients to record their blood pressure and pulse at the initial appointment. If a patient reports a history of hypertension, even if it is controlled by medication, the blood pressure should be monitored and recorded prior to and at the end of every dental appointment. The suggested norm for older adults has been 160/95 mmHg. It has been suggested that patients whose blood pressure is higher than these norms be referred to a physician for evaluation. Also, if a patient is being treated for hypertension, it has been suggested that the dentist consult with the patient's physician to find out the level at which their blood pressure has been stabilised.

If a patient is on anticoagulants (e.g. warfarin) or high doses of aspirin (> 2400 mg/day), and if deep scaling or minor oral surgery is to be carried out, the patient's physician needs to be consulted. Patients on warfarin should have their prothrombin time measured as international normalised ratio (INR). The suggested convention is that for deep scaling of multiple teeth, or for multiple extractions, the INR should not be more than 2.5. If a single tooth is to be extracted which allows for local haemostatic measure to be taken, the patient can have an INR of up to 3.5. Patients on high doses of aspirin or dipyridamole, which affect platelet aggregation, should have their bleeding time evaluated. If there is to be a surgical intervention in patients receiving chemotherapy, they may also have a bleeding problem and should also be evaluated.

A person with a recent myocardial infarction or cerebrovascular accident should not receive elective dental treatment for at least 6 months afterwards. Some cardiologists are evaluating their post-myocardial infarction patients with a stress test 6–8 weeks after the initial episode. These physicians may authorise elective dental treatment earlier than the usual 6 month time limit. However, if a dentist needs to treat such a patient earlier than the recommended time, the dentist must seek a consultation with the patient's cardiologist before commencing treatment. Patients who have coronary bypass surgery do not need prophylactic antibiotic coverage prior to dental care, having survived the immediate post-operative period of 2–3 weeks.

It has been reported that dental office equipment such as pulp testers, electrodesensitising, electrosurgery equipment, ultrasonic scaling devices or cleaner, and occasionally motorised dental chairs may be potential sources of electromagnetic interference. This electromagnetic force may adversely affect the functioning of certain types of cardiac pacemakers, although the newer versions seem to be less sensitive to electromagnetic interference. In a pilot study Foud et al. (1990) found that a pulp tester, a standard ultrasonic scaler, a piezoelectric ultrasonic scaler and an instrument for electrodental-anaesthesia did not interfere with pacemaker function in five patients using pacemakers.

The adrenal cortex of most normal adults secretes about 15–30 mg of hydrocortisone per day and increases in response to stress. Exogenous cortisone will cause a diminished ability of the adrenals to respond to stress such as pain or infection. The amount of suppression depends on the dosage, the duration and the route of administration of the drug. Patients on long-term corticosteroid therapy may need to have their steroid dosage increased for the day of the dental appointment and for the day following. The protocol, which has been suggested, is that any patient who has been on 5–15 mg/day of prednisolone or its equivalent in another corticosteroid continuously, for 3 weeks or more in the previous year, may require supplemental steroid for the duration of significant systematic stress. Consultation with the patient's physician may be required.

Care of functionally dependent older adults

Most patients who are homebound or in long-term care facilities (LTC) have multiple health problems that require the co-operation of many different types of providers. Dentists have a specific role in this process because they can improve the quality of life for the elderly by keeping them free of oral infection, by restoring their dentition so they can enjoy eating, and also by improving or restoring facial aesthetics.

Oral examinations

An effective oral health program within an LTC institution requires that a specific policy be developed. All residents should have a comprehensive oral examination as part of their admission evaluation. There is no reason why a physician cannot provide such an examination but, in fact, most physicians are not trained to evaluate the health of the oral soft tissues or to examine the individual teeth for the presence of caries and periodontal disease. Thus a comprehensive oral examination may be more appropriately carried out by a dentist. For individuals who are edentulous, yearly examination of the dentures and oral soft tissues should be adequate. For residents who have natural teeth, more frequent evaluations may be necessary, because most residents are at high risk of developing caries, especially root caries and periodontal problems. These oral examinations should also evaluate the oral tissues for malignant change, as described earlier.

Oral hygiene policy

The dentist or hygienist associated with an LTC institution should develop an individual oral hygiene plan for each resident. This plan should be part of the patient's record so that nursing staff are familiar with the resident's specific problems. It should also be reviewed at regular intervals and changed to accommodate the patient's current health and physical capabilities.

The nursing staff is primarily responsible for maintaining the oral health of the residents at an appropriate level. Often, due to lack of knowledge and training, or due to setting priorities and time constraints, daily oral hygiene is less than adequate. However, the consulting physician to an LTC should mandate that daily hygiene care for residents should include a thorough cleaning of teeth and all dental prostheses either by the resident or the staff.

An ultrasonic cleaner, a high frequency instrument that agitates and removes debris without damaging dentures, also can be used. This instrument is particularly useful in an institution where there are many residents with dentures. Each resident should have his or her own beaker, and enough tartar and stain remover should be poured into the beaker to cover the dentures. The dentures should be left for 5–10 minutes, then rinsed thoroughly under running tap water and brushed lightly with one of the following cleaning agents: dishwashing detergent, hand soap, baking soda or commercial denture cleanser. For residents with a remaining natural dentition, prevention requires that an adequate level of oral hygiene be maintained. For expediency in assessing potential oral problems and their treatability, individuals in institutions can be divided into three categories.

Category I

The category I group consists of residents who have sufficient neuromuscular skills and adequate vision and motivation to use a mechanical device (toothbrush or electric toothbrush) to clean their own teeth or dentures independently.

If a resident has had multiple sclerosis, a spinal cord injury, Parkinson's disease, severe arthritis or a cerebrovascular accident, he may be unable to control a toothbrush unless the size and weight of the brush handle can be increased. If a resident has limited arm movement at the shoulder, the length of the handle of a toothbrush can be increased. If a resident is wearing any kind of denture and has lost the use of one arm, independent cleaning of dentures is impossible. Suction cups attached to the base of a brush so that it can be fixed in position may help restore independence. In all these instances, once adequate oral hygiene levels have been attained, dental care becomes routine (see Figures 29.11(a) and (b)).

Category II

Residents in the category II group have poor or inadequate neuromuscular co-ordination and require daily assistance to maintain their oral hygiene at an acceptable level. If such a resident has a concerned or caring family member or reliable attendant to help with oral hygiene, dental care and treatment generally require no special considerations. However, the significant other or caregiver will need training in specific oral hygiene techniques applicable to that specific individual's needs.

Category III

The category III group consists of residents with poor or inadequate neuromuscular co-ordination who are unable to maintain their oral hygiene and who receive no regular help. The residents in this

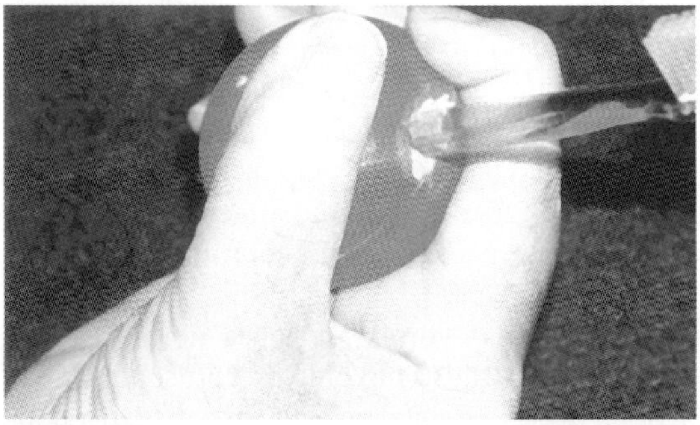

Figure 29.11(a) Toothbrush handle enlarged with a rubber ball for a patient with osteoarthritis of the fingers

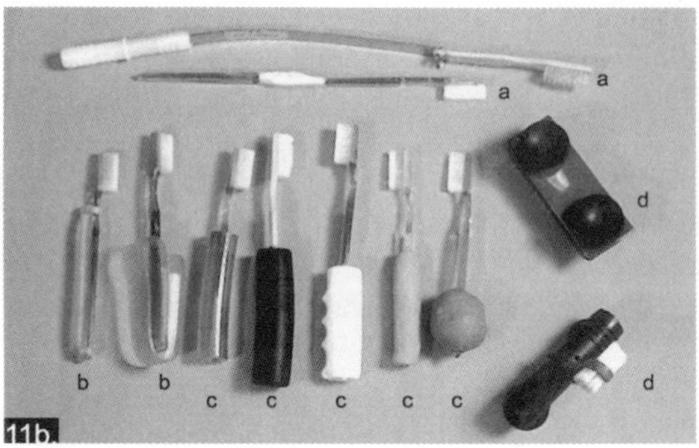

Figure 29.11(b) A variety of toothbrush handles are shown here:

- a how to elongate toothbrush handles for persons with limited arm movement
- b how to support toothbrushes for persons who cannot grip a brush
- c how to increase the size and weight of handles
- d how to add suction cups to the base of brushes so that they can be used in a washbasin full of water in order to allow a person who only has the use of one hand to clean dentures independently

group often have some congenital or acquired mental disabilities. Although with these residents it is easier to extract all teeth and place them on a soft diet, each individual should be assessed independently to evaluate the value of maintaining some sound teeth. Constructing complete dentures may not be possible for many of these residents. For selected individuals, an upper denture, if only to restore aesthetics, may be a great service.

Care of a prosthesis

Many residents within an LTC facility wear dentures. To wear a denture comfortably, the individual must:

1. have an adequate amount of bone left in the jaws to be able to support dentures
2. have healthy enough mucosal tissues to tolerate the low-grade trauma induced by the movements of every denture in function
3. have adequate oral neuromuscular skills to be able to control the denture.

Dentures should be removed during sleep when the lubricant saliva, whose production is diurnal, is reduced to practically zero. They also should fit adequately. Lower dentures in particular require good motor skills for successful use. When new dentures are made, an individual has to 'relearn' how to use them. Thus, patients with dementia, Parkinson's disease, or any other cognitive or neuromuscular disease will have difficulty adjusting and/or accommodating to new dentures. It is preferable in these situations to repair or reline the existing denture. It is important to avoid the loss of all natural teeth, especially on the lower arch, where a peripheral seal of the dentures is not possible and dentures are balanced between the muscles of the cheeks and lips and the tongue.

The loss of dentures is a constant hazard in an institution because residents may leave them on food trays or have them mixed up with laundry. The marking or identification of dentures becomes important not only because of replacement costs but also because many residents may not be able to accommodate new dentures. Unfortunately, the marking or identification of all oral prostheses with names or numbers is not compulsory. The most economical and effective method is to write the resident's name, initials or an identification number, using a marking pencil on a small area of the buccal flange that has been roughened with sand paper. The area can then be covered with two coats of clear nail varnish. The Identure (3M, St Paul, MN) denture marking system is a commercial version using a similar concept.

In-service training

It is necessary that the consulting physician of an LTC become knowledgeable about oral health care for institutionalised persons and be willing to help set oral health policies for the institution. Part of that oral health policy should be in-service training for the nurses and nurses aides on oral health care for residents and the recognition of potential oral problems. The consulting dentist or hygienist should be responsible for the content of the in-service programs. If such a program exists, the resident's quality of life and comfort will be greatly increased.

A physician or health care worker should be aware of certain conditions in a resident or patient (see Box 29.2).

In conclusion, if a physician or other health care worker sees any of these conditions, the resident/patient should receive an urgent dental/oral evaluation by a dentist.

Box 29.2 Signs and symptoms

General
- Orofacial pain
- Visible oral infection
- Difficulty chewing food
- Halitosis/dry/burning mouth
- Visible oral soft tissue lesions (white, red or ulcerated)

Tooth related
- Visible dental decay
- Loose or mobile teeth
- Bleeding or sore gums

Denture related
- Loose, ill-fitting or worn dentures
- Missing denture teeth
- Home repairs attempted

Bibliography and further reading

Arbes, S. J., Slade, G. D. & Beck, J. D. (1999), 'Association between extent of periodontal attachment loss and self-reported history of heart attack: An analysis of N Hanes III data', *Journal of Dental Research*, 78, pp. 1777–82.

Atkinson, J. C. & Wu, A. J. (1994), 'Salivary gland dysfunction: Causes, symptoms and treatment', *The Journal of the American Dental Association*, 125, pp. 409–16.

Banoczy, J. & Sugar, L. (1975), 'Progressive and regressive changes in Hungarian oral leukoplakias in the course of longitudinal studies', *Community Dentistry and Oral Epidemiology*, 3, pp. 194–7.

Bartlett, D. W., Evans, D. F. & Smith, B. G. N. (1996), 'The relationship between gastro-oesophageal reflux disease and dental erosion', *Journal of Oral Rehabilitation*, 23, pp. 289–97.

Beck, J. D. (1996), 'Periodontal implications: Older adults', *Annals of Peridontology*, 1, pp. 322–57.

Beck, J. D. & Offenbacher, S. (1998), 'Oral health and systemic disease: Periodontitis and cardiovascular disease', *Journal of Continuing Dental Education*, 62, pp. 859–70.

Bergman, J. D., Wright, F. A. C. & Hammond, R. H. (1991), 'The oral health of the elderly in Melbourne', *Australian Dental Journal*, 36, pp. 280–5.

Billings, R. J., Brown, L. R. & Kaster, A. G. (1985), 'Contemporary treatment strategies for root surface dental caries', *Gerodontics*, 1, pp. 20–7.

Dolan, T. A., Monopoli, M. P., Kaunich, J. & Rubenstein, L. Z. (1990), 'Geriatric grand rounds: Oral diseases in older adults', *Journal of the American Geriatics Society*, 38, pp. 1239–50.

Ettinger, R. L. (1992), 'Oral care for the homebound and institutionalized', *Clinics in Geriatric Medicine*, 8, pp. 659–72.

Ettinger, R. L. (1993a), 'Cohort differences among aging populations: A challenge for the dental profession', *Special Care in Dentistry*, 13, pp. 19–26.

Ettinger, R. L. (1993b), 'Management of elderly patients in the private practice system', *International Dental Journal*, 43, pp. 29–40.

Ettinger, R. L. (1996), 'Review: Xerostomia: A symptom which acts like a disease', *Age and Ageing*, 25, pp. 409–12.

Ettinger, R. L. & Hand, J. S. (1994), 'Factors influencing the future need for treatment of root surfaces', *American Journal of Dentistry*, 7, pp. 256–60.

Foud, A. F., Hobson, J. K., Martins, J. B. et al. (1990), 'Effects of electronic dental instruments on patients with cardiac pacemakers', *Journal of Endodontics*, 16, pp. 188–9 (abstr.).

Hand, J. S., Hunt, R. J. & Beck, J. D. (1988), 'Coronal and root caries in older Iowans: 36 month incidence', *Gerodontics*, 4, pp. 136–9.

Hand, J. S. & Whitehill, J. M. (1986), 'The prevalence of oral mucosal lesions in an elderly population', *The Journal of the American Dental Association*, 112, pp. 73–6.

Hurst, P. S. & Noblett, W. C. (1990), 'Geriatric dentistry', *Otolaryngologic Clinics of North America*, 23, pp. 1097–107.

Iacopino, A. M. & Wathen, W. F. (1992), 'Oral candidal infection and denture stomatitis: A comprehensive review', *The Journal of the American Dental Association*, 123, pp. 46–51.

Kinane, D. F. (1998), 'Periodontal disease's contributions to cardiovascular disease: An overview of potential mechanisms', *Annals of Periodontology*, 3, pp. 142–50.

Lewis, I. K., Hanlon, J. T., Hobbins, M. J. & Beck, J. D. (1993), 'Use of medications with potential oral adverse drug reactions in community-dwelling elderly', *Special Care in Dentistry*, 13, pp. 171–6.

Locker, D. (1992), 'The burden of oral disorders in a population of older adults', *Community Dental Health*, 9, pp. 109–24.

Moskona, D. & Kaplan, I. (1992), 'Oral lesions in elderly denture wearers', *Clinical Preventive Dentistry*, 14, pp. 11–14.

National Health Strategy (1992), 'Improve dental health in Australia', Background Paper No. 9, AGPS, Canberra.

Pindborg, J. J., Renstrup, G., Jolst, O. & Roed-Petersen, B. (1968), 'Studies in oral leukoplakia: A preliminary report on the period prevalence of malignant transformation in leukoplakia based on a follow-up study of 248 patients', *The Journal of the American Dental Association*, 76, pp. 767–71.

Ship, J. A. & Puckett, S. A. (1994), 'Longitudinal study on oral health in subjects with Alzheimer's disease', *Journal of the American Geriatrics Society*, 42, pp. 57–63.

Shuman, S. K. (1989), 'Ethics and the patient with dementia', *The Journal of the American Dental Association*, 119, pp. 747–8.

Shuman, S. K. (1990), 'A physician's guide to coordinating oral health and primary care', *Geriatrics*, 45, pp. 47–57.

Silverman, S., Gorsky, M. & Lozada, F. (1984), 'Oral leukoplakia and malignant transformation. A follow-up study of 257 patients', *Cancer*, 53, pp. 563–8.

Slade, G. D., Gansky, S. A. & Spencer, A. J. (1992), 'Two-year incidence of tooth loss among South Australians aged 60+ years', *Community Dentistry and Oral Epidemiology*, 25, pp. 429–37.

Slade, G. & Spencer, A. J. (1994), 'Social impact of oral conditions among older adults', *Australian Dental Journal*, 39, pp. 358–64.

Smith, R. G. & Burtner, A. P. (1994), 'Oral side-effects of the most frequently prescribed drugs', *Special Care in Dentistry*, 14, pp. 96–101.

Taylor, G. W., Burt, B. A., Becker, M. P. et al. (1996), 'Severe periodontitis and risk for poor glycemic control in patients with non-insulin dependent diabetes mellitus', *Journal of Peridontology*, 67, pp. 1085–93.

World Health Organization (1971), 'The economics of health and disease', *WHO Chronicle*, 25, pp. 20–4.

Xie, Q. & Ainamo, A. (1999), 'Association of edentulousness with systemic factors in elderly people living at home', *Community Dentistry and Oral Epidemiology*, 27, pp. 202–9.

Chapter 30

Assessment of nutritional status

IAN DARNTON-HILL, E. TERRY COYNE and MARK L. WAHLQVIST

Introduction

Health, nutrition and ageing

Many of the diseases acquired with age appear to have been preprogrammed many years previously. The hypothesis that the non-communicable, chronic diseases of adulthood, such as some heart diseases, hypertension and diabetes, are more likely to occur in people who were undernourished *in utero*, and possibly in infancy, is increasingly accepted. This is of course a good argument for ensuring adequate antenatal care and nutrition for expectant mothers, and especially in developing countries where the burden of both undernutrition and overnutrition is the most significant.

Attention to diet, exercise and health towards the end of the life cycle will improve the quality of life and lessen both the occurrence and the impact of diseases. Thus there are still benefits to maximising health behaviours. However, the earlier people adopt healthier lifestyles, the more likely they are to have relatively healthy and active lives in their later years.

Age-related changes in the elderly

Most physiological functions in the elderly are affected by the actual ageing process itself only to a minor extent. However, some functions do appear to decline progressively throughout adult life, such as mineralisation of the skeleton, host immunity and food intake in general. Most of these lead to a decrease in body weight due to their effect on systemic energy balance. Table 30.1 summarises age-related changes in body composition and physiological functions and the resulting impact on requirements for certain nutrients. Changes in body composition occur throughout adult life and can lead to a continuous decline in lean body mass, which tends to accelerate later in life and is greater in males. In addition to loss of active tissue mass, there is some reduction of function in many organs and tissues: for example, cellular enzymes for men fall on average by 15% over the 50 years to age 80; resting cardiac output by 30% and renal blood flow by 50%. However, even the magnitude of these changes is likely to be a result of reduced exercise and diet in later years as much as the inevitable effects of ageing in itself.

Table 30.1 Age-related changes that impact on nutritional needs

Change in body composition or physiological function	Impact on nutrient requirement
⇓ Muscle mass (sarcopenia)	⇓ Need for energy
⇓ Taste and olfactory acuity	⇑ Need for energy
⇓ Bone density (osteopenia)	⇑ Need for calcium, vitamin D
⇓ Gastric acid (atrophic gastritis)	⇑ Need for vitamin B_{12}, folic acid, calcium, iron, zinc
⇓ Skin capacity for cholecalciferol synthesis	⇑ Need for vitamin D
⇓ Calcium bioavailability	⇑ Need for calcium, vitamin D
⇓ Hepatic uptake of retinol	⇓ Need for vitamin A
⇓ Efficiency in metabolic utilisation of pyridoxal	⇑ Need for vitamin B_6
⇓ Immune function	⇑ Need for vitamin B_6
⇑ Oxidative stress status	⇑ Need for carotenoids, vitamin C, vitamin E and food polyphenolics
⇑ Levels of homocysteine	⇑ Need for folate, vitamin B_6, vitamin B_{12}

Source: Adapted from National Health and Medical Research Council (1999), *Dietary Guidelines for Older Australians*, Australian Government Printing Service, Canberra.

As the above metabolic functions progressively alter with ageing, nutrient needs change (Table 30.1). The rate of synthesis and breakdown of protein, expressed as per kilogram body weight, is significantly lower in older people of both sexes. Total body protein synthesis, body mass and bone mineralisation decreases, while the proportion of body fat increases. Tissue avidity for some nutrients (e.g. folate, zinc) appears to be reduced by ageing, and nutrient uptake may decrease. The relationship between physical activity, satiety and nutritional status is complex. A diminished ability to regulate food intake is an important subtle change that may affect dietary intake and hence nutritional status.

Immunological function is depressed by both ageing and by malnutrition, although the actual relationship is unclear and differs from one individual to the next. Although 25% of older individuals have immune responses as vigorous as those of young adults, elderly patients can develop deficiencies in host defences that may predispose to infections such as infectious diarrhoea. Nevertheless, the above changes can be relatively easily managed, and with small behavioural changes, older individuals can be healthy, and demonstrate adequate nutritional status.

Factors which influence nutritional status of the elderly

Specific risk factors can help identify elderly individuals who are especially likely to be malnourished or suffer other nutritional concerns. The factors leading to poor nutritional status can be broadly categorised as (Box 30.1):

1. social, such as inadequate dietary intake, isolation and poverty
2. physical/medical, including physiological reduction in utilisation of nutrients and reduced absorption, disease states, as well as difficulties with eating and dental problems
3. psychological and emotional factors, including depression, Alzheimer's disease and anorexia.

1. Social factors

Social isolation and poverty are major contributors to poor quantity and quality of food intake. Persons living alone and living in poverty may have limited access to food shopping and to transportation, limiting, among other things, their ability to attend meal programs. They may also lack adequate food preparation skills and food storage facilities. For the elderly living in the community, the degree of dependence is important. The more dependent the elderly are on being fed by others, the greater the risk of malnutrition. Living alone is related to decreased food intake among men, but not among women, and this has been reported in Australian, US and other studies. At all ages, people tend to eat more when eating with others.

Box 30.1 Major risk factors for nutritional conditions among the elderly

Social factors

- Poverty
- Isolation (living alone)
- Poor nutrition, food preparation or food safety knowledge
- Institutional factors
- Abuse of the elderly

Physical/medical factors

- Feeding or swallowing difficulties
- Poor dentition
- Diminished sense of smell or taste or xerostomia
- Dysphagia
- Drugs
- Malabsorption
- Increased metabolism
- Chronic disease or chronic infection
- Need assistance with feeding
- Need assistance with food shopping and meal preparation
- Severe visual deficit
- Physical disabilities/impaired basic activities of daily living

Psychological and emotional factors

- Widowed
- Depression
- Loneliness
- Dementia
- Alcoholism
- Eating disorders or diet phobias: choking, fat, salt, etc.
- Anorexia

Source: Adapted from J. E. Morley (1997), 'Anorexia of aging: Physiologic and pathologic', *The American Journal of Clinical Nutrition*, 66, pp. 760–73.

Dietetic assessment is needed to review appropriate choice and consistency of food to allow easier eating (although the latter is not an important issue with the majority of the elderly). Availability of fresh foods, sufficient variety, appropriate cooking and the attractive presentation of food are all factors which promote nutritious diets. Particularly for some older men living alone, knowledge of diet and food preparation may be important. Other aspects of diet that need to be assessed are food contamination or improper food handling, especially for those living alone and preparing food under less than ideal conditions, which may lead to infectious diarrhoea and which especially in the elderly lead to malnutrition.

2. Physical/medical factors

Most physiological functions in the elderly are affected by the ageing process per se only to a minor extent. However, there is a wide variation in the correlation between chronological and physiological ages among different persons. Underprivileged individuals often appear much older than their years, this variation being due more to socioeconomic conditions than to physiological processes. Physiologic changes that affect nutritional status and are directly associated with ageing are summarised in Table 30.1.

The decrease in energy intake common in elderly persons reflects, among other factors, a decline in basal metabolic rate, which is essentially due to a decrease in lean body mass. Some recent studies suggest that the early satiety in older persons may be caused by a nitric oxide deficiency, which decreases the adaptive relaxation of the fundus of the stomach in response to food. It has been observed that older men have a substantial reduction in their ability to maintain a constant energy balance compared with younger men and that age-related changes in food intake are observed in healthy older men and women, even when they do not report any problem with appetite. This may be due to diminished metabolic signals that drive adaptive variations in energy intake. A decrease in taste acuity and olfaction, as well as a variety of oral health problems, contribute to a declining energy intake in some elderly people.

Decreased energy intake may also accompany a decline in physical activity, which is sometimes a result of disabilities that limit movement. Usually, however, there are social and psychological factors that are responsible for loss of weight that accompanies the declining energy intake, and these are often amenable to modification.

The function of the gastrointestinal tract is essentially well preserved in ageing. One major change is in gastric function due to the prevalence of atrophic gastritis (20–50%) in elderly people. Atrophic gastritis causes a decrease in acid and intrinsic factor secretion and can cause vitamin B_{12} deficiency. Decreased gastric function is also associated with decreased absorption of folate, iron and zinc and reduced calcium bioavailability. The most important causal factor in the development of atrophic gastritis and ulcers is infection with *Helicobacter pylori*. If *H. pylori* infection is controlled, the prevalence of atrophic gastritis can be reduced.

Vitamin D deficiency is common in the elderly as sun exposure may decrease with age, especially in institutionalised or home-bound individuals, and there is a decreased ability of the ageing skin to convert 7-dehydrocholesterol to vitamin D_3. A reduction in kidney function can be responsible for a decrease in active vitamin D and thus reduced calcium absorption. There is also a reduced ability to secrete insulin in response to glucose challenges.

Eating and swallowing problems may occur at any age, but especially with ageing. The prevalence of eating disorders in nursing home residents may be as high as 50%, and are likely to be due to both physical and psychological factors. Common oral health problems that affect food intake in the elderly are summarised in Table 30.2. The lubricatory factors in saliva that soften and bind food material may decline with age. Saliva also affects taste, dissolving the parts of foods that taste and bringing them in contact with taste buds. The result of decreased olfactory and taste sensitivity often leads to decreased appetite, aggravated by any problems with the gums, teeth or dentures, particularly those that cause pain. The orofacial musculature atrophies with ageing, resulting in decreased biting force, slower chewing and denture problems.

Inflammation or burning of the tongue is often a complaint of elderly patients and may be secondary to nutritional diseases such as anaemia, or due to drug reactions, systemic infections or psychosomatic syndromes. Infections of the mucous membranes of the oral cavity, including burning mouth syndrome, candidiasis, contact stomatitis or ulcers can all cause pain and decrease the pleasure of eating. Dysphagia, which is most common in older adults, is often secondary to other conditions such as stroke, cancer, multiple sclerosis, parkinsonism and brain/spinal cord injuries.

Table 30.2 Oral health problems that affect the eating process

Oral function	**Problem**
Salivary glands	Reduction in secretion
Teeth	Attrition Dental caries Tooth hypersensitivity Tooth loss
Periodontium	Gingivitis Periodontitis
Alveolar bone	Bone loss/resorption
Temporomandibular joint (TMJ)	Dysfunction
Orofacial musculature	Atrophy
Tongue	Glossitis Glossodynia
Mucous membranes	Atrophy Burning mouth syndrome Candidiasis Contact stomatitis Oral cancer Traumatic ulcers
Dentures	Poor hygiene Stomatitis Ulceration Wearing

Source: Adapted from W. E. Martin (1995), 'The oral cavity and nutrition', in J. E. Morley, Z. Glick & L. Z. Rubenstein (eds), *Geriatric Nutrition: A Comprehensive Review*, 2nd edn, Raven Press, New York.

Some disease states can in themselves markedly affect nutritional status and these include wasting disorders such as cachexia, chronic obstructive pulmonary disease (COPD) and neoplastic disease. Attention to nutrition and diet in the management of these diseases will improve quality of life and may help slow the progression of the disease.

A further important cause of malnutrition in the elderly is the use of pharmaceuticals. A thorough history of current drug use, both prescribed and over-the-counter, is an important part of initial patient analysis and care. Hypertensive drugs adversely influence potassium and magnesium status, antibiotics affect intestinal absorption and hypnotics affect nutritional intake. More specifically, medication can produce:

- anorexia (e.g. digoxin, fluoxetine, hydralazine, psychotropics, quinidine, vitamin A)
- nausea (e.g. antibiotics, aspirin, theophylline)
- increased energy metabolism (e.g. theophylline, thyroxine)
- malabsorption (see below).

Withdrawal from certain drugs (e.g. alcohol, anxiolytics and psychotropics) may also be associated with weight loss.

3. Psychological and emotional factors

Psychological factors, such as recent loss of a spouse, depression, dementia, alcoholism and anorexia nervosa, have considerable impact on nutritional status in the aged. Bereavement, which is more common in women, is often associated with loss of interest in eating due to the loss of socialisation at meal times. It is estimated that approximately 5–10% of elderly persons living in the community suffer some form of depression. In elderly persons with depression, approximately 90% suffer weight loss, compared with 60% of young adults with depression. A common symptom of depression is a loss of desire to eat. Widowed, elderly men who live alone without a good support system are at risk of alcohol abuse, which in later life is often associated with weight loss, squalor syndrome and depression.

Persons with dementia or Alzheimer's disease are particularly at risk of malnutrition as they may forget to eat, make poor food choices, or become too disabled to be able to purchase or prepare food. Some patients with Alzheimer's disease develop constant wandering that may increase energy needs. Anorexia nervosa has been reported in older persons who were previously weight restrictors, and can lead to inadequate dietary intake, even in the face of normal energy requirements.

At all ages, the healthiest diet is one with enough variety to provide adequate micronutrients, and the appropriate amounts of energy, protein, carbohydrate and essential fatty acids (both omega-3 and omega-6). Although our knowledge of the exact requirements is imperfect, the approximate quantities are known, and there is some flexibility because of the range of the recommended intakes, and because of individual variation. The limited variety of foods in many geriatric diets has been identified as a factor in reduced nutrient intake.

Malnutrition

The term 'malnutrition' covers the three main areas of concern in the nutrition of elderly people: undernutrition, overnutrition and eating disorders. Although the last does appear to be of more significance in the older age group than usually thought (and should therefore be routinely sought out), only the first two will be considered in detail.

Undernutrition

Protein-energy malnutrition

While malnutrition in the elderly has often been described in the hospitalised and institutionalised elderly and those living in poor social circumstances, data on free-living, active elderly individuals has been less available. A recent study from Germany identified minimal changes in this population. However, a study in the US of institutionalised but ambulatory elderly patients concluded that malnutrition, both with and without accompanying disease, is relatively frequent, although a specific nutritional diagnosis is not made in many cases. While as many as 30–50% of institutionalised patients reportedly suffer from protein-energy malnutrition, even in non-institutionalised elderly individuals, significant unexplained weight loss becomes increasingly common after 65 years of age.

As noted previously, with advancing age there is generally a progressive decrease in energy intake as well as probably energy requirements. One study showed a progressive decrease in average daily intake from 11 300 kJ (2700 kcal) at 20–34 years to 8800 kJ (2100 kcal) at 75–90 years. One-third of this fall (840 kJ or 200 kcal) was accounted for by the reduction in basal energy metabolism consequent to reduced body cell mass, while the remaining 1680 kJ or 400 kcal were identified as the result of reduced activity. The sharp decline in the energy intake of the very old is often related to disability and chronic disease.

In most diets, as energy intakes fall, there is a very strong likelihood that the intake of other nutrients will also decrease. Protein inadequacy is frequently found in the diets of the elderly and contributes to increased susceptibility to infection. In the elderly, protein and energy status can go in opposite directions (unlike in young children). Box 30.1 lists the underlying causes of protein-energy malnutrition in the elderly.

Assessment/diagnosis

No screening battery has been shown to have both good sensitivity and specificity for identifying persons at risk for undernutrition. Weight loss remains the single best factor for predicting persons at risk for malnutrition. A body mass index (BMI): weight/height^2 of less than 20 kg/m^2 may suggest a problem. Mid-arm circumference or arm muscle circumference (which corrects for triceps skinfold thickness) can be useful in following muscle mass changes in persons with a fluid retention problem, whereas skin-fold thickness measurements have little diagnostic value in the elderly. In isolated communities, assessment can be done without biochemical tests and a manual has recently been published (by the London School of Hygiene and Tropical Medicine and HelpAge International) to this end.

However, in the absence of obvious malnutrition or obesity, in most cases a small battery of tests, such as a self-administered history (see Box 30.4), biochemical tests (see Table 30.4) and a simple combination of both (e.g. the SCALES protocol in Table 30.3) will be helpful. A simple check list may also help to ensure that nutritional status and undernutrition is actively considered in the analysis of every geriatric patient (Box 30.2).

In persons with wasting, serum albumin and haemoglobin levels, total iron-binding capacity, and tests of cell mediated immune function are usually normal. When hypoalbuminaemic protein-energy malnutrition occurs, anergy (failure to respond to common antigens) and oedema are often present. Serum albumin levels are generally < 35 g/L, and anaemia, lymphocytopenia and hypotransferrinaemia (as evidenced by a total iron-binding capacity < 45 mol/L) are likely. Albumin, which has a 21 day half-life, is a good measure of protein status. Healthy, ambulatory elderly people should have a serum albumin level > 40 g/L, while albumin levels < 32 g/L in hospitalised geriatric patients are highly predictive of subsequent mortality. Cholesterol levels < 4.0 mmol/L in residents of nursing homes have been reported to predict mortality, presumably because such levels reflect malnutrition (although acute disease associated with cytokine release can also lower cholesterol levels).

Table 30.3 'SCALES' protocol for evaluating risk of malnutrition in the elderly

Item evaluated	Assign 1 point	Assign 2 points
Sadness		
Yesavage Geriatric Depression Scale[a]	10–14	≥ 15
Clinical impression[b]	Moderate	Severe
Cholesterol level	< 4 mmol/L	
Albumin level	3.5–4g/dL	< 3.5g/dL
Loss of weight	1 kg (or 0.5 cm mid-arm circ.) in 1 month	3 kg (or 1 cm) in 6 months
Eating problems	Patient needs assistance	
Shopping and food preparation problems	Patient needs assistance	

(*a*) Yesavage, J.A., (1988), 'Geriatric depression scale', *Psychopharmacology Bulletin*, 24, p. 709.
(*b*) Has not been validated.
Note: A total score ≥ 3 indicates that the patient is at risk, and needs further assessment.
Source: The Merck Manual of Geriatrics, 2, Nutrition, 1999 (modified from J. E. Morley & D. K. Miller (1992), 'Malnutrition in the elderly', *Hospital Practice*, 27, pp. 95–116).

Box 30.2 History and quick check list

1. Weight change
   Current height ___________cm Weight ______________kg
   BMI ___________ $\frac{\text{wt (kg)}}{\text{ht (m)}^2}$
   Overall weight loss or weight gain in past 6 months _____________

2. Dietary intake change (relative to usual intake) or no change
   Type of change:
   - Suboptimal solid food
   - Hypocaloric liquids
   - Starvation
   - Supplement vitamin, mineral, energy

3. Gastrointestinal symptoms that persisted for more than 2 weeks
   None
   Nausea
   Vomiting
   Diarrhoea
   Pain at rest only on eating

4. Functional capacity
   No dysfunction
   Dysfunction Duration _______________days
   Type:
   - Working suboptimally
   - Ambulatory but not working
   - Bedridden

5. Disease and its relation to nutritional requirements
   Primary diagnosis __________________________
   Metabolic demand (stress)
   - No stress
   - Moderate stress
   - High stress (burns, sepsis, severe trauma)

6. Physical status
   Loss of subcutaneous fat
   - Muscle wasting
   - Oedema
   - Ascites
   - Mucosal lesions
   - Cutaneous/hair changes

Source: Adapted from K. N. Jeejeebhoy (1998), 'Nutritional assessment', *Gastroenterology Clinics of North America*, 27, pp. 347–69.

Treatment

The intensity of intervention clearly depends on the severity of the malnutrition and the cause. It may require no more than correcting the social isolation of the person by putting him in touch with a local support group through a social worker. With moderate malnutrition, a dietitian should analyse the diet and feeding patterns in detail and guide the nutritional intervention. In severe cases, aggressive intervention is required but would generally be in a hospital setting.

Some evidence indicates that the mortality rate for all hospitalised elderly patients would decrease if energy (kilojoule) supplements were given (e.g. hip fracture patients recovering; or in short-term tube-feeding patients when their serum albumin level drops below 30 g/L). Total parenteral nutrition should be reserved for severely undernourished persons (serum albumin < 20 g/L), and for those who cannot tolerate enteral feeding. The use of specific types of nutrient supplements has little scientific basis. In most cases, the choice of supplement should be based on the patient's preference. For tube feeding it should be the most cost effective.

When a malnourished elderly person is fed, food may induce side effects, including electrolyte abnormalities, hyperglycaemia and aspiration pneumonia, and can sometimes cause a significant drop in blood pressure, which can be associated with falls. Nevertheless, active food supplementation can save lives and is an important intervention. Identifying poor dietary habits or physical and social impediments is the most important first step in treatment. Correcting or modifying these is the next step.

Micronutrients

As indicated, many people eat less as they get older due to a combination of decreased activity and decreased lean body mass and decreased basal metabolic rate (BMR). The reduced food and energy consumption increases the risk of inadequate intake of micronutrients. If aggravated by disease, medications and economic, psychological and physical problems, the intake may be even lower. Tissue uptake of some nutrients (e.g. zinc) is reduced by ageing. Micronutrients identified as being particularly at risk include iron, thiamine, riboflavin and nicotinic acid. The most common deficiency in the elderly in both developing and industrialised countries is iron, important in resistance to infection and cognition.

Vitamin deficiencies

Vitamin deficiencies are common in institutionalised older persons. The deficiencies most commonly seen include riboflavin (B_2) and pyridoxine (B_6). There is no evidence that the absorption of B vitamins, other than folate, is affected by ageing. There is evidence of a decrease in the utilisation of polyglutamate forms of folacin from foods, although synthetic folic acid is well absorbed at all ages. Signs of vitamin B_2 deficiency include cheilosis, glossitis, angular stomatitis, seborrhoeic dermatitis and a magenta tongue. Evidence of vitamin B_6 deficiency include the sideroblastic anaemias. Thiamine deficiency occurs mainly in industrialised countries in people who have consumed excessive amounts of alcohol over a long period of time, often while consuming inadequate diets. The resulting Wernicke-Korsakoff syndrome, of which Australia has one of the highest prevalences in the world, is now seen more commonly in developing or transitional economies, as is niacin deficiency. Niacin deficiency can also occur in either patients receiving isoniazid or patients with the carcinoid syndrome. Characteristically the patient develops pellagra, comprising dermatitis (on areas exposed to the sun), dementia and diarrhoea.

Vitamin B_{12} deficiency can lead to dementia, megaloblastic anaemia, incontinence, orthostatic hypotension or posterior column disease (leading to loss of position and vibration sense). Up to 5% of persons over 80 years have vitamin B_{12} deficiency. The most common cause is pernicious anaemia, caused by a lack of intrinsic factor.

Vitamin C deficiency can be associated with increased bruising, poor wound healing and the development of pressure sores. It should be remembered that taking vitamin C at any dose can result in false-negative faecal and urinary occult blood tests. Ingesting megadoses can interfere with serum and urine glucose tests and may result in oxalate kidney stones, increased serum salicylate levels and rebound scurvy (bleeding after withdrawal). A British study reported that low intakes of vitamin

C in elderly men and low serum pyridoxine levels in elderly women were predictive of early mortality.

Mineral deficiencies

There is relatively little information on the non-institutionalised ambulatory population, although iron is consistently reported to be the micronutrient most at risk. Iron deficiency leads to tiredness, feelings of reduced 'energy', reduced productivity and a decrease in immune function.

Zinc deficiency occurs in institutionalised, closed in and ambulatory elderly persons. Zinc is lost in the urine of patients with diabetes, cirrhosis and alcoholism and in those using a diuretic, and can be associated with poor wound healing, impaired immune function, night blindness and hypogonadism. High doses of zinc have been reported to slow the progress of age-related macular degeneration. However, the taking of high doses is not recommended until further research has been done, partly due to caution being required to avoid secondary copper deficiency. Other food components, such as the carotenoids (pro-vitamin A), lutein and zeaxanthin, may be relevant to macular degeneration, although there are currently no clinical recommendations regarding these.

Antihypertensive drugs can influence potassium and magnesium status. The clinical picture of magnesium deficiency is often coloured by superimposed hypocalcaemia and/or hypokalaemia. This can be aggravated by a poor intake of potassium and magnesium due to anorexia and loop diuretics causing urinary magnesium loss. Magnesium depletion can be the result of severe diarrhoea, as is the case for potassium. Faecal magnesium excretion is related to the total water content of the stool. Much less commonly, selenium deficiency reportedly occurs in patients receiving long-term tube feeding and causes muscle weakness and pain. Copper deficiency is associated with anaemia and possibly mild glucose intolerance.

Other important nutrient and non-nutrient components in foods

Phytochemical deficiencies

Given the current interest in antioxidants and ageing, it is worth remembering that only a few of the food antioxidants available to humans are necessarily vitamins or minerals. Those that are vitamins or minerals are usually acting in metalloenzymes, such as glutathione peroxidase and superoxide dismutase. It is therefore a consideration that older people taking an inadequate diet may not be obtaining the antioxidants that would be beneficial. Phytochemicals, like the phytoestrogens, are usually multifunctional compounds with important health implications for older people, particularly their immune systems, and possibly have antimutagenic and anti-angiogenic properties. There is now good evidence that some sensory disorders characteristic of the elderly, such as maculopathy, can be ameliorated by the ingestion of carotenoids.

Essential fatty acids

In the aged, it is important to ensure adequate amounts of both omega-3 and omega-6 essential fatty acids are consumed because of their effects as anti-inflammatory and immunomodulatory nutrients; and in relation to central nervous functions they have a beneficial effect on mood and cognitive function. There is some evidence that omega-3 fatty acid deficiency can contribute to depression in some individuals and that exercise can alleviate the depressed mood.

Biochemical assessment

The biochemical tests useful in assessing nutritional status are shown in Table 30.4. It is rarely necessary to do an extensive assessment of the biochemical status of the micronutrients (or the other food components mentioned). Generally any treatment, apart from purely iron/folate interventions, is likely to be a multimicronutrient supplement. Thus precise baseline knowledge is not necessary, except where there are clinical signs or some aspect of the dietary history that might point to a particular problem. Exceptions would be iron, folate, vitamin B_{12} and occasionally vitamin B_6.

Iron deficiency, being the most commonly recognised deficiency, should be tested for routinely. In the aged, iron deficiency anaemia is more commonly due to blood loss—notably large bowel disease (haemorrhoids, diverticular disease, tumour or angiodysplasia)—and therefore requires active

Table 30.4 Biochemical tests used to assess nutritional status

Test	Nutritional problem	Normal range[(a)]	Levels considered to be high risk or require further investigation
Indicators of undernutrition or nutritional deficiencies			
Haemoglobin (g/L)	Anaemia	120–140	< 120 in males < 115 in females
Lymphocytopenia (× 10^9/L)	Weight loss/PEM[(b)]	1.0–4.0	< 1.0
Serum iron (μmol/L)	Anaemia/iron deficiency	11–32	< 11
Serum ferritin (μg/L)	Anaemia/iron deficiency	18–30	< 20
Plasma zinc (μmol/L)	Poor wound healing	11.5–18.6	< 12
Total iron-binding capacity (μmol/L)	Weight loss/PEM	45–82	< 45
Vitamin B_{12} (pmol/L)	Anaemia ('pernicious')	220–660	< 200
Red cell folate (nmol/L)	Anaemia, elevated homocysteine	450–1300	< 360
Plasma vitamin B_6 (μmol/L) (P5'P[(c)] nmol/L)	Sideroblastic anaemia	> 20 (> 30)	< 10 (< 20)
Serum albumin (g/L)	Weight loss/PEM	> 40	< 35
Serum cholesterol (mmol/L)	Weight loss/PEM	4.0–5.2	< 4.0
Indicators of overnutrition			
Homocysteine (μmol/L)	Risk factor for vascular disease	5–15	> 15
Fasting blood glucose (mmol/L)	Risk factor for diabetes mellitus	2.5–5.8	> 6.0
Serum cholesterol (total) (mmol/L)	Risk factor for heart disease	< 5.2	> 5.5
Serum high-density lipoprotein cholesterol (mmol/L)	Risk factor for heart disease	> 1.2	< 1.0

(*a*) Normal ranges can vary according to laboratory method, gender, age, etc.
(*b*) PEM = Protein-energy malnutrition.
(*c*) P5'P = is pyridoxal 5 phosphate.

investigation and not simply supplementation. As a first step, anaemia needs to be detected by measuring haemoglobin levels. In addition to measuring haemoglobin, in microcytic anaemia, measures of actual iron stores such as ferritin and serum iron should be tested to clarify the cause of low haemoglobin levels. Ferritin levels are affected by concomitant infection.

The presence of macrocytosis warrants the measurement of folate and B_{12} concentrations. The diagnosis of vitamin B_{12} deficiency is made by documenting a serum level < 200 pmol/L. However, 25% of persons with levels 200–300 pmol/L are also deficient, as demonstrated by elevated methylmalonic acid and homocysteine levels in the urine. These levels should be tested in those suspected clinically of having vitamin B_{12} deficiency. The Schilling test is not useful in diagnosing pernicious anaemia.

If there is apparent clinical evidence of other trace elements (which will be rare) then the clinical suspicion needs to be confirmed. Zinc is also likely to be a problem but the difficulties in measuring this trace element complicate the diagnosis; however, levels below 12 μmol/L are usually considered to indicate risk.

Elevated homocysteine

A wealth of epidemiological data now suggests that an increase in the serum homocysteine level is an important independent risk factor for vascular disease—specifically of the coronary arteries, cerebrovascular disease and peripheral vascular disease. A recent meta-analysis study estimated that 10% of coronary artery disease in the general population is associated with an elevation in homocysteine. High levels of homocysteine have been shown to be associated with decreased levels of folate, vitamin B_6 and vitamin B_{12}, and supplementation with these vitamins has resulted in decreased homocysteine levels. It is still unclear, however, whether interventions with these nutrients are effective in decreasing the risk of vascular disease. To date, only one randomised controlled clinical trial has shown a decrease in vascular disease outcome.

Evidence is now emerging that suggests that there may also be a link between elevated homocysteine levels, low levels of folate, vitamin B_{12} and Alzheimer's disease. The ranges for normal total homocysteine levels are shown in Table 30.4.

Treatment

Generally, treatment (excluding with vitamin B_{12}) and certainly prevention include increasing the dietary variety or introducing a multimicronutrient formulation. Any such supplement should include adequate levels of zinc (10–15 mg/day) and folate. Although vitamin deficiencies are common in institutionalised older persons, especially those having any degree of protein-energy malnutrition, most vitamin replacement studies have failed to show any major benefits, except for a decreased hip fracture rate with vitamin D replacement. Nevertheless, non-institutionalised persons in Newfoundland who took daily vitamin and mineral supplements had improved immune function compared to a control group. As with undernutrition in general, one needs to examine the elderly patient's socio-economic circumstances and diet, and modify these as appropriate. Concomitant disease that may be affecting absorption or utilisation of micronutrients, including side effects of prescribed drugs, should be excluded as possible causes, and corrected accordingly.

The elderly patient showing nutritional vulnerability should be given a multimicronutrient supplement that covers 100% of the recommended dietary intake (RDI) of the most common vitamins and minerals. As the dietary, non-nutrient constituents of food have other beneficial qualities (e.g. fibre, protection against some cancers, etc.) an aggressive attempt to improve the variety and quality of the diet should also be made. Given the relatively recent recognition of the phytochemicals and fatty acids, attention to improving dietary quality has become even more important.

Older persons who develop gastric achlorhydria may be able to absorb vitamin B_{12} that is not bound to food. Although oral vitamin B_{12} has been used to treat this deficiency, it is recommended that vitamin B_{12} 1000 μg be given intramuscularly (IM) monthly.

Increasing evidence indicates that free radical damage may play a role in the pathogenesis of many diseases in older persons, including atherosclerosis, cancer, arthritis and Parkinson's disease. This has re-opened the question of the pharmacological use of free radical scavengers (vitamins and minerals) to prevent a diverse group of degenerative diseases. However, there is presently inadequate information or scientific evidence to make recommendations, and pharmacological doses are not currently recommended for the elderly.

Overnutrition/obesity

Overweight and obesity in older adults appear to result from a decrease in physical activity, a decline in growth hormone, and for women, the loss of oestrogens. The major cause of overweight in the elderly, however, is an energy intake which exceeds energy output. Less common disorders, such as hypothyroidism, Cushing's syndrome and tumours of the ventromedial hypothalamus, should be excluded.

Obesity has been clearly associated in both the young and the elderly with a myriad of morbid conditions such as decreased longevity, coronary artery disease, hypertension, type II diabetes ('mature onset'), certain types of cancers, sleep apnoea, osteoarthritis, gall bladder disease, gout and poor wound healing and bed sores.

Assessment/diagnosis (WHO criteria)

The ranges of body mass index (BMI) classify underweight, overweight and obesity in most adults. These ranges indicate the higher risk of type II diabetes, hypertension and cardiovascular disease associated with higher BMI ranges, particularly when accompanied by increased waist circumference. However, with increasing age these ranges are less certain. Several large studies have shown that above the age of 74 years, higher body weight may be protective. A BMI range of 22–26 is acceptable for older Australians. It is generally agreed that for the obese elderly person, a reduction in BMI to 30 or below affords the healthiest long-term option. In terms of survival, older people can tolerate higher BMIs than their younger counterparts. However, quality of life in terms of movement, independence and proneness to chronic non-communicable disease is affected by total and abdominal obesity, and therefore requires some prevention, monitoring and management.

It is important to measure height as accurately as possible. Because loss of height in the elderly is commonly due to bone loss, stooped posture, etc., using 'usual height' to assess BMI will not be accurate. If height measurement in an upright position cannot be performed, there are several other alternatives: total arm span, half-arm span and mid-upper arm circumference are all possibilities but charts are needed for diagnosing risk (as, for example, in the London School of Hygiene and Tropical Medicine/HelpAge manual). Knee height can be measured in a recumbent position, but a knee height calliper is required. This instrument has two blades set at right angles to a measuring stick, and measures the distance between the base of the heel and the top of the thigh on a bended knee. The formula used to compute stature from knee height is:

$$\text{Stature for women} = (1.83 \times \text{knee height}) - (0.24 \times \text{age}) + 84.88 \text{ cm}$$

$$\text{Stature for men} = (2.02 \times \text{knee height}) - (0.24 \times \text{age}) + 64.19 \text{ cm}$$

Abdominal fat tends to increase with age. In women, this trend occurs after menopause. In men, there may be an increase in intra-abdominal fat with a decrease in subcutaneous abdominal fat compared with younger males. In both genders, increased waist circumference accounts for about 40% of the insulin resistance associated with ageing. Increased waist measurement is a sign easily recognised by both patient and doctor as indicative of overnutrition.

Food intake is an important part of any assessment of malnutrition (over-, under- or disordered). If at all possible, this assessment is best made by a trained dietitian or nutritionist. A good dietary assessment is essential for diagnosis, treatment and prevention.

Treatment

Weight management should be initiated in elderly persons whose BMI is > 30 kg/m^2 and in patients with diabetes whose BMI is > 27. Recommendations for appropriate weight management strategies in the elderly are summarised in Table 30.5. A weight management program that begins with increasing exercise is logical because decreased physical activity is the major aetiological factor in obesity for most older individuals. A walking program, beginning with 3–5 km per day 4 times a week and 1–2 km on the other days of the week, is attainable. Other types of physical activity, such as gardening, dancing, low impact aerobics, yoga or Tai Chi, can also be encouraged. Swimming or water aerobics are popular with older individuals, especially those with arthritis or conditions that affect movement of the lower extremities.

Strength (or resistance) training, which involves lifting a heavy load in rapid succession, will strengthen muscles and reduce muscle loss, and is also recommended for elderly individuals. Recent studies in older people have demonstrated that resistance training can result in a decline in the progress of sarcopenia, as well as decreased problems associated with type II diabetes, coronary

Table 30.5 Appropriate weight management techniques

Weight management technique	Appropriateness for elderly
Exercise	Yes
Diet: moderate energy restriction	Yes (if BMI greater than 27, or weight associated with diabetes mellitus)
Behaviour modification	Yes
Low and very low kilojoule diets	Potentially dangerous
Drugs (anorectic or thermogenic agents)	Rarely indicated
Gastric balloon	Not useful
Surgery: gastric restriction	Only when massive obesity is associated with sleep apnoea
Surgery: jejuno-ileal bypass	Never used

Source: Adapted from J. E. Morley & Z. Glick (1995), 'Obesity', in J. E. Morley, Z. Glick & L. Z. Rubenstein (eds), *Geriatric Nutrition: A Comprehensive Review*, 2nd edn, Raven Press, New York.

artery disease, hypertension, osteoporosis and obesity. Close follow-up or monitoring of the exercise program by a physician or therapist will result in greater long-term success.

Appropriate dietary recommendations for weight management in the elderly are outlined in the National Health and Medical Research Council's *Dietary Guidelines for Older Australians* (Box 30.3). Emphasis should be placed on increasing the consumption of nutrient dense foods, such as: vegetables; fruit; whole grain cereal; bread and pasta; low-fat dairy products; low-fat protein sources, such as dried beans and legumes; fish; poultry and lean meat. Elderly persons should be encouraged to limit (but not completely eliminate) food high in saturated fat and sugar. A moderate amount of alcohol (1–2 glasses per day) can help stimulate the appetite and provide a social and pleasant mealtime environment. It is vitally important that older people continue to enjoy meal times and not be overly restricted in their diet to the point of getting little satisfaction from eating.

Behaviour modification techniques such as self-monitoring and lifestyle changes have been used successfully with elderly persons. With the help of a skilled intervention team that includes a dietitian and a psychologist, elderly persons can learn techniques to limit the temptation to overeat and focus on positive outcomes, such as improved mobility and general wellbeing. Some successful weight management programs focus on improved eating habits and reduction of waist circumference rather than on weight loss alone. It is worth remembering that although through middle age there is a doubling of body fat, it is more typical for body fat to decrease after the age of 65 years, even in healthy individuals.

Low-energy diets (3350–4200 kJ or 800–1000 kcal/day) are not appropriate for weight management in the elderly. At this level of energy intake, micronutrient status is likely to be compromised. The use of pharmacological agents should be avoided, as there are few data on the effectiveness and safety of anorectic and thermogenic agents in the elderly.

Box 30.3 National Health and Medical Research Council Guidelines

Dietary guidelines for older Australians

1. Enjoy a wide variety of nutritious foods.
2. Keep active to maintain muscle strength and a healthy body weight.
3. Eat at least three meals every day.
4. Care for your food: prepare and store it correctly.
5. Eat plenty of vegetables (including legumes) and fruit.
6. Eat plenty of cereal, breads and pastas.
7. Eat a diet low in saturated fat.
8. Drink adequate amounts of water and/or other fluids.
9. If you drink alcohol, limit your intake.
10. Choose foods low in salt and use salt sparingly.
11. Include foods high in calcium.
12. Use added sugars in moderation.

Conclusion

At all ages, the healthiest diet is one that, through variety, provides adequate micronutrients and appropriate amounts of energy, protein and carbohydrate. The treatment goal is to empower the elderly person to develop a healthy lifestyle to reduce the risk of chronic diseases.

Studies have shown that the quality of life for the elderly is very much a subjective feeling and may be relatively unrelated to a more objective assessment. An ideal assessment scale would cover activities of daily living (including eating), communication, visual and hearing disability, cognitive function, depression, quality of life and assessment of social status. The family physician is suited to assessing his elderly patient's 'nutritional vulnerability', which covers physical health, food intake, socioeconomic status, disability, functional ability, family and social life, and psychological and emotional wellbeing.

The checklist in Box 30.4 is an outline for assessing the warning signs of poor nutritional health. Accurate nutritional assessment of the elderly is difficult, but should be kept as simple as possible to ensure it is actually done. The assessment involves taking a medical, dietary and social history; basic biochemical assessment; and further investigation when indicated. The most important factor in the nutritional assessment of the older patient is that the practitioner remains alert to the possibility of some degree of malnutrition (both under- and over-). As undernutrition, in particular, can be very subtle and develop over many years, a high degree of suspicion needs to be maintained.

Many countries have developed dietary guidelines specifically related to the elderly population. In Australia, the National Health and Research Council has published *Dietary Guidelines for Older Australians* (Box 30.3). These guidelines were designed to be used as a whole. The first four guidelines deal with general aspects of nutrition and lifestyle, while the remaining guidelines address issues related to specific foods and nutrients, and are ranked in approximate order of importance. Older persons should be encouraged to seek the advice of their physician, dietitian or other health or social service professional. There are a number of programs in most communities which provide nutritious meals in a social setting, a recognised positive factor in encouraging greater variety and quantity in the diet. Other programs, such as Meals-on-Wheels, offer meals delivered to the home by community volunteers.

Regular physical exercise, improving muscle strength and maintaining a healthy body weight, have all been shown to reduce the risk of several chronic diseases and premature death. Moderate physical activity has also been shown to promote a positive mental attitude and to promote stronger, healthier muscles, bones and joints. Research indicates that eating a wide variety of foods offers protection against major chronic diseases, such as coronary heart disease, hypertension, type II diabetes and some cancers. Eating a wide variety of foods also increases the likelihood of obtaining most of the essential nutrients.

It is encouraging that a national nutrition survey in Australia found that on average, older people actually eat better than their younger countrymen and women. Regular nutritional assessment and the awareness that this is needed will help maintain nutritional health and wellbeing as our society continues to age. The year 1999 was designated as the International Year of Older Persons. The UN Secretary-General described a society for all ages as 'one that does not caricature older persons as patients and pensioners', and one that 'seeks a balance between supporting dependency and investing in lifelong development'.

Editor's note

Box 30.4 is a mini-nutritional assessment (MNA), which is an 18 item instrument requiring only 20 minutes to complete. It incorporates anthropometric measures, data entry questions and health and functional status questions. The developers used discriminate analysis techniques applied to several cross-sectional samples to establish cut-off points for being 'at risk' of malnutrition and being undernourished. The instrument has been validated against the clinical judgment of nutritional status, dietary intake and biochemical measures. More importantly, predictive validity for weight loss, the occurrence of acute disease and the need for assistance has been documented.

Box 30.4 Mini-Nutritional Assessment

Last name: ______________ First name ______________ M.I. ______ Sex: _____ Date: ________

Age: __________ Weight (kg:) __________ Height (cm): __________ Knee height (cm): __________

Complete the form by writing the numbers in the boxes. Add the numbers in the boxes and compare the total assessment to the Malnutrition Indicator Score.

Anthropometric Assessment — Points

1. Body Mass Index (BMI) (weight in kg)/(height in m²)
   - a. BMI < 19 = 0 points
   - b. BMI 19 to < 21 = 1 point
   - c. BMI 21 to < 23 = 2 points
   - d. BMI > 23 = 3 points
2. Mid-arm circumference (MAC) in cm
   - a. MAC < 21 = 0.0 points
   - b. MAC 21 ≤ 22 = 0.5 points
   - c. MAC > 22 = 1.0 point
3. Calf circumference (CC) in cm
   - a. CC < 31 = 0 points
   - b. CC ≥ 31 = 1 point
4. Weight loss during last 3 months
   - a. weight loss greater than 3 kg (6.6 lb) = 0 points
   - b. does not know = 1 point
   - c. weight ooss between 1 and 3 kg = 2 points
   - d. no weight loss = 3 points

General Assessment

5. Lives independently (not in a nursing home or hospital)
   - a. no = 0 points b. yes = 1 point
6. Takes more than 3 prescription drugs per day
   - a. yes = 0 points b. no = 1 point
7. Has suffered psychological stress or acute disease in the past 3 months
   - a. yes = 0 points b. no = 2 points
8. Mobility
   - a. bed or chair bound = 0 points
   - b. able to get out of bed/chair but does not go out = 1 point
   - c. goes out = 2 points
9. Neuropsychological problems
   - a. severe dementia or depression = 0 points
   - b. mild dementia = 1 point
   - c. no psychological problems = 2 points
10. Pressure sores or skin ulcers
    - a. yes = 0 points b. no = 1 point

Dietary Assessment — Points

11. How many full meals does the patient eat daily?
    - a. 1 meal = 0 points
    - b. 2 meals = 1 point
    - c. 3 meals = 2 points
12. Selected consumption markers for protein intake
    - At least one serving of dairy products (milk, cheese, yogurt) per day ❑ Yes ❑ No
    - Two or more servings of legumes or eggs per week ❑ Yes ❑ No
    - Meat, fish, or poultry every day ❑ Yes ❑ No
    - a. 0 or 1 yes = 0.0 points
    - b. 2 yes = 0.5 points
    - c. 3 yes = 1.0 point
13. Consumes two or more servings of fruits or vegetables per day
    - a. no = 0 points b. yes = 1 point
14. Has food intake declined over the past 3 months due to loss of appetite, digestive problems, chewing or swallowing difficulties?
    - a. severe loss of appetite = 0 points
    - b. moderate loss of appetite = 1 point
    - c. no loss of appetite = 2 points
15. How much fluid (e.g., water, juice, coffee, tea, milk) is consumed per day? 1 cup = 220g)
    - a. less than 3 cups = 0.0 points
    - b. 3 to 5 cups = 0.5 points
    - c. more than 5 cups = 1.0 point
16. Mode of feeding
    - a. unable to eat without assistance = 0 points
    - b. self-fed with some difficulty = 1 point
    - c. self-fed without any problem = 2 points

Self-Assessment

17. Do they view themselves as having nutritional problems?
    - a. major malnutrition = 0 points
    - b. do not know or moderate malnutrition = 1 point
    - c. no nutritional problem = 2 points

continued

18. In comparison with other people of the same age, how do they consider their health status?
    a. not as good = 0.0 points
    b. do not know = 0.5 points
    c. as good = 1.0 point
    d. better = 2.0 points

Assessment Total (max. 30 points)

MALNUTRITION INDICATOR SCORE

≥ 24 points = well-nourished 17 to 23.5 points = at risk of malnutrition < 17 points = malnourished

Source: B. Vellas, Y. Guigoz, P. J. Garry et al. (1999), 'The Mini Nutritional Assessment (MNA) and its use in grading the nutritional state of elderly patients', *Nutrition*, 15(2), pp. 116–22.

Bibliography and further reading

Blumberg, J. (1997), 'Nutritional needs of seniors', *Journal of the American College of Nutrition*, 16(6), pp. 517–23.

Clark, R., Smith, A. D., Phil, D., Jobst, K. A., Refsum, H., Sutton, L. & Ueland, P. M. (1998), 'Folate, vitamin B_{12} and serum total homocysteine level in confirmed Alzheimer Disease', *Archives of Neurology*, 55, pp. 1449–55.

Darnton-Hill, I. (1995), 'Healthy aging and the quality of life', *World Health Forum*, 16, pp. 335–72.

Essama-Tjani, J.-C., Guilland, J.-C., Potier de Courcy, G., Fuchs, F. & Richard, D. (2000), 'Folate status worsens in recently institutionalized elderly people without evidence of functional deterioration', *Journal of the American College of Nutrition*, 19, pp. 392–404.

Expert Panel (1998), 'Clinical guidelines on the identification, evaluation, and treatment of overweight and obesity in adults: executive summary', *The American Journal of Clinical Nutrition*, 68, pp. 899–917.

Guo, S. S., Zeller, C., Cameron Chumlea, W. & Siervogel, R. M. (1999), 'Aging, body composition, and lifestyle: the Fels Longitudinal Study', *The American Journal of Clinical Nutrition*, 70, pp. 405–11.

Horwitz, A., Macfadyen, D. M., Schrimshaw, N. S., Munro, H., Steen, B. & Williams, T. F. (eds) (1989), *Nutrition in the Elderly*, Oxford University Press, Oxford.

Lehmann, M., Gottfries, C. G. & Regland, B. (1999), 'Identification of cognitive impairment in the elderly: homocysteine is an early marker', *Dementia and Geriatric Cognitive Disorders*, 10, pp. 12–20.

Marcus, E.-L. & Berry, E. M. (1998), 'Refusal to eat in the elderly', *Nutrition Reviews*, 56, pp. 163–71.

Miller, D. K., Morely, J. F. & Rubenstein, L. Z. (1995), 'An overview of aging and nutrition', in Morley, J. E., Glick, Z. & Rubenstein, L. Z. (eds), *Geriatric Nutrition: A Comprehensive Review*, 2nd edn, Raven Press, New York.

Posner, B. M., Jette, A. M., Smith, K. W. & Miller, D. R. (1993), 'Nutrition and health risks in the elderly: the Nutrition Screening Initiative', *American Journal of Public Health*, 83, pp. 972–8.

Riedel, W. J. & Jorissen, B. L. (1998), 'Nutrients, age and cognitive function', *Current Opinion in Clinical Nutrition and Metabolic Care*, 1(6), pp. 579–85.

Roberts, S. B. (2000), 'Energy regulation and aging: recent findings and their implications', *Nutrition Reviews*, 58, pp. 91–7.

Schneider, S. M. & Hebuterne, X. (2000), 'Use of nutritional scores to predict clinical outcomes in chronic diseases', *Nutrition Reviews*, 58, pp. 31–8.

Toth, M. J. & Poehlman, E. T. (2000), 'Energetic adaptation to chronic disease in the elderly', *Nutrition Reviews*, 58, pp. 61–6.

Trichopoulou, A., Kouris-Blazos, A., Wahlqvist, M. L., Gnardellis, C., Lagiou, P., Polychronopoulos, E., Vassilakou, T., Lipworth, L. & Trichopoulos, D. (1995), 'Diet and overall survival of the elderly', *British Medical Journal*, 311, pp. 1457–60.

Wahlqvist, M. (1997), 'Requirements in maturity and ageing', in Wahlqvist, M. (ed.), *Food and Nutrition: Australasia, Asia and the Pacific*, Allen & Unwin, Sydney.

Wahlqvist, M. L. & Briggs, D. R. (1998), 'Other biologically active substances in food', in Mann, J. & Truswell, A. S. (eds), *Essentials of Human Nutrition*, Oxford University Press, Oxford, pp. 245–56.

Wahlqvist, M. L. & Dalais, F. (1997), 'Phytoestrogens — The emerging multi-faceted plant compounds', Editorial, *The Medical Journal of Australia*, 167, pp. 119–20.

Wahlqvist, M. L. & Wattanapenpaiboon, N. (1999), 'Antioxidant nutrients', *Australian Prescriber*, 22, pp. 142–4.

Wahlqvist, M. L., Wattanapenpaiboon, N., Kannar, D., Dalais, F. & Kouris-Blazos, A. (1998), 'Phytochemical deficiency disorders: inadequate intake of protective foods', *Current Therapeutics*, July, pp. 53–60.

Chapter 31

Dysphagia

RANJIT N. RATNAIKE, SARAH HATHERLY and GABRIEL SUKUMAR

Dysphagia is difficulty in swallowing due to a variety of causes. It is important to have a heightened awareness that this is a common problem in older patients. Dysphagia may often be the presenting symptom of a range of conditions, from cerebrovascular accidents to external compression due to a mediastinal lesion. Patients with dysphagia frequently find solids, particularly bread, meat and potatoes, difficult to swallow. Dysphagia for *both* solids and liquids is usually due to a motor disorder of the oesophagus. Dysphagia initially for solids progressing to liquids suggests a progressive obstructive lesion narrowing the oesophageal lumen. Odynophagia is pain associated with swallowing.

Anatomical landmarks

The oral cavity leads to the oropharynx and the nasopharynx lies above the soft palate. The pharynx is bound superiorly by the nasal cavities and below by the oesophagus at the cricopharyngeal muscle, also referred to as the upper oesophageal sphincter (Figure 31.1).

The swallowing process

Swallowing is a complex process involving the coordinated activity of neural regulatory mechanisms in the medulla, the sensorimotor cortex and corticolimbic systems, and then mediated by cranial nerves V, VII, IX, X and XII in the pons and medulla oblongata.

Swallowing consists of three phases:

1. *The oral phase* constitutes: (a) lip closure to retain food or liquid in the mouth; (b) closure of the anterior and lateral sulci, and propelling food towards the tongue medially; (c) rotatory lateral jaw movements during mastication; (d) rotatory lateral tongue movement to control food in the mouth, mixing it with saliva; and (e) anterior bulging of the soft palate to prevent premature spillage of food from the oral cavity to the pharynx. The tongue then propels the prepared bolus of food along the palate to the faucial arches (the soft palate region above the fauces).
2. The involuntary *pharyngeal phase* begins with the triggering of the swallow response at the anterior faucial arches. The bolus stimulates the surface and deep receptors within the faucial arches, pharynx and base of the tongue. This

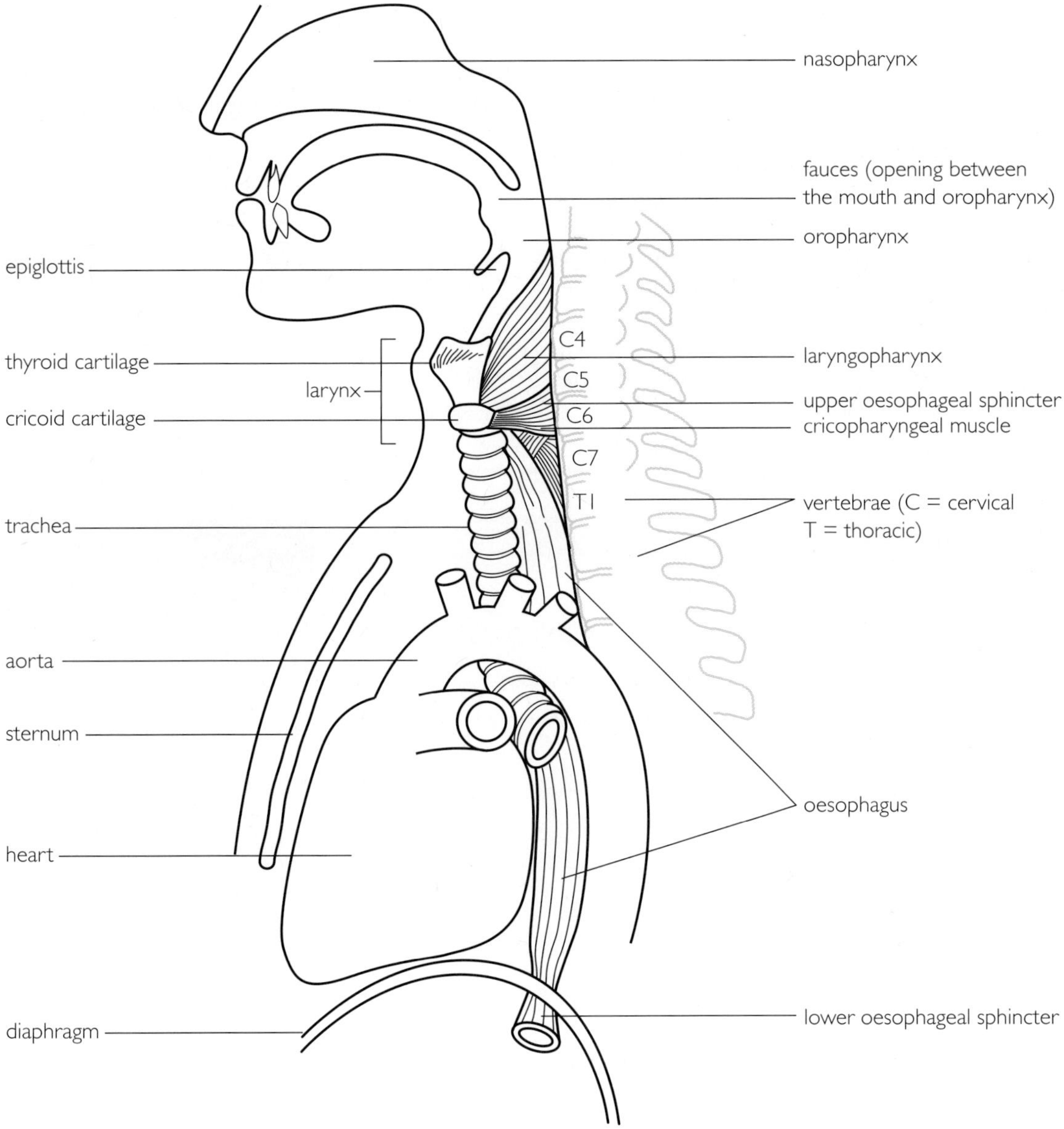

Figure 31.1 Schematic diagram showing structures in relation to the oesophagus. The laryngopharynx is a common passage that opens into the larynx and the oesophagus. The cricopharyngeal muscle attached to the cricoid cartilage forms the upper oesophageal sphincter. During the pharyngeal phase of swallowing, elevation of the larynx causes relaxation of the upper oesophageal sphincter, allowing food to enter the oesophagus

phase is characterised by a rapid co-ordinated sequence of events: (a) approximation of the soft palate to the pharyngeal wall; (b) elevation and anterior movement of the hyoid bone and larynx; (c) closure of the laryngeal inlet by the epiglottis, false vocal folds and true vocal folds; (d) initiation and progression of pharyngeal contraction as the bolus moves through the pharynx and to the cricopharyngeal muscle; and (e) relaxation of the cricopharyngeal muscle to allow the bolus to pass into the upper oesophagus. This phase normally takes 0.4–1.0 second in adults.

3. The *oesophageal phase* is also involuntary. The tube-like oesophagus, about 25 cm long, is in a 'collapsed' state and distends when liquid or food is ingested. Air swallowing also distends the oesophagus. Oesophageal peristalsis is a continuation of the contractions originating in the pharynx (Figure 31.2). The food bolus moves rapidly through the oesophagus via the lower oesophageal sphincter (LOS) into the stomach. The transit time of the oesophageal phase varies from 8 to 20 seconds.

The ageing swallow

Ageing affects swallowing because of changes in anatomical and physiological mechanisms, which result in:

- reduced salivary gland secretion
- increased mastication to prepare food
- increased time required to prepare the bolus
- a tendency to hold the bolus on the floor of the mouth initially
- reduced laryngeal and hyoid bone elevation due to a drop in resting laryngeal position
- slowing of pharyngeal contractions

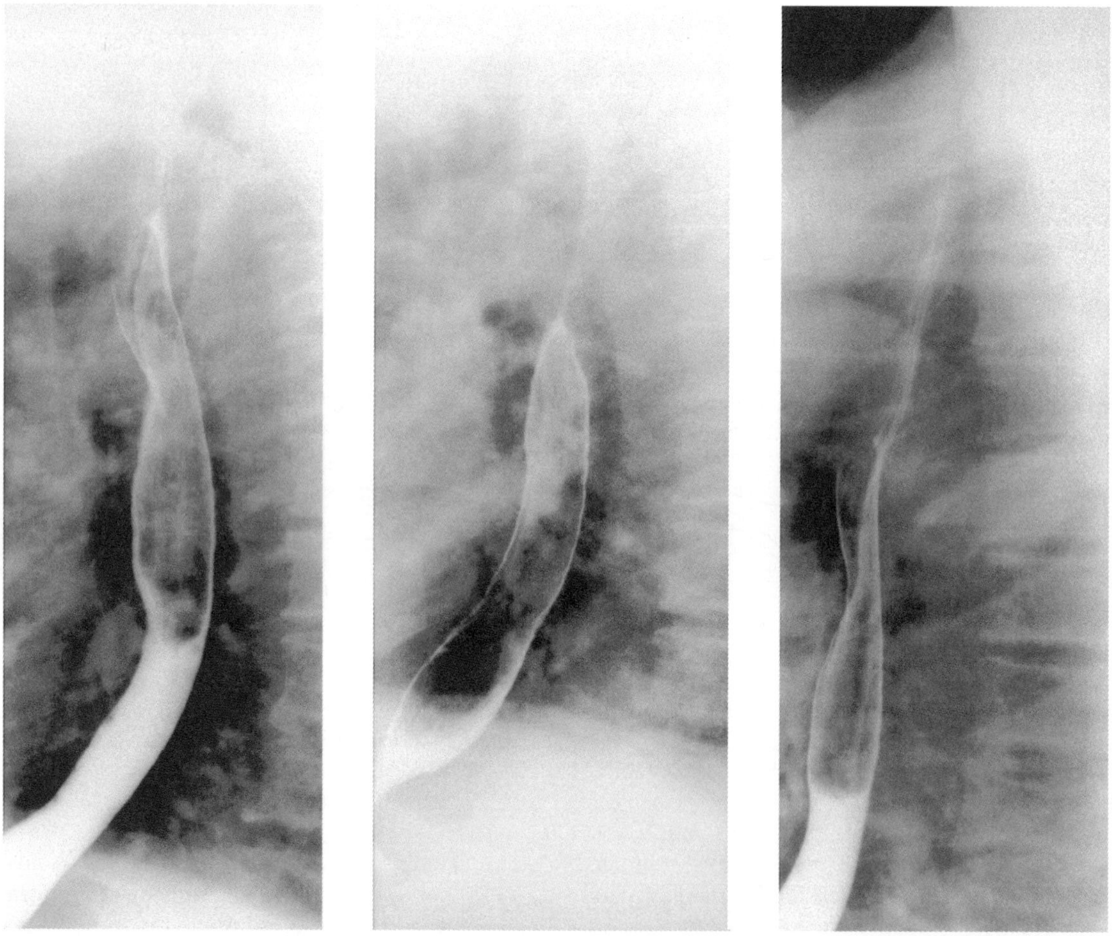

Figure 31.2 Normal barium swallow. Note the linear mucosal folds and peristalsis
Courtesy of Dr Anil B. Utturkar, Senior Radiologist, The Queen Elizabeth Hospital, Adelaide

- triggering of the pharyngeal phase more posteriorly
- delayed triggering of the pharyngeal phase of swallowing.

These changes may occur in 'normal' asymptomatic elderly individuals and do not lead to significant oropharyngeal dysphagia.

Disorders of swallowing

Dysphagia consists of two distinct entities:

1. *Oropharyngeal dysphagia* is the inability to initiate the act of swallowing or transferring food from the mouth to the upper oesophagus (Box 31.1).
2. *Oesophageal dysphagia* is due to problems experienced during the passage of food through the body of the oesophagus and the lower oesophageal sphincter (Box 31.2).

Box 31.1 Classification and aetiology of oropharyngeal dysphagia

Central nervous system
- Cerebrovascular accidents (especially involving the brain stem)
- Parkinson's disease
- Progressive supranuclear palsy
- Motor neuron disease
- Huntington's chorea
- Alzheimer's disease
- Myasthenia gravis
- Polymyositis and dermatomyositis
- Multiple sclerosis
- Neoplasia
- Guillain-Barré syndrome
- Myopathy
- Head trauma

Oropharyngeal causes
- Xerostomia (Sjogren's syndrome)
- Strictures
- Webs (Plummer-Vinson syndrome)
- Diverticula
- Radiation injury
- Drug-associated injury
- Neoplasia

Extrinsic causes
- Cervical osteophytes
- Neoplasia
- Thyromegaly
- Lymphadenopathy

Miscellaneous causes
- Thyrotoxic myopathy
- Diabetes mellitus

Box 31.2 Classification and aetiology of oesophageal dysphagia

Motility disorders
- Achalasia
- Diffuse oesophageal spasm
- Scleroderma
- Amyloidosis
- Diabetes mellitus
- Parkinson's disease

Oesophagitis
- Gastro-oesophageal reflux disease (GORD)
- Infectious causes
- Drug-associated injury (see Box 31.3)
- Radiation injury

Webs, rings and diverticula
- Strictures
- Neoplasia

Extra-oesophageal causes
- Aberrant right subclavian artery
- Massive thoracic aortic aneurism
- Mediastinal masses

Oropharyngeal dysphagia

In patients with oropharyngeal dysphagia, the problem may be in the mouth, pharynx or upper oesophageal sphincter. During attempts to swallow, muscular inco-ordination, depending on the severity, results in difficulty in initiating swallowing, regurgitation, aspiration, coughing or choking. A characteristic symptom is that repeated attempts are necessary to initiate swallowing. Dysarthria may also occur as some muscles used in swallowing are also employed in speech. Patients with oropharyngeal dysphagia may tend to localise food being 'stuck' in the throat or in the neck, although the exact location is often inaccurate. An example of a cause of oropharyngeal dysphagia is spasm of the cricopharyngeal muscle (Figure 31.3). In patients with symptoms of oropharyngeal dysphagia, the oropharynx must be carefully examined and a thorough neurological examination conducted. The investigations are discussed subsequently.

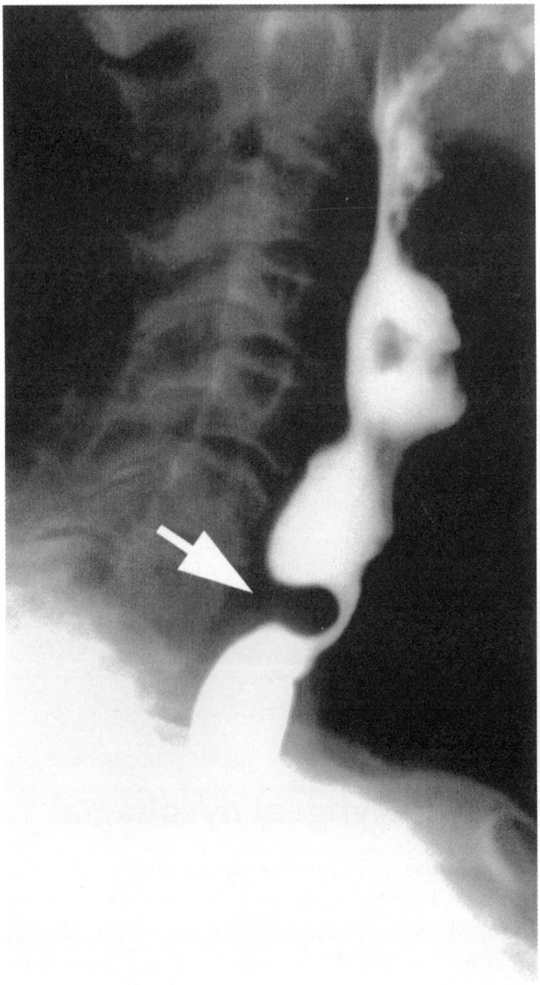

Figure 31.3 Cricopharyngeal spasm. Prominent thumbprint-like impression on the posterior aspect of the cricopharyngeal muscle situated at the level of the upper oesophageal sphincter, in association with gastro-oesophageal reflux

Courtesy of Dr Anil B. Utturkar, Senior Radiologist, The Queen Elizabeth Hospital, Adelaide

Neurological causes

Numerous neurological disorders of acute onset and of a progressive nature can result in swallowing disorders (Box 31.1). Many neurological causes of dysphagia listed under oropharyngeal dysphagia also involve the oesophagus. Swallowing problems are the causes of death in some of these neurological conditions due to aspiration and respiratory complications.

Cerebrovascular accidents

The most common cause of oropharyngeal dysphagia is a cerebrovascular accident, especially involving the brain stem. In these cases, patients may also experience difficulties in the initial oral phase of food preparation due to lingual paresis and in triggering the swallow response. In the pharyngeal phase, problems occur due to decreased pharyngeal contraction and impaired airway protection. In a transient cerebral ischaemic attack involving the vertebrobasilar territory, dysphagia may be the initial presentation, especially if the arterial supply to the pons and medulla oblongata is affected.

Parkinson's disease

A variety of swallowing problems are early manifestations of Parkinson's disease (see Chapter 14). About 50% of patients report dysphagia by 5 years. The dysphagia is progressive, affecting the oral, pharyngeal and oesophageal phases. Initiating the pharyngeal swallow requires repetitive tongue pumping. There is a delay in triggering the pharyngeal swallow and food residue remains in the pharynx due to reduced contractions.

Progressive supranuclear palsy

Progressive supranuclear palsy is a progressive degenerative extrapyramidal disease (Chapter 14) that often masquerades as Parkinson's disease. Dysphagia is an early manifestation, worsens as the disease progresses and is more severe than in Parkinson's disease.

Motor neuron disease

The degeneration of the upper and lower motor neurons in motor neuron disease (amyotrophic lateral sclerosis) frequently presents as oropharyngeal dysfunction. As the disease progresses, dysphagia occurs due to delayed triggering of the swallow response, decreased pharyngeal contraction and reduced laryngeal closure.

Huntington's chorea

Huntington's chorea is a rare autosomal dominant condition characterised by chorea and progressive dementia. The illness may develop with an initial subtle movement disorder that worsens to become disabling. Oropharyngeal dysphagia is a major problem and a consequence of this is aspiration pneumonia, which is a common cause of death.

Alzheimer's disease

In Alzheimer's disease (Chapter 15), the mechanism of dysphagia, a widely cited problem, is unclear. In a pilot study on eating changes in patients with mild-stage Alzheimer's disease, patients demonstrated significantly prolonged swallow 'durations' for the oral transit phase, pharyngeal response phase and total swallow duration.

Myasthenia gravis

Myasthenia gravis is an autoimmune disorder characterised by increasing fatigue with exertion. The majority of patients present with ptosis, diplopia, dysarthria and dysphagia. Myasthenia gravis is also a very rare complication of allogeneic bone marrow transplantation.

Polymyositis and dermatomyositis

Dysphagia may be a manifestation of polymyositis, which is an inflammatory muscle disease that is termed dermatomyositis when it occurs with a rash. The disease is characterised by symmetrical proximal muscle weakness that is insidious in onset and progressive. Pain is not a prominent feature, although tenderness may be present.

Multiple sclerosis

Dysphagia may occur as one of the many manifestations of multiple sclerosis, a condition notoriously difficult to diagnose at onset (or even subsequently). The symptoms and signs reflect multiple areas of neurological involvement. The diagnostic problem is compounded by the fluctuating nature of the illness. It is uncommon in older persons.

Neoplasia

Neoplasia can cause dysphagia by direct tissue involvement of the brain stem or by compression. Hemispheric lesions due to a neoplasm are also reported to cause dysphagia.

Guillain-Barré syndrome

The Guillain-Barré syndrome and other polyneuropathies can cause oropharyngeal or oesophageal dysphagia. The Guillain-Barré syndrome may rarely manifest after an episode of diarrhoea due to *Campylobacter jejuni* enteritis, possibly triggered by an autoimmune response directed against the cell-surface receptor ganglioside GM1. Molecular mimicry between GM1 and the lipopolysaccharide from *C. jejuni* appears to be the reason for developing autoantibodies with the potential to cause the Guillain-Barré syndrome.

Myopathy

Dysphagia of obscure aetiology may be due to thyroid disease. Both thyrotoxicosis and hypothyroidism are associated with a myopathy that may affect the muscles involved in swallowing.

Head trauma

In injuries involving the brain, brain stem and/or cranial nerves, changes in oropharyngeal swallowing may occur. The problem tends to resolve with neurological improvement.

Diverticula

Diverticula are sac-like outpouchings of one or more muscle layers. These abnormalities occur even in infants, but are more common in later years.

Zenker's diverticulum

Zenker's diverticula (Figure 31.4) are posterior hypopharyngeal diverticula located immediately above the upper oesophageal sphincter. They are

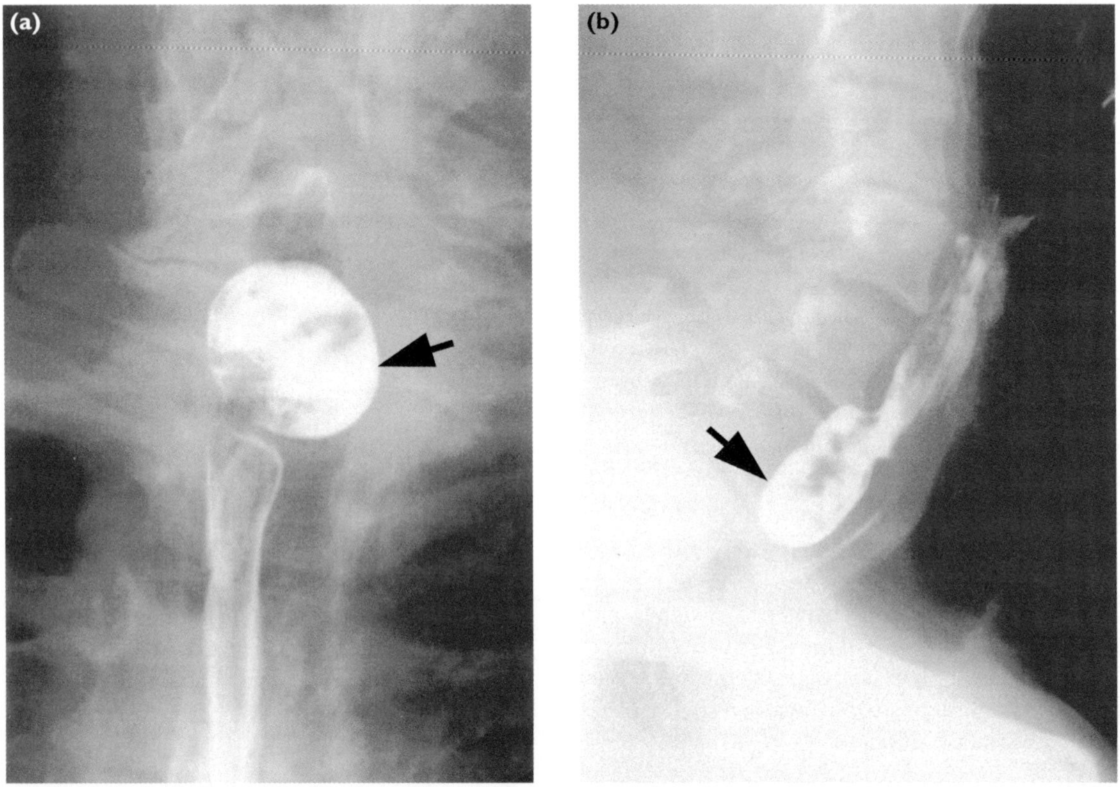

Figure 31.4 (a) Posterior-anterior and **(b)** lateral views of Zenker's diverticulum (with retained food material presenting as a superior mediastinal mass)
Courtesy of Dr Anil B. Utturkar, Senior Radiologist, The Queen Elizabeth Hospital, Adelaide

not true oesophageal diverticula but outpouchings of a weak posterior pharyngeal wall possibly caused by abnormal oesophageal motor activity generating excessive pharyngeal pressures. Dysphagia is a prominent symptom. Other symptoms and signs depend on the size of the diverticulum: after a meal or a drink, food retained in the pouch of the diverticulum may give rise to a feeling of fullness in the throat or a gurgling noise after meals; regurgitation of food and chronic pulmonary aspiration may occur. Halitosis is a common complaint. A very large Zenker's diverticulum may be felt as a mass in the throat. Rare complications are ulceration or perforation of the diverticulum during instrumentation or the development of neoplasm. Diagnosis is established by a barium swallow and upper oesophageal sphincter manometry. Treatment for symptomatic Zenker's diverticula is cricopharyngeal myotomy and diverticulopexy. A recent advance is endoscopic diverticulectomy.

Webs

The best known association of a web is with the Paterson-Kelly syndrome. The Paterson-Kelly syndrome (also called the Plummer-Vinson syndrome) consists of dysphagia due to a post-cricoid web that arises from the anterior and posterior portions of the hypopharynx, iron deficiency anaemia, glossitis and koilonychia. The dysphagia is oropharyngeal and of sudden rather than gradual onset. These patients should be treated for iron deficiency anaemia. Monitoring with endoscopy is important due to the possibility of developing a malignancy, although a rare occurrence. Figure 31.5 shows the presence of a cricopharyngeal web.

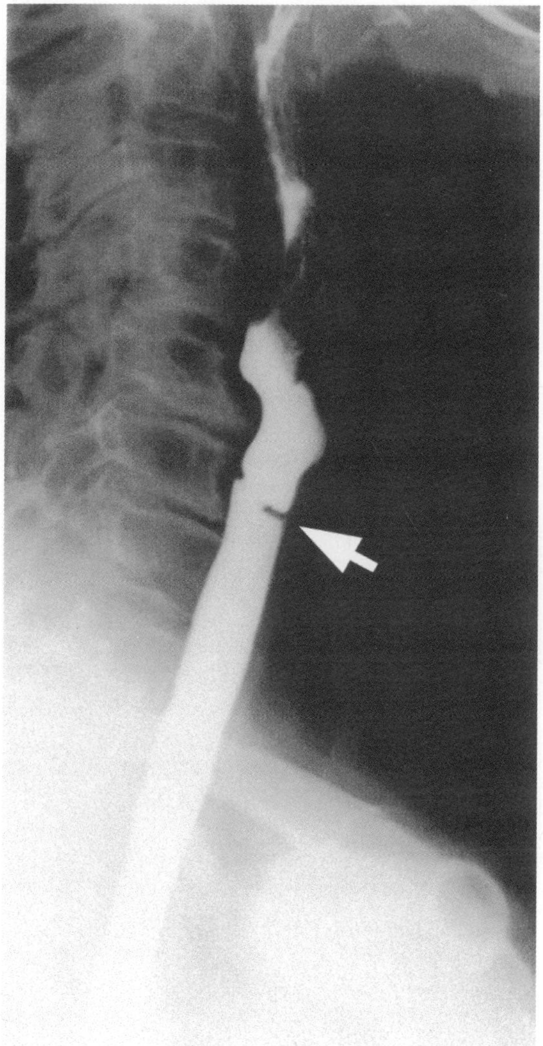

Figure 31.5 Cricopharyngeal web. Note the shelf-like web causing narrowing of the lumen in the cricopharynx
Courtesy of Dr Anil B. Utturkar, Senior Radiologist, The Queen Elizabeth Hospital, Adelaide

Therapeutic agents

Therapeutic agents can cause dysphagia. Neuroleptic drugs (antipsychotic drugs that influence cognition and behaviour characteristically producing a state of apathy and limited emotional range) alter neurotransmitter function and consequently extrapyramidal activity, which affects the oral and pharyngeal phases of swallowing. These medications also decrease salivary production. These effects, however, are reversible on withdrawal of the medication. Box 31.3 shows common medications that can cause dysphagia.

Box 31.3 Therapeutic agents that can cause oropharyngeal dysphagia

Neuroleptic drugs
- Haloperidol
- Trifluoperazine
- Loxapine (unavailable in Australia)

Infections

Infections such as pharyngitis and tonsillitis are frequent causes of oropharyngeal dysphagia. An abscess in the retropharyngeal space between the wall of the pharynx and the spine can present as dysphagia.

Oesophageal dysphagia

Oesophageal dysphagia may be caused by structural abnormalities that are either intrinsic (e.g. motor disorders, neoplasms, strictures, diverticula) or extrinsic (e.g. vascular compression, mediastinal adenopathy). Oesophageal dysphagia occurs when there is a problem related to the passage of food through the proximal striated portion or the distal smooth muscle portion of the oesophagus and/or the lower oesophageal sphincter. Patients may localise the swallowing problem to the neck or retrosternally.

A chest radiograph is an important initial investigation to identify extra-oesophageal causes of dysphagia. As the first oesophageal investigation, a barium swallow (Figure 31.2) is preferable to endoscopy. The barium swallow invariably detects an organic lesion and provides information on a motor abnormality. Endoscopy should also be performed as it enables the inspection of the mucosa and identifies any lesion undetected by the barium study. Importantly, a biopsy may be obtained. On occasion, more sophisticated investigations such as manometry may be necessary.

Motility disorders

Motility disorders of the oesophagus are due primarily to an intrinsic muscle or nerve disorder. In a motor disorder, dysphagia occurs with both solids and liquids. Patients often develop strategies to overcome dysphagia by repeated swallowing or by drinking a sufficient volume of fluid that acts as a 'hydrostatic ram'. Regurgitation of food is not a feature of a motor disorder. The association between emotional stress and dysphagia is strong. The two most important entities are achalasia and diffuse oesophageal spasm.

Achalasia

Achalasia is a primary motor disorder of the oesophagus due to degeneration of the ganglion cells in *Auerbach's plexus* (the myenteric plexus) in the wall of the mid and especially lower oesophagus (Figures 31.6 and 31.7). In time with further ganglion cell loss, the oesophagus becomes markedly dilated above the gastro-oesophageal junction. The aetiology is not known. A similar problem occurs in Chagas' disease, a condition prevalent in South America, where the ganglion cells are destroyed by the protozoan *Trypanosoma cruzi*.

In achalasia, dysphagia is due to three abnormalities:

1. the absence of oesophageal peristaltic contractions
2. a high resting pressure at the LOS
3. incomplete relaxation of the LOS.

The hallmark of the problem is progressive dysphagia for *both* liquids and solids. This is in contrast

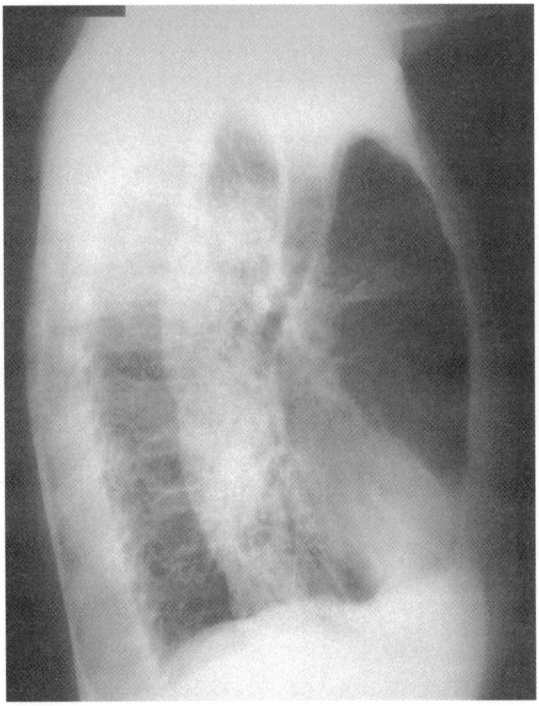

Figure 31.6 Achalasia evident on chest X-ray. The oesophagus is grossly dilated, featureless and contains a large amount of food material

Courtesy of Dr Anil B. Utturkar, Senior Radiologist, The Queen Elizabeth Hospital, Adelaide

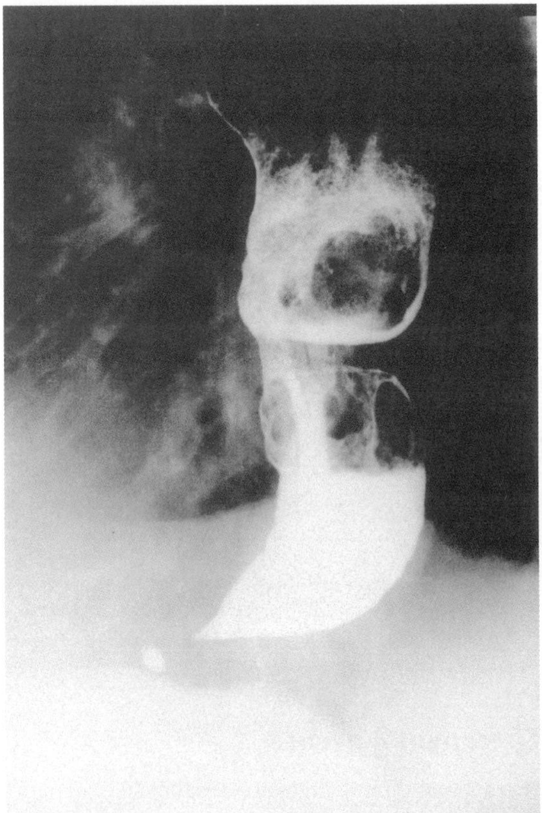

Figure 31.7 Achalasia. A barium swallow examination demonstrates a grossly dilated oesophagus with a large amount of retained food material. Note the classic beak-like narrowing at the lower end of the oesophagus due to the aganglionic segment

Courtesy of Dr Anil B. Utturkar, Senior Radiologist, The Queen Elizabeth Hospital, Adelaide

to obstructive lesions of the oesophagus, which decrease the oesophageal diameter, as in a carcinoma of the oesophagus, where dysphagia first occurs with solids and then liquids as luminal narrowing increases. In achalasia, progressive dilatation of the oesophagus occurs. Ingested solids and liquids do not reach the stomach. Consequently, nutritional problems ensue. Many patients have adopted techniques over time for the ingested material to pass into the stomach.

The barium swallow (Figure 31.7) shows a dilated oesophagus with absent peristalsis in the lower two-thirds, and failure of the LOS to relax. A characteristic feature is a smooth 'bird beak' tapering of the LOS (Figure 31.7). Manometry is an essential investigation to confirm the failure of the LOS to relax on swallowing. Endoscopic evaluation is valuable to rule out a malignancy that may have a similar presentation. Achalasia of long duration may be complicated by a malignancy.

The aim of therapy is to reduce the pressure at the level of the LOS. The treatment of achalasia is usually pneumatic dilatation of the hypertensive, non-functioning LOS, now performed with Rigiflex fixed diameter balloon dilators. Symptom improvement is reported in up to 90% of patients. Heller's myotomy is performed when pneumatic dilatation has failed. Invariably, since reflux may occur, a partial fundoplication is also performed. Intrasphincteric botulinum toxin is also used successfully in the treatment of achalasia, and is especially appropriate for older patients who are unsuitable for surgery or balloon dilatation. This is a safe and effective option that is particularly attractive in the elderly, but the benefits may be short lived.

Diffuse oesophageal spasm

Diffuse oesophageal spasm, a term widely used, is considered imprecise as it implies dysmotility of widely varying severity from a few inconsequential abnormal contractions to absence of normal peristaltic activity. The condition is closely linked to gastro-oesophageal reflux disease (GORD) due to the effects of acid reflux on the mucosa (Figure 31.8). Exercise can cause chest pain consequent on reflux and spasm. Dysphagia of variable severity may occur. A major symptom is central chest pain of

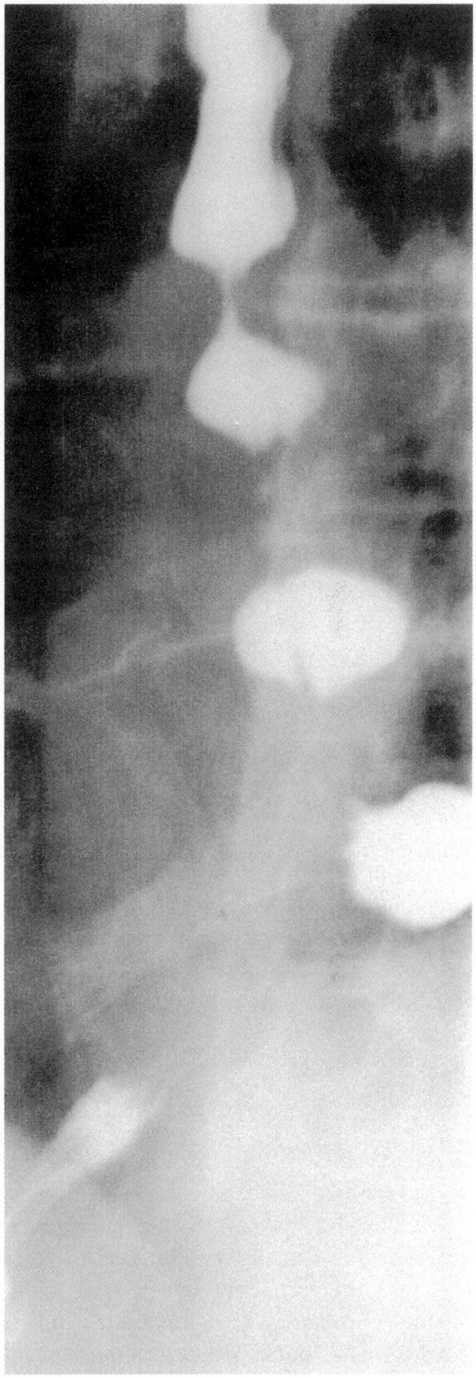

Figure 31.8 Diffuse oesophageal spasm, showing corkscrew-like appearance, is associated with chest pain and dysphagia

Courtesy of Dr Anil B. Utturkar, Senior Radiologist, The Queen Elizabeth Hospital, Adelaide

sufficient severity to suggest myocardial ischaemia. Pain radiates to sites similar to that in myocardial ischaemia, such as the neck and jaw, but less commonly to the arms.

The presence of dysphagia and the relief of symptoms with belching reported by many patients may help to distinguish oesophageal spasm from myocardial pain. However, the diagnosis of oesophageal spasm as the cause of chest pain, especially in the elderly, should be made with considerable caution. Patients with chest pain due to genuine myocardial ischaemia may, to their peril, be labelled as having oesophageal spasm.

The diagnosis, if facilities such as manometry are not available, may be one of exclusion of myocardial disease. Manometry reveals non-peristaltic, repetitive, simultaneous and multiphasic contractions of high amplitude. Radiological studies may show no abnormality or a 'corkscrew' oesophagus if diffuse spasm occurs during the examination (Figure 31.9). When oesophageal spasm occurs together with lower oesophageal sphincter dysfunction, the condition is termed 'variant achalasia'.

Treatment of oesophageal spasm involves dietary counselling to avoid reflux, and the use of nitrates and/or calcium channel blockers. In patients with GORD and severe chest pain, after exclusion of non-oesophageal causes, 12 weeks of therapy with a 'double dose' proton pump inhibitor is recommended. In these patients, endoscopy and/or 24-hour pH monitoring and/or motility studies are indicated.

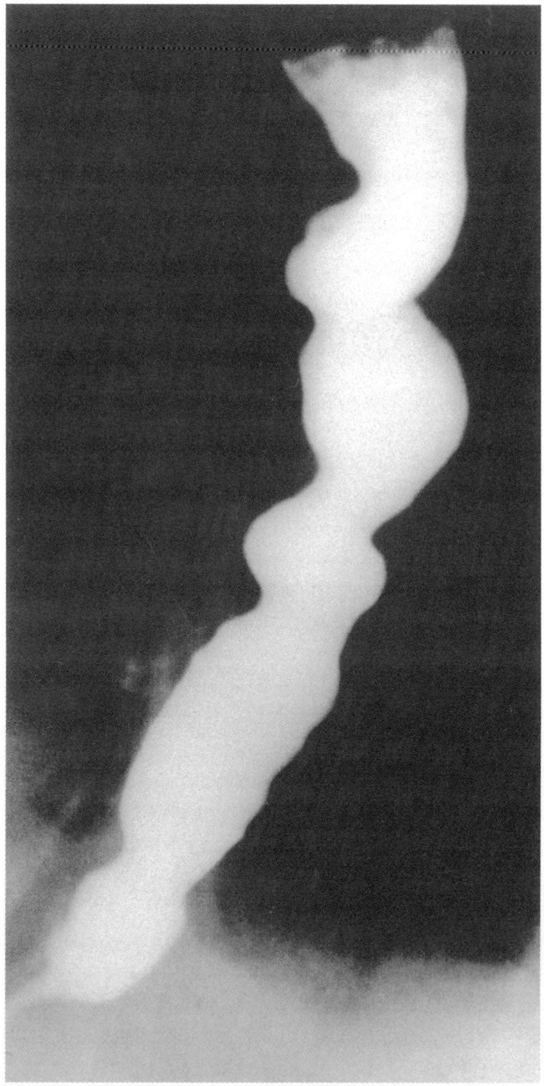

Figure 31.9 Corkscrew oesophagus. Note the ripple-like contraction of the oesophagus due to neuromuscular inco-ordination, as seen in elderly individuals

Courtesy of Dr Anil B. Utturkar, Senior Radiologist, The Queen Elizabeth Hospital, Adelaide

Oesophagitis

Gastro-oesophageal reflux disease

Gastro-oesophageal reflux disease occurs due to the reflux of stomach contents (usually gastric acid) into the oesophagus. There is no consistent evidence that GORD is more common in the elderly. However, the incidence of hiatus hernia increases with age and could predispose to gastro-oesophageal reflux disease. The mucosa of the oesophagus is protected by the lower oesophageal sphincter to prevent gastric acid regurgitation and GORD occurs when the tone of the LOS is compromised due to diverse aetiological factors. The LOS tone is decreased by calcium antagonists, β-blockers, prostaglandins, progesterone and diazepam. Other agents that contribute to reducing the LOS tone are tobacco, alcohol and caffeine.

The symptoms are retrosternal burning ('heartburn', 'pyrosis') rather than pain and in severe cases acid regurgitation into the mouth after longstanding reflux. Dysphagia with odynophagia results from severe oesophagitis and/or ulceration. Chest pain occurs as a discrete entity when oesophagitis develops. In cases of severe GORD, inflammation and fibrosis in time result in progressive luminal narrowing, causing a stricture and dysphagia.

The diagnosis is established by history, endoscopy and biopsy. In patients with serious reflux symptoms, 24-hour ambulatory pH monitoring is undertaken. Manometry is useful to determine if the reflux symptoms are due to conditions such as early achalasia, associated with a high pressure.

Treatment is initiated with patient education, emphasising simple measures such as weight loss if the patient is overweight, avoiding highly spiced foods, alcohol and caffeine, drinking less fluid with a meal (a period of acid secretion) to minimise acid regurgitation and avoiding tight clothing around the waist. Acid regurgitation during sleep is lessened or even prevented by not drinking fluids or having a meal immediately before going to bed, and by elevating the head end of the bed with two building bricks.

Medical therapy depends on the severity of symptoms. GORD is one of the few medical conditions that can be treated successfully with H-2 receptor antagonists, proton pump inhibitors or surgery. The initial therapy recommended is H-2 receptor antagonists. In cases of uncomplicated GORD, the first approach could be a trial of treatment. An endoscopy is indicated if initial therapy has failed and if non-compliance is not an issue.

Non-resolution of symptoms and/or severe oesophagitis warrants the use of proton pump inhibitors. In patients with GORD and severe chest discomfort (due to an oesophageal cause), therapy with a proton pump inhibitor for 8 weeks is indicated. In these patients, endoscopy and/or 24-hour pH monitoring and/or motility studies are warranted; some recommend a 12-week course with a higher dose. Surgery is considered when medical therapy has failed and continuing oesophageal symptoms affect quality of life, and there is evidence of oesophageal ulceration or strictures. When symptoms resolve, maintenance therapy is necessary using the drug that was most effective during the symptomatic stage.

The complications of persistent, severe long-standing GORD are Barrett's oesophagus, where the lower oesophagus is lined by metaplastic columnar epithelial cells which have replaced the normal squamous epithelium. Since Barrett's oesophagus is a pre-malignant condition, monitoring with endoscopy and biopsy is necessary. In cases of mild dysplasia, endoscopy is performed 3–6 monthly. If there is no dysplasia, endoscopy is necessary only every 2 years. The presence of severe dysplasia requires oesophagectomy. Oesophageal mucosal ablation is an alternative treatment if surgery is contraindicated. Adenocarcinoma may develop under the treated epithelium.

The extra-oesophageal complications of severe GORD are bronchial asthma, chronic cough due to aspiration that may even result in bouts of pneumonia and hoarseness due to posterior laryngitis.

Infectious causes

Oesophagitis due to infectious causes occurs most often in immunocompromised individuals or in patients receiving radiotherapy for malignancy. Inflammation of the oesophagus results in dysphagia and also odynophagia. The most common infectious agent is *Candida albicans*. The diagnosis is made on endoscopy, which shows white plaques in the oesophagus. In more severe cases, friability and ulceration may occur.

A rare but important cause of dysphagia is due to the neurotoxin of the anaerobic, spore-forming bacterium *Clostridium botulinum*. Interest in this potentially lethal condition has increased due to the possible use of botulinum toxin as a weapon of human destruction. Food is the most common source of transmission. The initial presentation is cranial nerve involvement, manifesting as visual disturbances such as blurred vision, and also as dysphagia and dysarthria. Subsequently, symmetric, descending, flaccid paralysis occurs. Botulism mimics myasthenia gravis, a cerebrovascular accident or the Guillain-Barré syndrome. The prognosis is good if, in conjunction with supportive measures, the trivalent equine antitoxin is administered promptly.

Drug-associated injury

Medication can cause oesophagitis, especially if a swallowing difficulty exists. Drugs that cause mucosal irritation, damage or even ulceration through long contact with the mucosa lead to significant dysphagia. In elderly patients, medications that may cause oesophageal damage should be given under supervision and with adequate instructions to the patient or carer. Ideally, patients must be instructed to take (all) medication while sitting if practicable. Lying down immediately after medication should be avoided. For example, with alendronate therapy for osteoporosis, the manufacturer's contraindications are important: 'delayed oesophageal emptying and inability to sit upright for at least 30 minutes'. Other medications leading to oesophagitis and stricture formation are listed in Box 31.4.

Box 31.4 Therapeutic agents causing oesophageal dysphagia

- Alendronate
- Aspirin
- Non-steroidal anti-inflammatory drugs (NSAIDs)
- Vitamin C
- Potassium chloride
- Quinidine

Radiation injury

Radiation injury to the oesophagus can cause oesophagitis and is discussed on page 454 under Strictures.

Systemic conditions

Patients with scleroderma often have oesophageal involvement characterised by smooth muscle atrophy and fibrosis, causing decreased oesophageal contractibility and poor LOS tone. These changes, in turn, lead to gastro-oesophageal reflux, chronic oesophagitis and oesophageal stricture formation. Treatment is to control the gastro-oesophageal reflux and dilate the stricture if present. The CREST syndrome consists of calcinosis, Raynaud's phenomena, oesophageal dysmotility, sclerodactyly and telangiectasia. Dysphagia may also occur with mixed connective tissue disorders. In patients with amyloidosis, dysphagia depends on the extent of oesophageal involvement. Autonomic neuropathy in patients with diabetes mellitus can lead to dysphagia.

In a study of patients with various stages of Parkinson's disease, the majority complained of, in addition to dysphagia, acid regurgitation and heartburn. In half the patients, non-cardiac chest pain and manometric abnormalities occurred. These consisted of repetitive contractions, simultaneous contractions, reduced LOS pressure, and high-amplitude contractions. In addition to oropharyngeal dysphagia, oesophageal motor abnormalities are also common in Parkinson's disease.

Webs, rings and diverticula

These structural abnormalities are usually detected in later life. Webs are very thin mucosal and submucosal membranes protruding a few millimetres into the lumen of the oesophagus. They do not occur at a specific location but are mostly in the upper one-third of the oesophagus. A ring is a band-like constriction typically located at the gastro-oesophageal junction. The best known is Schatzki's ring (Figure 31.10).

A typical presentation due to a web or ring is intermittent dysphagia to solids such as bread or meat, but not to liquids. Food may be regurgitated. Patients are able to continue eating after regurgitating a bolus of food. Rarely, food is impacted requiring endoscopic removal. Dysphagia may be episodic and not recur for decades. In time, patients learn to consume foods that do not cause dysphagia and thoroughly chew 'difficult food', such as meat, or swallow small portions of food with plenty of fluid. Chewing food well is an important preventative measure. The presence of a web or ring is confirmed by radiology. Treatment is by dilatation or by surgical intervention.

Diverticula are less common in the oesophagus than in the hypopharynx and are also less symptomatic. Traction diverticula are located in the mid oesophagus. They are usually asymptomatic and require no treatment. Pulsion diverticula (epiphrenic diverticula) are due to abnormal motor activity or a structural abnormality and are located most often in the mid oesophagus or just above the

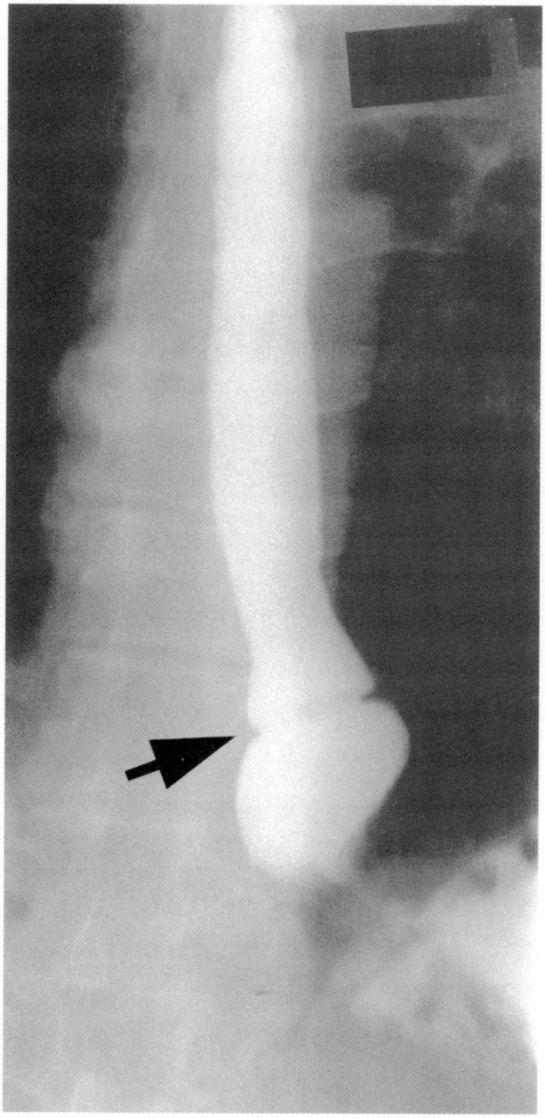

Figure 31.10 Schatzki's ring. Note the tight constriction at the lower oesophageal sphincter

Courtesy of Dr Anil B. Utturkar, Senior Radiologist, The Queen Elizabeth Hospital, Adelaide

LOS (Figure 31.11). The latter are occasional causes of dysphagia. The diagnosis is by radiology but a subsequent endoscopic examination is always prudent. An underlying muscular disorder may need to be excluded by oesophageal manometry. Treatment of symptomatic diverticula is diverticulectomy and surgical myotomy or dilatation.

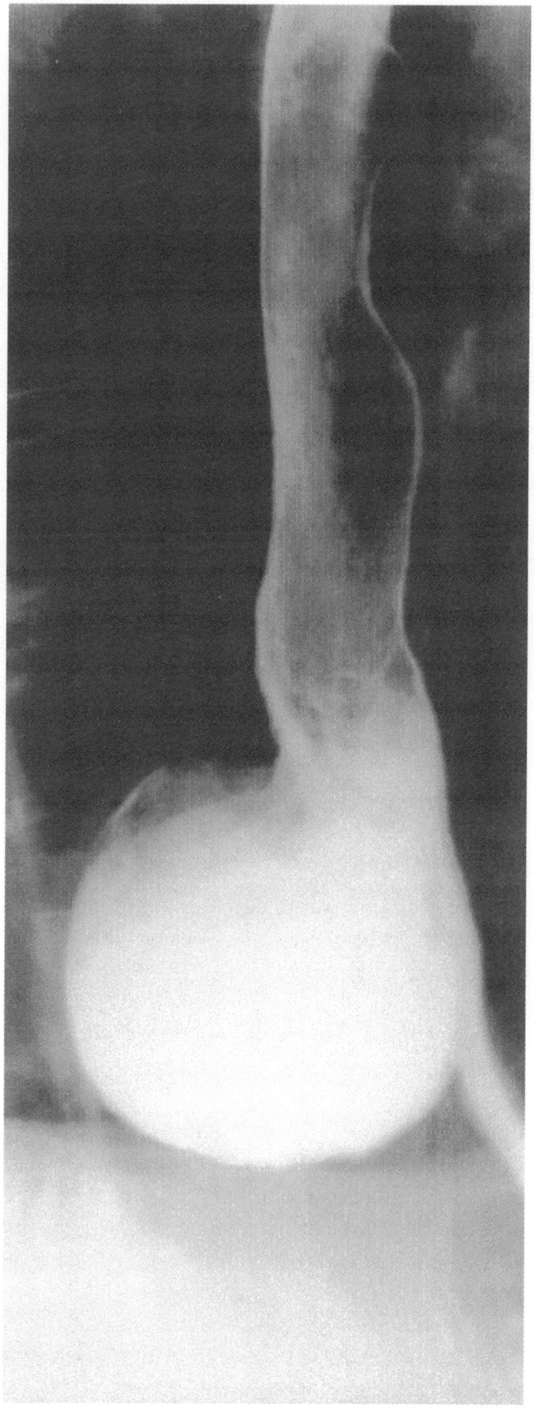

Figure 31.11 Large epiphrenic diverticulum above the diaphragm with retained food material

Courtesy of Dr Anil B. Utturkar, Senior Radiologist, The Queen Elizabeth Hospital, Adelaide

Strictures

Strictures may be benign or malignant. Benign strictures are usually the result of longstanding GORD, although other causes of inflammation or injury to the oesophageal mucosa can result in stricture formation. Corrosive agents, such as acids or alkalis, ingested accidentally or deliberately, invariably result in stricture formation. Radiation for head and neck malignancies increases the risk of both oesophageal stricture and, rarely, a malignancy of the oesophagus. Although infrequent, Crohn's disease can cause an oesophageal stricture. Severe narrowing of the lumen due to a constricting lesion can ultimately cause dysphagia to liquids as well.

The diagnosis is made by radiology and confirmed by endoscopy and biopsy. Malignant strictures are the result of neoplasia of the oesophagus. Radiology may be misleading when deciding whether a stricture is malignant or benign. Endoscopy with biopsy is essential. Treatment is directed to the cause and the stricture itself may require a series of dilatations. The most favoured intervention for benign stricture is endoscopic dilatation. A new technique is endoscopic mucosal injection of corticosteroid.

Neoplasia

Malignant tumours are more common than benign tumours, which are rare. The most common site for malignancy is the lower one-third of the oesophagus (Figures 31.12–31.14). The majority of tumours are squamous cell carcinoma. The aetiological factors associated with squamous cell carcinoma are cigarette smoking, a high alcohol consumption, untreated gluten sensitive enteropathy (coeliac disease), achalasia, mucosal damage from acids and alkalis and radiation therapy. A rare cause of adenocarcinoma of the oesophagus is the Paterson-Kelly syndrome. Barrett's oesophagus, discussed previously, leads to adenocarcinoma.

Direct invasion of the oesophagus may occur from the stomach, hypopharynx, thyroid and tracheobronchial tree. True metastatic carcinoma of the oesophagus occurs in about 1–3% of patients dying of carcinoma, and the largest proportion is due to lung and breast malignancy. Other malignancy sites resulting in metastatic carcinoma of the oesophagus are the pancreas, testis, eye, prostate, bone, cervix and endometrium.

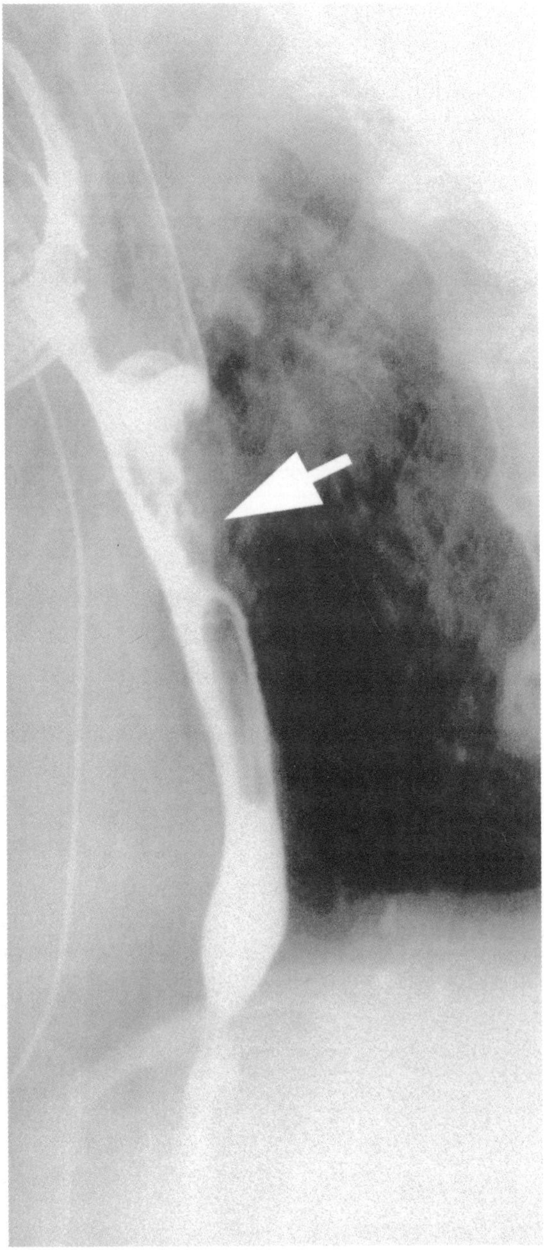

Figure 31.12 Carcinoma of the oesophagus

Courtesy of Dr Anil B. Utturkar, Senior Radiologist, The Queen Elizabeth Hospital, Adelaide

Treatment is directed to maintain a patent oesophageal lumen and includes dilatation, surgical

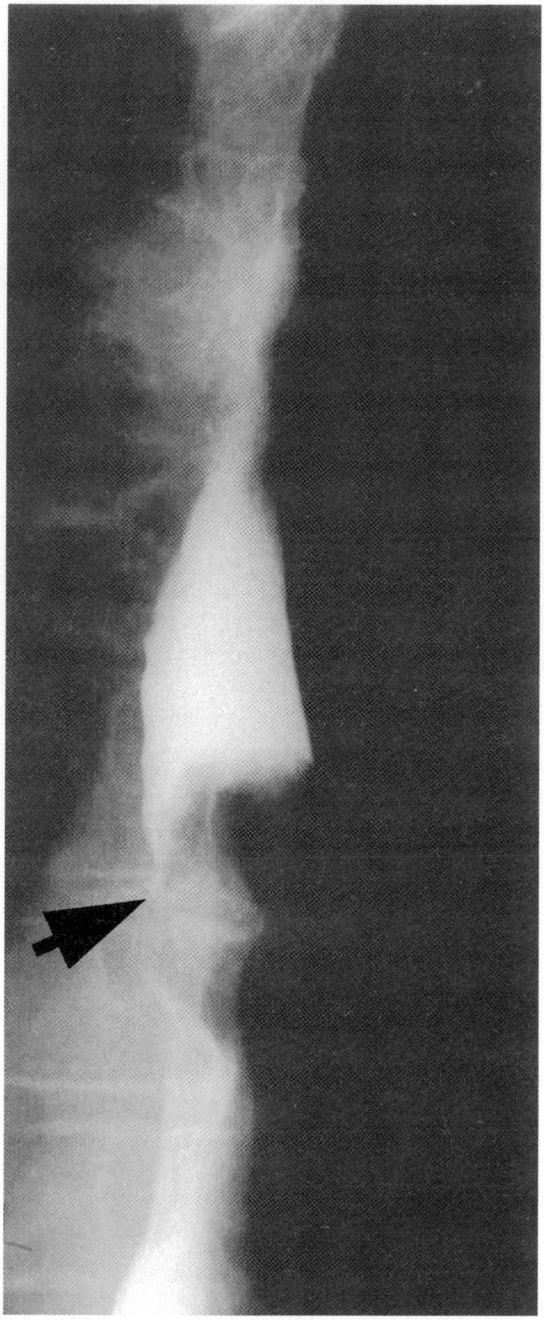

Figure 31.13 Carcinoma of the oesophagus

Courtesy of Dr Anil B. Utturkar, Senior Radiologist, The Queen Elizabeth Hospital, Adelaide

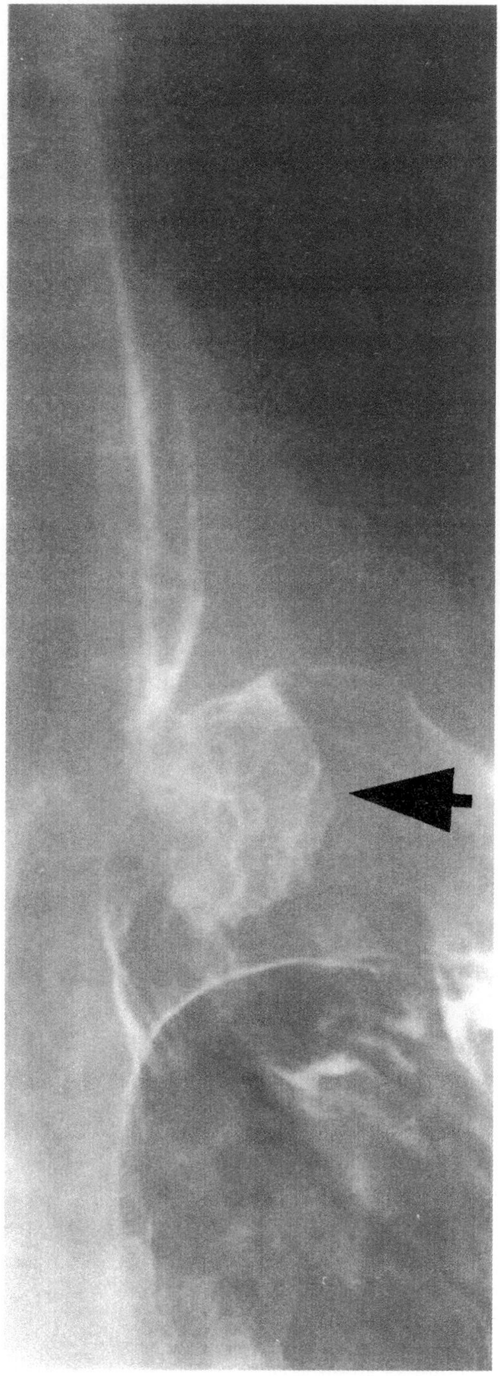

Figure 31.14 Carcinoma in a hiatus hernia: a moderate-sized polypoidal mass owing to a carcinoma within the hiatus hernia

Courtesy of Dr Anil B. Utturkar, Senior Radiologist, The Queen Elizabeth Hospital, Adelaide

resection, chemotherapy and/or radiotherapy, endoscopic laser therapy, bipolar electrocautery and stent placement. The choice of intervention is determined by factors such as the extent of the narrowing, and what resources and expertise are available in a particular institution. Modern self-expanding stents are particularly useful although expensive.

Extra-oesophageal causes

Since the oesophagus is relatively mobile and elastic, dysphagia occurs only if there is significant external compression.

Dysphagia may be the result of an aberrant right subclavian artery, known as dysphagia lusoria (Figure 31.15), where the artery appears to arise abnormally from the thoracic aorta, passing behind the oesophagus. Although this is a congenital anomaly, dysphagia may manifest in later life due to atherosclerotic changes 'stiffening' the artery. Radiological examination shows that the artery usually indents the oesophagus at the level of T3 or T4. The diagnosis is confirmed by angiography or computerised tomographic scan. Treatment consists of surgical reconstruction of the artery. Compression of the oesophagus can also be due to a thoracic aortic aneurysm or a mediastinal mass, including malignant lymphadenopathy as a result of a neoplasm of the respiratory tract, or lymphoma (Figure 31.16).

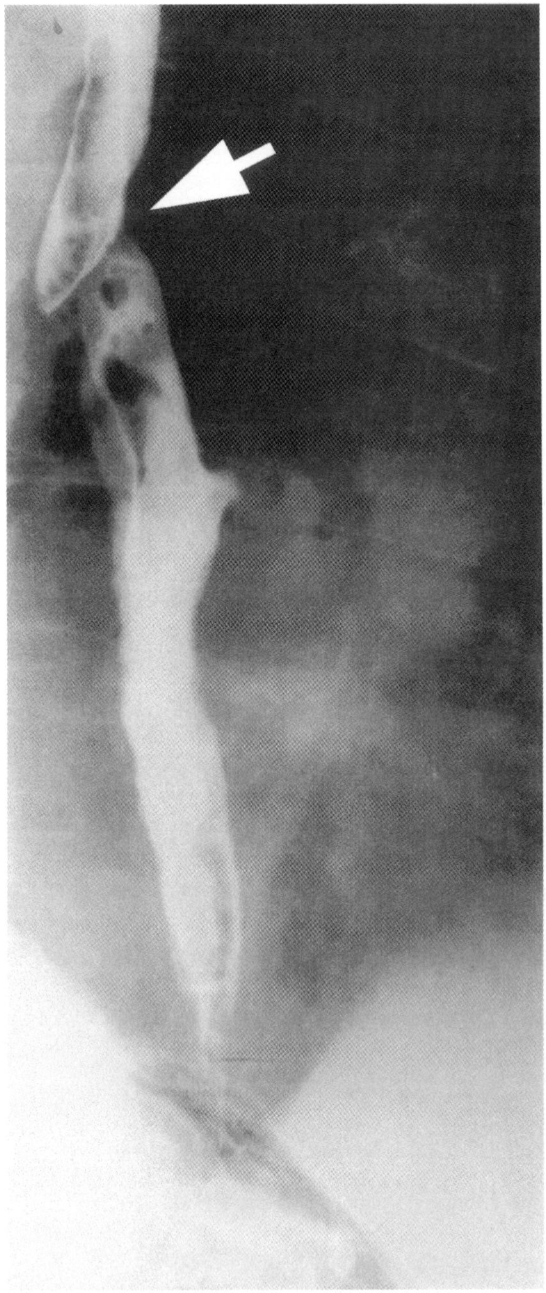

Figure 31.15 Dysphagia lusoria. A vascular impression on the upper oesophagus is causing compression. Also note the small oesophageal traction diverticulum

Courtesy of Dr Anil B. Utturkar, Senior Radiologist, The Queen Elizabeth Hospital, Adelaide

Issues of management

Dysphagia is frequently a complex and multifactorial problem that requires a multidisciplinary approach for optimal evaluation and management. The management team should include a speech pathologist. The indications for referral to a speech pathologist are:

- decreased mental status or alertness compromising feeding and nutritional status
- changes in approach to food, such as avoiding certain foods, modifying consistency, prolonged meal times
- impaired oropharyngeal function, such as dysarthria, dysphonia, coughing or choking

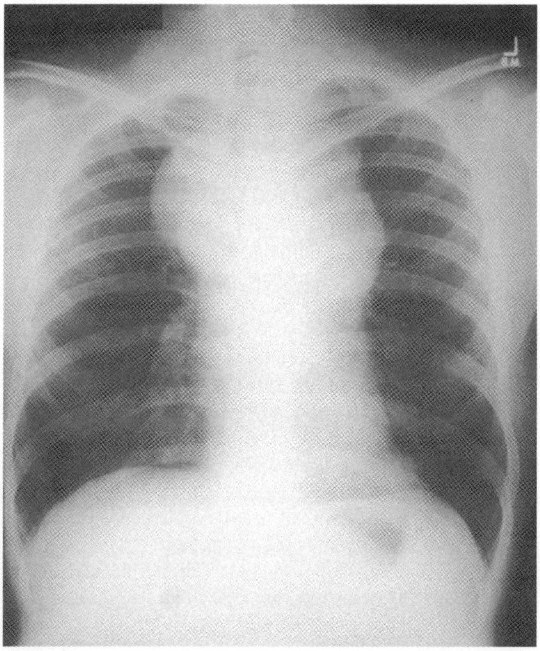

Figure 31.16 Mediastinal mass shown on chest X-ray. A lymphoma is causing obstruction by extrinsic compression of the oesophagus

Courtesy of Dr Anil B. Utturkar, Senior Radiologist, The Queen Elizabeth Hospital, Adelaide

- patient or caregiver reports of dysphagia, odynophagia, a sensation of sticking or regurgitation of food and/or fluid.

The assessment of dysphagia includes a detailed history of the problem and a systemic physical examination, especially of the central nervous system. It is essential that the speech pathologist undertakes the clinical swallowing examination. This involves assessing the motor and sensory systems, particularly oropharyngeal sensation, muscle function and airway protection that occurs during swallowing. The assessment of airway protection involves observing:

- phonation
- volitional cough
- the cough reflex.

Observing a patient's ability to swallow food and liquid enables postural adjustments to be made and manoeuvres to be suggested to assist with swallowing, alterations to food and liquid consistency and, if necessary, planning further investigations.

Further instrumental assessment is necessary and the frequently used assessments are videofluoroscopy and flexible endoscopy. Their use depends on the outcomes of the clinical examination, the availability of instrumentation and patient compliance.

Videofluoroscopy involves the dynamic radiographic examination of the swallowing mechanism using barium. The modified barium swallow is a variation of the standard barium swallow study in that it concentrates primarily on the oropharyngeal phase of the swallowing mechanism. The protocol includes both anterior-posterior and lateral views during the ingestion of a variety of graduated food and fluid consistencies. It is a vital tool for a comprehensive examination of oropharyngeal dysphagia. Forty per cent of patients with dysphagia after a cerebrovascular accident aspirate silently and videofluoroscopy enables such problems to be identified rapidly and comprehensively. It is also a valuable management tool enabling the speech pathologist to directly observe the patient using various swallowing strategies and to monitor the response to treatment.

Endoscopic assessment of swallowing (EAS) allows the direct visualisation of the hypopharynx and laryngopharynx during swallowing, providing specific information on the anatomy of the pharynx and larynx, assessment of laryngeal sensitivity, oropharyngeal secretion management and assessment of the pharyngeal phase. EAS is particularly sensitive in detecting aspiration. It also provides information on the effectiveness and/or response to therapeutic manoeuvres and interventions. EAS is convenient to the patient and therapist as it is a bedside examination that provides direct visual feedback to the patient about various swallowing manoeuvres and therapy techniques.

In patients with oesophageal dysphagia, the evaluation and management is similar to that of those with oropharyngeal dysphagia regarding the importance of a comprehensive history taking and physical examination, and ensuring that the management approach is multidisciplinary. A chest radiograph is an important preliminary investigation.

Endoscopy is a major diagnostic component. Suspected motor abnormalities of the oesophagus may require oesophageal manometry to complement radiological studies and endoscopy to document the nature and severity of the problem.

Issues to be taken into consideration in the management of dysphagia irrespective of aetiology include determining the cause, the safety of feeding and planning nutritional management (oral versus non-oral). When the patient is unable to take adequate oral nutrition, alternative feeding is recommended. Percutaneous endoscopic gastrostomy (PEG) is recommended when long-term alternative feeding is required. Other issues include the direct treatment of the underlying disease or process, possible surgical management, swallowing therapy and quality of life issues. In older patients, dysphagia is a common and important problem which should be actively sought and addressed to maintain optimal health status by preventing dehydration and nutritional problems.

Bibliography and further reading

Bassotti, G., Germani, U., Pagliaricci, S., Plesa, A., Giulietti, O., Mannarino, E. & Morelli, A. (1998), 'Esophageal manometric abnormalities in Parkinson's disease', *Dysphagia*, 13, pp. 28–31.

Beck, I. T., Champion, M. C., Lemire, S., et al. (1997), 'The Second Canadian Consensus Conference on the Management of Patients with Gastroesophageal Reflux Disease', *Canadian Journal of Gastroenterology*, 11 (suppl. B), pp. 7B–20B.

Bucholz, D. W. & Robbins, J. (1997), 'Neurologic diseases affecting oropharyngeal swallowing', in Perlman, A. L. & Schulze-Delrieu, K. (eds), *Deglutition and its Disorders: Anatomy, Physiology, Clinical Diagnosis and Management*, Singular Publishing, San Diego, pp. 319–42.

Feinberg, M. J., Knebl, J. K., Tully, J. & Segall, L. (1990), 'Aspiration and the elderly', *Dysphagia*, 5, pp. 61–71.

Groher, M. E. & Bukatinan, R. (1986), 'The prevalence of swallowing disorders in two teaching hospitals', *Dysphagia*, 1, pp. 3–6.

Logemann, J. A. (1990), 'Effects of aging on the swallowing mechanism', *Otolaryngologic Clinics of North America*, 23, pp. 1045–56.

Mackey, J. R., Desai, S., Larratt, L., Cwik, V. & Nabholtz, J. M. (1997), 'Myasthenia gravis in association with allogeneic bone marrow transplantation: clinical observations, therapeutic implications and review of literature', *Bone Marrow Transplantation*, 19, pp. 939–42.

Nagaya, M., Kachi, T., Yamada, T. & Igata, A. (1998), 'Videofluorographic study of swallowing in Parkinson's disease', *Dysphagia*, 13, pp. 95–100.

Narne, S., Cutrone, C., Bonavina, L., Chella, B. & Peracchia, A. (1999), 'Endoscopic diverticulotomy for the treatment of Zenker's diverticulum: results in 102 patients with staple-assisted endoscopy', *Annals of Otology, Rhinology and Laryngology*, 108, pp. 810–15.

Palmer, J. B. & DuChane, A. S. (1991), 'Rehabilitation and swallowing disorders due to stroke', *Archives of Physical Medicine and Rehabilitation Clinics of North America*, 2, pp. 529–46.

Priefer, B. A. & Robbins, J. (1997), 'Eating changes in mild-stage Alzheimer's disease: a pilot study', *Dysphagia*, 12, pp. 212–21.

Schofield, P. M., Whorwell, P. J., Jones, P. E., Brooks, N. H. & Bennett, D. H. (1988), 'Differentiation of "esophageal" and "cardiac" chest pain', *American Journal of Cardiology*, 62, pp. 315–16.

Shapiro, R. L., Hatheway, C. & Swerdlow, D. L. (1998), 'Botulism in the United States: a clinical and epidemiologic review', *Annals of Internal Medicine*, 129, pp. 221–8.

Sokoloff, L. G. & Pavlakovic, R. (1997), 'Neuroleptic-induced dysphagia', *Dysphagia*, 12, pp. 177–9.

Soykan, I., Sarosiek, I., Shifflett, J., Wooten, G. F. & McCallum, R. W. (1997), 'Effect of chronic oral domperidone therapy on gastrointestinal symptoms and gastric emptying in patients with Parkinson's disease', *Movement Disorders*, 12, pp. 952–7.

Trupe, E. H., Siebens, H. & Siebens, A. (1984), 'Prevalence of feeding and swallowing disorders in a nursing home', *Archives of Physical Medicine and Rehabilitation*, 65, pp. 651–2.

Chapter 32
Weight loss

MICHAEL WOODWARD

Introduction

Weight loss is a common problem in older people, yet frequently it is not recognised and is undertreated. It results from a combination of the illnesses that are more common in older people, the treatments for these illnesses and a physiological reduction in appetite with ageing. The most serious consequence of weight loss is the development of undernutrition, which in turn increases morbidity and mortality. Weight loss can be an important indication of underlying disease, and assessment must include a search for a potentially treatable cause. Too often older people are assessed in the community or in hospital and scant regard is paid to their nutritional status. It is not uncommon for older people to lose a large proportion of their body weight in institutional settings, including hospitals, and have no diagnostic work-up or intervention. Weight loss should be promptly recognised and assessed: earlier diagnosis and management will lead to a greater likelihood of a successful outcome.

The term 'malnutrition' refers to either under- or overnutrition. The term 'cachexia' is derived from the Greek words for bad (*kakos*) and condition (*hexis*) and refers to severe undernutrition. Overnutrition (obesity) will not be discussed in this chapter.

Aetiology and epidemiology

The maintenance of weight is determined by nutrient intake, absorption, energy expenditure and the formation and maintenance of body organs and tissues. Weight loss occurs when there is insufficient intake or absorption, or excess energy expenditure, of a significant duration. Often an illness affects several of these determinants. For instance, severe cardiac disease can lead to a wasting syndrome due to a combination of anorexia caused by early satiation and the effects of medications, combined with a protein-losing enteropathy and reduced liver protein synthesis. Alzheimer's disease can cause weight loss from reduced appetite (due to altered cerebral function) and excess activity from wandering and pacing. Parkinson's disease is associated with weight loss from a combination of reduced food intake, partly due to impaired swallowing and impaired ability to feed oneself, and to increased energy expenditure from tremor. Cancer causes weight loss through several mechanisms:

chemotherapy can cause anorexia; there is production of tumour necrosis factor (TNF) which causes a loss of muscle mass; and the tumour itself may affect swallowing (e.g. ENT tumours) or absorption (some bowel and pancreatic cancers).

Weight loss is not an inevitable consequence of ageing, but certain factors make weight loss more likely (see Table 32.1). Weight loss and malnutrition are particularly common in residential and institutional care.

Table 32.1 Risk factors for weight loss

Age related	Reduced taste Dry mouth Anorexia of ageing Hormonal changes
Social	Poverty Social isolation Inability to shop, prepare and cook food Bereavement Failure of institutions to cater for food preferences, including ethnic preferences Insufficient assistance with feeding Lack of knowledge of correct diet, including fad diets Cigarette smoking
Psychological	Depression Alcoholism Anorexia nervosa Paranoia Psychiatric medications
Medical	Cancer Dysphagia Poor diet Periodontal disease Parkinson's disease Stroke Essential tremor Malabsorption syndromes Medications (some) Infection AIDS Cardiac disease COPD Rheumatoid arthritis Diabetes Thyrotoxicosis Hyperglycaemia Phaeochromocytoma Renal disease Hepatobiliary disease

Prevalence and incidence

Prevalence figures are plagued by varying definitions of undernutrition. However, up to 15% of ambulatory older people in the community, 25–65% of acutely hospitalised older people and 25–60% of institutionalised older people are undernourished. Incidence figures for weight loss also vary with methodology. In the community, 13% of older persons have an annual weight loss of 4% of their body weight. Some 20% of acutely hospitalised patients have an average nutrient intake of less than 50% of their calculated maintenance energy requirements, and in medical wards the average daily caloric intake of older people has been calculated at 63% of maintenance requirements. A weight loss of 2.5 kg over 6 months has been found in 19% of nursing home patients.

Pathophysiology

There is a reduced food intake in older age. From age 20 to 80, average intake falls by 5530 kJ in males and 2633 kJ in females. This occurs mainly from reduced fat intake and occurs despite an increase in body mass index in middle age. Body mass index only starts to fall after the age of 75. The reduction in food intake is a response to the decrease in physical activity and reduced metabolic rate that occurs with ageing.

There are several causes of this anorexia of ageing. Taste is reduced with age. The gustatory papillae atrophy, taste thresholds increase and there is a reduction in smell, which accounts for much of taste. In addition, there are changes in neurotransmitters and peptide hormones. The endogenous opioid feeding drive is reduced with ageing, and there is decreased opioid receptor binding activity. Cholecystokinin, which is released when fat and protein pass through the gut, has an increased satiating effect in older age, and inappropriately elevated levels have been found in undernourished older people. Changes in other peptides with age may also contribute to the anorexia of ageing; these include neuropeptide Y, corticotrophin releasing factor and amylin.

Body fat regulates appetite through leptin, with increased fat causing more leptin secretion, which in turn reduces appetite and food intake. Thus the increase in adipose tissue in middle age may contribute to a relative anorexia through increased leptin production.

With advancing age, older people experience more satiation with a meal compared with younger people. This is related partly to changes in cholecystokinin effects, but also to decreased nitric oxide synthase activity, resulting in reduced relaxation of the fundus in response to food in the stomach.

Protein-energy undernutrition

Protein-energy undernutrition (PEU) is a serious syndrome characterised by weight loss associated with depletion of fat stores and muscle mass. There is a continuing spectrum of undernutrition from mild PEU to that of visceral organ failure resulting in gross peripheral oedema. Older people are particularly at risk of PEU. Other terms used to describe forms of PEU are 'marasmus' and 'kwashiorkor'. Marasmus occurs with energy depletion and is marked by weight loss and depletion of fat stores and muscle mass. Kwashiorkor occurs with protein depletion (despite reasonable total energy intake, usually from carbohydrates) and is characterised by depletion of visceral protein stores (muscle and albumin). However, clinically there is only limited value in distinguishing these subtypes.

Consequences

Weight loss and undernutrition can have serious health consequences for older people. Mortality is increased: a 90 day mortality of 50% has been demonstrated in patients admitted to hospital with PEU, compared to 16% in adequately nourished patients. Low body weight and hypoalbuminaemia increase hospital mortality. Severely malnourished medical patients have increased 1 year mortality, are more likely to be dependent in daily activities 3 months after discharge, and to spend more time in nursing homes during the year after discharge. Mortality following a hip fracture is strongly related to poor caloric intake and protein depletion.

In community studies, mortality rate doubles in women with a recent weight loss of greater than 15%. In men, both voluntary and involuntary weight loss of greater than 5% significantly increases mortality. Undernutrition also causes significant morbidity. It is a risk factor for fractured neck of femur, pressure ulcers, impaired immune responses and infections, and is associated with longer hospital lengths of stay.

Clinical tests

There are several tools with which to measure nutritional status. When there is marked cachexia, inspection is usually sufficient. However, for less malnourished patients, inspection alone is inaccurate. For example, some undernourished people, particularly those who are protein depleted, may not appear thin or wasted. Hypoproteinaemia related oedema can make an undernourished person appear well nourished.

There are five main methods of assessing nutritional status in older people. No single method is ideal, and it is often appropriate to commence with a screening test and, if indicated, proceed to a more detailed assessment.

1. Nutritional screening

Nutritional screening is the process of identifying the characteristics known to be associated with nutritional problems. One test is the Australian Nutrition Screening Initiative (ANSI—see Box 32.1). This checklist can be self-administered or used by health professionals to identify those older people living independently in the community who may be at risk of undernutrition. A related tool, the Nutritional Risk Index, consists of 16 items that tap into 5 dimensions for nutritional risk: mechanics of food intake, prescribed dietary restrictions, morbid conditions affecting food intake, discomfort associated with the outcomes of food intake, and significant changes in dietary habits.

2. Clinical evaluation

This is best standardised. The Subjective Global Assessment of Nutritional Status (see Box 32.2) consists of 11 items which incorporate a history of

Box 32.1 Australian Nutrition Screening Initiative

	Yes	No
I have an illness or condition that made me change the kind and/or amount of food I eat.	2	0
I eat at least 3 meals per day.	0	3
I eat fruit or vegetables most days.	0	2
I eat dairy products most days.	0	2
I have 3 or more glasses of beer, wine or spirits almost every day.	3	0
I have 6 to 8 cups of fluids (e.g. water, juice, tea or coffee) most days.	0	1
I have teeth, mouth or swallowing problems that make it hard for me to eat.	4	0
I always have enough money to buy food.	0	3
I eat alone most of the time.	2	0
I take 3 or more different prescribed or over the counter medicines every day.	3	0
Without wanting to, I have lost or gained 5 kg in the last 6 months.	2	0
I am always able to shop, cook and/or feed myself.	0	2
TOTAL		

Interpretation:
0–3: Minimal risk
4–5: Moderate risk
≥ 6: High risk

Source: P. S. Lipski (1996), 'Australian Nutrition Screening Initiative', *Australian Journal on Ageing*, 15, pp. 14–15.

weight loss, the presence of gastrointestinal symptoms, an assessment of muscle mass and an assessment of subcutaneous fat and oedema. While it has been validated for hospitalised elderly veterans, it has not so far been fully validated for older people. Other evaluation tools used in hospitalised patients include the Hospital Prognostic Index, the Prognostic Nutritional Index and Nutrition Risk Index. These use a mixture of clinical, arthropometric, biochemical and immunological tests.

3. Arthropometry

Arthropometric measures give an indication of body composition. More commonly used measures are shown in Table 32.2. Each measures a different aspect of nutritional status so they complement each other. Body mass index (BMI), arm circumference and triceps skinfold thickness (TSF) are measures of fat mass, but all are affected by hydration and TSF is affected by skin changes with ageing. Given the redistribution of body fat with age, measures of central adiposity (e.g. abdominal skinfold thickness) may be better measures of fat mass in older people, especially men. Serial skinfold circumference measurements may indicate changes in body composition that may not be detected with body weight alone, such as in the presence of oedema. All values are affected by age alone, even in the absence of significant undernutrition, and normative values are not available for those over the age of 75, limiting the usefulness of these measures in this age group.

Because of interobserver variability, the degree of training needed, and the wide range of variation in reference values for healthy older people, the best arthropometric measurement for nutritional screening is probably the BMI. Arm demispan can be used as a substitute for height, which can be difficult to measure in some older people (e.g. those with poor mobility or those who are bed-bound).

4. Laboratory tests

Measures of protein status such as levels of circulating proteins (albumin, prealbumin, transferrin and retinol-binding protein) can be markers of protein deficiency. Of these, albumin is the most widely used as it reflects chronic protein status, although its levels can be affected by other conditions such as acute sepsis. Other proteins have

Box 32.2 Subjective Global Assessment (SGA) of Nutritional Status

(Select appropriate category with a ✓, or enter numerical value where indicated by '#'.)

A. History

1. Weight change
   Overall loss in past 6 months = # _______ kg; % loss = # _______
   Change in past 2 weeks: _______ increase
   _______ no change
   _______ decrease
2. Dietary intake change (relative to normal)
   _______ no change,
   _______ change: _______ duration = # _______ weeks
   _______ type: _______ suboptimal solid diet _______ full liquid diet
   _______ hypocaloric liquids _______ starvation
3. Gastrointestinal symptoms (that persisted for > 2 weeks)
   _______ none _______ nausea _______ vomiting _______ diarrhoea _______ anorexia
4. Functional capacity
   _______ no dysfunction (e.g. full capacity)
   _______ dysfunction: _______ duration = # _______ weeks
   _______ type: _______ working suboptimally
   _______ ambulatory
   _______ bedridden
5. Disease and its relation to nutritional requirements
   Primary diagnosis (specify): _______________________
   Metabolic demand (stress): _______ no stress _______ low stress
   _______ moderate stress _______ high stress

B. Physical (for each trait specify: 0 = normal, 1+ = mild, 2+ = moderate, 3+ = severe)
   # _______ loss of subcutaneous fat (triceps, chest)
   # _______ muscle wasting (quadriceps, deltoids)
   # _______ ankle oedema
   # _______ sacral oedema
   # _______ ascites

C. SGA rating (select one)
   _______ A = Well nourished
   _______ B = Moderately (or suspected of being) malnourished
   _______ C = Severely malnourished

Note: Final SGA rating is subjective, not using a numerical rating scale.
Source: A. S. Detsky, J. R. McLaughlin, J. P. Baker, N. Johnston, S. Whittaker, R. A. Mendelson, & K. N. Jeejeebhoy (1987), 'What is Subjective Global Assessment of Nutritional Status?', *Journal of Parenteral and Enteral Nutrition*, 11, pp. 8–13.

shorter half-lives than albumin and reflect more acute changes in protein status.

Micronutrient levels may also be markers of undernutrition. Vitamins such as folate, the B group, C, D, E and A may be reduced. Trace elements such as zinc, selenium and cobalt may be reduced, but low levels may have other causes. For instance, zinc is redistributed to inflamed areas around skin wounds, and a low serum level may reflect this redistribution rather than a true deficiency.

Table 32.2 Arthropometric measures

Measure	Significance	Calculation	Evidence of undernutrition
Body mass index (BMI)	Overall body fat	Weight (kg) divided by square of height (m)	< 22
Skin-fold thickness	Subcutaneous fat	Measured using a calliper—e.g. over triceps (TSF)	< 4 mm (male) < 9 mm (female)
Mid-arm muscle area (MAMA)	Skeletal muscle mass	$\frac{MAMC^2}{4\pi}$ where MAMC (mid-arm muscle circumference) $= MAC\ (cm) - \pi \frac{TSF\ (mm)}{10}$ and MAC (mid-arm circumference) is measured with a tape	< 16

Low or falling serum cholesterol may also be a marker of undernutrition, and is associated with higher 1 year mortality.

Antigenic challenge often fails to provoke an immune response in undernourished people. This failure can be used as a marker of undernutrition. Delayed cutaneous hypersensitivity to a panel of antigens, including *Candida albicans*, mumps, tuberculosis and streptokinase/streptodornase, can be sought. Other markers include reduced total lymphocyte count and reduced T and B cell function. However, such measures are not specific; reductions also occur with severe sepsis and disseminated cancer.

5. *Measures of nutritional intake*

Diet recall is performed by asking subjects to recollect the foods they have eaten during a given time frame, usually 24 hours. Memory related measurement errors can occur. Best results are obtained when dietitians perform this task. The 24 hour recall appears to perform as well as actual food weighing or longer periods of diary recording for estimating the mean nutrient intake for a group. Variation in individual diets makes a single 24 hour recall an inaccurate measure of a single person's usual intake. Generally 7–14 days should be recorded to estimate an individual's intake, and longer periods to estimate intake of specific dietary components (e.g. cholesterol, vitamins).

Food records can be more accurate, but are more burdensome for the individual. During a specified time frame, the individual records all the food she eats, either estimated or by weighing. A less burdensome approach is pre- and post-meal photography of the food, especially helpful in hospitals and other institutions.

Diet histories are performed during interviews, usually by dietitians, and consist of open-ended questions that attempt to ascertain the person's usual food intakes. They take at least an hour and are therefore impractical as screening tools.

Food frequency questionnaires attempt to estimate the customary dietary intake over a specified period of time (e.g. 1 year). The individual reports on her usual frequency and portion size of various foods from a predetermined list. These are used to estimate nutrient intake in groups and are lengthy to administer, requiring a trained person, such as a dietitian, so are not suitable as screening tools.

Diagnosis: The common causes of weight loss

Conditions causing reduced food intake

Decreased appetite

Apart from anorexia of ageing, several illnesses can suppress appetite. Peptic ulceration, gastric carcinoma, post-gastrectomy syndrome, biliary disease, mesenteric ischaemia, severe constipation and colitis can all cause anorexia. Systemic diseases that can suppress appetite include cancer, infections, alcoholism, liver dysfunction, renal impairment, chronic lung disease and congestive cardiac failure. The latter two conditions can also cause dyspnoea on eating, further reducing oral intake. Hypercalcaemia and zinc deficiency have also been associated with anorexia. Cigarette smoking is also a cause of anorexia. Psychiatric causes of reduced appetite include depression, anxiety, paranoia, dementia and anorexia nervosa—all of which can be associated with reduced appetite or failure to remember to eat.

Many medications can suppress appetite. Table 32.3 summarises the more common ones, but almost all medications can cause anorexia. Older people have altered pharmokinetic characteristics, predisposing them to drug toxicity, and toxic levels of drugs are most prone to suppress appetite. Examples of drugs that normally do not cause anorexia but do when toxic levels develop include phenytoin, carbamazepine, valproate and aminoglycosides.

Oral disease

Mouth diseases are a relatively uncommon cause of weight loss in older people, although cancers of the

Table 32.3 Medications that can cause anorexia

Antibiotics	All, but especially: Metronidazole Griseofulvin
Antineoplastics	All
Antirheumatics	Non-steroidal anti-inflammatory drugs COX-2 inhibitors Penicillamine Prednisolone
Analgesics	Opiates (morphine, codeine) Dextropropoxyphene
Cardiovascular agents	Amiodarone Digoxin Frusemide Spironolactone
CNS agents	Haloperidol Phenothiazines (e.g. thioridazine) Selective serotonin reuptake inhibitors (SSRIs—e.g. sertraline, paroxetine, fluoxetine) Venlafaxine Levodopa Lithium
Gastrointestinal agents	Cimetidine Psyllium
Cholinergic agents	Donepezil Rivastigmine
Nutritional supplements	Iron sulphate Potassium salts Tocopherol (vitamin E)—in excess Cholecalciferol (vitamin D)—in excess
Metabolic agents	Metformin
Pulmonary agents	Theophylline

tongue, gingiva and floor of the mouth may present late, at a stage which can interfere with mastication. In addition, surgical resections of these conditions tend to be quite radical, reducing the ability to chew and swallow. Mouth ulcers and oral conditions can also impair oral intake. Although the majority of older people do not have their own teeth, this only affects oral intake if they do not have dentures, or if the dentures are loose-fitting or associated with ulcers. Severe periodontal disease may also be responsible for reduced oral intake.

Older people are more prone to dry mouth from reduced salivary gland excretion and this can affect chewing. This is most pronounced in Sjögren's syndrome or when strong anticholinergic agents such as tricyclic antidepressants or oxybutynin are being used.

Neuromuscular diseases of the pharynx and oesophagus

Dysphagia after a stroke is common and can cause severe weight loss, as well as aspiration if oral intake of inappropriate consistency is used. Other neurological conditions that can cause dysphagia include motor neurone disease and Steele-Richardson syndrome (progressive supranuclear palsy). In Parkinson's disease, dysphagia is mainly due to difficulty with the oesopharyngeal phase of swallowing, which is not levodopa responsive. Oesophageal achalasia can be acquired in older people. Oesophageal mobility disorders such as diffuse oesophageal spasm are a relatively common cause of swallowing difficulties in older people.

Structural lesions of the pharynx and oesophagus

Carcinomas of these organs most commonly present with dysphagia, pain and weight loss. Benign oesophageal strictures and webs, oesophageal pouches and an oesophageal diverticulum can also impair swallowing and cause weight loss.

Social

The major social cause of weight loss is poverty, which can limit access to foods. Poverty may be partly iatrogenic: when physicians prescribe expensive medications or other treatments, this may use money that would otherwise be put towards food. Unsubsidised drugs such as donepezil used in Alzheimer's disease can be a factor here. Social isolation may reduce access to shops or cooking facilities. Also, people are less inclined to prepare well balanced meals when cooking only for themselves, and may eat less when dining alone.

In institutional settings, there may be a failure to attend to ethnic or other dietary food preferences. Shortages of staff may limit carers' ability to assist older disabled people with their meals, and older people may not be able to open extensively packaged food. Budgetary constraints may also reduce the attractiveness and variety of food in these settings.

Decreased food absorption

Decreased food absorption due to acute and chronic diarrhoeal diseases and malabsorption is accompanied by weight loss and is discussed in detail in Chapter 34. Malabsorption of food is accompanied by weight loss and often also by diarrhoea and steatorrhoea. In addition, there may be abdominal symptoms such as pain and distension. The malabsorption may extend to all components of the diet or may be isolated to specific nutrients. Fat malabsorption is confirmed by an increased 3 day faecal fat, while consuming a relatively fatty diet. The diet and collection may prove difficult in older people. Carbohydrate malabsorption can be confirmed by a xylose absorption test, although this is rarely performed. Micronutrient malabsorption is confirmed by a low level on an appropriate blood test.

Pancreatic disease

Chronic pancreatitis accounts for half of all cases of steatorrhoea in older people. Undernutrition can be both a cause and a consequence. The most common identifiable causes include alcohol abuse, impacted gallstones, pancreatic carcinoma and cancer of the sphincter of Oddi. The condition can be difficult to diagnose and treat. Suggestive symptoms include central abdominal pain and diarrhoea. Diabetes may be a secondary complication of pancreatic disease. The diagnosis can be made by abdominal CT scan or ERCP.

Coeliac disease

Fewer than 10% of patients with coeliac disease are first diagnosed when over 65 years of age. Clinical features include weight loss, weakness and symptoms of micronutrient deficiency such as bone pain and fractures from osteomalacia, or anaemia from iron or folate deficiency. Diagnosis is by demonstrating villous atrophy on intestinal biopsy. The condition is associated with dermatitis herpetiformis and if untreated, longstanding coeliac disease may result in lymphoma of the small bowel.

Bacterial overgrowth

This is a common cause of malabsorption in the elderly but is frequently undiagnosed. Small bowel bacterial overgrowth can occur due to a variety of causes and is discussed in Chapter 34. The consequences are diarrhoea, caused by bacterial degradation of bile acids, leading primarily to fat malabsorption, and bacterial utilisation of nutrients that leads to deficiencies—for example, vitamin B_{12}. Common presentations are therefore diarrhoea, steatorrhoea, weight loss and anaemia. The diagnosis can be made by culturing pathogenic organisms from a small bowel aspirate, or from a ^{14}C bile acid breath test. Bowel imaging through a barium study or other radiological approaches can also establish an anatomical abnormality that may be responsible for bacterial overgrowth.

Inflammatory bowel disease

Crohn's disease has a bimodal age incidence, with a second peak occurring between the ages of 60 and 80. As in the younger age group, about half the cases involve the terminal ileum but distal colonic disease is relatively common in older people. The major differential diagnosis is ulcerative colitis, which can also occur in older people. The clinical presentation can include abdominal pain, diarrhoea, anaemia, perianal disease and weight loss. Pyoderma gangrenosum, an inflammatory skin ulcer usually on the lower limb, arthritis and liver disease are recognised complications of both forms of inflammatory colitis. The diagnosis is by colonoscopy with colonic biopsy.

Bowel ischaemia

Occlusion to mesenteric vessels from atheroma can cause chronic abdominal pain, worsened by food intake. Weight loss is due both to avoiding food and to malabsorption. There is usually widespread atheromatous disease, which strongly suggests the diagnosis. Colonoscopic biopsy can be diagnostic. Acute ischaemia can be life-threatening and usually is not associated with weight loss.

Short bowel syndrome

This causes malabsorption, diarrhoea and weight loss through insufficient absorptive surface being available. Small bowel resection is usually performed for chronic mesenteric ischaemia, Crohn's disease, volvulus or bowel infarction from acute ischaemia or abdominal hernia.

Other causes of malabsorption

Cardiac failure can contribute to malabsorption by causing mucosal oedema, but better medical management has now made this a rare complication of cardiac disease. Many medications, including some that also cause anorexia, can cause malabsorption. These medications either damage the small bowel mucosa, bind bile salts, promote bacterial overgrowth or alter intestinal motility. Examples include broad-spectrum antibiotics, cytotoxic agents, cholestyramine, laxatives, anticholinergic agents and colchicine.

Increased energy expenditure

Several diseases can increase energy expenditure and thus lead to weight loss.

Neurological diseases

Essential tremor can contribute to weight loss. Indeed, even 'acquired tremor' through constant foot tapping and gum chewing have been known to considerably increase energy expenditure. Parkinson's disease is associated with weight loss through several mechanisms, including anorexia (partly from the medications used to treat it), dysphagia and increased energy expenditure from tremor.

However, the bradykinesia may reduce energy expenditure.

Malignancy

Malignant diseases may cause anorexia and malabsorption, as may the medications used to treat them. In addition, many cancers have profound metabolic effects that can contribute to cachexia. Significant weight loss and undernutrition is found in almost half those with cancer even before advanced disease occurs. Cancer has been shown to account for between 16% and 36% of older people with weight loss. While with some cancers the actual mass of the tumour, which is using energy substrates such as glucose, is the explanation, in most cases it is the humoral agents with catabolic effects that are produced by the cancer which are responsible. These agents include the interleukins and TNF, which can also contribute to anorexia.

Infective illnesses

Chronic infections such as bacterial endocarditis, osteomyelitis, lung abscesses and tuberculosis are associated with weight loss. The mechanisms are similar to those that cause weight loss in malignant disease—humoral agents and the effects of medications used to treat the infection. Severe weight loss can further impair immune responses, making elimination of the infections more difficult.

Thyrotoxicosis

This is associated with an increase in the basal metabolic rate through the direct effects of increased thyroxine. The associated tremor may also contribute, but is often absent in older people with thyrotoxicosis.

Diabetes mellitus

Although this most commonly presents with obesity, in older people it may present in the same aggressive manner that typifies insulin dependent diabetes in a younger patient, with polyuria, lethargy and weight loss. The weight loss is mainly due to fat and water depletion.

Rheumatoid arthritis and other inflammatory conditions

Patients with rheumatoid arthritis have increased resting energy expenditure, with associated weight loss. The mechanism seems to be humoral, with increased circulatory levels of TNF and interleukins. This is probably the explanation of weight loss in other inflammatory conditions such as polymyalgia rheumatica, polymyositis, systemic lupus erythrematosis and polyarteritis nodosa. In each of these conditions, steroid therapy can be associated with fat and fluid weight gain, but ongoing loss of muscle mass.

Treatment

To achieve the best outcome, weight loss and undernutrition should first be detected, then a reversible cause sought and managed appropriately. Early diagnosis and management are more likely to lead to a favourable outcome. In addition to the treatment of the cause, or where such treatment is not likely to be curative or is delayed, several direct nutritional approaches may be appropriate.

Improving food intake

Reduced oral intake can be attenuated by offering people an unlimited choice of their favourite foods until appetite returns. Flavour enhancers (salt, spices, sauces) may also be required to counteract the effects of reduced taste and smell. However, added salt may be contraindicated. Assistance with feeding is often essential in maintaining an adequate food intake in institutionalised people with dementia or functional disabilities. This requires sufficient dedicated staff time, or the assistance of visiting relatives and volunteers. People with dementia may need to be repeatedly reminded to swallow after each mouthful. A central dining area in institutions can assist oral intake through socialisation, and allow one staff member to assist several people with their feeding. At home, dining with a friend or relative may also improve intake. Delivered meals are appropriate for older people at home who have difficulties acquiring or preparing food. These approaches are shown in Box 32.3.

Box 32.3 Approaches to improve dietary intake

- Increase food choice
- Provide favourite food more often
- Use flavour enhancers such as salt, spices, sauces
- Ensure food is appropriate temperature and not dried out
- Reduce unnecessary packaging, or assist in unpacking
- Serve food in a social environment
- Provide assistance with eating for those with physical disability or severe dementia
- Provide delivered meals (e.g. Meals On Wheels)

Oral nutritional supplements

Where normal diet alone is insufficient, supplements can be added to the diet. Although they are widely used, there is a lack of data about the benefits of oral caloric supplements in older undernourished patients. These supplements have been associated with decreased mortality in undernourished older people admitted to hospital, but other studies have shown no benefits. There is evidence that oral supplements improve the outcomes in people with hip fractures and in those with pressure ulcers, but again the results are inconsistent. Patients hospitalised with chest infections achieve a better functional status 3 months later if given a 1255 kJ supplement each day of hospitalisation. Despite conflicting data, oral supplements should be strongly considered for older people with current undernutrition or at risk of developing this, particularly in hospitals and other institutional settings.

There are numerous commercial oral nutritional supplements in a range of prices. Supplements should be given between meals, at least 2 hours before the next meal. Liquid caloric supplements, because of the more rapid gastric emptying time, are preferred to more solid supplements such as biscuits or bread. Alternatively, milk based supplements can be prepared and are considerably cheaper. It is often necessary to try many different types of supplements to identify one that the patient finds most acceptable. Preparations suitable for diabetics and those intolerant of cow's milk or other ingredients are available. Dietary supplementation is best done in conjunction with a dietitian who can tailor the supplement appropriately.

Supplementation should begin early and continue until premorbid functional status has been regained. There is a tendency for patients to reduce their normal food intake when taking supplements, but this can be prevented with appropriate timing of supplements.

Micronutrient supplements

The current recommended daily intake (RDI) of vitamins and minerals may be too low for older people and cannot be relied upon to exclude the need for vitamins and mineral supplements. However, the routine use of supplements in well nourished people is of unproven benefit. Where weight loss and undernutrition are present, such supplements should be considered.

Vitamin deficiency in older people is usually multifactorial with low dietary intake, disease and reduced activity all often playing a role. Overt deficiency syndromes should always be treated, but using large doses of vitamins in the absence of a definite deficiency is of no proven benefit.

Older people are prone to vitamin D deficiency, particularly if they are house-bound or confined to institutions. This can contribute to osteoporosis and can cause osteomalacia. Supplementation should be with oral vitamin D, ensuring there is also a sufficient intake of calcium. The use of calcitriol and calcium has been shown to reduce hip factures in institutionalised older people, including those without low levels of vitamin D.

Low levels of vitamin B_{12} and folate should always be treated, even in the absence of haematological effects. When both levels are low, vitamin B_{12} replacement should begin first to avoid precipitating subacute combined degeneration of the spinal cord. Vitamin B_{12} is usually given as a parenteral preparation as gut absorption is often impaired, but high oral doses have been shown to be as effective.

Vitamin C deficiency can cause skin and perifollicular haemorrhages, bleeding from the gums (but not in edentulous people), slow wound healing and joint pains. This syndrome, scurvy, is still found in severely malnourished older people. Oral supplementation is well tolerated.

Thiamin deficiency can precipitate cardiac failure (wet beri beri) or neurological signs (dry beri beri) such as amnesia and ophthalmaplegia (Wernicke-Korsakoff syndrome). It is particularly common in alcohol dependent people but is also correlated with poverty and institutionalisation. Oral replacement is well tolerated and should be commenced before caloric supplements, as such supplements may utilise the last remaining thiamine stores.

Correcting trace element deficiencies such as hypomagnesaemia is important. Low serum zinc levels may not reflect true zinc deficiency, but supplementation is appropriate if there are conditions present which are associated with zinc deficiency, such as slow-healing skin ulcers.

Enteral feeding

Enteral feeding should be considered when swallowing is difficult, or unsafe, or when oral intake is safe but not sufficient. This approach requires an intact absorption system (bowel). The main methods are nasogastric and either gastric or jejunal via a percutaneous endoscopic gastrostomy (PEG). A fine bore tube, although it is more difficult to insert and requires an X-ray to confirm its position, is preferable for nasogastric feeding as it is more comfortable. Nasogastric tubes are easily dislodged and not aesthetic, so should be avoided if long-term enteral feeding is required. PEG tubes require a gastroscopy to insert but their use has increased dramatically over the last 5 years.

Situations where enteral feeding is frequently used include unsafe swallowing after stroke, ongoing weight loss despite adequate attempts to improve oral intake, and to increase nutrition in undernourished people rapidly after acute problems such as a fractured neck of femur. As with nutritional supplements, there is still a lack of data on the effectiveness of enteral feeding in improving outcomes. The initial weight gain frequently seen from enteral feeding is mainly from water and fat retention.

Enteral feeding can be associated with numerous complications, as shown in Box 32.4. Both types of tubes can become infected at the insertion site, but this is more common with PEG tubes, probably as they breach the skin and stay in longer. Bleeding can occur at the insertion site or, rarely, in the bowel from effects of the tube itself. No enteral feeding approach prevents aspiration, and nasogastric tubes in particular may increase the risk of aspiration. A more distal site for the tip of the tube (duodenal for nasal route or jejunal for a PEG) may reduce the risk of aspiration of gastric contents.

Box 32.4 Risks of enteral feeding

- Local irritation
- Infection (PEG site most commonly)
- Bleeding
- Aspiration
- Vomiting
- Diarrhoea
- Hyperglycaemia
- Dehydration
- Electrolyte imbalance

Diarrhoea may be troublesome but is more commonly related to medications or infection than the osmotic content of the feeding formula. An isotonic formula may be better tolerated if other causes of diarrhoea are excluded. Glucose abnormalities may occur in diabetics requiring enteral feeding, requiring adjustments to both the feeding and to the diabetic therapy. Occasionally, glucose levels will become high in an apparent non-diabetic: this may be the first evidence of diabetes in that person. Dehydration can occur with enteral feeding due to diarrhoea, insufficient volume of feeding formula, the formula having insufficient water content (too hypertonic) or from hyperglycaemia with polyuria. Electrolyte disturbances are common and serum electrolytes should be regularly checked.

Ethical issues should be addressed prior to commencing enteral feeding. Its use in severely demented older people, or older people with a very poor prognosis from other illnesses, is ethically complex. Most clinicians, competent patients and carers are comfortable avoiding enteral feeding when the prognosis is very poor. On the other hand, enteral feeding should not be denied to those who could benefit from it.

Parenteral feeding

Parenteral nutrition is most appropriate for patients with diseases of the gastrointestinal tract that prevent enteral feeding. It may be appropriate for those who have acute gastrointestinal stasis, such as after abdominal surgery. One study demonstrated reduced infections and better outcomes in severely malnourished elderly people fed parenterally after surgery. However, parenteral feeding has a limited role in older people as it is associated with numerous complications, and is very expensive. It is rarely appropriate for long-term use. The use of a peripheral rather than a central route of administration may be associated with fewer complications.

Medications for treating anorexia

Drugs that stimulate appetite and assist with weight gain are not a first line therapy in undernourished older people. There are very few studies that show any efficacy of this approach. Most studies concentrated on patients with cancer or AIDS and were not carried out exclusively in older people.

Corticosteroids promote appetite and weight gain in patients with cancer. Much of the weight gain is due to fluid and fat. Their use is limited by numerous adverse effects, including oedema, delirium, proximal myopathy, indigestion, osteoporosis, hypokalaemia, hyperglycaemia, suppression of immune response and adrenal cortical insufficiency.

Small amounts of alcohol (less than 10 g) can stimulate appetite. This has been shown to increase total energy intake in men but in women this is offset by a reduced sugar intake, leading to no net energy gain. In larger amounts, alcohol can cause undernutrition and weight loss.

Growth hormone administration has been trialled to combat the large reduction in growth hormone level that occurs with ageing ('growth hormone menopause'). Studies of growth hormone administration generally show no beneficial effects in older people and are associated with a range of adverse effects, including carpal tunnel syndrome and gynaecomastia. Short-term use may be beneficial in severely malnourished patients, but therapy is extremely expensive.

Megestrol causes weight gain in those with cancer or AIDS related cachexia. It has also been trialled in undernourished nursing home residents but completion of therapy was reduced because of adverse effects, including delirium, constipation and oedema. Other adverse effects include hyperglycaemia and venous thromboembolism. Cyproheptadine is an antiserotonin and antihistamine shown to increase weight in advanced cancer. It decreases nausea and vomiting, but increases sedation and dizziness. Tetrahydrocannabinol produces weight gain in those with cancer or AIDS, but causes dizziness, somnolence and cognitive impairment so is generally inappropriate in older people.

Prokinetic medications such as metoclopramide and cisapride have been used to treat early satiation and anorexia due to nausea. Metoclopramide can cause extrapyramidal and dystonic effects and is best avoided in older people. Cisapride can cause abdominal discomfort and, rarely, cardiac arrhythmias but is generally well tolerated.

Other tonics and related preparations are of no proven benefit for the treatment of undernutrition, although some practitioners continue to prescribe them.

Prognosis

Early treatment and prevention of weight loss and undernutrition is associated with the best prognosis. Once significant weight loss has occurred, complete restoration of body weight is very difficult, and mortality can be high. A high index of suspicion is needed for early recognition. Despite this, many undernourished people in hospitals and institutions are not diagnosed, and treatment is not commenced. One study showed 50% of undernourished hospitalised patients were not recognised and had no nutritional information recorded. Improved awareness of malnutrition among medical and other health professionals is essential in improving detection and thus the prognosis for individual patients.

A major challenge for the future is the development of well validated and practical screening tools that will help clinicians identify malnourished patients. We also need more effective nutritional supplement regimens—and we need to utilise current regimens more extensively. More effective community intervention to improve whole-population nutrition is also needed if older people are to avoid being undernourished even before illness ensues.

Bibliography and further reading

Australian Society for Geriatric Medicine, Position Statement number 6 (1997), 'Nutrition in the elderly', available from the ASGM, 145 Macquarie Street, Sydney.

Covinsky, K. E., Martin, G. E., Beyth, R. J. et al. (1999), 'The relationship between clinical assessments of nutritional status and adverse outcomes in older hospitalised medical patients', *Journal of the American Geriatrics Society*, 47, pp. 532–8.

Detsky, A. S., Smalley, P. S. & Chang, J. (1994), 'Is this patient malnourished?', *Journal of the American Medical Association*, 271, pp. 54–8.

Incalzi, R. A., Capparella, O., Genima, A. et al. (1998), 'Inadequate caloric intake: A risk factor for mortality of geriatric patients in the acute-care hospital', *Age and Ageing*, 27, pp. 303–10.

Incalzi, R. A., Landi, F., Cipriani, L. et al. (1996), 'Nutritional assessment: A primary component of multidimensional geriatric assessment in the acute care setting', *Journal of the American Geriatrics Society*, 44, pp. 168–74.

McWhirter, J. P. & Pennington, C. R. (1994), 'Incidence and recognition of malnutrition in hospital', *British Medical Journal*, 308, pp. 945–8.

Morley, J. E. (1996), 'Anorexia in older persons: Epidemiology and optional treatment', *Drugs and Aging*, 8, pp. 134–55.

Morley, J. E. & Kraenzle, D. (1994), 'Cause of weight loss in a community nursing home', *Journal of the American Geriatrics Society*, 42, pp. 583–5.

Reuben, D. B., Greendale, G. A. & Harrison, G. G. (1995), 'Nutrition screening in older persons', *Journal of the American Geriatrics Society*, 43, pp. 415–25.

Sullivan, D. H., Sun, S. & Walls, R. C. (1999), 'Protein-energy undernutrition among elderly hospitalised patients', *Journal of the American Medical Association*, 281, pp. 2013–19.

Wahlqvist, M. L., Savige, G. S. & Lukito, W. (1995), 'Nutritional disorders in the elderly', *Medical Journal of Australia*, 163, pp. 376–81.

Wallace, J. I., Schwartz, R. S., La Croix, A. Z. et al. (1995), 'Involuntary weight loss in older outpatients: Incidence and clinical significance', *Journal of the American Geriatrics Society*, 43, pp. 329–37.

Whitehead, C. & Finucane, P. A. (1997), 'Malnutrition in elderly people', *Australian and New Zealand Journal of Medicine*, 27, pp. 68–74.

Chapter 33
Gastrointestinal bleeding

RICHARD. D. KIMBER and IAN. C. ROBERTS-THOMSON

Introduction

Bleeding from the gastrointestinal tract is a common clinical problem in geriatric practice. The presentation varies widely from an acute haemorrhage with overt upper or lower gastrointestinal bleeding to an obscure presentation with iron-deficiency anaemia or positive results from faecal occult blood tests. The site of bleeding also varies widely, although the proportion of patients with bleeding from the lower gastrointestinal tract increases with advancing age. This is largely due to an association between advancing age and potential bleeding disorders such as diverticulosis, angiodysplasia, haemorrhoids and colonic neoplasms.

There is only limited data on the incidence of various forms of gastrointestinal bleeding. The most common, however, is the intermittent detection of blood in stools. This has been reported to have an annual incidence of approximately 800 per 100 000 population in community studies. Most of these patients do not require admission to hospital. In contrast, most patients with gross gastrointestinal bleeding require hospitalisation. Annual rates have been estimated at 35–100 patients per 100 000 population for gross upper gastrointestinal bleeding and 20 per 100 000 population for gross lower gastrointestinal bleeding. Iron-deficiency anaemia has been estimated to affect up to 10% of the world's population but in only a minority of cases is it due to gastrointestinal bleeding. More important causes include low dietary levels of haem and non-haem iron and iron losses associated with menstruation and pregnancy.

Mortality rates from gastrointestinal bleeding vary with the mode of presentation and the cause of bleeding. In cases of acute bleeding, mortality rates of 3–7% are common and tend to be higher in elderly subgroups, perhaps largely because of co-existing medical disorders. While mortality from acute upper gastrointestinal bleeding has remained relatively constant, mortality from lower gastrointestinal bleeding has fallen, hopefully because of improved diagnostic methods and therapeutic procedures.

This chapter provides an overview of the causes and management of gastrointestinal bleeding in elderly patients. It focuses on common problems relevant to a general practice setting rather than complex problems, such as bleeding oesophageal varices, which often require specialised management in tertiary referral centres.

Minor rectal bleeding

The identification of blood in stools is an important symptom of colorectal cancer. Because of this, health messages to the community have encouraged people to consult doctors with minor rectal bleeding and, in some circumstances, to have regular faecal occult blood tests in the absence of symptoms. A positive faecal occult blood test result in the latter setting is called occult gastrointestinal bleeding and is addressed separately below.

Symptoms

A careful history and examination is central to the evaluation of patients with minor rectal bleeding. For example, it is important to know whether blood is bright or dark, is mixed within the stool or largely on the outside of the stool and whether most of the bright blood is on the toilet paper or drips into the toilet bowl. Other symptoms are also relevant, including the presence or absence of anal pain, perianal lumps and a change in bowel habit. Anal examination is sometimes helpful and may reveal disorders such as external haemorrhoids or features of an anal fissure. A list of common causes of minor rectal bleeding is shown in Table 33.1.

Investigations

Surprisingly, few studies have evaluated the diagnostic yield of various investigations for minor rectal bleeding. A minimum protocol, however, would involve a rectal examination and rigid sigmoidoscopy. This should detect a variety of common conditions, including haemorrhoids, anal fissures, rectal neoplasms and ulcerative proctitis. This may be sufficient in patients with typical symptoms of haemorrhoids or an anal fissure. In some patients, additional investigations will be necessary, such as a barium enema X-ray, flexible sigmoidoscopy or colonoscopy. Symptoms that highlight the need for further evaluation include blood that is mixed in with the stool, a change in bowel habit, anaemia and the presence of rectal blood at the time of sigmoidoscopy. The choice of investigation will be determined by factors such as age, co-existing medical disorders and an estimate of the likelihood of colonic neoplasia. For example, a barium enema X-ray may be the most appropriate investigation in patients over 75 years of age who are considered to be at lower risk for colonic neoplasia. This approach reduces hospitalisation (since barium enema X-rays can be performed in an outpatient setting) and reduces the inconvenience and morbidity of the more vigorous purgative regimens associated with colonoscopy. In contrast, flexible sigmoidoscopy or colonoscopy are the preferred methods of investigation for patients with a higher probability of neoplasia, such as those with blood mixed with stool and those who have rectal blood at the time of sigmoidoscopy.

Table 33.1 Common causes for minor rectal bleeding in elderly patients with an estimate of the frequency of each diagnosis[(a)]

Diagnosis	Percentage of total diagnoses
Haemorrhoids	75
Anal fissure	5
Colorectal adenoma	5
Colorectal carcinoma	5
Colitis (ulcerative, Crohn's disease)	3
Diverticulosis	2
Other	5

(*a*) Individual diagnoses can become more or less likely depending on the characteristics of the bleeding.

Management

The management of minor rectal bleeding depends on the cause and the extent of bleeding. For example, bleeding is due to haemorrhoids in at least 75% of patients. These arise because of dilatation of haemorrhoidal veins and can involve the superior venous plexus (internal haemorrhoids) or inferior venous plexus (external haemorrhoids). Apart from bleeding, complications include thrombosis (usually associated with significant anal pain) and prolapse of internal haemorrhoids, occasionally associated with strangulation.

The majority of patients with small haemorrhoids do not require therapy, perhaps apart from measures to soften stools and reduce straining at defecation. Such measures may include an increase in dietary fibre or the use of a bulk-forming supplement. Referral to a specialist will be necessary if bleeding persists or other complications arise. Treatment by band ligation is suitable for many patients but other options include injection sclerotherapy and haemorrhoidectomy.

Anal fissures may account for bleeding in approximately 5% of patients, particularly if bleeding is associated with significant anal pain. An anal fissure is a linear tear or ulcer in the anal canal and is usually located posteriorly. A minority of fissures (10%) are associated with bowel disorders such as Crohn's disease, ulcerative proctitis and rectal cancer. Some fissures heal either spontaneously or with measures to improve constipation. However, additional measures will be necessary in the majority of patients with 'chronic' fissures that have been present for several weeks. Options include the local use of nitrates to dilate the internal sphincter, injections of botulinum toxin to relax the internal sphincter, and disruption of the internal sphincter by dilatation (Lord's procedure) or sphincterotomy. The latter option appears to be the procedure of choice for patients with recurrent fissures.

Occult gastrointestinal bleeding

Occult gastrointestinal bleeding is, by definition, bleeding that is not recognised by inspection of the stools. Occult bleeding can be suspected because of the development of iron-deficiency anaemia or because screening occult blood tests are found to give positive results. Whether bleeding is occult or overt depends on a variety of factors, including the rate of bleeding and the anatomical site of bleeding. For example, ingestion of at least 200 mL of blood is required to consistently produce melaena in volunteers. In contrast, as little as a few drops of blood may be visible as a bright streak on the surface of the stool or on the toilet paper in patients with anorectal lesions such as haemorrhoids.

The mode of presentation, either as anaemia or a positive faecal occult blood test result, has some influence on the probability of various diagnoses and, subsequently, on management. An additional consideration relevant to faecal occult blood tests is the nature of the test system. Guiac-based tests, such as Hemoccult (Smith Kline Diagnostics), are simple and inexpensive but are not specific for blood. False-positive results can occur after the ingestion of animal foods containing haem (red meat) and plant foods rich in peroxidases. Furthermore, guiac-based tests give positive results for lower rates of colonic bleeding (0.5 mL per day) than for bleeding from the upper gastrointestinal tract (10–20 mL per day). In contrast, immunochemical tests rely on antihaemoglobin antibodies to detect the presence of human haemoglobin. As haemoglobin is degraded by proteases in the bowel lumen, positive test results almost always indicate the presence of colorectal bleeding, usually greater than a daily rate of 0.1–0.7 mL. A third assay system marketed as HemoQuant is a fluorometric assay of haem and haem-derived porphyrins. The assay is quantitative and is of higher sensitivity for the detection of proximal gastrointestinal bleeding than either guiac-based or immunochemical tests. Disadvantages of the HemoQuant test include the need for dietary modification (particularly the avoidance of red meat) and more complex assay methods, which require transfer of specimens to a reference laboratory. The radiochromium-labelled erythrocyte method is accepted as the gold standard for the measurement of gastrointestinal blood loss. However, as at least three days of stool collections are required, the test is usually reserved for research studies or for more complex patients where management may be influenced by a more accurate assessment of blood loss.

Investigations

In Western countries, bleeding from the gastrointestinal tract appears to account for iron-deficiency anaemia in 60–70% of elderly patients. In some circumstances, however, other possibilities need to be considered, including diets deficient in iron, iron malabsorption and extra-intestinal bleeding such as gross haematuria. It should also be remembered that iron studies may be difficult to interpret when anaemia occurs in chronic inflammatory disorders such as rheumatoid arthritis.

The choice and sequence of investigations should be influenced by the mode of presentation (iron-deficiency anaemia or positive faecal occult blood test result), by the test system used for faecal occult blood (guiac-based or immunochemical) and by any co-existing gastrointestinal symptoms. Typical diagnoses in patients subjected to both upper gastrointestinal endoscopy and colonoscopy for positive faecal occult blood test results (guiac-based) and iron-deficiency anaemia are shown in Tables 33.2 and 33.3, respectively. Some of these diagnoses are illustrated in Figures 33.1–33.7. In general, there is a higher frequency of endoscopic abnormalities in patients with iron-deficiency anaemia than in those with positive faecal occult blood test results. Furthermore, abnormalities are more likely to be identified at upper gastrointestinal endoscopy than at colonoscopy. However, more cancers are identified by colonoscopy than by upper gastrointestinal endoscopy. If faecal occult blood test results are positive by the immunochemical method, investigations should focus on the large bowel since the frequency of upper gastrointestinal abnormalities is much lower than that shown in Table 33.2.

Table 33.2 Gastrointestinal findings in elderly patients with positive faecal occult blood test results[a] with an estimate of the frequency of each diagnosis

Diagnosis	Percentage of total diagnoses
Oesophagitis	10
Gastric/duodenal ulcer	9
Gastritis/duodenitis	5
Upper GI cancer	2
Colorectal adenoma (> 1 cm)	12
Colorectal cancer	5
Colonic angiodysplasia	2
Colitis (ulcerative/Crohn's disease)	2
Miscellaneous (upper or lower)	3
No cause for bleeding	50

(*a*) Based on the results of upper gastrointestinal (GI) endoscopy and colonoscopy in patients with positive guiac test results but without iron-deficiency anaemia or overt bleeding. Abnormalities are found in approximately 50% of patients. When immunochemical tests are positive, the frequency of upper gastrointestinal disorders is much lower.

In patients with positive faecal occult blood test results (without anaemia) who have normal upper gastrointestinal endoscopy and colonoscopy, further investigation is usually unnecessary. This may also apply to patients with iron-deficiency anaemia, since at least 80% respond to orally administered iron with a low recurrence rate of anaemia over the subsequent 2 years. Those cases with persistent or recurrent anaemia can be categorised as 'obscure gastrointestinal bleeding' and are discussed later in this chapter.

Table 33.3 Gastrointestinal findings in elderly patients with iron-deficiency anaemia with an estimate of the frequency of each diagnosis[a]

Diagnosis	Percentage of total diagnoses
Oesophagitis	15
Gastritis/duodenitis	10
Gastric/duodenal ulcer	9
Upper GI cancer	6
Colorectal cancer	10
Colorectal adenoma (> 1 cm)	10
Colonic angiodysplasia	2
Colitis (ulcerative, Crohn's disease)	2
Miscellaneous (upper or lower)	4
No cause for bleeding	32

(*a*) Based on results of upper gastrointestinal endoscopy and colonoscopy in Western countries. Most studies have shown significant gastrointestinal disorders in 60–70% of patients.

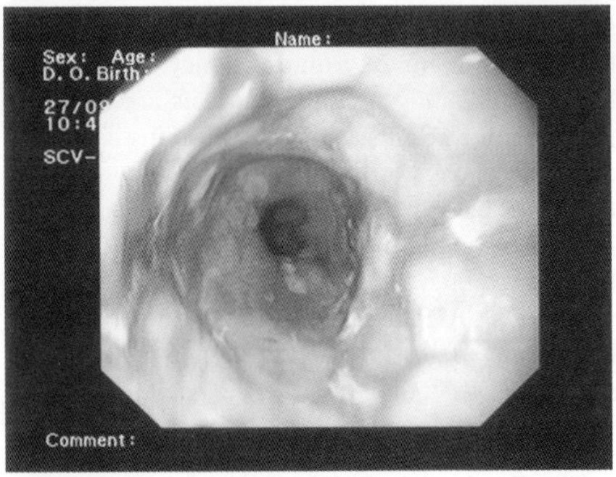

Figure 33.1 Oesophageal ulceration and inflammation due to reflux oesophagitis in an elderly man with iron-deficiency anaemia

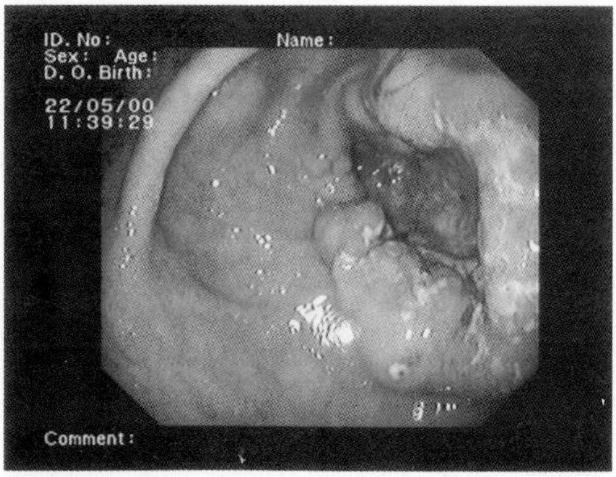

Figure 33.2 An ulcerating cancer in the antrum of the stomach in an elderly woman with iron-deficiency anaemia

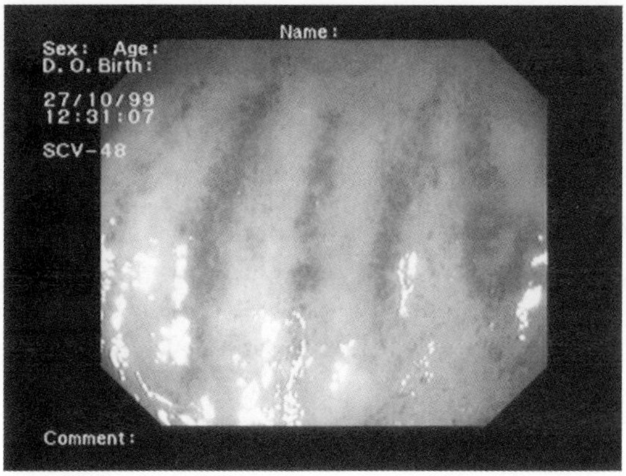

Figure 33.3 Red streaks radiating from the pylorus due to gastric antral vascular ectasia in an elderly man with iron-deficiency anaemia

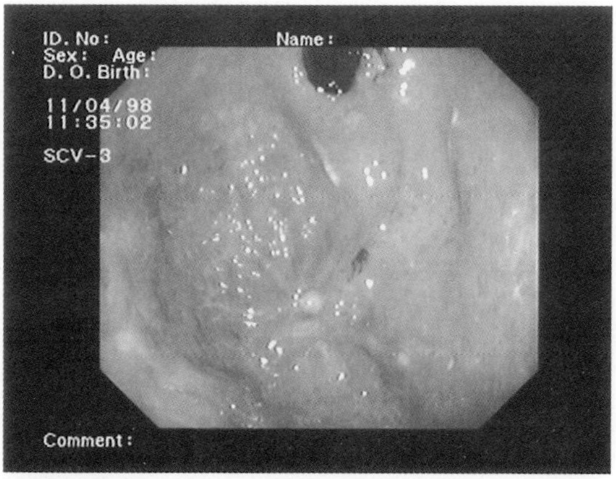

Figure 33.4 Small chronic ulcer in the fundus of the stomach in an elderly woman taking non-steroidal anti-inflammatory drugs who developed iron-deficiency anaemia

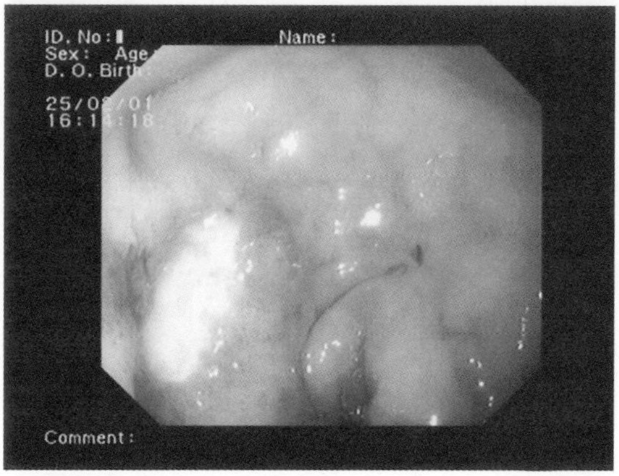

Figure 33.5 Chronic ulcer on the anterior wall of the duodenal cap in an elderly woman with a positive faecal occult blood test result

Acute upper gastrointestinal bleeding

Overt bleeding from the upper gastrointestinal tract is usually associated with haematemesis, melaena or both symptoms. With haematemesis, blood may be bright or dark depending on the rate of bleeding and the time interval between bleeding and vomiting. Melaena denotes the passage of black, tarry stools, which are often loose and malodorous. On rare occasions, active bleeding from the upper gastrointestinal tract can be associated with the presence of bright rectal blood.

Emergency assessment

Most patients with haematemesis and melaena are referred for assessment in an emergency service. This will include an estimate of blood loss, establishment of intravenous access and the administration of intravenous fluids. Blood samples will be sent for typing and cross-matching and additional

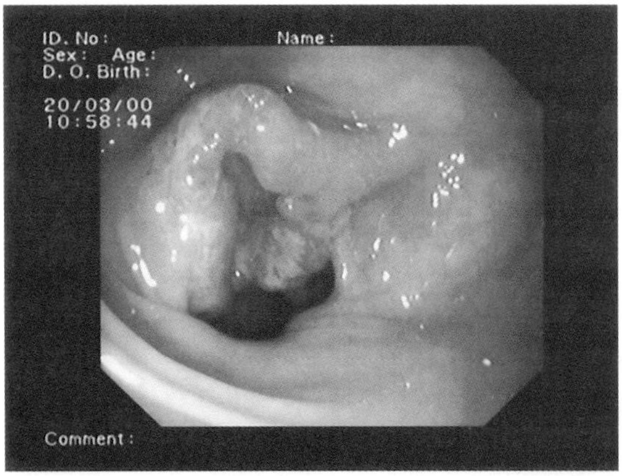

Figure 33.6 Ulcerating cancer of the caecum in an elderly woman with iron-deficiency anaemia

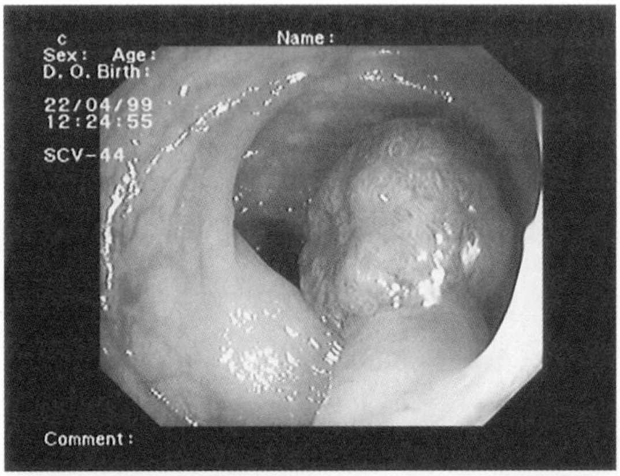

Figure 33.7 Large polyp in the sigmoid colon in an elderly man with positive faecal occult blood test results

samples will be sent for a complete blood count (particularly haemoglobin or haematocrit) and for plasma concentrations of electrolytes and creatinine. A history and clinical examination may then provide clues as to the cause of bleeding. For example, there may be a previous history of chronic peptic ulceration, use of non-steroidal anti-inflammatory drugs (NSAIDs) or clinical features of chronic liver disease.

Patients with major upper gastrointestinal bleeding are usually nursed in special high-dependency areas or in a fully-equipped intensive care unit. This will normally include the administration of intravenous fluids and blood as well as supplements of oxygen. Monitoring will include vital signs, urine output, evidence of continued bleeding (e.g. melaena) and, in some patients, monitoring of central venous pressure. In general, packed red blood cells are the preferred form of blood transfusion. Coagulation factors, such as fresh frozen plasma and platelet transfusions, may be appropriate if coagulation tests are abnormal, as in some patients with cirrhosis. It may also be helpful to have a nasogastric tube in place if there is doubt as to the presence of continued bleeding.

Endoscopy

Endoscopy has become central to the management of patients with upper gastrointestinal bleeding. The procedure not only establishes the presence and site of bleeding but often permits the application of various therapeutic measures that may stop the bleeding. Patients with life-threatening bleeding require urgent endoscopy. In most patients, however, endoscopy is performed after a period of resuscitation but usually within 24 hours. Relative contraindications to endoscopy include a confused and unco-operative patient and serious co-existing cardiac and pulmonary disorders.

A list of common causes of upper gastrointestinal bleeding in elderly patients is shown in Table 33.4. Patients with chronic duodenal or gastric ulceration may have a non-bleeding ulcer, a non-bleeding ulcer with a visible vessel, an ulcer with an adherent clot or an ulcer with evidence of minor or arterial 'spurting' bleeding. Ulcers with evidence of active bleeding and ulcers with visible vessels are at higher risk for continued bleeding and rebleeding. Most authors recommend endoscopic treatment for actively bleeding ulcers and for non-bleeding visible vessels, particularly if the visible vessels are elevated. Adherent clots should be aggressively washed off in patients with major bleeds but can probably be left intact in those with minor bleeds. Endoscopic options for the management of bleeding chronic ulcers include thermal methods and injection methods. The latter includes injections of vasoconstrictors such as adrenaline (1:10 000) and sclerosing agents such as alcohol and ethanolamine. Thermal methods include the use of a heater probe, multipolar electrocoagulation and the neodymium-yttrium-aluminium-garnet (Nd:YAG)

Table 33.4 Common causes for acute upper gastrointestinal bleeding in elderly patients with an estimate of the frequency of each diagnosis

Diagnosis	Percentage of total diagnoses
Duodenal ulcer	25
Gastritis/gastric erosions	20
Gastric ulcer	20
Oesophageal varices	9
Mallory–Weiss tear	6
Oesophagitis	5
Erosive duodenitis	5
Upper GI cancer	3
Other	7

laser. Various comparative studies indicate that both thermal and injection therapies are equally effective. Furthermore, some endoscopists use combination therapy with an initial injection of adrenaline followed by electrocoagulation.

Although oesophageal varices only account for approximately 10% of patients with upper gastrointestinal bleeding, such patients make a significant contribution to mortality rates. For example, the risk of death from each episode of variceal bleeding is of the order of 20–30%. Almost all patients with oesophageal varices (95%) have cirrhosis. Unusual causes for varices in the absence of cirrhosis include thromboses of the portal or splenic vein and vascular abnormalities involving the portal vein. In many patients, endoscopy is performed as an emergency procedure to confirm the presence of bleeding varices and to initiate endoscopic therapy, either band ligation or injection sclerotherapy. Endoscopic therapy is often supplemented by intravenous infusions of octreotide or vasopressin to reduce the pressure in the portal vein. Balloon tamponade may also be used in patients with catastrophic bleeding and in those who have persistent bleeding despite the above measures. Other forms of therapy include the infusion of various coagulation factors and the creation of a shunt between the portal vein and hepatic vein, a technique usually performed by radiologists called a transjugular intrahepatic portosystemic shunt (TIPS).

Although diagnoses such as gastric erosions, Mallory–Weiss tears, oesophagitis, duodenitis and neoplasms are important causes of upper gastrointestinal bleeding, it is uncommon for bleeding to be major and life-threatening. In most of these patients, bleeding settles spontaneously, occasionally after endoscopic therapy, such as injection treatment for a Mallory–Weiss tear.

Non-endoscopic therapy

The increased use of endoscopic techniques for bleeding lesions has resulted in a substantial fall in the need for emergency surgery. In the 1970s, for example, emergency surgical rates were often in the order of 15–40%. Current surgical rates are approximately 5%, with operations largely restricted to patients with persistent or recurrent bleeding from large gastric or duodenal ulcers. For chronic gastric ulcers, the most common surgical procedure is a partial gastrectomy (including the ulcer) with a Billroth I or Billroth II anastomosis. For duodenal ulcers, surgical options include direct suture of the ulcer base, suture of the base associated with pyloroplasty and vagotomy, and excision of the ulcer with antrectomy, vagotomy and often a Billroth II anastomosis. If bleeding is controlled by direct suture, the patient should subsequently be given an eradication regimen for *Helicobacter pylori*.

In bleeding oesophageal varices, surgical procedures remain controversial, largely because of high mortality rates (50%). However, in special circumstances, patients may be considered for an urgent portosystemic shunt or for transection of the lower oesophagus using a staple gun technique.

Rarely, radiological techniques may be used to diagnose and treat upper gastrointestinal bleeding due to causes such as vascular malformations and false aneurysms. However, these techniques are more likely to be applied to lower gastrointestinal bleeding and are discussed in more detail below.

Predictors of mortality

Despite the advent of endoscopic therapy, mortality rates for upper gastrointestinal bleeding have remained relatively constant at between 3% and about 7%. In most clinical surveys, at least 50% of deaths are due to cirrhosis with bleeding varices.

The remainder largely occur in elderly patients, often after emergency surgery.

In ulcer disease, clinical factors associated with a higher mortality rate include higher transfusion requirements (> 5 units), advanced age (> 70 years), rebleeding in hospital, hypotension at the time of presentation and the presence of serious co-existing medical problems. Endoscopic features predictive of higher mortality include a 'spurting' vessel, a visible vessel in the base of the ulcer and large chronic ulcers (> 2 cm).

Acute lower gastrointestinal bleeding

Acute lower gastrointestinal bleeding has a lower incidence than acute upper gastrointestinal bleeding. The typical patient presents with the frequent passage of bright blood per rectum. Initially, this may be mixed with stools but, if bleeding persists, stools are largely composed of bright blood and clots. In the case of slow but persistent bleeding from the right colon, stools may have the appearance of melaena.

Most patients with acute lower gastrointestinal bleeding are referred to an emergency service. Initial assessment is similar to that for patients with upper gastrointestinal bleeding and includes an estimate of blood loss, administration of intravenous fluids and cross-matching of blood for a possible blood transfusion. Patients will normally be nursed in special high-dependency areas to facilitate regular observations.

A history and clinical examination may provide clues as to the cause of bleeding. For example, co-existing abdominal pain, particularly in the left upper quadrant, may suggest the diagnosis of ischaemic colitis. Other patients may have a previous history of ulcerative colitis, Crohn's disease or pelvic irradiation. Acute lower gastrointestinal bleeding due to neoplasms is uncommon but such patients may describe a change in bowel habit, abdominal pain or weight loss. Abdominal masses may be present in some patients with Crohn's disease and colon cancer. A list of common causes of lower gastrointestinal bleeding in elderly patients is shown in Table 33.5.

Table 33.5 Common causes of acute lower gastrointestinal bleeding in elderly patients with an estimate of the frequency of each diagnosis

Diagnosis	Percentage of total diagnoses
Diverticulosis	35
Angiodysplasia	15
Undetermined	15
Neoplasia (cancer/polyp)	15
Radiation colitis	5
Ulcerative colitis/Crohn's disease	5
Ischaemic colitis	4
Anorectal disorders (e.g. haemorrhoids)	2
Other	4

Investigations

The sequence of investigations for patients with acute lower gastrointestinal bleeding is likely to vary from patient to patient depending on factors such as the rate of bleeding, the presumed cause of bleeding and the availability of specialised investigations, such as mesenteric angiography and nuclear medicine scans. For most patients, the first investigation will be rigid sigmoidoscopy. This will confirm the presence of bright blood in the rectum and may indicate whether bleeding is from the anorectal region or more proximally. Rarely, bleeding may arise from a rectal neoplasm or from haemorrhoids.

Fortunately, bleeding settles spontaneously in the majority of patients. In this setting, colonoscopy would normally be performed during the inpatient admission, usually within 2 or 3 days. This approach may identify blood clots in the region of diverticula or, less commonly, vascular abnormalities consistent with angiodysplasia. A more cautious approach may be adopted if bleeding is thought to be due to disorders such as severe inflammatory bowel disease or ischaemic colitis, where vigorous purgation and colonoscopy may result in complications such as toxic megacolon and progressive ischaemia, respectively. For these patients, alternative approaches include flexible sigmoidoscopy without vigorous purgation or perhaps a barium enema X-ray. It should be remembered, however, that use of a barium enema X-ray will compromise urgent angiography and may delay subsequent colonoscopy.

For patients with persistent bleeding, options include early mesenteric angiography, nuclear medicine scans and colonoscopy. For major episodes of bleeding, most authors favour urgent mesenteric angiography (Figure 33.8). This technique is able to detect bleeding rates of 0.5–1 mL/min, mostly with accurate localisation of the site of bleeding. The cause of bleeding may also be determined if there are characteristic radiological changes of angiodysplasia. An additional benefit of angiography is the possibility of therapeutic intervention using selective catheterisation of small vessels followed by the infusion of vasoconstrictors (vasopressin) or obstruction of the vessels using a variety of devices, including coils. The ability to catheterise and obstruct small vessels has resulted in a much lower frequency of complications such as bowel ischaemia.

When bleeding is persistent but not life-threatening, helpful information may be obtained from urgent colonoscopy or a nuclear medicine scan. For urgent colonoscopy, bleeding sites can be identified in about 50% of patients, particularly when bleeding is arising from neoplasms, diverticula, inflammatory bowel disease and ischaemic colitis. Angiodysplasia is only identified at colonoscopy in a minority of patients but localisation of the site of bleeding may permit therapeutic approaches, including the injection of adrenaline and alcohol, and the application of thermal methods, such as a heater probe. Endoscopic injections may also be helpful when bleeding is arising from diverticula. Nuclear medicine scans using technetium-99m labelled red blood cells have been reported to detect bleeding rates down to 0.1 mL/min. Because of this, positive scans are more common than with angiography. However, nuclear medicine scans take some hours to perform, may be misleading as to the site of bleeding and do not include a therapeutic component. Nevertheless,

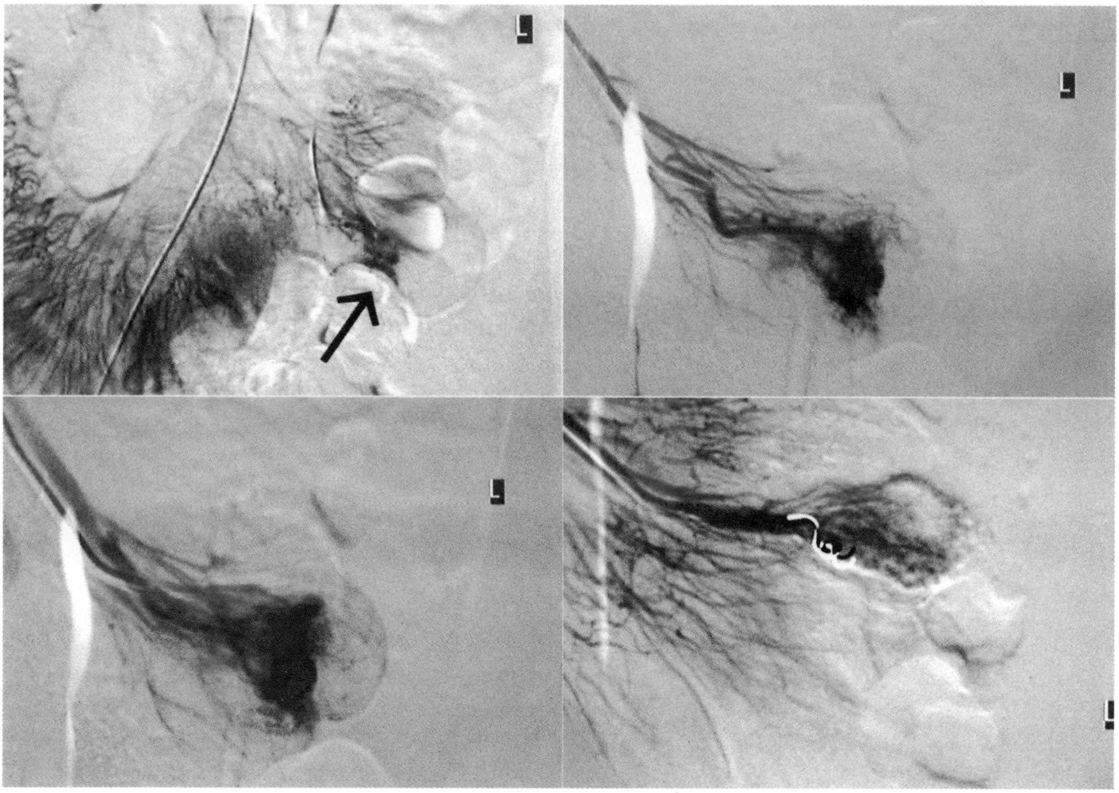

Figure 33.8 Superior mesenteric angiogram in an elderly woman with acute lower gastrointestinal bleeding. An abnormal area was identified (arrow, upper left). A selective angiogram showed an abnormal vascular pattern (upper right) and contrast in the bowel lumen (lower left). Bleeding ceased after placement of a coil in the feeding artery (lower right)

such scans have a useful role in patients with minor but persistent bleeding, particularly when other investigations are unhelpful.

Surgical therapy

Because of therapeutic endoscopy and angiography, the need for urgent surgery is now uncommon (< 5% of patients). Nevertheless, emergency surgery may be required for catastrophic bleeding or for bleeding that fails to respond to other therapeutic measures. If the bleeding site remains unclear despite preoperative investigations and surgical exploration, some authors have advocated a subtotal colectomy. Others have favoured a right hemicolectomy since at least 70% of major bleeds arise from the right colon, often from angiodysplasia. Typical surgical mortality rates are of the order of 5–10%.

Obscure gastrointestinal bleeding

Obscure gastrointestinal bleeding shares some features with occult bleeding: both are associated with slow intermittent or chronic bleeding from various disorders of the gastrointestinal tract. One definition of obscure bleeding is that of bleeding of unknown origin that persists or recurs after negative upper gastrointestinal endoscopy and colonoscopy. The manifestations of bleeding may include visible blood in stools, recurrent positive faecal occult blood test results and/or iron-deficiency anaemia. It may also be important to define subgroups of patients with obscure bleeding since those disorders that result in overt rectal bleeding may be different from those that result in positive faecal occult blood test results or iron-deficiency anaemia. For example, gastrointestinal causes for anaemia are found in most patients with overt rectal bleeding although this may reflect the outcome of more extensive investigations. Small bowel disorders that may be responsible for overt bleeding or recurrent anaemia are listed in Box 33.1.

Box 33.1 Small bowel lesions in elderly patients which may explain overt bleeding or recurrent anaemia

- Angiodysplasia[a]
- Erosions/ulcers (largely with NSAIDs)
- Stromal cell tumour
- Carcinoid tumour
- Carcinoma/lymphoma
- Aorto-enteric fistula
- Dieulafoy's lesion
- Vascular fragility syndromes
- Ruptured pancreatic pseudocyst

(*a*) Angiodysplasia appears to account for bleeding in at least 50% of patients.

In patients with obscure bleeding, serial faecal occult blood tests may confirm the presence of bleeding and may suggest a site in either the upper or lower gastrointestinal tract. If occult blood tests are unhelpful, options include repeat endoscopy and various barium studies, including a small bowel follow-through X-ray, small bowel enteroclysis and enema X-ray. In most studies, repeat endoscopy has been more helpful than repeat colonoscopy. Significant lesions that may be missed during upper gastrointestinal endoscopy include erosions associated with large hiatus hernias (Cameron's erosions), peptic ulcers and angiodysplasia. Small bowel enteroclysis differs from small bowel follow-through X-ray in that a small bowel tube is placed in the proximal small bowel either directly or facilitated by endoscopy. With small bowel X-ray series, significant abnormalities are detected in fewer than 10% of patients but the yield from enteroclysis appears to be greater than that of a follow-through X-ray. Small bowel series are abnormal in most patients with small bowel cancer but abnormalities are rare in patients with small bowel angiodysplasia.

More recently, long endoscopes (enteroscopes) have been used to examine the upper small bowel, largely the jejunum. The diagnostic yield of these 'push enteroscopes' varies from 30% to 70% with a relatively low frequency of complications. Abnormalities identified at enteroscopy include angiodysplasia, benign tumours and malignant tumours. The terminal ileum is difficult to view with a push enteroscope but may be visualised with a standard colonoscope or colonoscopy using a small bowel enteroscope. However, terminal ileoscopy appears to be associated with a low diagnostic yield (< 5%). Another technique, currently in the developmental phase, is that of visualisation of the small bowel by ingestion of a wireless video-capsule system propelled by peristalsis and not requiring air insufflation.

Other investigations may include nuclear medicine scans, mesenteric angiography and exploratory laparotomy. The diagnostic yield of labelled red blood cell scans in obscure rectal bleeding remains unclear. However, scans may be helpful in patients with intermittent overt rectal bleeding, as shown in Figure 33.9. Bleeding from ulcers associated with Meckel's diverticula are a rare cause of obscure bleeding in elderly patients but the use of 99m-technetium-pertechnetate (Meckel's scan) has been reported to have a sensitivity of 75–100%. Angiography may also be helpful even in the absence of active bleeding by demonstrating typical vascular patterns of angiodysplasia or neoplasia. For angiodysplasia, the most common finding is slow-filling of a vein that persists after other mesenteric veins have emptied. Additional features may include a vascular 'tuft' during the arterial phase and an early filling vein. Efforts to improve the yield of angiography have included the administration of anticoagulants and vasodilators to aggravate or precipitate bleeding. Finally, a small number of patients with obscure bleeding and recurrent anaemia may proceed to laparotomy and intraoperative endoscopy. The majority of these patients have been found to have angiodysplasia of the small bowel.

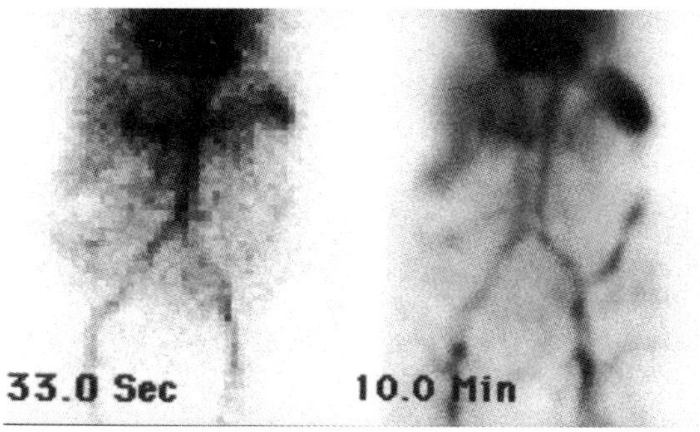

Figure 33.9 Labelled red blood cell scan in a patient with obscure rectal bleeding showing isotope in the transverse colon at 33 seconds with passage into the descending colon at 10 minutes

Medical therapy may be considered for patients with bleeding vascular lesions who are considered to be at higher risk for a surgical procedure. One option is hormonal treatment using a combination of oestrogen and progesterone. This appears to be helpful in some patients with angiodysplasia, hereditary haemorrhagic telangiectasia and von Willibrand's disease. Another option is that of octreotide given subcutaneously, which has been reported to reduce blood loss from intestinal angiodysplasia.

The outcome of patients with obscure gastrointestinal bleeding is generally good as malignant tumours are uncommon and it is rare for patients to have a series of minor bleeds followed by a major episode of bleeding. Endoscopic treatment for presumed causes of bleeding appears to be helpful in some studies, while others suggest that results of endoscopic and pharmacological therapy are similar to those of no intervention. The long-term success rates of surgery guided by intraoperative endoscopy have varied from approximately 40% to 70%.

Bibliography and further reading

Allison, J. E, Tekawa, I. S., Ransom, L. J., et al. (1996), 'A comparison of fecal occult-blood tests for colorectal-cancer screening', *New England Journal of Medicine*, 334, pp. 155–9.

Fijten, G. H., Blijham, G. H. & Knottnerus, J. A. (1994), 'Occurrence and clinical significance of overt blood loss per rectum in the general population and in medical practice', *British Journal of General Practice*, 44, pp. 320–5.

Hardcastle, J. D., Chamberlain, J. O., Robinson, M. H. E., et al. (1996), 'Randomised controlled trial of faecal-occult-blood screening for colorectal cancer', *Lancet*, 348, pp. 1472–7.

Kerlin, P., Reiner, R., Davies, M., et al. (1979), 'Iron deficiency anaemia—a prospective study', *Australian and New Zealand Journal of Medicine*, 9, pp. 402–7.

Kronborg, O., Fenger, C., Olsen, J., et al. (1996), 'Randomised study of screening for colorectal cancer with faecal-occult-blood test', *Lancet*, 348, pp. 1467–71.

Levin, B., Hess, K. & Johnson, C. (1997), 'Screening for colorectal cancer. A comparison of 3 fecal occult blood tests', *Archives of Internal Medicine*, 157, pp. 970–6.

Longstretch, G. F. (1995), 'Epidemiology of hospitalization for acute upper gastrointestinal hemorrhage: a population-based study', *American Journal of Gastroenterology*, 90, pp. 206–10.

Longstretch, G. F. (1997), 'Epidemiology and outcome of patients hospitalized with acute lower gastrointestinal hemorrhage: a population-based study', *American Journal of Gastroenterology*, 92, pp. 419–24.

Mandel, J. S., Bond, J. H., Church, T. R., et al. (1993), 'Reducing mortality from colorectal cancer by screening for fecal occult blood', *New England Journal of Medicine*, 328, pp. 1365–71.

Rockey, D. C., Koch, J., Cello, J. P., et al. (1998), 'Relative frequency of upper gastrointestinal and colonic lesions in patients with positive fecal occult-blood tests', *New England Journal of Medicine*, 339, pp. 153–9.

Yavorski, R. T., Wong, R. K. H., Maydonovitch, C., et al. (1995), 'Analysis of 3294 cases of upper gastrointestinal bleeding in military medical facilities', *American Journal of Gastroenterology*, 90, pp. 568–73.

Zuckerman, G. R. & Prakash, C. (1999), 'Acute lower intestinal bleeding. II: Etiology, therapy, and outcomes', *Gastrointestinal Endoscopy*, 49, pp. 228–38.

Zuckerman, G. R., Prakash, C., Askin, M. P., et al. (2000), 'AGA technical review on the evaluation and management of occult and obscure gastrointestinal bleeding', *Gastroenterology*, 118, pp. 201–21.

Chapter 34

Diarrhoea

RANJIT N. RATNAIKE

Introduction

Diarrhoea is an important cause of morbidity and mortality in older persons. It is potentially life-threatening due to the greater impact of severe dehydration and electrolyte loss on diminished physiological reserves compared to younger persons. Even a single episode of acute diarrhoea may lead to a rapid and significant deterioration in nutritional status. Those most vulnerable are the frail elderly, those with co-morbidities and residents in long-term care and in acute care facilities. Diarrhoea and its complications can significantly affect the patient's and carer's quality of life.

Diarrhoea as a problem is sometimes underestimated and its consequences minimised by patients, carers and even medical and allied health practitioners who may regard diarrhoea as an inconsequential manifestation of ageing. This may in part be due to the term 'diarrhoea' having a range of connotations. Diarrhoea describes a single loose bowel action that may resolve within hours without treatment, and also a debilitating acute episode of bloody loose motions, or weeks or months of loose bowel actions as in malabsorption or inflammatory bowel disease.

Terminology

The World Health Organization defines diarrhoea as 3 or more unformed bowel actions in 24 hours. Acute diarrhoea is a diarrhoeal episode that lasts less than 2 weeks, while persistent diarrhoea is an episode that lasts for 2 weeks or longer. Chronic diarrhoea is defined as diarrhoea of at least 3–6 weeks' duration.

'Dysentery' is a term that refers to diarrhoea with blood and mucus due to severe colonic infection. The bowel actions are frequent, of small volume with pus, mucus and often blood. Tenesmus, urgency, cramping and infra-umbilical abdominal pain are prominent features. Constitutional symptoms such as pyrexia may be present. Faecal leucocytes are an important feature.

Predisposing and risk factors

Compared to younger people, in the elderly a number of factors predispose to diarrhoea. Increased hospitalisation and institutionalisation significantly increase the risk of infections that include exposure to nosocomial infections, common source outbreaks such as food borne epidemics and person-to-person spread of infection. Sharing toilets with patients with infective diarrhoea (especially those with faecal incontinence) increases the risk of infection. In both the institutional and home setting, cognitive impairment and physical incapacity decreases personal and domestic hygiene, especially food hygiene. Drug therapy, radiation therapy and surgery on the gastrointestinal tract (discussed below) predispose to diarrhoea. Systemic diseases are more common in older people and some directly involve the gastrointestinal tract to cause diarrhoea. Decreased systemic defences, physiological reserves, undernutrition, malnutrition, general debility and co-existing illnesses all contribute to increasing the risk of diarrhoea.

Gastrointestinal tract defences

Immune mechanisms

In the small intestine, the local immune response is mediated by secretory immunoglobulin A (IgA), a dimer that, unlike the monomeric systemic IgA, has greater antibody specificity to respond to the diverse antigenic material in the upper small intestine. Secretory IgA prevents adherence to and colonisation of intestinal epithelial cells by binding directly to bacteria such as *Vibrio cholerae.* Secretory IgA also neutralises bacterial toxins, inhibits viral replication and binds dietary antigens. Data on the effect of ageing alone on secretory IgA production in the small intestine is not yet available in humans. Secretory IgA is highly T cell (particularly T_4) dependent. Immunosuppressive agents used in malignant disease affect secretory IgA production through their effects on lymphocyte populations. Since the quality and proportion of T-helper and T-suppressor subpopulations decrease with age, older persons may experience a decreased primary immune response.

Non-immune defences

The non-immune defences are the gastric acid barrier, the motility of the stomach and the small intestine, and the commensal bacteria of the large intestine. Both ageing and iatrogenic interventions can significantly influence these, leading to diarrhoea, as discussed below.

Gastric acid

Decreased gastric acidity is associated with increased pathogens in the stomach that may lead to small bowel bacterial overgrowth (discussed below). The usual gastric acid pH is below 4 and prevents the survival of viruses, bacteria and intestinal parasites—for example, *Giardia lamblia.* At a pH of 3.0 the stomach is virtually sterile. At a pH of 4–5, bacteria in saliva are present in the stomach, and at a pH greater than 5, bacteria, viruses and protozoa survive.

Gastric acid production decreases with age. Medical conditions associated with decreased gastric acidity that are more prevalent in older persons are:

- gastric carcinoma
- chronic atrophic gastritis
- pernicious anaemia
- WDHA syndrome (watery diarrhoea, hypokalaemia and achlorhydria).

Gastric acid production is decreased by therapeutic agents used in peptic ulcer disease, severe gastroesophageal reflux and the Zollinger-Ellison syndrome, and by surgical procedures such as total gastrectomy and vagotomy.

Gastric motility

Gastric motility, by mixing gastric contents (which may contain pathogens) with gastric juice, decreases growth and survival of pathogens. Decreased contact between gastric acid and pathogens occurs when gastric emptying increases due to gastric surgery, pancreatic exocrine deficiency, 'early' non-insulin dependent diabetes mellitus and prokinetic agents (discussed subsequently).

Small bowel motility

Normal small bowel motility cleanses the lumen of pathogens preventing mucosal invasion and mucosal adherence. Decreased intestinal motility may lead to bacterial overgrowth (see below).

Bacterial deconjugation of bile salts leads to a secretory diarrhoea discussed subsequently. Bile salt deconjugation may also cause fat malabsorption due to a decrease in the critical micellar concentration necessary for optimal fat absorption.

Intestinal flora

The commensal bacteria of the colon form a complex, well balanced ecological system that defends the host against harmful pathogens. Protection occurs by the modification of bile acids; stimulation of peristalsis; induction of immunologic responses; depletion of essential substrates from the environment; competition for adhesion sites; creation of restrictive metabolic environments; and elaboration of antibiotic-like substances. Antibiotics often breach this colonic line of defence.

Table 34.1 Common secretagogues

Class	Agent
Enteropathogens	*Staphylococcus aureus* *Bacillus cereus* *Clostridium perfringens* *Vibrio cholerae* *Vibrio parahaemolyticus* Enterotoxigenic *Escherichia. coli* (ETEC) *Yersinia enterocolitica* *Aeromonas* species *Shigella* species *Cryptosporidium* species
Therapeutic agents (see also Table 34.4)	Laxatives Prostaglandin E2 analogues
Humoral agents	Vasoactive intestinal peptide Glucagon Secretin Calcitonin Bradykinin
Endogenous agents	Long chain fatty acids Dihydroxy bile acids

Mechanisms of diarrhoea

Each day the small intestine converts about 10 L of fluid and digested food into approximately 1.5–2 L of ileal content. This volume is then transformed into about 200 g of solid stool by fluid absorption in the colon. Diarrhoea occurs when the balance between the absorptive capacity of the intestine and its secretory function is disrupted. Despite many aetiological factors, the basic mechanisms that cause diarrhoea are few.

Secretory diarrhoea

Secretory diarrhoea occurs due to intracellular changes induced by a secretagogue (e.g. cholera toxin) which binds to surface receptors on intestinal epithelial cells. This increases the concentrations of cAMP (or less commonly cGMP) that activate adenylate cyclase in the cytoplasm. There is then active secretion of anions (Cl^- and HCO_3^-), the passive efflux of Na^+, K^+ and H_2O and the inhibition of Na^+ and Cl^- entry into cells. The outcome is a net fluid loss. Table 34.1 lists common secretagogues.

Osmotic diarrhoea

Osmotic agents (e.g. sorbitol) generate high osmolality in the lumen to cause diarrhoea by interfering with the normal intestinal function of initiating and maintaining a water gradient. This results in fluid retention in the lumen and fluid secretion into the lumen. An essential diagnostic feature is that diarrhoea ceases when the osmotic agent is not ingested.

Na^+–K^+ exchange pump

In the intestine the Na^+–K^+ exchange pump regulates water and electrolyte transport by generating a potential difference across the epithelial cell membrane. This provides an electrochemical gradient for the (electrogenic) entry of sodium and water from the intestinal lumen into the cell. The energy for this pump is from the breakdown of ATP by ATPase that may be inhibited by therapeutic agents discussed below.

Mucosal damage

Mucosal damage in the small and large intestine occurs due to many aetiological agents discussed subsequently in this chapter. Damage to either the small or large intestinal mucosa causes diarrhoea by disrupting the mechanisms of absorption and secretion. In the small intestine, mucosal damage leads to villous atrophy of varying severity. Severe malabsorption causes steatorrhoea characterised by frothy, foul-smelling faeces that are difficult to flush away, and a film of oil may be present in the toilet pan even after flushing.

In the large intestine, mucosal damage results in colitis of varying severity. The clinical features are diarrhoea with mucus (the large intestine is well endowed with mucus glands) and, if severe, blood, iliac fossa pain and tenesmus.

Aetiology of diarrhoea

The aetiology of diarrhoea in the elderly differs from younger persons in that the incidences of some conditions are more common (see Box 34.1).

Box 34.1 Common causes of diarrhoea in the elderly

- Iatrogenic causes
- Faecal incontinence
- Infections
- Irritable bowel syndrome
- Malabsorption
- Inflammatory bowel disease
- Neoplasms
- Metabolic causes

Iatrogenic causes

Drug therapy

Drug therapy is a frequent cause of diarrhoea (see Table 34.2). Diarrhoea is more often dose related than due to idiosyncratic drug reactions. Drug consumption increases with age and about 85% of older persons consume therapeutic agents for one or more diseases. Table 34.3 lists the frequency of the types of drugs used by older persons.

The drugs that cause diarrhoea can be conveniently classified in the context of the mechanisms of diarrhoea. Table 34.4 lists drugs that act as secretagogues. Box 34.2 lists drugs causing osmotic diarrhoea (undigested monosaccharides and, more commonly, disaccharides also act as osmotic agents as discussed below under 'Lactose intolerance'). Sorbitol is a compound frequently used alone or in combination as a laxative and has replaced lactulose, a synthetic disaccharide used in the management of constipation (see Chapter

Table 34.2 Drugs associated with diarrhoea

Class of drug	Drug
Cardiovascular drugs	Methyldopa, digoxin, quinidine, propranolol, hydralazine, ACE inhibitors, procainamide
Gastrointestinal drugs	Laxatives, lactulose, antacids (magnesium salts), H-2 receptor antagonists, proton pump inhibitors, cholestyramine, chenodeoxycholic acid, olsalazine, misoprostol, enprostil, cisapride
Musculoskeletal drugs	Colchicine, indomethacin, auranofin, naproxen, phenylbutazone, mefenamic acid
Central nervous system drugs	Anticholinergic agents, levodopa, alprazolam, lithium, fluoxetine, donepezil (Aricept), tacrine
Endocrine system drugs	Oral hypoglycaemic agents, clofibrate, thyroxine
Miscellaneous	Antibiotics: clindamycin, amoxycillin, ampicillin, cephalosporins, neomycin Antimetabolites: 5-fluorouracil, methotrexate Osmotic cathartics: magnesium-containing antacids, lactulose, sorbitol, acarbose, propranol

Table 34.3 Frequency of drug consumption in the elderly

Drug type	Frequency of use (%)
NSAIDs	15.0–45.0
Cardiac glycosides	6.0–60.0
Diuretics	12.0–36.0
Analgesics	6.0–17.0
Cardiovascular	10.0–73.0
Psychotropic	6.5–57.0
Gastrointestinal	3.5–18.5

Table 34.4 Drugs that cause secretory diarrhoea

Laxatives	Bisacodyl Dioctyl sodium sulfosuccinate (Docusate Sodium) Phenolphthalein Castor oil Ricinoleic acid Senna Anthraquinone cathartics
Prostaglandin E2 analogues	Misoprostol Enprostil
Miscellaneous	Irinotecan hydrochloride Olsalazine

35) as it is less expensive. Lactulose is now reserved for preventing and treating portal systemic encephalopathy. Other osmotic agents that may cause diarrhoea are antacids containing magnesium trisilicate or magnesium hydroxide. Acarbose, an α-glucosidase inhibitor used to treat type 2 diabetics who are on maximal doses of oral antidiabetic agents (Chapter 41), inhibits small intestinal enzymes that digest disaccharides, oligosaccharides and polysaccharides, but not monosaccharides. The undigested, non-absorbed carbohydrates accumulate and ferment in the small intestine to cause osmotic diarrhoea. Propranolol infrequently causes osmotic diarrhoea. Antibiotics may alter the colonic bacterial flora and decrease the colonic fermentation of carbohydrates, resulting in osmotic diarrhoea.

Some drugs decrease Na^+–K^+-ATPase exchange pump activity. Digoxin was second only to antibiotics as the most common cause of diarrhoea in a study of 100 elderly inpatients. Diarrhoea due to the oral gold preparation auranofin (used in rheumatoid arthritis) may occur in 30–40% of patients in the first 6 months and at 18–24 months in about 10%. At least one episode of diarrhoea was reported by 74% of patients. Diarrhoea declines with time in most patients but in 8–14% of patients the severity requires the drug to be discontinued. Colchicine, used for gout and in recurrent polyserositis (familial Mediterranean fever) and more recently advocated in the treatment of constipation, and olsalazine affect Na^+–K^+-ATPase activity.

Drugs causing mucosal damage are shown in Table 34.5. In the small intestine, mucosal damage results in villous atrophy and this leads to diarrhoea and even significant malabsorption. In the large intestine drugs cause colitis and diarrhoea (Table 34.5). Gold administered parenterally may result in serious enterocolitis within 3 months of therapy and occurs more often in females. The diarrhoea is severe and unrelated to dosage. Auranofin-induced diarrhoea can cause enterocolitis and may persist despite drug withdrawal.

Box 34.2 Agents that cause osmotic diarrhoea

- Magnesium-containing antacids
- Lactulose
- Sorbitol
- Acarbose
- Propranolol
- Antibiotics
- Irinotecan hydrochloride
- Glycerol
- Mannitol
- Magnesium sulphate (Epsom salts)
- Sodium sulphate (Glauber's salt)
- Sodium citrate
- Disaccharides—see 'Lactose intolerance'

Alterations in motility

Alterations in motility occur with various drugs (see Table 34.6). Drugs that have cholinergic activity

Table 34.5 Drugs that cause mucosal damage

Location of action	Drug
Small intestine	Neomycin Colchicine Antimetabolite cancer chemotherapeutic agents
Large intestine (colitis)	NSAIDs Gold salts (including Auranofin) Antimetabolite cancer chemotherapeutic agents Penicillamine Methyldopa Antibiotics Flucytosine

Table 34.6 Causes of altered gastrointestinal motility

Action	Cause
Decreased motility	*Systemic causes* Diabetic autonomic neuropathy Hypothyroidism Amyloidosis Scleroderma Myotonia dystrophica (an hereditary condition characterised by myotonia, muscular wasting, cataracts, testicular atrophy and frontal baldness) *Local causes* Lymphoma Intestinal pseudo-obstruction Radiation enteritis Drugs: propantheline, benztropine
Increased motility	*Cholinomimetics (mimic the parasympathetic effects of acetylcholine)* Tacrine hydrochloride Donepezil (Aricept) *Inhibitors of acetylcholine* Irinotecan hydrochloride Propantheline Benztropine *Enhancers of interdigestive and post-prandial small bowel motor activity* Cisapride Misoprostol Castor oil

(cholinomimetics) mimic the parasympathetic effects of acetylcholine either by acting directly upon acetylcholine receptors or by inhibiting the enzyme acetylcholinesterase. The accumulated acetylcholine in the parasympathetic nerve synapses excites gastrointestinal tract muscles causing increased motility and diarrhoea. Tacrine hydrochloride and donepezil (Aricept) in Alzheimer's disease reversibly bind with and inactivate acetylcholinesterase, resulting in diarrhoea. Irinotecan hydrochloride also inhibits acetylcholinesterase, causing a cholinergic-like syndrome. Diarrhoea may be of sudden onset and severe enough to be life-threatening. Cisapride, a prokinetic agent used in gastroparesis and in gastroesophageal reflux disease, induces diarrhoea by increasing interdigestive and post-prandial small bowel motor activity. However, diarrhoea is usually mild and in most patients requires no intervention.

Anticholinergic drugs may decrease intestinal motility and cause bacterial overgrowth that leads to diarrhoea, although constipation is the most frequent side effect. Common anticholinergic agents include propantheline for urinary incontinence and benztropine for Parkinson's disease. Nursing home patients on drugs with strong anticholinergic effects are reported to require long-term laxative usage. Spurious diarrhoea may be a consequence of constipation (see Chapter 35).

Alterations to gastrointestinal tract defences

As previously discussed, both the immune and non-immune defences are vulnerable to many therapeutic agents. The defence offered by the commensal colonic bacteria is often breached by antibiotics. The diarrhoea is due to a temporary alteration of the bacterial population that is usually mild and self-limiting. Antibiotics are used more frequently in the elderly and are probably the most common iatrogenic cause of diarrhoea.

However, superinfections occur frequently with *Clostridium difficile* and rarely with *C. perfringens*, *Salmonella* and *Shigella*. Pseudomembranous colitis is not inevitable but is the most serious consequence of *C. difficile* infection. It occurs with virtually all antibiotics, including vancomycin and metronidazole used in treating *C. difficile* infection. Clindamycin, lincomycin, ciprofloxacin, amoxycillin, ampicillin and cephalosporins are most often responsible, reflecting their widespread use. Other predisposing factors to *C. difficile* infection are hospitalisation, long-term care facilities, chemotherapy for malignancy, feeding tubes, urinary and faecal incontinence, and the presence of three or more underlying diseases. In mild cases of pseudomembranous colitis, antibiotic therapy is unnecessary. In severe diarrhoea (5–6 motions a day associated with blood, tenesmus and abdominal pain), oral vancomycin, bacitracin or metronidazole are the drugs of choice. Metronidazole is the preferred antibiotic due to the emergence of vancomycin resistant enterococci, the equivalent efficacy and relapse rates and lower cost. It is not unusual for relapses to occur. In patients who are severely ill or immunocompromised or with multisystem disease, vancomycin is recommended. Antidiarrhoeal agents are contraindicated: toxic mega colon may occur. In institutions standards of hygiene should be urgently reviewed since the spores of *C. difficile* survive for up to 5 months and have been isolated from sources such as bedding and bedpans.

Some drugs cause diarrhoea by multiple mechanisms. In ulcerative colitis 12–25% of patients on olsalazine develop diarrhoea. Olsalazine inhibits sodium dependent bile acid transport into the ileum and bile acids reach the colon, acting as powerful secretagogues to cause diarrhoea. Another mechanism may involve the inhibition of Na^+–K^+-ATPase activity.

Colchicine causes diarrhoea by mucosal damage and also by diminishing the activity of the Na^+–K^+-ATPase pump. Misoprostol increases motor activity to cause diarrhoea and also acts as a secretagogue. Castor oil increases intestinal motility to cause diarrhoea and ricinoleic acid, a metabolite of castor oil, acts as a secretagogue.

Chemotherapy with irinotecan hydrochloride can cause diarrhoea through two separate mechanisms: (1) by affecting motility by inhibition of acetylcholinesterase; and (2) by causing osmotic and secretory diarrhoea through its active metabolite SN-38.

Laxative abuse

Laxative abuse among older people, whether intentional or inadvertent, is a prominent cause of diarrhoea. Besides diarrhoea, the presentation may include eating or psychiatric disorders. Screening for laxatives is widely available.

Infectious causes

The elderly are at an increased risk of acquiring infectious diarrhoea caused by the risk factors discussed. The pathogens can affect either the small or large bowel.

Secretagogue production

Bacteria and protozoa that produce toxins which act as secretagogues to effect secretory diarrhoea are:

- *Staphylococcus aureus*
- *Bacillus cereus*
- *C. perfringens*
- *Vibrio cholerae*
- *Vibrio parahaemolyticus*
- Enterotoxigenic *E. coli* (ETEC)
- Enteroadhesive *E. coli* (EAEC)
- *Yersinia enterocolitica*
- *Aeromonas* species
- *Shigella* species
- *Cryptosporidium* species.

Cytotoxin production

Many bacteria secrete a cytotoxin that causes cell injury and cell death, resulting in diarrhoea. These bacteria are:

- *Shigella* species
- *Shigella dysenteriae 1*
- *Shigella sonnei* (some strains)
- *Shigella flexneri* (some strains)
- *C. difficile*
- Enterohaemorrhagic *E. coli* (EHEC)
- *Campylobacter jejuni.*

Mucosal invasion

Cell *invasion* is the primary event and then a cytotoxin is produced. Invasion, intracellular replication and, in some instances, submucosal invasion cause tissue death and diarrhoea. The diarrhoeal stool consists of an inflammatory exudate, sloughed cells and cell debris, copious mucus from goblet cells, pus and blood—the essential features of dysentery.

The bacteria responsible for mucosal invasion are:

- Enteroinvasive *E. coli* (EIEC)
- *Salmonella* species
- *Shigella* species
- *C. jejuni*
- *Y. enterocolitica*
- Enterohaemorrhagic *E. coli* (EHEC)
- Enteroaggregative *E. coli* (EAggEC).

Food borne illness and food poisoning and bacterial diarrhoea

The term 'food borne illness' now includes the term 'food poisoning'. Food poisoning infers the presence of a toxin in food elaborated by a pathogen. Symptoms are due to the toxin and not the pathogen. A food borne disease outbreak occurs if the following criteria are met:

1. Two or more people experience the same symptoms, usually referable to the gastrointestinal tract, after the consumption of the same dietary item.
2. A dietary item is implicated as the common source by epidemiological investigation. Food poisoning is diagnosed when nausea, vomiting and diarrhoea occurs after 2–3 persons have consumed the same food or drink contaminated by a preformed toxin elaborated by a pathogen. The incubation period is short and the onset of symptoms is abrupt. Bacteria commonly implicated are:
   - *S. aureus*
   - *Bacillus cereus*
   - *C. perfringens*
   - *V. parahaemolyticus*

Viruses such as the Norwalk agent produce an identical clinical picture.

Parasitic causes of diarrhoea

Parasitic infection of the gastrointestinal tract causing diarrhoea is common in states of immunosuppression. The parasites which are most often associated with diarrhoea are listed in Table 34.7.

Table 34.7 Parasites most often associated with diarrhoea

Protozoa	*G. lamblia* *Entamoeba histolytica* *Cryptosporidium* species *Isospora belli* Microsporidia *Sarcocystis hominis* *Balantidium coli* *Blastocystis hominis*
Nematodes (round worms)	*Strongyloides stercoralis* *Trichuris trichura* *Capillaria philippinensis* *Trichinella spiralis*
Trematodes (flukes)	*Schistosoma mansoni* *Schistosoma japonicum*

In the Western world *G. lamblia*, a flagellate protozoan, is the most common parasite to infect the small intestine. Diarrhoea is due to mucosal damage. Outbreaks of giardiasis have occurred in visitors to the snowfields in Aspen and Boulder, Colorado in the US, to New Zealand and St Petersburg, Russia. Dogs and cats act as reservoirs of infection. Ingesting as few as 10 cysts can cause infection. The symptoms occur about 2 weeks after infection and include abdominal discomfort, distension, flatulence and diarrhoea. Diarrhoea may occur acutely, intermittently or be chronic due to malabsorption. Reinfection is frequent.

Cryptosporidium causes diarrhoea by elaborating a secretagogue. *Strongyloides stercoralis* invades the mucosa of the small intestine and is associated with a high eosinophil count. *Entamoeba histolytica* invades and extensively damages the large intestinal epithelial cells.

Viral diarrhoea

A viral cause of diarrhoea is not uncommon in older persons and epidemics of viral diarrhoea have occurred. Viral diarrhoea is more common in patients when a chronic carrier state is reactivated as a result of immunosuppression—for example, cytomegalovirus (CMV). Rotavirus infection is a common viral cause of diarrhoea in healthy adults. Diagnostic clues are a history of contact with a young child with diarrhoea, vomiting for about 36 hours and watery diarrhoea (for 3–8 days). Norwalk virus infection occurs predominantly during winter and, since vomiting is severe, has been called the 'winter vomiting disease'. The illness lasts for 1–2 days.

Traveller's diarrhoea

Travel abroad is increasingly popular among older persons. The risk of acquiring traveller's diarrhoea depends on the destination of travel, with different geographical areas having different potential risks for visitors.

Common bacterial causes of traveller's diarrhoea are:

- Enterotoxigenic *E. coli*
- Enteroadherent *E. coli*

- Enteroinvasive *E. coli*
- *Salmonella* species
- *Shigella* species
- *C. jejuni*
- *Aeromonas hydrophila.*

Rotavirus is the most frequent viral agent identified in traveller's diarrhoea. Common parasitic causes are *G. lamblia, E. histolytica, Cryptosporidium* and *S. stercoralis*.

In traveller's diarrhoea most diarrhoeal episodes are self-limiting. Antibiotics should be used cautiously. Antibiotics are indicated in dysentery, especially if symptoms such as fever, chills, headache and myalgia are present or if the diarrhoea persists for more than 48 hours. Ciprofloxacin and norfloxacin have a broad spectrum of activity. Before antibiotic treatment, a parasitic cause should be ruled out. Diarrhoea during travel may be due to a non-infective cause—for example, overindulgence of alcohol, and exotic and spicy food.

Whipple's disease

Whipple's disease is now known to occur in the elderly and is not confined as previously thought to the middle aged. The disease is uncommon, although lethal if not treated. The causative organism has been identified: *Tropheryma whippelii*, derived from the Greek words *trophe* (nourishment) and *eryma* (barrier) and George Whipple's surname. The organism, although predominantly affecting the small intestine and leading to malabsorption, frequently affects other systems. Diarrhoea, weight loss, abdominal pain and arthralgia are the most frequent but not invariable manifestations. Arthritis or arthralgia may be the only presenting symptom, predating other manifestations by years. The characteristic histopathological features in the small intestine are diagnostic: distension of the normal villous architecture by an infiltrate of foamy macrophages with a coarsely granular cytoplasm that stains a brilliant magenta colour with PAS, and variable villous atrophy. A recent important diagnostic test is the polymerase chain reaction of the 16S ribosomal RNA of *Tropheryma whippelii*. Treatment consists of an adequate regimen of antibiotics as relapses are common.

Tropical sprue

Tropical sprue is a primary malabsorption syndrome in residents or visitors to certain areas of the tropics. An infective aetiology is most likely. Unlike coeliac disease, the entire small intestine is involved and therefore both folate and vitamin B_{12} absorption (due to terminal ileal involvement) occurs. The symptoms are malaise and easy fatigability, weight loss, diarrhoea and abdominal discomfort. Bowel movements are typical of steatorrhoea. Small intestinal biopsy shows villous atrophy and an inflammatory infiltrate of the lamina propria.

In making the diagnosis it is important to exclude parasitic causes of malabsorption, especially giardiasis. As with all malabsorption syndromes, treatment should focus on correcting the nutritional consequences of malabsorption. The specific treatment for tropical sprue is a combination of folic acid and tetracycline, usually for several months until histological improvement of small intestine morphology occurs.

Small bowel bacterial overgrowth

Small bowel bacterial overgrowth (blind loop syndrome, stagnant loop syndrome) associated with diarrhoea and even malabsorption is common in older subjects. Aetiological factors are diverticulae, strictures, fistulas, blind loops and conditions discussed earlier that decrease motility. However, the aetiology is often unknown. Diarrhoea is due to bacterial deconjugation of primary bile salts to dihydroxy bile acids (predominantly deoxycholic acid) which cause net fluid and electrolyte secretion in the colon. Bile salt deconjugation also impairs micelle formation and may lead to steatorrhoea.

The definitive diagnosis is by a bacterial count greater than 10^5 colony forming units (CFU) per millilitre, or counts of aerobic bacteria exceeding 10^4 CFU per millilitre in a sterile aspirate of duodenal or jejunal fluid. A more convenient diagnostic test is the ^{14}C-xylose breath test.

The underlying condition which predisposes to bacterial overgrowth should be treated if practicable. If there is no demonstrable cause, as in many elderly patients, a course of antibiotics is recommended, given in cycles to prevent further bacterial overgrowth and antibiotic resistance. Tetracycline and erythromycin are commonly used. Antibiotic therapy ultimately resolves the problems of malabsorption and undernutrition.

HIV infection

In patients with HIV infection, more so during the advanced stages of the illness, diarrhoea associated with a wide variety of infections is common. These include protozoa, helminths (*Strongyloides stercoralis*), bacteria and viruses. The most common pathogens are listed in Table 34.8.

Table 34.8 Pathogens commonly found in patients with HIV

Pathogen	Agent
Protozoal	*Cryptosporidium* species
	Microsporidia
	Cyclospora
	Isospora
	G. lamblia
Bacterial	*Mycobacterium avium* complex
	Salmonella/Shigella
	Campylobacter species
Viral	Cytomegalovirus

Malabsorption

Malabsorption refers to both maldigestion and malabsorption of nutrients. The malabsorption syndrome encompasses the many consequences of the malabsorption of fats, carbohydrates, protein, vitamins and minerals. Fat malabsorption is the hallmark of the malabsorption syndrome, and may be attributable to fat maldigestion due to a pancreatic cause, or a small intestinal problem preventing fat absorption. Less commonly, fat malabsorption is due to inadequate bile salts. The consequence of fat malabsorption is steatorrhoea, the passage of abnormal quantities of fat in the faeces, characterised by loose, bulky, extraordinarily foul-smelling stools that are difficult to flush and often leave a film of oil in the toilet pan.

Small bowel malabsorption

The aetiology of small bowel malabsorption is extensive and is shown in Box 34.3. Coeliac disease is discussed below, and Tropical sprue, Whipple's disease and giardiasis, which also cause malabsorption, are discussed in the section on 'Infectious diarrhoea'. The consequences of malabsorbed vitamin, mineral and protein may manifest as anaemia, a bleeding diathesis, peripheral neuropathy, osteomalacia or oedema.

Coeliac disease

Coeliac disease (gluten sensitive enteropathy; coeliac sprue) is not confined to children and may occur for the first time in an older person. It is a common cause of malabsorption in the West. Diarrhoea may not be a constant feature. Older patients may present only with the manifestations of vitamin and mineral deficiency and hypoproteinaemia. In coeliac disease since ileal damage is rare, B_{12} malabsorption is uncommon. In longstanding, untreated coeliac disease, malignancies of the small intestine such as lymphoma and adenocarcinoma, or malignancies of the pharynx and oesophagus, may occur.

Currently the most effective method of diagnosis is by obtaining 2–3 biopsies during endoscopy from the second part of the duodenum and demonstrating villous atrophy on morphology. Anti-endomysial antibodies and, more recently, antitransglutaminase antibodies are advocated as a sensitive non-invasive screening test for coeliac disease. Dietary gluten restriction results in villous architecture reverting to normal. A rechallenge with gluten is perhaps unnecessary in the elderly.

HIV enteropathy

HIV enteropathy is associated with malabsorption, diarrhoea and weight loss and other manifestations of malabsorption. The aetiology is obscure: although infectious agents are implicated, no opportunistic infection is evident in up to 30% of patients with symptoms of malabsorption. Small intestine mucosal abnormalities include villous atrophy with and without crypt hyperplasia of varying severity, inflammation of the lamina propria and enterocyte cytoplasmic vacuolation. In the lamina propria CD4 lymphocytes and macrophages may show HIV. In addition, HIV has been isolated from small bowel enterocytes. Antiretroviral therapy improves the enteropathy.

Box 34.3 Small bowel causes of malabsorption

Anatomical causes
Short bowel syndrome
- Small bowel resection
- Congenital

Arterial insufficiency and intestinal ischaemia

Mucosal causes
Coeliac disease and related entities
Tropical sprue
Eosinophilic gastroenteritis
Regional enteritis (Crohn's disease)
Whipple's disease
Therapeutic agents
- Neomycin
- ColchicineMethotrexate
- Microvillus inclusion disease

Abetalipoproteinaemia
Acrodermatitis enteropathica
Macroglobulinaemia
Radiation injury
Infections
- Acute
  - Bacterial
  - Viral
  - Fungal
  - Parasitic
- Chronic
  - Tuberculosis
  - Tropical sprue
  - Whipple's disease
- Miscellaneous
- Malnutrition
- Zollinger-Ellison syndrome

Submucosal causes
Infiltrative conditions
- Amyloidosis
- Systemic mastocytosis
- Lymphoma

Fibrosis
- Radiation enteritis
- Systemic sclerosis

Lymphatic obstruction
- Intestinal lymphangiectasia
  - Primary

– Secondary

Vascular
- Atherosclerosis
- Vasculitides
- Radiation injury

Motility disorders
Endocrine and metabolic causes
- Diabetes mellitus
- Hyperthyroidism
- Hypothyroidism
- Hypoadrenalism (Addison's disease)
- Hypoparathyroidism
- Pseudohypoparathyroidism

Infiltrative conditions
Intestinal pseudo-obstruction
Therapeutic agents
- Anticholinergics
  - Propantheline
  - Benztropine
- Tricyclic antidepressants

Fibrosis
- Radiation enteritis
- Systemic sclerosis

Source: Modified from R. N. Ratnaike. & A. H. Barbour (2000), 'Maldigestion and malabsorption', in R. N. Ratnaike (ed.), *Small Bowel Disorders*, Edward Arnold, London, pp. 302–15.

Pancreatic causes of malabsorption

Steatorrhoea is most frequently caused by pancreatic insufficiency in elderly patients. Alcoholic and idiopathic pancreatitis comprise about 95% of cases of chronic pancreatitis. A subtype of non-alcoholic pancreatitis, termed 'idiopathic senile chronic pancreatitis', is common in older persons. Pancreatic carcinoma as a cause of steatorrhoea is rare as steatorrhoea occurs only when about 90% of pancreatic secretory capacity is lost.

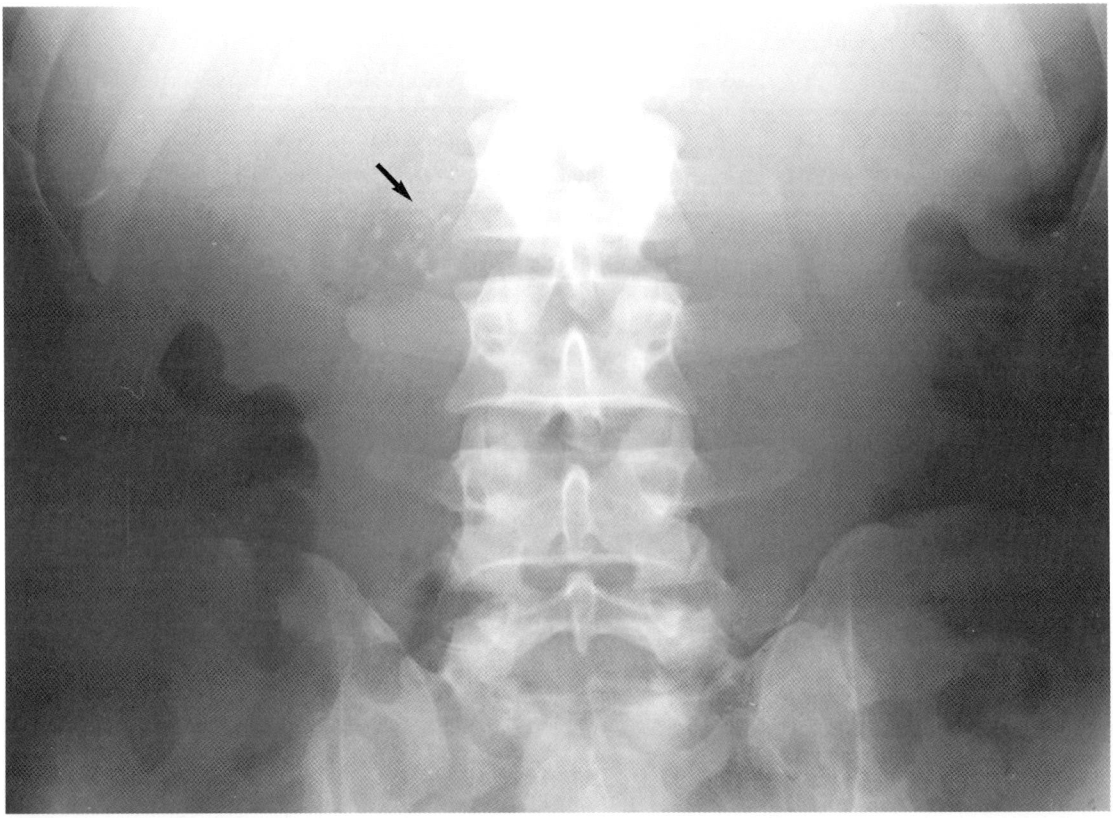

Figure 34.1 Calcification in the pancreas in chronic pancreatitis REPRINTED FROM RATNAIKE (1999) WITH PERMISSION OF THE PUBLISHER, CAMBRIDGE UNIVERSITY PRESS

A diagnosis of chronic pancreatitis should be considered in patients with a history of recurrent upper abdominal pain (located in the epigastrium and frequently referred to the back; the intensity of the pain varies with posture and is relieved by bending forward), and diarrhoea associated with steatorrhoea, weight loss and diabetes mellitus. Pancreatic calcification (see Figure 34.1) and a normal small bowel biopsy virtually establish a pancreatic cause of diarrhoea. Pancreatic enzyme replacement therapy is the principal treatment for steatorrhoea.

Lactose intolerance

Lactose intolerance is the most common cause of carbohydrate malabsorption, due to an absence or deficiency of the enzyme lactase in the small intestine. Lactase deficiency is primary or secondary. The incidence of lactase deficiency in older persons is not known. It is likely that secondary lactose intolerance, rather than the congenital primary form, is more common. Secondary lactose intolerance, which is mild and temporary, is due to damage to small intestinal villi from infection, radiation therapy or a primary mucosal disorder such as coeliac disease.

$$\text{Lactose glucose} \xrightarrow{\text{lactase}} \text{galactose}$$

In lactose intolerance undigested lactose reaches the colon unchanged and is metabolised by colonic bacteria:

$$\text{Lactose} \xrightarrow{\text{colonic bacteria}} \text{acetic, propionic and butyric acids}$$

These organic acids—acetate, propionate and butyrate—act as osmotic agents, causing diarrhoea. The clinical features are explosive watery diarrhoea, cramping abdominal pain, abdominal distension and flatulence after the ingestion of milk or milk products. Interestingly, yoghurt may be consumed with no ill effects since bacterial lactase in yoghurt is activated at body temperature. In adults the diagnosis is made by the hydrogen breath test. A cheap, rapid visual screening test developed by Buttery et al. (1994) is now available.

Irritable bowel syndrome

Irritable bowel syndrome (IBS) is not as common in the elderly compared to younger persons. The prevalence of IBS in a study from Denmark in a sex stratified random sample of 70-year-olds was 3–18% among men and 6–32% among women. IBS is defined as: 'chronic or recurrent symptoms attributable to the intestines and occurring in varying but characteristic combinations of abdominal pain, bloating (distension) and symptoms of disordered defecation, especially urgency, straining, feeling of incomplete evacuation and altered stool form and frequency'. The dominant symptoms are abdominal pain and/or disordered bowel function.

The strong association of IBS with psychosomatic factors is relevant in older persons who experience significant life events such as bereavement of a spouse, ill health, physical and mental incapacity, relocation from the family home, or dependence on a carer.

In a random cohort of 734 Italian subjects over 70 years, a significant association between reduced functional ability and IBS was documented, and a diffuse disorder affecting both smooth and striated muscles was postulated.

A positive diagnosis of IBS can be made by history taking alone. However, in elderly patients it is prudent to obtain at least a haematological and biochemical profile, an abdominal ultrasound and perform a sigmoidoscopy. Therapy is directed towards relief of pain (antispasmodic drugs), diarrhoea (loperamide, diphenoxylate) and constipation if present. The latter may require advice on a diet with adequate if not a high content of fibre and fluid of at least 1.5 L a day and, depending on the response, laxatives such as normacol and/or an osmotic laxative—for example, sorbitol (Chapter 35).

Radiation enteropathy

Diarrhoea is a common side effect of radiation therapy for carcinoma of the cervix, uterus, rectum and prostate—malignancies common in the elderly. Diarrhoea may occur during treatment, shortly afterwards or, in a small number of patients, even after 20 or 30 years. The availability of supravoltage radiation that causes minimal or no skin damage despite high doses of radiation has increased the occurrence of diarrhoea. The small intestine is most vulnerable due to the rapid turnover of epithelial cells, and malabsorption may result. Diarrhoea may also be due to stricture formation, especially in the less mobile duodenum and terminal ileum, leading to bacterial overgrowth. Damage to the colon, the caecum and recto sigmoid, which are fixed in the pelvis, causes diarrhoea in about 50% of patients.

Surgical intervention

Bowel resection is the most common cause of diarrhoea secondary to surgical intervention for mesenteric ischaemia, Crohn's disease, radiation enteritis, trauma, volvulus and malignancy. Bowel adaptation can occur in adults with more than 60 cm of small bowel, or 30 cm of small bowel *and* an intact ileocaecal valve. The short bowel syndrome is defined as malabsorption secondary to significant and extensive small bowel resection, such that the small bowel is unable to functionally compensate.

Carcinoma of the colon

In Australia colorectal cancer is the most frequent non-cutaneous cancer. In 1995 there were 4508 deaths in 10 615 cases in a population of approximately 20 million. The lifetime risk in Australia of developing colorectal cancer before the age of 75 is approximately 1 in 18 for men and 1 in 26 for women; and the median age at diagnosis is 70 years. A colonic malignancy (see Figure 34.2) should be suspected in instances of iron deficiency anaemia with no obvious cause, sudden weight loss or a change in bowel habit. Diarrhoea, or diarrhoea alternating with constipation, is not uncommon. Alterations in bowel patterns associated with bleeding or melaena strongly suggest a malignancy. Pain is an uncommon symptom except in advanced disease.

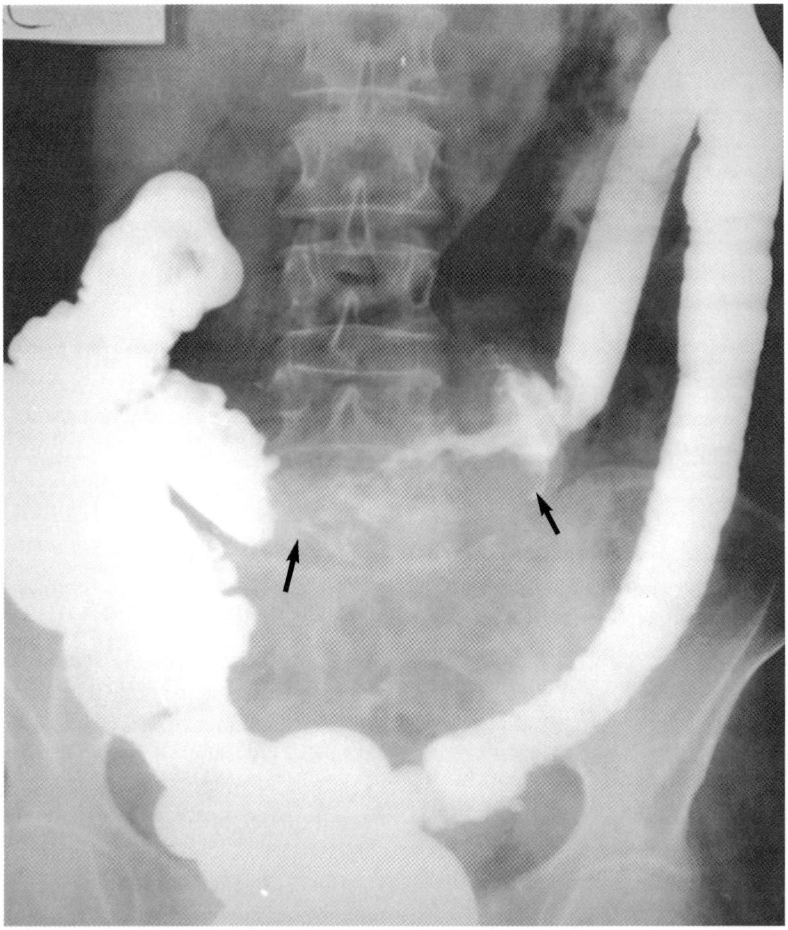

Figure 34.2 Carcinoma of the colon. An 'apple core' lesion in the transverse colon

Physical examination must include a rectal examination. Faecal occult blood may be tested by a laboratory or by individuals with a commercial kit carefully following the manufacturer's instructions. Patients with a positive test should be referred for further investigations to visualise the lower gastro-intestinal tract.

Faecal incontinence

A common problem of older persons is faecal incontinence (spurious diarrhoea; overflow diarrhoea). About 10% of elderly persons in institutional care experience this problem at least once a week. The prevalence is 42% in geriatric wards. The most common cause of faecal incontinence is faecal impaction secondary to constipation (Chapter 35). Spurious diarrhoea may also result from a partial obstruction due to an obstructive lesion of the colon or rectum, or with impaired rectal sensation and reservoir capacity, impaired puborectalis function or cognitive impairment.

Diverticular disease

The risk of developing diverticula of the colon (see Figure 34.3) increases with age (Chapter 37). Diarrhoea is associated with acute or chronic inflammation due to a mechanical obstruction within the diverticula. The clinical picture of diverticulitis is a

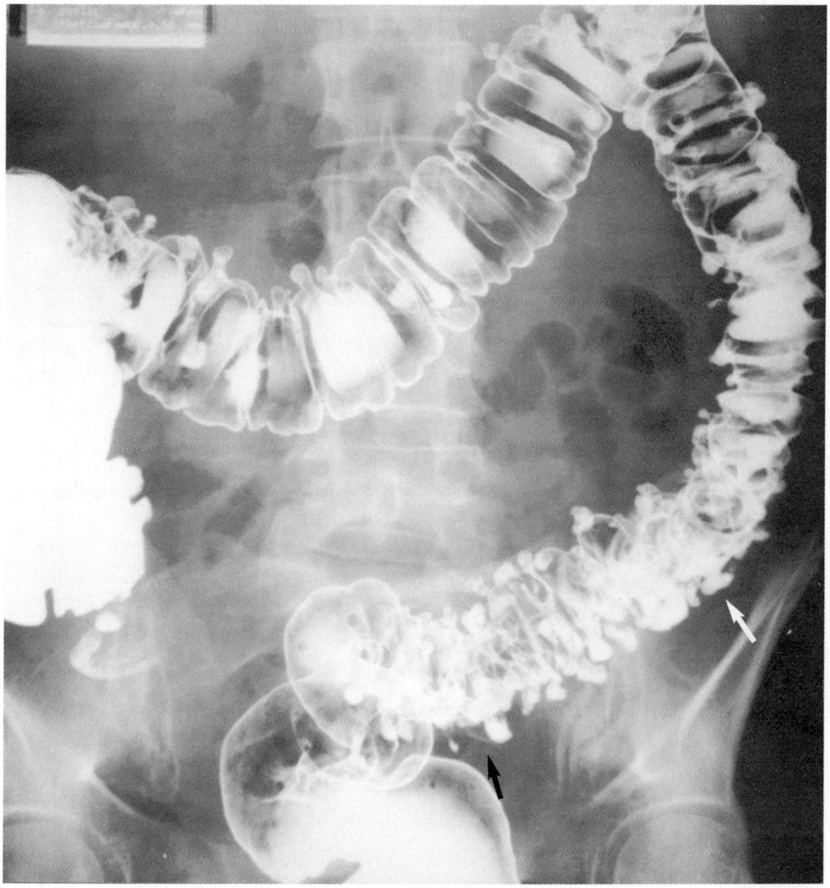

Figure 34.3 Diverticular disease. Multiple flask-like outpouchings of the colon. Note hypertrophy of the circular muscle folds and accentuation of the haustral pattern REPRINTED FROM RATNAIKE (1999) WITH PERMISSION OF THE PUBLISHER, CAMBRIDGE UNIVERSITY PRESS

febrile illness with bloody diarrhoea, lower abdominal pain, tenderness and a possible mass due to an abscess.

Ischaemic colitis

Atherosclerosis, polycythaemia, diabetes mellitus, arteritis and digitalis preparations increase the risk of ischaemic colitis. The presentation may be acute or chronic with diarrhoea, cramping lower (usually left-sided) abdominal pain and the passage of frank blood or clots. If pain after food is the only symptom, the focus of investigation may often shift to the upper gastrointestinal tract and the diagnosis of ischaemic colitis could be delayed or not made. Evidence of other manifestations of vascular disease are important pointers. The diagnosis is based on the typical barium enema findings of 'thumb printing', or 'saw tooth' indentations (see Figure 34.4).

Inflammatory bowel disease

It is not unusual for Crohn's disease and ulcerative colitis to occur for the first time in the elderly. Two peaks of incidence occur in ulcerative colitis: the first in the third and fourth decade and the second in the eighth decade. In older persons the illness profile and response to treatment in both conditions is no different to that in younger persons.

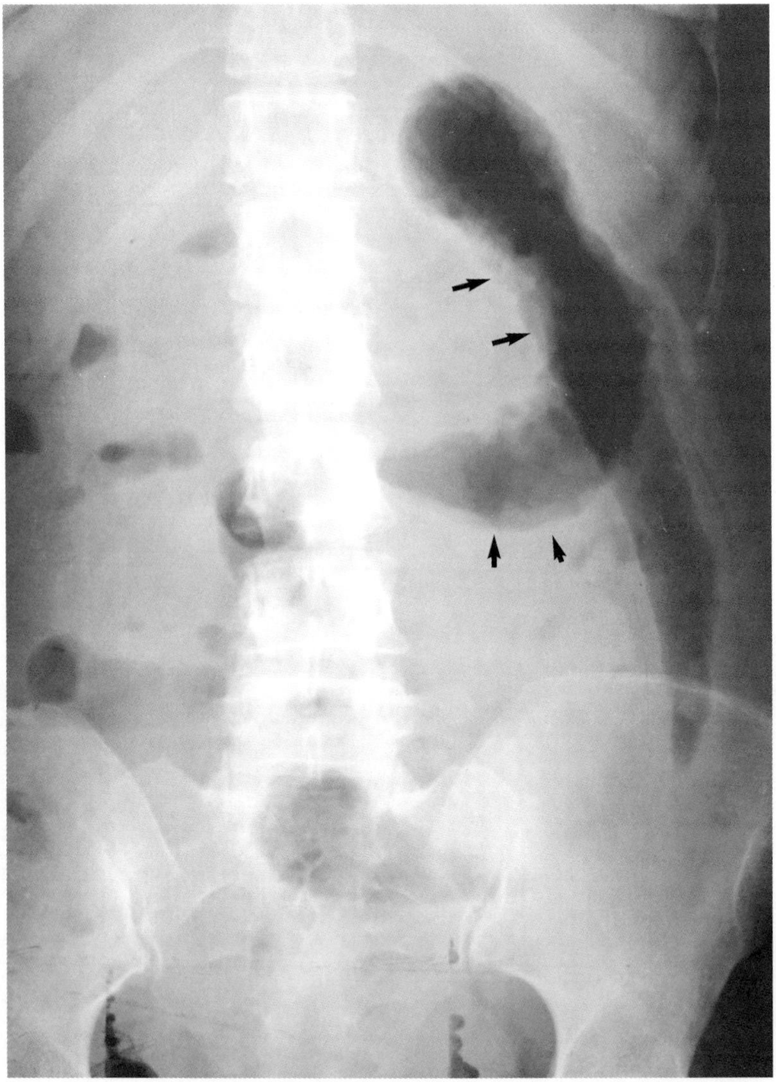

Figure 34.4 'Thumb printing' in ischaemic colitis REPRINTED FROM RATNAIKE (1999) WITH PERMISSION OF THE PUBLISHER, CAMBRIDGE UNIVERSITY PRESS

Collagenous colitis and lymphocytic ('microscopic') colitis

These two conditions are recognised with increasing frequency. Patients present with chronic watery diarrhoea. Colonoscopy and barium studies are normal. In collagenous colitis a band of subepithelial collagen is seen on biopsy. Microscopic colitis is now thought to be an entity distinct from collagenous colitis. The surface epithelium of the colon shows damage and infiltration by large numbers of lymphocytes. Lymphocytic colitis is suggested as a more appropriate term.

Endocrine and metabolic causes

Diarrhoea is associated with a variety of endocrine and metabolic causes. In thyroid disease, both hyperthyroidism and hypothyroidism, the mechanism of diarrhoea is altered motility. Older patients may present with apathetic thyrotoxicosis characterised by lethargy and apathy and the absence of eye signs and tachycardia.

Diarrhoea may be a problem in patients with diabetes mellitus, especially those on insulin and with evidence of peripheral vascular disease and neuropathy. The mechanism of diarrhoea is possibly multifactorial, including both 'rapid and decreased' transit time, the latter leading to bacterial overgrowth. Treatment with α_2-adrenergic agonists (e.g. clonidine) are beneficial, although side effects on the central nervous system and cardiovascular system preclude extensive use. α_2-adrenergic agonists occupy the post-synaptic adrenergic receptors on the enterocyte and decrease cyclic AMP concentrations, which ultimately results in net water and electrolyte retention.

Other less common endocrine and metabolic causes of diarrhoea are due to the Zollinger-Ellison syndrome, gastrinoma, carcinoid tumours, thyroid carcinoma, somatostatinoma, glucagonoma and vipomas such as ganglioneuroma, ganglioblastoma and phaeochromocytoma.

Diagnosis, management and prevention

Despite the extensive aetiology of diarrhoea, 'diagnostic directions' can be mapped out by a good history, a thorough physical examination and a logical choice of investigations. At the clinical interview it is essential to establish at the onset:

- the patient's usual bowel habit
- what is meant by diarrhoea
- if the problem is spurious (overflow) diarrhoea due to constipation
- if there is faecal incontinence
- what medication the patient is on (including over-the-counter medication).

History taking from many older patients requires a change in style and tempo. History taking is an art, not a science, and this is particularly true in the setting of the older patient. The 'poor historian' is more often the physician and not the patient. Denial or minimising the problem of diarrhoea, especially faecal incontinence, is not uncommon. Constipation may be regarded as 'normal'. The time of onset of diarrhoea and its duration may not be recalled as they may not be important events to the patient.

Determining if the diarrhoea is drug related obviates unnecessary investigations, expense and inconvenience. A comprehensive drug history may require information from a relative or carer, the patient's physician or pharmacist. Sighting all drugs consumed, including over-the-counter medication and products from health shops, is rewarding. Polypharmacy, self-medication and the possibility of surreptitious laxative abuse should not be ignored. Patients and carers should be given clear verbal (and perhaps written information) on drug side effects such as diarrhoea.

Suggested guidelines on when patients and carers and health professionals should seek medical attention are:

- bloody diarrhoea
- evidence of dehydration
- abdominal pain and tenderness, rectal pain, tenesmus
- persistent vomiting and inability to retain fluids for a 6 hour period
- fever
- more than 5–6 bowel actions in 24 hours
- patients with current medical problems
- patients on drug therapy.

The patient (and/or caregiver) should be instructed about the importance of increased fluid intake and a plan regarding further intervention should be agreed on. Guidelines for advice during an episode of diarrhoea at home are:

- Decrease physical activity.
- Stay indoors on a hot day.
- Drink plenty of fluids (up to 3 L per day, unless there is a contraindication).
- Avoid milk and alcohol.
- Do not stop eating solids; eat what can be tolerated.
- Avoid milk products, high-fibre food, spicy food, raw food.
- Take a drug such as loperamide if recommended by your physician.
- Avoid home remedies unless they are first discussed with your doctor.

- Wash your hands frequently, especially after going to the toilet, before eating and handling oral medication.

An initial diagnostic approach to diarrhoea is to establish whether it is acute or chronic. Is it iatrogenic? Is diarrhoea a manifestation of a disease intrinsic to the gastrointestinal tract or secondary to a systemic illness?

A viral infection, for example, rotavirus, is suggested by significant vomiting, low-grade fever, myalgia, malaise, headache and contact with a very young child with diarrhoea. Diarrhoea due to food poisoning has a sudden onset, with vomiting being a prominent feature. The clustering of cases strengthens the diagnosis of food borne illness. The onset of diarrhoea may be associated with a particular type of food and specific bacteria often contaminate a particular type of food: *Bacillus cereus* with fried rice; *Vibrio parahaemolyticus* with seafood; enterohaemorrhagic *E. coli 0156:H7* with minced beef in fast foods; *Campylobacter jejuni* with poultry; *Trichinella spiralis* with pork.

If the diarrhoea is chronic (over 3 weeks' duration), the most useful approach is to decide if the small or large intestine is involved. Chronic small bowel diarrhoea is most often due to malabsorption secondary to a small intestinal or pancreatic problem with steatorrhoea.

The optimal method to exclude a small intestinal cause of malabsorption, such as coeliac disease, is an endoscopic small bowel biopsy for histopathological examination. Upper gastrointestinal tract radiology is of value to demonstrate anatomical abnormalities such as diverticula, fistulae, tumours, surgical procedures and terminal ileal lesions.

Large bowel diarrhoea may be associated with the passage of blood and mucus. In the elderly a neoplasm must always be considered, especially if stools are bloody. In these circumstances rectal examination is essential. Sigmoidoscopy should precede a barium enema and be performed in all patients with diarrhoea with blood and mucus and with chronic diarrhoea. A carcinoma of the recto-sigmoid area should be diagnosed by the clinician and not the radiologist when the enema tube is inserted. Especially in older patients, colonoscopy for examination of the large intestine is a more comfortable procedure than a double contrast barium enema and has higher diagnostic accuracy. The CT scan and ultrasound of the abdomen are useful investigations to demonstrate intra- and extraluminal masses.

Stool examination for leucocytes, widely popular in North America, is advocated to identify an infective aetiology. Microscopic examination of faeces with concentration for cysts and ova is an important preliminary screening test for protozoal and helminth infections. Informing the laboratory staff of the suspected diagnosis when bacterial culture and sensitivity are requested enables selection of appropriate enrichment and isolation techniques to reach a rapid diagnosis.

A haematological screen provides useful information in the diagnosis of diarrhoea. Low haemoglobin can occur due to malabsorption, chronic blood loss or in association with an increased reticulocyte count caused by acute blood loss (from the large intestine). In the peripheral blood film Howell-Jolly bodies (nuclear remnants in erythrocytes) occur in coeliac disease with splenic atrophy. Macrocytosis occurs with folate or vitamin B_{12} deficiency. Folate levels are invariably abnormal when the proximal small intestine, the site of folate absorption, is involved. Low vitamin B_{12} concentrations reflect severe and extensive ileal damage. Upper small bowel pathology may also manifest as decreased concentrations of albumin, calcium, zinc and magnesium. In diagnosing steatorrhoea the ^{14}C-triolein breath test is more convenient than the 3 day faecal fat estimation. The breath hydrogen test is an accurate, relatively simple and rapid method of diagnosing lactose intolerance. Bacterial overgrowth can be diagnosed by the ^{14}C-xylose breath test, although the ^{14}C-cholyglycine breath test is also widely used.

The initial objective in the management of diarrhoea is to prevent dehydration and electrolyte loss. The conventional symptoms and signs (reduction of skin turgor, increased thirst, decreased peripheral perfusion, postural hypotension, low jugular venous pressure, patient sensations of thirst and dryness, tachycardia and temperature) are not strong correlates of dehydration in the elderly. This may be due to normal age related changes in these variables, differences in physiological responses to dehydration between the elderly and younger patients caused by, for example, postural hypotension independent of the state of hydration or autonomic dysfunction or drug therapy.

In older persons Gross et al. (1992) describe seven signs and symptoms that strongly correlate with dehydration but are independent of significant, age related change:

- dry tongue
- longitudinal tongue furrows
- dry mucous membranes of nose and mouth
- eyes that appear recessed in their sockets
- upper body muscle weakness
- speech difficulty
- confusion.

Treatment of dehydration should initially centre on oral rehydration that can effectively replace fluid and electrolyte loss. Older patients often need continual encouragement to take sufficient fluids. The decreased fluid intake is due mainly to:

- a decreased perception of thirst
- inability to ask for fluids due to dementia or altered consciousness
- physical inability to obtain fluids
- inability to drink because of dysphagia and/or
- reluctance to drink because of fear of nocturia or incontinence.

A large (fluid) osmotic load should be avoided—for example, Coca-Cola (680 mOsm per kg), apple juice (870 mOsm per kg), orange juice (935 mOsm per kg) and grape juice (1170 mOsm per kg). Commercially available oral rehydration solutions in adequate quantities replenish fluid and electrolyte loss. Drinks containing caffeine have a diuretic action and should be avoided.

The nutritional status of the patient should be assessed. Diarrhoea can lead to decreased food intake and impaired nutrient absorption. Undernutrition or even malnutrition may result, as discussed previously. Fasting is inadvisable and patients should be encouraged to eat food that can be tolerated but to avoid food with a high fat or high roughage content, spicy food and raw food.

If the aetiology is known, treatment should be directed to the specific cause of diarrhoea. Most mild episodes of diarrhoea are self-limiting. Symptomatic treatment with fluid repletion and antimotility drugs are usually sufficient. Loperamide is the antimotility drug of choice superior to placebo, diphenoxylate and bismuth subsalicylate in terms of side effects and efficacy. The drug is not recommended in inflammatory bowel disease, infective diarrhoea with features of dysentery, if fever or systemic toxic symptoms are present or if the diarrhoea lasts more than 48 hours. In traveller's diarrhoea adsorbents that are solid compounds which absorb fluid and perhaps bacterial toxins are advocated in the US. Examples are kaolin and bismuth subsalicylate (Pepto-Bismol). Concurrent ingestion of aspirin is not advised.

Antibiotic use depends on the severity of diarrhoea and the patient's current clinical circumstances and should take into account the potential side effects. Antibiotics are indicated in dysentery, especially if systemic symptoms such as fever, chills, headache and myalgia are present. Trimethoprim-sulphamethoxazole, norfloxacin or, if systemic symptoms are prominent, ciprofloxacin may be used. Parasitic causes of dysentery, such as *Entamoeba histolytica*, should be ruled out before antibiotic treatment is initiated.

In patients with secretory diarrhoea (high fluid output) octreotide, an analogue of somatostatin, is widely used.

Prevention of diarrhoea

Preventive aspects of diarrhoea range from personal, domestic and institutional hygiene to food preparation and storage. During cooking, care should be taken to prevent the cross-contamination of cooked and fresh food, such as salads, from kitchen implements, utensils or surfaces used to prepare, for example, uncooked poultry, with the potential to harbour enteric pathogens. Immunosuppressed patients, who are at the greatest risk of acquiring diarrhoea, should avoid consuming raw milk and uncooked animal products.

If an outbreak of diarrhoea occurs, public health authorities should be notified immediately to document the outbreak, determine the source and mode of transmission, identify, if possible, the aetiological agent and help with control measures. Controlling the spread of diarrhoea in a single ward or area of occupancy is often difficult, especially if there are overcrowding, incontinent patients, inadequate staff and inadequate shared toilet facilities. Measures to stop the spread of diarrhoea to other wards should be paramount. It is suggested that all patients and staff from the 'infected ward' be restricted from entering other wards. A health education program directed towards patients and staff should be implemented and it should focus on:

- thorough cleaning of toilets
- meticulous disposal of faeces and soiled linen
- increased ward cleaning
- increased hand washing with soap especially after visiting the toilet and before eating and handling medication and
- optimal food-handling practices.

Other precautions are to locate patients with diarrhoea near toilets. Staff with diarrhoea should be advised not to attend work, preferably until the pathogen which caused diarrhoea is no longer present in 2 consecutive stool samples.

In older persons diarrhoea may be a significant problem of greater prevalence than appreciated by health professionals. The quality of life of both patient and carer can often be preserved by education regarding prevention and management.

Acknowledgment

I am grateful to Mr Austin Milton for his excellent assistance in the preparation of this chapter.

Bibliography and further reading

Belitsos, P. C., Greenson, J. K., Yardley, J. H., Sisler, J. R. & Bartlett, J. G. (1992), 'Association of gastric hypoacidity with opportunistic enteric infections in patients with AIDS', *Journal of Infectious Diseases*, 166, pp. 277–84.

Buttery, J. E., Ratnaike, R. N. & Chamberlain, B. R. (1994), 'A visual screening method for lactose maldigestion', *Annals of Clinical Biochemistry*, Vol. 31, pp. 566–7.

Forston, W. C. & Tedesco, F. J. (1984), 'Drug induced colitis: A review', *American Journal of Gastroenterology*, 79, pp. 878–83.

Garibaldi, R. A. & Nurse, B. A. (1986), 'Infections in the elderly' [Review], *American Journal of Medicine*, 81, pp. 53–8.

Gross, C. R., Lindquist, R. D., Woolley, A. C., Granieri, R., Allard, K. & Webster, B. (1992), 'Clinical indicators of dehydration severity in elderly patients', *Journal of Emergency Medicine*, 10, pp. 267–74.

McEvoy, A., Dutton, J. & James, O. F. W. (1983), 'Bacterial contamination of the small intestine is an important cause of occult malabsorption in the elderly', *British Medical Journal*, 287, pp. 789–93.

Neil, G. A. & Weinstock, J. V. (1991), 'Gastrointestinal manifestations of systemic diseases', in Yamada, T. (ed.), *Textbook of Gastroenterology*, Vol. II, J. B. Lippincott Co., Philadelphia, pp. 2135–57.

Ratnaike, R. N. (ed.) (1999), *Diarrhoea and Constipation in Geriatric Practice*, Cambridge University Press, Cambridge.

Ratnaike, R. N. (2000a), 'Non immunological defence mechanisms', in Ratnaike, R. N. (ed.), *Small Bowel Disorders*, Edward Arnold, London, pp. 68–76.

Ratnaike, R. N. (ed.) (2000b), *Small Bowel Disorders*, Edward Arnold, London. Co-published in New York by Oxford University Press.

Ratnaike, R. N. (2000c), 'Whipple's disease', *Postgraduate Medical Journal*, 76, pp. 760–6.

Ratnaike, R. N. & Barbour, A. H. (2000), 'Maldigestion and malabsorption', in Ratnaike, R. N. (ed.), *Small Bowel Disorders*, Edward Arnold, London, pp. 302–15.

Ratnaike, R. N., Milton, A. G. & Nigro, O. (2000a), 'Drug associated diarrhoea and constipation in older people. I. Diarrhoea', *Australian Journal of Hospital Pharmacy*, 30, pp. 165–9.

Ratnaike, R. N., Milton, A. G. & Nigro, O. (2000b), 'Drug associated diarrhoea and constipation in older people. II. Constipation', *Australian Journal of Hospital Pharmacy*, 30, pp. 210–13.

Thorens, J., Froehlich, F., Schwizer, W., Saraga, E., Bille, J., Gyr, K. et al. (1996), 'Bacterial overgrowth during treatment with Omeprazole compared with Cimetidine: A prospective randomised double blind study', *Gut*, 39, pp. 54–9.

Tobin, G. W. & Brocklehurst, J. C. (1986), 'Faecal incontinence in residential homes for the elderly: Prevalence, aetiology and management', *Age and Ageing*, 15, pp. 41–6.

Weber, J. R. & Ryan, J. C. (1993), 'Effects on the gut of systemic disease and other extraintestinal conditions', in Feldman, M., Scharschmidt, B. F. & Sleisenger, M. H. (eds), *Sleisenger and Fordtran's Gastrointestinal and Liver Disease*, Vol. I, W.B. Saunders Co., Philadelphia, pp. 411–38.

Welborn, T. A. (1998), 'Acarbose, an alpha glucosidose inhibitor for non-insulin dependent diabetes', *The Medical Journal of Australia*, 168, pp. 76–8.

World Health Organization, The Management and Prevention of Diarrhoea (1993), *Programme for Control of Diarrhoeal Diseases*, 3rd edn, World Health Organization, Geneva.

Chapter 35
Constipation

RANJIT N. RATNAIKE

Constipation is one of the most common problems faced by older persons. The enormity of the problem is reflected by the number of laxatives and over-the-counter medications that are available for the treatment of the constipated patient. The manufacture of laxatives is a burgeoning business and of the over-the-counter medications used by older persons in the US, laxatives are second only to analgesics, generating sales of over $400 million. This high expenditure on laxatives may reflect equating good health with good bowel evacuation. Despite the extent of constipation, both patients and carers may regard it as a problem of little consequence—a burden of old age to be carried with stoicism. Even some health professionals (unless they themselves have experienced constipation) have an attitude of benign neglect. This may reflect the importance given to the topic during their training. Indeed, a highly regarded textbook of medicine with the word 'Essentials' in its title does not mention constipation in the index nor in the section on gastrointestinal disease.

One hundred years ago the importance of constipation was recognised in another medical text: 'There is no more troublesome symptom in the derangements of the digestive organs, nor any more difficult to overcome, than habitual constipation.'

Definition and normal bowel action

There is no precise, universal definition of constipation, as there is considerable variation regarding what 'normal' bowel habits are. On a typical Western diet the normal frequency of bowel motions is between 3 times a day and 3 times a week. The most widely accepted definition of constipation is 'a chronic condition of over 6 weeks' duration with the passage of hard stools and/or a frequency of bowel action less than 3 times a week'. 'Constipation' is a term widely interpreted and may mean the infrequent passage of stools associated with straining, the passage of 'hard' stools or a sense of incomplete evacuation unrelated to the frequency or consistency of bowel actions.

Many people hold strong views that may not be negotiable regarding the number of bowel motions a day they should have, and those who are more obsessional dwell on colour, shape, consistency and quantity. But the perfect stool—'not too hard, not too soft, pointed at both ends and swirling twice round the pan'—is elusive.

Prevalence

Among older persons the prevalence of constipation is high compared to younger people and increases dramatically after the age of 65. Constipation is more common among the institutionalised elderly, in up to 60–70%, and is also widespread in acute care facilities.

Constipation occurs more often in:

- women than men
- non-Caucasians than Caucasians
- low socioeconomic groups and
- less educated people.

The frequent complaints of constipation in older persons are attributed by some to their alleged preoccupation with bowel habits. Although a degree of introspection into bodily functions is understandable, many younger and older people fear 'autointoxication' if their bowels are not regular. Obsessional people of any age often elaborate on their bowel habits and rituals. Many older people live alone with limited or no opportunities to stimulate their mind and therefore avoid introspection.

This high prevalence of constipation in older persons is not due to normal ageing alone and there is no conclusive evidence that colonic transit time is altered in older persons compared with younger age groups. In a study of 30 ambulatory elderly patients with constipation, colonic transit time was normal in 8, increased in 5, and a delay in evacuating faeces from the rectum occurred in 17. Information available suggests that constipation in ambulatory elderly patients is primarily due to distal colonic and/or anorectal dysfunction. In chronically constipated older persons there is some evidence of decreased motility in the rectosigmoid region. However, regardless of age, major predisposing factors are a low-fibre diet, inadequate fluid intake, lack of exercise and suboptimal toilet habits.

Faeces formation, colonic and anorectal function

The balance between the processes of absorption and secretion in the gastrointestinal tract ensures a well formed stool. About 90% of the 10 L of fluid from dietary sources and salivary, gastric, small intestinal, pancreatic and biliary secretions is absorbed daily. The jejunum, which has the largest surface area, absorbs most of the fluid. A lesser quantity of 3–5 L is absorbed by the ileum.

The colon avidly absorbs the remaining 1–2 L of fluid, converting digested food in a liquid phase into solid faeces. This function is not uniform along its length, reflecting the different embryological origins of the colon. The region up to the junction of the proximal two-thirds of the transverse colon develops from the mid-gut and has the primary function of absorbing fluids and electrolytes facilitated by non-propulsive contractions between the colonic haustra. These movements are predominantly up and down (rather than forward and propulsive). Throughout this area of the colon continuous fluid absorption results in the formation of increasingly solid faeces. The distal colon initiates forward propulsive contractions to push the solid faeces to the rectum helped by mucus from goblet cells.

The colon is innervated both intrinsically and extrinsically. The intrinsic innervation is termed the 'enteric nervous system'. This consists of myenteric neuronal layers in both the mucosa and the submucosa. The enteric nervous system functions through amine and peptide neurotransmitters that include acetylcholine, opioids, norepinephrine, serotonin, somatostatin, cholecystokinin, substance P, vasoactive intestinal polypeptide (VIP) and neuropeptide Y. The enteric nervous system co-ordinates both smooth muscle function and the important colonic processes of water and electrolyte absorption.

Extrinsically the proximal colon is innervated by the vagus. The distal colon, internal anal sphincter and the motor activity of the rectosigmoid are controlled by the pelvic nerve arising from the sacral region of the spinal cord. The external anal sphincter and the muscles of the pelvic floor are innervated by the pudendal nerves that also arise from the sacral segments of the spinal cord.

Normal defecation is a well co-ordinated activity. Peristalsis spreads from the proximal colon to the rectum. The effectiveness of peristalsis determines the extent to which the diaphragm and abdominal muscles are utilised. They raise the intrapelvic pressure and relax the pelvic floor, causing it to descend. On contact with faeces, receptors in the upper anal canal trigger the urge to evacuate stools. The internal anal sphincter relaxes. Sitting or squatting and full hip flexion stretches the anal canal.

Normally the puborectalis muscle of the pubic floor is contracted to maintain the anorectal angle. This specifically prevents the passage of faeces into the anal canal from the rectum. The anal sphincters also provide a barrier to the external movement of faeces. During defecation the puborectalis relaxes, straightening the anorectal angle, and concurrently the external anal sphincter relaxes. It is not unusual for faeces to be present in the rectum without the urge to defecate.

The term 'dyschezia' refers to difficulty in defecation. This suggests that the problem lies in the evacuation of formed faeces. In this situation the cause may be due to an anorectal disorder or lesion, discussed below. Anismus (anal dyssynergia) is a condition in which the striated muscles of the pelvic floor contract instead of relaxing when attempting to defecate.

Further colonic and anorectal function studies, especially in patients with chronic constipation refractory to treatment, and data on age-related changes in circulating neuroendocrine agents involved in gastrointestinal motility would help clarify unresolved issues in regard to constipation (see also Chapter 36).

Box 35.1 Therapeutic agents that cause constipation

- Opioids (e.g. codeine, pethidine, morphine, fentanyl, oxycodone)
- Antacids (e.g. calcium and aluminium compounds)
- Antispasmodics (e.g. dicyclomine)
- Antidepressants (e.g. imipramine, amitriptyline)
- Antipsychotics (e.g. clozapine, chlorpromazine)
- Anti-parkinsonian medications (e.g. benztropine)
- Antidiarrhoeal agents
- Antihypertensives (e.g. methyldopa, clonidine, propranolol, and calcium antagonists verapamil, diltiazem, dihydropyridines, nifedipine and felodipine)
- Anticonvulsants (e.g. phenytoin, clonazepam)
- Anti-inflammatory agents
- Anorectic agents (e.g. clophentermine, phenmetrazine, phenfluramine)
- Minerals
  - Aluminium (e.g. antacids, sucralfate)
  - Calcium compounds
  - Iron compounds
  - Lead, arsenic (poisoning)
  - Barium sulphate
- Other compounds
  - Polystyrene resins
  - Cholestyramine
  - Oral contraceptives
  - Octreotide

Source: Modified from R. N. Ratnaike, A. G. Milton & O. Nigro (2000), 'Drug associated diarrhoea and constipation in older people. II. Constipation', *Australian Journal of Hospital Pharmacy*, 30, pp. 210–13.

Aetiology

The extensive aetiology of constipation ranges from dietary and systemic causes to metabolic disturbances and, especially in an ageing population, malignancy and drug therapy (see Box 35.1).

Idiopathic constipation

When a medical cause cannot be identified, the term 'idiopathic' or 'simple constipation' is used. Studies on colonic transit times have not as yet provided a definitive pattern of dysmotility in specific areas of the colon. There is evidence that in a subset of patients small bowel transit is also delayed, although it is unclear if these patients have a generalised dysmotility affecting the entire gastrointestinal tract. Common remediable causes of idiopathic constipation are insufficient intake of dietary fibre (a predominant cause), inadequate fluid intake, inadequate exercise and poor toilet habits. Constipation may also arise as a result of the patient ignoring the urge to defecate.

Central nervous system

Constipation is linked to a number of problems of the central nervous system. In older persons cerebrovascular accidents are common (see Chapter 17) and, depending on the site of the lesion, weakness of the abdominal and pelvic muscles and hypomotility of the large bowel can occur, resulting in constipation. In Parkinson's disease (Chapter 14), constipation results from prolonged colonic transit and may be worsened by drug side effects. A community study in the UK showed that more than half the patients experienced constipation.

Depression, dementia and confusional states (Chapters 9, 15 and 16) are important causes of constipation. Patients with cognitive impairment, especially in unfamiliar surroundings (such as a hospital), often find locating the toilet (especially if signage is inadequate) a problem and may suppress the urge to defecate and constipation may occur. This is an important reason to avoid transferring patients with dementia from one ward to another or from one ward bay to another unless it is absolutely essential. Patients who are depressed or confused are more likely to develop constipation from the medications they are receiving. Elderly patients with anxiety and depression may distort or exaggerate their symptoms of constipation.

A variety of spinal cord lesions can result in an adynamic bowel. These include trauma (e.g. secondary to osteoporotic vertebral crush fractures), malignancy, ischaemia and spinal cord stenosis. Spinal cord lesions above the sacral segments result in the loss of parasympathetic innervation, with colonic tone decreased or lost in response to a meal so that retention of faeces occurs. Factors such as inactivity and weakness of abdominal muscles contribute to constipation.

Drug related constipation

Drugs are a common and increasingly important cause of constipation, more common than the many illnesses that cause constipation. Box 35.1 lists the therapeutic agents associated with constipation. The mechanisms by which many of these therapeutic agents act are not known. Some drugs may indirectly cause constipation. For example, confusion is a recognised side effect of many medications, especially benzodiazepines, tricyclic antidepressants, antipsychotics and opioids and the side effect of constipation due to the drugs may be compounded by ignoring the urge to defecate or being unable to locate the toilet.

Opioid induced constipation

Constipation occurs in up to 95% of patients on opioid analgesia and is thought to be dose related. The primary mechanism of constipation is significantly extended gut transit times. Other contributory factors are a reduction in gastrointestinal secretions and an increase in intestinal fluid absorption. Some, if not all, of these effects may be mediated by a local effect on the opioid receptors in the gastrointestinal tract, since the use of oral naloxone (an opioid antagonist) alleviates opioid induced constipation without loss of analgesic effects. In long-term methadone therapy, 58% of patients experience constipation of varying severity. This side effect of opioids should be anticipated and preventive measures, such as initiating laxative use, taken. The constipation may be of sufficient severity to require the use of enemas.

Anticholinergic effects

Constipation is a frequent side effect of many drugs with anticholinergic properties. These compounds antagonise acetylcholine and the decreased intestinal tone and motility result in constipation. Examples of such compounds are some anti-parkinsonian drugs (e.g. benztropine), tricyclic antidepressants and antipsychotic agents. Of the tricyclic antidepressants, the tertiary amines (e.g. imipramine, amitriptyline, clomipramine) may have the greatest anticholinergic effects. Among the antipsychotics, the phenothiazines (predominantly thioridazine) have the most potent anticholinergic effect. Clozapine, a newer generation antipsychotic, is a particularly prominent cause of constipation.

Miscellaneous compounds

Verapamil, a widely used calcium channel blocker, commonly causes constipation. The exact mechanism is unknown. Some evidence suggests verapamil delays transit in the colon. This increases mucosal contact time, allowing for greater fluid absorption and resulting in constipation.

Vincristine, a cytotoxic vinca alkaloid, invariably causes constipation. Vincristine therapy may also lead to other gastrointestinal side effects such as an adynamic ileus, megacolon and abdominal pain. A major complication is damage to the autonomic nervous system and/or the enteric nervous system, causing disordered gastrointestinal function. Constipation is a consequence.

Antacids that contain aluminium may cause constipation due to the astringent effect of aluminium. High doses of these compounds may even cause intestinal obstruction. Long-term stimulant laxative abuse (see below) causes loss of smooth muscle tone and contractility, worsening the problem of constipation. The excessive use of antidiarrhoeal agents may also cause constipation.

Constipation may occur with the use of many drugs that affect fluid balance. Diuretics can cause constipation due to fluid loss, especially in situations of restricted fluid intake, such as in cardiac failure. In particular, commercially available bulking agents in the absence of sufficient oral fluids may worsen constipation.

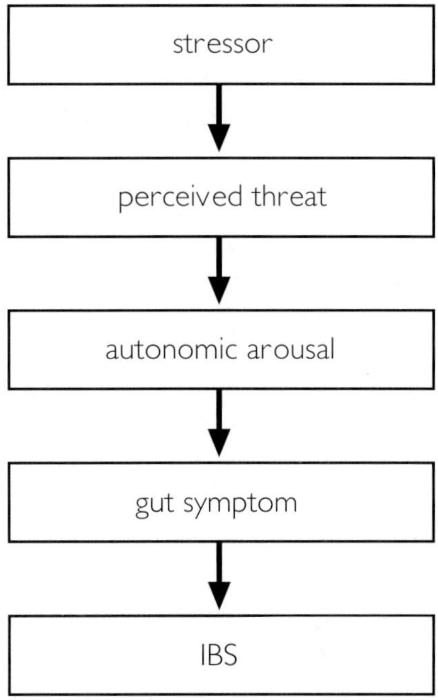

Figure 35.1 A possible mechanism between perception of a psychosocial stressor and IBS

Alimentary tract

Irritable bowel syndrome (IBS) (Chapter 34) is a common cause of constipation. It is defined as at least bi-weekly non-menstrual abdominal distress with diarrhoea, constipation, or alternation between the two, over at least 3 months, for which no organic cause can be found. Other symptoms are combinations of abdominal pain, bloatedness (distension) and symptoms of disordered defecation, especially urgency, straining, feelings of incomplete evacuation and altered stool form and frequency. Although there is no conclusive evidence linking specific personality patterns with IBS, an association may exist between psychosocial stressors and IBS (see Figure 35.1). In patients with irritable bowel syndrome in whom constipation is the dominant problem, a fibre intake of at least 12 g a day is recommended.

Another common cause of constipation is painful defecation due to anorectal pathology, particularly haemorrhoidal itching and bleeding, or anal fissures. A frequent sequence of events is straining to overcome constipation which results in a fissure or tear, causing pain and spasm, and then a reluctance to defecate, worsening constipation. Other anorectal causes are rectal prolapse, rectocoele and, rarely, a solitary rectal ulcer. In females a weak pelvic floor from hormonal changes during pregnancy and trauma at childbirth may be associated with difficulty in passing faeces.

Among the elderly, it is especially important to exclude the possibility that a change in bowel habits may be due to gastrointestinal tract malignancy. Tumours of the gastrointestinal tract comprise nearly half of all cancers. The sudden onset of constipation or worsening of chronic constipation heightens the suspicion of malignancy, as does constipation alternating with diarrhoea. Appropriate tests are examination of stools for occult blood, rectal examination, proctoscopy, flexible sigmoidoscopy and, if indicated, colonoscopy or radiology.

Constipation in Hirschsprung's disease may not occur until adulthood. In this condition intramural ganglion cells are absent in the submucosal and myenteric plexuses. The diagnosis is usually established during infancy and confirmed by rectal biopsy.

Diverticulae are present in the large intestine of about half the population aged over 50. While about 90% of cases are symptom-free, constipation or loose bowel actions may be a feature if diverticulosis develops (Chapter 37).

Metabolic and endocrine disorders

Most patients with hypothyroidism experience constipation, but this resolves with thyroid hormone replacement. Both hypercalcaemia (Table 35.1) and hypokalaemia are associated with constipation. Although the condition is uncommon, porphyria is also a cause of constipation.

Complications

An important consequence of constipation is continued fluid absorption from stools which then leads to faecal impaction. Faecal impaction in turn could result in spurious diarrhoea (overflow diarrhoea). Spurious diarrhoea may be the presenting complaint masking constipation. It is not uncommon for patients with spurious diarrhoea to be investigated vigorously for diarrhoea or, worse still, treated for diarrhoea. Faecal impaction is a common problem in older persons. Among those in institutional care, approximately 10% experience this problem at least once a week. The prevalence is 42% in geriatric wards. Faecal impaction can also lead to intestinal obstruction. Faecal impaction can cause urinary retention due to distension of the rectum and pelvic floor, resulting in parasympathetic inhibition of the bladder. In addition, the faeces may physically obstruct the bladder outlet, causing irritation, urinary retention and overflow.

Many other complications are associated with constipation, including abdominal pain, infections, pyrexia, toxic megacolon and volvulus of the sigmoid colon (see Figure 35.2). The latter condition presents as abdominal distension, cramping abdominal pain, vomiting and obstipation (severe constipation). Straining at stools can cause rectal tears, bleeding and haemorrhoids. An extremely rare complication is stercoral ulceration (colonic ulceration due to pressure and irritation from retained faeces) and even perforation. Cardiovascular symptoms such as myocardial ischaemia may be precipitated by straining at stools.

History and examination

The search for the underlying cause of constipation should not be abandoned, even if the problem is chronic. A comprehensive history based on a knowledge of the likely pathogenesis of constipation may suggest a primary, remediable cause and prevent unnecessary investigations, treatment and inconvenience. The patient's own understanding

Table 35.1 Hypercalcaemia associated with constipation

Common causes	Less common causes
Malignancy	Thiazide diuretics
• Neoplasia with bony metastases	Lithium
• Humoral hypercalcaemia of malignancy	Theophylline
Multiple myeloma	Vitamin D toxicity
Sarcoidosis	Thyrotoxicosis
Primary hyperparathyroidism	Paget's disease
	Addison's disease
	Phaeochromocytoma
	Milk-alkali syndrome (extremely rare)

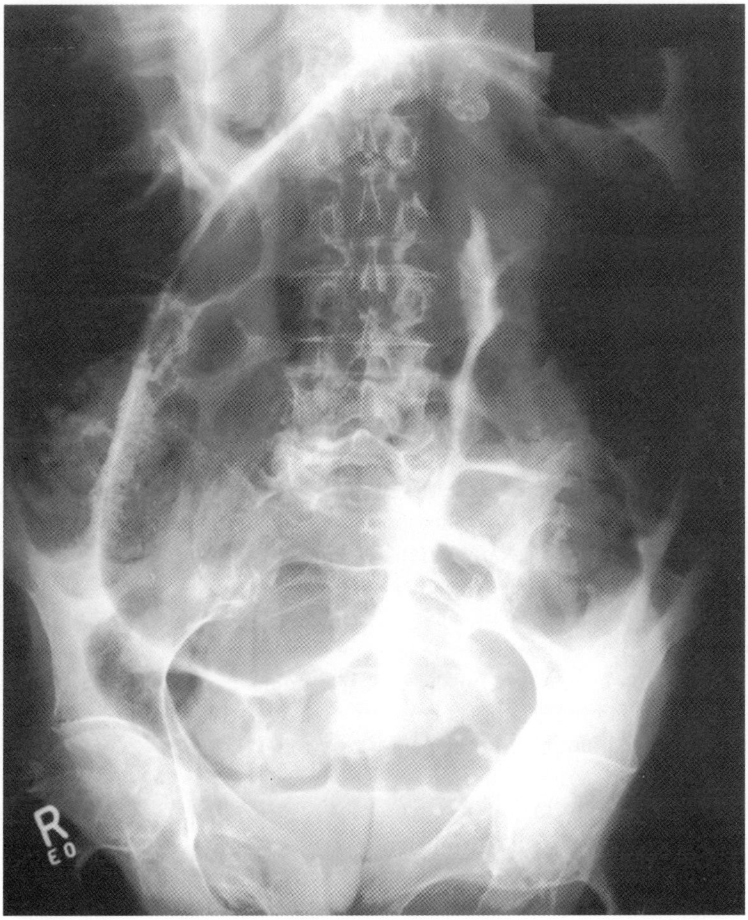

Figure 35.2 Sigmoid volvulus COURTESY OF DR SUZANNE LE P. LANGLOIS, DEPARTMENT OF RADIOLOGY, ROYAL ADELAIDE HOSPITAL, ADELAIDE, SOUTH AUSTRALIA

of constipation should be carefully established, especially if the patient is elderly with problems of cognition. It is essential to determine if constipation is of recent or sudden onset and if there is blood in the stools or bleeding per rectum or a recent sensation of incomplete evacuation and the need to strain at stool. These features require urgent intervention rather than a wait-and-see approach, and malignancy should always be suspected and excluded. Another important question to ask is whether the patient has manually removed faeces. Soiling of underwear in a patient with constipation suggests faecal incontinence due to faecal impaction.

Therapeutic agents are so often associated with constipation. Information on and sighting of *all* medication is essential. This should include proprietary and over-the-counter medications from a pharmacy, health food store or herbalist. If a drug related cause of constipation is suspected, information on medication may also have to be sought from carers, health professionals or the local pharmacist. Ask about the regular use of laxatives and check for possible complications of constipation. These may not be confined to the gastrointestinal tract. Document a detailed history of concurrent and past illnesses and consider their possible link to constipation.

Physical examination

A thorough physical examination is essential. The examination should be systematic to detect neurological causes, endocrine causes (such as hypothyroidism) and the features of hypercalcaemia, such as anorexia, lassitude, anxiety, depression and increased thirst. Examine the mouth to detect any cause that would deter an adequate intake of food (Chapter 29). Abdominal palpation may reveal a faecal mass. A malignancy may also be palpable. Auscultate for bowel sounds.

In every patient with constipation a rectal examination and proctoscopy are essential. Visual examination of the perineal area may show external haemorrhoids, fissures or a rectal prolapse. Most rectal tumours are within reach of the examiner's finger during a rectal examination. Digital examination also helps to assess sphincter tone, areas of tenderness, puborectalis muscle function and faecal impaction. It is important to note that an inability to detect impacted faeces on puborectal examination does not rule out faecal impaction. During the digital rectal examination, if the puborectalis muscle is intact, the patient should be able to bear down and expel or attempt to expel the examiner's finger. A normal 'anal wink' occurs when there is reflex contraction of the anal canal after a pin prick in the perineal area. This reflects the integrity of the lower sacral nerve roots. Local anal and rectal lesions such as a tear, ulceration or inflammation should be sought during proctoscopy. Proctoscopy may also reveal a proctocele (rectocele) which may or may not be the cause of constipation. Sigmoidoscopy should be considered, especially if there is a history of passage of blood per rectum or if blood is present in stools. Other investigations should include a complete blood examination, thyroid function tests, serum calcium and electrolytes, especially potassium.

A plain radiograph of the abdomen would show the extent of faecal loading in the colon and whether the colon is dilated. Other invasive investigations such as a barium enema or colonoscopy should be requested depending on the particular diagnostic probabilities.

Management

The effective management of constipation requires a commitment by both patient and health professional. This is particularly so if the problem is chronic. Resolution of the problem may be neither easy nor rapid. An integral part, as with any treatment, is to spend time explaining to the patient (and carer if necessary) what is being done and why it is being done. Head down and prescription writing with mumbled directions to no one in particular is unhelpful. Good communication is essential in any circumstance, but more so with many older patients whose understanding may be clouded by medications and whose hearing may be impaired. Increasingly, data now shows that elderly patients prefer written instructions. If no obvious pathology is established, the primary therapeutic measure is patient education. The concept that constipation is a normal and acceptable part of ageing, held by many older persons and their carers, should be strongly refuted. Constipation can be resolved in time by the informed patient following a simple plan of action. The essential components of such a plan relate to:

- diet
- fluids
- exercise
- toilet habits.

Diet

Fibre is the most important component of a well balanced diet designed to maintain regular bowel actions and prevent constipation (Table 35.2). Fibre is derived from plant cell walls containing cellulose, hemicellulose, pectins, lignins and waxes resistant to digestion. In most Western countries the fibre intake is inadequate. The recommended daily fibre intake is 30–35 g. Ten grams of dietary fibre is equivalent to about 1 oz of bran, 3 oz of shredded wheat or 4 slices of wholemeal bread. The major natural sources of dietary fibre are cereals and green vegetables. Common dietary sources of fibre are:

- fruits, green vegetables and legumes
- bran
- wholegrain or wholemeal bread
- cereals, pastas and rice, especially brown rice
- seeds and nuts.

Methylcellulose and psyllium preparations are non-dietary sources of fibre. 'Roughage' is a widely used colloquial term for dietary fibre.

Table 35.2 Selected dietary items with a high fibre content

Serve	Source	Fibre/ serve (g)
Fruits		
1 cup	Mixed dried fruit	9.8
1 medium	Pear, fresh	4.3
1 medium	Apple, fresh with skin	3.1
1 medium	Banana, peeled fresh	3.1
5 medium	Prunes, dried	3.0
1 medium	Orange, peeled fresh	2.4
Vegetables/legumes		
½ cup	Kidney beans	9.7
½ cup	Baked beans, canned	6.6
½ cup	Peas	5.8
½ cup	Corn	2.6
½ cup	Broccoli, boiled	2.5
Grains and cereals		
⅓ cup	All Bran	8.4
1 cup	Wheaties	3.5
1 cup	Cornflakes	1.0
1 tsp	Unprocessed bran	3.0
½ cup	Muesli, Swiss-style	8.1
½ cup	Muesli, toasted	4.8
1 bar (30 g)	Muesli bar	2.8
1 roll	Wholemeal roll	5.1

Dietary fibre increases faecal mass (both solid residue and water content) and increases bowel motility, facilitating bowel actions. In addition to their host protective role discussed in Chapter 34, the commensal colonic bacteria have a role in faeces formation. Fibre provides a substrate for these bacteria to produce gases, predominantly methane and some hydrogen sulphide, and short chain fatty acids that increase stool bulk. Bacteria also contribute to stool bulk, stimulating colonic motility.

The patient's daily fibre intake should be estimated. If the fibre intake is inadequate it is important to determine the reason(s) for this, which may relate to ignorance about the role of fibre, lack of benefit from previous fibre ingestion, issues of cost, problems with dentition (Chapter 29) or the side effects of dietary fibre. These side effects are due to intestinal gas formation in the colon by bacterial degradation of the long-chain carbohydrates causing excessive flatulence (normal persons pass wind about 15 times a day), bloating and abdominal discomfort. Irregular bowel movements may occur. These side effects are most noticeable during the first 2–3 weeks of fibre intake and decrease with time.

In patients with pre-existing intestinal stenosis, ulceration or strictures, bulk-forming agents such as bran may cause intestinal obstruction. Phytic acid in crude bran may decrease calcium absorption—an important consideration in the older patient.

Fluids

Adequate fluid intake is an essential part of the management of constipation. The minimum fluid intake should be 1.5 L a day. Encouraging increased fluid intake is not easy, especially in older persons because thirst perception decreases with age and, despite being dehydrated, older patients may not recognise the need for more fluids. In older patients with cognitive problems greater supervision of fluid intake is essential. A jug of fluid at the bedside helps to remind the patient to drink fluids and also helps carers determine the fluid intake.

Exercise

The relationship between constipation and a sedentary lifestyle is well documented. Exercise need not be vigorous nor the duration prolonged. Even a minimal amount of exercise helps prevent constipation.

Toilet habits

There is an optimal time to go to the toilet for a bowel motion. This parallels periods of high gut motility which occur in the morning after sleep and after meals and may explain why most people go to the toilet for a bowel action in the morning after waking up or after breakfast. On consuming a meal, or mechanically distending the stomach for about 2 hours, colonic contractility results in the urge to defecate. Although no evidence is available, it is recommended that going to the toilet at a regular time each day helps to establish a regular bowel pattern. Using the same toilet helps. Feelings of frustration or self-condemnation should not be generated if there is a failure to have a motion.

The reasons for ignoring the call to stool vary with individuals. A frequently heard claim is that there is insufficient time to go to the toilet in the morning and constipation results from chronically suppressing or postponing the urge to defecate. Avid fluid absorption in the intestine causes faeces to undergo dehydration and the stool hardens. Many persons who complain of constipation do not spend an adequate amount of time in the toilet to have a bowel action. Behaviour patterns may need to be reviewed and altered. These problems of lack of time and impatience are best addressed by the patient waking up earlier. This commonsense approach is preferable to laxative use. Constipation may be situational—for example, having to share a toilet, lack of privacy, or being confined to bed—or be due to enforced reduced physical activity as in a hospital. Not using a toilet in an unfamiliar environment and trying to spend the minimal time in a toilet which may not meet with one's own standards of hygiene promotes constipation. In hospital, embarrassment or difficulty using a bedpan is a common cause of constipation. Having a bowel action in a cloistered 6-bed bay of a hospital ward shared with sick but perhaps vigilant patients is a challenging experience for all concerned. In some older patients the inability to communicate the need to defecate is not uncommon. A major problem with many elderly patients in hospitals is the inability to locate the toilet.

Box 35.2 Laxatives

Bulk-forming agents
Bran, psyllium, ispaghula, frangula, sterculia, methylcellulose

Stool softeners
Bisacodyl, docusate sodium, coloxyl and senna

Lubricants
Paraffin oil

Osmotic laxatives
Lactulose, sorbitol, lactitol, mannitol, glycerol, polyethylene glycol, magnesium-containing salts, sodium phosphate

Secretagogues
Phenolphthalein, bisacodyl, castor oil, anthraquinones (senna and cascara sagrada), danthron, docusate sodium

Suppositories and enemas
Glycerol, soap and water, bisacodyl

Laxatives

About 30% of healthy elderly people use laxatives regularly, although 55% are not constipated. The cure rate with placebo in self-reported constipation is 60%. Laxatives can be grouped into several categories, including bulk-forming laxatives, stool softeners, lubricants, secretagogues, suppositories and enemas (see Box 35.2).

Bulk-forming agents

Bulking agents act by increasing faecal mass and water content of faeces. Their action is not immediate and may take 2–3 days to be effective. The fibre content should be increased gradually. Up to 6–8 g per day is well tolerated by patients.

If lifestyle measures relating to diet, fluid, exercise and toilet habits are unsuccessful, bulk-forming agents are the preferred laxatives. Bulking agents from food sources like bran, cereals and high-fibre bread are more palatable and thus preferable.

Natural non-dietary preparations include psyllium, which also lowers cholesterol levels, and isphagula (both from various plantago species), frangula (from the bark of *Rhamnus frangula*) and sterculia (the gum obtained from *Sterculia urens* and other sterculia species). Methylcellulose is a synthetic compound. The non-dietary sources are not as popular as dietary compounds and may lead to non-compliance or to using a more convenient but less preferable laxative. However, bulking agents are valuable treatment options and are safe to use with no long-term side effects.

These bulking agents absorb considerable quantities of fluid. Therefore they must be consumed with an adequate fluid intake to avoid worsening constipation and leading to faecal impaction. Fibre should not be prescribed if there is bowel obstruction due to faecal impaction or any other cause.

Stool softeners

Although not strictly laxatives, compounds such as bisacodyl and docusate sodium soften stools, thereby preventing straining by easing evacuation. Stool softeners increase the entry of water into the stool by acting as surfactants to maintain the moisture of faecal material. An adequate fluid intake should be maintained when these compounds are used. Although stool softeners such as docusate salts are widely used, especially in the institutionalised elderly, there is no evidence that they are superior to placebo. These compounds should not be used to treat chronic constipation.

Stool softeners are often combined with an irritant laxative. Combinations of bisacodyl with docusate sodium and docusate sodium with sennosides (the dried leaflets or legumes of *Cassia acutifolia* or *C. angustifolia*) are widely available as coloxyl and senna.

Lubricants

Lubricants such as paraffin, a hydrocarbon, merely coat the stools. The side effects include faecal incontinence, pruritus ani and malabsorption. These agents are sometimes combined with a stimulant laxative such as phenolphthalein (Agarol). These agents are *not* recommended for older patients and are contraindicated in patients with dysphagia or oesophageal motility disorders, or if diverticula (such as Zenker's diverticulum) or severe gastroesophageal reflux are present because of the danger of lipid pneumonia from aspiration. If used at all, agents such as paraffin should be given between meals.

Osmotic laxatives

Osmotic agents are increasingly popular in chronic constipation and are regarded as the laxatives of choice. They include lactulose, sorbitol, mannitol, glycerol (in suppository form) and polyethylene glycol, magnesium sulphate, magnesium hydroxide, magnesium citrate, and sodium and magnesium phosphates. They act by increasing fluid in the lumen of the colon and increasing motility in the ascending colon.

Lactulose was originally widely and exclusively used to treat constipation until, in 1964, the suggestion was made that it may be beneficial in portal systemic encephalopathy. Lactulose is a synthetic disaccharide (β-1-4 galactosido-fructose) that reaches the colon unchanged as it is not broken down by the disaccharidase enzymes in the small intestine. In the colon lactulose is converted by bacteria to form lactic, acetic and formic acids with the liberation of carbon dioxide. Due to its cost, lactulose is now restricted to patients with hepatic encephalopathy and sorbitol is used instead in constipation. Sorbitol is a polyhydric sugar alcohol with half the sweetening power of sucrose. It occurs naturally in many fruits and vegetables and is prepared commercially by the reduction of glucose. Sorbitol has an osmotic effect similar to lactulose, is very much cheaper than lactulose and is the agent of choice. The recommended dose of sorbitol is 20–30 mL 3 or 4 times a day, but this should be monitored, depending on the patient's response. Lactitol is a disaccharide analogue of lactulose, available at present in the UK and Europe, with a similar mode of action in treating constipation. It has the advantage over lactulose of not affecting blood sugar levels and is thus suitable in diabetic patients.

Polyethylene glycol is a potent hyperosmolar agent used for bowel cleansing before colonoscopy and to treat faecal impaction. It has also been included in commercially available preparations to treat chronic constipation.

A variety of salts, listed below, are used as laxatives. Although they are referred to as 'saline laxatives', this term is incorrect. Saline, which is sodium chloride, is not used as a laxative as it is absorbed. The salts listed are not absorbed and act as osmotic agents in the intestinal lumen. The osmotic effect is created by the non-absorbable anions and cations of the salts. Cardiac failure, renal impairment or decompensated liver disease may limit their use. The compounds used are:

- magnesium hydroxide (milk of magnesia)
- magnesium citrate
- magnesium sulphate
- magnesium phosphate
- sodium phosphate.

Magnesium salts, especially magnesium sulphate, are powerful osmotic agents and a vigorous bowel action of large volume usually occurs within about 3 hours. Cholecystokinin concentrations are also increased by magnesium, thus aiding gut motility. Cramping abdominal pain is an immediate side effect, and dehydration and hypermagnesaemia occur with chronic use. Therefore, magnesium based agents should not be used in patients with renal failure.

Secretagogues

Secretagogues, or irritant/stimulant laxatives, comprise 25% of laxative sales in the US. These compounds include phenolphthalein and phenolphthalein derivatives, bisacodyl, castor oil, anthraquinones such as senna and cascara sagrada (dried bark of aloe), danthron and docusate sodium. Secretagogues act in a manner similar to cholera toxin. They increase intracellular concentrations of cyclic AMP which, through a series of chemical reactions in the cell, affects intraluminal secretion of water and electrolytes.

These compounds may also act by:

- increasing permeability of the mucosa at the tight junctions, enabling fluid to leak into the lumen
- increasing synthesis of prostaglandins to increase fluid and electrolyte secretion; and
- increasing colonic motility.

The long duration of action of phenolphthalein is due to about 15% being absorbed by the small intestine and then undergoing enterohepatic circulation. Significant adverse effects include cramping and vomiting, erythema multiforme and photosensitive bullous skin lesions. A widely used compound is senna. A trial of a combination of senna and fibre was a cost effective and well accepted treatment in constipation. In elderly patients with rectal dyschezia (difficulty in the passage of stool) bisacodyl suppositories are effective.

Long-term use of secretagogues may cause electrolyte disturbances and malabsorption of fat and the fat soluble vitamins A, D, E and K. Because of their side effects, they are not the laxatives of choice, especially in older persons.

Suppositories and enemas

Both types of compound are introduced rectally and act by softening hard stools and/or stimulate peristalsis to help evacuate stools from the rectum.

Suppositories

Suppositories act through a variety of mechanisms. These agents are particularly useful if the patient is unable to evacuate stools present in the rectum. Some cause mucosal irritation and rectal distension, initiating the urge to defecate. Others, such as glycerol, are hyperosmolar and increase intraluminal fluid, resulting in softening of the stool. Mucosal irritants—such as soap, saline or bisacodyl—should be avoided. Glycerol suppositories do not cause mucosal irritation and are safe to use as often as once daily.

Enemas

Enemas act through mechanical distension and by a lavaging effect, leading to the evacuation of faeces. They may also stimulate peristaltic movement. Glycerol and water enemas are effective and without side effects. These are prepared by mixing equal parts (90–100 mL) of glycerol, olive oil and water at a temperature of 36°C before administration. Soap and water enemas are irritant to the mucosa and should not be used.

Fluid and electrolyte loss and mucosal irritation of the rectum are potential side effects of the recurrent use of most enemas. Improper enema techniques may result in perforation of the rectum. Prolonged use of enemas leads to decreased rectal tone.

Laxative abuse

The chronic use of laxatives is common and can generate a cascade, requiring ever-increasing quantities and stronger laxatives. The adverse effects of prolonged laxative abuse include atonic bowel (the cathartic colon) and hypokalaemia associated with muscle weakness. Other possible dangers are fluid loss, especially in the frail elderly. 'Melanosis coli' (a term coined by Virchow) is the brown or black pigmentation seen in the colon due to chronic use of anthracene-containing laxatives (cascara sagrada, senna, frangula).

Recent advances in treatment

Colchicine is reported to be effective in chronic refractory constipation. The recommended oral dose is 0.5 mg tds. The suggested mechanism of action is multifactorial, including increased motility, intestinal secretion and prostaglandin secretion. Colchicine induced malabsorption may be a contributory mechanism. The long-term use of colchicine, as in familial Mediterranean fever, is reported to be relatively safe. It is essential that the drug is taken strictly as prescribed and the dose not increased by the patient if the constipation does not resolve.

Another therapeutic agent advocated is misoprostol, a synthetic prostaglandin E_1 analogue. Its mechanism of action may be increased fluid accumulation in the intestine and increased intestinal motor activity.

Four stage management plan

In constipation of long duration, the emphasis should be on patient education rather than numerous investigations. However, the sudden onset or sudden worsening of longstanding constipation warrants careful assessment.

Stage I

Initially, several key issues should be resolved:

- Is there evidence of faecal impaction? If so, this needs to be addressed immediately (see stage IV).
- Is the dietary intake of fibre adequate?
- Is fluid intake adequate?
- Is the patient taking regular exercise (if this is a realistic goal)?
- Is medication(s) causing constipation?

The patient and carer, if relevant, should be educated about the causes of constipation and the benefits of appropriate diet, fluid intake, adequate exercise and optimal toilet habits. All medications, including over-the-counter preparations, should be checked. Asking for *all* the medications that the patient and his spouse use is a rewarding exercise. The accidental ingestion of drugs prescribed to others is not uncommon. The use of these simple measures in preference to therapeutic agents should be emphasised. This approach should not be abandoned because a health professional, patient or carer is impatient for quick results. A 1 month trial at least should be followed. An encouraging change in bowel habit may occur in as little as 2 days.

Education should also focus on possible side effects of laxatives, especially their long-term use and abuse. Some patients may be constipated despite being chronic laxative users (or abusers). Their choice of laxative may not be the most suitable one. It is often necessary to wean patients off laxatives that could be injurious. However, this issue should be dealt with diplomatically. Insistence on discontinuing the favourite laxative or changing to a more user friendly product may be resisted and may damage the patient–doctor relationship. The preferred approach would be to compromise initially on the frequency of use (e.g. 3 times a week instead of daily) and then persuade the patient to accept the treatment plan suggested.

If the patient's main problem is difficulty in evacuation, resulting in straining at stools, using a faecal softener in the form of a suppository is appropriate. This is best administered after breakfast.

Stage II

After about a month it is important to determine if the management initiatives discussed in stage I are being followed. Stage I initiatives should be continued and re-emphasised. Evidence of faecal impaction should again be sought. Laxatives may prove necessary, despite the measures in stage I being adhered to, but efforts should be made to curtail their duration of use. Bulk-forming laxatives are the mainstay of treatment. The major goal at this stage is to plan on as short a period of laxative use as possible. If necessary, consider adding an osmotic agent such as sorbitol, 20–30 mL up to 4 times a day. Magnesium sulphate is an alternative but should not be used in patients with impaired renal function.

Stage III

Compliance with the management initiatives discussed in stages I and II should be reviewed and re-emphasised. Serious consideration should be given to why the constipation is not resolving. The common underlying aetiological factors should be re-examined. Are further investigations necessary? Additional agents that can be used are suppositories and/or enemas.

Stage IV

Faecal impaction may be present and should be examined for. If so, the use of suppositories and then enemas are indicated. Regimens used to cleanse the lower bowel for radiological studies or endoscopy are extremely effective. A variety of compounds are available and some regimens are less burdensome than others. It is important, especially in older patients, to prevent dehydration by advising the patient to drink plenty of fluids during these procedures.

If faecal impaction does not resolve, it may be necessary to perform a manual evacuation. This is an unpleasant procedure and may need to be carried out over a period of time (e.g. over a day rather than as a single procedure). A local gel anaesthetic should be used liberally. Manual evacuation requires complete sphincter relaxation. It is important to note that dilation of any sphincter may result in potent vagal stimuli leading to bradycardia or, rarely, cardiac arrest. In addition, sphincter dilation is extremely painful. Since considerable dilation is necessary to perform a manual evacuation successfully, a general anaesthetic may be required.

Once the immediate problem of faecal impaction has been dealt with, vigorous preventive measures should be initiated as outlined previously. Long-term sorbitol use may be necessary in order to prevent impaction. Persistent or recurrent faecal obstruction raises the possibility of a colonic obstruction such as a malignancy.

Bibliography and further reading

Adverse Drug Reactions Advisory Committee (ADRAC) (1999), 'Constipation—It can be severe with clozapine', *Australian Adverse Drug Reactions Bulletin*, 18, p. 14.

Andorsky, R. & Goldner, F. (1990), 'Colonic lavage solution (polyethylene glycol electrolyte lavage solution) as a treatment for chronic constipation: A double-blind, placebo-controlled study', *American Journal of Gastroenterology*, 85, pp. 261–5.

Camilleri, M. & Ford, M. J. (1998), 'Review: The pathophysiology of colonic disorders', *Alimentary Pharmacology and Therapeutics*, 12, pp. 287–302.

Castle, S. C. (1989), 'Constipation: Endemic in the elderly? Gerontopathophysiology, evaluation and management', *Medical Clinics of North America: Geriatric Medicine*, 73, pp. 1497–509.

DeLuca, A. & Coupar, I. M. (1996), 'Insights into Opioid action in the intestinal tract', *Pharmacology and Therapeutics*, 69, pp. 103–15.

Harari, D., Gurwitz, J. H. & Minaker, K. L. (1993), 'Constipation in the elderly', *Journal of the American Geriatric Society*, 41, 130–40.

Heaton, K. W. (1988), 'Functional bowel disease', in Pounder, R. E. (ed.), *Recent Advances in Gastroenterology*, Churchill Livingstone, Edinburgh, pp. 291–312.

Hope, A. K. & Down, E. C. (1986), 'Dietary fibre and fluid in the control of constipation in a nursing home population', *Medical Journal of Australia*, 144, pp. 306–7.

Johanson, J. F., Sonnenberg, A. & Koch, T. R. (1989), 'Clinical epidemiology of chronic constipation', *Journal of Clinical Gastroenterology*, 11, pp. 525–36.

Krevsky, B., Maurer, A. H., Niewiarowski, T. & Cohen, S. (1992), 'Effect of verapamil on human intestinal transit', *Digestive Diseases and Sciences*, 37, pp. 919–24.

Lederle, F. A., Busch, D. L., Mattox, K. M., West, M. J. & Aske, D. M. (1990), 'Cost-effective treatment of constipation in the elderly: A randomized double-blind comparison of sorbitol and lactulose', *American Journal of Medicine*, 89, pp. 597–601.

MacMahon, D. G. (1999), 'Parkinson's disease nurse specialists: An important role in disease management', *Neurology*, 52(7 Suppl. 3), pp. S21–5.

McIlkerssen, M., Andersson, H., Bosaeus, I. & Falkheden, T. (1983), 'Intestinal transit time in constipated and nonconstipated patients', *Scandinavian Journal of Gastroenterology*, 18, pp. 593–7.

Moore, A. R. & O'Keeffe, S. T. (1999), 'Drug-induced cognitive impairment in the elderly', [Review] *Drugs and Aging*, 15, pp. 15–28.

Mullins, M. E., Carrico, E. A. & Horowitz, B. Z. (2000), 'Fatal cardiovascular collapse following acute colchicine ingestion', *Journal of Toxicology — Clinical Toxicology*, 38, pp. 51–4.

Mykyta, L. J. (1999), 'Faecal incontinence', in Ratnaike, R. N. (ed.), *Diarrhoea and Constipation in Geriatric Practice*, Cambridge University Press, Cambridge, pp. 70–8.

Passmore, A. P., Wilson-Davies, K., Stoker, C. & Scott, M. E. (1993), 'Chronic constipation in long stay elderly patients: A comparison of lactulose and a senna-fibre combination', *British Medical Journal*, 307, pp. 769–71.

Ratnaike, R. N., Milton, A. G. & Nigro, O. (2000), 'Drug-associated diarrhoea and constipation in older people. I. Diarrhoea', *Australian Journal of Hospital Pharmacology*, 30, pp. 165–9.

Sandler, R. S., Jordan, M. C. & Shelton, B. J. (1990), 'Demographic and dietary determinants of constipation in the US population', *Journal of Public Health*, 80, pp. 185–9.

Thompson, W. G. (1980), 'Laxatives: Clinical pharmacology and rational use', *Drugs*, 19, pp. 49–58.

Verne, N. G., Eaker, E. Y., Davis, R. H. & Sninsky, C. A. (1997), 'Colchicine is an effective treatment for patients with chronic constipation: An open-label trial', *Digestive Diseases and Sciences*, 42, pp. 1959–63.

Whitehead, W. E., Drinkwater, D., Cheskin, L. J., Heller, B. R. & Schuster, M. M. (1989), 'Constipation in the elderly living at home. Definition, prevalence, and relationship to lifestyle and health status', *Journal of the American Geriatric Society*, 37, pp. 423–9.

Wright, B. A. & Staats, D. O. (1986), 'The geriatric implications of fecal impaction', *Nurse Practitioner*, 11, pp. 53–8, 60, 64–6.

Woodward, M. C. (1999a), 'Constipation: Aetiology and diagnosis', in Ratnaike, R. N. (ed.), *Diarrhoea and Constipation in Geriatric Practice*, Cambridge University Press, Cambridge, pp. 187–93.

Woodward, M. C. (1999b), 'Constipation: Issues of management', in Ratnaike, R. N. (ed.), *Diarrhoea and Constipation in Geriatric Practice*, Cambridge University Press, Cambridge, pp. 194–200.

Yuan, C. S., Foss, J. F., O'Connor, M., Moss, J. & Roizen, M. F. (1998), 'Gut motility and transit changes in patients receiving long-term methadone maintenance', *Journal of Clinical Pharmacology*, 38, pp. 931–5.

Chapter 36
Faecal incontinence

WEI MING SUN and CHUNG OWYANG

Constipation is the thief of time: diarrhoea waits for no man.

Nicholas W. Read 1989

Introduction

Abnormal anorectal and/or pelvic floor function accounts for a large number of older patients seeking medical advice for abnormalities that are sufficiently stressful to cause social withdrawal and also reduce their quality of life.

Aetiology and epidemiology

There is no universally accepted definition of faecal incontinence. In general, faecal incontinence is defined as continuous or recurrent uncontrolled passage of faecal material for at least 1 month. More stringent criteria also include the occurrence in the last 3 months and at least 3 times a week at the time of diagnosis. Clear mucus secretion must be excluded by careful questioning. Uncontrolled passage of flatus only may represent an early sign of dysfunction of continence.

Faecal incontinence, although a common condition, is rarely discussed even between doctors and patients unless specific questions are asked. It occurs more often in two groups in the general population: children and the elderly. The largest surveys available suggest that faecal incontinence occurs in about 1.5% of children aged 7 years. Among children, faecal incontinence occurs more frequently in boys than in girls by a ratio of approximately 4:1. Among adults, the gender difference tends to reverse, with women outnumbering men. The occurrence is relatively low at about 4.2 per 1000 adults aged 15–64 years, but it triples to 12.1 per 1000 in those aged over 65 years. The prevalence of faecal incontinence rises sharply to 26–60% in geriatric wards. Fifty per cent of elderly residents of long-term care facilities suffer from faecal incontinence. The prevalence is about 31% in psychiatric wards, although some of these patients suffer from dementia rather than psychiatric problems.

In children, the strongest risk factor for faecal incontinence is constipation. This also holds true for incontinent elderly patients. In both cases, there is an association of faecal impaction, overflow diarrhoea and incontinence. The irritable bowel syndrome is also a recognised risk factor: an estimated 22% of patients with irritable bowel syndrome report at least occasional faecal soiling. Less common illnesses such as ulcerative colitis and other colonic conditions that are associated with urgency are also associated with faecal incontinence. Among the elderly, other risk factors for faecal incontinence are cognitive impairment and reduced mobility.

Pathophysiology

Faecal continence depends on the social awareness of the need to control the contents of the rectum until it is appropriate to evacuate in a controlled manner. It is a conscious function reflecting the exquisite sensitivity of the distal rectum and the anal canal and the resistance to the passage of faeces provided by anal sphincter contraction and the acute angulation of the anus and rectum caused by the contraction of the puborectalis muscle (Figure 36.1). Impairment of this process may therefore cause dysfunction in defecation. Box 36.1 lists the common causes that contribute to faecal incontinence in the general population.

Faecal incontinence can be divided into minor incontinence, in which partial soiling or occasional incontinence of liquid stool occurs, and major incontinence, with loss of control of stools of normal consistency. Faecal incontinence may even occur in normal subjects with diarrhoea when the normal continence mechanism is inadequate to cope with the large volumes of stool.

Childbirth

Childbirth is the most common cause of faecal incontinence in women, caused by damage to the anal sphincters and pudendal nerves. Factors that correlate with a reduction in the external sphincter function are a prolonged second stage, related to the time spent pushing, and the weight of the baby, with increased weight correlating inversely with

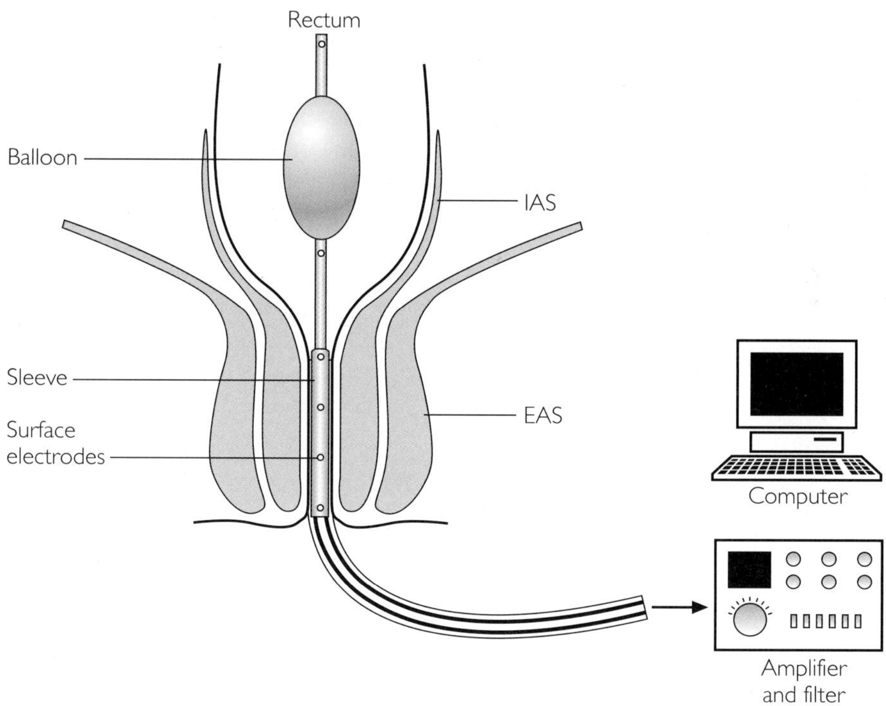

Figure 36.1 Diagram of the anal canal showing the different muscle components and the catheter used to measure pressure in multiple sites in the rectum and anal canal. The balloon is used for rectal distension and the intraluminal surface electrodes are used for recording electrical activity. The sleeve sensor situated in the anal canal is particularly useful for ambulatory recordings (IAS = internal anal sphincter, EAS = external anal sphincter)

Box 36.1 Common causes of faecal incontinence

Trauma
- Obstetric injury
- Surgery
- Injury
- Radiation

Pudendal neuropathy
- Prolonged labour
- Prolonged straining at stool
- Perineal descent
- Injury

Neurological and psychological diseases
- Multiple strokes
- Diabetic autonomic neuropathy
- Dementia
- Injury
- Neoplasms
- Psychological illness
- Scleroderma
- Amyloidosis
- Multiple sclerosis
- Degenerative diseases

Irritable bowel syndrome

Inflammatory bowel disease

Congenital abnormality
- Spina bifida
- Myelomeningocoele
- Imperforate anus

Prolapse

Constipation
- Faecal impaction
- Drugs

squeeze pressures, and the circumference of the head of the baby. The effects of traumatic delivery are not always apparent immediately, as many women present many years after delivery with a relatively short history of incontinence.

One study selected 125 primiparous women for investigations after delivery. They included patients with a history of a large number of interventions due to a difficult delivery. Thirty-seven were delivered without intervention, 37 with forceps, 20 by Ventouse extraction, 10 were breech, six had elective Caesarean section, and 15 had emergency Caesarean section. At 6 months after delivery, 99 returned for follow-up. Thirty-two (32%) had urgency of defecation, representing 26% of the whole group. However, patients with these symptoms were more likely to return for follow-up. Eighteen per cent complained of varying degrees of faecal incontinence. Sixteen had both urgency and loss of control. Fourteen of the 22 with faecal incontinence had forceps deliveries, compared with only two after Ventouse extraction. Thus, 14 of 37 (38%) women with delivery by forceps developed varying degrees of incontinence compared with only two of 20 (10%) with delivery by Ventouse extraction. Whether the latter mode of delivery can replace the former needs to be determined, but obstetricians have to be aware of the deleterious consequences of forceps usage. Twenty-six women had perineal tears—11 were second degree and 15 third degree—out of 104 women with vaginal deliveries. Of the 15 women with tears involving the sphincters, seven had deliveries with forceps, two used Ventouse extraction, and six had spontaneous vaginal deliveries.

In another study, further evidence of the adverse effects of forceps delivery was that the outcome of a tear with forceps was worse than a tear associated with a spontaneous vaginal delivery. Thus, 6 of 9 patients who sustained a third-degree tear during forceps delivery developed incontinence, whereas only 1 of 6 were incontinent after a non-instrumental delivery associated with a similar tear. In all these studies it is likely that endoanal ultrasonography may have revealed an even higher incidence of tears.

Pudendal nerve damage

The external sphincter is innervated by the pudendal nerve, which is relatively fixed as it passes through the pudendal canal. Thus, perineal descent will stretch the nerve and may lead to irreversible damage. Childbirth is the most potent cause of neurogenic injury to the external sphincter. Several studies show that immediately following delivery there is prolongation of the pudendal nerve terminal motor latency but this has invariably recovered 6 months after delivery. Repeated injury during further deliveries or as a result of chronic defecatory straining or simply as a result of ageing results in a weakened sphincter, manifesting signs of chronic partial denervation. Biopsies of these sphincters show changes consisting of atrophy, hypertrophy and fibre grouping that are characteristic of chronic partial denervation. Electromyographic studies are consistent with a neurogenic cause and nerve conduction studies have shown a delay in the latency of transmission of terminal impulses along the pudendal nerve. These studies support the view that the sphincter mechanism has been denervated. The pudendal latency prolongation is consistent with denervation in incontinence, and suggests nerve entrapment, possibly within the pudendal canal. The most obvious cause for these neurogenic changes is trauma sustained during delivery, resulting in injury to the pudendal nerve or direct injury to the sphincter musculature.

Anal sphincter damage

Anal ultrasonography enables accurate definition of defects in the internal anal sphincter (IAS) and external anal sphincter (EAS) and provides a qualitative assessment of the muscle. This has altered the understanding of faecal incontinence, as well as its investigation and management. Anal ultrasonography studies have shown a high incidence of structural defects affecting the sphincters and therefore cast some doubt on the overall importance of neurological factors in the pathogenesis of faecal incontinence.

To determine the incidence of sphincter damage after childbirth, a study was conducted in 202 consecutive pregnant women before and after delivery, and repeated 6 months later if abnormalities were detected. Thirty-five per cent of primiparous women developed a sphincter defect affecting either the internal or external sphincter or both. This damage persisted at 6 months. Thirteen per cent of primiparous women developed symptoms of anal incontinence, such as flatus and urgency, after delivery. There was no correlation of bowel symptoms with nerve latency. The same study showed that 8 of 10 women who had forceps deliveries sustained a tear compared to none of the 5 women who had deliveries assisted by vacuum extraction.

Relative importance of the pudendal nerve and anal sphincter

Pudendal nerve denervation has been central to our understanding of the pathophysiology of faecal incontinence, but the advent of anal ultrasound scanning has shown that many more patients have tears than was formerly recognised. This has generated debate over the role of denervation in these patients.

Early postpartum incontinence is usually the result of a direct injury to the anal sphincters. Patients who present with incontinence many years after a traumatic injury almost certainly have a different cause. They have lived and coped with the sphincter injury apparently without ill effects. It is likely that these women present when denervation leads to progressive sphincter weakness. They may also benefit from surgery, but denervation explains why the results of a repair are less satisfactory.

Neurological and psychological diseases

All diseases that involve the central nervous system may cause incontinence. Incontinence of faeces is a common manifestation of senile dementia and all forms of psychotic illness.

Diabetes mellitus

Anorectal dysfunction leading to faecal incontinence occurs in up to 20% of unselected patients with diabetes mellitus. In diabetic patients, incontinence is due to multiple anorectal motor and sensory dysfunctions. IAS and EAS pressures are reduced, the IAS is frequently unstable and rectal sensation may be impaired. It is thought that faecal incontinence in diabetes mellitus is caused by irreversible autonomic neuropathy. Recent studies indicate that the blood glucose concentration may have a major, reversible effect on motor and sensory function in the anorectum. This suggests that optimisation of blood glucose control is an important component of treatment.

Irritable rectum

Irritable rectum is not confined to the irritable bowel syndrome. The physiological features of irritable rectum are also present in patients with inflammatory bowel diseases, ulcerative colitis and solitary rectal ulcer syndrome. During physiological tests, such patients feel a desire to defecate, experiencing urgency and pain at much lower rectal volumes than normal subjects. The rectal compliance in these patients is also reduced. Also, the rectal contractile response to rectal distension and the rectoanal reflex are abnormally enhanced, making the anal sphincter incapable of maintaining continence.

Constipation

Constipation is a major cause of faecal incontinence in elderly patients (Chapter 35). The frequency of bowel movements is not decreased with normal ageing, nor does ageing alone slow intestinal transit. However, constipation is common among the elderly population. Factors contributing to the development of constipation in elderly persons include chronic disease, medication, decreased mobility, dietary habits and decreased fluid intake (Box 36.2). Endocrinological or metabolic disturbance or drugs also predispose to constipation.

Faecal impaction occurs often in the elderly, especially in bed-bound patients, and is the most common cause of faecal incontinence in this group of patients. Some drugs may also cause constipation and lead to overflow incontinence (Chapter 35).

Diagnosis and clinical tests

Extra-gastrointestinal causes of anorectal dysfunction should be excluded, for example, autonomic neuropathy and spinal lesions.

The anorectal examination is an important part of the evaluation. Some diagnoses can be made readily after a routine physical examination; on the other hand, some conditions will not be diagnosed unless more sophisticated tests are used. Most of the time, physical examination reveals the direction of further testing.

Inspection of the perineum

Once the patient is properly positioned, examination begins with inspection of the perineum. Evidence of deformity and previous surgery should be looked for. Faecal or mucus soiling, excoriation or chronic skin changes give clues to the underlying disease processes. Skin tags, anal fissures and prolapsing haemorrhoids are easily identified. Anal gaping may be seen upon slight retraction of the buttocks in severe cases of external sphincter dysfunction.

Incontinent patients or constipated patients with a history of excessive straining at defecation may show perineal descent. This is best demonstrated by asking the patient to cough during the inspection of the perineum or during straining that simulates defecation. The perineum will be seen to bulge towards the examiner. The extent of perineal descent can be measured in relation to the plan of the ischial tuberosities using a device called a perineometer.

Box 36.2 Common causes of constipation

Mechanical obstruction

- Tumour (colon cancer or external compression)
- Stricture (post-ischaemic or diverticular disease, radiation)
- Surgery
- Prolapse
- Haemorrhoids

Neurological and psychological diseases

- Cerebrovascular disease
- Diabetic autonomic neuropathy
- Dementia
- Injury
- Neoplasms
- Psychological illness
- Parkinson's disease
- Amyloidosis
- Multiple sclerosis
- Degenerative diseases

Irritable bowel syndrome

Metabolic conditions

- Hypothyroidism
- Hypercalcaemia
- Hypokalaemia
- Uraemia
- Heavy metal poisoning
- Porphyria

Drugs

Digital examination

A digital examination can exclude organic disease of the rectum. Digital examination may detect stool in the rectal ampulla in patients with constipation, but stool may also be present in some normal subjects. The main purpose of digital examination in anal examination is to assess the tone and the strength of the anal sphincter. The correlation between the anal tone estimated by the anal examination and that measured by manometry is still not clear. Digital assessment gives an 'on the spot' impression of the strength of the anal muscle. However, it is not able to distinguish as to which component of the sphincter is weak, whether the intrinsic rectoanal reflex is intact, and whether spinal reflex or functions of other higher centres (e.g. spinal cord, cerebral cortex) are normal (see below). Furthermore, there is evidence that stretching of the sphincter by digital examination may cause a subsequent manometric recording to be less accurate in patients with an extremely weak sphincter.

Anal gaping immediately upon withdrawing the finger from the anal canal may suggest denervation of the external sphincter. Similarly, the lack of anal 'wink', a reflex contraction of the anal sphincter after pinprick of the perianal area, may also suggest abnormal neurologic function of the perineal areas.

Anal ultrasonography and magnetic resonance imaging

It is important that anatomical anomalies be excluded during the process of making a diagnosis. For example, occult muscle tears occur frequently during vaginal delivery and appropriate early recognition and prompt repair is vital to maintaining anal function in the long term.

Both anal endosonography and magnetic resonance imaging (MRI) can directly image the anal sphincters. The concordance between these two techniques has been poor until an internal coil that can be inserted into the anal canal was used. Nevertheless, anal ultrasonography is the most practical method to use in a clinic as it is easy to use and cheap to run. The main difference between anal and rectal ultrasonography is the probe. In the former method, the rotating head of the probe is protected by a plastic capsule (outer diameter approximately 2 cm) which is filled with water.

Submucosal structure and the IAS and EAS can be visualised by anal ultrasonography. Due to its resolution, it is mainly used to detect the integrity of both the IAS and the EAS and to measure their thickness. Recently, it has been used to inspect the submucosa. With the aid of a computer, a three-dimensional reconstruction of the anal sphincters can be made. However, many parameters can be measured by conventional techniques.

A better image of the anal sphincter and epithelial structures can be obtained when the probe is placed in the vagina. Although some patients may find this less acceptable, it may nevertheless be useful in the diagnosis of anovaginal sepsis and malignancy.

Anal sensation

The anoderm (the lining of the anal canal immediately inferior to the dentate line) is heavily innervated with sensory fibres. In normal subjects, it precisely defines a variety of sensations, for example, touch, temperature, pain and movement within the anal canal. Qualitative assessment using electrical stimulation has been developed. With increases in current across the electrodes, patients perceive stimulation as a burning or tingling sensation. Although the sensations elicited are not natural and it is not known which sensory fibres are stimulated, this technique does give useful information about sensory nerve innervation. Quantitative measurement of anal temperature sensation has also been used.

Manometric assessment of anorectal function

The anorectal canal has a complicated mechanism. Disorders of defecation, either constipation or incontinence, may result from defects in several different components of the anorectal mechanism. The purpose of anorectal manometry is to test the integration of this functional unit, including motor and sensory activities. From these measurements it is possible to assess the expulsion force, resistance to bowel contents, the anorectal sensory response to the arrival of bowel contents and their nervous control under conditions that mimic defecation or challenge the continence mechanism.

Techniques for assessment

A number of techniques have been or are being used to measure anal sphincter pressure. Each technique has particular advantages and disadvantages to influence the pressure recorded.

Water perfused system

An assembly that incorporates multiple side-hole sensors is the most commonly used recording device for anorectal manometry (Figure 36.1). This method is inexpensive, versatile and effective. The pressure recorded in each catheter is an index of the resistance to flow of fluid out of the catheter. Closely spaced sensors can generate a pressure profile along the rectum and anal canal with great accuracy and discriminate between external and internal sphincter activity. They may be combined with a sleeve sensor. This technique can be combined with other functional tests, such as rectal distension and dynamic functional assessment of anorectal function (see below). Perfused side holes are less useful to record pressures in large, hollow organs such as the rectal ampulla unless the contractions occlude the lumen.

With this technique, a vectogram using a three-dimensional, computer-generated representation of the pressure profile of the anal sphincter can be made. However, its accuracy (or the detail in the image) is limited by the number of perfusion side holes and the ability of the sensors to detect pressure deficiency, indicating potential structural abnormality. Radially arranged solid state transducers can also be used (see below) for the same purpose. However, structural abnormalities are better demonstrated by endosonography.

1. *Sleeve.* The properties of the sleeve sensor (Figure 36.1) make it ideal for prolonged or ambulatory recordings of anal sphincter pressure due to its relative tolerance of sphincter movement. It records contractions anywhere along its length as an increased resistance to the flow of perfused water. Therefore, it usually does not localise the site of the resistance (i.e. the highest pressure point in the anal canal), apart from when the contraction happens at the site of perfusion hole, but measures the net resistance of the entire sphincter to the flow of fluid.
2. *Balloon.* The first device using a balloon technique to measure EAS and IAS activity was developed by Schuster. Anal pressures were measured by two balloons placed in the anal canal, with the inner one measuring IAS pressure and the outer one EAS pressure. The interpretation of the data is limited due to the overlap of the two sphincters in the anal canal. Subsequently, a microballoon technique was developed to overcome drawbacks associated with the use of large balloons.
3. *Microballoon.* This device avoids stretching of the sphincter and radial pressure asymmetry. Anal pressure is measured with a 1 cm balloon, and because of this, only limited sampling sites are possible.

Microtransducer

Although the use of transducers offers high fidelity, the number of recording sites are limited by their physical size and cost. Recent designs of solid state catheters incorporate four radially arranged transducers (90° apart), which detect the radial anal pressures along the anal canal. When doing a pull-through, it is also possible to generate a vectogram of the anal canal. A defect in an anal sphincter is indicated when a low anal pressure is recorded in one quadrant.

Sphincter functions

The anal canal is about 2–4 cm long, depending on which definition is used. The 'anatomical' or 'embryological' definition is that the anal canal is approximately 2 cm in length extending from the anal valves to the anal margin. The 'clinical' or 'surgical' definition is that the anal canal is about 4 cm long and is called the 'long' canal. The termination of the 'long' canal is usually at the level of the anorectal ring or the levator ani. This corresponds to the distal end of the dilated, or ampullary, part of the rectum, and the acute angle of the perineal flexure. The angle between the rectum and anal canal is maintained by active contraction of the puborectalis loop. These factors lend support to the claim that the 'long' canal is a useful physiological concept, even though its proximal limit is not marked by any apparent epithelial or developmental boundary.

Internal anal sphincter

The IAS, a smooth muscle, is 0.15–0.5 cm thick. The smooth muscle cells are smaller than those in the rectum, and the thickness of the IAS is due to the increased number of muscle cells. Cellular and intracellular arrangements also differ between rectal and IAS muscles.

Anal pressure can be recorded using manometric methods. The resting pressure in the anal canal undergoes regular fluctuations consisting of slow waves (amplitude, 5–25 mmHg; frequency, 6–20 contractions/min) and much larger amplitude, ultra-slow waves (amplitude, 30–100 mmHg; frequency, < 3 contractions/min). The frequency of the IAS slow wave is higher in the lower canal than in the upper canal. This inwardly directed contraction gradient possibly causes small amounts of material in the anal canal to move back into the rectum.

Ultra-slow waves are associated with particularly high resting pressures. They occur in about 40% of normal subjects but only when the resting pressure is above 100 mmHg. Other studies have reported ultra-slow waves in only 5% of normal subjects, but in 30–45% of patients with haemorrhoids and 67–80% of patients with anal fissures. Resting sphincter pressure is often very high in both of these conditions.

Resting anal pressure is reduced in patients with meningocoele, spinal shock and spinal anaesthesia and patients who have had a sacral resection with ablation of sacral nerves on one or both sides. It is not, however, lowered in long-term paraplegics.

The activity of the IAS is modulated by the sympathetic nervous system. Stimulation of the distal end of the hypogastric nerves induces sphincter contraction. Blockade of the sympathetic outflow with high spinal anaesthesia reduces resting anal pressure more than with low spinal anaesthesia or with pudendal block. Finally, the tone of the IAS is reduced by about 50% after using a selective α-adrenoceptor blocker, phentolamine. These results are contradicted by recent reports that high-frequency stimulation of the presacral nerves reduces anal pressure. However, it seems likely that the presacral outflow contains functionally mixed nerves rather than just adrenergic fibres, and high-frequency electrical stimulation might selectively excite the inhibitory nerves.

External anal sphincter

The EAS is a thick striated muscle. The EAS can usually be divided into three layers and there are some gender differences in the structure.

1. *Pressure recorded during voluntary contraction.* Phasic contraction of the EAS is under voluntary control and is usually associated with contraction of the puborectalis sling. Voluntary contraction elevates the pressure throughout the anal canal, but the pressure rise is maximal in the lower canal where the bulk of the EAS is situated (Figure 36.2).
2. *High pressure zone.* The length of the high pressure zone determined by the pull-through technique is 2.5–5 cm and is longer in males than females. The functional sphincter length is increased during conscious contraction of the sphincter and reduced when the rectum is distended.

   The EAS contributes to 15–20% of the resting anal pressure. Anal pressure is increased in an upright posture and is associated with increased electrical activity in the external sphincter. Coughing or increases in intra-abdominal pressure also increase the EAS activity, possibly by stimulation of tension receptors in the pelvic floor.

   Resting pressures in women, particularly those who have had several children, are lower than those in men, and also in elderly subjects compared to younger subjects. Patients with spinal lesions usually have low resting anal pressures.
3. *Responses to increases in intra-abdominal pressure.* Increases in intra-abdominal pressure, brought about by asking subjects to blow up a balloon, are associated with a compensatory increase in activity of the EAS, causing the sphincter pressure to increase above the rectal pressure and maintaining continence. This response is thought to be triggered by receptors

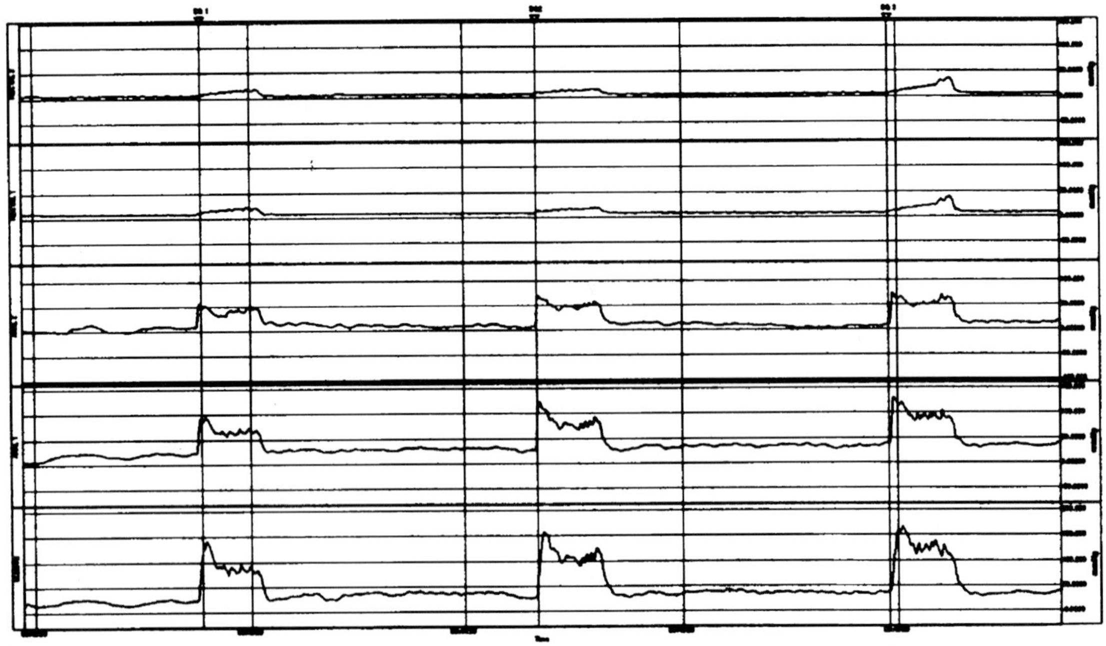

Figure 36.2 Recording of anorectal pressure changes in a normal subject before and during conscious contraction of the EAS (squeeze). The tracing shows the resting pressure, maximum and maximum plateau or sustained pressure responses

in the pelvic floor acting through a spinal reflex. If subjects are asked to strain, as if to defecate, many abolish activity in the EAS, lowering sphincter pressure and facilitating defecation. This activity is under cortical control and in patients with high spinal lesions there is no discrepancy between the two manoeuvres.

4. *Reciprocal contraction of the IAS and the EAS.* The relationship between contraction of the IAS and the EAS in the preservation of continence is poorly understood because of the difficulty in recording the function of both muscles simultaneously in human subjects. Although both muscles relax during defecation, they contract in a reciprocal manner during attempts to maintain continence. For example, rectal distension and contraction relax the IAS, but contract the EAS, while micturition is associated with relaxation of the EAS and contraction of the IAS. This reciprocal activity may explain why patients who have weakness of both the IAS and the EAS tend to be more incontinent than patients who have EAS weakness alone.

Rectal motor function

The rectum is 12–15 cm long. The general distribution of smooth muscle in the rectum is typical for the gut. The longitudinal muscle, however, is derived from the colonic taeniae that fan out to form the longitudinal muscle layer. The caudal end is the junction with epithelium of the anal canal, the dentate line. The rectum is not straight but is S-shaped in the sagittal plane and has three flexures in the coronal plane.

Rectal pressures

The rectum is often quiescent under normal resting condition and exerts a basal pressure of about 5 mmHg. Arrival of faecal material or gas in the rectum may stimulate rectal contraction. Three major types of rectal contractile activity have been described:

1. runs of simple contraction, occurring at a frequency of 5–10 contractions/minute
2. slower contractions, occurring at a frequency of about 3 contractions/minute and attaining amplitudes of up to 10 mmHg

3. slow contractions of similar characteristics that appear to propagate through the rectum, lasting 80–90 minutes during the day and 50–60 minutes during the night.

This periodic activity in the rectum is disrupted by the ingestion of food for approximately 150–180 minutes. The runs of rectal contractions have been compared to the phase III activity of the migrating motor complex (MMC) of the small intestine and named the 'rectal motor complex' (RMC). However, the RMC does not migrate but only occurs at one site in the rectum; the period between consecutive runs varies from 10 to 260 minutes, and there is no temporal relationship with the phases of the migrating motor complex of the small intestine or with the REM/non-REM sleep cycle. Therefore, it has been suggested that such variable phenomena be termed 'periodic motor activity' (PMA). The normal patterns of rectosigmoid colon motor activity remain poorly understood.

Responses to rectal distension

1. *Rectal accommodation*. The reservoir function of the rectum plays an important role in maintaining continence. The initial rectal filling induces rectal contraction, followed by a decrease in pressure to pre-distension level. This is known as the 'accommodation response', a receptive relaxation of the rectal ampulla to accommodate the bowel contents. The rectum can often tolerate more than 300 mL with no increase in rectal pressure. The nature of the capacity and distensibility of the rectum is reflected in this compliance. The higher the compliance, the lower the resistance to distension or the higher the distensibility, and vice versa.

   The phasic contractile response to rectal distension is reduced or absent in patients with lesions involving the low spinal cord, suggesting that it is mediated by a spinal reflex. Rectal tone is increased and compliance reduced in patients with high spinal lesions, while in patients with low spinal lesions rectal tone is reduced and compliance increased.
2. *Rapid intermittent distension*. Rapid intermittent distension (Figure 36.3), carried out with a hand-held syringe, is used to mimic the rapid arrival of faecal material in the rectum. The initial rectal response is the normal response described above. As the distending volume increases, the phasic rectal pressure response increases in amplitude and duration and the steady-state pressures increase. Eventually the rectum fails to accommodate the new volume and a large increase in steady-state pressure is observed as the balloon is distended. This increase in pressure is often associated with pain. Other specific rectal sensations are also experienced by subjects, ranging from perception of the distension to gas in the rectum and a desire to defecate.

Rectoanal co-ordination

Rectoanal inhibitory reflex ('sampling reflex')

The rectoanal inhibitory reflex, previously commonly called the 'sampling reflex', consists of an anal pressure decrease in response to intermittent distension of the rectum. This is associated with suppression of IAS electrical oscillations but not those of the EAS. As the rectal balloon is distended with larger volumes, the amplitude and duration of the relaxation increases (Figure 36.3). A proportionately greater reduction in pressure is observed in the upper than in the lower anal canal, until the pressure in the upper anal canal equals that in the rectum. This allows the rectal contents to be sampled by receptors in the upper anal canal, which plays a role in discriminating between flatus, liquid and solid faeces. Recently it has been suggested that sensitivity to temperature change may be an important factor in the discrimination between gas, liquid and solid faeces.

Upon deflating the balloon, the anal pressure often exceeds the values observed immediately before inflation. The rebound increases in pressures are always associated with increases in the amplitude of the IAS slow wave, but only transient increases in the activity of the EAS. It should also be recognised that distension of the more proximal region of the colon may cause IAS relaxation. Episodes of 'spontaneous' IAS relaxation can be recorded in 17–50% of healthy subjects and are usually associated with an increase in electrical activity of the EAS.

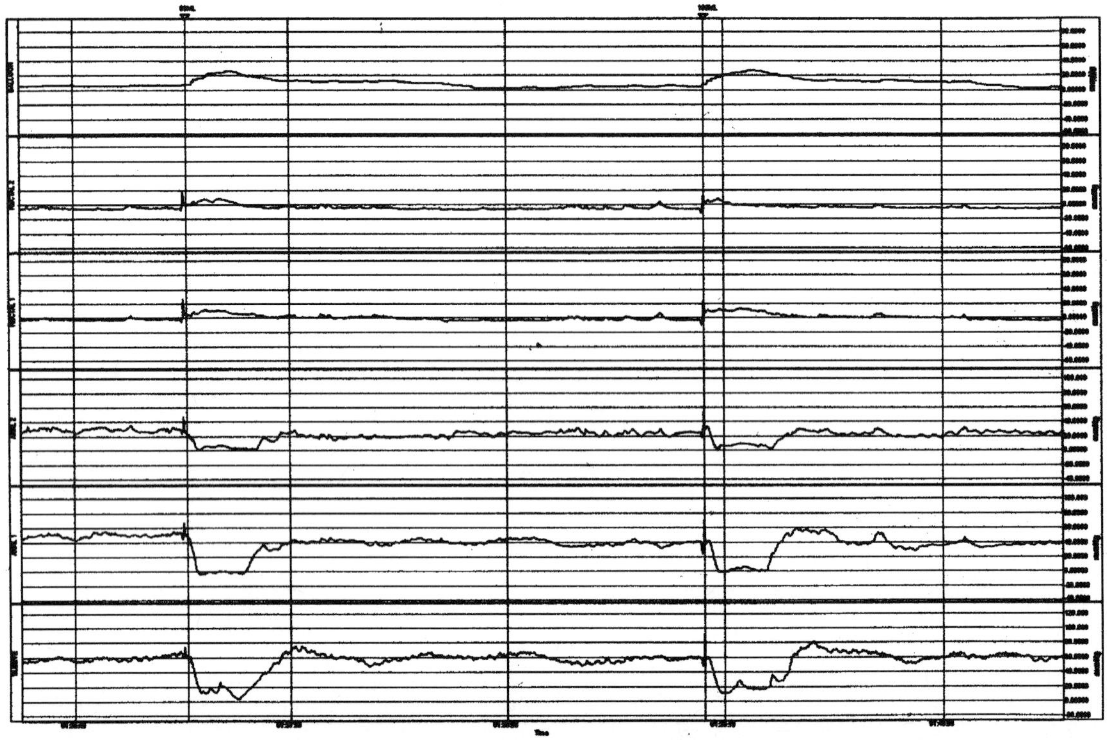

Figure 36.3 Recording of anorectal pressure in the typical normal subject during rectal distension with 60 mL and 100 mL of air, showing an increase in rectal volume and a simultaneous decrease in anal pressure

This reflex is strongly bound to intrinsic innervation. Firstly, it occurs normally in patients with transection of the high spinal cord and can be observed in patients with sectioned hypogastric nerves or with a lesion of the sacral spinal cord. Secondly, it is absent in patients with Hirschsprung's disease, in whom nitric oxide synthetase is absent in the enteric ganglia. Lastly, it is abolished by section, followed by an end-to-end anastomosis, of the distal rectal wall, although recent studies show that this reflex recovers after a period of time, presumably due to nerve regrowth into the distal rectal transection zone.

EAS excitatory response to rectal distension

Intermittent distension of the rectal balloon induces a transient increase in anal pressure, which is associated with an increase in the electrical activity of the EAS. The electrical activity of the EAS reduces to a steady state that increases in amplitude and duration as the rectal volume increases. Very high levels of rectal distension can be associated with an abolition of EAS activity causing a profound reduction in anal pressure.

During slow rectal distension, the electrical activity of the EAS remains at basal levels as long as rectal distension has not been perceived. The perception of the balloon increases the electrical activity of the EAS, and this increase is maintained or increased as the rectal volume increases. The onset of each new sensation is associated with a burst of the electrical activity of the EAS.

The initial EAS response to rectal distension is most likely a spinal reflex because it is preserved in patients with complete high spinal lesions but diminished after a posterior rhizotomy (afferent nerve). This is also absent in patients with low spinal lesions. However, the secondary, prolonged response involves a conscious mechanism because of its close temporal relationship to the conscious perception of the rectal sensation. In patients with complete high spinal lesions the secondary response is absent.

Electrophysiological assessment of anorectal function

There are three major reasons why an electrophysiological assessment should be performed. Firstly, electromyography (EMG) can be used as a functional test of muscle activity. It quantitatively measures electrical activity in the EAS or puborectalis muscle. Secondly, measurement of the amplitude during a number of phases of motor unit action potentials provides information about the innervation and function state of individual motor units within the muscle. Thirdly, EMG of the EAS and IAS greatly facilitates the interpretation of the pressure recordings because of the overlap of the two muscles (except, perhaps, in the distal anal canal, where there is only an EAS recording).

The techniques used to record EMG activity include bipolar wire electrodes, surface electrodes, monopolar electrodes, concentric needle electrodes, single fibre electrodes and intraluminal electrodes (Figure 36.1).

Dynamic assessment of anorectal function

Standard anorectal manometry provides clinicians with almost instant information regarding the anorectal/pelvic floor function by simultaneous measurement of rectal and anal pressures in the resting state, during conscious contraction of the anal sphincter, during increases in intra-abdominal pressure and during rectal distension. Rectal distension, in particular, mimics the arrival of faecal material, revealing information about rectal sensation and compliance and the interaction of the rectum with anal sphincters. This study is easy to perform and repeat if necessary. However, it may not supply all of the information that is sometimes needed for diagnosis, or is not sufficiently sensitive to diagnose certain abnormalities (e.g. volume load incontinence, and anismus—the inappropriate contraction of the EAS). Other techniques have been developed that complement or supplement standard anorectal manometry.

Saline continence test

This is usually done at the end of standard anorectal manometry. While the anorectal catheter is still in situ, an additional perfusion tube is introduced anally into the rectum. The rectum is then slowly distended with saline pre-warmed to 37°C. This mimics the situation where the sphincter is trying to retain a large volume of liquid faeces in the rectum. Apart from pressure changes in the anorectum, rectal sensations can be recorded, and the minimum volume at which the first leakage of the infused fluid occurs and the maximum volume of retention of fluid can be calculated. The test is sensitive enough to detect minor compromised sphincter function. By adding very small amounts of bile acid into the infusate, the volume that healthy volunteers can tolerate reduces significantly. This test can also be used as an indicator of improved anorectal function after treatment.

Defecometry

This test is commonly used to examine the defecation function and detect obstructive constipation. It is usually performed with a pressure sensor in the rectum and bipolar wire electrodes in the anal sphincter, so that the expulsion force and whether or not there is paradoxical contraction of the external sphincter can be assessed. Studies done in both healthy subjects and patients with constipation show that more effort is required to expel stools if they are small and hard than if they are large and soft. Patients have more difficulty in evacuating simulated stools than healthy subjects. Although it is difficult to interpret the data, when combined with pressure measurement in the anal canal, defecometry may be a more logical test of anismus.

Defecography

This technique radiographically images the rectum and, indirectly, its surrounding structures. The process of expelling the contrast agent is recorded on a video tape. The test has been further developed by combining intrarectal pressure sensing and anal sphincter EMG. Defecography provides information on the anorectal angle, pelvic floor descent, the length of the anal canal, time to achieve maximal dilatation of the anal canal, maximum anteroposterior diameter of the anal canal, time taken to evacuate completely and the presence of rectocoeles. This technique provides useful information about whether a patient can pass the rectal contents and whether the above-mentioned parameters are within normal range. However, the technique is complex and involves radiation, and interpretation of results remains controversial.

Scintigraphy

Radionuclear methods can be used to measure the entire gastrointestinal tract transit. When used to assess rectal function, this is usually included as part of the colonic transit test. By measuring the counts in the visually created 'region of interest', the time course of radioisotope transit through different regions is quantitated. Scintigraphic studies may also give some information about rectal volume and its relationship to the pelvic floor. As an alternative to radiological methods, a balloon filled with technetium-99m labelled water can be used to measure the anorectal angle. A recent study shows that in healthy subjects the mean percentage segmental evacuation was right colon 20%, left colon 32% and rectum 66%. This suggests that colonic emptying occurs during defecation and that defecation is not a process of rectal evacuation only. Although rectal scintigraphy has potential advantages as a diagnostic test in terms of quantitation and decreased radiation exposure, the inability of the test to distinguish patients with slow-transit constipation and defecatory complaints makes the potential utility of this test of uncertain value in clinical and investigative settings.

Summary of investigations

There is no general consensus about what tests should be done and in which order to investigate abnormal anorectal function. Disorders of defecation and continence are usually associated with defects in several components of an integrated system. An ideal test should identify these causes and provide guidance for treatment. Unfortunately, there is no single test that satisfies these criteria. Our experience suggests that combined *multiport manometry*, *electrophysiology* and *sensory testing* is a set of tests useful for clinicians.

If a problem is associated with a weak anal sphincter, then EAS electromyography or measurement of pudendal nerve terminal motor latency may identify the pathophysiology. If the pudendal nerve conduction is normal, then the lesion may be in the spinal cord, and this may be identified by electrical stimulation of the brain or the spinal cord and by measuring the latency of the EAS response. In order to test the efferent nerve function specifically, evoked potential recording may be a useful test to choose. Imaging techniques can provide objective evidence as to whether defecatory function is normal or not but need specialised equipment and involve radiation, and the interpretation of data is usually difficult. However, one particular technique may be sensitive to a specific abnormality and a clinician should choose the most informative test according to the patient's symptoms and possible underlying mechanism.

Treatment

Medical treatment

When diarrhoea is complicated by faecal incontinence, the first priority is to control the diarrhoea and then determine if the patient has a treatable cause of incontinence. The first line of treatment for diarrhoea is the use of opiate-like antidiarrhoeal agents (loperamide, lomotil and codeine phosphate). These inhibit the local nervous reflexes responsible for both intestinal propulsion and secretion and increase the tone of the IAS. Loperamide (Imodium) is the most potent of these, and unlike codeine phosphate, does not cross the blood–brain barrier. As many as 12 tablets of loperamide (8 mg tds) may be taken per day with no obvious unwanted side effects. It is important to exclude diarrhoea due to intestinal stasis with bacterial overgrowth (Chapter 34) since loperamide will only exacerbate the intestinal stasis.

Rapid intestinal transit sufficient to cause diarrhoea is often associated with bile acid malabsorption (Chapter 34). Alan Hoffman of the Mayo Clinic has termed bile acids as nature's laxatives. They stimulate colonic secretion and propulsion and when absorption is impaired by rapid intestinal or ileal resection or when there is a chronic leak of bile acids into the gut consequent on cholecystectomy, they may be responsible for copious diarrhoea and urgency. In severe diarrhoea that is resistant to loperamide and associated with urgency, incontinence and evidence of bile acid malabsorption, treatment with the bile-acid-binding resin, cholestyramine (Questran), given in association with loperamide can be dramatically effective. Bile acids are released in association with a meal. Therefore, it is essential that the patient be instructed to take Questran half an hour before meals and to titrate the dose to the size of the meal. We usually commence with a small dose, two sachets (8 g) before dinner in the evening and one (4 g) before lunch, but the clinician should enlist the patient's co-operation to find the most appropriate dose according to the patient's pattern of eating and response to treatment.

Since there is evidence that diabetic diarrhoea and nocturnal incontinence may be related to sympathetic neuropathy, it is not surprising that α-2 adrenergic agonists, such as clonidine, have been advocated and shown to be effective in the management of diabetic diarrhoea associated with evidence of neuropathy. Clonidine artificially restores the sympathetic tone, enhancing salt and water absorption and reducing propulsive contractions. Recent studies demonstrate that clonidine can modulate human colonic motor and sensory function in healthy subjects. It also seems probable that clonidine may help to restore IAS stability and tone, although this has yet to be tested. Clonidine should always be considered in the management of patients with nocturnal incontinence. The dose is similar to that employed to treat hypertension and although it may not necessarily lower a normal blood pressure, considerable caution should be exercised in treating neuropathic patients with postural hypotension and nocturnal incontinence.

Faecal incontinence even in the presence of a normal or nearly normal bowel action requires further investigation and treatment for anorectal dysfunction. Loperamide should always be tried in such patients since it reduces rectal sensitivity and reflex activity, enhances sphincter tone and has been shown to reduce urgency and incontinence, even in patients who do not have frank diarrhoea.

Obstetric causes for faecal incontinence are at least as common in diabetics as they are in non-diabetics and can be treated by surgery. Defects in the sphincter ring caused by previously undetected tears can respond to an overlap sphincter repair. It may well be important to ascertain that the remaining muscle is active by carrying out measurements of myoelectrical activity before surgery. Obstetric trauma also weakens the pelvic floor and causes perineal descent and pudendal neuropathy. The progression of this may be halted and the mechanical function of the pelvic floor improved by a procedure known as post-anal repair, where the pelvic floor is strengthened with a darn or a graft. This procedure may also help in the management of urinary incontinence. The results of post-anal repair are poor if perineal descent has caused severe neuropathic weakness of the sphincter or pudendal neuropathy due to compression, and tension is exacerbated by diabetic microangiopathy. Alternative procedures, such as the use of the gracilis or gluteus muscle to construct a new sphincter or the more experimental artificial sphincter devices, have inconclusive results. When somebody is suffering from continuous soiling that does not respond to treatment, a permanent colostomy may prove to be the only reasonable solution.

Faecal impaction with overflow is usually treated by evacuation using digital extraction and enemas followed by a regular regimen of bulk laxatives and toilet training (Chapter 35).

Biofeedback training (operant reconditioning) is a useful method for treating incontinence of all types, probably by increasing external sphincter strength, rectal sensation and improving co-ordination between rectal perception and external sphincter contraction. The sphincter activity during conscious contraction of the external sphincter is displayed to patients visually. Patients are encouraged to improve the response in both strength and duration. Co-ordination between rectal perception and pelvic floor contraction improves by training the patient to recognise and react promptly to progressively smaller volumes of air introduced into a rectal balloon by contracting the external sphincter. Studies show impressive responses to biofeedback training in patients with idiopathic faecal incontinence. However, when tested for the 'active principle' by removing the feedback, patients still did well. Therefore, the beneficial effects of biofeedback might be related to establishing confidence through the nature of the relationship between the patient and the therapist.

Surgical treatment

Treatment of patients who have sustained a tear of the sphincter muscle is surgical. Several options are available.

Primary repair

Primary repair of the sphincter is often inadequate since half the patients who have sustained a tear continue to have symptoms of incontinence and urgency, and sonographic defects can be identified in 85% of those who have sustained a third-degree tear compared to 33% of controls who did not.

Acute sphincter injuries are best treated by primary repair whenever possible. Direct apposition of the severed sphincter muscles without tension or with slight overlap using prolene sutures may achieve satisfactory results in skilled hands. When appropriate skills are not available, the management depends on the extent of the injury. With a substantial defect of the sphincter the most appropriate course of action is to carry out a loop colostomy to divert the faecal stream until the patient can be referred for elective reconstruction.

Secondary repair

Many incontinent patients have to be treated after the primary repair has failed due to sepsis, haematoma, faulty technique or because the injury was simply not recognised.

Secondary repairs should be performed only after all contaminated wounds have healed and inflammation has completely subsided. This generally requires about three months following injury. Routine preoperative care includes complete bowel preparation and prophylactic antibiotic therapy. The use of a colostomy is not often necessary. The repair options include a direct overlapping approach that may or may not be combined with levatorplasty. The purpose of adding this in such injuries is to strengthen and lengthen the anal canal with the theoretical objective of improving continence.

In a series of 55 women with incontinence, EAS damage was delineated preoperatively. Eighty per cent became continent postoperatively. Improvement correlated with restoration of normal anatomy. In the failures, defects were still present. The above results need to be assessed at 5 years and beyond to ascertain if such improvements are sustained.

Plication repair

In less severe injuries it may be evident that the muscle is not completely divided but rather attenuated anteriorly. In this instance, rather than dividing the splayed out but intact muscle, a plication of the intact muscle and scar is achieved using horizontal mattress sutures instead of the conventional overlapping repair. After the sphincters have been reconstructed with one of these three procedures, the vaginal wall and perineum is usually repaired with interrupted absorbable sutures. This may require V-Y-plasty or Z-plasty to achieve adequate skin cover. Sometimes the wounds are left open to heal by secondary intention.

Post-anal repair

Post-anal repair is based on Park's observation that many incontinent patients have an intact but poorly functioning sphincter with a wide anorectal angle. He proposed redirection of the apparent abnormality by performing a posterior levatorplasty to tighten the anorectal angle and lengthen the anal canal. The initial high rate of success (83%) has not been reproduced in other centres and the post-anal repair may actually lead to progression of neurogenic damage. Lengthening and tightening of the anal canal may be of some value in some patients. A combined anterior and posterior levatorplasty has been advocated in selected patients. Analysis of the results from several series suggests the operation is of little help in improving continence to liquid stool but may improve continence to solid stools in 77% of patients.

Synthetic encirclement procedures

Thiersch wiring is now obsolete but Dacron-impregnated Silastic sheets have been advocated by some to reinforce weakened sphincters. The concept of a totally implantable artificial bowel sphincter is particularly attractive for the patient not suited to other options. An artificial urinary sphincter has been used in over 4000 patients since 1972. The septic and failure rates are acceptably low with this device. There is limited experience using a similar device for anal incontinence with reasonable results in the majority of patients in the small series reported.

Muscle transfer techniques

Gracilis muscle transposition has been used to reconstruct the anal sphincter. It is not as effective as anticipated because it consists mostly of type II fibres. However, a 1990 technique developed the concept of using electrical stimulation of the gracilis muscle to transform it from a fast twitch (type II) to a slow twitch (type I) muscle, capable of sustained tonic contractility. Stimulating electrodes are sutured to the gracilis muscle before transposition and their leads are connected to a permanent pacemaker device implanted in the chest wall. Once satisfactory function has been obtained, continence rates have been excellent.

Prognosis

Faecal incontinence in the elderly population is not an isolated disease entity but it is part of, or the consequence of, other disease processes. Clinical management should focus on the correctable or reversible causes; for example, change of mental status caused by infection or medication, or alteration of bowel function caused by dietary factors or drugs. Only if the attempt at correcting these causes fails, should one try to correct the faecal incontinence itself.

Bibliography and further reading

American Gastroenterological Association (1999), 'American Gastroenterological Association Medical Position Statement on anorectal testing techniques', *Gastroenterology*, 116, pp. 732–60.

Dent, J. (ed.) (1991), *Gastrointestinal Motility*, Balliere's Clinical Gastroenterology, Balliere Tindall Ltd, London, pp. 5.

Parks, A. G. (1975), 'Anorectal incontinence', *Proceedings of the Royal Society of Medicine*, 68, pp. 681–90.

Rao, S. S. C. & Sun, W. M. (2001), 'Manometric assessment of anorectal function', *Gastroenterology Clinics of North America*, 30, pp. 15–32.

Ratnaike, R. N. (ed.) (1999), *Diarrhoea and Constipation in Geriatric Practice*, Cambridge University Press, Cambridge.

Read, N. W., Abouzekry, L., Read, M. G., Howell, P., Ottewell, D. & Donnelly, T. C. (1985), 'Anorectal function in elderly patients with faecal impaction', *Gastroenterology*, 89, pp. 959–66.

Read, N. W. & Sun, W. M. (1992), 'Anorectal manometry', in: Henry, M. & Swash, M. (eds), *Coloproctology and Pelvic Floor*, 2nd edn, Butterworths, London, pp. 119–45.

Romero, Y., Evans, J., Fleming, K. & Phillips, S. (1996), 'Constipation and fecal incontinence in the elderly population', *Mayo Clinic Proceedings*, 71, pp. 81–92.

Schuster, M. M., Hookman, P. & Hendrix, T. R. (1965), 'Simultaneous manometric recording of internal and external anal sphincter reflexes', *Bulletin of Johns Hopkins Hospital*, 116, pp. 79–88.

Sun, W. M., Donnelly, T. C. & Read, N. W. (1992), 'Utility of a combined test of anorectal manometry, electromyography, and sensation in determining the mechanism of "idiopathic" faecal incontinence', *Gut*, 33, pp. 807–13.

Wald, A. (1994), 'Colonic and anorectal motility testing in clinical practice', *American Journal of Gastroenterology*, 89, pp. 2109–15.

Chapter 37
Diverticular disease

PER-ANDERS LARSSON

Introduction

Diverticulae are outpouchings of the intestinal wall. There are two different types: the first is called 'true diverticulae' and contains all layers of the intestinal wall. Such diverticulae exist mostly as isolated lesions, can be found at all levels of the gastrointestinal tract and represent congenital structures. The other type of diverticulae is mostly serial outpouchings located in the distal part of the colon. These 'false' or 'pseudo-' diverticulae are herniations of mucosa through the colon muscle and are presumably acquired lesions. This chapter will focus on the latter type of diverticulae, as well as the symptoms and complications related to their presence in the colon.

'Diverticulosis' is a morphologic term and refers to the existence of diverticulae that may or may not be associated with any symptoms. Diverticulosis is mostly a harmless condition and only 1 out of 5 patients with diverticulosis develops any symptoms from the bowel. On rare occasions, however, the complications related to diverticulosis can be extremely severe and accompanied by significant mortality. Diverticular disease embraces both the existence of diverticulae in the colon—that is, diverticulosis—and complications to diverticulosis. The most common complications to diverticulosis are inflammation, perforation and bleeding. Symptoms related to uncomplicated diverticulosis are pain and motility disorders, but the aetiological relationship between diverticulosis and these symptoms is obscure. Diverticulitis is an inflammatory condition that involves diverticulae, mostly in the left colon. It must be emphasised that even if the existence of diverticulae is a pathological condition, it is primarily the complications of diverticulae that create the clinical problem, diverticular disease. Both the prevalence of diverticulosis and the incidence of complications related to diverticulosis are increased in elderly people.

Aetiology and epidemiology

Diverticular disease of the sigmoid and left colon is an acquired disease and the general opinion is that it is related to insufficient stool volume and high pressure in the colon. The hypermotility of the colon in the patients developing diverticulosis can frequently be identified in the sigmoid colon on contrast radiography even before the development of diverticulae.

Sigmoid diverticular disease was rare until the 20th century, but the epidemiological data available before the 20th century are limited to the complicated cases, as uncomplicated diverticulosis was unrecognised before the advent of contrast radiography. The incidence of diverticular disease has increased in the industrialised world throughout the 20th century. However, there are several remaining problems in epidemiological studies of diverticular disease that are related to the fact that the pathological state in the colon exists already in the early forms of the disease, but most epidemiological studies will only find patients with symptomatic forms of the disease. The first problem is the lack of definitions of the early forms of diverticular disease. Studies on resected specimens show that there is a change in protein composition of the longitudinal muscle layer of the colon, which initially renders the circular muscle layer less able to relax, and then splits into bundles. When the circular layer splits it enables outpushings of the mucosa beyond the bowel wall. It is when these outpushings are visible on X-ray examinations that we know that diverticulae exist. Then arises the second problem: how many diverticulae need to be present to justify the label of diverticulosis? A third problem in epidemiological studies of diverticular disease is how many symptoms need to be present to justify the label of diverticular disease. In clinical practice it is convenient to apply a broad definition of diverticulosis and label any number of diverticulae as diverticulosis, but restrict the term 'diverticular disease' to patients with defined complications such as bleeding or inflammation.

The presence of diverticulae in the left colon is strongly correlated to age. When the prevalence of diverticulosis has been estimated in the healthy population, the prevalence is negligible in people below the age of 20 and diverticulae are seldom identified in individuals below 40. The prevalence of diverticulae in developed countries increases to 30% in individuals above 50, and more than 65% in octogenarians. These estimations of the prevalence of diverticulae are based either on autopsy reports or X-ray examinations. Both methods are flawed by the fact that they are only applied to individuals with symptoms of disease and the estimations are based on individuals both with and without symptoms of the disease. The true prevalence of diverticulae in healthy individuals is unknown.

Despite the fact that diverticulosis is frequent in the elderly population and in the elderly requiring hospital care, it is a rare cause of mortality. Studies from the US reveal that less than 0.5 of 100 000 deaths in the population younger than 64 years and between 2.7 and 6.5 per 100 000 in individuals 64–75 years old are due to diverticular disease.

The current concept that diverticular disease is a disease of the elderly population is closely related to the lack of epidemiological evidence of the preclinical forms of the disease. However, the clinical presentation of the disease provides evidence that diverticular disease is a health problem in the ageing population. Studies from the US on health care spending due to various chronic disorders reveals a remarkable prevalence of colon diverticulosis as a cause of hospitalisation in patients aged 65 and over. One study found that 17% of all hospitalisations for digestive disease in this group of patients were due to diverticular disease of the colon. This study also revealed that 4% of all hospital discharges in the patients of age 65 and over had a diagnosis of diverticulosis.

The prevalence of diverticulosis varies in different cultures and populations. Diverticular disease is closely related to Western countries and even in Europe it was a rare disease before the 20th century. Epidemiological studies have emphasised the increasing incidence and prevalence of diverticulosis when a population changes its lifestyle from rural to urban. Diet has been regarded as the most important lifestyle factor in these studies. Longitudinal studies from North America and Western Europe show prevalence figures around 10% in the beginning and between 25 and 40% in the second half of the 20th century. Studies from Israel performed in the 1970s have revealed prevalence figures of 17% in Aschenazi Jews and substantially lower figures in both Sephardic-oriental Jews (3.8%) and the Arab population (0.7%). In studies from the late 1980s these figures had risen to 12.3% in Sephardic-oriental Jews and 5.4% in the Arab population. The influence of cultural and temporal trends in lifestyle and diet has also been supported by data from South African and Chinese studies. Although several authors have presented huge differences in the prevalence of diverticular disease between different ethnic groups, it seems to be clear that these differences are more related to lifestyle and diet than racial differences. The difference between different populations in the distribution of diverticulae in the colon does not seem to be affected by lifestyle differences in the same manner. Oriental populations mostly have a few right-sided diverticulae in the colon, whereas European and white populations mostly have numerous sigmoid and left-sided colon diverticulae when their disease is related to symptoms. It is important, however, to remember that differences in the prevalence of diverticular disease may not only be attributed to changes in dietary habits along the course of social and economical development of the society but also to the effect of technical advances in medical diagnostics. The development of barium enema and colonoscopy has enabled us to detect the disease in large groups of patients, which was impossible in the 19th century.

It has been proposed that a lack in bulk and fibre intake can account for the difference in prevalence between various populations. Another important factor, which may reflect the incidence of diverticulosis, is that people a century ago had a much shorter life expectancy and that diverticulae today reflect a natural age related development of the colon. However, diverticulae arise in gaps of the musculature where the vasa recta penetrates the intestinal wall. Such gaps have been observed also in experimental studies on young rats that were fed a low-fibre diet. These findings do not exclude, rather they contradict, that the bowel wall weaknesses that predispose to mucosal outpouchings should be an effect of ageing only. These experimental studies in rodents have been systematically performed and reveal that rats on a high-fibre diet have a low incidence of diverticulae and that they also survive significantly longer than rats on an almost fibre-free diet of which 50–55% develop diverticulae. These studies strongly support a role of fibre in the aetiology, but studies in humans confirming the importance of fibre for counteracting the developments of diverticulae are lacking.

Pathophysiology

Both dietary and hereditary factors have been identified in the pathogenesis of diverticulosis and complications to diverticulosis. The most important theories about diverticula formation have been focused on the strength, activity and function of the muscular layers of the bowel wall. Several studies have reported abnormal tension in the bowel wall and high pressure in the colon lumen in patients with diverticulosis. Early stages of diverticular disease are characterised by a muscular hyperactivity which can be demonstrated as a serrated appearance of the bowel profile on barium contrast X-ray examinations. Patients with diverticular disease are also characterised by abnormal pressure responses in their colon when provoked by alimentary stimuli. A vicious circle has been described in which tension in the muscular wall results in an increased intraluminal pressure. Further increase in muscular activity and further narrowing of the lumen leads to a segmental occlusion of the lumen and creation of closed compartments between the haustrae, which further increases the intraluminal pressure. Diverticulae are then formed as herniations—that is, protrusions of mucosa through the weakest points of the muscular layer.

The muscular layer of the colon wall is composed of two layers: the internal layer in which the smooth muscle fibres are arranged in a circular fashion, and an outer layer, which is condensed into three taenias. These structures running along the colon consist of longitudinally arranged smooth muscle fibres. The circular muscle layer is only covered with serosa—that is, visceral peritoneum between the taenias. As the outer longitudinal layer of colon muscle is arranged in taenias, the inner circular layer also has the tendency to form a lattice, which concentrates tensile strength to specific parts of the colon wall and makes other portions weaker. The wall is especially weak where the vasa recta passes from the outside into the submucosa. These foramina of the bowel wall are the weak points where the mucosa is pushed outwards by the intraluminal pressure and diverticulae are formed.

Epidemiological studies have indicated that a low-residue diet is related to a high incidence of diverticular disease; the pathophysiologic mechanisms beyond this relation are less well understood. Experimental data from a large randomised study in rats indicate that the incidence of diverticulae varies with the intake of dietary fibre. In this study 45% of the rats fed on a fibre-free diet developed diverticulae, whereas only 9% of the rats on a fibre supplemented diet developed diverticulae. The fibre intake in the latter group of rats was calculated to be equivalent to a daily intake of 100 g fibre in humans. There are no such experimental studies of sufficient duration in humans proving a causative relationship between low fibre intake and diverticula formation. On the other hand there are plenty of studies of transit time, faecal weight and colonic intraluminal pressure in subjects on high and low-residue diets. Since these physiologic factors are related to diverticula formation, there is indirect evidence for a relation between diet and diverticulosis, but this relation is obscure. The pathophysiology of complications to diverticulosis is based on the previous formation of mature diverticulae and progression of the pathological process within these diverticulae in different directions, depending on the interaction between the diverticula and the bowel content.

Although the aetiology of diverticulitis is obscure, one generally accepted theory is that oedema of the neck of the diverticula causes entrapment of faeces. Uncontrolled bacterial growth and inflammatory reaction in the occluded diverticula and surrounding tissues follows. The inflammation spreads through the mucosa and laterally in the serosa of the sigmoid. This has also been called perisigmoiditis although all layers of the intestinal wall are afflicted at this stage. The pathophysiology of the serious complications to inflammatory diverticular disease is the aggressive inflammation in the bowel wall, which results in a phlegmon and microabscesses of the intestinal wall. When the inflammatory process proceeds it will either result in a necrosis and perforation of the bowel wall or the formation of a larger abdominal abscess.

The pathophysiological background to the late complications of inflammatory diverticular disease is the progression of the inflammatory process in the bowel wall. In the case of strictures, the chronic inflammation results in fibrosis of the bowel wall, which leads to a narrowing of the lumen. The emergence of fistulas is explained by drainage of a pericolic abscess into an adjacent hollow organ such as the vagina or the bladder.

The pathophysiology of bleeding in diverticular disease is related to the aetiology of diverticulae which arise where the small branches from the mesenteric blood supply reach the colon and enter the wall of the colon. Thus diverticulae are located in close connection to these vessels and the neck of the mature diverticular sac will be immediately adjacent to such a major vessel of the colon. It is postulated that the passage of stools through the colon induces decubital ulceration on the distal side of the neck, which ultimately penetrates into the vessel lumen, resulting in major bleeding.

Clinical tests

At least 80% of diverticulosis never presents clinically. In these cases the presence of diverticulae will only be detected when morphological examination is performed for other clinical conditions. On the other hand, morphologic demonstration of diverticulae by either colonoscopy or barium enema is necessary for the diagnosis of diverticular disease. They can replace each other and they are equally efficient with regard to sensitivity and specificity in the diagnosis of diverticulosis. In the case of a distal stricture there may be an advantage in using the barium contrast enema in examination of the proximal colon if the stricture is impossible to pass with the colonoscope. Adequate preparation of the colon prior to examination is extremely important before both examinations. These preparations are frequently problematic and unpleasant for elderly patients. In the case of weak and circulatory unstable patients, these preparations may also be dangerous. Colon preparation for endoscopic or barium enema examinations can be performed with either enemas or oral purgatives that have mechanical or chemical effects on the colon. Despite the differences between these cleaning methods, most of them are equally effective and yield excellent results when applied properly. Patient compliance may be a problem with the most complicated methods as well as with methods requiring oral intake of large amounts of fluids. The judgment of further therapeutic options and the impact of the diagnostic yield for the choice between therapeutic options in elderly patients must be carefully assessed before they are referred for either colonoscopy or contrast X-ray examinations.

For the diagnosis of inflammatory diverticular disease, additional diagnostic criteria must be fulfilled which, in addition to the clinical presentation, also require blood chemistry for demonstration of inflammatory parameters such as C-reactive protein and leucocytosis. CT scans and ultrasound are essential in the diagnosis of complicated diverticulitis. Their specific advantages and drawbacks will be described later in relation to the inflammatory complications of diverticular disease. Additional examinations in complicated diverticulitis are plain abdominal X-ray, which in the case of free perforation will demonstrate intra-abdominal gas and fistulography in the pre-operative investigation of fistulas.

Diagnosis, treatment and prognosis

Diverticulitis

The diagnosis of diverticulitis is based on the combination of clinical symptoms and the presence of diverticulae in the left colon. However, barium contrast enemas and colonoscopy are contraindicated in the initial phase of the disease, as the risk of perforation is substantial in these patients. The diagnosis can then only be established on clinical and laboratory findings.

The most important differential diagnosis is appendicitis. The clinical symptoms in both appendicitis and diverticulitis are low abdominal pain and tenderness in combination with fever. The sigmoid colon as well as the appendix is mostly situated intraperitoneal and mobile in the abdomen, which may obscure the localisation of symptoms to the right or left side of the midline. One important differentiating feature is that appendicitis does not respond to conservative therapy—that is, antibiotics and bowel rest with intravenous fluids.

Other differential diagnoses are ulcerative colitis, Crohn's disease, radiation induced colitis, endometriosis and gynaecological infections. Ulcerative colitis and gynaecological problems are less frequent in the geriatric patients whereas Crohn's disease, especially when it is localised to the rectum, has a clinical appearance, which may closely mimic the symptoms of diverticulitis. Although the clinical diagnosis is not always unequivocal, it is mostly sufficient for clinical management of the patients. It is mandatory to perform a colonoscopy or a sigmoidoscopy in combination with a barium enema, after 3 or 4 weeks. The rationale for this diagnostic work-up is to rule out or find a colorectal cancer, which is the most important differential diagnosis. A few recent publications report a higher incidence of left side colorectal cancers in patients with a previous history of diverticulitis compared to the general population. It is even more important to perform these examinations in the elderly after a suspected episode of diverticulitis, as the incidence of colorectal cancer is high in this group of patients. In patients with frequent recurrences of diverticulitis, these examinations should be repeated. There are no unequivocal data on how frequently X-ray or colonoscopy examinations need to be repeated but a practical policy is to perform a new examination after a new attack of diverticulitis if the previous examination was done more than 4 years before.

The clinical management of patients with diverticulitis is straightforward when the diagnosis is unequivocal, but mostly it is not. It is therefore wise to admit these patients as inpatients and observe them as undiagnosed abdominal emergencies. The standard treatment is conservative and relies on intravenous fluid resuscitation, restricted oral intake and antibiotics. It is of the utmost importance to observe these patients carefully to avoid or promptly handle further complications of the disease.

If the patient's general condition is unaffected and the diagnosis is established, it is acceptable to treat the patient as an outpatient. It is then recommended to prescribe oral antibiotics and adherence to a low-residue diet. Most patients improve during the first 24–48 hours with these regimens and hospital inpatients can gradually resume oral intake and continue as outpatients with oral antibiotics. The total length of antibiotic treatment is usually

7–10 days and the antibiotics are chosen to cover a spectrum of the most common Gram-negative aerobic species and anaerobic species as the bacteroides strains which are suspected in the aetiology of the disease. Spasmolytic drugs, which can relieve discomfort in painful diverticular disease, have no place in the treatment in uncomplicated diverticulitis since the intestinal lumen obstruction in these cases are induced by bowel wall inflammation and oedema and not muscular activity. Dietary fibres—that is, high-residue diet and stool softeners—are important in other stages of the disease but are contraindicated in acute diverticulitis.

These practical guidelines are widely accepted as standard treatment but the scientific evidence for them is weak. Controlled randomised studies should be valuable but they are almost impossible to perform since patients with suspected diverticulitis seldom have a clear diagnosis when they present but rather when the disease gradually resolves. A few scientific reports have indicated that both antibiotics and restricted oral intake can be omitted but there are no modern randomised studies with untreated diverticulitis patients in the control group.

Complicated diverticulitis—abscess, sepsis and peritonitis

A number of patients will develop serious complications of diverticulitis, such as peridiverticular abscess, purulent peritonitis and faecal peritonitis. However, these complications are rare in patients who are treated with antibiotics and bowel rest in hospitals. The clinical course of these complications is rapid and these complications are usually evident when the patient initially presents. It is only a minority of these patients who have a previous history of uncomplicated diverticulitis.

The occurrence of inflammatory diverticular disease is due to the aggressive inflammation in the bowel wall, which initially results in a phlegmon and micro-abscesses and may proceed to necrosis and perforation of the bowel wall. If the perforation occurs adjacent to the peritoneal surfaces of the pelvis, the abdominal cavity, the intestines or the mesentery, it will be closed and the perforation will result in an abscess. The abscess may subsequently burst and result in a purulent peritonitis. The most serious development is when the aggressive inflammation in the bowel wall results in significant necrosis and a faecal leak into the free peritoneal cavity—that is, faecal peritonitis.

The symptoms in patients with acute phlegmon and peridiverticular abscess are more pronounced and it may be possible to palpate a mass in the left iliac fossa. Bowel rest and medical treatment with antibiotics may not always be sufficient to cure or improve the condition in patients with complicated diverticulitis. Diagnostic work-up in patients with suspected complicated forms of acute diverticulitis relies mainly on ultrasound examinations and computerised tomography. Magnetic resonance imaging (MRI) could also be useful, but its value is not as well defined in the literature. CT scans give pictures, which are easier to compare and are well suited to follow the clinical course. One of the main advantages with ultrasound is the availability of therapeutic accessories for drainage of abscesses, which can be performed directly at the time of diagnosis. A disadvantage of CT is the need for oral contrast intake, which can be difficult due to the impairment of bowel movements in these patients.

When there is a free perforation with purulent or faecal peritonitis, the clinical diagnosis of peritonitis is clear and no further examinations should delay the laparotomy, which must be performed immediately. Laparotomy will also be a diagnostic procedure in these patients if the cause of peritonitis is not known.

Acute phlegmon of the bowel should be treated with prolonged bowel rest, intravenous fluid resuscitation and antibiotics. Most patients are cured after a week with this treatment. Bowel resection may be necessary if medical treatment continues to be ineffective or if the diagnostic work-up with double contrast barium enema or colonoscopy fails or is suspicious of a colorectal neoplasm.

Acute diverticulitis can also be complicated by a walled off diverticular abscess. Percutaneous drainage and antibiotics, in combination with bowel rest, is the treatment of choice in these cases. This treatment is also effective in most cases, even when septicaemia is present initially. The cavity must be completely emptied of all pus. This can be done either by leaving a catheter in the cavity for prolonged drainage or by carefully rinsing the cavity with saline. Only a few patients with abscess phlegmon and local peritonitis will require surgical treatment, although some surgeons may argue that resection with a primary anastomosis should be the treatment of choice in these cases.

Both faecal and purulent peritonitis are serious conditions, frequently complicated by septicaemia and shock. The mortality is high and different figures have been mentioned for different subpopulations of patients. The mortality is dependent on the type of peritonitis—that is, faecal, 35%; purulent, 6%—but the mortality in this condition is also dependent on the patient's age, type of treatment and concomitant disease. Mortality figures as high as 70% in elderly patients have been presented in some studies. The main therapeutic principle is that a patient with peritonitis should immediately be referred to emergency surgery. However, in geriatric practice it is extremely important to ensure that the patient is capable of undergoing surgery. The high mortality, the treatment associated morbidity both with surgery and in intensive care units, and the prolonged suffering these patients are exposed to before they can resume normal activities makes the choice between a curative or a palliative approach to these patients pivotal. The choice must be based on the patient's present physical condition and expectancy to survive the surgical treatment as well as the patient's life expectancy.

The laparotomy in these cases aims to identify the reason for peritonitis, clear the abdominal cavity of contamination and relieve the septic condition. The inflammatory process—that is, the diverticulae affected part of the colon—should be resected. This can be done either at the emergency laparotomy or in a subsequent surgical procedure when theoretically the patient would be in a better condition.

There are three main surgical procedures for perforated diverticulitis. The initial emergency laparotomy in a 'three stage procedure' consists of clearance of the abdominal cavity of contamination, drainage of the area around the perforation, closure of the perforation and construction of a stoma proximal to the perforation to deviate the faecal stream to protect the diseased bowel. The second stage is performed when the patient has recovered, and judged to be in an optimal condition for the surgical procedure. A complete resection of the diseased part of the intestine is performed and an anastomosis is constructed. The proximal deviating stoma is left in place for a month to protect the anastomosis before it is closed.

Hartmann's procedure is considered the standard procedure today. It is a 'two stage procedure', and the abdominal cavity is cleaned and a resection of the perforated colon segment is performed in the first emergency operation. The proximal colon is deviated through a stab wound in the left ileac fossa and a stoma is constructed. The distal colon is closed blindly. The second stage of this procedure is performed after some months when the inflammatory process in the abdominal cavity has healed and the patient has recovered. The second stage is optional and the patient can be with a stoma if he is not fit enough for a second operation or is satisfied with the colonostomy. If a limited resection was performed at the initial emergency, supplementary resections of the distal sigmoid and proximal sigmoid and descending colon can be performed at the time of reconstruction of bowel continuity.

Resection of the perforated colon and primary anastomosis as a 'one stage procedure' can be performed in selected cases. Both resection and reconstruction of intestinal continuity are performed during the emergency operation. Healing of the anastomosis requires optimal conditions, which means that the patient must be in a good general condition and that the colon must be completely clean. As pre-operative purgatives are impossible to use in these critically ill patients, a per-operative lavage of the colon is performed on the table. An optional deviating ileostomy can be constructed.

It is rare that the above mentioned conditions can be met in the case of generalised peritonitis. The one stage procedure with primary anastomosis is most commonly applied in elective surgery and in cases of localised peritonitis. The choice of an optimal surgical procedure in complicated diverticulitis continues to be an issue for debate among colorectal surgeons. Hartmann's procedure is today the most frequently employed operation in perforated diverticulitis with generalised peritonitis when it is technically feasible to perform a resection. The three stage procedure makes the first step a gentle and atraumatic operation, which could be an advantage in individuals in poor health. It is a disadvantage, however, not to attend to the inflammatory focus. Although the only controlled randomised study in the literature shows an advantage in terms of lower post-operative mortality in patients with purulent peritonitis, the majority of retrospective case series reveals an advantage for patients when resection is performed during the initial emergency operation. The total morbidity and days in hospital will also be lower in patients operated on with a one or two stage strategy compared to when a three stage procedure is employed. Whenever the resection is performed it must be emphasised that the distal line of bowel is on the rectum in order to clear the distal sigmoid colon completely to avoid the risk for residual disease.

Late and chronic complications of diverticulitis—colon obstruction and fistulas

Strictures are characterised by prolonged symptoms and afflict 5% of the patients after a primary attack of diverticulitis and 7% of patients who have experienced two or more episodes of acute diverticulitis. Strictures can also present as the initial manifestation in patients with discrete symptoms of inflammation. These patients present with obstructive symptoms or change in bowel habits. Colonoscopy or barium contrast examinations must then be performed. When the presence of a stricture is revealed, the two main goals of examination are to define the level of the stricture and the pathology. The emphasis in this diagnostic work-up is to differentiate between benign and malignant strictures. Benign strictures caused by diverticulitis are more elongated and spindle-shaped on X-ray compared to the typical apple core appearance of a colon cancer. Strictures related to diverticulitis differ from malignant tumours in that they are covered with normal mucosa when found at colonoscopy. In rare cases patients may present with a complete obstruction of the colon, requiring an emergency laparotomy. The treatment is a resection of the stricture or an intestinal bypass or a deviating stoma. These strictures may also be accessible to endoscopic treatment with stents. However, resection is frequently mandated for two reasons: cancer cannot be ruled out, despite endoscopic evaluation, and also because the stricture disables the patient. The most frequent procedure in elective surgery is resection and primary anastomosis. If an emergency resection must be performed it is on most occasions feasible to perform a primary anastomosis after lavage—that is, cleansing of the proximal colon by antegrade rinsing on the operating table.

Another late complication is fistulas, which arise in 2% of patients with diverticulitis. Fistulas are also the primary indication for 20% of the operations for diverticular disease in Western Europe. Colovesical fistulas are the most common, followed by colovaginal fistulas in the female, especially in women who have been subjected to hysterectomy. Colo-enteric fistulas are seldom related to diverticular disease but more to Crohn's disease. These fistulas present with diarrhoea. The subsequent dehydration and electrolyte imbalance can be hazardous, especially to the elderly patients. Colocutaneous fistulas are mostly the results of surgical procedures.

The pathophysiology of fistulas is also progression of an inflammatory process in the bowel wall and hollow organs that are situated in direct connection with the inflammatory process. When the inflammatory process forms an abscess that breaks through into the hollow organ, and drains itself, a fistula is formed. The patient will then also experience an improvement in his clinical condition. This will also obviate the necessity of emergency surgery. A significant proportion of the patients presenting with fistulas do not report any previous experience of diverticulitis—that is, the diverticulitis has been completely subclinical in these patients until it presents as a fistula. Colovesical fistulas are recognised as gas and faeces in the urine, but these patients may also present with recurrent low urinary tract infections.

The diagnostic work-up in fistula patients includes contrast X-ray examinations, but cystography is mostly negative in these cases and barium enemas of the colon will only show diverticulitis. CT scans may be beneficial for estimation of the size of the inflammatory process. The patient's history will in some cases be the only clue to the diagnosis. A simple test is to give the patient an oral dose of inorganic carbon. In 24 hours the urine will turn black if a fistula is present. The primary treatment of fistulas is resection of the part of the colon where the fistula originates. The complete segment of the colon that is involved in the diverticulitis process must be resected, and reconstruction of intestinal continuity is mostly feasible at the primary operation. When a fistula ends in the bladder, a partial resection of the bladder wall should be performed and the bladder closed. When a fistula ends in the vagina, a simple resection of the vaginal wall is enough, and small defects in the vagina do not require closure.

Recurrent uncomplicated diverticulitis—treatment and prognosis

A striking feature of uncomplicated diverticulitis is its tendency to recur. A significant portion (25%) of patients who respond to medical treatment and in whom the inflammatory symptoms resolve completely will have a new attack of the disease. Almost 50% of these patients experience a new attack within a year after their first attack has subsided. When calculated according to the actuarial method, the annual risk of having a recurrent attack is 3% in patients whose initial attack resolved completely without surgical intervention. A British audit on complicated diverticular disease revealed a significant mortality in patients who were not operated on for sigmoid resection after their first attack of complicated diverticulitis. These results prompted the conclusion that a sigmoid resection was indicated in these patients. Sigmoid resections in patients who have recovered from a previous uncomplicated diverticulitis have also been advocated, especially in the American literature. The objective would then be to avoid new attacks of the disease with potential risk of complications. However, a Swedish study from the 1970s did not find any risk for peritonitis or death during subsequent attacks of diverticulitis in these patients if the first attack was uncomplicated. Several retrospective reports have also shown that especially young people, patients with immunosuppressive diseases and patients using corticosteroids and other immunosuppressive drugs should be evaluated for surgery after the first attack of diverticulitis, since a more aggressive course of the disease has been reported in these subgroups.

Despite the lack of firm evidence for a low-fibre diet as an aetiological cause in diverticular disease, there is emerging evidence that changes in dietary habits may have resulted in a plateau of hospital admissions due to diverticulitis. This has been found in certain subgroups of the population in the industrialised world who have changed their dietary habits with a higher intake of vegetables and other sources of dietary fibre. Uncontrolled studies from the 1970s also revealed that daily intake of bran controlled symptoms in 60% of the patients. However, these studies did not differentiate patients with diverticulitis from patients with painful diverticular disease. More recent placebo controlled randomised studies have not been able to show any differences in symptom control when patients with uncomplicated diverticulitis were supplemented with bran or isphagula, despite improvements in bowel habits. It has been shown in several studies that a high-fibre diet will reduce the risk of recurrent symptoms and the need for surgical interventions in these patients fourfold. The impact of these findings is difficult to assess.

Antispasmodics and agents acting on the smooth muscle layers of the intestinal wall have been of no proven value against diverticulitis or the complications of diverticulitis. Furthermore, these drugs may be accompanied by a plethora of side effects such as dry mouth, urinary retention and impaired visual accommodation that are especially problematic in elderly patients. Thus bulking agents or fibre supplementation is the only available medical prophylaxis today to prevent recurrent attacks of diverticulitis.

The available evidence suggests that both fibre supplementation and sigmoid resection may be beneficial for patients with recurrent diverticulitis, but which of these treatment modalities is superior to the other is not known. A randomised study must be performed to resolve this issue. However, available data are sufficient to state that patients who recover after conservative treatment of complications to diverticulitis should be offered either surgical resection or lifelong treatment with bulk regulators or a fibre supplemented diet.

The optimal prophylaxis for geriatric patients who have recovered from an initial attack of diverticulitis without being subjected to emergency surgery is unknown. It seems wise to adopt a more conservative approach in the elderly patients than in patients younger than 50. The general advice should then be that elderly patients who recover completely clinically after their first or any subsequent attack of uncomplicated diverticulitis should be left with medical treatment—that is, bulk laxatives, high-fibre or high-residue diet. If the elderly patient has persistent clinical symptoms—that is, complicated disease—a resection is advised if the patient is fit enough and the surgical risk is acceptable. The practitioner, the surgeon and the patient must undertake this evaluation together. If endoscopy or barium enema reveals a stricture in a patient who has completely recovered from the first or a subsequent attack of diverticulitis, the risk of malignancy should be ruled out. If this can be done the indication for resection is less strong; if a malignant aetiology of the stricture cannot be ruled out and the patient is fit enough for surgery, the indication for resection is absolute.

Diverticular bleeding

Bleeding occurs in 3–5% of patients with diverticulosis. Despite this low frequency of bleeding from diverticulae, they are one of the two most frequent causes of lower gastrointestinal bleeding, which is explained by the high frequency of diverticulosis in elderly people. It is estimated that 30–60% of all cases of massive low gastrointestinal tract bleeding are from diverticulae. As diverticulae are located in close connection with a rich network of blood vessels, the neck of the mature diverticular sac is immediately adjacent to a major vessel of the colon—the vasa recta. It is postulated that the passage of stools may induce decubital ulceration on the distal side of the neck, which ultimately penetrates the vessel lumen.

Haemorrhage from colon diverticulae is major and affects principally older patients without previous symptoms from their diverticulosis. Bleeding from diverticulae usually occurs without warning and the patient experiences a sudden onset of cramping in the abdomen and the urge to defecate. Patients pass a large volume of old blood with a dark maroon to bright red colour. When bleeding is massive, symptoms of hypovolaemia will result if the patient is not promptly resuscitated or the bleeding does not cease spontaneously. Bleeding from colon diverticulae regularly recurs every couple of days until spontaneous resolution occurs. Seventy-five per cent of these patients experience only one episode of colon bleeding, but a majority of those who experience a second diverticular bleed subsequently have further bleeding episodes. It is unlikely that anaemia or positive test for blood in faeces is caused by diverticulosis in the absence of massive bleeding. If stool samples stain positive for occult bleeding, other causes apart from diverticulosis must be suspected.

Diverticular bleeding may be evaluated and identified at colonoscopy or by extravasation of contrast visible at arteriography. The clinical evaluation of the bleeding source in these patients can be extremely intriguing. When bleeding resolves spontaneously, an endoscopic examination of the colon can be performed after regular bowel preparation in a stable patient. If the patient is unstable and continues to bleed, urgent intervention with an arteriography and selective injection of contrast in the mesenteric vessels is warranted. This requires no further bowel preparation and blood loss exceeding 0.5 mL per minute can be identified. Modern radiological techniques also allow treatment of bleeding vessels by the use of coils and injection of vasoactive drugs. An alternative procedure in the case of massive lower gastrointestinal tract bleeding is to perform an emergency colonoscopy. In the case of bleeding from a vessel on the distal side of a diverticular neck, obtaining a good view and treating the bleeding source may be more difficult than in the case of bleeding vascular ectasias of the right colon.

If emergency angiography and intervention is not successful and the bleeding does not stop spontaneously, surgery is warranted. The preferred operation is segmental colectomy according to the same principles as in surgery for inflammatory diverticular disease. Resection of the bleeding segment and extension of the distal resection line is carried out so the anastomosis will be created as a colorectal anastomosis. The proximal resection line should be chosen at level proximal to the majority of diverticulae to avoid further episodes of bleeding. In those cases when a massive haemorrhage from the colon ceases spontaneously, a subsequent diagnostic work-up must be performed and the defined bleeding sources attended to in due course. A complete colonoscopy is the preferred procedure. If this reveals diverticulosis as the most probable bleeding source, the issue of undertaking elective resection or not must be resolved. Although firm epidemiological evidence is lacking, the majority of patients do not experience more than one episode of bleeding during their lifetime. The dominant opinion among colorectal surgeons is therefore that elective resections should not be undertaken for this reason. In those very rare cases when a patient suffers from recurrent episodes of massive diverticular bleeding, an elective resection may be warranted

Painful diverticular disease

Painful diverticular disease has been an elusive entity in the literature during the last decades. The question whether it is a clinically and pathologically distinct entity is still unresolved. Several authors and specialists in the field regard it as just a mixture of painful symptoms due to various disorders in individuals with colon diverticulae visible at X-ray or endoscopy. Others have defended painful diverticular disease as a clinical entity.

The clinical symptoms are colicky or steady abdominal pain localised in the left lower quadrant. It is usually initiated or worsened by meals and improved after passage of flatus or stools. There are no reports of specific physical signs or abnormalities in blood chemistry of these patients besides the existence of colon diverticulae. If any such signs are present, it is unlikely that painful diverticular disease is the aetiology of these signs. It is then more probable that diverticulitis or a more serious condition is responsible for the symptoms. The major differential diagnosis is irritable bowel syndrome, which has the same clinical features and the same absence of objective signs of disease.

Bibliography and further reading

Cheskin, L. & Lamport, R. (1995), 'Diverticular disease. Epidemiology and pharmacological treatment', *Drugs and Aging*, 6(1), pp. 55–63.

Cho, K., Morehouse, H., Alterman, D. & Thornhill, B. (1990), 'Sigmoid diverticulitis: Diagnostic role of CT—comparison with barium enema studies', *Radiology*, 176, pp. 111–15.

Elliot, T. B., Yego, S. & Irvin, T. T. (1997), 'Five year audit on the acute complications of diverticular disease', *British Journal of Surgery*, 84, pp. 535–9.

Farmakis, N., Tudor, R. G. & Keighley, M. R. B. (1994), 'The 5-year natural history of complicated diverticular disease', *British Journal of Surgery*, 81, pp. 733–5.

Haglund, U., Hellberg, R., Johnsén, C. & Hultén, L. (1979), 'Complicated diverticular disease of the sigmoid colon, an analysis of short and long term outcome in patients', *Annales Chirurgiae et Gynaecoliae*, 68, pp. 41–6.

Hultén, L., Haboubi, N. Y. & Schofield, P. F. (1999), 'Diverticular disease', *Colorectal Disease*, 1, pp. 128–36.

Hyland, J. & Taylor, I. (1980), 'Does a high fibre diet prevent the complications of diverticular disease?', *British Journal of Surgery*, 67, pp. 77–9.

Khan, A., Ah-See, A., Crofts, T., Heys, S. & Eremin, O. (1995), 'Surgical management of the septic complications of diverticular disease', *Annals of the Royal College of Surgeons (England)*, 77(1), pp. 16–20.

Leahy, A., Ellis, R., Quill, D. & Peel, A. (1985), 'High fibre diet in symptomatic diverticular disease of the colon', *Annals of the Royal College of Surgeons (England)*, 67, pp. 173–4.

Munson, K., Hensien, M., Jacob, L., Robinson, M. & Liston, W. (1996), 'Diverticulitis. A comprehensive follow up', *Diseases of the Colon & Rectum*, 39(3), pp. 318–22.

Painter, N., Truelove, S. & Ardran, G. (1965), 'Segmentation and the localization of intraluminal pressures in the human colon, with special reference to the pathogenesis of colonic diverticula', *Gastroenterology*, 49, pp. 169–77.

Parks, T. (1969), 'Natural history of diverticular disease of the colon, A review of 521 cases', *British Medical Journal*, 4, pp. 639–45.

Roberts, P., Abel, M., Rosen, L. et al. (1995), 'Practice parameters for sigmoid diverticulitis—supporting documentation. Prepared by The Standards Task Force American Society of Colon and Rectal Surgeons', *Diseases of the Colon and Rectum*, 38(2), pp. 125–32.

Stefansson, T., Ekbom, A., Sparén, P. & Påhlman, L. (1993), 'Increased risk of left sided colon cancer in patients with diverticular disease', *Gut*, 34, pp. 499–502.

Part VIII

Renal and endocrine conditions

Chapter 38
Chronic renal failure

GEORGE T. JOHN

Introduction

The proportion of the elderly population (> 65 years) is about 15% in developed nations and is steadily increasing. The prevalence of chronic renal failure (CRF) increases with ageing. In the coming years health personnel will encounter a larger number of patients with CRF in this age group. It is imperative that the disease is recognised early, complications prevented and rational decisions facilitated when renal replacement therapy (RRT) is considered.

Pathophysiology

There is a natural decline in all the elements of the ageing kidney. There is thickening of the glomerular and tubular basement membrane, glomerular sclerosis, gradual loss of tubule length and volume and increased interstitial fibrous tissue. The remaining glomeruli show compensatory hypertrophy, hyperfiltration and increased intraglomerular pressures.

This natural decline occurs at the rate of 1% per year from 40 years of age—that is, at 80 years of age the glomerular filtration rate (GFR) is 60 mL/m^2/min. An increasing number of survivors of renal insults among the aged would mean a larger proportion of patients with renal dysfunction. Ageing brings in its train diseases such as hypertension, diabetes mellitus, atherosclerosis, myocardial dysfunction, vasculitides and malignancy which compromise renal function. The elderly, being twice as often exposed to multiple drugs, have a higher risk of renal compromise.

Aetiology

The aetiology of CRF in the elderly can be broadly defined (see Table 38.1). Correctible disorders, although relatively few, merit attention.

Table 38.1 Aetiology of CRF

Aetiology	%
Nephrosclerosis	41.0[(a)]
Diabetes mellitus	23.0
Tubulointerstitial disease	13.5
Obstructive uropathy	10.9
Glomerular disease	10.6
Polycystic disease	2.0

(*a*) Small contracted kidneys.

A large proportion of patients present with renal failure, small contracted kidneys and non-nephrotic range proteinuria—an entity called nephrosclerosis, which is characterised by slow progression. There is a group of patients masquerading under this label with significant bilateral renovascular disease. Diabetes mellitus type 2 is a common disorder and, with the passing years, a larger number of ageing kidneys fall prey to diabetic nephropathy, resulting in CRF. Tubulointerstitial disorders are the end result of an assortment of afflictions, including ischaemic renal disease, reflux nephropathy and renal parenchymal infections. Primary and secondary glomerular disorders present with nephrotic illness. The most common of primary glomerular diseases in the elderly is membranous nephropathy. A few patients with membranous nephropathy subsequently manifest a malignancy—usually a solid neoplasm—and some may have associated hepatitis B virus infection. The rest have idiopathic disease. Apart from diabetes mellitus, vasculitides, amyloidosis and multiple myeloma contribute to a significant proportion of secondary glomerular disorders.

Clinical tests for CRF

When does one consider the possibility of CRF in the elderly? The diagnosis of early CRF depends on clinical suspicion (see Box 38.1). The symptoms of early CRF mimic many of the symptoms that the elderly commonly voice, but persistent symptoms require evaluation.

What are the clinical features of CRF (see Box 38.2)? These clinical features are appreciated only in a third of patients with asymptomatic patients with CRF but manifest in a larger number of patients suffering from uraemia.

Box 38.1 Clinical suspicion of CRF

1. Failure to thrive
2. Accelerated hypertension
3. Unexplained anaemia
4. Symptoms of bladder outflow tract obstruction
5. Worsening of pre-existing symptoms of systemic disease

Box 38.2 Clinical features of CRF

1. Half and half nails (distal half of the nail discoloured)
2. Coarse, brittle hair
3. Sallow complexion
4. Features of uraemia (e.g. uraemic fetor, asterexis, clouded mentation and pericardial rub)

Clinical evaluation should also consist of assessment of nutrition, the presence of anaemia, vascular disease, osteodystrophy, variation of blood pressure with position, enlargement of kidneys, bladder, prostate and auscultation of flanks for bruits. The best location to hear bruits is the area above and lateral to the umbilicus on either side.

Laboratory measurements and careful clinical assessment form the basis for diagnosis of CRF. The essential laboratory tests (see Table 38.2) are available to most physicians. The initial screen to rule out CRF should consist of blood urea, serum creatinine along with urine microscopy and dipstick tests for protein and sugar. Care must be taken to avoid multiple blood samplings to ensure

Table 38.2 Laboratory diagnosis of CRF

Type of test	Test
Blood tests	Serum creatinine Blood urea Electrolytes Blood sugars Calcium, phosphate Uric acid Electrophoretic strip[a]
Urine tests	Urine microscopy on a freshly voided sample Urine phase contrast microscopy Urine dipstick examination 24 hour urine protein measurement
Ultrasound examination	Renal size, corticomedullary differentiation, post-void residue in bladder Doppler study of renal arteries[a]

(a) If indicated.

continuing compliance in the elderly. Subsequent tests are planned based on ultrasound findings and the degree and type of renal failure. Serial observations are mandatory in patients who present with renal failure, haematuria and proteinuria to swiftly act upon a rapidly progressive renal failure.

Persistently elevated urea and serum creatinine forms the hallmark of CRF. However, in the elderly, decreasing muscle mass offsets the natural decline in GFR and attendant increase in serum creatinine. Poor dietary intake of protein in the elderly decreases the urea generation. Thus renal ageing is hidden from the clinician under the guise of normal serum creatinine. Despite a drop of GFR to 60 mL/m^2/min, serum creatinine does not alter, signifying that in patients with initially higher filtration rates, stable serum creatinine does not necessarily reflect a stable disease state. However, at stable serum creatinine > 2 mg/dL (176 mmol/L), the tubular secretion processes are saturated and it would be unlikely that renal damage is occurring.

In interpreting serum creatinine values, age, muscle mass and gender are important as exemplified by the Cockroft and Gault Formula:

Creatinine clearance (mL/min) = (140 − age) × Ideal body weight (kg)/72 × serum creatinine (mg/dL)

(In women, multiply the value by 0.85)

If this formula is used to calculate GFR for the serum creatinine 1.4 mg/dL (124 mmol/L) in a 20-year-old, 80 kg male, the GFR is 101 mL/min, while for an 80-year-old 40 kg woman, it is 20 mL/min. This calculation is only as accurate as an informed assessment of the GFR considering these variables in a stable clinical state, but demonstrates the declining function of glomerular senescence hidden within normal serum creatinine levels. Creatinine clearance calculated from timed collections of urine is not reliable, particularly in the elderly, and should be used only for specific indications.

Management of chronic renal failure

The general management of the patient with chronic renal disease involves the following:

- Look for and treat reversible causes of CRF.
- Prevent or slow down the progression of CRF.
- Treat the complications of CRF.
- Identify and prepare the patient who requires renal replacement therapy (RRT).

Reversible causes of renal dysfunction

In addition to exacerbation of their original renal disease, patients with CRF with a recent decrease in renal function may suffer from an underlying reversible process which, if identified and corrected, may result in the recovery of function (see Box 38.3).

Decreased renal perfusion

Hypovolaemia (with vomiting, diarrhoea, diuretic use, bleeding), hypotension (due to myocardial dysfunction or pericardial disease), infection (sepsis) and the administration of drugs which lower the GFR (such as non-steroidal anti-inflammatory drugs (NSAIDs) and ACE inhibitors) are common causes of potentially reversible declines in renal function. Superimposition of a pre-renal process on CRF may not result in the expected low values of spot urine sodium. Hypovolaemia in these patients remains a clinical diagnosis of weight loss, dry skin, sunken eyes and postural drop in blood pressure. Fluid repletion may result in the return of renal function to the previous baseline. Renovascular disease, commonly due to atherosclerosis in the elderly, exaggerates the effects of fluid depletion and renal failure manifests with trivial losses of body fluids. Bruit at the flanks, especially with a diastolic component to it, increases the chance of finding a renal artery stenosis, as does the presence of vascular disease in a smoker affecting the extremities, visceral organs, the brain or the heart. Renovascular

Box 38.3 Treatable causes of CRF in the elderly

- Decreased renal perfusion
- Administration of nephrotoxic drugs
- Urinary tract obstruction
- Rapidly progressive renal failure
- Renal parenchymal infection

disease on ultrasound shows up with asymmetric kidneys with fairly well preserved internal echoes.

Renal venous thrombosis occurs in association with proteinuric states—in particular, membranous nephropathy. Heritable disorders such as antithrombin III deficiency, protein C and protein S deficiency or acquired antiphospholipid syndromes (e.g. systemic lupus erythematosus) are important causes. Malignancies of the testes, the pancreas or the liver and paroxysmal nocturnal haemoglobinuria also cause renal venous thrombosis. Early recognition of the disease offers some hope of recovery. Doppler ultrasound done by an experienced radiologist on a co-operative patient is a good non-invasive test to rule out renal venous thrombosis. While conventional angiogram remains the gold standard, magnetic resonance angiography and carbon dioxide angiography are being used in situations such as with the elderly, where the risk for contrast nephrotoxicity is significant.

Administration of nephrotoxic drugs

The administration of drugs or diagnostic agents which adversely affect renal function are a frequent cause of worsening renal failure and metabolic abnormalities (see Table 38.3). Among the elderly with CRF, common offenders include aminoglycoside antibiotics (particularly with unadjusted doses), NSAIDs and radiographic contrast material, particularly in diabetics. The administration of such drugs and compounds should therefore be avoided or used with caution in patients with underlying CRF.

Urinary tract obstruction

Urinary tract obstruction should always be considered in the patient with unexplained worsening renal function although, in the absence of prostatic disease, it is less common than decreased renal perfusion. Prostatic hyperplasia is present in 50% of patients after the age of 50 years and in 90% of patients in their 90s. Pelvic pathology causes obstruction in women while bilateral nephrolithiasis or retroperitoneal fibrosis is responsible for obstruction in some individuals. Patients with slowly developing obstruction typically have no changes in the urinalysis, no symptoms referable to the kidney, and initially maintain their urine output. Renal ultrasonography, which is a highly sensitive test, will have to be performed to exclude urinary tract obstruction in patients with an unexplained elevation in the serum creatinine.

Table 38.3 Common drugs that can cause renal failure

Class of drug	Examples
Antibiotics	Aminoglycosides
Anti-inflammatory	NSAIDS
Antihypertensives	Angiotensin-converting enzyme inhibitors
	Angiotensin II receptor blockers
	Diuretics
Anticancer agents	Cisplatin

Rapidly progressive renal failure

A remarkably high incidence of crescentic glomerulonephritis (39%) followed by other forms of glomerulonephritis (19%) was found in an elderly population presenting with a rapid worsening of renal functions subjected to a renal biopsy. Among the conditions associated with rapidly progressive glomerulonephritis, both the idiopathic and anti-glomerular basement membrane (anti-GBM) associated glomerulonephritis are relatively common in older patients. The presence of oliguric acute renal failure was associated with a poor renal prognosis. Older patients with any form of crescentic glomerulonephritis have a poorer prognosis. The relative risk of death is 5.3 times higher in the elderly. However, intensive immunosuppression in both age categories is associated with a better preservation of renal function. A trial with pulse corticosteroids and immunosuppressive agents is warranted in the elderly patient presenting early with non-oliguric, rapidly progressive glomerulonephritis.

Renal parenchymal infection

Upper tract infection associated with obstruction and/or stones destroys renal tissue and leads to permanent loss of function if early treatment is not instituted. Obstruction increases the potential for renal damage, including papillary necrosis and severe bacterial nephritis. Subacute obstruction may become complete due to the inflammatory oedema associated with infection. An obstructed and infected system predisposes to life-threatening septicaemia and can lead to perinephric abscess. Large staghorn calculi due to recurrent infection, particularly with *Proteus mirabilis*, obstruct or destroy the kidney tissue by their size. Diabetes mellitus, sickle-cell disease or trait, NSAID abuse or upper tract infection increase the potential for sloughing of papillae, which may in turn lead to obstruction and should alert the clinician to the potential for further damage if infection persists or recurs.

Bacterial infection of the kidneys in patients with normal upper tracts and no associated disease is usually easily treated and leaves no sequelae. Acute oliguric or non-oliguric renal failure is an uncommon complication of metastatic infection and rarely of ascending infection, occurring in association with risk factors such as stones, obstructive uropathy, diabetes mellitus or with pre-existing tubulointerstitial disease. It produces severe multifocal bacterial interstitial nephritis with or without septicaemia. Severe focal or multifocal infection produces cortical scars, which may compromise the already declining renal function in the elderly. Occasionally diabetics without obstruction to urine flow present with an insidious loss of renal function. Mycobacterial infection of the kidneys, if not managed appropriately, causes permanent damage.

Preventing or slowing the progression of renal disease

The administration of angiotensin-converting enzyme (ACE) inhibitors slows the progression of CRF in diabetic nephropathy and also in non-diabetic chronic renal diseases. This has the greatest benefit if it is initiated relatively early in the course, before the serum creatinine concentration exceeds 1.5–2 mg/dL (132–176 μmol/L). At this point, most patients have already lost more than one-half of their GFR. It is not advisable to use ACE inhibitors when the serum creatinine is > 3 mg/dL in the elderly.

Treatment of hypertension is essential at any stage of the disease, preferably beginning with an ACE inhibitor, diltiazem or amlodipine. A β-blocker can be added if necessary and concurrent diuretic therapy is indicated in patients with fluid overload. A diastolic pressure of 80 mmHg (mean arterial pressure of 98 mmHg in the absence of systolic hypertension) should be targeted in previously hypertensive patients excreting 1–2 g of protein per day. A lower diastolic pressure of 75 mmHg (mean arterial pressure 92 mmHg) should be the target in patients who are normotensive or excreting more than 2 g of protein per day. However, in the elderly, the blood pressure should be lowered gradually, with frequent measurements to determine if a significant postural drop in blood pressure has occurred.

Antihypertensive therapy also diminishes protein excretion by at least half, and this is probably due to reduced intraglomerular pressure and improved glomerular permeability and selectivity. ACE inhibitors achieve this when there is concomitant salt restriction. Restriction of dietary salt has to be recommended with care in the elderly, who are prone to hyponatraemia. Even normotensive patients should be treated with ACE inhibitors and gentle restriction of salt if they have proteinuria, which is a marker for haemodynamically mediated glomerular injury.

The optimal level of protein intake has also not been determined in the elderly, but it may be reasonable to restrict intake to 0.8–1.0 g/kg of high biologic value protein, with the lower value used in patients with progressive renal failure and in patients with adequate nutrition.

Treatment of the complications of renal dysfunction

These include not only disorders of fluid and electrolyte balance—such as volume overload, hyperkalaemia, metabolic acidosis and hyperphosphataemia—but also hypertension, anaemia, malnutrition, hyperlipidaemia, bone disease and pericarditis which are abnormalities related to hormonal or systemic dysfunction.

Volume overload

Until the GFR falls below 15 mL/min, sodium and intravascular volume homeostasis is maintained. However, the elderly patient with moderate decline in GFR, despite being in relative volume balance, is less able to respond to rapid infusions of sodium and is therefore prone to fluid overload. A detailed drug inventory, including those of over-the-counter medications, occasionally helps unravel the mystery of fluid retention. NSAIDs, liquorice, steroids, oestrogens, minoxidil, β-blockers and calcium channel blockers are common culprits in the elderly. However, patients generally respond to the combination of dietary sodium restriction and diuretic therapy, usually with a loop diuretic (frusemide) given twice daily.

Hyperkalaemia

Hyperkalaemia usually develops in the patient who is oliguric or who has an additional problem such as a high potassium diet, increased tissue breakdown or hypoaldosteronism (in some cases due to the administration of an ACE inhibitor) and in elderly diabetics who have type 4 renal tubular acidosis. Hyperkalaemia due to ACE inhibitor therapy is most likely to occur in patients in whom the plasma potassium concentration is elevated or in the high normal range prior to therapy. In this setting, a low-potassium diet or concurrent use of a loop diuretic (to increase urinary potassium losses) often decreases hyperkalaemia. In selected patients—that is, those without a history of diverticulitis, chronic constipation or colonic pathology—low dose Resonium (5–10 g with each main meal) lowers the plasma potassium concentration without the side effects of nausea and constipation associated with larger doses. If constipation occurs, patients should receive a laxative to prevent reverse exchange of potassium, or caecal necrosis, a rare complication, from taking place.

Prevention of hyperkalaemia includes ingestion of a low-potassium diet and avoiding, if possible, the use of drugs that raise the plasma potassium concentration such as NSAIDs, ACE inhibitors, angiotensin II-R blockers, amiloride, spironolactone, lithium, trimethoprim and heparin. Non-selective β-blockers cause a post-prandial rise in the plasma potassium, especially in poorly controlled diabetics, but do not produce persistent hyperkalaemia.

Metabolic acidosis

CRF leads to a progressive metabolic acidosis with the plasma bicarbonate concentration tending to be between 12 and 20 mmol/L. Metabolic acidosis also causes catabolism by enhancing the proteolytic pathways. Treatment of metabolic acidosis decreases renal osteodystrophy and uremic myopathy. Sodium bicarbonate (0.5–1 mmol/kg per day) can be used, but careful attention should be paid to prevent exacerbation of volume expansion and hypertension.

Hyperphosphataemia

Phosphate balance and a normal plasma phosphate concentration are maintained in patients with a GFR of greater than 30 mL/min with a trade-off for secondary hyperparathyroidism and renal osteodystrophy. Dietary phosphate restriction may limit the development of secondary hyperparathyroidism in patients with CRF. An intake of about 800 mg/day may be desirable by limiting protein intake, which is possible only in patients with good nutritional status. Once the GFR falls below 25–30 mL/min, the addition of oral phosphate binders are usually required to prevent hyperphosphataemia. Calcium carbonate or acetate, taken with meals, binds dietary phosphate. The dose of calcium carbonate (2.5–5 g/day) is increased gradually until the plasma phosphate falls to between 4.5 and 5.5 mg/mL (1.5 and 1.8 mmol/L) or hypercalcaemia ensues.

Hypercalcaemia (particularly in patients also treated with calcitriol) and constipation are common complications; both these problems assume special significance in the elderly. Aluminium hydroxide is best avoided due to aluminium toxicity and magnesium-containing antacids (such as magnesium hydroxide), because of the risk of hypermagnesaemia and diarrhoea. For those patients with hyperparathyroidism who cannot tolerate vitamin D_3, newer analogues—for example, 22-oxycalcitriol, which inhibits parathormone but does not cause hypercalcaemia—will soon be available.

For patients who cannot tolerate calcium carbonate (e.g. due to hypercalcaemia or constipation) or who have persistent hyperphosphataemia, sevelamer hydrochloride (RenaGel) which contains neither calcium nor aluminium can be used as a phosphate binder.

Renal osteodystrophy

Osteitis fibrosa, osteomalacia and adynamic bone disease are important variants of renal osteodystrophy. Osteitis fibrosa results from secondary hyperparathyroidism. Prevention and treatment of this disease in patients with CRF is primarily based upon active or passive exercises along with phosphate-binding antacids and calcitriol to directly suppress the secretion of parathyroid hormone. Low-dose calcitriol (0.25 µg/day) is used in patients with CRF who have increased plasma parathyroid hormone levels or hypocalcaemia that persists despite correcting hyperphosphataemia. Vitamin D should not be given until hyperphosphataemia is controlled, since it enhances intestinal phosphate absorption. Adynamic bone disease is frequent among the elderly and is preventable in a proportion of these patients by avoiding/restricting aluminium based antacids.

Hypertension

Hypertension is present in approximately 80% of elderly patients with CRF. Blood pressure control can usually be safely achieved with combined therapy, best begun with an ACE inhibitor or angiotensin receptor antagonists (also given to slow disease progression), calcium channel blocker or a diuretic. Volume expansion, often in the absence of overt oedema, contributes to the elevation in blood pressure in most forms of CRF. As a result, before other medications are added, the dose of diuretics should be increased gradually until the blood pressure is normalised or the patient has attained 'dry weight' (weight at which further fluid loss will cause fatigue or orthostatic hypotension). A loop diuretic in small, divided doses is recommended. The thiazide diuretics in conventional dosage are less effective when the GFR falls below 20 mL/min and may produce hyponatraemia. In cases of refractory oedema, a combination of loop diuretics and thiazides have an additive effect. ACE inhibitors should be introduced gradually, starting with short-acting agents such as captopril or enalapril, after being reasonably certain of the absence of renovascular disease. Reasonable certainty of renovascular disease is based on the absence of flank bruit, peripheral vascular disease and asymmetric kidneys. Renal biochemistry should be checked in the elderly within 24–48 hours and subsequently after a few days to ensure there is no deterioration in GFR. These drugs can worsen renal anaemia, produce angioedema (leucopoenia with captopril) and cough in a small proportion of patients. Angiotensin receptor antagonists are similar in utility and tolerability but have the advantage of not causing cough or angioedema. Calcium channel blockers, particularly the non-dihydropyridine group, are a good choice in patients who cannot be on ACE inhibitors. Troublesome ankle oedema occurs in a few patients. The elderly patient and/or carers must be educated and motivated to continue treatment; side effects and inconveniences of treatment should be minimised to ensure compliance.

Anaemia

Many elderly patients with CRF suffer from anaemia that begins to develop when the serum creatinine concentration climbs above 2–3 mg/dL (177–265 µmol/L). The anaemia of CRF is normocytic and normochromic, and is due primarily to relatively reduced production of erythropoietin (EPO) by the kidney and to shortened red cell survival. In a significant proportion, the anaemia is due to iron deficiency. The blood picture shows microcytes, low levels of ferritin and serum iron. Microcytic anaemia without iron deficiency must bring to mind the possibility of aluminium toxicity due to prolonged ingestion of aluminium-containing antacids.

If untreated, the haematocrit of patients with CRF normally stabilises at approximately 25% (Hb 8 g). Further lowering of haematocrit mandates correction with transfusions and/or EPO. Although primarily used in those with end stage renal disease on dialysis, EPO also corrects the anaemia in patients with CRF with specific indications like angina precipitated by anaemia, or severe anaemia with transfusion iron overload. EPO therapy requires co-administration of either oral or intravenous iron, preferably prior to EPO.

Hyperlipidaemia

In patients with CRF, hypercholesterolaemia and hypertriglyceridaemia contributes to the accelerated atherosclerosis commonly seen in end stage renal disease. Dietary modification may be helpful, and a statin (HMG coA reductase inhibitor) can effectively and safely lower the plasma cholesterol concentration. This group of drugs has a good safety profile apart from occasional cases of muscle injury. Statins such as simvastatin, pravastatin and atorvastatin have not been evaluated in patients with CRF with normal lipids and are not indicated in the elderly unless there is persistent hypercholesterolaemia, unresponsive to dietary modification.

Uraemic bleeding

An increased tendency to bleeding occurs in CRF due primarily to impaired platelet function. This problem assumes greater importance in elderly patients with gut pathology. Correction of the platelet dysfunction is desirable in patients who are actively bleeding, who are at risk of bleeding—for example, due to a gastrointestinal tract lesion—or who require a surgical or invasive procedure. A number of different modalities can be used in this setting, including the correction of anaemia to above 10 g of haemoglobin, the administration of IV dDAVP (desmopressin), cryoprecipitate and the initiation of dialysis.

Malnutrition

Malnutrition is common in elderly patients with advanced CRF because of anorexia and subsequent poor food intake, decreased intestinal absorption, and metabolic acidosis. There is a strong correlation between malnutrition and death in maintenance dialysis patients. It is therefore important to monitor the nutritional status of patients with CRF. A low plasma concentration of albumin and/or serum creatinine (which varies with muscle mass as well as glomerular filtration rate) may be indicative of malnutrition. The benefits of slowing progressive renal failure with marked dietary protein restriction is not recommended in the elderly, who are prone to malnutrition. The maintenance of adequate nutrition in patients with CRF gains precedence over attempts to slow the progression of renal dysfunction with the use of a low-protein diet. It is reasonable to prescribe an intake of 0.8–1.0 g/kg (of ideal body weight) of high biologic value protein. This level of restriction avoids protein malnutrition and may slow progressive disease. Overall, the diet of most patients with CRF should provide approximately 125–146kJ/kg of ideal body weight per day.

Preparation and initiation of renal replacement therapy (RRT)

It is important to identify patients who may eventually require RRT since adequate groundwork can decrease morbidity and perhaps mortality. This involves discussions with the patient, his family members/caregivers and the nephrologist regarding the various options that are available. Early identification and referral enables dialysis to be initiated electively through a functioning long-term vascular access. The survival rates for patients with equal risks with different dialytic modalities are similar, although the choice of a particular technique has to be made with great care. In addition, the elderly patient's acceptance of the requirement of lifelong RRT is often diminished if the issue of RRT is addressed too close to the actual event. If the patient is fit for renal transplantation, early referral also allows for the evaluation of family members as prospective volunteers for kidney donation before the need for dialysis arises (pre-emptive transplantation).

However, CRF progresses variably in different individuals, making prediction of time to end stage renal failure difficult. In addition, many elderly patients waver when RRT is offered till the onset of uraemia pushes the reluctant uncertain elderly patient to make a decision.

Early referral to nephrologists

Patients with CRF should be referred to nephrologists early in the course of their disease. These specialists are trained to counsel the patient and family in choósing the optimal RRT and to manage the many complex issues associated with CRF. Patients may be able to visit a dialysis unit and talk with elderly patients already undergoing RRT before making up their minds about being on such treatment. An occasional patient may benefit from a trial of dialysis before a decision for long-term dialysis can be made. Early referral reduces costs and decreases morbidity.

Indications for RRT

The decision to initiate dialysis in a patient with CRF involves the consideration of subjective and objective parameters by the physician, nephrologist, the patient and relatives/caregivers. These parameters are often modulated by the patient's perception of her quality of life and by possible anxiety about starting new therapy that is technologically complex. On occasion, there may be a difference in the perception of quality of life by the patient and the assessment of others involved in decision making. In such situations, the patient's opinion should gain precedence.

There are a number of absolute clinical indications to initiate maintenance dialysis (see Box 38.4). These are important to the general practitioner in that the referral to the nephrologist must occur well before these indications present themselves.

Psychosocial aspects of RRT in the elderly

A life of dependence on a never-ending treatment option needing multiple hospital visits for repetitive procedures involving, in turn, several medical/nursing/dialysis staff and advanced electronic instruments, can be depressing for many elderly patients. On the other hand, most patients accept the changes as inevitable and a small price to pay for staying alive. A good number come to enjoy newfound social contacts, new challenges, opportunities and a fresh lease of life.

Box 38.4 Indications for dialysis

1. Persistent nausea and vomiting, worsening nutritional status
2. Fluid overload or pulmonary oedema refractory to diuretics
3. Accelerated/refractory hypertension
4. Progressive uraemic encephalopathy/neuropathy
5. Uraemic bleeding
6. Pericarditis
7. Serum creatinine concentration above 12 mg/dL (1060 μmol/L) or blood urea nitrogen (BUN) greater than 100 mg/dL (36 mmol/L); persistent hyperkalaemia (potassium > 6.0 mmol/L)

Bibliography and further reading

Appel, G. (1991), 'Lipid abnormalities in renal disease', *Kidney International*, 39(1), pp. 169–83.

Choudhury, D., Raj, D. S. C., Palmer, B. F. & Levi, M. (2000), 'Effect of aging on renal function and disease', in Brenner, B. M. (ed.), *The Kidney*, WB Saunders Company, Philadelphia, pp. 2187–215.

Delmez, J. A. & Slatopolsky, E. (1992), 'Hyperphosphatemia: Its consequences and treatment in chronic renal failure', *American Journal of Kidney Diseases*, 19, pp. 303–17.

Disney, A. P. S. (1990), 'Dialysis treatment in Australia 1982 to 1988', *American Journal of Kidney Diseases*, 25(5), pp. 402–9.

Fournier, A., Morinière, P., Ben Hamida, F. et al. (1992), 'Use of alkaline calcium salts as phosphate binder in uremic patients', *Kidney International*, 38(Suppl.), p. S50–61.

Hamdy, N. A., Kanis, J. A., Beneton, M. N. et al (1995), 'Effect of alfacalcidol on natural course of renal bone disease in mild to moderate renal failure', *British Medical Journal*, 310, pp. 358–63.

Hruska, K. A. & Teitelbaum, S. L. (1995), 'Mechanisms of disease: Renal osteodystrophy', *The New England Journal of Medicine*, 333, pp. 166–74.

Lazarus, J. M., Bourgoignie, J. J., Buckalew, V. M. et al (1997), 'Achievement and safety of a low blood pressure goal in chronic renal disease. The Modification of Diet in Renal Disease Study Group', *Hypertension*, 29, pp. 641–50.

Lewis, E. J., Hunsicker, L. G., Bain, R. P. & Rohde, R. D. (1993), 'The effect of angiotensin-converting enzyme inhibition on diabetic nephropathy', *The New England Journal of Medicine*, 329, pp. 1456–62.

McCarthy, J. T. (1999), 'A practical approach to the management of patients with chronic renal failure', *Mayo Clinic Proceedings*, 74, pp. 269–73.

Mathew, T. H., D'Apice, A. J. F. & Kincaid-Smith, P. S. (1983), 'Selection of patients and integration between dialysis and transplantation, the quality of life of the patients', in Drukker, A., Parsons, F. M. & Maher, J. F. (eds), *The Replacement of Renal Function by Dialysis*, 2nd edn, Nijhoff, Dordrecht, pp. 280–9.

Peterson, J. C., Adler, S., Burkart, J. M. et al. (1995), 'Blood pressure control, proteinuria, and the progression of renal disease. The Modification of Diet in Renal Disease Study', *Annals of Internal Medicine*, 123, pp. 754–62.

Revicki, D. A., Brown, R. E., Feeny, D. H. et al (1995), 'Health-related quality of life associated with recombinant human erythropoietin therapy for predialysis chronic renal disease patients', *American Journal of Kidney Diseases*, 25, pp. 548–54.

Roy, A. T., Johnson, L. E., Lee, D. B. N., Brautbar, N. & Morley, J. E. (1990), 'Renal failure in older people', *Journal of the American Geriatric Society*, 39, pp. 239–53.

Slatopolsky, E., Berkoben, M., Kelber, J. et al (1992), 'Effects of calcitriol and non-calcemic vitamin D analogs on secondary hyperparathyroidism', *Kidney International*, 38(Suppl.), pp. S43–9.

Slatopolsky, E. A., Burke, S. K., Dillon, M. A. & the RenaGel study group (1999), 'RenaGel, a nonabsorbed calcium- and aluminum-free phosphate binder, lowers serum phosphorus and parathyroid hormone', *Kidney International*, 55, pp. 299–307.

Widmer, B., Gerhardt, R. E., Harrington, J. T. & Cohen, J. J. (1979), 'Serum electrolyte and acid-base composition: The influence of graded degrees of chronic renal failure', *Archives of Internal Medicine*, 139, pp. 1099–102.

http://www.uptodate.com

Chapter 39

Female urinary incontinence

ALISTAIR CAMERON-STRANGE

Introduction

The management of urinary incontinence in the elderly female may appear to be a daunting problem for the busy family practitioner, but with an understanding of bladder function and the types and causes of urinary incontinence, many of these patients can be helped, if not cured. Incontinence in the elderly is often a complex problem with associated impaired mental status, restricted mobility, neurologic disorders and medical problems making the precise diagnosis more difficult.

Epidemiology

Urinary incontinence is a significant problem in the elderly female with regular episodes of incontinence occurring in more than 16% over the age of 85 years. This figure is even higher in long-stay geriatric wards. In the US the fastest growing sector of the population is in those over 80 years with a more than 50% chance of being institutionalised. Once this happens more than 40% will develop incontinence. Urinary incontinence will have a significant impact on the elderly woman, resulting in loss of self-esteem, social immobility and depression. The cost burden to the community is significant.

It is vital that the patient's practitioner have a basic understanding of the diagnosis and management of urinary incontinence if she is to help to resolve this clinical problem.

The anatomy of micturition

The pelvic outlet with the symphysis pubis anteriorly, the ischiopubic rami laterally and the coccyx posteriorly is spanned by a fasciomuscular sheet called the pelvic floor. Similarly, the respiratory diaphragm spans the bottom of the rib cage. The urogenital diaphragm is perforated, from anterior to posterior, by the urethra, vagina and rectum. This complex fasciomuscular sheet is innervated by the pelvic floor nerves, and it can therefore be appreciated that damage to the pelvic floor or its nerve supply will result in disorders of structure and function to the urethra, bladder, vagina and rectum. Damage to pelvic floor muscles may contribute to urinary incontinence and, in some, to faecal incontinence.

The urethra is a 3–4 cm muscular tube supported by the urogenital diaphragm. Beneath the urethral mucosa is a rich blood supply which promotes urethral coaptation and therefore a seal against urine loss. The urethral epithelium is hormonally sensitive and consists of stratified squamous epithelium in the distal urethra and transitional epithelium proximally.

Urine constantly drips in to the urinary bladder at a rate of 50–100 mL an hour, depending on the fluid intake. The first desire to void occurs at about 180 mL and a strong desire to void at 500 mL. The bladder has the unique ability to accept increasing volumes of urine without an increase in detrusor pressure. The person is therefore able to defer voiding until a convenient time. During bladder filling the detrusor pressure remains at less than 15 cm of water, regarded as stable pressure. The pressure normally rises only when the patient voids, reaching pressures of 30–40 cm of water. Voiding occurs by relaxation of the pelvic floor muscles and contraction of the detrusor muscle. These events must be co-ordinated so that voiding occurs through an unobstructed outlet. If the bladder contracts and the pelvic floor does not relax, urine will pass in spurts—so-called detrusor sphincter dyssynergia. People with normal bladder function should be able to defer voiding for 3–4 hours but this may vary with alterations in fluid intake and in urine production.

Micturition is controlled by a series of three reflex arcs called Bradley's loops. Nerve fibres run from the frontocortical centre in the brain to the pontine centre and then to the sacral micturition centre housed within the vertebral bodies T12–L1. Fibres from the micturition centre pass out through S2–S4 to the urinary bladder. The process of voiding reaches consciousness in the frontocortical centre. It is from this centre that continence is acquired by developing the ability to inhibit a reflex detrusor contraction.

Damage or dysfunction to any of these centres will result in voiding dysfunction. Damage to the cord above T12–L1 will result in an upper motor neurone type lesion with a spastic bladder. Damage to the cord below this level will result in a flaccid bladder or lower motor neurone type lesion.

Receptors are present in the bladder wall and the urethra. Cholinergic receptors predominate in the bladder wall while adrenergic receptors are present in the bladder neck. Anticholinergic agents will cause a reduction in detrusor contractility and possibly urinary retention. Cholinergic drugs are disappointing, however, in that they do not tend to increase detrusor contractility. Adrenergic agents will stimulate bladder neck closure and may precipitate urinary retention, while α-adrenergic blocking agents can cause relaxation of the bladder neck fibres, resulting in stress incontinence.

Physiological changes in the elderly

The integrity of the bladder and urethra are dependent to a large degree on adequate levels of oestrogen. In elderly women, urogenital atrophy occurs as a result of inadequate oestrogenisation, with the tissues becoming thin, less elastic and blood supply to the urethral and bladder mucosa inadequate. The submucosal blood supply in the urethra plays an important role in helping maintain urethral closure, but with decreased oestrogen levels urethral closure is impaired and incontinence may occur. Senile vaginitis may be accompanied by symptoms of dysuria. The normal defence mechanisms against infection may be impaired, resulting in recurrent urinary tract infections. Those women who have had forceps delivery or prolonged second stage labour may have dysfunction of the pelvic floor due to neuropathy, as well as functional changes seen in those who have previously had a hysterectomy or pelvic radiotherapy.

Changes in normal bladder function are frequently seen in the elderly (see Table 39.1). These include a reduction in bladder capacity, a reduction in bladder compliance, impaired detrusor contractility, unstable detrusor contractions and an increase in post-void residuals. In some patients impaired detrusor contractility may co-exist with high pressure unstable contractions, a condition known as detrusor hyperreflexia with impaired contractility (DHIC). This is frequently seen in the elderly without any evidence of neurologic dysfunction, although it does occur in association with dementia, Parkinson's disease and stroke.

Table 39.1 Effects of ageing on the female urinary tract

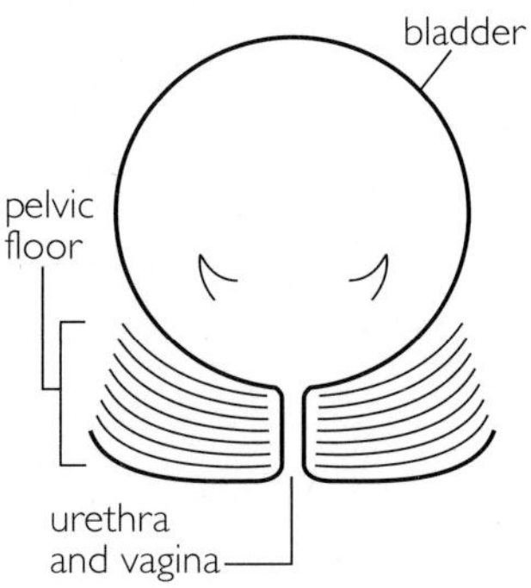

Site	Symptoms
Bladder	
Reduced capacity	Urinary frequency
Impaired contractility	Slow, incomplete voiding
Reduced bladder compliance	Frequency
Unstable bladder contractions	Urgency, urge incontinence
Increased post-void residual	Urinary retention, infections
Pelvic floor	
Urogenital atrophy	Thin inelastic tissues Irritative voiding Stress incontinence
Urethra and vagina	
Atrophic urethritis and vaginitis	Stress incontinence Irritative voiding

The normal stable relationship between bladder filling, storage and emptying may therefore be disturbed by hormonal changes, pelvic floor dysfunction (both physiologic and neurologic), as well as the imposition of other co-existing morbidity such as cardiovascular disease, dictating the need for diuretics or drugs which affect bladder and urethral function. Respiratory disorders may result in a chronic cough and therefore worsen stress incontinence. Pelvic malignancy or fistula should not be forgotten in these patients and may be overlooked. Vesicocolic fistula may present with recurrent urinary tract infections. Neurologic disorders such as stroke, Parkinson's disease and dementia are frequently associated with disturbances of bladder function.

Types of incontinence

Urinary incontinence is the involuntary loss of urine, and may be classified as:

- stress incontinence
- urge incontinence
- mixed incontinence—where both stress and urge incontinence co-exist
- overflow incontinence
- unconscious incontinence.

Stress incontinence (SI)

This is the involuntary loss of urine on coughing, straining or exercise and is present in 30–45% of women over 65 years of age. A history of stress incontinence is easily elicited by direct questioning. SI may be worsened by co-existing medical problems such as a chronic cough or the use of α-adrenergic blocking drugs such as minipres that cause bladder neck relaxation.

Urge incontinence (UI)

This is caused by detrusor overactivity. It is the loss of urine due to a sudden unwarranted detrusor contraction that the patient is unable to inhibit.

The history is one of the patient saying that the urge to void comes on so suddenly that she cannot get to the toilet on time and the urine simply comes out. This is uncontrollable and usually large volume incontinence as compared to stress incontinence which tends to be of small volume. Although unstable detrusor contractions tend to increase with age for no known reason, urge incontinence is the type of leakage one sees in patients with upper motor neurone type lesions.

Detrusor overactivity is the predominant cause of incontinence in the institutional setting.

Mixed incontinence

When both stress incontinence and urge incontinence occur, it is called mixed incontinence. It may be present more often than one thinks when trying to sort out if the patient has pure SI or pure UI, as they frequently co-exist. The precise diagnosis can only be made by urodynamic testing.

Overflow incontinence

When the bladder fails to empty with each contraction it gradually enlarges, with the detrusor muscle becoming weaker and weaker. With the ever-increasing residuals, the urine starts to trickle out. This often occurs during the night—so-called nocturnal enuresis. Eventually these patients present with chronic urinary retention and, in a very small percentage, chronic renal failure.

Unconscious incontinence

This is where urine loss is unaccompanied by either stress or urge incontinence. It may be due to bladder disorders, sphincter disorders, a combination of both or possibly a urinary fistula such as a vesicovaginal fistula.

Diagnosis

To diagnose the precise cause of incontinence in this age group without sophisticated urodynamic testing is often difficult. However, in the elderly, urodynamic testing is often extremely inconvenient, especially if the patient is bed-bound. It is reasonable to make an educated clinical decision as to the primary cause of the patient's incontinence. If the patient complains predominantly of urge incontinence then one would treat the patient for detrusor instability. If stress incontinence is predominant, this component is treated. Many patients may have both stress incontinence and urge incontinence, making clinical diagnosis difficult. One can, however, try empirical treatment.

When assessing this problem it is important to familiarise yourself with the patient's current medical problems and be aware of the impact of the drugs prescribed for that particular condition on the urinary tract.

The first step is to decide whether the incontinence is of acute onset. The mnemonic 'MAIDS' (see Box 39.1) is a simple way of classifying frequently found reversible disorders of urinary incontinence in elderly females.

Box 39.1 Reversible causes of incontinence—'MAIDS'

M Mobility disorders
A Atrophic vaginitis and urethritis
I Infected urine
D Drugs, delirium and depression
S Stool impaction

Mobility

If an elderly patient has restricted mobility, in the event of a sudden uncontrollable urge to void it is unlikely that she will be able to get to the toilet. It is important therefore that mobility is maintained in the elderly wherever possible. Simple measures such as raising the height of the patient's chair may be helpful, as may having a commode within easy reach. Dressing in easily removed clothing may also help.

Atrophic vaginitis and urethritis

This is common and due to the lack of oestrogen in post-menopausal women. It may result in dysuria and irritative voiding symptoms. Provided there is no past history of hormonal dependent cancers (endometrial or breast cancer), oestrogen in oral, topical or transdermal form may be beneficial.

Infected urine

Urinary incontinence may be the sole indicator of underlying urinary tract infection in this age group. If present, treatment with the appropriate antibiotic may resolve the incontinence. Recurrent urinary infection should be treated with the appropriate antibiotic followed by Hiprex (a urinary antiseptic) and vitamin C, which may help to maintain urinary sterility. An ultrasound of the urinary tract should also be obtained in those with recurrent infection as upper tract disorders such as a stone or hydronephrosis may be causative.

Drugs, delirium and depression

Drugs may impair detrusor contractility (anticholinergics), stimulate bladder neck closure (α-adrenergic agents), relax the bladder neck (α-blockers) or cause a sudden increase in urine output (diuretics). Drugs which compromise patient mobility or cause postural hypotension should be considered (see Table 39.2).

Stool impaction

Impaction and distension of the rectum and pelvic floor may cause parasympathetic inhibition of the bladder, resulting in urinary retention. Appropriate measures should be taken to treat this and also to prevent this in the future.

Aetiology

The three major factors to consider in assessing incontinence are:

P **P**rolapse of the anterior vaginal wall and the position of the urethra (see Figure 39.1)
U Intrinsic **u**rethral function
B Intrinsic **b**ladder function.

This can be remembered by the acronym 'PUB'. Often all three factors are present.

Prolapse

A cystocoele and rectocoele are commonly found in those women who have had vaginal deliveries. The endopelvic fascia may be disrupted and support for the bladder neck and urethra is lost, resulting in prolapse of the anterior vaginal wall. Deep to the bulge seen on the anterior vaginal wall is the urinary bladder. This loss of support is one of the major factors responsible for stress incontinence. The presence of a cystocoele does not mean that the patient necessarily has stress incontinence, as many women, even with large cystocoeles, are completely dry (see Figure 39.1).

Intrinsic urethral function

The urethra is a muscular tube closed at rest. At the proximal end is the bladder neck which is richly supplied with α-adrenergic receptors, while at the distal end is the external sphincter which is under voluntary control. Beneath the submucosa is an

Table 39.2 Drugs used in the treatment of urinary incontinence

Drug	Site of action	Mechanism	Effect	Side effects
Minipres	Bladder neck	α-blocker	Stress incontinence	Hypotension
Pseudoephedrine	Bladder neck	α-stimulant	Reduces SI	Hypertension
Oxybutynin	Bladder wall	Anticholinergic	Reduces UI	Dry mouth, urinary retention, constipation
Probanthine	Bladder wall	Anticholinergic	Reduces UI	Dry mouth, urinary retention, constipation
Imipramine	Bladder wall and bladder neck	Anticholinergic α-stimulant	Reduces bladder contractility Reduces SI	
Oestrogen	Urethral mucosa	Increases vascularity	Reduces SI	

Depression should be treated. Delirium and confusional states may result in incontinence.

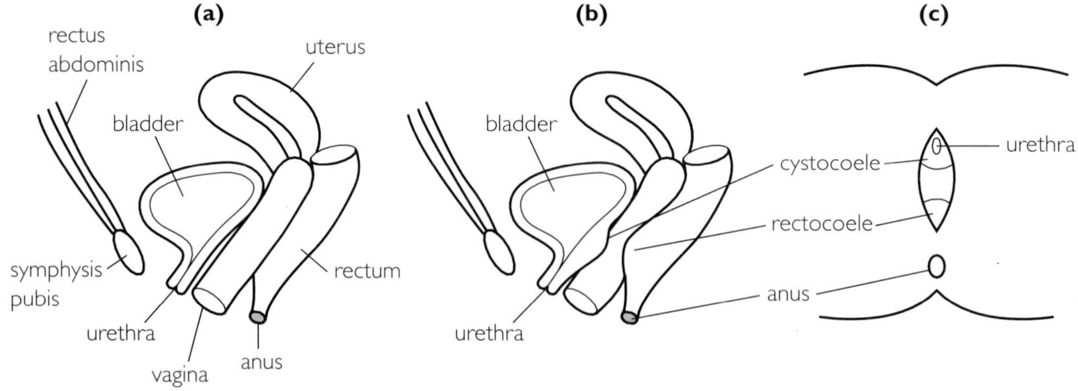

Figure 39.1 The anatomical relationship between the bladder, vagina and rectum: **(a)** normal, **(b)** and **(c)** prolapse with development of cystocoele and rectocoele

oestrogen dependent vascular plexus which provides bulk to help maintain urethral coaptation. It can be appreciated that α-blocking drugs, oestrogen deficiency and loss of normal tissue elasticity can all contribute to stress incontinence.

Intrinsic bladder function

The function of the bladder is to store urine until the desire to void (DTV) arises. The first desire to void occurs after approximately 180 mL of filling, with an urgent desire to void at 500–600 mL. The onset of a DTV will vary with fluid intake and the use of diuretics. Under normal circumstances, the bladder fills with a stable detrusor pressure of less than 15 cm of water. In some patients, however, the bladder generates a sudden contraction which, if of high enough pressure, will result in urine loss—so-called urge incontinence.

Patients who exhibit urgency and urge incontinence are usually suffering from an unstable bladder. Where a patient has had a stroke affecting the bladder this may indeed occur. The bladder pressure may be even higher and the bladder capacity low. The unstable bladder is a common form of incontinence in the elderly.

Examination

Once the reversible causes of incontinence have been excluded, a general medical examination as well as abdominal, neurological and pelvic floor examinations should be performed.

Abdominal examination

An abdominal examination is performed to exclude an abdominal mass, such as a chronically overdistended bladder arising from the pelvis, in the midline and not infrequently up to the level of the umbilicus. Ovarian masses as well as a renal malignancy may also be detected. If a mass is felt, this should be investigated further by an abdominal ultrasound. A rectal examination will reveal faecal impaction.

Neurological examination

This is most important in this age group. Perform a screening neurological examination to exclude any unknown underlying neurological disorders.

Pelvic floor examination

Inspect the introitus for signs of senile vaginitis. Examination of the urethra may reveal a urethral caruncle. Ask the patient, preferably with a full bladder, to cough. Look for urinary leakage from the urethra. If there is no leakage this does not necessarily mean that stress incontinence does not exist. If possible, repeat this test with the patient standing. Ask the patient to bear down. A mucosal bulge arising from the anterior vaginal wall is called a cystocoele, while a bulge arising posteriorly is typically a rectocoele.

Special investigations

Urine culture

A urine culture should be done on every patient presenting with urinary incontinence, and infection, if present, treated with the appropriate antibiotic. Both macroscopic and microscopic haematuria need to be evaluated further by upper tract imaging and a cystoscopy.

Ultrasound

An abdominal ultrasound should be performed in patients with recurrent urinary infections, a palpable abdominal mass or haematuria, in which case a cystoscopy is also indicated. A large post-void residual (PVR) will alert one to chronic urinary retention as the cause of incontinence but this should be repeated on three occasions, preferably without preloading the patient with water to confirm the accuracy of the PVR. A PVR of < 75 mL is usually acceptable.

Time and volume voiding chart

This is a simple and particularly helpful way of assessing a patient's urinary incontinence. The amount of fluid and the time of ingestion, as well as the time and volume of each void, should be documented. Incontinent episodes should be recorded, as well as whether it was preceded by a sudden desire to void or by coughing.

Cystometry

While complex urodynamic testing will reveal the cause of incontinence in the majority of patients, this is not readily available in nursing homes and transporting a patient to a facility where this is available may present special difficulty. Simple bedside cystometry will give helpful clues to the underlying cause and therefore enable initiation of first line management. It is important that the test reproduce the symptoms of which the patient complains. The pretest residual will give a clue to possible chronic urinary retention. If the patient gives a history of urgency and urge incontinence you would expect leakage of water around the catheter at any time during bladder filling, usually preceded by the sudden desire to void which the patient is unable to inhibit. This would indicate detrusor instability or detrusor hyperreflexia. If the patient is seen to leak on coughing after the bladder has been filled and the catheter removed, then this is indicative of stress incontinence. Both of these conditions frequently co-exist, however.

Treatment

Successful treatment outcomes are achieved by defining the precise cause of urinary leakage. After a thorough medical examination the reversible causes of incontinence should be addressed (MAIDS).

Mobility problems may be helped by having a commode close at hand, and ensuring that the patient's attire can be conveniently removed when she gets to the bathroom or on to the commode. Urogenital atrophy should be treated with oestrogen and urinary infection with the appropriate antibiotic. Careful attention should be given to the drug regimen and the timing and use of diuretics. The use of those drugs with side effects on the urinary bladder deserves special consideration. Faecal impaction may in some cases require manual disimpaction but usually stool softeners will suffice. The patient's diet should be assessed with the intent to minimise the chance of recurrence of this problem. The next step is to treat the type of incontinence.

Stress incontinence (SI)

The initial treatment for SI should be a course of pelvic floor exercises, although patient compliance may present a problem in this age group. This will require ongoing follow-up by an experienced and enthusiastic continence nurse specialist. Co-existing conditions, such as chronic cough, which aggravate SI should be treated. It is also important to exclude α-blocking drugs from the drug regimen as these cause bladder neck incompetence and therefore stress incontinence. α-adrenergic stimulants such as Sudafed (pseudoephedrine) may prove successful in stimulating bladder neck closure and therefore reduce or cure SI. The patient's blood pressure should be monitored, however.

Where conservative treatment fails and the patient is fit enough to undergo surgery, this should be considered. It is most important that a urodynamic evaluation be done first to confirm that the diagnosis of pure stress incontinence is the correct one. The standard Burch colposuspension should be considered, while in some patients injection of periurethral collagen may suffice.

Urge incontinence

In this group of patients it is most important not to forget the possibility of underlying bladder malignancy as a cause of urinary urgency. Provided the urine is cell free and sterile, urinary tract ultrasound is normal and there is no history of gross haematuria, it is reasonable to assume malignancy is not present. Urgency can be either sensory or motor. Sensory urgency is due to infection, the urethral syndrome or, occasionally, malignancy. The urethral syndrome is a symptom complex of frequency, urgency and dysuria in the absence of documented urinary infection, interstitial cystitis or carcinoma in situ. Not infrequently one finds on endoscopic examination inflammatory change on the trigone which can be a contributory factor. The precise cause of the urethral syndrome is not known. Motor urgency that manifests as a sudden desire to void with leakage is due to a bladder contraction. The cause of this is often idiopathic but may be due to neurological causes—for example, stroke or Parkinson's disease.

Bladder training may be helpful in some patients. Techniques involve deferring voiding to increase bladder capacity, using pelvic floor contractions to help control and inhibit an unstable detrusor contraction and keeping a time and volume voiding diary. The patient needs to record the time and volume of all oral fluid intake and the time and volume of each void. Each episode of incontinence must be documented and the nature of the leakage noted—whether it was of the urge or the stress type.

Where altering fluid regimes and bladder retraining have failed, the use of anticholinergic medication will need to be considered (see Table 39.2). Ditropan should be tried first in low dosage, after warning the patient of the common side effect of dry mouth. Other problems may be the precipitation of urinary retention, an intraocular crisis in those with narrow angle glaucoma or constipation. The dosage of 2.5 mg twice daily, half an hour before meals, should be prescribed. This should be increased gradually, on a weekly basis, increasing the dose to 2.5 mg tds, then qid. If this does not cause significant improvement the dose should be increased until the desired therapeutic response is achieved. For example, 5.0 mg, 2.5 mg, 2.5 mg and 5.0 mg on a daily basis. These doses can be changed according to the patient's response. Always remember the possibility of the patient quietly going into urinary retention: she should be monitored clinically by palpation or with an ultrasound of the bladder.

Overflow incontinence

This is due to a chronically distended and poorly contractile bladder. A residuum of more than 1 L may be found. A pelvic mass should be excluded with ultrasound examination, as it may be the cause of chronic urinary retention. Chronic constipation should also be considered and treated. Frequently this type of bladder does not respond well to conservative measures and catheterisation, intermittent or permanent, may need to be instituted.

Catheterisation

While the use of catheters is the least favourable option and should only be considered as a last resort, the reality is that in certain situations where all attempts at trying to prevent urinary leakage have failed, catherisation of the bladder is infinitely better than a wet, miserable patient. The bladder can be catheterised transurethrally or by the suprapubic route. A suprapubic catheter is far more comfortable for the patient than a urethral catheter and the infection rate is lower. A 16 Fr silastic catheter should be used and replaced every 5–6 weeks. Inevitably the bladder will become colonised with bacteria but this should not be treated with antibiotics unless the patient becomes symptomatic of a urinary tract infection, in which case the catheter should also be changed. To treat asymptomatic bacteriuria with antibiotics will, in time, result in a urinary cocktail of multiresistant organisms.

Intermittent catheterisation

In those patients with a decompensated or acontractile bladder, clean intermittent self-catheterisation (CISC) is a useful technique. It requires meticulous attention to aseptic technique and also manual dexterity and co-ordination. This may prove impossible in some elderly patients with poor vision, arthritis of the hands or obesity but in those patients capable of performing this technique it is far superior to a permanent catheter. In those unable to perform CISC, this could be done by the nursing staff 2–3 times a day.

Box 39.2 Indications for urologic referral

- Failure of conservative treatment
- Marked symptomatic pelvic prolapse
- Urinary fistula
- Gross haematuria
- Unexplained microhaematuria
- Where surgery is an option
- For diagnostic urodynamic evaluation

Surgery

The place of surgery in urinary incontinence should not be forgotten in the elderly. Where conservative treatment has failed to alleviate or cure the problem, surgery should be considered if the patient is fit enough to undergo this. Surgery should not be withheld on the basis of age alone.

Successful surgical outcomes are achievable in patients with SI. The operations include the standard Burch colposuspension performed through an open surgical incision or laparoscopically. Transvaginal procedures may also be performed but the long-term outcomes are not as good. If surgery is contemplated, urodynamic evaluation should always be performed preoperatively.

Urge incontinence can, if refractory to drugs, be difficult to treat. The only procedure that may be helpful in those with urodynamically proven UI is transvaginal phenol injection in which phenol is injected into the paraureteric space to obliterate the pelvic parasympathetic nerves to the bladder. While this may result in urinary retention, it can often lead to a dramatic reduction in UI and therefore a marked improvement in quality of life.

A urinary fistula will require major surgical intervention (see Box 39.2) if continence is to be achieved.

Bibliography and further reading

Brocklehurst, J. C. (1986), 'The ageing bladder', *British Journal of Hospital Medicine*, 35, pp. 8–10.

Cameron-Strange, A. (1999), 'Female urinary incontinence', *Current Therapeutics*, 40, pp. 17–24.

Diokno, A. C., Wells, T. J. & Brink, C. (1987), 'Urinary incontinence in elderly women: Urodynamic evaluation', *Journal of the American Geriatrics Society*, 35, pp. 880–2.

Kursch, E. D. & McGuire, E. J. (1994), *Female Urology*, J. B. Lippincott Company, Philadelphia.

Resnick, N. M. & Yalla, S. V. (1987), 'Detrusor hyperactivity with impaired contractile function', *The Journal of the American Medical Association*, 22, pp. 3076–81.

Tapp, A. J. & Cardozo, L. (1986), 'The postmenopausal bladder', *British Journal of Hospital Medicine*, 35, pp. 20–3.

Wall, L. L., Norton, P. A. & DeLancey, J. O. (1993), *Practical Urogynecology*, Williams & Wilkins, Baltimore, MA.

Wells, T. J., Brink, C. A. & Diokno, A. C. (1987), 'Urinary incontinence in elderly women: Clinical findings', *Journal of the American Geriatrics Society*, 35, pp. 933–9.

Wyman, J. F., Choi, S. C., Harkins, S. W. et al. (1988), 'The urinary diary in the evaluation of incontinent women: A test-retest analysis', *Obstetrics and Gynecology*, 71, pp. 812–17.

Chapter 40
Male urinary incontinence

LAURA C. MAZZENGA and WADE BUSHMAN

Introduction

Urinary incontinence (UI) is defined as the involuntary loss of urine in sufficient amount to constitute a social or hygienic problem. UI is not a normal occurrence of the ageing process. It is a significant health issue that predisposes the affected individual to loss of hygiene, skin breakdown, embarrassment, social isolation, loss of self-esteem and decreased quality of life. It burdens caregivers and increases the likelihood of institutionalisation. In fact, UI is the single most common reason for admission to a long-term care facility. This text will help the primary care provider to initiate the evaluation and treatment of men with UI.

Epidemiology and aetiology

The reported overall prevalence of UI in men ranges from 3% to 11%. In the US, prevalence rates of 1.5–5% have been reported for men 15–64 years of age. The prevalence of UI correlates with increasing age, tripling for men over age 60 to a rate of 15–18%, and may overlap with symptoms of prostatism (Figure 40.1). The true prevalence of UI may be underestimated because of a reluctance of men to broach the subject with their providers; as UI receives increased attention in the media, the reported incidence may increase.

Many elderly men may be continent but experience bothersome and progressive voiding symptoms. It is critically important for the community practitioner to recognise bothersome voiding symptoms and/or UI as an important health issue and be

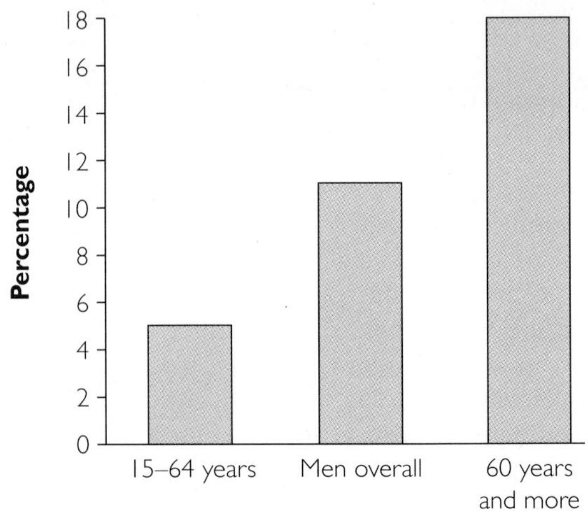

Figure 40.1 Prevalence of incontinence in men in the US

Box 40.1 International Prostate Symptom Score

The International Prostate Symptom Score (I-PSS) is based on the answers to seven questions concerning urinary symptoms. Each question allows the patient to choose one of five answers indicating increasing severity of the particular symptom. The answers are assigned points from 0 to 5. The total score can therefore range from 0 to 35 (asymptomatic to very symptomatic). Furthermore, the International Scientific Committee (SCI) recommends the use of only a single question to assess the quality of life. The answers to this question range from 'delighted' to 'terrible' or 0 to 6. Although this single question may or may not capture the global impact of benign prostatic hyperplasia (BPH) symptoms or quality of life, it may serve as a valuable starting point for a practitioner–patient conversation. The SCI strongly recommends that all health-care providers who counsel patients suffering from symptoms of prostatism utilise these measures not only during the initial interview but also during and after treatment to monitor treatment response.

The SCI, under the patronage of the World Health Organization (WHO) and the International Union Against Cancer (UICC), has agreed to use the symptom index for BPH, which has been developed by the American Urologic Association (AUA) Measurement Committee, as the official worldwide symptoms assessment tool for patients suffering from prostatism.

Patient name	Not at all	Less than 1 time in 5	Less than half the time	About half the time	More than half the time	Almost always	Your score
Incomplete emptying Over the past month, how often have you had a sensation of not emptying your bladder completely after you finished urinating?	0	1	2	3	4	5	
Frequency Over the past month, how often have you had to urinate again less than 2 hours after you finished urinating?	0	1	2	3	4	5	
Intermittency Over the past month, how often have you found you stopped and started again several times when you urinated?	0	1	2	3	4	5	
Urgency Over the past month, how often have you found it difficult to postpone urination?	0	1	2	3	4	5	

Box 40.1 International Prostate Symptom Score *(continued)*

Weak stream Over the past month, how often have you had to push or strain to begin urination?	0	1	2	3	4	5	
Straining Over the past month, how often have you had to push or strain to begin urination?	0	1	2	3	4	5	
	None	1 time	2 times	3 times	4 times	5 times or more	
Nocturia Over the past month, how many times did you most typically get up to urinate from the time you went to bed at night until the time you got up in the morning?	0	1	2	3	4	5	
Total I-PSS score							

Quality of life due to urinary symptoms	Delighted	Pleased	Mostly satisfied	Mixed—about equally satisfied and dissatisfied	Mostly dissatisfied	Unhappy	Terrible
If you were to spend the rest of your life with your urinary condition just the way it is now, how would you feel about that?	0	1	2	3	4	5	6

Add the score for each question above, and write the total in the space to the right.
Symptom score = 1–7: Mild; 8–19: Moderate; 20–35: Severe.

prepared to take the initial steps in addressing a problem that is often curable or effectively managed. Useful screening measures include a few simple questions (see below) and the International Prostate Symptom Score (I-PSS) (Box 40.1).

- Do you ever leak or lose control of your urine?
- Do you ever find yourself wet?
- Do you use any pads or other type of protection?

UI may result from a variety of causes: urologic disease (e.g. benign prostatic hyperplasia); neurologic disease; anatomical defects; medication side effects; or from peripheral nerve injury from radical pelvic surgery. In some men, a combination of factors may be at work, while in others a clear aetiology is never determined.

Pathophysiology

Normal micturition

Normal bladder control is a neurologically mediated process involving the cerebral cortex, the spinal cord, and the lower urinary tract. It is characterised by voluntary (cortical) control over an organ system primarily innervated by the autonomic nervous system. The component of voluntary control is what differentiates the bladder and lower urinary tract from other visceral organs, such as the stomach, heart and intestines. Bladder function is comprised of two phases: filling and storage, then relaxation and voiding (Table 40.1).

The filling and storage phase entails low-pressure bladder filling and sphincteric continence. During filling, sympathetic outflow induces β-adrenergic receptor-mediated relaxation of the detrusor muscle. This allows the bladder to accommodate an increasing volume while maintaining low pressure. Continence is maintained by a combination of sympathetic stimulation of α-adrenergic receptors in the bladder neck and somatic-nerve-mediated tone in the external sphincter and pelvic floor. Sensations of fullness are detected by stretch receptors in the bladder detrusor muscle and communicated to the cortical centres. The micturition reflex is voluntarily inhibited until a socially acceptable time and place are achieved. At that time, voiding is initiated by cessation of the inhibitory cortical outflow and a pontine-mediated switch from the filling and storage phase to the relaxation and voiding phase.

In the relaxation and voiding phase, sympathetic outflow is turned off and parasympathetic outflow is activated. Stimulation of cholinergic receptors causes contraction of the detrusor muscle, while inhibition of sympathetic outflow facilitates opening of the bladder neck, and inhibition of signalling through the somatic nerves causes relaxation of the distal sphincter and striated muscles of the pelvic floor (Figure 40.2). This reorganisation of neural outflow initiates voiding and is maintained until the bladder has emptied. At the conclusion of micturition, the pattern of neural outflow reverts to the filling and storage phase. The micturition cycle is normally executed 4–8 times per day and is under strict voluntary control. For those with UI, this cycle is punctuated by the involuntary loss of urine. There are 6 identifiable types of UI: urge, stress, mixed, overflow, functional and reflex incontinence (Table 40.2).

Table 40.1 Normal micturition cycle

Phase	Description
First	Filling and storage • Closure of bladder neck and distal sphincter • Low pressure filling of the bladder • Inhibition of detrusor contraction
Second	Relaxation and voiding • Relaxation of bladder neck and distal sphincter • Sustained detrusor contraction

Types of incontinence

Urge incontinence is the involuntary loss of urine associated with an abrupt desire to urinate. It is the most common form of incontinence in the elderly male and results from an involuntary contraction of the detrusor muscle. Patients often report generalised urgency with risk of leakage if urination is delayed. Incontinence often occurs on the way to the toilet. The volume of urine leakage is variable, ranging from just a few drops to the entire volume of the bladder. Urge incontinence can result from a specific neurologic cause, such as stroke or Parkinson's disease. Commonly, urge incontinence is associated with non-neurologic conditions, such as bladder outlet obstruction, infection, bladder stones or even bladder cancer. Most commonly, it is idiopathic and is suspected to result from degenerative changes in the detrusor muscle. The terminology of uninhibited detrusor activity is confusing, with detrusor hyper-reflexia and detrusor instability used to designate uninhibited contractions of neurogenic and non-neurogenic origin, respectively. One broad term, which encompasses both and is equally correct, is detrusor hyperactivity.

Detrusor hyperactivity is often associated with impaired detrusor contractility (detrusor hyperactivity/impaired contractility: DHIC). Because of diminished contractility, incomplete bladder emptying occurs. Affected individuals may strain in the effort to empty their bladders and often have an

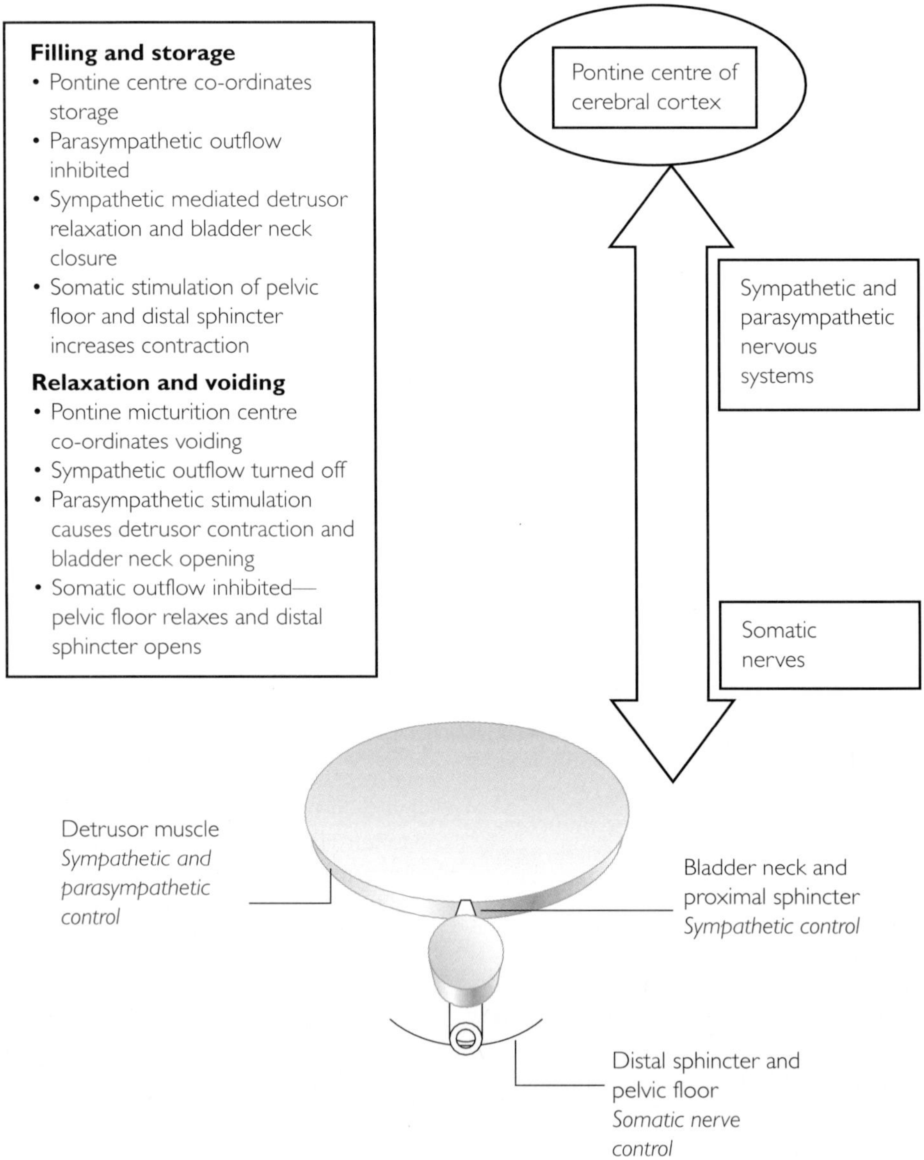

Figure 40.2 Cycling phases of continence

elevated post-void residual (PVR). This can reduce the functional capacity of the bladder and aggravate the symptoms of frequency and urgency. The frequent association of detrusor hyperactivity with impaired contractility hints at a generalised dysfunction of the detrusor muscle affecting both filling and voiding phases. DHIC can co-exist with and be exacerbated by an associated component of bladder outlet obstruction.

Stress incontinence results from a deficiency of urethral sphincter function. Leakage is provoked by activities that increase abdominal pressure, such as coughing, laughing, sneezing, changing position, lifting or straining. Stress incontinence is uncommon in men, in contradistinction to its prevalence in women. Stress incontinence occurs in men only when the sphincter is damaged or its neurologic regulation is disturbed. Sphincter damage can occur

Table 40.2 Symptoms and types of urinary incontinence

Type of UI	Definition	Pathophysiology	Symptoms and signs
Urge	Involuntary loss of urine associated with a strong sensation of urinary urgency.	Involuntary detrusor (bladder) contractions.	Loss of urine with an abrupt and strong desire to void; usually loss of urine on way to the toilet.
Stress	Leakage associated with increased intra-abdominal pressure.	Urethral sphincter deficiency due to surgery or trauma.	Small amount of urine loss during coughing, sneezing, laughing or other physical activities.
Mixed	Combination of urge and stress incontinence.	Involuntary detrusor (bladder) contractions and urethral sphincter deficiency due to surgery or trauma.	Combination of urge and stress incontinence. One symptom (urge or stress) often more bothersome to the patient than the other.
Overflow	Bladder overdistension.	Acontractile or hypotonic detrusor secondary to drugs, faecal impaction, diabetes or neurologic disease. Obstruction due to prostatic hyperplasia, prostatic carcinoma or urethral stricture.	Frequent or constant dribbling, urge or stress incontinence.
Functional	Chronic impairments of physical and/or cognitive functioning.	Chronic functional and mental disabilities.	Urge incontinence or overflow incontinence.
Unconscious or reflexive	Neurologic dysfunction.	Reflex detrusor contractions during bladder filling, most often associated with spinal cord injury or disease. Decreased bladder compliance secondary to radiation cystitis, inflammatory bladder conditions or radical pelvic surgery.	Continual incontinence or episodic leakage without perceived urge or provocative manoeuvre.

with pelvic trauma, transurethral surgery, radical prostatectomy and/or radiation therapy for prostate cancer. Neurologic injury that affects sphincter function may occur with damage to the pelvic nerves by radical pelvic surgery or with disease affecting the spinal cord. A common form of incontinence in ageing men is post-void dribbling. This may be due to a loss of co-ordination in closure of the bladder neck and external sphincter, which can trap urine between the sphincter mechanisms, and/or loss of peristaltic activity in the bulbous urethra, which normally completes the process of evacuation.

Mixed incontinence is the combination of urge and stress incontinence. This pattern of incontinence results from a combination of detrusor hyperactivity and deficient sphincter function. This is sometimes observed in men following surgery or radiation therapy for prostate cancer.

Overflow incontinence is leakage from a chronically overdistended bladder. Leakage comes from uninhibited detrusor contractions that produce urge-type incontinence and/or from stressful manoeuvres that increase intravesical pressure and produce stress-type incontinence. Patients may complain of frequent to constant dribbling, urgency, urge incontinence and leakage with straining. The distinguishing feature of overflow incontinence is the failure of the bladder to empty and thus remain chronically overdistended. This may result from either outlet obstruction or from a hypotonic or acontractile detrusor muscle. Benign prostatic hypertrophy is the most common cause of overflow incontinence in the elderly male. Other less common causes of outlet obstruction are prostate carcinoma and urethral stricture. Detrusor hypocontractility or acontractility may occur secondary to medication effects, faecal impaction, diabetes, or neurologic disease.

Functional incontinence is leakage that is due to impairments of physical and/or cognitive function that interfere with bladder control. Patients leak because they lack either the ability or the motivation to control their bladder. Limited mobility, severe cognitive impairment or emotional problems are the most common causes. A contributing factor may be the lack of a readily accessible toilet. Functional incontinence may co-exist with and exacerbate other forms of incontinence.

Reflex incontinence is leakage occurring without a sensation of urgency or in the absence of a provocative manoeuvre. It is a type of UI often associated with neurologic dysfunction from spinal cord injury or disease, where leakage results from uninhibited contractions of the detrusor muscle during bladder filling, and sensation of urgency is blunted or absent. Another cause of reflex incontinence is diminished bladder compliance, which may occur with radiation cystitis, inflammatory bladder conditions or radical pelvic surgery. A progressive rise in intravesical pressure occurs with filling and eventually results in dribbling leakage across the closed sphincter.

Diagnosis

The diagnostic evaluation of UI begins with a clinical assessment that pays particular attention to the pattern of voiding behaviour and incontinence, identifies relevant historical features, and distinguishes those patients who are appropriately managed at the primary care level from those who merit referral to a specialist.

History

Particular attention should be paid to reversible conditions (Table 40.3) and medications (Table 40.4) that effect micturition. The acronym DRIP is a useful reminder:

- **D**elirium
- **R**estricted mobility
- **I**nfection, inflammation, impaction
- **P**olyuria, pharmaceuticals.

Table 40.3 Reversible conditions

Condition	Impact	Management
Urinary tract infection (UTI)	Symptomatic infection with urgency and dysuria may cause urge incontinence. Asymptomatic UTI generally not associated with incontinence.	Treat symptomatic UTI with antibiotics, then reassess.
Stool impaction	Urge or overflow incontinence.	Disimpact, stool softeners, increase fibre, bulk adding agents, increase fluid intake, laxatives.
Metabolic (hypercalcaemia, hyperglycaemia, diabetes insipidus) Excess fluid intake Volume overload	Polyuria can precipitate urge incontinence or overdistension.	Treat the underlying condition.

Table 40.4 Medications and effects

Medications	Effects on urinary incontinence
Alcohol	Polyuria, frequency, urgency, cognitive dysfunction, immobility
α-Adrenergic agonists	Retention
Antihistamines	Retention, overflow incontinence, faecal impaction
Decongestants	Retention
Diuretics	Polyuria, frequency, urgency
Narcotic analgesics	Retention, faecal impaction
Psychotropics	Retention, overflow incontinence, faecal impaction, immobility
Sedatives and hypnotics	Muscle relaxation, cognitive dysfunction, immobility

Any history of abdominal, lumbosacral or pelvic surgery, injury or trauma is relevant. A voiding diary (Box 40.2) is an excellent source of information. Most practitioners have patients record their intake and voiding behaviour for at least 3 days to obtain an accurate picture of a patient's symptoms and pattern of UI. As a prelude to any treatment efforts, patients should be asked which symptom is most bothersome to them and whether or not they desire treatment. The I-PSS questionnaire (Box 40.1) can be used to quantify voiding symptoms and to monitor treatment success.

Physical assessment

The physical examination is conducted with a focus on the abdominal, genitourinary, rectal, and sacral–neurological region. Assess for organomegaly, masses or bladder distension. Assess the genitals and perineum for skin breakdown. Check for

Box 40.2 A voiding diary

Name: ______________________ Date: ______________

Instructions:

Place a check in the appropriate column next to the time you urinated in the toilet or when an episode of urine leakage occurred. Note the reason for the leakage (e.g. toilet not close by, coughing) and describe your liquid intake (e.g. coffee, water) and estimate the amount (e.g. one cup, half a litre).

Time interval	How many times urinated in toilet?	Any episodes of leakage or incontinence?	How much urine leakage (e.g. small, moderate, large)?	What type of activity were you doing (e.g. coughing, walking)?	What type of fluid did you drink and how much?
Sample	2	1	Moderate	Walking upstairs	Coffee: 2 cups
6–7 a.m.					
7–8 a.m.					
8–9 a.m.					
9–10 a.m.					
10–11 a.m.					
11 a.m.–12 noon					

Box 40.2 A voiding diary *(continued)*

12 noon–
1 p.m. ____________________

1–2 p.m. ____________________

2–3 p.m. ____________________

3–4 p.m. ____________________

4–5 p.m. ____________________

5–6 p.m. ____________________

6–7 p.m. ____________________

7–8 p.m. ____________________

8–9 p.m. ____________________

9–10 p.m. ____________________

10–11 p.m. ____________________

11 p.m.–midnight ____________________

12–1 a.m. ____________________

1–2 a.m. ____________________

2–3 a.m. ____________________

3–4 a.m. ____________________

4–5 a.m. ____________________

5–6 a.m. ____________________

Number of pads used today?____________ Number of incontinence episodes?____________

Comments:____________________

____

Adapted from: J. A. Fantl, D. K. Newman, J. Colling, et al. (1996), *Managing Acute and Chronic Urinary Incontinence. Clinical Practice Guideline. Quick Reference Guide for Clinicians*, no. 2, 1996 update, Department of Health & Human Services, Public Health Service, Agency for Health Care Policy & Research, Rockville, MD (AHCPR pub. no. 96-0686).

evidence of urine loss when coughing or using the Valsalva manoeuvre. On rectal examination, note abnormalities of the prostate, abnormal anal sphincter tone or faecal impaction. Test the integrity of perineal sensation. The sacral, S2–S4, reflex arc may be assessed by compressing the glans penis with a fingertip in the rectum to elicit the bulbocavernous reflex. Abdominal examination should be performed after the patient voids to rule out a markedly elevated PVR. A palpable, distended bladder indicates a significant impairment of bladder emptying. If a more accurate measure is desired, then either urethral catheterisation or ultrasound of the bladder may be performed. If the PVR is markedly elevated, hydronephrosis may result and the risk of urinary tract infection (UTI) may be increased.

Laboratory studies

An examination of the urine is essential. If haematuria (> 5 red blood cells/high power field) is present, then urologic evaluation, including cystoscopy, is recommended to rule out bladder stones or malignancy. If pyuria is present, a urine culture should be obtained and documented infection treated. Pyuria that exists in the absence of bacteriuria (negative culture) merits urologic consultation to exclude other aetiologies, such as bladder stones or tumour. Blood tests should include a basic chemistry analysis with glucose, blood urea nitrogen (BUN) and creatinine tests, and prostate specific antigen (PSA).

Imaging studies

Imaging studies are not a standard component of the evaluation of incontinence. Office-based ultrasound of the bladder is useful to determine the PVR in a non-invasive manner but it is not generally available. Ultrasound of the kidney and bladder is used selectively to rule out hydronephrosis and screen for stones. Intravenous pyelogram (IVP) is the radiologic study of choice in the evaluation of haematuria.

Urodynamic studies

Urodynamic studies evaluate the function of the lower urinary tract. The following urodynamic studies are generally obtained by a specialist as part of a detailed investigation.

Uroflowmetry measures urine flow. A diminished peak flow rate may indicate the presence of outlet obstruction. A *cystometrogram* assesses compliance and capacity of the bladder. This study can identify diminished compliance, abnormally small or large bladder capacity, impaired sensation to bladder filling, and the presence of involuntary detrusor contractions. *Pressure-flow studies* combine a cystometrogram with uroflowmetry performed with a small-diameter pressure catheter in the bladder. This study provides information on the behaviour of the detrusor muscle during voiding, which is helpful in determining the presence of outlet obstruction or detrusor hypocontractility. When combined with fluoroscopy (video urodynamics), the pressure flow study provides a comprehensive test of bladder and sphincter function and is the test of choice for patients with complicated forms of incontinence. In addition to these tests, a urologist may perform cystoscopy to identify the location of obstruction revealed by urodynamic studies as well as rule out tumours, stones or other lesions of the bladder.

Triage

The goal of the initial assessment is to identify men with UI who may be managed in the primary care setting and to distinguish those who require evaluation by a specialist (Box 40.3). Three types

Box 40.3 Initial triage and management

Triage

Initial assessment aims to identify 3 groups of men suitable for initial management:

- those with *post-micturition dribble*
- those with symptoms of *frequency/urgency* with or without urge incontinence
- those with *post-prostatectomy incontinence.*

Patients with incontinence associated with *haematuria, pain* or *recurrent infection,* or who are known to have, or who are thought to have, *poor bladder emptying* are recommended for *specialised management.* Poor bladder emptying may be suspected from symptoms, physical examination or if imaging has been performed by X-ray or ultrasound after voiding.

Management

Post-micturition dribble requires *no assessment* and can usually be effectively treated by pelvic floor exercises and manual compression of the bulbous urethra at the end of micturition.

Urge incontinence and *post-prostatectomy stress incontinence* should be treated by *non-invasive* means initially:

- pelvic floor exercises
- bladder training
- antimuscarinic drugs for detrusor hyperactivity.

Adapted from P. Abrams, S. Khoury & A. Wein (eds), (1999), *Incontinence*, Health Publication, Jersey, UK.

of incontinence are appropriately managed by the primary care physician: post-micturition dribble, urge incontinence, and mild post-prostatectomy stress incontinence. Patients with more severe stress incontinence, mixed incontinence, overflow incontinence or reflex incontinence should be referred to a specialist. Patients with functional incontinence may be referred selectively. Patients with haematuria, pain or recurrent urinary tract infection should also be referred for specialised evaluation and management (Figure 40.3).

Treatment

Many elderly men complain of a post-void dribbling of urine from the penis that stains their clothes. Men with this complaint should be instructed to take a few extra seconds to ensure that the voiding act is completed and to then compress the region of the bulbous urethra and 'strip' the urethra toward the glans to milk out the small volume of pooled urine. Patients with urge incontinence without significant impairment of bladder emptying are treated with a

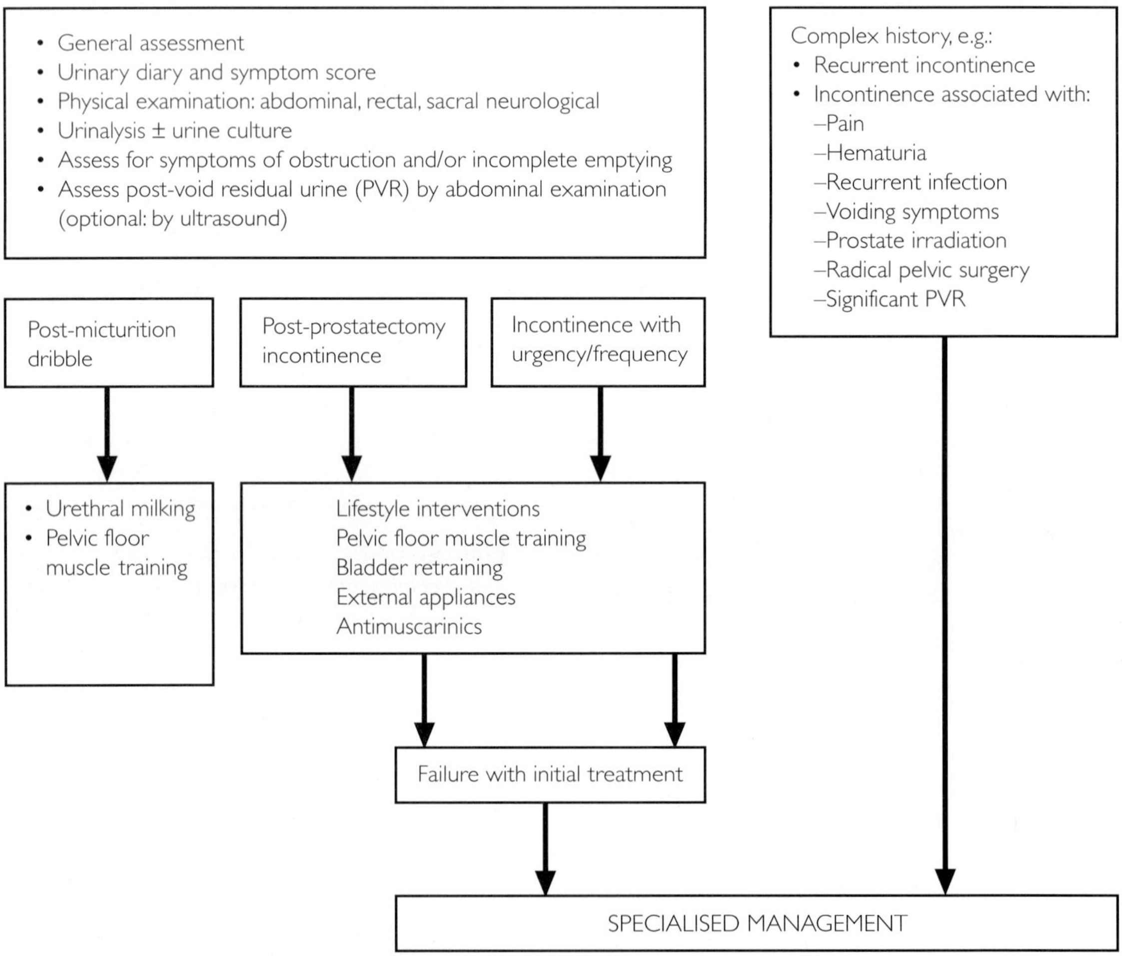

Figure 40.3 Initial triage and management of urinary incontinence in men

Adapted from P. Abrams, S. Khoury & A. Wein (eds), (1999), *Incontinence*, Health Publication, Jersey, UK.

combination of modalities. Lifestyle interventions, such as moderating fluid intake and a regimen of regular toileting, may reduce the frequency of episodes of urgency and leakage. Pelvic floor exercises and bladder training may be used to develop the patient's ability to control the bladder, resist urgency and prevent leakage. The use of antimuscarinic medications will increase functional bladder capacity and reduce urgency and urge incontinence. However, these agents should, as a rule, not be used in patients who may have outlet obstruction. For those with outlet obstruction, antimuscarinics can impair emptying and cause urinary retention. For men with mild post-prostatectomy stress incontinence, pelvic floor muscle strengthening exercises may improve their ability to prevent leakage with certain specific manoeuvres such as coughing, sneezing or bending.

If initial treatment efforts do not provide adequate resolution, then referral to specialised care is indicated. The specialist will usually offer those with stress, mixed or urge incontinence management strategies or interventions based on a detailed investigation of their symptoms (Box 40.4). For those with sphincteric incompetence, bulking agents (collagen), artificial sphincter or sling procedures may be done. Men with severe detrusor hyperactivity may be treated with combinations of medications to modulate bladder function, offered neurostimulation or considered candidates for surgical bladder augmentation. Patients with bladder outlet obstruction and an underactive bladder may be treated with clean intermittent catheterisation (CIC), α-blockers, neurostimulation or correction of anatomic bladder outlet obstruction (Figure 40.4).

Conclusion

Urinary incontinence is a health problem that can be effectively managed. The first step is identifying its presence. The second step is working towards a diagnosis, then offering assistance and assessing the effectiveness of treatment. The simple act of identifying UI can bring much needed relief to an anxious patient.

Box 40.4 Specialised management in men

Assessment

Patients referred directly to specialised management are likely to require urodynamic testing, cystourethroscopy and urinary tract imaging.

Treatment

Non-invasive treatment tailored on the basis of a detailed evaluation is tried first. When a comprehensive effort of conservative management with patient compliance has been attempted and the patient's symptoms persist, and the incontinence markedly disrupts his quality of life, then invasive therapies should be considered.

- For *sphincter incompetence*, the recommended option is the *artificial urinary sphincter, bulking agents (collagen)* or *male urethral sling*.
- For *urge incontinence* the recommended therapies are *sacral nerve stimulation*, *bladder augmentation* and *urinary diversion*.
- When *overflow incontinence* due to obstruction persists despite efforts at medical therapy (e.g. α-blockers), *surgical treatment* may be directed towards alleviating bladder outlet obstruction. If *poor bladder emptying* is due to detrusor hypocontractility, as shown by urodynamic studies, it may be managed by *intermittent catheterisation*.
- For *reflex incontinence*, specialised intervention, such as *bladder augmentation* or *urinary diversion* may be offered.

Adapted from P. Abrams, S. Khoury & A. Wein (eds), (1999), *Incontinence*, Health Publication, Jersey, UK.

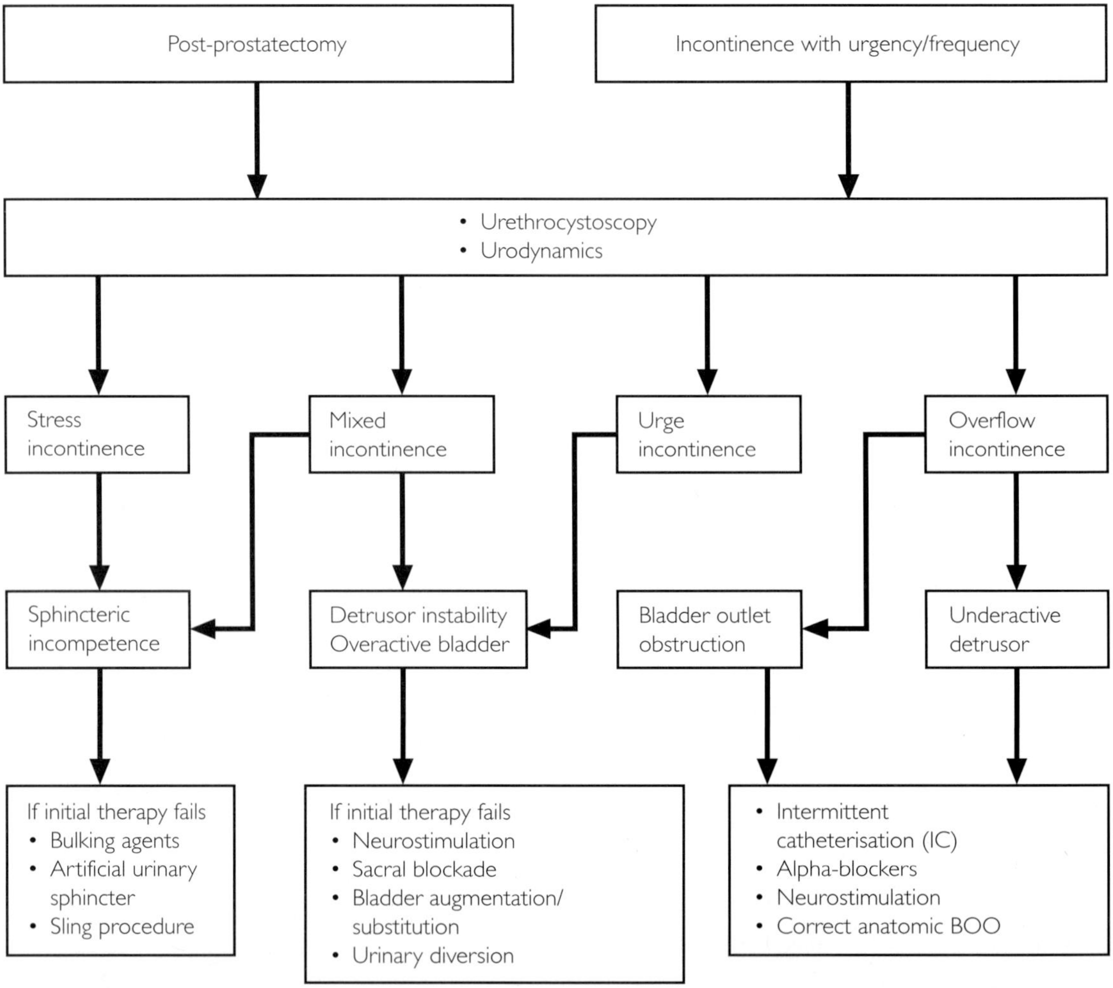

Figure 40.4 Specialised management of urinary incontinence in men

Adapted from P. Abrams, S. Khoury & A. Wein (eds), (1999), *Incontinence*, Health Publication, Jersey, UK.

Bibliography and further reading

deGroat, W. C. (1997), 'Central nervous system control of micturition', in O'Donnell, P. D. (ed.), *Urinary Incontinence*, Mosby, St Louis, pp. 33–47.

Dmochowsk, R. R. & Leach, G. E. (1996), 'Bladder dysfunction and urinary incontinence', in Noble, J. (ed.), *Textbook of Primary Care Medicine*, Mosby, St Louis, pp. 1772–82.

Fantl, J. A., Newman, D. K., Colling, J., et al. (1996), *Managing Acute and Chronic Urinary Incontinence. Clinical Practice Guideline. Quick Reference Guide for Clinicians*, no. 2, 1996 update, US Department of Health & Human Services, Public Health Service, Agency for Health Care Policy & Research, Rockville, MD (AHCPR pub. no. 96-0686).

Fonda, D., Benvenuti, F., Castleden, M., et al. (1999), 'Management of incontinence in older people', in Abrams, P., Khoury, S. & Wein, A. (eds), *Incontinence*, Health Publication, Jersey, UK, pp. 731–73.

Ghoniem, G. M. (1996), 'Pharmacologic therapy for urinary incontinence', *Urologic Nursing*, 16(2), pp. 55–8.

Kane, R. C., Ouslander, J. G. & Abrass, I. B. (1999), 'Incontinence', in Kane, R. L., Ouslander, J. G. & Abrass, I. B. (eds), *Essentials of Clinical Geriatrics*, McGraw-Hill, New York, pp. 181–230.

Karlowicz, K. A. & Meredith, C. E. (1995), 'Adult voiding

dysfunction', in Karlowicz, K. A. (ed.), *Urologic Nursing: Principles and Practice*, W. B. Saunders, Philadelphia, pp. 377–407.

Kondo, A., Hedlund, H., Sirolcy, M., et al. (1999), 'Conservative treatments in men', in Abrams, P., Khoury, S. & Wein, A. (eds), *Incontinence*, Health Publication, Jersey, UK, pp. 669–89.

O'Donnell, P. D. (1998), 'Special considerations in elderly individuals with urinary incontinence', *Urology*, 51(suppl. 2A), 20–3.

Payne, C. K. (1998), 'Epidemiology, pathophysiology and evaluation of urinary incontinence and overactive bladder', *Urology*, 51(suppl. 2A), 3–10.

Ratchik, S. D. & Resnick, M. I. (1998), 'The epidemiology of incontinence in the elderly', *British Journal of Urology*, 82(suppl. 1), 1–4.

Romanzi, L. J. & Blaivas, J. G. (1997), 'Office evaluation of incontinence', in O'Donnell, P. D. (ed.), *Urinary Incontinence*, Mosby, St Louis, pp. 48–54.

Sirls, L. T. & Choe, J. M. (1997), 'The incontinence history and physical examination', in O'Donnell, P. D. (ed.), *Urinary Incontinence*, Mosby, St Louis, pp. 54–63.

Steers, W. D., Barrett, D. M. & Wein, A. J. (1996), 'Voiding dysfunction: diagnosis, classification and management', in Gillenwater, J. Y., Grayhack, J. T., Howards, S. S. & Duckett, J. W. (eds), *Adult and Pediatric Urology*, Mosby, St Louis, pp. 1220–325.

Stone, A. R. & Nelson, R. J. (1999), 'Evaluation and management of male urinary incontinence', *Digital Urology Journal*, www.duj.com/Article/Stone/Stone.html.

Wagg, A. & Malone-Lee, J. (1998), 'The management of urinary incontinence in the elderly', *British Journal of Urology*, 82(suppl. 1), pp. 11–17.

Chapter 41
Diabetes mellitus

BERNARD A. ROOS and L. FERNANDO SAMOS

Introduction

Diabetes mellitus is a very common disease, characterised by disturbance of the intermediary metabolism and marked by elevated blood glucose. The disease affects at least 6.6% of the population (by the criterion of the 75 g oral glucose tolerance test) and is caused by inadequate insulin secretion, action or a combination of both. Most diabetes cases divide into two categories: type I and type II diabetes.

Type I diabetes is characterised by the absence or severe deficit of insulin in the pancreatic β-cell; it has a strong autoimmune basis and usually presents during the first 2–3 decades of life in the form of diabetic ketoacidosis. Type II diabetes, on the other hand, does not have an immune basis; its underlying mechanism implies deficient peripheral action of insulin, or insulin resistance, and it usually occurs in persons older than 30 years and usually in a gradual and subtle manner. Almost 90% of all diabetics, including older diabetics, have type II diabetes.

Diabetes is a very costly disease, in both humanistic and monetary terms, carrying with it the direct costs related to acute glycaemic care and chronic complications and the indirect costs related to disability and premature mortality.

Epidemiology

As the number of older patients rapidly increases, the prevalence and burden of chronic diseases like diabetes mellitus also grow. The prevalence rate of diabetes increases significantly with age: in the US diabetes affects less than 2% of the population between the ages of 20 and 39, 7% between ages 40 and 49, 12% between ages 50 and 59, and about 20% of all persons 75 and older. The disease shows little gender preference, with men and women similarly affected. In some subpopulations the disease tends to be even more common; the number of elderly Mexican-Americans affected by diabetes approaches 30%, a prevalence nearly twice that of the general population.

After excluding persons who meet the criteria for diabetes, the prevalence of impaired glucose tolerance (IGT; 2-hour post-challenge glucose > 140 but < 200 mg/dL) and impaired fasting glucose (IFT; fasting glucose > 110 but < 126 mg/dL) (1997 ADA guidelines) also increases with age. When the incidence rates for both diabetes and IGT/IFT are considered together, more than 40% of the elderly population in the US is affected.

Macrovascular complications in the form of coronary artery disease, cerebrovascular disease and peripheral vascular disease are a serious complication for older diabetics and the main cause of death. Microvascular problems, like renal disease and retinopathy, and neuropathy cause major morbidity and disability. Compared with the rates for older persons without diabetes, the disease increases tenfold the risk of lower extremity amputation; doubles the risk of myocardial infarction, stroke and renal disease; and increases the risk of blindness by nearly 50%. About 30% of the diabetics between 65 and 74 years old are hospitalised each year, a third higher rate than that of elderly individuals without diabetes, and the group of elderly diabetics incurs about two-thirds of the total attributable medical costs for diabetes.

There are studies suggesting that poor glycaemic control may synergistically interact with other age-related pathology to accelerate diabetic complications, so that the time needed, in years, to develop a chronic complication might be shortened in the diabetic. In a cross-sectional study of type II diabetics, logistic regression analysis showed a significant increase in the prevalence of retinopathy with ageing, independent of the effects of metabolic control, duration of disease and other risk variables. Age was also associated with the prevalence of peripheral neuropathy, hypertension and impotence. Another study, of type I and type II diabetics, found independent associations of age with renal insufficiency, macrovascular complications and sensory neuropathy.

Pathophysiology

By far the most prevalent form of diabetes is type II, which includes cases of diabetes secondary to other conditions like pancreatic disease, Cushing's syndrome, acromegaly or drug-induced diabetes (Box 41.1). It is clear that several carbohydrate metabolism changes and peculiarities are related to age in older individuals. Many studies found elevations in both fasting and predominantly postprandial glucose levels that correlate directly with age. In lean elderly diabetics, insulin deficiency appears to predominate over resistance; on the other hand, obese diabetics have significant resistance and relative insulin deficiency.

Box 41.1 Medications that increase glycaemia

- Glucocorticoids
- Thiazides
- Nicotinic acid
- Growth hormone
- Megestrol
- Pentamidine
- β-blockers[a]
- Calcium channel blockers[a]
- Oestrogen/progesterone compounds
- Phenytoin
- NSAIDs[a]
- Caffeine

(*a*) Data regarding glycaemic effect are less well established.

Insulin clearance studies have demonstrated a modest increase of insulin half-life, from 11 minutes in the young to 13 minutes in the elderly. Nonetheless, insulin resistance and relative insulin deficiency mark the ageing process. Although the relative importance of the several mechanisms that cause impaired glucose and carbohydrate metabolism is not fully clarified, the causes for such impairment are clearly multifactorial.

The glucose-sensing–insulin-release regulatory loops appear altered in older subjects, with a delay/decrease of the glucose-induced insulin release. There is also delayed insulin-induced suppression of the hepatic glucose output, which contributes to the increase in fasting blood glucose. An important role is concurrently played by the impaired insulin-mediated glucose uptake (resistance) in skeletal muscle and adipose tissue. The increased adiposity of older patients is accompanied by declining lean body mass; middle-aged obese diabetics also have an increase in adipocyte mass, but with preservation of lean body mass.

Despite the finding that insulin's peripheral action is impaired, no major changes are seen in insulin membrane receptors in target cells. It is thought that impairment in the insulin-sensitive transporter, GLUT4, may be responsible for the decreased response to insulin. Exercise in middle-aged subjects has been shown to elevate the levels of GLUT4 in muscle, with accompanying improvement in insulin sensitivity, and a similar phenomenon might underlie the post-exercise improvement in glucose tolerance of older persons who exercise.

Other important factors that contribute to glucose metabolism changes with ageing are co-existing illnesses and multiple medications in this elderly group, physical inactivity, genetics and possibly 'β-cell ageing', with higher proinsulin–insulin molar ratios that could affect the peripheral effectiveness of insulin (Figure 41.1).

Diagnosis

Diagnosis is based on documenting elevated circulating glucose. Although increased insulin resistance marks the ageing process, the diagnostic criteria for older individuals are the same as those used for the population in general. Efforts to establish age-specific diagnostic criteria have generally proven impractical. Thus, diabetes diagnostic criteria, as is the case for hypertension and hypercholesterolaemia, have not yet been adjusted for age. In 1997 the American Diabetes Association (ADA) revised the diagnostic criteria (summarised in Box 41.2), which lowered the fasting level required to diagnose diabetes, from 140 to 126 mg/dL.

Epidemiological studies have found a very strong correlation between diabetic complications and a 2-hour value of 200 mg/dL or more on the oral glucose tolerance test (OGTT). These studies also demonstrated that diagnosing diabetes by the criterion of a fasting glucose level of 140 or more misses a significant number of persons with abnormal OGTT results, which was a fundamental reason why the fasting diagnostic level was lowered to 126 mg/dL. Therefore, OGTT is not very useful clinically, both because it is cumbersome and, under the new fasting criteria, often redundant; the fasting cut-off of 126 mg/dL and the random value of 200 mg/dL if

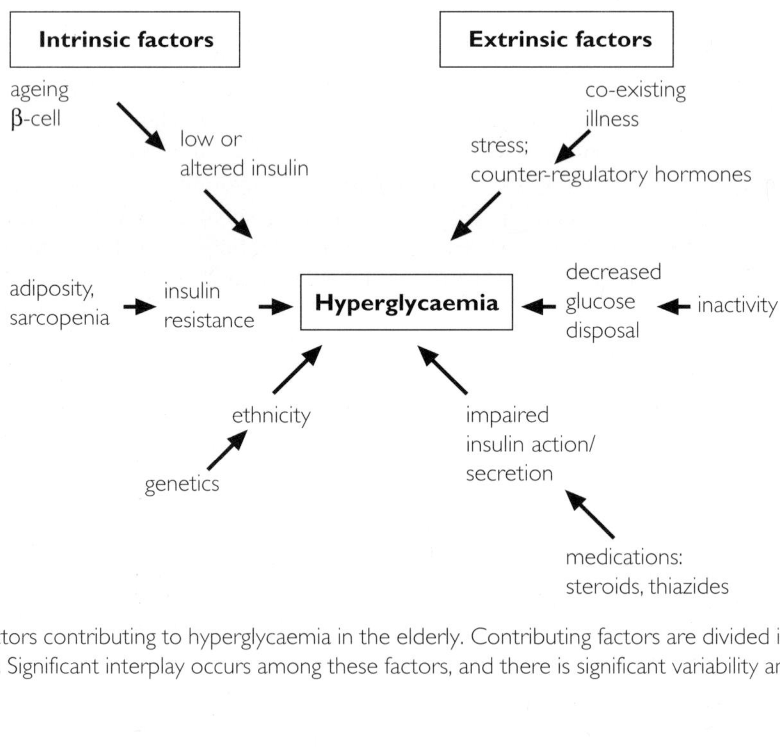

Figure 41.1 Factors contributing to hyperglycaemia in the elderly. Contributing factors are divided in this figure for didactic purposes. Significant interplay occurs among these factors, and there is significant variability among diabetic individuals

Box 41.2 Diagnostic criteria for diabetes mellitus and impaired glucose tolerance

Diabetes mellitus, if any of the following is present:

- Fasting plasma glucose ≥ 126 mg/dL (7.0 mM), on at least 2 separate days
- Classic symptoms of diabetes and a random plasma glucose of ≥ 200 mg/dL (11.1 mM)
- Plasma glucose ≥ 200 mg/dL 2 hours after a glucose load (OGTT)

Impaired glucose tolerance (IGT), if:

- Glucose ≥ 140 mg/dL (7.9 mM) but < 200mg/dL during OGTT

Impaired fasting glucose (IFG), if:

- Fasting glucose ≥ 110 mg/dL (6.1 mM) and < 126 mg/dL

symptoms occur are the most useful clinical measures. There are no criteria for the use of haemoglobin A_{1c} as a diagnostic tool due to the lack of standardisation and the low sensitivity and specificity of the test.

Testing of older adults

The ADA recommends testing all individuals aged 45 and older for diabetes, using a fasting glucose level. The rationale for the ADA recommendation is the high frequency of undetected diabetes mellitus reported in population studies. The ADA also advises that normal tests should be repeated every 3 years, while yearly testing should be considered for high-risk groups, such as overweight people (body mass index > 27 kg/m^2), people with a diabetic first-degree relative, persons with hypertension or hyperlipidaemia, and those with prior impaired fasting glucose. In addition, some ethnic groups with higher incidence of diabetes overall, such as African-Americans, Hispanics and Native Americans, should be considered for more frequent testing.

Clinical manifestations of diabetes in the elderly

Although elderly persons can present with typical diabetic complaints, such as polyuria, polydipsia, dry mouth and blurred vision, they more often present with atypical and variable complaints that might be mistakenly attributed to other organ system problems. Such non-specific complaints are more frequent in the frail elderly patient, who often has difficulty in clearly expressing his complaints. The overall reason for the frequent atypical manifestation of diabetes in an elderly patient can be better understood when one recognises that some organ systems might be functioning only at borderline capacity in this age group at the time when diabetes impacts on them to produce overt clinical symptoms.

Urinary incontinence can be a presenting diabetic symptom, which could be mistaken for a urological sign. The polyuria caused by diabetes could easily overwhelm the urinary bladder that might already be handling an increased post-void residual volume in a man suffering from prostatic hypertrophy. This polyuria also affects older women, who have an increased frequency of cystocele and relaxation of the pelvic muscles; like men they can experience dysmotility of the detrusor muscle, which could lead to incontinence aggravated by diabetes.

Weight loss and *weakness* might be inaccurately attributed to a malignant process, if one does not take into account that these symptoms may be due to loss of glucose and kilojoules in the urine, plus some degree of volume depletion and impaired general homeostasis from chronic hyperglycaemia.

Older persons often have a deficient thirst drive, with functional hypodipsia even in the presence of hyperosmolality. This condition contributes to the development of a hyperglycaemic hyperosmolar non-ketotic state. Decreased thirst together with polyuria can lead to volume depletion, which results in hypotension, especially in the setting of autonomic neuropathy, and renders older patients more prone to falls, bruises, fractures and head trauma. Hypovolaemia and hypo-osmolarity can also lead to *confusion* and even *delirium* as presenting complaints. Elderly diabetics also exhibit an increased frequency of *depression*, which is likely to be associated with worsening glycaemic control and decreased compliance with treatment. It is therefore important to inquire about depressive symptoms and even apply tests such as the Geriatric Depression Scale if needed.

Several neuromusculoskeletal syndromes and complaints occur preferentially in older diabetics: for example, painful shoulder periarthrosis, which can limit the range of motion of the glenohumeral joint, at least temporarily, occurs in up to 10% of patients. *Diabetic amyotrophy* is a dramatic syndrome consisting of asymmetric weakness and pain and wasting of the pelvic girdle and thigh muscles without much sensory change. This condition happens mainly in older men and, although difficult to manage, often resolves spontaneously within a year. *Diabetic neuropathic cachexia* is a classical syndrome also affecting mainly older men and characterised by painful peripheral neuropathy, weight loss and depression. This disorder also generally resolves within a year. The therapeutic approach for both syndromes is to control the glycaemia and employ pain control, antidepressants (if needed) and supportive therapy.

Older patients also are more susceptible to *hypothermia*, due to the combination of low metabolic heat production, decreased muscle mass, decreased shivering, diminished peripheral blood flow, high surface–body mass ratio and impaired autonomic nervous system function. Older diabetics also might not be able to mount an appropriate febrile reaction in response to serious *infections*, which can delay the diagnosis of entities like *malignant otitis externa* due to *Pseudomonas aeruginosa* or the polymicrobial *necrotising fasciitis* that tends to be seen more in older patients. Diabetics who reside in long-term care institutions may also be at a higher risk for tuberculosis. Another condition documented in patients older than 70 is *bullous diabetic dermopathy of the feet*, which also tends to resolve spontaneously. Because of the high frequency of secondary infections, this skin condition is especially problematic in elderly diabetics.

Acute complications

Older diabetics can present with any acute diabetic complications, including diabetic ketoacidosis (DKA), but two conditions merit special consideration in the elderly: hyperglycaemic hyperosmolar non-ketotic state and hypoglycaemia.

Hyperglycaemic hyperosmolar non-ketotic state

The hyperglycaemic hyperosmolar non-ketotic (HONK) state is a syndrome more specific to the elderly, characterised by severe dehydration and a blood glucose > 600 mg/dL, serum osmolality > 320 mOsm/kg, a serum pH over 7.3 and a bicarbonate of > 20 mEq/L, together with an anion gap of 15 or less. Ketones are usually absent but can be mildly positive. The most frequent predisposing event is an acute infection (in half the cases), with pneumonia being the most common (representing half the infections). Other events such as stroke, myocardial infarction or even medications like glucocorticoids can also be predisposing factors. Mortality can be as high as 35%.

In HONK states, most individuals with type II diabetes have just enough residual insulin to suppress lipolysis and ketogenesis (therefore avoiding DKA), but not enough to inhibit hepatic glucose production. Key factors for the development of HONK include decreased thirst sensation (hypodipsia) of elderly patients, impaired maintenance of serum osmolality, and decreased access to water, especially in frail patients with decreased mobility and sensory deprivation. Human survivors of hyperosmolar coma exhibit subnormal osmoregulated thirst and fluid intake and increased arginine vasopressin (AVP), suggesting the concept of an 'ageing osmoreceptor' that may cause hypodipsia.

The onset of HONK can be preceded by days or even weeks of polyuria, polydipsia and weakness. Patients present with severe dehydration, hypotension, tachycardia and sometimes with cardiovascular collapse. Patients may be confused, lethargic or comatose. Focal neurologic deficits, seizures and central hyperthermia may be present. Leucocytosis is a characteristic feature, with counts up to 50 000/mm^3. When HONK occurs in the elderly, up to half the time diabetes has not been diagnosed or treated before.

Treatment of the HONK state requires very careful and frequent monitoring, with the following goals:

1. restore volume
2. correct electrolyte abnormalities

3. lower glycaemia towards normal
4. diagnose and treat the precipitating events.

If circulatory collapse or severe hypotension is present, normal saline is given initially; if these conditions are not present, half-normal saline is preferred because it will more rapidly correct the free water deficit. Three to four litres of fluid may be needed in the first 12 hours, but it is important to be cautious in the elderly, whose cardiac reserve may not accommodate aggressive fluid replacement. In most cases, insulin and intravenous fluids can be started together, with the exception of patients with hypokalaemia or hypotension, who should receive intravenous fluids before they receive insulin in order to prevent the worsening of these conditions that can result from insulin moving potassium, glucose and water into the cells.

Less insulin is needed in HONK than in DKA; as a general rule, 0.1 unit of insulin per kilogram of body weight is given initially as an intravenous bolus, followed by an infusion of regular insulin at 0.1 unit/kg body weight/hour, until blood glucose levels drop to about 250 mg/dL; at that time, dextrose is added to the intravenous fluids, and insulin infusion is decreased to 0.05 unit/kg body weight/hour. In general, a decrease of about 10% of serum glucose per hour is reasonable. Body potassium is usually depleted despite a normal potassium level, so that potassium chloride can be added early, even in the presence of normal serum potassium, as long as urine production is maintained.

Hypoglycaemia

The glucose transport system in peripheral tissues like fat and muscle depends on insulin, but brain glucose uptake does not. Therefore, the brain does not have to compete for glucose with peripheral tissues under basal circumstances, such as after an overnight fast when insulin levels are low. Peripheral tissues do become a major competitor of the brain when glucose transport is activated by insulin and glucose is lowered. Older patients tend to have more limited central nervous system reserve, which makes hypoglycaemia a more serious consideration for older persons.

The defence against hypoglycaemia depends on a series of events generated by counter-regulatory hormones. Glucagon is the first line of defence against acute hypoglycaemia; when glucagon responses fail, epinephrine and then cortisol and growth hormone become major defences against prolonged/severe hypoglycaemia. Epinephrine and other stress hormones are also important for symptom recognition. However, in the elderly, recognition of hypoglycaemia is more difficult because of decreased catechol and autonomic nervous system responses. Elderly persons may no longer exhibit symptoms like tremors, anxiety, sweating and palpitations that are induced normally in younger persons.

Diminished glucagon secretion has also been documented in older patients, which can significantly impair the efficiency of the counter-regulatory process. Sensory impairment, motility dysfunction, cognitive deficits and medications like β-blockers can all contribute to the greater severity of hypoglycaemia and its consequences in the elderly.

Chronic complications

Tissue damage from chronic complications derives from complex interactions involving chronic exposure to hyperglycaemia and many other factors, which can be either intrinsic to the individual, such as altered or normal metabolic pathways, or extrinsic or environmental, such as exposure to cigarette smoke. Many diseases like hypertension and hyperlipidaemia can also interact with diabetes in a synergistic manner to cause chronic complications.

Evidence indicates that diabetes alone tends to promote accelerated ageing through modifications of tissue function and structure. When the clinical course and complications of diabetes are considered together with the degenerative changes of ageing, both the course of the disease in older diabetics and its management are significantly altered due to the shortening of the period from disease onset to the beginning of structural tissue damage.

One mechanism by which hyperglycaemia could lead to diabetes complications is through the interaction of glucose with proteins in a process called glycation, a term used to describe the non-enzymatic bonding of glucose with primary amino groups of proteins. This reaction causes permanent modifications in proteins, changing not only their physical–chemical characteristics, but also their biological function. The modified molecules that result from glycation are called advanced glycation end products, or AGEs (Figure 41.2).

Numerous investigations in recent years have pointed out the critical role of non-enzymatic glycation in the mechanisms involved in complications associated with normal ageing and with diabetes mellitus. This non-enzymatic glycation, also called the Maillard reaction, begins with the spontaneous formation of the easily reversible Schiff base, which is the combination of an aldehyde group in a carbohydrate (glucose) and a primary amino group in a protein. Within days the Schiff base undergoes rearrangement, leading to the formation of a more stable molecule called Amadori product. Over several weeks the Amadori products undergo a series of intermolecular and intramolecular rearrangements that result in the formation of a heterogeneous mix of end products, which as a group are yellow-brown in colour, fluorescent, and have stable inter- and intramolecular cross-links (AGEs). The extent of formation and characteristics of this mix of end products depend on a number of factors, including pH, temperature, protein half-life and blood glucose levels.

Because glucose is a ubiquitous molecule in normal tissues, AGE formation is physiologically diverse. In the lens proteins, AGEs contribute to the formation of cataracts, which tend to develop even in otherwise healthy, non-diabetic older individuals. In the case of diabetics, where AGE formation occurs at an accelerated pace, many signs of accelerated ageing can be seen, including early cataract formation. Thus it has been suggested that the interaction between diabetes and ageing might hasten the course of chronic diabetic complications in geriatric patients, especially in the presence of multiple organ disease so frequently encountered in the elderly. Chronic hyperglycaemia can also lead to the accumulation of products of the aldose reductase system, primarily sorbitol, and to the depletion of myoinositol in some tissues. Both mechanisms also contribute to the long-term complications of diabetes (Table 41.1).

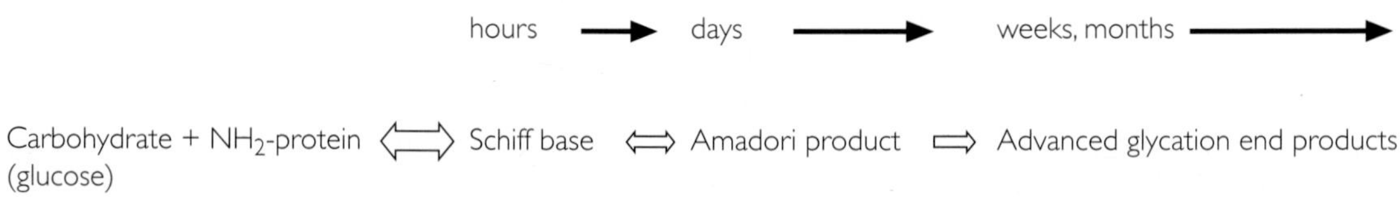

Figure 41.2 Advanced glycation end products. Glycation may take months to years to progress to completion. The more advanced the process, the more irreversible the products it renders. The larger double arrow represents easy reversibility (i.e. the products can proceed both ways). The smaller double arrow represents only limited reversibility. Advanced glycation end products are irreversibly formed

Table 41.1 Complications of diabetes

Macrovascular	Microvascular	Neuropathy
Coronary artery disease Myocardial infarction	*Retinopathy* Proliferative Non-proliferative	*Autonomic* Gastroparesis Orthostatic hypotension
Cerebrovascular disease Stroke	*Nephropathy* Renal insufficiency Proteinuria	*Peripheral* Paresthesias, pain Lack of sensation in feet
Peripheral vascular disease Ischaemia in lower extremities Claudication		

Central nervous system changes, dementia and diabetes

A good outcome in diabetes treatment plans requires active patient participation, involvement and understanding. The patient must be able to follow a prescribed diet, co-ordinate medication intake with meals and activity, and monitor glucose levels—all activities that require cognitive skills and a dependable memory. Thus cognitive dysfunction challenges treatment efforts and tends to modify treatment plans and interventions.

Several studies have pointed out the increased frequency of cognitive impairment in older diabetics and have also linked declining cognitive function with worsening glycaemic control. Although multiple factors may lower cognition in diabetics (depression, hypertension and cerebrovascular disease), it appears that hyperglycaemia by itself may account for lower brain function. A review of evidence of cross-sectional and prospective associations between type II diabetes and cognitive impairment both in memory and executive function reveals an elevated risk of vascular dementia and Alzheimer's disease, although with strong interaction of other diabetes-associated factors like hypertension, hyperlipidaemia and apolipoprotein E phenotype.

Diffuse cerebral and cortical atrophy has been found in association with diabetes, allowing for the effects of age, hypertension and cerebrovascular disease. Many studies have demonstrated an association between cognitive function and indices of long-term glycaemic control. A few studies have shown that cognitive impairment is exacerbated by increased duration of diabetes and that cognitive impairment may be associated with peripheral neuropathy, which is a specific complication associated with the duration of the disease and with the degree of glycaemic control. A prospective cohort study by Gregg et al. (2000), of more than 9000 community-dwelling women 65 years and older, found that diabetics had lower baseline scores in the Mini-Mental State Examination as well as in the Digit Symbol (memory) and the Trail B tests (psychomotor performance). They also showed that diabetes for more than 15 years was associated with a 57–114% greater risk of cognitive decline than that experienced by non-diabetic women.

Recent investigations identified a potential role of AGEs in Alzheimer's disease. Amyloid plaques (a hallmark of Alzheimer's) in non-diabetic brains were assessed for the presence of AGEs. Alzheimer's brains were found to have 3 times more AGEs than the brains of age-matched controls. This finding, together with the finding that *in vitro* glycation of soluble β-amyloid peptides markedly increases deposition of insoluble fibrillar β-amyloid, suggests that AGEs may participate in amyloid plaque formation and deposition and thus be associated with Alzheimer's. Therefore, maintaining euglycaemia in the elderly might also reduce dementia risk.

Management

Older diabetics are more likely as a group than non-diabetics to develop acute and chronic illness, to be hospitalised and to develop disability. Older patients are subject to social, medical, psychological and economic circumstances that can affect diabetes treatment and control. Before care planning, a comprehensive assessment must be performed of the geriatric patient to establish functional and cognitive level, unmask depression and inquire about socioeconomic circumstances and support needed (Box 41.3). The Diabetes Control and Complications Trial (DCCT) demonstrated that reducing glycaemia lowers complications in type I diabetics, thereby establishing the benefit of tight control in that group of patients. Although the study found only a trend for risk reduction in macrovascular disease, it showed a 54% risk reduction for nephropathy, 76% for retinopathy (microvascular disease) and 60% for neuropathy.

Despite earlier uncertainty, we know now that improved glycaemia decreases the risk for complications in type II diabetes patients. A prospective study that followed 110 individuals for 6 years found that better glycaemic control (haemoglobin A_{1c} = 7.1%) through multiple insulin injections significantly reduced the incidence of microvascular

Box 41.3 Assessment of the older diabetic

1. Cognitive assessment (capacity to understand instructions)
2. Estimation of life expectancy and co-morbidities
3. Psychological assessment
   (a) Depression
   (b) Anxiety
4. Social evaluation
   (a) Support system
   (b) Financial issues
5. Functional evaluation: ADLs, IADLs and sensory assessment
6. Review of medications
7. Patient preferences

complications when compared with conventional treatment (haemoglobin A_{1c} = 9.4%).

Conclusive evidence of the benefits of tight control in type II diabetes has emerged from the United Kingdom Prospective Diabetes Study (UKPDS). This landmark study, which enrolled more than 5000 newly diagnosed type II diabetics and followed them for 10 years, established the benefit of lowering blood glucose levels for reducing retinopathy and nephropathy and, to a lesser extent, neuropathy. The difference in haemoglobin A_{1c} was 0.9 g%—from 7.9 g% in the conventionally treated to 7.0 g% in the intensively treated group. Epidemiological analysis showed that for every 1 g% point reduction in haemoglobin A_{1c} there was about a 35% reduction in the risk of microvascular complications, similar to the reduction seen in the DCCT per gram percentage decrease in haemoglobin A_{1c}.

The UKPDS also showed a 16% reduction in the risk of combined fatal and non-fatal myocardial infarction and sudden death, but the number was not quite statistically significant. The intensively treated groups received either insulin, sulphonylurea (chlorpropramide or glyburide) or metformin, and the benefits were seen across all groups regardless of the agent used, indicating that the key factor is reduction of the glycaemic level. This study also documented the large benefits of lowering blood pressure to a mean of 144/82 mmHg, which significantly reduced strokes, diabetes-related deaths, heart failure, microvascular complications and visual loss. Both of the antihypertensives used—captopril (an ACE inhibitor) and atenolol (a β-blocker)—were equally effective. Thus, if both diabetes and hypertension are present, additive benefits for improved microvascular and macrovascular outcomes can be expected if both glycaemia and hypertension are treated more aggressively.

The incidence of major hypoglycaemic events was 2.3% in those receiving insulin, 0.6% in the glyburide (glybenclamide) group and 0.4% in the chlorpropramide group. Based on the cited results, there is no doubt that middle-aged adults with type II diabetes should be treated more aggressively, but can this intensive approach be applied to the elderly? It is important to point out that the UKPDS was not designed to study the elderly: the oldest enrolled patient was 65 years old, and geriatric and frailty issues were not part of the study. For an optimal outcome in an older diabetic, an interdisciplinary and individualised approach should be implemented, with dietitians, social workers, educators, nurses and physicians with the experience and training to recognise changing demographics, frailty and prospects for complications and their prevention.

Although ADA guidelines recommend a fasting blood glucose level of between 80 and 120 mg/dL, a bedtime value of between 100 and 140, and a haemoglobin A_{1c} within 1 g% of the upper limit of normal, these numbers may not be feasible or appropriate for a number of geriatric patients. It is important to avoid hypoglycaemia in the frail elderly, who could be at risk for serious consequences like hip fractures after a fall due to hypoglycaemia, and in patients who still live independently but may not be able to help themselves if they develop hypoglycaemia.

The benefits of good blood glucose control are many, but some that should be emphasised for the elderly diabetic are:

1. less polyuria, hypovolaemia and nocturia and better sleep
2. fewer infections and hospital admissions

3. better wound healing
4. slower progression of retinopathy, cataracts, neuropathy and nephropathy
5. better control of dyslipidaemia and cardiovascular disease.

Diet

Diet management is an integral component of diabetes care. Kilojoule requirements depend on physical activity, which is often limited in the elderly. Provision of enough nutrients like vitamins and minerals is important, and a protein intake of 0.8 g/kg body weight is recommended. Difficulties in food preparation and shopping as well as changes in chewing, swallowing and appetite may favour the consumption of unrefined carbohydrates, which will have a negative impact on blood glucose. Older patients may also present changes in taste perception and oral health and may suffer from xerostomia, which can significantly affect their eating pattern. It is therefore extremely important to take a dietary history and remain vigilant about the possibility of undernutrition.

Exercise

Exercise is essential to the therapy of diabetes. During exercise muscle uses glucose, triglycerides and free fatty acids at a greatly increased rate, thus decreasing their circulating levels. Studies have demonstrated that moderate intensity physical activity could be associated with 30–60% lower incidence of type II diabetes over 4–14 years and 15–25% lower glycosylated haemoglobin over 3–4 months in type II diabetics. Exercise enhances insulin sensitivity via an increase in GLUT4, often deficient in ageing.

Before an elderly person begins an exercise program, a careful and detailed evaluation should be done. It is important to screen for the presence of macrovascular and microvascular problems that could be aggravated by exercise. Coronary artery disease (macrovascular) and proliferative retinopathy (microvascular) could be contraindications to certain types of exercises, such as vigorous resistance training. The presence and severity of peripheral neuropathy should be investigated, since exercise on insensitive feet could lead to trauma and ulcerations; non-weight-bearing exercises should be recommended for those patients. Exercise appears beneficial even in non-ambulatory and paraplegic patients who are capable of upper body exercises.

Drug therapy

The recent availability of several new antidiabetic drugs, while complicating the decision-making process, also offers a variety of ways of meeting the needs of particular patients. Drug therapy in type II diabetes is a rapidly evolving field, where lines of treatment will continue to change and evolve.

For the most part, the same common treatment principles that apply to younger diabetics also hold true for elderly diabetics. But in this special population, several age and frailty factors must be considered:

1. *individual characteristics*, such as functionality, degree of frailty, body mass, co-existence of medical illnesses, and specific diabetic complications
2. *pharmacological properties*, especially side effects and interaction with other medications
3. *pharmacokinetic changes*, like changes in hepatic metabolism and distribution
4. *degree of hyperglycaemia*, because some agents have greater glucose-lowering capacity than others. In marked hyperglycaemia, insulin should be used, at least temporarily.

Several groups of agents are discussed in the following sections (summarised in Table 41.2).

Sulphonylureas stimulate insulin secretion through the closing of an adenosine-triphosphate-dependent potassium channel, leading to depolarisation of the β-cell, with subsequent calcium influx and secretion of insulin. These agents are often used as first-line drug therapy after diet and exercise fail; however, they are also effective when added to regimens started with biguanides or α-glucosidase inhibitors (see below). There is some tendency towards weight gain, and hypoglycaemia is a potential side effect. Among the first-generation sulphonylureas, chlorpropramide has a half-life of up to 72 hours, is metabolised in the liver to active

Table 41.2 Diabetic medications in the elderly

Medications by class	Advantages	Disadvantages
Sulphonylureas *First generation* Tolbutamide (Orinase) Chlorpropamide (Diabenese) Glipizide (Glucotrol) Glyburide (Diabeta, Micronase) *Second generation* Glimepiride, glicazide	Low cost Second-generation medications have fewer drug interactions than first generation medications	May cause hypoglycaemia Tendency to cause weight gain Chlorpropamide not recommended for the elderly (half-life up to 72 hours, ADH activity, disulphiram-type interaction with alcohol)
Biguanides Metformin (Glucophage)	Does not cause hypoglycaemia Does not promote weight gain Positive effect on lipids	Potential for causing lactic acidosis Use with caution in the elderly Cannot use in renal insufficiency May cause nausea and diarrhoea
α-glucosidase inhibitors Acarbose (Precose) Miglitol (Glyset)	No serious side effects No hypoglycaemia Acarbose is not absorbed	Low potency as blood-glucose-lowering agents Some patients develop flatulence and diarrhoea Titrate dose up gradually
Thiazolidinediones Rosiglitasone (Avendia) Pioglitazone (Actose)	No hypoglycaemia Lower insulin resistance	Troglitazone was associated with liver injury and withdrawn from the market
Meglitinides Repaglinide (Prandin)	Release of insulin appears to depend on glucose level	Short duration of action Must be taken with meals
Insulin	Universal agent; can be used in any type of diabetes and with any patient No interactions No contraindications	May cause hypoglycaemia Must be injected; requires dexterity

metabolites, and is renally excreted; because of several serious side effects, this drug should not be used in the elderly. Tolbutamide is a more acceptable first-generation sulphonylurea. However, in older patients, second-generation agents are preferred because they have less interaction with medications and tend to have a shorter half-life, which lessens the risk of hypoglycaemia. Among the second-generation agents, glyburide (glybenclamide) has been reported to cause as much hypoglycaemia as chlorpropamide; it is also metabolised to active metabolites and must be used with great caution, if at all, in the elderly. Glipizide is a preferable agent, because of its shorter half-life and lack of active metabolites. The starting dose in the elderly is 5 mg/day 30 minutes before breakfast; when doses higher than 15 mg/day are required, the doses should be divided and given before meals.

Metformin is the most commonly used *biguanide*. They inhibit hepatic gluconeogenesis by interfering with lactate oxidation and uptake and enhancement of the insulin sensitivity of muscle, which may be explained by increased insulin receptor tyrosine kinase and GLUT4 activity. Unlike sulphonylureas, biguanides do not cause hypoglycaemia and may be associated with weight loss; they can cause loose bowel movements in some patients, which could be advantageous in older individuals who often suffer from constipation. Metformin has favourable effects on lipids, reducing triglyceride levels and low-density lipoprotein (LDL) cholesterol and slightly increasing high-density lipoprotein (HDL) levels. Adverse effects, including nausea, vomiting, diarrhoea, and anorexia, occur in 20% of the patients.

While therapeutic doses of metformin reduce

lactate uptake by the liver, the serum lactate level rises minimally, if at all, unless there is impaired kidney function and therefore decreased lactate clearance; a creatinine of more than 1.4 is contraindication for its use. States of hypoxia, such as severe cardiovascular or respiratory disease or liver failure, can also contribute to elevated lactate levels and thus contraindicate metformin. Metformin should be used with caution in the elderly due to the high frequency of renal insufficiency in the elderly and the other conditions noted above. Metformin should be withheld when the patient is undergoing contrast studies. The agent could be combined with sulphonylureas, insulin, glucosidase inhibitors or repaglinide, depending on the clinical scenario. The usual dose range is 1–2 g/day.

The *α-glucosidase inhibitors* act by inhibiting intestinal α-glucosidase enzymes (maltase, isomaltase, sucrase and glucoamylase), which break down oligosaccharides and disaccharides into monosaccharides. This inhibition delays the digestion of carbohydrates and decreases their rate of absorption. These agents are effective in reducing postprandial glycaemia and can achieve small but significant haemoglobin A_{1c} reduction (0.5–1%). Alpha-glucosidase inhibitors do not cause hypoglycaemia by themselves. The two most commonly used inhibitors are acarbose and miglitol. Acarbose is not absorbed, and no systemic side effects should be expected, but as the dose is increased intestinal side effects emerge, including flatulence, soft stools, diarrhoea and abdominal discomfort due to the undigested carbohydrates. The key to successful use of these drugs is having the patient titrate the dose, starting with a dose of 25 mg twice a day with the first bite of food and working up gradually to a dose in the range of 100 mg 3 times a day. Miglitol has a similar side effect profile and is more potent than acarbose; the starting dose is 25 mg once a day with meals, with gradual titration to the maximal dose that suits the patient, at most around 300 mg daily. These agents can be used in combination with sulphonylureas and metformin when the target glucose level is not reached.

Thiazolidinediones act as insulin sensitisers in peripheral tissues and decrease hepatic gluconeogenesis. They reduce hyperglycaemia, hyperinsulinaemia and hypertriglyceridaemia and increase HDL levels, although there are some reports that these agents can increase LDL levels. The mechanism of action requires the presence of insulin and involves stimulation of a family of transcription factors called peroxisome proliferator activated receptor gamma (PPAR-γ), which are believed to increase the expression of glucose transporters GLUT1 and GLUT4. Insulin levels are not increased, and thus there is no concern about hypoglycaemia.

Because these agents attack the insulin resistance that marks early type II diabetes, there is increasing enthusiasm for using thiazolidinediones early in the pharmacological management strategy. However, this enthusiasm was recently dampened when the first of these agents, troglitazone, was withdrawn from the market due to its association with liver injury. The newer agents, rosiglitazone and pioglitazone, appear to be at least as effective as troglitazone and may cause fewer hepatic side effects. However, until more data are available, the use of a thiazolidinedione requires monitoring of the liver function test during therapy, especially throughout the first year of treatment.

Repaglinide is currently the only agent in the new class of drugs termed *meglitinide analogs*. This drug is a non-sulphonylurea insulin secretagogue that requires the presence of glucose for its action and works by closing ATP-dependent potassium channels in β-cells. Repaglinide increases insulin levels postprandially, and compared to sulphonylureas, it has a rapid onset of action and rapid clearance. Because of this short duration of action, dosing must be timed to meals and should not be taken on a regular schedule. Repaglinide can be used in combination with metformin. The starting dose is 0.5 mg before meals, with a maximum daily dose of 16 mg. Side effects include mild hypoglycaemia and gastrointestinal symptoms.

Insulin therapy is a universal treatment for all types of diabetes and patients (it is essential for sustaining life in type I diabetes), and there are virtually no contraindications for its use and no interactions. Nonetheless, the initiation of insulin treatment can be a stressful event in older people. This treatment requires needles and injections, and patients and caregivers must become familiar with injection techniques and insulin formulations. The fact that insulin needs to be injected to be effective can be a tremendous obstacle in older patients; there is not only the psychological fear of the injections but also the real concern of dosing errors due to cognitive or visual impairment. Older patients must also have the manual dexterity for self-injection and self-monitoring; given that many older individuals have arthritis, tremors and rigidity or suffer the consequences of a stroke, their lack of adequate manual skills may make hypoglycaemia a significant concern. Especially in the frail patient who lives independently, undertreatment is a likely event. Hence, a thorough assessment of the patient's clinical condition and circumstances is critically important in order to plan for necessary education and support.

The patient should be started on insulin therapy when treatment goals are not met with maximal oral agent therapy, although insulin could be started before oral agents if there is the need to bring a symptomatic patient under control rapidly. Insulin is indicated if there is marked fasting hyperglycaemia (> 250–280 mg/dL) or if the patient is very symptomatic. There is substantial individual variation in the total daily dose required, but it may be possible to start therapy with a single dose of 10–15 units of an intermediate-acting insulin (NPH or lente) before breakfast. Once the single morning dose reaches approximately 30 units, it is a good idea to add a second dose before dinner. In many instances the addition of a short-acting insulin is required, and some patients may benefit from splitting the daily dose into three administration intervals.

Prospects for the future

Changing demographics—the ageing of the population in much of the world—will continue to contribute to the creation of complex challenges in the treatment of older diabetics. Increased survival and increasing numbers of older diabetics, together with philosophical and practical changes in medical care and new diagnostic and therapeutic possibilities, are forming the basis of a new understanding of diabetes mellitus in old age. The advancement of the concepts of 'geriatric diabetology' is creating a referral field and discipline within geriatric medicine that offers longitudinal, long-term follow-up to elderly diabetics. The treatment modalities for elderly diabetics are evolving rapidly and in the future are likely to focus on better diabetes control, with targets closer to euglycaemia, especially in the less frail elderly. It is also probable that more intervention will be undertaken very early in the disease, when impaired glucose tolerance or impaired fasting glucose first occurs.

Bibliography and further reading

American Diabetes Association (1999), 'Implications of the United Kingdom Prospective Diabetes Study', *Diabetes Care*, 22, pp. 527–31.

American Diabetes Association (2000a), 'Diabetes mellitus and exercise', *Diabetes Care*, 3(suppl. 1), pp. S50–4.

American Diabetes Association (2000b), 'Standards of medical care for patients with diabetes mellitus', *Diabetes Care*, 23(suppl. 1), pp. S32–42.

Amos, A. F., McCarty, D. J. & Zimmet, P. (1997), 'The rising global burden of diabetes and its complications: estimates and projections to the year 2010', *Diabetic Medicine*, 14, pp. S7–85.

Davidson, M. B. & Peters, A. L. (1997), 'An overview of metformin in the treatment of type II diabetes mellitus', *American Journal of Medicine*, 102, pp. 99–110.

DeFronzo, R. A. (1999), 'Pharmacologic therapy for type II diabetes mellitus', *Annals of Internal Medicine*, 131, pp. 281–303.

Elias, P. K., Elias, M. F., D'Agostino, R. B., Cupples, L. A., Wilson, P. W., Silbershatz, H. & Wolfe, P. A. (1997), 'NIDDM and blood pressure as risk factors for poor cognitive performance. The Framingham Study', *Diabetes Care*, 20, pp. 1388–95.

The Expert Committee on the Diagnosis and Classification of Diabetes Mellitus (1997), 'Report of the Expert Committee on the Diagnosis and Classification of Diabetes Mellitus', *Diabetes Care*, 20, pp. 1183–97.

Greene, D. A. (1986), 'Acute and chronic complications of diabetes mellitus in older patients', *American Journal of Medicine*, 80(suppl. 5A), pp. 39–53.

Gregg, E. W., Yaffe, K., Cauley, J. A., Rolka, D. B., Blackwell, T. L., Narayan, K. M. V. & Cummings, S. R., for the Study of Osteoporotic Fractures Research Group (2000), 'Is diabetes associated with cognitive impairment and cognitive decline among older women?', *Archives of Internal Medicine*, 160, pp. 174–80.

Halter, J. B. (1999), 'Diabetes mellitus', in Hazzard, W. R., Blass, J. P., Ettinger Jnr, W. H., Halter, J. B. & Ouslander, J. G. (eds), *Principles of Geriatric Medicine and Gerontology*, 4th edn, McGraw-Hill, New York, pp. 991–1011.

Lalau, J. D., Vermersch, A., Hary, L., Andrejak, M., Isnard, F. & Quichaud, J. (1990), 'Type II diabetes in the elderly: an assessment of metformin (metformin in the elderly)', *International Journal of Clinical Pharmacology, Therapy and Toxicology*, 28, pp. 329–32.

Lee, A. T. & Cerami, A. (1996), 'Glycation', in Birren, J. E. (ed.), *Encyclopedia of Gerontology. Age, Aging, and the Aged*, vol. 1, Academic Press, Los Angeles, pp. 605–9.

McKenna, K., Morris, A. D., Azam, H., Newton, R. W., Baylis, P. H. & Thompson, C. J. (1999), 'Exaggerated vasopressin secretion and attenuated osmoregulated thirst in human survivors of hyperosmolar coma', *Diabetologia*, 42, pp. 534–8.

Meneilly, G. S., Cheung, E. & Tuokko, H. (1994), 'Counterregulatory hormone responses to hypoglycemia in the elderly patient with diabetes', *Diabetes*, 43, pp. 403–10.

Nowak, F. V. & Mooradian, A. D. (1996), 'Endocrine function and dysfunction', in Birren, J. E. (ed.), *Encyclopedia of Gerontology. Age, Aging, and the Aged*, vol. 1, Academic Press, Los Angeles, pp. 477–91.

Samos, L. F. & Roos, B. A. (1998), 'Diabetes mellitus in older persons', *Medical Clinics of North America*, 82, pp. 791–803.

Scheen, A. J. & Lefebvre, P. J. (1998), 'Oral antidiabetic agents: a guide to selection', *Drugs*, 55, pp. 225–36.

Sinclair, A. J. (1998), 'Diabetes mellitus', in Pathy, M. S. J. (ed.), *Principles and Practice of Geriatric Medicine*, 3rd edn, vol. 2, John Wiley & Sons, New York, pp. 1321–40.

Turner, R., Cull, C. & Holman, R. (1996), 'United Kingdom Prospective Diabetes Study 17: a 9-year update of a randomized, controlled trial on the effect of improved metabolic control on complications in non-insulin-dependent diabetes mellitus', *Annals of Internal Medicine*, 124, pp. 136–45.

UK Prospective Diabetes Study Group (1998a), 'Intensive blood-glucose control with sulphonylureas or insulin compared with conventional treatment and risk of complications in patients with type II diabetes (UKPDS 33)', *Lancet*, 352, pp. 837–53.

UK Prospective Diabetes Study Group (1998b), 'Tight blood pressure control and risk of macrovascular and microvascular complications in type II diabetes: UKPDS 38', *British Medical Journal*, 317, pp. 703–13.

UK Prospective Diabetes Study Group (1998c), 'Efficacy of atenolol and captopril in reducing risk of macrovascular and microvascular complications in type II diabetes: UKPDS 39', *British Medical Journal*, 317, pp. 713–20.

UK Prospective Diabetes Study Group (1998d), 'Cost effectiveness analysis of improved blood pressure control in hypertensive patients with type II diabetes: UKPDS 40', *British Medical Journal*, 317, pp. 720–6.

Chapter 42
Thyroid disorders

CHRISTOPHER R. STRAKOSCH

Introduction

The population of all industrialised Western societies is becoming older both in absolute numbers of older persons and in relative increase of the elderly to younger persons. Thyroid disorders are more common in older persons, and may differ in clinical manifestations and require different management to thyroid disorders in younger persons. In older persons thyroid disorders are often more subtle in their presentation and clinical findings, and presentation may be due to unmasking of other illnesses. Intercurrent illnesses may also result in changes in thyroid function tests, and some clinical manifestations of thyroid disorders in the elderly may be confused with the ageing process itself.

The aim of this chapter is to assist in the management of thyroid disease in the elderly so that early detection of these disorders results in not only a healthier older population but also decreased costs. Intercepting thyroid disorders before progression to hospitalisation, either due to the disorder itself or decompensation of intercurrent illnesses, will result in a decreased burden on ever more stretched national health budgets. The initial part of this chapter looks at changes in the thyroid gland itself, thyroid hormone levels and metabolism in older persons, while later sections discuss clinical manifestations and management of the major thyroid disorders: hypothyroidism, hyperthyroidism and neoplastic nodular thyroid disease in the elderly.

Anatomy and histology

Human and animal studies indicate that the thyroid gland increases in size in older persons. On a smaller scale, thyroid follicles increase in size with increased colloid and the lining epithelial cells decrease in height. There is an increased amount of extrafollicular fibrous tissue. Autoradiographic studies show frequent occurrence of hypofunctioning micronodules in these persons. Macronodular thyroid disease also becomes more frequent in the elderly in proportion to age, such that by the eighth decade about 80% of older persons will have ultrasonographically detectable thyroid nodules which could therefore be thought to be an essentially normal part of ageing. These changes result in the thyroid gland in older persons being somewhat easier to palpate and having a firmer consistency than the soft fleshy texture of the thyroid gland in younger persons.

Thyroid hormone levels in the elderly

Earlier studies suggested that changes in thyroid function were a normal process of ageing and, indeed, when thyroid hormone levels are looked at in a cross-section of older patients there are changes noted. When patients with other illnesses are excluded, however, and thyroid hormone levels are looked at only in healthy older persons, they are essentially normal. There is a decreased production of thyroxine (T4) and a decreased peripheral conversion of T4 to triiodothyronine (T3), but there is also a decrease in hepatic metabolism of both these thyroid hormones, resulting in serum free T4 levels being essentially normal in older persons and serum free T3 levels being 10–20% below the average levels in younger persons. Eighty per cent of T3 found in the bloodstream is obtained by peripheral conversion of T4 to T3, and T4 may be converted to the metabolically inactive reverse T3, but when only healthy elderly patients are studied there is in fact no increase in reverse T3 to explain the small decrease in T3. Serum thyroid stimulating hormone (TSH) levels are also normal in healthy elderly patients, although thyrotropin-releasing hormone (TRH) stimulation tests may show a decreased TSH response in both males and females.

Radioactive iodine uptake decreases in older persons but there is also a decreased metabolic clearance of iodine, and when this is corrected for, radioactive iodine uptake remains essentially normal with ageing. Metabolic rate also declines in older persons but this is accounted for by relative increase in fat to lean body mass; when corrected for fat free mass, the metabolic rate remains essentially normal in older persons as well.

In summary, although there are some changes in all levels of thyroid hormone production and metabolism, in general thyroid function is well maintained in healthy older persons.

Disorders of thyroid function

Management of disordered thyroid function in the elderly requires assessment of:

1. the cause of the disorder, since this influences the likelihood of the thyroid levels worsening, remitting or remaining stable; and
2. the significance of the disorder in the particular patient, since a mild abnormality in a patient with serious non-thyroidal illness may be more significant than a more marked abnormality in an otherwise healthy older person.

From these two may be derived the decision as to whether or not to recommend treatment.

Hypothyroidism

Causes of hypothyroidism in the elderly

Hashimoto's thyroiditis

First described by Hashimoto, a Japanese surgeon, in 1912, the condition classically consists of hypothyroidism in a patient with a large firm goitre. The aetiology was unknown in Hashimoto's time but now it is recognised as being due to an organ specific autoimmune disorder with high serum levels of antithyroid antibodies and thyroid histology showing round cell infiltrate. Some patients still present with the classical signs, but the condition is often less pronounced, with thyroid hormone levels still normal or only slightly abnormal and thyroid size normal or only slightly enlarged. Thyroid antibodies may sometimes be normal. Some authorities feel the diagnosis of Hashimoto's thyroiditis may only be made in patients with classical signs, but I feel there is little to be gained by dividing patients into groups which do not affect clinical management. I treat all patients with hypothyroidism as having Hashimoto's thyroiditis, unless another cause is apparent. Hashimoto's thyroiditis is so common in the elderly, particular elderly women, that a case can be made for routine annual measurement of levels of TSH and thyroid antibody. In one British study, the prevalence of thyroid antibodies increased with age, with 10.3% of women and 2.7% of men being positive. Patients may have positive thyroid antibodies with completely normal T4 and T3 levels, but have an elevated TSH, a situation sometimes called 'subclinical hypothyroidism'. Other patients may have an elevated TSH, with low levels of T4 and T3, and usually also with positive thyroid antibodies, so-called clinical hypothyroidism.

Iatrogenic causes of hypothyroidism in the elderly

Amiodarone

See the section on 'Amiodarone associated thyroid disorders'.

Lithium

As well as increasing the risk of autoimmune thyroid disease, lithium has an effect on intrathyroidal enzymes, worsening hypothyroidism.

Patients on lithium and amiodarone should have thyroid function tests and thyroid antibodies checked every 6 months.

Other iatrogenic causes

Other iatrogenic causes, which the patient may not recall, include a previous hemithyroidectomy for thyroid nodular disease years in the past or radioactive iodine used to treat Graves' hyperthyroidism. Radioactive iodine treatment for hyperfunctioning thyroid nodules (Plummer's disease) can also result in a slow decline in function of normal thyroid tissue many years later. Elderly patients may not recall the reason for some of their medication and it is not uncommon for thyroxine medication to be ceased accidentally when a patient is transferred, say, from home to nursing care because of inability to cope.

Clinical features of hypothyroidism

Hypothyroidism is very difficult to diagnose in the elderly by clinical means alone, since symptoms of hypothyroidism are very similar to those complained of in a euthyroid geriatric population and, to further complicate matters, thyroid disease may come on slowly over decades. Both euthyroid and hypothyroid patients may complain of tiredness, fatigue, declining mental agility with low level depression, vague arthralgia, dry skin, hair loss, cold intolerance and weight gain.

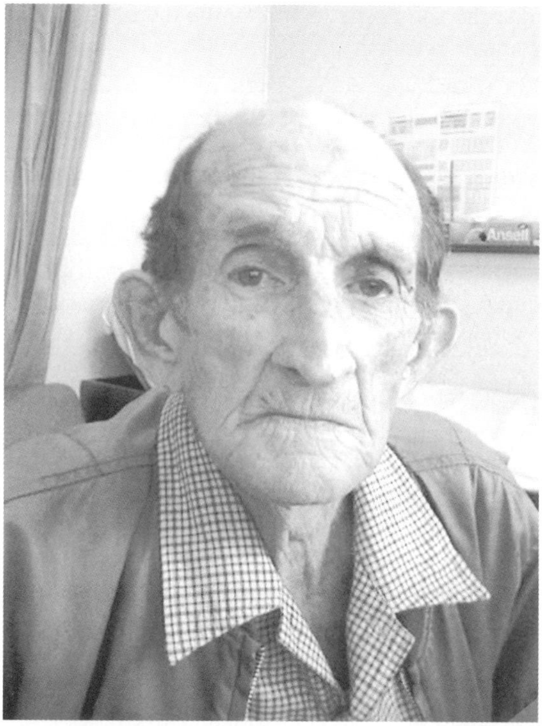

Figure 42.1 Elderly man with severe hypothyroidism. He looks little different from other euthyroid geriatric men

Box 42.1 Clinical features of hypothyroidism in the elderly

Subtle, difficult to distinguish from general geriatric population:

- slow, tired, vague, unsteady
- cold, dry skin, hoarse voice
- bradycardia, slow reflexes

All elderly patients should have a routine annual check of TSH and thyroid antibody levels.

A variety of metabolic abnormalities are reflected in biochemical changes in patients with hypothyroidism. Decreased free water clearance may cause hyponatraemia and decreased lipid clearance elevation in cholesterol and triglyceride levels. About 15% of patients will have a microcytic hypochromic anaemia, partly explained by decreased iron absorption seen in hypothyroidism. The hypochlorhydria, found in up to half of patients with hypothyroidism, will further decrease iron absorption.

The prevalence of thyroid abnormalities varies greatly between studies and between countries but does seem to be more common in areas that are iodine replete. Iodine itself may be involved in the aetiology of autoimmune thyroid disease. Women are 7 times more likely than men to have thyroid abnormalities that are more common in Asian women than Caucasian women, who, in turn, have more disorders than African women. Other risk factors include a family history of thyroid disease or other autoimmune disorders, especially pernicious anaemia and coeliac disease. The overall prevalence of hypothyroidism, both subclinical and clinical, in the elderly varies between studies but can be up to 5% in men and 15% in women. A history of smoking also may predispose persons to thyroid hypofunction, since the production of thiocyanic acid residues interferes with intrathyroidal peroxidase enzyme activity, and smoking also seems to predispose to autoimmune disorders in its own right. Lithium treatment for bipolar disorder is associated with increased prevalence of autoimmune thyroid disease.

Treatment of hypothyroidism

Now commonplace and taken for granted, the successful treatment of hypothyroidism is one of the triumphs of Western medicine. A potentially fatal condition is completely reversed by a 'natural' treatment which is active by mouth, long-lasting and has no side effects. Although the treatment was first described by British physician George Redmayne Murray in 1891, we have never done better.

Treatment of clinical hypothyroidism

Patients with clinical hypothyroidism—elevated TSH and low serum free T4 and T3 levels—should be treated even though symptoms may differ little from those expressed by the general geriatric population. Patients may attribute such symptoms to the ageing process itself and often don't realise they were unwell until they feel better with treatment. More marked hypothyroidism is associated with decrease in mental ability with increased risk of falls and fractures. In younger persons the dose of thyroxine is on average 1.6 μg/kg and may be instituted immediately without problems. In older patients, however, this approach may result in decompensation of ischaemic heart disease with worsening angina, and the treatment is usually instituted more slowly. The final thyroxine dose is, on average, 25% less than that in a younger person, being around 1.2 μg/kg. A dose of 25 μg is commenced and increased by 25 μg every 4 weeks until the final dose is reached. Thyroxine is well absorbed from the gastrointestinal tract, but is slightly inhibited by food so the dose is usually given before breakfast. Thyroxine should not be given with iron supplements since this combination may result in the thyroxine being precipitated in the gut with diminished absorption. Thyroxine has a half-life of approximately 1 week, so if the dose on one day is accidentally omitted, a double dose may be given the next day. The long half-life of thyroxine also permits it to be given in an average dose—for example, 114 μg/day may be obtained by giving 100 μg on 5 days in the week and 150 μg on, say, Wednesday and Sunday. In the US this is not necessary since many tablet strengths—for example, 112 μg—are available, whereas in Australia thyroxine is only produced in 50, 100 and 200 μg tablets. It is usual to monitor elderly patients clinically and not repeat thyroid function tests until about 8 weeks after the final dose has been reached in order to allow time for TSH to stabilise. The aim is to get a TSH around 1.0 mU/L. TSH and free T4 and free T3 tests are then repeated in 3 months, and if the levels are stable, then only every 12 months. An easy to remember regimen is to check the thyroid function tests near the patient's birthday.

Treatment of subclinical hypothyroidism

Patients with subclinical hypothyroidism—elevated TSH but with free T4 and free T3 still in the normal range—may have no specific symptoms or signs of hypothyroidism, but treatment with thyroxine has been associated with improvement in both reported wellbeing and other parameters, such as cholesterol level. A recent Dutch study found subclinical hypothyroidism to be a strong

Box 42.2 Thyroxine regimens in the elderly

Go slow, start low.

- Average thyroxine dose 1.2 μg/kg is 25% less than for younger persons.
- Start 25 μg a day, increase by 25 μg a month to final dose.
- Monitor dosage clinically, check thyroid function tests 8 weeks after final dose.
- Dosage may be averaged over the week e.g. 114 μg/day = 100 μg on 5 days and 150 μg Wednesday and Sunday.
- Should be given before meals in single dose.
- Aim to get TSH to about 1.0 mU/L.

predictor of atherosclerosis and myocardial infarction in elderly women. Since the patients are not clinically hypothyroid, the dosing regimen can be more vigorous than in clinical hypothyroidism and start, for example, at 50 μg/day with an increase in 4 weeks to the final dose with thyroid function tests then being repeated 8 weeks later.

Situations in which the dosage requirements of thyroxine may vary

Some patients seem to require higher doses of thyroxine than expected. Causes may include decreased absorption as with coeliac disease or concurrent treatment with cholestyramine or iron supplements, or increased clearance as with phenytoin treatment. Patients with other non-thyroidal illness may have normal TSH and serum free T4, but low free tertroxine, indicating a disorder of T4 to T3 conversion. This phenomenon may be seen also in patients treated with amiodarone and β-blockers.

Why don't some patients feel better after thyroxine therapy?

This is a controversial area. To the great disappointment of the treating doctor, some patients who had significant symptoms and signs of hypothyroidism do not report any improvement in wellbeing despite thyroid function tests having been returned to normal. Underlying causes could include:

- a continuing depression. Untreated hypothyroidism has been associated with depression, and hypothyroidism interferes with the efficacy of antidepressant medication. Indeed, triiodothyronine has been used with some success as an adjuvant therapy in patients with depression resistant to other medication. Hypothyroidism has been associated also with rapid-cycling bipolar disorder
- another autoimmune disorder. Coeliac disease is present in some 5% of patients with Hashimoto's thyroiditis. Many of these patients with coeliac disease are not aware of the disease being present, since symptoms are either absent, at low level and attributed to something else or not recognised as the typical coeliac symptoms of postprandial bloating and diarrhoea. Pernicious anaemia is another autoimmune disorder associated with Hashimoto's thyroiditis, as is Addison's disease. Decreased absorption of thyroxine can occur due to small bowel disease associated with malabsorption, due to a variety of causes (see Chapter 35)
- non-specific effects of the autoimmune process itself mediated by leucocyte release of lymphokines, giving the body the injury signal. There is no effective treatment for this. Some patients of their own accord may try increasing the dose of thyroxine and sometimes feel somewhat better with thyroid hormone levels above the normal range. In elderly patients, however, this can cause problems, with a decrease in bone density in the long term and an increased risk of cardiac arrhythmias in the short term.

Euthyroid sick syndrome

Thyroid hormone levels tend to be abnormal in patients with severe non-thyroidal illness, with the level of abnormality varying with the severity of the illness. There is evidence of a central suppression of the hypothalamic pituitary thyroid axis, resulting in a decrease in TSH and free T4 levels, and there is also a decrease in peripheral T4 to T3 conversion with an even lower free T3 (and elevated reverse T3). It remains controversial as to whether patients thought to have euthyroid sick syndrome should be treated or not. Some authorities feel, however, that although it is probably a defence mechanism to conserve energy, it does represent a genuine hypothyroid state and should be treated. The calculated replacement dose is commenced immediately. One of the major abnormalities seen is a T4–T3 conversion block, and some authorities recommend the use of triiodothyronine. Triiodothyronine has a shorter half-life of approximately 1 day and should be given in a divided dose. The 20 μg triiodothyronine tablet is approximately equal to the 100 μg thyroxine tablet. The small tablet size, difficulty in dividing the tablet and the short half-life make precise dosage difficult, and triiodothyronine is usually only used as a temporary measure in severely ill patients.

Myxoedema coma

Although fortunately rare, myxoedema coma is a medical emergency that carries a high mortality rate even if treated appropriately. This severe form of hypothyroidism is usually of insidious onset, with symptoms often being disregarded by patients and attending staff alike. Patients become ever more lethargic and drowsy and slip gently into coma. Signs include bradycardia, hypothermia, hypoventilation, hypotension and the finding of hyponatraemia and possible hypoglycaemia. In some cases, the onset is more rapid and is precipitated by infection, with the fever often masked by hypothermia, or by other major events such as myocardial infarction or general anaesthetic. Treatment consists of vigorous resuscitation with intravenous fluids, intravenous glucocorticoids at full stress dose of 100 mg 8 hourly and the management of any decompensating factors. The thyroid replacement regimen remains controversial. Thyroxine is given intravenously, if possible, to avoid probable diminished absorption if given by nasogastric tube. An initial loading dose of 200–500 μg, depending on the patient's size, is used initially, followed by 50–100 μg per day. Some authorities recommend using triiodothyronine as well to avoid problems of T4 to T3 conversion. Triiodothyronine is absorbed, even in the presence of gastric atony, and may be given by nasogastric tube at a dose of 10–20 μg 8 hourly. When the patient regains consciousness, the usual dose of thyroxine is given orally. Passive warming with a space blanket is preferable to active warming, which may worsen hypotension due to vasodilation.

Hyperthyroidism

Although the terms 'hyperthyroidism' and 'thyrotoxicosis' are often used interchangeably, hyperthyroidism is a more general term and refers to the finding of elevated thyroid hormone levels in the bloodstream, whereas thyrotoxicosis should be reserved for the clinical picture of significant symptoms and signs resulting from hyperthyroidism. These persons have been rendered toxic by their hyperthyroidism.

Hyperthyroidism is more common in the elderly population than in younger persons, with a prevalence between 0.5% and 2.5%, depending on studies carried out in various places of the world. The increased prevalence is mainly due to a more frequent finding of low levels of hyperthyroidism, whereas the higher thyroid hormone levels associated with typical symptoms of thyrotoxicosis are relatively less common than in younger persons.

Causes of hyperthyroidism

Graves' disease

First described by Anglo-Irish physician Robert Graves in 1835, Graves' disease is the most common

Box 42.3 Hyperthyroidism in the elderly

Patients may be apathetic rather than hyperdynamic.

- Graves' hyperthyroidism is relatively less common than in young persons.
- Autonomous thyroid nodules are relatively more common.
- Even mild 'subclinical' hyperthyroidism may have significant effects.
- Hyperthyroidism in the elderly should be treated.

cause of hyperthyroidism in younger persons, but is relatively less common in the elderly. It is an autoimmune disease in which the thyroid is subject to attack by the humoral and cellular arms of the immune system. It is a very unusual autoimmune disorder, in that instead of being destroyed, the thyroid is stimulated by an antibody directed against the TSH (thyrotrophin) receptor—thyrotrophin receptor antibody or TRAb. The destructive antibodies, antithyroglobulin and antimicrosomal antibodies, are often elevated, although not usually as much as is seen in Hashimoto's thyroiditis.

Graves' hyperthyroidism is 7 times more common in women than men and may be precipitated by major life events such as a death in the family or moving house. It is also more common in areas of iodine excess.

Patients often have a family history of thyroid or other autoimmune disorders. Graves' ophthalmopathy, the second part of the Graves' trilogy—the third being the rather rare Graves' infiltrative dermopathy (pretibial myxoedema)—is less common in the elderly than in younger persons, but when present is more severe. The management of Graves' ophthalmopathy is beyond the scope of this chapter, but its presence indicates the cause of accompanying hyperthyroidism. Patients with Graves' hyperthyroidism should be screened for pernicious anaemia and coeliac disease, two other autoimmune disorders which may accompany Graves' disease, but which are frequently clinically silent.

About 50% of patients with Graves' hyperthyroidism will have a spontaneous remission of hyperthyroidism within 12 months, although may relapse at any time.

Hyperfunctioning thyroid nodules (Plummer's disease)

Hyperthyroidism due to hyperfunctioning thyroid nodules is relatively more common in elderly patients than in younger persons. These nodules are more common in persons coming from areas of low iodine intake. Iodine deficiency is associated with endemic multinodular goitres and hyperplasia of thyroid follicular cells and, over time, the nodules may become autonomous, perhaps as a result of mutations in the TSH receptor gene. Plummer's disease does not go into remission, so treatment needs to be long term.

Amiodarone associated hyperthyroidism

See the section on 'Amiodarone associated thyroid disorders'.

Less common causes of thyrotoxicosis in the elderly

Silent thyroiditis

Silent thyroiditis is a temporary autoimmune phenomenon where elevated thyroid levels are due to release from a damaged gland. In weeks to months, levels return to normal and in about 40% of cases there is a temporary hypothyroid phase before levels return to normal once more. In the hyperthyroid phase, a radionuclidic thyroid scan shows suppressed uptake. It is rare for patients to have a continuing hypothyroidism. The hyperthyroid phase may be treated expectantly or β-blockers may be used to control cardiac symptoms. Steroids are not useful in this situation.

Subacute thyroiditis

An uncommon problem in elderly persons, subacute thyroiditis is a response of the thyroid to a viral infection. It is thought to be not due to an actual infection of the thyroid by a virus, but a condition where any of several viruses may attach to the thyroid, which is damaged in the ensuing antiviral assault. Again there is a biphasic pattern of thyroid hormone levels, with elevated thyroid levels seen for some weeks followed by return to euthyroid state. In about 40% of cases there is a hypothyroid phase with patients almost always returned to the euthyroid state. In the thyrotoxic phase, a radionuclidic thyroid scan will show suppressed uptake. Subacute thyroiditis is usually associated with severe thyroid pain in younger persons, although in elderly persons this may not be such an obvious symptom. Treatment may be with aspirin to control pain and β-blockers to control cardiac symptoms and signs. If the pain is too severe, a course of steroid, starting at prednisone 40 mg and decreasing to 0 mg over 2 weeks is dramatically effective. Occasionally patients will relapse when the steroid dose is decreased so quickly. The prednisone is then increased again and the dosage decreased more slowly.

Thyrotoxicosis factitia

Elevated thyroid hormone levels and suppressed radionuclidic thyroid scan can be due to ingestion of thyroxine. This may be inadvertent where the treating physician, and the elderly patient, are unaware that thyroxine is being administered, or it may be deliberately taken by persons in an attempt to, say, control weight. Serum thyroglobulin is suppressed in this situation, whereas it is elevated in the other conditions that cause high thyroid hormone levels.

Hashimoto's thyroiditis

Hashimoto's thyroiditis may present in a thyrotoxic phase before the condition goes on to hypothyroidism. This is often difficult to differentiate from Graves' hyperthyroidism, particularly since TRAb may be low positive in this situation. Treatment is initially the same—that is, with carbimazole—but the dose is rapidly decreased as the thyroid hormone levels fall and the patient progresses to thyroxine replacement.

Management of hyperthyroidism in the elderly

Mild hyperthyroidism, sometimes known as subclinical hyperthyroidism

This condition, in which TSH is suppressed with free T4 and free T3 still in the normal range, is quite common and may be found in 5–6% of the elderly population. It is usually due to a mild Plummer's disease with autonomously functioning thyroid nodules. Graves' hyperthyroidism is not usually stable and tends to progress to more active disease, but may be present at a chronically low level. Although usually asymptomatic in younger persons, elderly persons tolerate even mild hyperthyroidism very poorly and there is a markedly increased risk of cardiac arrhythmias, particularly atrial fibrillation. One study showed that a person is 3 times as likely to develop atrial fibrillation within 10 years of the finding of suppressed TSH but normal thyroid hormone levels as is a person with normal TSH levels. There is at least some evidence that bone density decreases at a rate of about 1.0% per year in subclinical hyperthyroidism. A recent Dutch study found subclinical hyperthyroidism to be associated with an increased rate of dementia in elderly women. Because of these findings, subclinical hyperthyroidism should be treated in older persons.

Clinical hyperthyroidism

In this chapter clinical hyperthyroidism refers to the finding of suppressed TSH and elevated thyroid hormone levels. Some patients, especially those with Graves' hyperthyroidism, may exhibit the typical symptoms and signs of thyrotoxicosis with a staring appearance, tremor, tachycardia, hyperphagia and weight loss. It is more common, however, for elderly patients to have more subtle non-specific symptoms such as lethargy, weight loss due more to anorexia than to hyperphagia, depression, arthralgia and muscle weakness. This constellation has been known for many years as 'apathetic thyrotoxicosis'. In younger persons, hyperthyroidism due to hyperfunctioning thyroid nodules (Plummer's disease) accounts for only about 12% of patients with hyperthyroidism, the majority having Graves' hyperthyroidism. In elderly patients, however, Plummer's disease is relatively more common. Plummer's disease usually is of slow onset and rarely results in full blown thyrotoxicosis with markedly elevated thyroid function tests. On the other hand, Graves' disease typically comes on more rapidly and is associated with a more florid clinical constellation of symptoms and signs. In some patients, Graves' disease may supervene on a multinodular goitre, so the finding of elevated thyroid function tests in a patient with a multinodular goitre does not necessarily give the diagnosis of Plummer's disease. Because of the increased incidence of non-specific symptoms, more subtle signs and the more frequent finding of Plummer's disease, elderly patients with hyperthyroidism usually require more vigorous investigation to make the diagnosis than is the case with younger patients who might have obvious Graves' disease.

Investigations

The recommended list of investigations of hyperthyroidism in elderly patients is:

- serum TSH, free T4, free T3
- TRAb, antithyroglobulin and antimicrosomal antibody
- parietal and gliadin antibody (in patients with Graves' disease)
- radionuclidic thyroid scan (Figure 42.2). Although radionuclidic thyroid scans may not be necessary in young persons who have typical symptoms and signs of Graves' hyperthyroidism with Graves' ophthalmopathy, in elderly persons, radionuclidic thyroid scans are useful for differentiating between Graves' disease, Plummer's disease and Graves' disease supervening on a multinodular goitre. In Graves' hyperthyroidism, the radionuclidic thyroid scan will show a diffusely increased uptake. In Plummer's disease there are one or more areas of nodular hyperfunction, with the rest of the thyroid being suppressed. The scan picture of Graves' disease supervening on a multinodular goitre shows increased uptake, with areas of decreased uptake corresponding with nodules on ultrasound, whereas in Plummer's disease the nodules seen on ultrasound are associated with increased uptake in the radionuclidic thyroid scan.

Management of hyperthyroidism in the elderly

Since even mild or 'subclinical' hyperthyroidism can cause problems in elderly persons, it is recommended that treatment be offered until thyroid hormone levels and TSH levels reach the mid-normal range. The usual treatment is with carbimazole (Neomercazole) which inhibits organification of tyrosine and the coupling of iodotyrosines and therefore causes decreased production of thyroxine. The other thionamide drug available, propylthiouracil, is sometimes used, but it has a shorter half-life of 75 minutes compared with about 5 hours for carbimazole and a much shorter biological duration of action. It is also a weaker agent, so higher doses are needed with a resulting increased risk of side effects.

Dosing regimen

Carbimazole is usually given in higher doses to begin with and the dose tailed off when the thyroid hormone levels are normalised. For example, a patient with moderately elevated thyroid levels may be commenced on carbimazole 5 mg ii bd with thyroid function tests checked in 4 weeks, and the dose then halved to i bd or ii mane if levels are then in the normal range. In general, lower doses may be used because of decreased metabolism of the agent in older persons. Once a stable dose has been reached, it is continued until there is a remission if the patient has Graves' disease, or indefinitely if the patient has Plummer's disease. The major side effect of carbimazole and propylthiouracil is agranulocytosis. Fortunately, this is a rare problem, occurring in about 1 in 200 persons, but it can have most serious consequences. Patients should be warned to contact the prescribing doctor if they develop a fever or severe sore throat, and this warning should be documented. Less serious but more common side effects are pruritic skin rash, arthralgia, nausea or vomiting, especially with propylthiouracil. The skin rash may be managed with antihistamines and often remits as the dosage of the agent is decreased. The other thionamide may be substituted if side effects occur, but there is a cross effect in about 50% of patients.

If at the end of 12 months there is no sign of remission in patients with Graves' disease, or for patients with Plummer's disease who cannot expect a remission, another option is radioactive iodine. In some parts of the world, radioiodine is the initial treatment of choice in patients with both Graves' hyperthyroidism and Plummer's disease. Radioactive iodine has been available since World War II, does not cause increased rates of malignancy and is in general very safe. Originally it was hoped that a small dose of radioiodine in patients with Graves' hyperthyroidism would suppress the thyroid to normal function, but in time it appears that all persons will continue on to hypothyroidism over years. It is probably best to use a dose of radioiodine which will render the patient hypothyroid at the start. The patient is then commenced on thyroxine long term. The major problem associated with the use of radioiodine in patients with Graves'

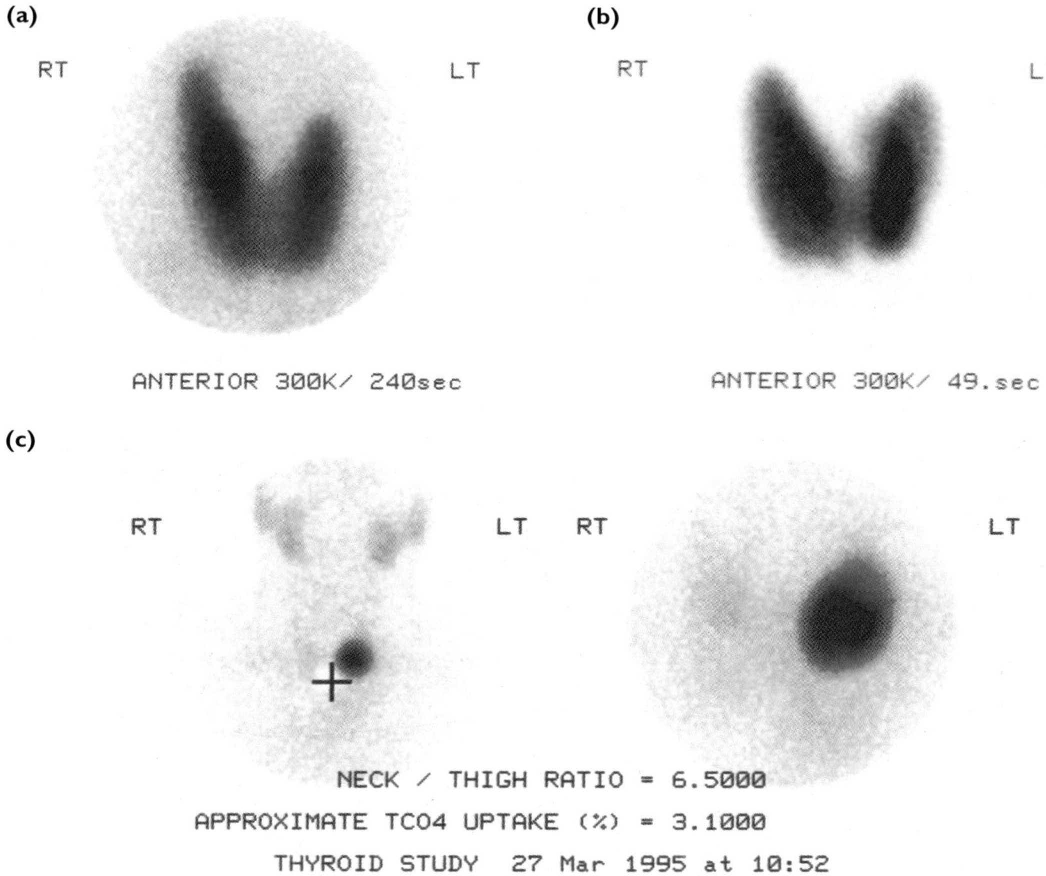

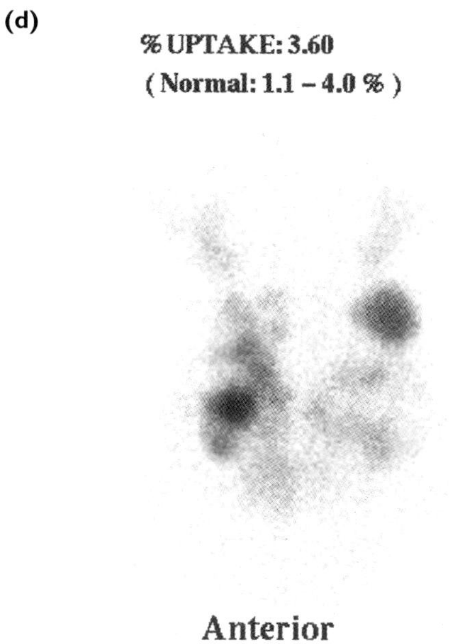

Figure 42.2 Radionuclidic thyroid scans in: **(a)** a normal scan; **(b)** a patient with Graves' hyperthyroidism; **(c)** a patient with a hyperfunctioning thyroid nodule; and **(d)** an elderly patient with a multinodular goitre and the typical patchy thyroid scan

hyperthyroidism is a 15% chance of worsening Graves' ophthalmopathy. Because of this and the general concern in society about the use of radioactive materials (in Japan, radioiodine is not used much at all), there is a tendency to continue with carbimazole indefinitely as the treatment of Graves' hyperthyroidism.

If radioiodine is to be used, carbimazole is ceased in patients with Graves' hyperthyroidism 3 days before the dose is given to unblock organification of iodine, so the radioiodine is taken up into thyroglobulin. The penetration of the damaging ray (a β-particle) is only 2 mm. Radioiodine also releases a penetrating γ-ray which has not been shown to be of any harm to the patient, let alone any bystander. However, patients should probably stay away from babies and pregnant women for a week, the biological half-life of the radioiodine. Patients with Plummer's disease should cease the carbimazole several weeks before the dose is given to allow thyroid hormone levels to rise and to suppress the normal thyroid tissue in order to keep it out of harm's way. In Plummer's disease the hyperfunctioning thyroid nodules are ablated and the remaining thyroid tissue is able to take over and prevent permanent hypothyroidism. The suppressed tissue, however, may still take up small amounts of the radioiodine and the patient may drift into hypothyroidism decades after the dose is given. Despite this and because the alternative is to keep the patient on carbimazole indefinitely, radioiodine is the treatment of choice in Plummer's disease.

Amiodarone associated thyroid disorders

Amiodarone is a cardiac medication used quite frequently in elderly patients to treat refractory arrhythymias. Amiodarone has a very long half-life of, on average, 50 days. It is 37.2% by weight organic iodine and a 200 mg tablet will release approximately 6 mg of iodine into the circulation every day, compared with the average iodine ingestion in elderly persons in the West of about 0.5 mg a day. Amiodarone has a very complicated effect on thyroid function, which is still not fully understood. The major effect is to block conversion of T4 to T3 with the result that almost all patients will have changes in thyroid function tests. Free T3 levels fall by up to 30% in the first few weeks, with a slight compensatory rise in TSH. Much of this elevation of TSH is due to a decrease in T4 to T3 conversion in the pituitary gland with a decrease in the feedback signal. Free T4 levels may increase by about 30% in the first few weeks in response to this increased TSH. The TSH and T4 levels then slowly fall to pretreatment levels, although T3 levels remain decreased. As well, some patients progress to more marked thyroid abnormalities.

Abnormalities of thyroid function or development of frank disease are not, in themselves, reasons for discontinuation of amiodarone. It is an effective treatment for otherwise refractory arrhythymias; it has a long half-life, so that even if stopped, effects will continue for months; and the thyroid abnormalities, with occasional exceptions, are easily and effectively treated.

Amiodarone associated hypothyroidism

As well as the above minor increase in TSH with increase in T4, about 20% of patients will have a further increase of TSH and a fall in T4. About half of these, especially women and persons with a family history of autoimmune disorders, will

Box 42.4 Amiodarone induced thyroid disorders

- 20% patients develop low level hypothyroidism, a few autoimmune thyroiditis; thyroxine dosage may need to be higher to normalise TSH
- 3% patients develop hyperthyroidism
  - Type I autoimmune hyperthyroidism—treated with carbimazole
  - Type II thyroiditis treated with steroids, cease amiodarone
- Type II thyroiditis excepted, if the patient requires amiodarone for cardiac problems, should stay on it

develop Hashimoto's thyroiditis with positive antithyroid antibodies. It is usually very difficult to decide if early symptoms are due to the thyroid abnormality or to the underlying condition. If TSH is only mildly elevated and T4 levels are normal with T3 only a little down, treatment may be withheld. But if thyroid antibodies are present, rather than wait until symptoms become severe, treatment should be commenced to normalise thyroid hormone levels. If the hypothyroid state is of recent duration and has been detected before the patient has become severely hypothyroid, thyroxine treatment may be commenced at full dose rather than slowly increasing the dosage as would normally be the case in the elderly.

Amiodarone associated hyperthyroidism

Up to 9% of patients will develop amiodarone associated hyperthyroidism, especially in areas of iodine deficiency. Two types of hyperthyroidism have been described as being associated with amiodarone, although they may represent the ends of a spectrum:

- *Type 1* This is the more usual form of hyperthyroidism, being a version of iodine induced or 'Jod-Basedow' hyperthyroidism, and follows a similar course to Graves' hyperthyroidism. Amiodarone may also induce a flare up in activity of autonomously functioning thyroid nodules. Treatment is with carbimazole, which may need to be continued long-term. Radioactive iodine may not be used because of suppression of uptake by the enormous iodine load from the amiodarone.
- *Type 2* This is an amiodarone induced thyroiditis which is more difficult to treat. Patients may have a tender thyroid on palpation. Elevated thyroid hormone levels are due to release of hormones from a damaged thyroid gland. Levels remain elevated for weeks to months before returning to the euthyroid state or returning to normal. In about 40% of cases there is a further hypothyroid phase, but again over weeks to months thyroid levels return to normal. Treatment is either expectant if symptoms are not too severe, or with steroids using, say, prednisone 50 mg day decreasing to 0 mg over 4–6 weeks in more severe cases. An intermediate course is to use low level β-blockade only while patients have elevated thyroid hormone levels. A few patients develop a severe thyroiditis that does not respond to steroids and may need urgent thyroidectomy. In all cases of suspected type 2 hyperthyroidism, the amiodarone should be ceased.

It may be difficult, however, to differentiate between the two types of amiodarone induced hyperthyroidism and, in these cases—particularly if the patient is severely thyrotoxic—carbimazole and steroids should be used together. It has been suggested that colour flow Doppler sonography be used to assist in differentiation, since patients with type 1 are said to have increased vascularity in the thyroid and with type 2 decreased vascularity.

Monitoring patients treated with amiodarone

Patients being commenced on amiodarone should be questioned about any personal or family history of thyroid disorders. Thyroid function tests and thyroid antibody levels should be checked 3 months after commencement and then every 6 months of treatment. Since the autoimmune types of amiodarone induced thyroid dysfunction, Hashimoto's thyroiditis and type 1 hyperthyroidism may come on months to years after cessation of the amiodarone, patients should be checked for several years.

Nodular thyroid disorders

As noted above, thyroid volume normally increases in the older person, with an increase in follicular size and a decrease in the height of lining epithelial cells. Extrafollicular fibrous connective tissue increases in amount, so the thyroid normally feels more nodular in older persons. Ultrasonographic examination of the thyroid in older persons reveals that there is a steadily increasing prevalence of detectable thyroid nodules, with a rough correlation with age, such that by the seventh decade about

70% of normal persons will have nodules and by the eighth decade, 80%, with men being somewhat less likely to have nodules than women. If only clinically significant nodules are counted (those more than 1.0 cm in diameter), still about 5% of persons over the age of 60 will be included. Nodular goitres are often noted incidentally in persons having neck imaging for other purposes—for example, Doppler studies of the carotid, or even routine chest X-rays in which tracheal deviation is noted. Risk factors for nodular goitre include:

- increasing age
- areas of iodine deficiency. There is evidence that iodine levels in older persons in Australia may be lower than previously thought
- family history of goitre. A low level intrathyroidal peroxidase deficiency may predispose to development of multinodular goitre
- history of radiation exposure in childhood. Radiation therapy was used in the past to treat several medical conditions, including acne and chronic tonsillitis. Persons who may have been exposed to nuclear fallout from atomic tests, or military personnel more directly involved in the atomic programs, are now reaching older age.

Multinodular goitre

Multinodular goitre refers to benign nodular enlargement of the thyroid due to a variety of endogenous or exogenous factors. The initiating process may be a deficiency of the intrathyroidal enzyme peroxidase, rendering the thyroid less efficient in production of thyroid hormone with resulting reactive enlargement, thereby avoiding hypothyroidism. Persons with a relatively low level of deficiency may not have a goitre at all. In areas of chronic iodine deficiency, these adaptive processes will be compromised, causing endemic goitre in persons with any peroxidase deficiency at all. The term 'endemic goitre' is used if more than 15% of the population are affected.

Patients may present with symptoms of pressure in the neck, dysphagia or just be concerned with the cosmetic appearance. The natural history of multinodular goitre in individuals is unclear since the several large studies were cross-sectional and looked at changes in overall prevalence of goitres with time. Treatment is conservative if possible. In the past, it was felt that using thyroxine to suppress TSH would result in a decrease in goitre size, but this approach is marginally effective, if at all. Iatrogenic suppression of TSH is problematic in elderly persons who tolerate even borderline hyperthyroidism very poorly: there is an increased risk of cardiac arrhythmias and the elevated thyroid hormone levels may result in a decrease in bone density over time. If local neck symptoms are too troublesome, the only effective treatment is surgery in the hands of an experienced surgeon. Often one lobe of the thyroid is more affected than the other, leading to hemithyroidectomy being performed. This is probably not the best approach, since the underlying process causing the goitre is present on both sides and the remaining gland may well increase in size over time, even if the patient is being treated with thyroxine. A second surgical approach is much more difficult because of scarring from the first operation. If surgery is contemplated, it is best to go to an almost total thyroidectomy, leaving some thyroid tissue to protect the parathyroid glands. The patient is then commenced on thyroxine in a dose adjusted to give a TSH in the mid- to low-normal range. The amount of thyroxine needed is a little less than that used in younger persons and is usually about 1.2 μg per kg body weight.

Solitary nodules or dominant nodules in multinodular goitres

Single nodules, which are greater than 1.0 cm in diameter, or nodules that are much larger than other nodules in a multinodular goitre, should be investigated for malignancy. About 5–6% of such nodules are malignant, meaning that thyroid cancer is quite common in older persons, recalling that 5% of the older population have significant nodules—a prevalence of about 1 in 400. The annual death rate from thyroid cancer, however, is only 4 per million. Most thyroid cancers pursue a fairly benign course, with the exception of a few aggressive types. The excess 7% of elderly patients who die within 5 years of diagnosis, compared with an age adjusted population, is mainly due to these more malignant tumours.

Clinical features of thyroid nodules, which increase suspicion of malignancy, are:

- rapid increase in size of a nodule. Sudden painful increase, however, is probably due to a haemorrhage into a nodule and may be relieved with aspiration
- masses which are firm and attached to overlying structures and which do not move much with swallowing, or which are associated with a hoarse voice.

The investigation of choice is fine-needle aspiration. Provided a good sample is obtained (more than 5 groups of follicular cells), a negative result virtually rules out thyroid malignancy. Nodules do not become malignant: they either are or are not at onset. Thyroid ultrasonography may be used to guide the needle, but thyroid ultrasound itself is not a cost-effective way of investigating thyroid nodules. Radionuclidic thyroid scans are not useful in this situation either, since functioning or 'warm' nodules may still be malignant. Hyperfunctioning nodules, with suppressed TSH, on the other hand, are virtually never malignant.

Thyroid malignancy in the elderly

Although the incidence of differentiated (papillary and follicular) thyroid carcinoma does not seem to increase with age, the frequency of the different types of cancer does vary. Papillary carcinoma, the major malignancy in younger persons, is relatively less common in older persons and the anaplastic carcinoma, fortunately uncommon, is virtually only seen in persons over the age of 65 years. All types of thyroid malignancy, however, are said to carry a worse prognosis in older persons.

Papillary carcinoma

Although relatively less common than in younger persons, papillary carcinomas are still the most common thyroid malignancy seen in older persons. They tend to be more aggressive than in younger persons, with a greater tendency to early local metastases, but still carry a favourable prognosis. The tumours are 2–4 times more frequent in women than men, are non-encapsulated and feel firm on palpation, and sometimes enlarged cervical lymph nodes may be detected, indicating metastases. Psammoma bodies, areas of interstitial calcification, are virtually only ever seen in papillary carcinoma and may show up as stippling in X-rays of the neck. Diagnosis is finally made on histological grounds. Patients with a mixed follicular and papillary pattern are now classified as papillary rather than follicular carcinomas. Autopsy studies of thyroid glands in older patients show that there is a 10–20% prevalence of small, < 1.0 cm diameter, 'occult' papillary carcinomas. These are seen as often in men as women, unlike the clinical papillary carcinomas, and seem to represent a different, quite benign, disorder.

Follicular carcinoma of the thyroid

Follicular carcinoma is relatively more common in older persons, with the peak incidence being between 60 and 70 years of age. Women are more commonly affected than men, and the tumours are more common in areas of iodine deficiency. Presentation is usually as a firm thyroid nodule and some 40% will have distant metastases at the time of diagnosis, usually to lung or bone. Follicular carcinomas may be difficult to differentiate from benign follicular adenomas on histopathology, and a careful search needs to be undertaken for microvascular invasion. A promising line of research has found that there are certain tumour markers, which are expressed only in malignant tissue. If confirmed, this will assist in differentiating adenomas from carcinomas in tissue obtained from fine-needle aspiration. Follicular carcinomas were said to have a worse prognosis than papillary carcinomas, mainly due to the tendency to widespread metastases at presentation. If this is corrected for, some studies have shown little difference between the two types. However, there is a poorly differentiated subtype known as 'insular carcinoma', which carries a significantly worse prognosis. Inclusion of this subtype in the main group of follicular carcinomas may account for some of the increase in reported mortality. Apart from the presence of metastases, increasing patient age, size of tumour and the presence of local invasion are associated with a worse outcome. Men with follicular carcinoma of the thyroid do a little worse than women.

Treatment of differentiated thyroid carcinoma

Treatment of differentiated thyroid cancer in the elderly is essentially the same as that in younger persons. If the carcinoma is of significant size (more than 1.0 cm in diameter), the patient undergoes a total thyroidectomy with ablation of residual thyroid tissue by high dose radioactive iodine. The patient is then placed on a dose of thyroxine, adequate to just suppress the TSH, indefinitely. Once functioning tissue has been ablated, patients can be followed up with measurement of serum thyroglobulin. Undetectable or very low levels of thyroglobulin make presence of metastases very unlikely. If there is suspicion of local recurrence of the malignancy or of metastases, the patient undergoes a whole-body radioiodine scan after thyroxine replacement has been withdrawn for several weeks to maximise TSH levels. The high dose radioiodine both detects and treats the recurrence.

Anaplastic carcinoma of the thyroid

Anaplastic carcinoma, the most aggressive of the thyroid cancers, is virtually only seen in patients over the age of 65. The female to male ratio is 2.4:1. Presentation is usually with a rapidly enlarging mass in the neck with dysphagia and neck tenderness. Radiotherapy and chemotherapy are not useful and the best chance of prolonging life is with vigorous surgical intervention. The average survival, however, is only some months.

Bibliography and further reading

Burman, K. D. (ed.) (1995), 'Thyroid cancer I', *Endocrinology and Metabolism Clinics of North America*, 24(4).

Burman, K. D. (ed.) (1996), 'Thyroid cancer II', *Endocrinology and Metabolism Clinics of North America*, 25(1).

Collin, P. (1994), 'Autoimmune thyroid disorders and coeliac disease', *European Journal of Endocrinology*, 130, pp. 137–40.

De Groot, L. J. (1999), 'Dangerous dogmas in medicine: the nonthyroidal illness syndrome', *Journal of Clinical Endocrinology and Metabolism*, 84, pp. 151–64.

Hak, A. E., Pols, H. A., Visser, T. J., Drexhage, H. A., Hofman, A. & Witteman, J. C. (2000), 'Subclinical hypothyroidism is an independent risk factor for atherosclerosis and myocardial infarction in elderly women: the Rotterdam Study', *Annals of Internal Medicine*, 15, 132(4), pp. 270–8.

Iudica-Souza, C. & Burch, H. B. (1999), 'Amiodarone-induced thyroid dysfunction', *The Endocrinologist*, 9, pp. 216–27.

Jordan, R. M. (1995), 'Myxedema coma. Pathophysiology, therapy, and factors affecting prognosis', *Medical Clinics of North America*, 79, pp. 185–94.

Kalmijn, S., Mehta, K. M., Pols, H. A., Hofman, A., Drexhage, H. A. & Breteler, M. M. (2000), 'Subclinical hyperthyroidism and the risk of dementia. The Rotterdam Study', *Clinical Endocrinology* (Oxf), 53(6), pp. 733–7.

Loh, K. C. (2000), 'Amiodarone-induced thyroid disorders: a clinical review', *Postgraduate Medical Journal*, 76, pp. 133–40.

Mariotti, S., Franceschi, C., Cossarizza, A. & Pinchera, A. (1995), 'The aging thyroid', *Endocrine Reviews*, 16, pp. 686–715.

Robuschi, G. et al. (1987), 'Hypothyroidism in the elderly', *Endocrine Reviews*, 8, pp. 142–53.

Part IX

Haematological and malignant conditions

Chapter 43
Anaemia

KAREN E. CHARLTON and INGRID C. SCHLOSS

Introduction

Twenty-four per cent of persons over the age of 65 years seeking medical attention are anaemic, with an estimated prevalence between 27% and 40% in all men aged 85 years and older and between 16% and 21% in women of the same age. Institutionalised elderly or those with cognitive impairment may show a prevalence of anaemia of 30–50% in men and 25–40% in women. There is a paucity of data on the prevalence of anaemia in elderly populations in developing countries, although some cross-sectional studies have demonstrated a similarly high prevalence. A South African study found that 1 in 7 of the older subjects studied was anaemic (14% of the population). Consistent with studies conducted in America and Europe, iron deficiency predominated in the South African study, followed by folate deficiency and finally vitamin B_{12} deficiency.

Numerous components of red blood cells facilitate the transport and delivery of oxygen around the body. These include protein (globin of haemoglobin), iron, vitamin B_{12} (cobalamin) and folate. A deficiency of any one of these parameters may result in a reduction in the concentration of haemoglobin or number of red blood cells leading to anaemia, which causes fatigue and, in some instances, cardiovascular complications. Causes of micronutrient deficiencies in the elderly are usually multifactorial. Physiological changes that affect iron, folic acid and vitamin B_{12} status include achlorhydria and lowered secretion of intrinsic factor, chronic disease and inflammation, chronic polypharmacy, gastrointestinal bleeding as well as poverty, physical inability to prepare food, alcoholism and inadequate dietary intake.

It is likely, however, that the most common cause of anaemia in the elderly is that associated with chronic disease. Anaemia of chronic disease may result from underlying conditions such as cancer, rheumatoid arthritis or chronic infections. A defect in iron release and ineffective recycling of iron from ageing red blood cells results in an insufficient supply of iron delivered to the bone marrow for incorporation into newly forming erythrocytes.

Haemoglobin is the most often used indicator of anaemia; however, there has been much debate regarding the use of a single cut-off value for haemoglobin (Hb) to define anaemia in older adults. This is partly due to the marked overlap in the frequency distribution curves of anaemic and normal individuals, together with an apparent decline in Hb concentrations with age, particularly in men. In the US, data from the NHANES II study suggests Hb reference values for the definition of anaemia in men and women older than 65 years to be 12.6 g/dL and 11.7 g/dL, respectively. The World Health Organization (WHO) criteria for anaemia are Hb values below 13 g/dL and 12 g/dL for adult men and women, respectively, and no separate reference values are given for older adults. Recently, Izaks and colleagues (1999) demonstrated that anaemia, defined using WHO criteria, was associated with an increased risk of 10 year mortality in persons aged 85+ years. These authors concluded that WHO reference values for Hb in adults are appropriate for use in the elderly, and that Hb levels even slightly below normal may be indicative of disease in this age group.

As with any understanding of a clinical problem, the diagnosis of anaemia requires a careful history and a meticulous physical examination, as anaemia may be the symptom of an underlying cause. Anaemia may be overlooked, especially in cases where it is already advanced, as the patient may present with non-haematologic symptoms such as congestive cardiac failure. Despite recognised symptoms of anaemia such as pallor, fatigue and shortness of breath, among others, indices of the red blood cell, such as structure and form, assist in diagnostic confirmation and provide clues for management. However, this does not indicate a battery of tests for all anaemic patients. A discerning evaluation of the investigation should allow for an accurate but simple procedure. The rest of the chapter will

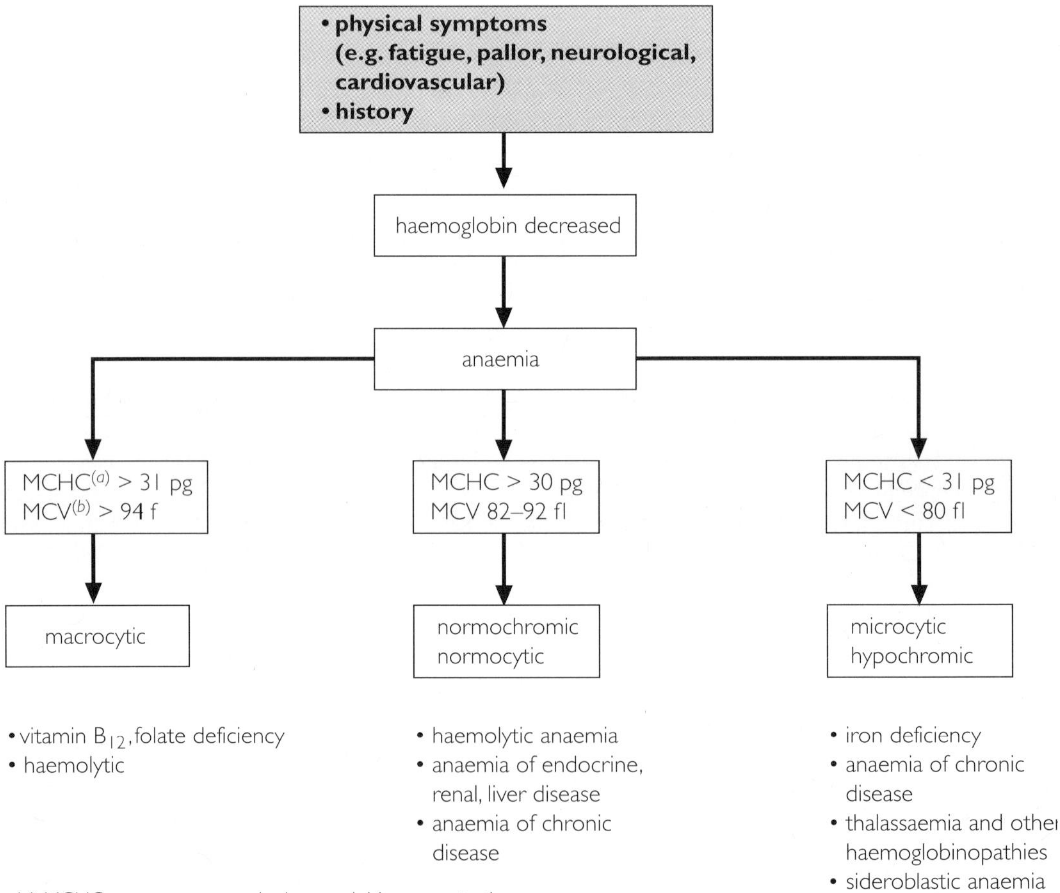

(*a*) MCHC = mean corpuscular haemoglobin concentration.
(*b*) MCV = mean corpuscular volume.

Figure 43.1 Algorithm for morphological classification ADAPTED FROM LEE ET AL. (1999)

present each of the anaemias based on their morphological characteristics (see Figure 43.1).

Microcytic hypochromic anaemia

Refer to Figure 43.2. These anaemias are linked not only by their morphology but also by their haemoglobin concentration, which is generally reduced. The degree of microcytosis and hypochromia is proportional to the severity of the anaemia.

Iron deficiency anaemia

Iron deficiency anaemia can present in up to 20% of elderly persons seeking medical attention, with an overall prevalence in older adults of 8.3%.

Iron status is determined by the balance achieved between absorption and the sum of excretion, the

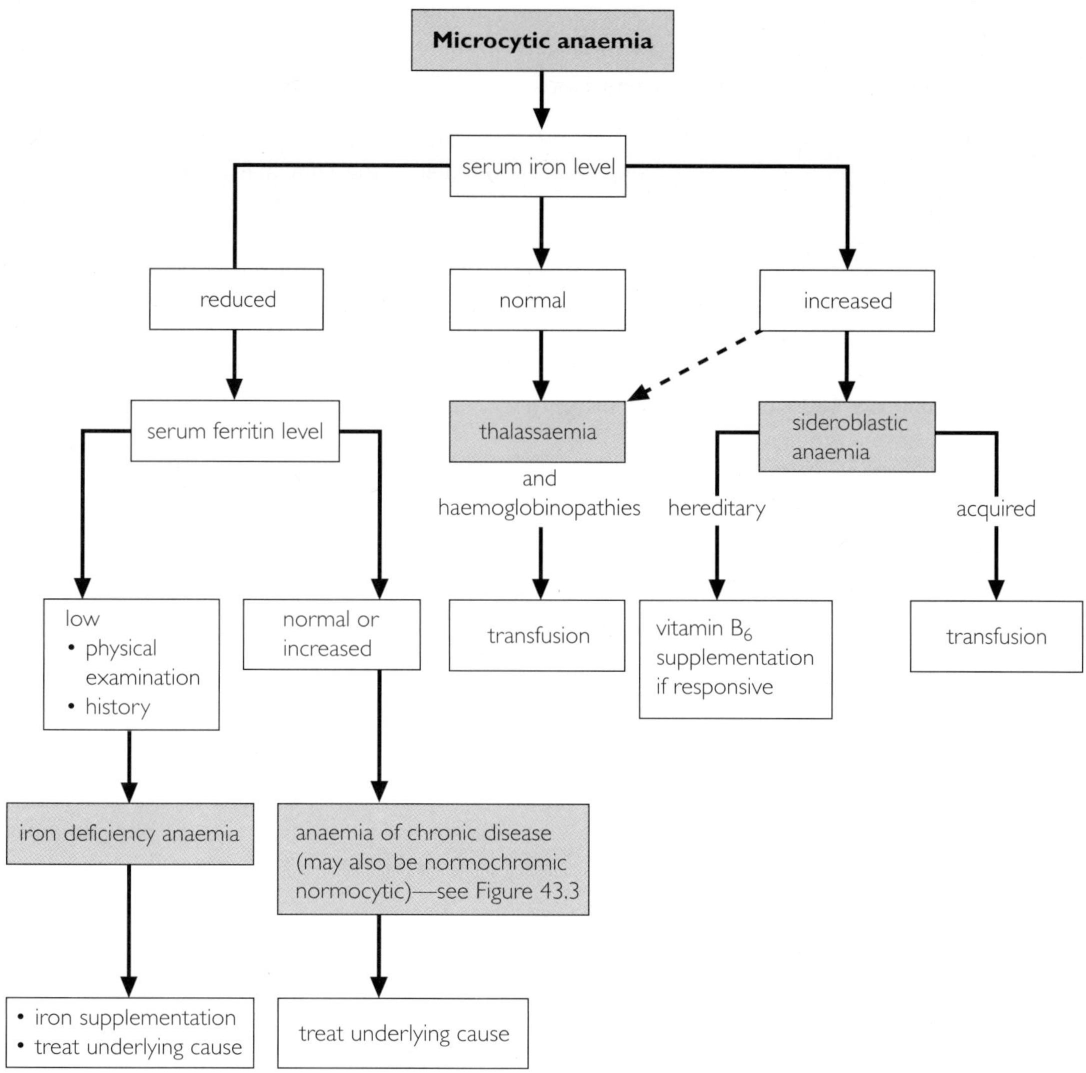

Figure 43.2 Algorithm for microcytic anaemia differentiation and management ADAPTED FROM LEE ET AL. (1999)

requirements for growth and development in children, and menstrual losses or the demands of pregnancy and lactation in women. Since excretion is relatively fixed and limited, iron balance is achieved through the regulation of absorption. The intestinal mucosa modifies absorption as an inverse function of body stores, so that any change in body absorption must be interpreted in the context of iron balance. In the elderly, therefore, the body's need for iron is determined primarily by the rate of excretion.

There is conflicting data regarding changes, if any, that occur in iron absorption with ageing. There is some evidence that iron absorption decreases with age, but only with non-haem dietary sources from a mixed meal. This may be related to hypochlorhydia or the negative feedback effects of gradually increasing iron stores. Sixty per cent of body iron is within Hb in the circulating red cells. The iron stores of healthy men aged 20–50 years average about 1000 mg, and those of women of the same age only about 300 mg, due to losses associated with menstrual blood losses. After menopause in women and after the age of 50 years in men, body iron stores begin to increase. By age 70 years, a woman's average iron reserve is 800 mg, while a man's is 1200 mg. Consequently, unlike with infants and young women where iron deficiency is a consequence of increased requirements and decreased intake, nutrition related iron deficiency occurs in less than 5% of the elderly population and is predominantly the result of blood loss due to underlying disease or medication.

Iron metabolism

Iron is an essential constituent for haemoglobin and therefore erythropoeisis. Iron is consumed in two forms: non-haem iron and haem iron. Haem iron is rapidly absorbed, transported and absorbed intact. Non-haem iron has a slower absorption rate and is often tightly bound in organic molecules (e.g. amino acids, fructose) in the form of ferric iron (Fe^{3+}). Non-haem iron needs to be transformed into the more soluble ferrous iron state (Fe^{2+}) for absorption. All the iron in grains and vegetables and about 60% of the iron in animal food sources is non-haem iron; the remaining portion of iron (40%) in meat, poultry and fish is the haem type. Milk, cheese and eggs do not contain haem iron. Iron is absorbed mainly proximal to the jejenum, and the gastrointestinal environment has important effects on the absorption of non-haem iron. Only about 5–10% of total dietary iron intake is of the haem type, although this will be absorbed 5 times more effectively than non-haem sources. A number of factors either promote or inhibit iron absorption, particularly the non-haem type.

Promoters

- Ascorbic acid (vitamin C) is well known for aiding the absorption of iron due to its excellent reducing effect on ferric form (Fe^{3+}) to ferrous form (Fe^{2+}), as well as its ability to bind to iron to form a more absorbable complex. Reducing substances must be consumed at the same time as non-haem iron to be effective (e.g. orange juice taken with breakfast cereal).
- Certain animal proteins found in meat, fish and poultry (MFP) enhance the absorption of iron, although the exact factor is not known. The release of amino acids and polypeptides probably forms absorbable complexes with non-haem iron.
- An adequate amount of calcium helps bind and remove inhibiting agents (see below).

Inhibitors

- Phytates (found in unrefined cereals and soybeans), phosphate, fibre and oxalate may bind with iron, rendering it non-bioavailable.
- Tannin in tea, as well as EDTA, a food preservative, can cause a 50% reduction in the absorption of non-haem iron.
- Iron in egg yolk is poorly absorbed because of the presence of phosvitin (a phosphoprotein isolated from vitellin in egg yolk).

Iron transport and storage

After absorption, iron is transported from the intestine to the tissues by the transport protein, transferrin. Specific receptors for transferrin are found on the cell membranes of target tissues that bind the transferrin-iron complex with subsequent release of iron into the cell. Iron supply is therefore indicated by the degree of saturation of the transferrin, where a low saturation indicates a low supply. Iron is stored in the form of ferritin and haemosiderin which are present in the bone marrow, liver and reticuloendothelial cells.

The causes and development of iron deficiency anaemia

Iron deficiency anaemia, accompanied by a drop in haemoglobin, is usually the end result of a long period of negative iron balance and progressive depletion of iron stores until deficiency results (see Table 43.1). A characteristic set of distinctive stages of iron deficiency exist whereby ferritin levels become reduced prior to changes in haemoglobin concentration. Patients who present with symptoms compatible with anaemia, but who have a normal haemoglobin level, should have their ferritin levels checked to determine early signs of deficiency.

Factors that contribute to iron deficiency are listed in Box 43.1. Iron deficiency in the elderly is almost exclusively due to blood loss from the gastrointestinal tract, but may also be caused by impaired iron absorption associated with hypochlorhydria, partial/complete gastrectomy, or reduced gastric acidity due to chronic use of some medications (see Table 43.2).

Diagnosis

A diagnosis is usually possible based on a physical examination, history and haematological evaluation described below.

Clinical features

Due to the delayed insidious nature of iron deficiency, it may take years before patients will seek medical attention, during which time they may have adapted to suboptimal physical function. The manifestations of iron deficiency anaemia listed below may be masked or co-exist with the signs and symptoms of an underlying disease. The common manifestations are as follows:

- fatigue, irritability, palpitations, dizziness, breathlessness, headache
- pallor associated with anaemia can characteristically be seen as a pinkish colour in the mucosal membranes of the mouth, conjunctiva, lips or nail beds
- nails: brittle, thinning, flattened and concave (koilonychia)
- tongue: atrophic, sore, burning sensation, glossitis
- dysphagia: Plummer-Vinson syndrome in which a 'web' of mucosa develops between the pharynx and oesophagus

Table 43.1 Stages of iron deficiency anaemia

Parameter	Iron replete	Iron depletion		Iron deficiency anaemia	
	Normal	***Pre-latent***	***Latent***	***Early***	***Late***
Haemoglobin level	Normal	Normal	Normal	Low (8–14 g/dL)	Low (< 8 g/dL)
Iron stores (serum ferritin level)	Normal	Diminished	Depleted (< 12 μg/L)	Depleted (< 12 μg/L)	Depleted (< 12 μg/L)
Serum iron level	Normal	Normal	Diminished	Diminished	Diminished
MCV	Normal	Normal	Normal	Normal or ↓	Normal or ↓
Transferrin saturation	Normal	Normal	Low (< 16%)	Low (< 16%)	Low (< 16%)

Box 43.1 Causes of iron deficiency in the elderly

Chronic blood loss

1. Gastrointestinal bleeding
   (a) Neoplasm (e.g. colon cancer)
   (b) Upper intestinal bleeding (oesophageal)
   (c) Haemorrhoids
   (d) Diverticular disease
   (e) Coeliac disease (patients over the age of 60 years constitute 19% of the adult coeliac population)
   (f) Hiatus hernia
   (g) Peptic ulcer
   (h) Biliary tract
   (i) Inflammatory bowel disease
   (j) Chronic gastritis
   (k) Alcohol
   (l) Parasites
   (m) Vascular anomalies
   (n) Drug induced (see Table 43.2)
2. Non-gastrointestinal bleeding
   (a) Respiratory tract infections (carcinoma)
   (b) Genitourinary tract (e.g. kidney or uterine carcinoma)

Impaired absorption

1. Achlorhydria
2. Gastrectomy
3. Drug induced (see Table 43.2)

Decreased dietary intake

Congenital disorders

- stomach: gastritis due to mucosal atrophy, with associated reduction in gastric secretion, pepsin and intrinsic factor
- impaired cardiovascular function (oedema)
- slightly enlarged spleen
- impaired muscle performance and work tolerance
- impaired ability to maintain body temperature when exposed to a cold environment
- immunity and infection: It has been suggested that proneness to infection is increased due to defective cell mediated immunity and impaired bactericidal activity by phagocytes. Data is conflicting, as it is well known that decreased iron supply may help prevent proliferation of invading organisms that are deprived of this mineral.

Haematological indicators

• Serum Hb concentration	< 13 g/dL (8.1 mmol/L) in men and < 12 g/dL (7.5 mmol/L) in women
• Microcytosis	MCV < 80 fl; MCH < 26 pg
• Serum iron (decreased)	< 40 μg/dL
• TIBC (increased)	350–460 μg/dL
• Transferrin saturation levels (decreased)	< 16%
• Serum transferrin (increased)	> 375 μg/dL
• Serum ferritin level	< 12 μg/L 12–20 μg/L suggests iron deficiency but is not diagnostic. Red blood cell ferritin level is a more reliable indicator, as it appears to be less influenced by inflammation.

If facilities are available, or for the purposes of research, the following indicators may also be used; however, further studies are required to evaluate their efficacy in clinical diagnosis of anaemia.

• Reticulocytes	Normal or slightly increased
• Transferrin receptors (TfR)	Increased

The most reliable diagnostic criterion is a normalisation of haematological parameters in response to oral iron therapy.

Investigating the underlying causes of iron deficiency

Gastrointestinal loss

As many as 44% of adults with iron deficiency anaemia will have gastrointestinal lesions capable of causing chronic blood loss. A careful screening procedure should always be followed with these

Table 43.2 Drugs implicated in anaemia

	Drug	Mechanism
Folate	Primidone, carbamazepine, phenobarbitone, phenytoin (anticonvulsants)	Change in gut environment (reduced pH)
	Ethanol	Affects vitamin metabolism; direct toxicity on bone marrow
	Metformin (oral hypoglycaemic)	Not known
	Cholestyramine (bile acid sequestrant)	Intraluminal interaction of drug and nutrients
	Sulphasalazine (intestinal anti-inflammatory)	Affects intestinal transport
	Methotrexate (antineoplastic)	Vitamin antagonist
	Pyrimethamine (antimalarial)	Affects transport mechanism (vitamin antagonist)
	Triamterene (diuretic)	Vitamin antagonist
	Isoniazid (tuberculosis agent)	Complexes with nutrients
Vitamin B_{12}	Para aminosalicylic (PAS) (tuberculosis agent)	Affects intestinal transport
	Colchicine (antigout)	Drug induced damage to brush border
	Neomycin (antibiotic)	Drug induced damage to brush border
	Ethanol	Affects vitamin metabolism; direct toxicity on bone marrow
	Metformin (oral hypoglycaemic)	Not known
	Nitrous oxide (anaesthetic)	Vitamin antagonist
	Cholestyramine (bile acid sequestrant)	Intraluminal interaction of drug and nutrients
Iron	Indomethacin (anti-inflammatory)	Gastric erosion
	Aspirin (analgesic)	Gastric erosion
	Cimetidine (H-2 blocker)	Changes acid environment in stomach
	Omeprazole (proton pump inhibitor)	Changes acid environment in stomach
	Neomycin (antibiotic)	Drug induced damage to brush border

patients so that the appropriate intervention can be implemented.

- *A complete and thorough medical and physical examination* should be made, with further questioning relating to gastrointestinal (GI) symptoms such as abdominal pain, constipation or diarrhoea; previous or present disease; surgery; medication (see Table 43.2); social and dietary details. If gastrointestinal symptoms are present, the positive predictive value for upper GIT lesions is 60%, compared to 35% for lower GIT pathology.
- *A faecal occult blood test* is traditionally used as a preliminary investigation to determine GIT bleeding. The sensitivity of this test in suspected GI blood loss is shown to be low, at 50–55%, and in particular shows a poor site specificity. The positive predictive values of faecal occult blood for upper and lower GIT lesions are 17–43% and 16–26%, respectively. Even when colonoscopic investigations are negative, it has been shown that as many as 37% of patients with positive faecal occult blood tests prove to have upper gastrointestinal sources of blood loss. It appears that prediction of the site of gastrointestinal blood loss by either standardised questionnaire regarding symptomology and/or the use of faecal occult blood tests is limited. The investigation of choice in the lower bowel is therefore a colonoscopy.
- *Lower gastrointestinal examination*, preferably by colonoscopy, otherwise with flexible sigmoidoscopy and barium enema to determine colonic malignancy or inflammatory conditions.
- *Upper gastrointestinal tract endoscopy* to determine lesions in the oesophagus, stomach and upper intestine. GIT lesions appear to be twice as frequent in the upper GI; however, there is a much higher prevalence (9–29%) of malignancy in lesions of the lower gut. The co-existence of malignant colorectal pathology with benign lesions of the upper GIT needs to be ruled out in this age group. A lesion of the upper GIT may be an incidental finding and the patient may have a

far more sinister neoplasm of the colon, which may go undiagnosed.

It has also been suggested that patients who have iron deficiency, but who have not yet developed anaemia, would also benefit from endoscopic examinations.

Non-gastrointestinal blood loss

Genitourinary investigation may be important to pursue if no clear gastrointestinal source of bleeding has been determined.

Helicobacter pylori infection

Helicobacter pylori infection in the stomach seems to be a possible diagnostic indicator of iron deficiency anaemia. It has been shown that *H. pylori* causes a considerable decrease in the concentration of ascorbic acid in gastric juice (which can be reversed by eradication of the infection), thus inhibiting iron absorption. *H. pylori* may also lead to an imbalance of body iron homeostasis by increasing iron demand. The bacterium has been shown to contain an iron-binding protein resembling ferritin, with a binding capacity for haem iron in erythrocytes.

Infection by *H. pylori* has been identified as a cause for iron deficiency anaemia in 16% of 189 adult patients referred to a gastroenterology department in an Italian hospital. Treatment of *H. pylori* bacteria with two antibiotics (amoxicillin and metronidazole), in the absence of iron replacement therapy, resulted in recovery from anaemia and replete ferritin levels in 75% of these patients at 6 months.

Tests to determine presence of *H. pylori* include the following:

- *Breath test* *H. pylori* contains a urease enzyme that breaks urea down to carbon dioxide. The patient has a pre-urea breath test before consuming radioactively labelled urea. The labelled carbon dioxide can then be determined. (This test is not always readily available.)
- *Blood test* Antibodies to *H. pylori* can be confirmed by a simple blood test (does not necessarily confirm *present* infection).
- *Gastric endoscopy* During endoscopy a biopsy can be obtained and a urease test performed on the biopsy sample.

Further research is required to determine whether detection and treatment of *H. pylori* is a valid treatment method for the alleviation of iron deficiency.

Even after intensive investigation, as many as 40% of patients aged > 50 years may have no identifiable underlying cause of iron deficiency. The cost implications of the numerous diagnostic tests mentioned above need to be considered in this age group, who may have limited financial means. In terms of improved management of anaemia, the cost–benefit ratio of undertaking sophisticated tests should be carefully considered.

Management

1. Where possible, treat the underlying cause.
2. Restore haemoglobin to normal and replenish body stores of iron with iron therapy:
   (a) Oral iron therapy of 120–200 mg elemental iron, taken as ferrous sulphate, is indicated in iron deficiency anaemia, depending on the severity of the anaemia. As the elderly may have reduced iron absorption, a larger dose may be necessary. Administration of the supplement with food markedly reduces iron absorption. However, if iron is taken on an empty stomach, some patients experience adverse gastrointestinal side effects, such as heartburn, nausea, abdominal pain, constipation or diarrhoea. Patients should be advised initially to take the tablets 1 hour before meals, unless symptoms become too troublesome. A gradual increase in dosage, as well as dividing the dosage into 3 smaller doses over the day, may help alleviate adverse effects.
   (b) Patients should be pre-warned that iron supplementation causes a black colouration of the faeces. Constipation, and other gastrointestinal adverse effects mentioned previously, are the main underlying reasons for non-compliance. Constipation should especially be monitored in the elderly, because if prolonged it may lead to faecal impaction.

(c) Supplementation should not be taken with medication such as antacids or H-2 antagonists, as the efficacy of both agents will be affected. If necessary, H-2 antagonists can be taken at night or, alternatively, the treatment of the iron deficiency should only follow once the ulcer has resolved.
(d) Following normalisation of haemoglobin, treatment should be continued for a further 3–6 months to allow for repletion of iron stores.
(e) Ascorbic acid supplements can be used, although at least 200 mg is necessary for each 30 mg of iron administered and they may increase the side effects of the iron therapy. Dietary sources of ascorbic acid consumed at the same time as the iron source may improve iron absorption.
(f) It is essential that a good dietary intake of iron be encouraged (see Table 43.3) to prevent future recurrence of iron deficiency anaemia. However, oral intake from dietary sources alone will not replenish stores.
(g) Accidental iron toxicity can occur with doses of 3–10 g or more, leading to severe gastrointestinal symptoms and possible dyspnoea. Immediate gastric lavage using deferoxamine is required in this instance.
(h) Parenteral iron therapy is effective but more dangerous, expensive and painful for the patient. It is indicated when the patient:
   (i) is unable to tolerate oral supplementation
   (ii) is incapable of compliance
   (iii) has had rapid blood loss
   (iv) demonstrates intestinal malabsorption
   (v) is unable to maintain iron balance due to haemodialysis.

Dosage of iron to be injected = ((15 – patient's Hb (g/dL)) × body weight (kg) × 3), using a 50 mg iron per mL of solution given intramuscularly (buttock) or intravenously. Adverse effects of parenteral therapy are associated with allergic reactions, including anaphylaxis, fever, leucocytosis and tachycardia. After checking for hypersensitivity, a maximal recommended dose of 2 mL (i.e. 100 mg iron) is given. Parenteral iron supplementation results in rise of ferritin to normal and this is sustained for a month.

Course and prognosis

1. Physical symptoms such as headache and fatigue may abate after a few days. Other symptoms should be resolved within 3–6 months of therapy, provided that gastritis has been excluded.
2. Supplementation is normally required for 3–6 months to return serum and red cell ferritin, as well as saturation of transferrin, to normal (depending on the original severity of initial anaemia). The stores will fill more slowly as the degree of absorption drops with the replenishing stores. Haemoglobin can be expected to rise by 2 g/dL every 3 weeks until fully corrected by 8–16 weeks, regardless of the starting

Table 43.3 Dietary sources of iron, folate and vitamin B_{12}

	Iron	**Folate**	**Vitamin B_{12}**
Recommended dietary allowance (RDA) or dietary reference intake (DRI)	10 mg	400 μg	2.4 mg
Good food sources	Liver, shellfish, beef, fish, chicken (haem); legumes, dried fruit, fortified cereals (non-haem)[(a)]	Liver, yeast, dark green leafy vegetables, pulses, a few fruits, including oranges	Animal only: liver, kidney, seafood, fish, meat and, to a lesser degree, milk, cheese and eggs
Effect of cooking	None	70–100% loss	10–30% loss

(*a*) Good sources of vitamin C for facilitating iron absorption include: citrus fruits, guavas, kiwifruit, strawberries, mangoes, blackcurrants, tomatoes, green vegetables and potatoes eaten with the skin.

level. In some elderly patients, it may take at least a month for an increase of 1 g/dL.

3. Failure to respond to therapy may indicate inappropriate diagnosis, complicating illness (including folate and B_{12} deficiency), non-compliance, insufficient supplement dosage, continuing blood loss or malabsorption.
4. Prognosis is excellent if the underlying cause of the deficiency is benign, the bleeding is under control and the supplementation has been sufficient to fully replenish stores.

Anaemia of chronic disease

Anaemia of chronic disease is predominantly (40–70%) normochromic normocytic; however, as the pathophysiology and diagnostic tools are similar to those for iron deficiency, it has been considered under this section (see Figures 43.2 and 43.3). Anaemia of chronic disease is an important cause of anaemia in the elderly and individuals known to have a chronic infection or malignant disease (see Box 43.2) should be haematologically assessed on a regular basis.

Box 43.2 Conditions associated with anaemia of chronic disease

Chronic infections
- Pulmonary (tuberculosis, pneumonia)
- Subacute bacterial endocarditis
- Osteomyelitis
- Chronic urinary tract infections
- Meningitis
- Human immunodeficiency virus (HIV)

Chronic, non-infectious complications
- Rheumatoid arthritis and fever
- Systemic lupus erythematosus
- Severe trauma, including thermal injury
- Vasculitis

Malignant disease
- Carcinoma
- Hodgkin's disease
- Leukaemia
- Multiple myeloma

Miscellaneous
- Alcoholic liver disease
- Congestive cardiac failure
- Thrombophlebitis
- Ischaemic heart disease

Idiopathic

Source: Adapted from G. R. Lee et al. (1999), *Wintrobe's Clinical Hematology*, Vol. 2, 10th edn, Williams & Wilkins, Baltimore, MD.

Pathophysiology

This is a moderate anaemia associated with a decreased erythrocyte count and a reduced serum iron level. It is associated with many different conditions, therefore the symptoms that manifest are wide-ranging. The anaemia generally develops 1–2 months into the illness and the severity of the anaemia seems to be related to the severity of the chronic illness. After 2 months, a new balance is established between red cell production and red cell destruction, and the haemoglobin stabilises (Hb concentrations normally range from 7 g/dL to 11 g/dL).

There is a shortened red blood survival (20–30% reduction) which causes a demand on the marrow to produce more red blood cells. However, due to limited iron availability and a blunted erythropoeitin response, the marrow is unable to accommodate this demand. It is thought that cytokines, such as tumour necrosis factor and interferons, which are produced as a result of the chronic disorder, may result in the production of other mediators that have a role in erythropoeitin suppression. A decreased serum iron concentration is probably a combination of poor dietary iron intake, poor absorption, shunting of iron away from transferrin to storage and poor release of haemoglobin from old red blood cells. The presence of a low serum iron level despite adequate iron stores indicates the severe disturbance in iron metabolism.

Diagnosis

Anaemia of chronic disease differs from iron deficiency anaemia mainly in that iron ferritin stores are present or increased but flow to plasma is partially blocked, resulting in a drop of serum iron and an accumulation in the macrophages (see Table 43.4).

Serum ferritin is an acute phase protein that is typically elevated in infection, inflammation and malignancy. When iron deficiency therefore *co-exists* with chronic disease, serum ferritin may be falsely raised and a concurrent iron deficiency may remain undiagnosed. In this case, ferritin levels are not likely to be higher than 20–100 μg, with the exception of liver disease (see 'Anaemias of renal, liver or endocrine disease') where the ferritin level should exceed 200 μg before iron deficiency anaemia can be ruled out.

Management

Management of anaemia associated with chronic disease or inflammation primarily requires adequate treatment of the underlying disease process. The anaemia itself is not an important clinical problem as the haemoglobin level is usually only moderately decreased. Some of the following therapies have been used, however.

- Recombinant erythropoeitin is effective and safe but expensive. This should probably be reserved only for severe cases. (Intravenous or subcutaneous dosage = 100–150 U/kg 3 times a week; dosage adjusted according to the response.)
- Parenteral iron therapy is not recommended as the risks outweigh the benefits. Oral iron replacement is likely to be useful only in patients who have concurrent iron deficiency.

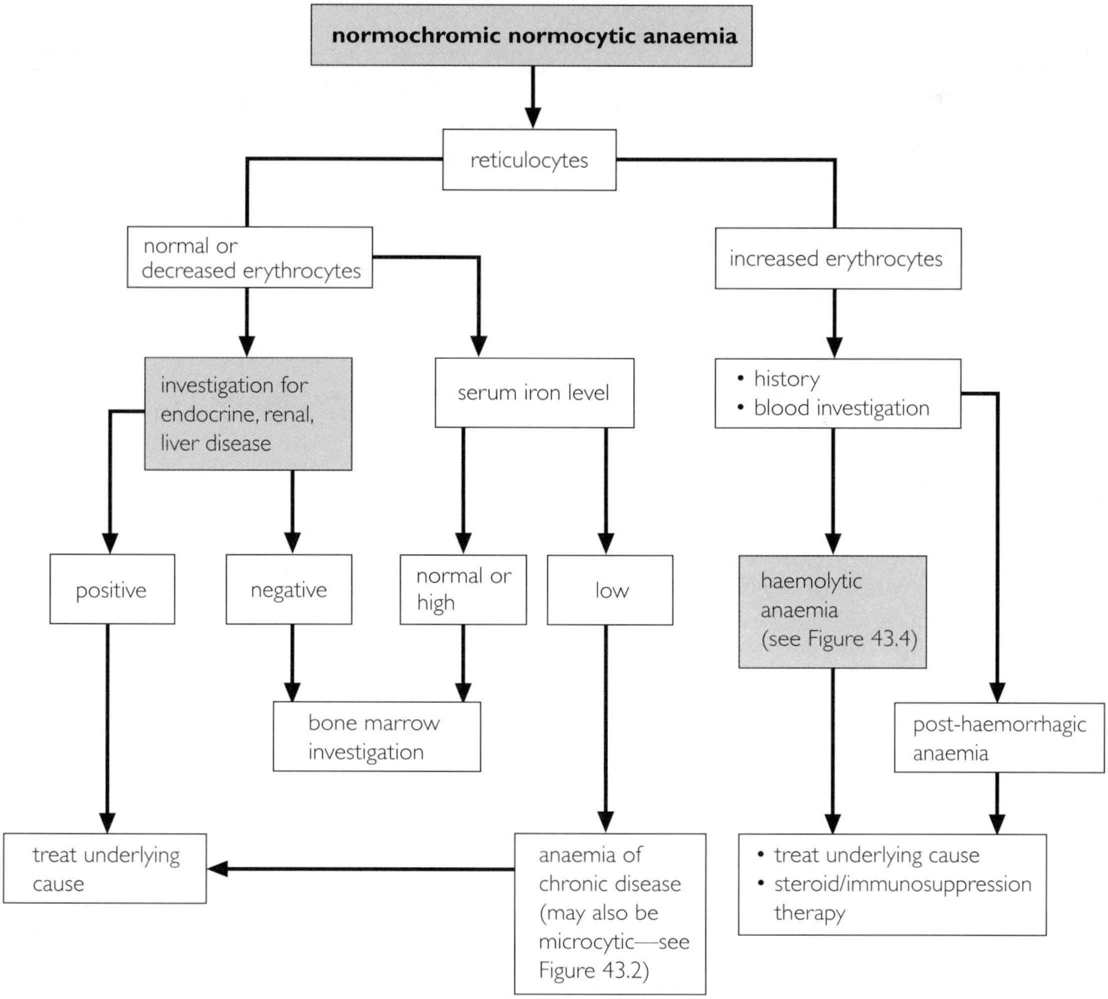

Figure 43.3 Algorithm for normochromic normocytic differentiation and management ADAPTED FROM LEE ET AL. (1999)

Table 43.4 Haematological parameters in iron deficiency anaemia and the anaemia of chronic disease

Parameter (normal range)[a]	Iron deficiency anaemia	Anaemia of chronic disease
Serum Hb level (women: 12 g/dL) (men: 13 g/dL)	< 12 g/dL (women) < 13 g/dL (men)	< 12 g/dL (women) < 13 g/dL (men)
Serum iron level (70–200 μg/dL)	< 40 μg/dL	< 60 μg/dL
Transferrin level (200–380 μg/dL)	> 375 μg/dL	< 250 μg/dL
Transferrin saturation (20–45%)	< 16%	< 16%
Serum ferritin level (women: 10–200 ng/mL) (men: 20–500 ng/mL)	< 12 ng/mL	> 100 ng/mL

(a) Reference values may vary from laboratory to laboratory.

Thalassaemia and other haemoglobinopathies

Refer to Figure 43.2.

The thalassaemias are a group of inherited disorders often found in individuals of Mediterranean origin. In mild forms of the disease (thalassaemia mild), hypochromia and microcytosis may be mild with or without anaemia. However, in more severe thalassaemic disorders (including β-thalassaemia), the anaemia may be severe. Red blood cells are short-lived as the synthesis of one of the normal polypeptide chains of globin is severely deficient.

Thalassaemia is characterised by an increased erythrocyte count (> 5000×10^{12}/L), despite low haemoglobin, and a consistently low MCV value (60–70 fl). Iron deficiency does not present with such a high erythrocyte count and is seldom associated with MCV concentrations as low as those seen in thalassaemia, other than in advanced iron deficiency anaemia. Clinical manifestations can include jaundice, splenomegaly and skeletal changes.

Management

Transfusion therapy, or even splenectomy, is required for severe anaemia found in many of these individuals.

Thalassaemia is associated with increased iron absorption and therefore iron supplementation should be avoided (unless iron deficiency is documented biochemically), as iron overload may result. Most patients with thalassaemia die from complications of iron overload as a result of intractable cardiac failure caused by multiple transfusions. Iron-chelating agents (e.g. desferrioxamine) are therefore essential in helping to deal with these complications.

Sideroblastic anaemia and other disorders of porphyrin synthesis

Refer to Figure 43.2.

The sideroblastic anaemias are a diverse group of disorders characterised by the classic triad of red cell dimorphism, elevated serum iron levels and red blood cell mitochondrial iron deposition. They result in defective iron utilisation, ineffective erythropoiesis and a marrow that contains a large number of abnormal normoblasts with abundant haemosiderin granules known as sideroblasts. This condition is more common in old age than anaemias of defective globin synthesis (thalassaemias). It is suggested that the problem lies within the mitochondrial transport of ferrous iron for conjugation with protoporphyrin, resulting in insufficient haem generation. Sideroblastic anaemia can be either hereditary or acquired (idiopathic or reversible). Both hereditary and idiopathic sideroblastic anaemias show increased transferrin saturation and serum ferritin levels, as well as a susceptibility towards iron overload. This is particularly the case in the hereditary type where virtually all patients exhibit manifestations of iron overload. One-third of patients with hereditary sideroblastic anaemia respond to pyridoxine (vitamin B_6) administration to varying degrees, while only a few patients with idiopathic acquired sideroblastic anaemia respond.

Reversible acquired sideroblastic anaemia is often associated with conditions such as alcoholism, copper deficiency or as a result of medication (e.g. antituberculosis drugs that are pyridoxine antagonists). This form of sideroblastic anaemia tends to be progressive, with normal transferrin saturation and ferritin levels, although this may vary depending on the underlying condition. It is seldom responsive to pyridoxine therapy.

Management

- As one-third of all cases of hereditary sideroblastic anaemia are responsive to pyridoxine, all patients in this category should be administered with 50–200 mg of oral pyridoxine per day. Among patients who respond, the response is variable but maintenance treatment is normally necessary.
- In severely ill anaemic patients and/or those not responding to pyridoxine therapy, periodic blood transfusions are necessary, often accompanied with the administration of an iron-chelating agent, such as desferrioxamine.
- A therapeutic trial of 50–200 mg of pyridoxine per day can be administered to patients with idiopathic acquired sideroblastic anaemia, although most patients don't respond. Fortunately, these patients are not significantly incapacitated by the anaemia. Follow-up medical examinations are, however, indicated and the presence of iron overload should be monitored if blood transfusions become necessary.
- Acquired sideroblastic anaemia often resolves with management of the underlying cause.

It is often difficult to differentiate between the microcytic anaemias described in this section. Although certain haematological indicators are diagnostic (see Table 43.5), these may not always be consistent and consultation with a specialist haematologist may be required.

Table 43.5 Comparative haematological indicators in microcytic anaemia and anaemia of chronic disease (range in brackets)

Indicator (normal values)[(a)]	Iron deficiency	Anaemia of chronic disease	Thalassaemia	Sideroblastic anaemia
Serum Hb level (men: 13 g/dL) (women: 12 g/dL)	Decreased (4–13 g/dL)	Moderately decreased (8–13 g/dL)	Variable: Minor (9–13 g/dL) Major (2–7 g/dL)	Variable: Hereditary (4–10 g/dL) Acquired/ idiopathic (7–12 g/dL)
Serum iron level (70–200 μg/dL)	Decreased	Decreased	Increased	Increased
Transferrin saturation (20–45%)	Decreased	Decreased	Normal or increased	Normal or increased
TIBC (250–435 μg/dL)	Increased	Normal or decreased	Normal or decreased	Normal or decreased
Serum ferritin level (men: 20–500 μg/dL) (women: 10–200 μg/dL)	Decreased	Normal or increased	Normal or increased	Increased

(a) Reference values may vary from laboratory to laboratory.

Normocytic normochromic anaemias

Despite a lowered haemoglobin, this type of anaemia presents with normal MCV and MCHC levels. Many anaemias can have variable values for MCV—anaemia of chronic disease or, as in iron deficiency anaemia, where the full morphological and haematological picture presents only when the deficiency is advanced.

With reference to Figure 43.3, normocytic normochromic anaemia is related either to a low rate of erythropoiesis suggestive of underlying endocrine, renal or liver diseases or to an increased rate of erythropoiesis which would suggest haemolytic or post-haemorrhagic anaemia. It is only necessary to perform a bone marrow aspirate and biopsy if no underlying disease is apparent after screening.

Severe protein-calorie malnutrition can be associated with reduced erythropoietin and a mild normocytic anaemia may result, making assessment of the nutritional status of the elderly important.

Anaemias of renal, liver or endocrine disease

Anaemias associated with renal, liver or endocrine diseases also have normal or decreased erythrocyte production and their haematological indicators should be regularly assessed. Anaemia of chronic renal failure is due, in part, to erythropoietin deficiency. Anaemia of liver disease may show an increased serum iron and percentage saturation which is increased, while the total iron-binding capacity (TIBC) is normal or decreased. In general TIBC is normal or decreased in anaemia of chronic disease and in renal, liver or endocrine disease, but increased in iron deficiency.

Macrocytic anaemias

Megaloblastic anaemia in a previously healthy, well-nourished elderly individual is most likely due to pernicious anaemia (see Figure 43.4). Megaloblastic anaemia may also be a result of vitamin B_{12} or folate deficiencies. Using intermediate metabolites, such as raised plasma homocysteine or methylmalonic acid (MMA) concentrations as markers of these micronutrient deficiencies, the prevalence may be as high as 39–68%.

Megaloblastic anaemias: folate and vitamin B_{12} deficiency

Megaloblastic anaemia is caused predominantly by folate and/or vitamin B_{12} deficiency and rarely by inherited or drug induced disorders. It occurs as a result of slowed DNA synthesis due to failure to convert homocysteine to methionine, with a consequent decrease in purine synthesis. Megaloblastic anaemias usually develop slowly with mild symptoms, so that at diagnosis, the anaemias are often severe, with haemoglobin concentrations less than 8 g/dL. Folate tissue stores may drop after 3–4 months of deprivation. Stores of vitamin B_{12} last for much longer, namely years rather than months.

Determination of the serum levels of vitamin B_{12} and folate in the serum is essential for distinguishing between these two causes of megaloblastic anaemia, as their haematological manifestations are otherwise essentially identical (see Figure 43.4). It is also useful to take a careful history, including a dietary assessment, as folate deficiency in the elderly can be due to inadequate dietary intake and excessive alcohol consumption, whereas these causes are unlikely in vitamin B_{12} deficiency. Neurological side effects are seen frequently in vitamin B_{12} but not in folate deficiency.

Vitamin B_{12} (cobalamin) deficiency

The true prevalence of cobalamin deficiency in the elderly is unclear, and is reported to range from 3% to 44%, depending on which reference values are used. Vitamin B_{12} is a co-factor for two reactions in higher animals, namely the conversion of L-methylmalonyl-CoA to succinyl-CoA, and the methylation of homocysteine to methionine. Vitamin B_{12} deficiency can cause numerous clinically important manifestations, including subacute degeneration of the spinal cord; neuropsychiatric disorders such as dementia, peripheral neuropathy and psychosis; as well as gastrointestinal problems such as glossitis and, rarely, malabsorption.

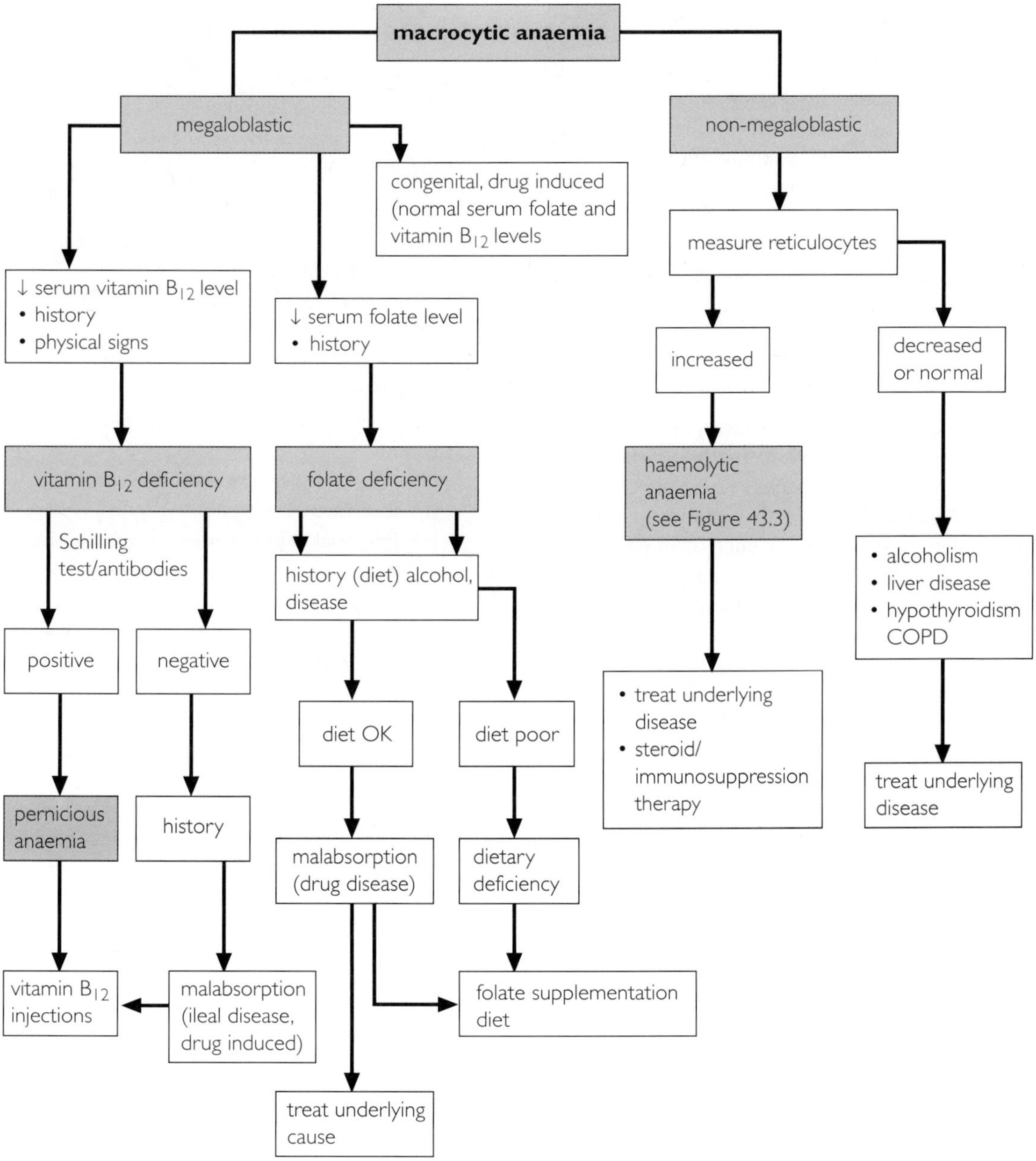

Figure 43.4 Algorithm for macrocytic anaemia differentiation and management ADAPTED FROM LEE ET AL. (1999)

Pathophysiology

In normal vitamin B_{12} metabolism, cobalamin is released from food by proteases and acids in the stomach, where it binds with cobalophilins (glycoproteins). These complexes are digested in the upper intestine by pancreatic enzymes, and cobalamin is transferred to a protein produced in the stomach, known as intrinsic factor (IF). The cobalamin-IF complex attaches to receptors in the ileum from which the vitamin is released into the circulation for uptake by body systems. Vitamin B_{12} in bile is highly efficiently conserved via the enterohepatic cycle; its half-life is approximately 4 years. Thus, deficiency from an inadequate intake takes between 2 and 6 years to develop. Clinical manifestations only become evident when haemoglobin levels drop below 8 g/dL. Iron deficiency and vitamin B_{12} deficiency may co-exist due to the effect of atrophic gastritis on both these vitamins. In these cases, vitamin B_{12} deficiency may be masked and result in a microcytic, hypochromic anaemia.

Box 43.3 Vitamin B_{12} deficiency

Inadequate intake

1. Dietary deficiency (rare)
   (a) Strict vegetarianism/vegans
   (b) Poverty

Inadequate absorption

1. Gastric disorders—absent or inadequate intrinsic factor
   (a) Pernicious anaemia
   (b) Gastric surgery
2. Food-cobalamin malabsorption (mild cobalamin deficiency)
3. Small intestinal disorders (affecting the ileum)
   (a) Inflammatory bowel disease
   (b) Intestinal resection
   (c) Bacterial overgrowth
   (d) Fish tapeworm *Diphyllobothrium latum*
   (e) Lymphoma
   (f) Tuberculosis
   (g) Whipple's disease
   (h) Gluten enteropathy
   (i) Tropical sprue
4. Drug-induced malabsorption (see Table 43.2)
5. Other
   (a) Zollinger-Ellison syndrome, pancreatic disease (poor alkaline environment in ileum)
   (b) Familial vitamin B_{12} malabsorption
   (c) Haemodialysis

Causes of cobalamin deficiency

Causes of vitamin B_{12} deficiency include factors which decrease absorption, including pernicious anaemia, atrophic gastritis, certain medications, disorders of the small intestine, inadequate dietary intake and increased losses, such as in patients on haemodialysis (see Box 43.3). Inadequate dietary intake of vitamin B_{12} is generally only seen in individuals who have been strict vegetarians or vegans for a long period of time.

Pernicious anaemia is defined as vitamin B_{12} deficiency due to loss of intrinsic factor secretion by the stomach. It occurs in about 2% of free-living elderly persons and is particularly common among individuals of Scandinavian, English and Irish ancestry, in whom the incidence is reported to be between 9% and 17%. Type A gastritis, a phenomenon caused by antiparietal cell antibody immune activity, together with acquired gastritis, may account for up to 90% of cases of pernicious anaemia in older persons. As well as reduced intrinsic factor secretion, other gastric secretions (e.g. pepsin, hydrochloric acid) are reduced to about 10% of normal. Gastritis may also result from injury to the stomach mucosa, nutritional deficiency (e.g. iron), endocrinological insufficiency, as well as genetic and other autoimmune abnormalities.

Given adequate treatment, the prognosis of pernicious anaemia is good. Relapses occur as a result of the patient's reluctance to continue with lifelong therapy. Relapse can occur from 21 months to 10 years, depending on the individual patient. The most serious long-term complication of pernicious anaemia is carcinoma of the stomach, with an incidence 2–5 times that of the general population. Chronic atrophic gastritis is generally considered a precursor for stomach cancer and the higher pH may result in increased vulnerability of the stomach to carcinogenic pathogens. There is some evidence that these patients may also have an increased risk for colon cancer, especially in the first 5 years after diagnosis. Annual or 2 yearly endoscopy and gastric biopsy examination for malignancy should therefore be encouraged in patients with pernicious anaemia.

Mild cobalamin deficiency/low cobalamin status

The clinical significance of low to low-normal serum vitamin B_{12} levels, which are commonly found in up to 13% of geriatric medical patients, is controversial. These patients may have levels within the lower reference range of normal (i.e. < 175 pmol/L (237 pg/mL)) and, despite having a normal full blood count, may have neuropsychiatric disorders thought to be due to vitamin B_{12} deficiency. The value used to diagnose vitamin B_{12} deficiency is < 100 pmol/L; a megaloblastic marrow is commonly found in patients with a level < 115 pmol/L (155 pg/L).

Mild cobalamin deficiency appears to be due to food-cobalamin malabsorption. The disorder is described as the inability to absorb food-bound or protein-bound vitamin B_{12} in a person who is fully capable of absorbing free vitamin B_{12}. The Schilling test cannot detect this problem, as it measures only the ability to absorb free vitamin B_{12}. It is currently difficult to measure this cause of low cobalamin status, although routine tests may become available in future. In a study of older Dutch subjects, mild cobalamin deficiency could be explained by atrophic gastritis in only a quarter of cases, and in the majority of cases no explanation was apparent. The malabsorption of protein-bound cobalamin is apparent only in subjects with severe atrophic gastritis; however, older adults with mild to moderate atrophic gastritis may be at risk of developing vitamin B_{12} deficiency as atrophic gastritis progresses. Gastric surgery or drugs that suppress gastric acid secretion, such as H-2 antagonists, are well known causes of this form of malabsorption.

Patients with mild cobalamin deficiency respond well to treatment with intramuscular hydroxycobalamin (i.e. show a significant fall in MCV and rise in Hb). It has been recommended that elderly patients with serum vitamin B_{12} levels < 175 pmol/L (237pg/mL) should be assumed to have suboptimal cobalamin status, even if their full blood count is normal. However, consensus has not been reached regarding the description of mild cobalamin deficiency: values ranging from below 260 pmol/L (352 pg/L) to below 175 pmol/L (237 pg/mL) have been proposed.

Available evidence to date suggests that mild cobalamin deficiency should be viewed as potentially treatable in older adults, even in patients without clinical signs of overt vitamin B_{12} deficiency.

Diagnosis

Clinical indicators

- General appearance: when severe, the skin has a lemon-yellow tint resulting from pallor and mild icterus. The sclerae can also be yellowish. Skin may be hyperpigmented, dry and inelastic.
- Loss of appetite occurs in up to 65% of patients and results in considerable weight loss.
- A sore, fiery red or smooth, shiny, atrophic tongue is symptomatic (glossitis). Patients may have burning and pain on swallowing, as well as a loss of taste.
- Weakness and fatigue.
- A fifth of patients complain of fever in the absence of infection.
- Diarrhoea may result from changes to the gastrointestinal epithelia.
- Neurological changes, such as mild confusion, apathy, depression, cognitive impairment, paraesthesia and peripheral neuropathy, may be present. Neurological symptoms do not necessarily relate to the severity of the condition, although if the condition continues undiagnosed, neurological disease can progress. The white matter of the spinal cord and the cerebral cortex are affected due to the decrease in myelin synthesis.
- The patient most commonly complains of pins and needles in all 4 limbs or a feeling of numbness or coldness. In the more advanced stage, evidence of dorsal column involvement is clear and the patient may complain that his gait is unco-ordinated, with position and vibration sense also being affected. Later, a scissor or spastic gait may develop, and tendon reflexes may be reduced. The combination of peripheral neuropathy with corticospinal tract signs, such as ataxia, is known as subacute combined degeneration. Some patients with this condition may exhibit cerebral manifestations such as depression, loss of memory, and in very severe cases, delusional outbursts and reduction in the level of consciousness.

- Co-morbidity may complicate the identification of clinical manifestations such as diabetes mellitus, peripheral vascular disease, osteoarthritis, Alzheimer's disease and other dementias which can also cause paraesthesias, sensory loss, neuropathy, gait disturbances, other pain disturbances of the legs as well as cognitive dysfunction. It would probably be advisable to supplement all psychogeriatric patients with water soluble vitamin preparations that contain folate and vitamin B_{12}.

Biochemical and haematological indicators

- Macrocytic erythrocytes with a distinctly oval shape.
- Megaloblasts in the bone marrow.
- Serum vitamin B_{12} < 100 pg/mL (74 pmol/L) (normal range, 200–300 pg/mL). Serum vitamin B_{12} values < 175 pmol/L (237 pg/mL) are generally considered to indicate mild cobalamin deficiency. (*Note:* Vitamin B_{12} levels may be subnormal in patients with folate deficiency; see Table 43.6.)
- Earliest changes in vitamin B_{12} status are seen with a decrease in serum holotranscobalamin II (holoTCII) (< 50 pg/mL), a circulating protein that delivers vitamin B_{12} to all DNA synthesising cells. This indicator can precede a drop in serum cobalamin by weeks or even months. It has therefore been suggested as a screen for early deficiency in adults between 50 and 90 years.
- Elevated plasma concentrations of two vitamin B_{12} metabolites, methylmalonic acid (MMA) (> 0.32 μmol/L) and total homocysteine (> 19.9 μmol/L) may also be useful early indicators of low cobalamin status or vitamin B_{12} deficiency. Elevated urinary MMA levels > 20 mg/L may also be used. Further, MMA assessment enables the practitioner to distinguish between vitamin B_{12} and folate megaloblastic anaemias, since MMA levels are not increased in the latter unless renal failure or volume depletion is present.
- Pernicious anaemia is diagnosed by a positive Schilling test. A 24 hour urine sample is collected following 2 doses of radiolabelled B_{12}, one with intrinsic factor and one without. The relative ratio between the 2 isotopes allows for the determination of intrinsic factor deficiency. This test cannot detect food-cobalamin malabsorption as it measures only the ability to absorb free cobalamin.
- Approximately 50–60% of patients with pernicious anaemia have intrinsic factor antibody in their plasma. Although not a sensitive test, it has good specificity (i.e. patients without pernicious anaemia will not show a positive result). If this test is available, it should be used together with haematological evidence of megaloblastic anaemia and low serum vitamin B_{12} (or a raised urinary MMA) to diagnose pernicious anaemia without the need for a time-consuming Schilling test.
- Plasma pepsinogens A and C indicate the severity of atrophic gastritis.
  - Ratio of pepsinogen I (PGI) to pepsinogen II (PGII) < 1.6, combined with a PGI concentration ≥ 17 μg/L, indicates mild to moderate atrophic gastritis.
  - PGI:PGII ratio < 1.6, combined with a PGI concentration < 17 μg/L, indicates severe atrophic gastritis.

Management

1. Treat the underlying cause of the anaemia, where possible.
2. Review medication status for drug–nutrient interactions (see Table 43.2).
3. Treatment of pernicious anaemia associated vitamin B_{12} deficiency and that caused by atrophic gastritis in the elderly conventionally consists of 250–1000 μg (depending on severity of complications from deficiency) intramuscular or deep subcutaneous injections on alternate days for 1–2 weeks. This is followed by 250 μg weekly until blood count is normal and thereafter maintenance doses of 1000 μg at monthly or, in some instances, 3 monthly intervals for life. Higher dosages may be required to reverse the deficiency in certain cases.

Two forms of vitamin B_{12} are commercially available—cyanocobalamin and hydroxycobalamin. The latter is initially better retained, is more bioavailable, and one dose may last slightly

Table 43.6 Haematological indicators in megaloblastic anaemia

		Vitamin B_{12} deficiency			
	Normal range[a]	Cobalamin deficiency	Pernicious anaemia	Mild cobalamin deficiency	Folate deficiency
Serum vitamin B_{12} level	200–900 pg/mL	< 100 pg/mL (74 pmol/L)	< 100 pg/mL	< 237 pg/mL (see text)	May co-exist
Serum folate level	6–21 μg/L	Normal	Normal	Normal	< 3 μg/L
RBC folate level	160–640 μg/L	Normal	Normal	Normal	< 140 μg/L (haemolysis may result in falsely elevated values)

(a) These values may vary from laboratory to laboratory.

longer (allowing 2–4 monthly, instead of once monthly, injections). Hydroxycobalamin is only available as intramuscular (IM) preparations, unlike cyanocobalamin, which is available as oral supplements. The potential benefits of hydroxy- compared with cyanocobalamin are of particular interest to patients with pernicious anaemia who are smokers, as hydroxycobalamin is an important cyanide antagonist, whereas cyanocobalamin is not. In all cases there should be regular vitamin B_{12} monitoring.

It has been suggested that large doses of vitamin B_{12} given orally (300–2000 μg/day) may also be effective as intramuscular injections for the treatment of pernicious anaemia. About 1% of orally administered vitamin B_{12} is absorbed via mass diffusion, without intrinsic factor. This route is useful for patients who refuse parenteral injections or in whom it may be hazardous to do so. Closer supervision is required with oral vitamin B_{12} supplementation in elderly persons with cognitive impairment because the chances of forgotten or omitted treatment may result in increased relapse.

4. In elderly persons with gastric atrophy, oral vitamin B_{12} supplementation can be given as a prophylaxis, provided it is consumed either 1 hour before or 1 hour after meals, in order to prevent binding of cobalamin with food proteins.
5. Mega-doses of vitamin C (> 500 mg) should not be consumed with vitamin B_{12} as it adversely affects the availability of vitamin B_{12} from food. Persons taking vitamin C in doses ≥ 1 g/day may develop vitamin B_{12} deficiency in the absence of any other underlying causes.
6. Vitamin B_{12} should be administered at least 24 hours prior to folate to ensure there is no masking of B_{12} neurological side effects.
7. Patients respond well to treatment with alleviation of symptoms within 2 weeks, or in the case of neurological symptoms, within 1–3 months. Some neurological manifestations may be irreversible.
8. Blood transfusions are not normally required unless the anaemia is very severe. It is important to avoid circulatory overload in older patients, especially those with evidence of cardiac disease, such as myocardial ischaemia or cardiac failure.
9. The following guide is suggested for the screening and treatment of mild cobalamin deficiency:
   (a) Serum vitamin B_{12} = 200–300 pg/mL and normal MMA: repeat the test in 6–12 months.
   (b) Serum vitamin B_{12} = 200–300 pg/mL and mildly elevated MMA: repeat MMA in 3–6 months and consider low dose B_{12} supplementation.
   (c) Serum vitamin B_{12} = 200–300 pg/mL and markedly elevated MMA: treat with B_{12} and determine cause of deficiency.
10. Although inadequate dietary vitamin B_{12} intake is unlikely, sources of this vitamin are included in Table 43.3.

Folate deficiency

Folic acid deficiency, described as either a low serum or red blood cell folic acid concentration, is common in older adults, with reported prevalences ranging from 11% to 28% among institutionalised and cognitively impaired elderly patients. Deficiency in elderly individuals living at home is reportedly lower at 9%.

Pathophysiology

Folic acid is vital for many methylation and nucleotide biosynthetic reactions. Folate, like vitamin B_{12}, is also conserved via the enterohepatic cycle. Absorption of folate (polyglutamates) occurs in the jejunum after conversion to monoglutamates. Once absorbed, most folic acid is reduced and methylated in the liver to form N-methyltetrahydrofolate, which is the main storage and transport form of folate. Methyl folate can only become available to the body with the assistance of an enzyme requiring vitamin B_{12} that removes a methyl group from methyl folate. The methyl group is delivered to homocysteine while tetrahydrofolic acid is regenerated and used for thymidylate synthesis. A deficiency of vitamin B_{12} will trap methyl folate, thus making it unavailable.

Folate, unlike vitamin B_{12}, has stores that remain adequate only for 2–4 months. Folate deprivation results in a decrease in serum folate after only 2 weeks, but this is not a sensitive indicator of tissue stores. Red blood cell (RBC) folate is a more useful indicator, as folate accumulates and remains in the erythrocyte during the life of the RBC. A deficiency of folate is thus evident in RBCs after about 17 weeks. The marrow may become megaloblastic within 18 weeks, leading to anaemia by 20 weeks. The stages involved in folate deficiency include the following:

- Early negative folate intake results in a fall in serum folate to 3 ng/mL while RBC folate remains unchanged.
- Low serum folate is accompanied by a reduction in RBC folate to $<$ 160 ng/mL.
- Folate deficient erythropoiesis is indicated by defective DNA synthesis, manifesting later as macrocytosis and anaemia.

Causes

Numerous factors, including underlying gastrointestinal disease, polypharmacy and inadequate dietary intake due to poverty and chronic alcoholism, contribute to folic acid deficiency in the elderly (see Box 43.4). Excessive alcohol intake may impair folate metabolism by impaired storage in the liver, excessive urinary folate loss, inhibition of absorption of folate (alcohol inhibits the enzyme responsible for converting polyglutamate to monoglutamate) as well as a direct toxic effect on the bone marrow.

Diagnosis

Clinical indicators

- Fatigue and dyspnoea.
- Loss of appetite with weight loss.
- Sore tongue, glossitis.
- Gastrointestinal symptoms (diarrhoea).
- Folate deficiency may show cognitive disorders (forgetfulness, irritability) but is differentiated from vitamin B_{12} deficiency by the absence of neurological deficits.

Box 43.4 Causes of folate deficiency

Inadequate intake

1. Dietary deficiency (rare)
   (a) Poverty
2. Chronic alcoholism

Inadequate absorption

1. Small intestinal disorders (affecting ileum)
   (a) Gluten enteropathy
   (b) Tropical sprue
   (c) Inflammatory bowel disease
   (d) Intestinal resection
2. Drug induced malabsorption (see Table 43.2)
3. Chronic disease
4. Congenital folate malabsorption and inherited disorders of DNA synthesis

Increased loss

1. Haemodialysis

Haematological indicators

- Macrocytic erythrocytes with distinctly oval shape.
- Megaloblasts in the bone marrow.
- RBC folate levels < 140 μg/L (317 nmol/L) or low serum folate levels (< 3 μg/L).

Management

- A careful diagnosis must be made. Treating a patient with vitamin B_{12} deficiency may provide haematological improvement but the neurological side effects of vitamin B_{12} deficiency will continue to become more severe.
- Folate deficiency can be corrected with oral folic acid supplementation of 5 mg/day for 3–4 months. Maintenance will depend on the underlying cause of the deficiency. If the underlying cause is unlikely to resolve, then a 0.25–0.5 mg dose of folic acid per day as a prophylaxis should be encouraged.
- In patients taking chemotherapeutic folate antagonists, folinic acid is given intramuscularly at a dosage of 3–15 mg until treatment is finished.
- Good sources of dietary folate should be encouraged to maintain stores and especially if inadequate intake was an underlying cause of the deficiency (see Table 43.3).

Macrocytic non-megaloblastic anaemia

This type of anaemia can be caused by various mechanisms including alcohol, liver disease, hypothyroidism, certain neoplastic disorders, other anaemias and cytotoxic drugs. Haemolytic anaemia is relatively rare in the elderly, with one study of anaemic hospitalised geriatric patients demonstrating a prevalence of haemolytic anaemia of less than 1%. Haemolytic anaemia is caused by a shortened red cell survival due to peripheral destruction or increased rate of red cell destruction and the bone marrow is unable to respond. It can be either inherited or acquired. In the inherited form, abnormalities in the red blood cell membrane or in haemoglobin structure and synthesis occur. The acquired type is more common in the elderly and is normally mediated by immune or non-immune mechanisms. Drugs, including antimicrobials (e.g. penicillin, rifampicin), antirheumatics and tranquillisers, should always be considered as a cause of haemolysis in the elderly. Other non-immune causes include infection with malaria and certain bacteria or liver disease. Patients with liver disease have large, thin macrocytes. Alcoholism produces mild macrocytosis in 40–96% of individuals, with or without anaemia, as a result of the direct effects of alcohol on the bone marrow.

Diagnosis

Clinical manifestations vary according to the type of haemolytic disorder but include jaundice, splenomegaly, cholelithiasis and skeletal abnormalities.

Haematological indicators

- Specific morphological characteristics (e.g. sickle-cell anaemia).
- Increased haem catabolism (e.g. increased bilirubin level), increased serum lactate hydrogenase, reduced glycosylated haemoglobin.
- A fall in haemoglobin at a rate > 1.0 g/dL per week.
- Coombs' test is positive for antibodies to the red cell surface (immunohaemolytic anaemia).
- Increased reticulocytes.

Management

- Treat or prevent further exposure to the underlying cause.
- Steroid or immunosuppression therapy.
- Splenectomy.

Conclusion

Anaemia in all patients is a challenge to medical practitioners, but particularly in the elderly who manifest with a wide range of potential underlying diseases and a complexity of physiological and psychosocial issues that compound their problems. Anaemia in this age group will result in a decreased level of both physical and cognitive functioning, thus increasing dependency levels and resulting in an overall reduced quality of life. As well as influencing morbidity, anaemia has been shown to be associated with an increased risk of mortality. In a sample of 755 subjects aged 85 years and older, the presence of anaemia was associated with a greater than twofold risk of mortality at 10 years of follow-up, compared with persons who had a normal Hb concentration at baseline.

In the older adult, anaemia is likely to be due to disease and should not be considered a normal consequence of ageing. Thorough investigation of the underlying cause is indicated in all elderly patients presenting with anaemia.

In the case of prophylaxis for the prevention of iron deficiency anaemia, the potential for harm needs to be considered. Concerns for iron deficiency and iron deficiency anaemia frequently overshadow that for iron overload, despite the documented prevalence of the latter in 7% of the adult (20–74 years) population of the US. Iron overload has been reported in 22% of an elderly population in Glasgow. Whereas optimal iron status is accepted to be of considerable importance for normal neurological and immune function, an association between iron overload and ischaemic heart disease, as well as cancer, has been suggested.

The importance of an optimal vitamin B_{12} and folate status, together with vitamin B_6 status, in the elderly has only recently been appreciated. Much work has been conducted around the role of these B vitamins in the metabolism of homocysteine, a sulphur-containing amino acid, which has been shown to be an independent risk factor for vascular disease and stroke. Deficiencies of folate, vitamin B_{12} or vitamin B_6 slow the conversion of homocysteine to methionine and lead to an accumulation of homocysteine in the blood.

At least in the case of vitamin B_{12}, there appears to be a shifting paradigm with regard to maintaining optimal serum concentrations and body stores, rather than merely preventing clinical deficiency states. The clinical significance of suboptimal or even borderline vitamin deficiencies, with regard to physical and cognitive functioning, as well as risk of chronic, degenerative disease in the elderly, will become evident with future intervention studies in this age group.

Bibliography and further reading

Ahluwalia, N., Lammi-Keefe, C. J., Bendel, R. B., Morse, E. E., Beard, J. L. & Haley, N. R. (1995), 'Iron deficiency and anemia of chronic disease in elderly women; a discriminant-analysis approach for differentiation', *The American Journal of Clinical Nutrition*, 61, pp. 590–6.

Annibale, B., Marignani, M., Monarca, B., Asntonelli, G., Marcheggiano, A., Martino, G., Mandelli, F., Caprilli, R. & Delle Fave, G. (1999), 'Reversal of iron deficiency anemia after *Helicobacter pylori* eradication in patients with asymptomatic gastritis', *Annals of Internal Medicine*, 131, pp. 668–72.

Carmel, R. (1997), 'Cobalamin, the stomach, and aging', *The American Journal of Clinical Nutrition*, 66, pp. 750–9.

Charlton, K. E., Kruger, M., Labadarios, L., Wolmarans, P. & Aronson, I. (1997), 'Iron, folate and vitamin B_{12} status of an elderly South African population', *European Journal of Clinical Nutrition*, 51, pp. 424–30.

Fineman, Z., Gurerich, V., Coscas, D., Kopleman, Y., Segal, A. & Sternberg, A. (1999), 'Results of gastrointestinal evaluation in 90 hospitalized iron deficiency anaemia patients', *The Israeli Medical Association Journal*, 1, pp. 232–5.

Holyoake, T. L., Stott, D. J., McKay, P. J., Hendry, A., MacDonald J. B. & Lucie, N. P. (1993), 'Use of plasma ferritin concentration to diagnose iron deficiency in an elderly patient', *Journal of Clinical Pathology*, 46, pp. 857–60.

Izaks, G. J., Westendorp, R. G. J. & Knook, D. L. (1999), 'The definition of anemia in older persons', *Journal of the American Medical Association*, 281, pp. 1714–17.

Jolobe, O. M. P. (2000), 'Does this elderly patient have iron deficiency anaemia, and what is the underlying cause?', *Postgraduate Medical Journal*, 79, pp. 195–8.

Joosten, E., Ghesquiere, B., Lindthoudt, H., Krekelberghs, F., Dejaeger, E., Boonen, S., Flamaing, J., Pelemans, W., Hiele, M. & Gevers, A. (1999), 'Upper and lower gastrointestinal evaluation of elderly inpatients who are iron deficient', *American Journal of Medicine*, 107, pp. 24–7.

Lee, G. R., Foerster, J., Luken, J., Parashevas, F., Greer, J. P. & Rodgers, G. M. (1999), *Wintrobe's Clinical Hematology*, Vol. 2, 10th edn, Williams & Wilkins, Baltimore, MD, pp. 897–1405.

Sayer, J. M., Donnely, M. T., McIntyre, A. S., Barton, J. R., Grundman, M. J., Vicary, F. R. & Long, R. G. (1999), 'Barium enema or colonoscopy for the investigation of iron deficiency anaemia?', *Journal of the Royal College of Physicians London*, 33, pp. 543–8.

Stabler, S. P., Lindenbaum, J. & Allen, R. H. (1997), 'Vitamin B-12 deficiency in the elderly: Current dilemmas', *The American Journal of Clinical Nutrition*, 66, pp. 741–9.

Stott, D. J., Langhorne, P., Hendry, A., McKay, P. J., Holyoake, T., Macdonald J. & Lucie, N. (1997), 'Prevalence and haemopoietic effects of low serum vitamin B_{12} levels in geriatric medical patients', *The British Journal of Nutrition*, 78, pp. 57–63.

Van Asselt, D. Z. B, de Groot, L. C. P. G. M, van Staveren, W. A., Blom, H. J, Wevers, R. A., Biemond, I. & Hoefnagels, W. H. L. (1998), 'Role of cobalamin intake and atrophic gastritis in mild cobalamin deficiency in older Dutch subjects', *The American Journal of Clinical Nutrition*, 68, pp. 328–34.

Chapter 44

Haematological effects of systemic disorders

NICHOLAS WICKHAM

Introduction

Changes in the blood and blood cells are a sensitive but not necessarily specific indicator of systemic disease. Blood is a complex fluid consisting of cells suspended in plasma. With the exception of completely avascular tissues such as dental enamel, blood maintains an intimate relationship with all organs of the body. Systemic disease may produce changes in blood cells and/or plasma of a varying degree of subtlety. If a patient has a normal blood count, with a normal differential count, normal morphology on examination of the film and an erythrocyte sedimentation rate within the normal range, then serious organic illness can be excluded. The purpose of this chapter is to delineate the changes that may occur in the blood in relation to systemic disease, the significance of these changes and how they may be utilised as a guide to further investigation.

Aetiology and epidemiology

Changes in the blood associated with systemic disease may be produced directly or indirectly and these changes may be quantitative or qualitative. The aetiology and epidemiology of such changes are therefore best considered together with the particular system involved and its relevant pathophysiology in the context of the ageing process. However, one popular misconception, that should be discounted at the outset, is that low blood counts may be attributed to a consequence of ageing. Although bone marrow cellularity does decrease somewhat with age, this is a late event, occurring gradually after the age of 60 years; it is in the order of a 15% decrease in overall cellularity in the very elderly. This does not translate into correspondingly lower blood counts, although it is true that the haemopoietic reserve is less substantial than in a younger person, partly due to diminished numbers of stem cells and reduced bone marrow cytokine production, particularly in patients over the age of 65.

Pathophysiology

Skin

Senile purpura

Increased capillary fragility and thinning of the skin is a consequence of ageing, and the somewhat disconcerting but accurately named complaint of senile purpura is common. On occasion it causes distress more because of its appearance than because of any other concern. It may be exacerbated by low-dose aspirin which many patients may be taking for vascular or ischaemic disease. It occurs particularly on the upper limbs, wrists and back of the hands, and results in large superficial skin bruising which occurs spontaneously or with minimal trauma. Treatment is reassurance and, for those concerned about aesthetics, cosmetics may be used to disguise discoloured areas of skin.

Thrombocytopenic purpura

Purpura secondary to low platelets occurs initially in dependent areas and therefore is often most prominent in the skin of the lower limbs. It usually commences as a fine rash. It may be associated with gingival, nasal, gastrointestinal and retinal haemorrhage. The causes are outlined in Box 44.1. A detailed discussion of thrombocytopenic purpura falls outside the scope of this chapter, but drug-induced immune thrombocytopenia, myelodysplastic syndrome (MDS), acute leukaemia and malignant infiltration should be considered particularly in the elderly. Elderly patients are more likely to be taking medication, and the incidence of both MDS and malignancy increase with age. Urgent referral for expert haematological review is the correct management.

Box 44.1 Causes of thrombocytopenic purpura

1. Bone marrow failure
   (a) Aplastic anaemia
   (b) Myelodysplastic syndromes/acute leukaemia
   (c) Malignant infiltration
   (d) Severe haematinic deficiency
2. Peripheral consumption
   (a) Immune thrombocytopenia (idiopathic)
   (b) Immune thrombocytopenia (drug induced)
   (c) Thrombotic thrombocytopenic purpura
   (d) Diffuse intravascular coagulation
3. End-stage liver disease

Non-thrombocytopenic purpura

Vasculitides may present with purpuric lesions that resemble closely those due to low platelet counts, but in fact are due to immune complexes causing capillary damage; platelet counts are within the normal range. Another rarely seen cause of non-thrombocytopenic purpura which should be considered, especially in the elderly and malnourished patient, is scurvy. Vitamin C deficiency causes capillary fragility due to defective connective tissue production, resulting in purpura and gingival haemorrhage. It may be diagnosed by performing a vitamin C loading test which measures the amount of vitamin C excreted in the urine after a test loading dose of vitamin C.

Burns

Full-thickness burns that cover an appreciable amount of body surface area result in a microangiopathic haemolytic anaemia due to fibrin strands in damaged blood vessels that damage red cells. This results in the appearance of poikilocytes, spherocytes and, characteristically, microspherocytes in the blood film.

Cardiovascular system

Valve replacement and macroangiopathic haemolytic anaemia

Significant mechanical haemolysis may be associated with artificial heart valves. This is more likely to occur with artificial valves inserted on the high pressure side of the heart (i.e. aortic mitral valves) than with pulmonary or tricuspid valves. This problem only presents if there is dysfunction of the valve due to incompetence or a peripheral leak, resulting in small high-pressure jets that damage red cells, leading to their intravascular destruction. The diagnosis is suspected in patients with recurring anaemia after valve replacement surgery with an increased reticulocyte count, red cell fragments on the blood film and other markers of haemolysis, such as low serum haptoglobin, and raised lactate dehydrogenase (LDH) and bilirubin levels. The presence of urinary haemosiderin will confirm intravascular haemolysis and echocardiography will confirm the faulty valve function. Treatment is by further surgical intervention.

Hypertension and red cell anomalies

In high blood pressure similar damage to red cells may occur but to a lesser extent. This will manifest as a low grade intravascular haemolysis with red cell fragments and poikilocytes on the blood film and increased reticulocytes. It is not of sufficient severity to result in anaemia.

Cardiac bypass surgery and platelet dysfunction

A patient undergoing cardiac bypass will not infrequently suffer from bleeding, despite only a moderately reduced or normal platelet count and normal coagulation studies. This is secondary to platelet activation during their passage over the artificial surfaces of the bypass circuit. This results in platelet degranulation and hence their subsequent inability to aggregate appropriately at the wound site on their return to the normal circulation. Platelets should therefore be made available for patients undergoing bypass surgery in whom postoperative capillary ooze is a problem, despite what would normally be considered adequate platelet counts (bleeding times are not usually affected until platelet counts fall below 90×10^9/L).

Cardiac ischaemia and antiplatelet drugs

The factors leading to coronary atherosclerosis and ischaemic heart disease involve a complex interplay between the coagulation system, lipid metabolism, vascular wall biology, monocyte-macrophage function and platelet aggregation. Antiplatelet drugs include blockers of prostaglandin metabolism such as aspirin, inhibitors of other platelet metabolic pathways and inhibitors of platelet activation that decrease the risk of subsequent ischaemic events as well as limit the damage that such events may cause.

Respiratory system

Hypoxia, secondary polycythaemia and blood viscosity

Chronic hypoxia results in stimulation of erythropoietin production from the kidney and an increase in the number of red cells. This results from primary lung disease, cor pulmonale, living at high altitudes, sleep apnoea and by the regular practice of complex hatha yoga postures which restrict the ability of the lungs to ventilate adequately. It is interesting that hatha yoga was recommended in traditional yoga practice as being beneficial for the treatment of anaemia.

For individuals who have cardiorespiratory failure, although the body has seemingly responded appropriately by increasing red cell mass to improve oxygen delivery to the tissues, the corresponding increase in whole blood viscosity results in increased cardiac work. Beyond a certain point the increased cardiac work (and therefore oxygen consumption) diminishes severely any advantage that might have been gained from the polycythaemia. This results in a vicious cycle of increasing hypoxia and decreasing cardiorespiratory efficiency, provoking further inappropriate red cell production. This cycle can only be broken by venesection to lower blood viscosity to a level where the heart can cope with the extra work load, without compromising the improvement in oxygen-carrying capacity due to the extra red cells.

Patients with haematocrits above 50% suffer an increasing risk of cerebrovascular accident or thrombosis and this risk is significant with haematocrits above 55%. Thus in patients with primary polycythaemia or that secondary to non-cardiorespiratory causes, it is recommended that haematocrits are kept below 50%. However, patients with respiratory insufficiency require higher haematocrits than would normally be recommended. The aim with venesection in these patients is to achieve a balance that diminishes the risk of stroke or thrombosis and allows more efficient cardiac function without depriving them of the extra oxygenation associated with a higher haemoglobin. Great care has to be taken with venesection in patients who will undergo cardiac decompensation if venesection is instigated in a cavalier fashion. No more than 1 unit of red cells should be removed at one session and preferably an equal volume of normal saline should be given as replacement fluid so that the patient remains isovolaemic. The precise haematocrit to be achieved has to be assessed on clinical grounds for each patient, although one aims for the lowest haematocrit that can be tolerated. Many such patients will not tolerate a reduction of their haematocrit below 60% or even higher.

Sleep apnoea

Sleep apnoea is now a recognised and well documented condition that can give rise to polycythaemia with an haematocrit of over 55% or higher. Diagnosis depends on excluding other causes of polycythaemia and confirming sleep apnoea in a sleep laboratory where overnight monitoring of respiratory function is possible. Treatment is now available with the provision of positive airways pressure oxygen masks worn during sleep which, by removing the nocturnal hypoxic drive responsible for excess red cell production, may obviate the need for venesection. If the patients who do not have cardiorespiratory disease cannot tolerate nocturnal oxygen therapy, then venesection to maintain an haematocrit below 50% would be recommended.

Pneumonia/sepsis and leucocytosis

Pneumonia and other severe sepsis may result in extremely high white cell counts (i.e. 80×10^9/L) with a neutrophilia and may provoke concern whether the patient has chronic myeloid or myelomonocytic leukaemia. Severe sepsis may stimulate the release of immature precursors into the peripheral blood, but review of the blood film will usually be sufficient to reassure the physician and the patient that the white cell changes are reactive. It is important to have an expert review the blood film, however, as patients with myelodysplastic syndromes such as chronic myelomonocytic leukaemia or leukaemia are at increased risk of infection and lobar or bronchopneumonia may be a presenting feature of other haematological malignancies, such as non-Hodgkin's lymphoma or multiple myeloma.

The response of the bone marrow to infectious and inflammatory stimuli as well as to drugs and other chemicals is complex and is often reflected in changes in the differential white cell count. An overview of changes in the differential white cell count is provided in Tables 44.1, 44.2 and 44.3.

Gastrointestinal system

Liver disease and red cell anomalies

Cirrhosis and liver failure lead to a variety of changes which affect the red cells in particular. The triglyceride and lipid profile in the plasma is different in patients with liver disease and some of these lipids are freely interchangeable with those in the red cell membrane. This results in an altered lipid composition in the red cell membrane which alters its flexibility and results in changes in morphology, producing both large flat red cells, referred to as leptocytes, as well as target cells.

End-stage liver disease, coagulopathy, thrombocytopenia and hypersplenism

Liver failure results in a decrease in all the proteins manufactured by the liver. This results in a prolonged prothrombin time, prolonged activated partial thromboplastin time (APTT) and a prolonged thrombin time due to a decrease in all clotting factors produced by the liver. It is important to note that this differs from the effect, with normal liver function, of warfarin which blocks the vitamin K dependent carboxylation of the coagulation factors II, VII, IX and X (as well as the anticoagulant factors protein C and protein S). With normal hepatic function these factors are still produced by the liver and are known as PIVKA (proteins in vitamin K absence). The administration of exogenous vitamin K will restore normal function, overcoming the carboxylation block. In hepatic failure, however, there is an absolute decrease in all clotting factors, not just the vitamin K dependent factors, and vitamin K will not reverse the clotting abnormalities. Vitamin K is still administered to such patients to ensure that there is not also an associated lack of vitamin K due to malabsorption or antibiotic use (which will decrease vitamin K production by organisms normally synthesising this in the gut). Treatment for the coagulopathy requires replacement of coagulation factors with both fresh frozen plasma and cryoprecipitate. Cryoprecipitate, which is high in fibrinogen, as well as fibronectin and von Willebrand factor, is necessary in particular for the replacement of fibrinogen, as adequate levels cannot be attained with fresh frozen plasma without infusing excessive

Table 44.1 White cell responses

White cell	Disorders causing an increase	Disorders causing a decrease
Neutrophil	*Physiological stress* Exercise, food, emotion, pregnancy, labour, parturition Epileptic convulsion, left ventricular failure, paroxysmal tachycardia *Haemorrhage/haemolysis* *Infection* Pyogenic cocci (especially) Non-pyogenic organisms: diphtheria, polio, cholera Typhus Zoster *Necrosis* Myocardial infarction, burns, rheumatoid arthritis Polyarteritis nodosa, hepatic necrosis *Metabolic* Gout, diabetes mellitus, uraemia *Malignancy* Myeloproliferative disorder: chronic granulocytic leukaemia (CGL), polycythaeonia rubra vera (PRV) myelofibrosis Carcinoma of lung, liver, colon and bladder; melanoma *Drugs/poisons* Digitalis, quinine, phenacetin, lithium, adrenaline Growth factors: G-CSF, GM-CSF Steroids, mercury, potassium chlorate, lead, venoms *Hypersensitivity* Serum sickness, rheumatic fever, acute glomerulonephritis	*Physiological* Ethnic neutropenia with white blood cell count around 3.0 and neutrophils of 1.5×10^9/L Afro-Caribbean and Middle Eastern people who are otherwise well *Infection* Enteric fevers, rickettsia, protozoa, viral, especially influenza and hepatitis Tuberculosis, especially miliary, typhoid, overwhelming Gram-negative infections *Drugs* Analgesics: amidopyrine, phenylbutazone, oxyphenbutazone Antibiotics: tetracycline, chloramphenicol, penicillins Anticonvulsants: phenytoin Antidiabetics: tolbutamide, chlorpropamide, carbutamide Antihistamines: chlorpheniramine, promethazine, mepyramine Antituberculosis: isoniazid, periodic acid Schiff (PAS), streptomycin Antithyroid: carbimazole, propylthiouracil Antiviral: azidothymidine, gancyclovir Diuretics: chlorothiazide, frusemide, ethacrynic acid Tranquillisers: barbiturates, promazines, trichlor/trifluperazine Miscellaneous: interferon, chemotherapy, allopurinol, phenindione, penicillamine, gold salts *Bone marrow impairment* Infiltration: carcinoma, lymphoma, leukaemia Myelofibrosis ± hypersplenism Starvation, anorexia nervosa, alcohol excess Aplastic anaemia, paroxysmal nocturnal haemoglobinuria Congenital disorders: reticular dysgenesis, chronic idiopathic neutropenia, benign cyclical neutropenia *Immune* Systemic lupus erythematosus, Felty's syndrome, multiple blood transfusions Haemodialysis: may be associated with complement activation Hypersensitivity: anaphylaxis, endotoxin exposure *Endocrine* Myxoedema, hypopituitarism

volumes. The total protein load in hepatic failure has to be carefully assessed in the light of clinical need and overall assessment of the patient's condition, as portal systemic encephalopathy may be precipitated.

Thrombocytopenia is commonly seen in end-stage liver failure and was previously attributed to increased platelet sequestration in a chronically enlarged spleen. However, thrombopoietin, or

Table 44.2 White cell responses

White cell	Disorders causing an increase	Disorders causing a decrease
Lymphocyte	*Acute viral infections* Pertussis, rubella, mumps, infectious hepatitis, cytomegolavirus Infectious mononucleosis, infectious lymphocytosis *Chronic infections* Tuberculosis, syphilis, toxoplasmosis, brucellosis *Malignancy* Chronic lymphocytic leukaemia, prolymphocytic leukaemia, lymphocytic lymphoma, Waldenstrom's macroglobulinaemia *Thyrotoxicosis* Variable: often only relative increase	*Stress* Steroids/adrenocorticotropic hormone (ACTH) *Drugs* Antilymphocyte globulin Anti-T-cell monoclonal antibodies (i.e. Campath) Immunosuppressant cytotoxics: azathioprine *Ionising radiation* *Immune deficiency* Acquired immune deficiency (AIDS) Congenital: agammaglobulinaemia, severe combined immune deficiency *Bone marrow failure/impairment* Aplastic anaemia, Hodgkin's disease
Monocyte	*Infections* Bacterial: tuberculosis, syphilis, brucellosis, subacute bacterial endocarditis, typhoid, paratyphoid, *Listeria monocytogenes* (rarely) Protozoa: malaria, leishmaniasis, trypanosomiasis Rickettsia: typhus, Rocky Mountain fever *Malignancy* Acute myelo-monocytic and monocytic leukaemia (M4, M5) Chronic myelo-monocytic leukaemia Hodgkin's disease (30% cases) Carcinomas: may provoke a reactive monocytosis *Connective tissue disease* Systemic lupus erythematosus, rheumatoid arthritis *Inflammatory bowel disease* Crohn's and ulcerative colitis *Chronic skin disease* Psoriasis, neurodermatitis *Sarcoidosis* *Poison* Tetrachloroethane	*Malignancy* Hairy cell leukaemia Chronic myeloid leukaemia

megakaryocyte growth and differentiation factor (MGDF), is produced by the liver; in end-stage liver failure, low circulating levels also contribute to a decrease in the platelet count. There are several synthetic thrombopoietic hormones under development and in the near future these may be of use in raising the platelet count in such situations, although early trials of one such drug in haematological conditions have been disappointing to date.

Table 44.3 White cell responses

White cell	Disorders causing an increase	Disorders causing a decrease
Eosinophil	*Allergy* Angioneurotic oedema, asthma *Parasites* Bilharzia, filaria, hookworm, hydatid, etc. *Pulmonary eosinophilia* Loeffler's syndrome, Tropical eosinophilia, polyarteritis nodosa *Skin diseases* Dermatitis herpetiformis, eczema, exfoliative dermatitis Pemphigus, psoriasis, prurigo, scabies *Malignancy* Hodgkin's disease; myeloproliferative disorders, especially CGL Eosinophilic leukaemia Carcinoma, especially with necrotic metastases *Haematological* Pernicious anaemia, post-splenectomy, post-chemotherapy Post-bone marrow transplant, especially in regenerating phase *Infections* Scarlet fever, erythema multiforme, cytomegalovirus Acute infectious lymphocytosis, chorea *Drugs/chemicals* Liver extract, streptomycin, penicillin, PAS, hydralazine Nitrofurantoin, sulphonamides, mephenesin, nickel *Other eosinophilic syndromes* Familial eosinophilia, hyper-eosinophilic syndrome Churg-Strauss, Schuller-Christian, Letterer-Siwe diseases	*Drugs* Steroids, ACTH, adrenaline *Stress* Severe infection, trauma, burns Following electroconvulsive therapy Strenuous exercise *Endocrine* Cushing's syndrome Acromegaly *Connective tissue disease* Systemic lupus erythematosus
Basophil	*Chronic myeloid leukaemia* Especially accelerated phase/transformation to acute leukaemia *Uncommonly seen in* Hypothyroidism, chronic haemolysis, PRV, cirrhosis Chronic inflammation, chickenpox and smallpox	*May decrease occasionally in* Rheumatic fever Lobar pneumonia Thyrotoxicosis Steroid therapy Stress

Malabsorption and myelodysplasia

Malabsorption is of particular importance in the elderly. They may suffer subtle degrees of malabsorption relating to pernicious anaemia or occult blind loop syndrome. Macrocytosis is a clue to the presence of folate, vitamin B_{12} deficiency or thyroid dysfunction, but can also be an early sign of myelodysplasia. Myelodysplasia is a myeloproliferative condition, the incidence of which increases with age, and it is associated with refractory anaemia and cytopenias, which can also be part of severe vitamin B_{12} or folate deficiency. Review of the blood film may detect other signs of myelodysplasia such as abnormal, dysplastic neutrophils. The cause of vitamin B_{12} deficiency and folate deficiency will depend on further inquiry and investigations, which may include a Schilling test and small bowel biopsy. Where vitamin B_{12} deficiency has been detected, from whatever cause, then it is important to pre-treat with parenteral vitamin B_{12} for at least 2 weeks prior to performing a Schilling test, as severe vitamin B_{12} deficiency also causes changes in the epithelial cells of the gut which result in a secondary malabsorption and thus may result in an incorrect diagnosis. Combined deficiencies of iron as well as vitamin B_{12} and/or folate may mask each other's changes of macrocytosis and microcytosis. In the more extreme cases of malabsorption and debility, patients may present with low haemoglobin values of 60 g/L (6 g/dL) or less. In elderly patients, this degree of anaemia may easily provoke ischaemic cardiac or other symptoms, and cautious blood transfusion to bring the haemoglobin up to and maintain it above 90 g/L may be necessary. Large volume transfusion to completely reverse a low haemoglobin to normal values will result in cardiovascular overload and decompensation, and is contraindicated. If patients are not suffering symptoms and are stable, then normal enteral/parenteral supplements will be sufficient to permit a gradual return to normal haematological values.

Starvation and anorexia

In these patients, pancytopenia is associated with extreme wasting. They may have profound suppression of their bone marrow and require hospitalisation for investigation and treatment. Bone marrow examination will reveal the classical appearance of reduced cellularity associated with an amorphous eosinophilic deposit due to degradation of the normal supporting tissue ground substance. Management is complicated by the metabolic derangement present in severely malnourished patients, who require cautious and balanced supplementation, sometimes with intensive care support.

Inflammatory bowel disease

Inflammatory bowel disease is a potent bone marrow stimulant, as inflammation, bleeding and infection all provoke a leucocytosis and in combination may produce a leukaemoid response in acute toxic episodes. The platelet count, which varies normally between 150 and 400×10^9/L, is affected in the acute phase response to bleeding and inflammation. It mirrors the erythrocyte sedimentation rate and other markers of inflammatory bowel disease and may be useful as a monitor of response to therapy. Marked thrombocytosis ($> 1000 \times 10^9$/L) has also been reported in Whipple's disease. Conversely, thrombocytopenia and leucopenia are seen as side effects of immunosuppressive (and myelosuppressive) medication, but there are also reports of immune thrombocytopenias occurring as part of an extraintestinal autoimmune dysregulation in inflammatory bowel disease. Iron deficiency may result from the chronic blood loss and may be difficult to document in early stages due to the acute phase response. Although the serum ferritin is the best single guide to total body iron, it is also an acute phase response protein and therefore has to be interpreted in this light. For example, a cut-off (lower limit of normal) of 50 μg/L has been suggested instead of 15 μg/L in patients with inflammatory bowel disease, in whom the diagnosis of iron deficiency is often associated with evidence of undernourishment.

Colorectal cancer

A moderate rise in the platelet count should alert the physician to look for occult blood in the stools, as thrombocytosis may be a marker for iron deficiency secondary to chronic gastrointestinal blood loss. If positive, endoscopic or radiological investigations are mandatory to exclude malignancy or ulceration. However, patients may not be anaemic, as a fall in haemoglobin is an end-stage response to depleted total body iron stores; patients may be developing iron deficiency due to occult blood loss, but may not actually be anaemic because the haemoglobin doesn't fall until their iron stores are exhausted. Anaemia is a late development in iron deficiency.

Genitourinary system

Uraemia/chronic renal failure

Patients with impaired renal function develop anaemia that, by and large, is proportional to the degree of renal failure and secondary to a corresponding decrease in the production of erythropoietin. Complicating factors include other inflammatory conditions and malabsorption of water soluble vitamins in particular. In these patients, the anaemia of chronic disease (due to ineffective erythropoiesis secondary to the effect of inflammatory cytokines on the bone marrow) and iron deficiency can increase the severity of the anaemia. Red cells in patients with uraemia are classically crenated due partly to changes in lipid composition within the plasma and partly to changes in water distribution between the red cell and the plasma. In most cases the anaemia is normochromic and normocytic, but may also be hypochromic and microcytic. It can be difficult to determine from iron studies in some patients if an associated iron deficiency exists. Serum ferritin is a sensitive acute phase protein and may be raised well into the normal range by associated inflammation. In such cases, a bone marrow examination is the most direct way of assessing iron stores and scrutinising haematopoiesis for signs of other problems such as myelodysplasia or occult malignant infiltration.

Many renal patients with moderate renal impairment, not requiring dialysis, may tolerate a subnormal haemoglobin down to around 100 g/L. At values below this, there is a definite reduction in a sense of wellbeing. In the past, intermittent transfusion was offered to patients on dialysis with severe anaemia and this resulted in problems of iron overload and the risk of exposure to viral infections. At present recombinant erythropoietin, administered regularly according to patient response, can reverse the anaemia of chronic renal failure. The suggestion that there may be a myelosuppressive element associated with uraemia is not correct. Patients who respond poorly to erythropoietin may be iron deficient, and iron supplementation either orally or parenterally will ensure a satisfactory response.

Central nervous system

Transient ischaemic attacks

Low-dose aspirin (50–100 mg a day) undoubtedly has a role to play in the prevention of arterial platelet thrombus formation which is responsible for transient ischaemic attacks. Other antiplatelet drugs, as discussed above in relation to cardiac ischaemia, may be appropriate and effective agents in this situation.

Stroke

Patients with hemiplegic stroke have a more than sixfold increase in the risk of deep vein thrombosis in the paralysed limb compared to the mobile limb and are also at increased risk therefore of pulmonary embolism (Chapter 26). Early treatment of thrombotic cerebrovascular events with low molecular weight heparin has not been shown to be of convincing benefit, despite some studies supporting this approach. Long-term prophylactic anticoagulation with warfarin for patients with stroke has to be judged on the basis of a risk–benefit assessment for the individual patient.

Endocrine

Thyroid disease

Hyperthyroidism may rarely present with severe iron deficiency anaemia secondary to malabsorption as a result of intestinal hurry. This results in both decreased iron absorption and excess loss of iron due to the increase in gut epithelial cell turnover and excretion. Further problems may be encountered once antithyroid treatment has been commenced, the chief of these being drug-induced neutropenia, particularly associated with the use of carbimazole.

Hypothyroidism results in macrocytosis and in some cases abnormal 'gingerbread man'-shaped red cells may be detected on the blood film. Depending on how severe and longstanding the decrease in thyroid function has been, further abnormalities such as folate and/or iron deficiency may be apparent once thyroid replacement therapy has commenced. Hypothyroidism can unmask malabsorption when treatment has increased the metabolic rate and therefore marrow function returns to normal. Furthermore, as both hypothyroidism and pernicious anaemia share an autoimmune basis, an associated vitamin B_{12} deficiency is occasionally also identified.

Adrenal failure/panhypopituitarism

Failure of adequate corticosteroid synthesis, whether due to primary adrenal failure or secondary to pituitary dysfunction, may present with a normochromic normocytic anaemia for which no other obvious cause may be found. Failure of the pituitary-adrenal axis should always be considered as a cause in older patients with otherwise unexplained anaemia. Other clues are low blood pressure or electrolyte abnormalities which are often attributed to other factors or drugs.

Diabetes mellitus

Diabetic patients tend to have higher plasma fibrinogen levels and less deformable red cells, factors that both contribute to diabetic vascular problems because of increased viscosity and decreased flow in the microvasculature. Haemoglobin allows for a ready assessment of diabetic control by providing a direct measure of damage to proteins caused by chronically raised glucose levels in the form of the assay for the end-glycosylation product—haemoglobin A_1c.

Metabolic disorders

Many metabolic disorders may involve abnormal infiltration of the bone marrow as well as other tissue with products of defective metabolism. Most of these are more relevant to the paediatric population, but two disorders of metabolism, one congenital and one acquired, should be considered in relation to older patients.

Gaucher's disease (type I) and anaemia and thrombocytopenia

Gaucher's disease type 1 (as opposed to types 2 or 3) is an autosomal recessive disorder which accounts for 99% of cases and may rarely present in late adult life with fatigue and easy bruising due to anaemia and thrombocytopenia with hepatosplenomegaly and bone pain. It is caused by a deficiency of acid β-glucosidase which results in a progressive accumulation of glycolipids, especially glucosylceramide, in reticuloendothelial cells. This leads to bone marrow infiltration, hepatosplenomegaly and bony lesions. Bone marrow biopsy will confirm the presence of Gaucher cells (histiocytes laden with glycolipids) that stain positive with periodic acid Schiff (PAS). (Figure 44.1). Treatment until recently was supportive with transfusions and splenectomy (for hypersplenism or cardiac decompensation). Enzyme supplementation with recombinant glucosidase is currently being trialled in a limited number of patients (due to cost and availability) and is expected to eventually lead to an effective treatment.

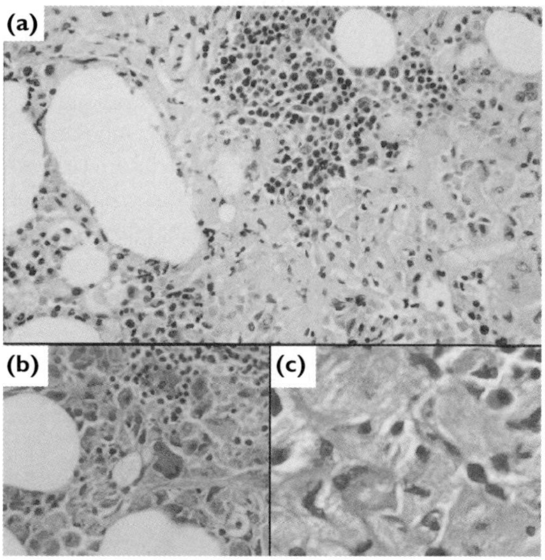

Figure 44.1 Extensive infiltration in the bone marrow in a patient with Gaucher's disease. **(a)** An H & E stain of the large abnormal Gaucher cells surrounding a small island of normal haematopoiesis. **(b)** The glucocerebroside in the Gaucher cells staining positively with PAS. **(c)** High power, showing the fibrillary nature of the cytoplasm in the Gaucher cells

Amyloidosis and abnormal coagulation

Amyloidosis is due to the deposition of insoluble fibrous amyloid proteins in the extracellular spaces of tissues. There are several different protein precursors, but all the amyloid proteins share a similar fibrillar nature. Amyloid deposition may be symptomless or result in serious disability. The most common form of amyloidosis, primary or AL amyloidosis, is associated with Bence Jones proteins or light chains. However, only 20% of such patients will have multiple myeloma, and amyloid deposition is only discovered in about 5% of multiple myeloma cases during life but may be found in up to 10% of myeloma patients at post-mortem.

Amyloidosis may present in many ways, but infiltration and enlargement of the heart, liver, spleen and tongue are common in AL amyloidosis. Splenomegaly due to amyloidosis is thought not to be associated with cytopenias, but instead amyloidosis protein may have an adverse affect on the clotting system. Low fibrinogen, increased fibrinolysis and deficiencies of other clotting factors may occur. Factor X deficiency in particular may occur due to binding to polyanionic amyloid fibrils. Splenectomy, by removing a large mass of amyloid, can reverse factor X deficiency caused by this mechanism. Treatment for AL amyloidosis involves using anti-myeloma drugs such as melphalan and prednisolone plus colchicine (which interferes with the production of the fibrils), and this combination has been shown to prolong life. High dose therapy with stem cell transplantation has also produced some excellent anecdotal responses. An anthracycline derivative, iododoxorubicin, binds to AL amyloid and promotes its resorption, and has shown some promise in small preliminary trials.

Malignancy

Apart from the gross effect of tumours on the body and its function, malignant cells may infiltrate the bone marrow (Figure 44.2). Classically, established malignant infiltration in the bone marrow produces a degree of anaemia with the presence of tear drop poikilocytes on the blood film. In addition to these red cell shape changes, the blood film will show nucleated red cells and primitive myeloid precursors in the so-called leuco-erythroblastic blood film (Figure 44.3). The response of the white blood cells and platelets is variable. They may initially be stimulated by low level infiltration, but will ultimately be suppressed, especially if severe myelofibrosis supervenes or if the infiltrate is so extensive that it supplants normal bone marrow. Myelofibrosis is a

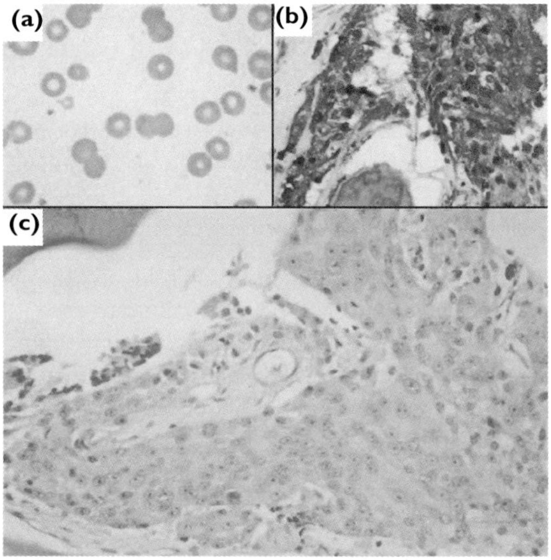

Figure 44.2 Malignant infiltrate in the bone marrow. **(a)** Tear drop poikilocytes in the peripheral blood, which are associated with abnormal marrow infiltration. **(b)** A bone marrow trephine with a heavy infiltrate of large monomorphic cells with prominent nucleoli. **(c)** These cells are strongly positive when stained for the tumour marker prostate specific antigen, confirming a prostatic origin for this malignant infiltrate. The patient presented with panycytopenia and did not have classic signs of metastatic prostatic carcinoma

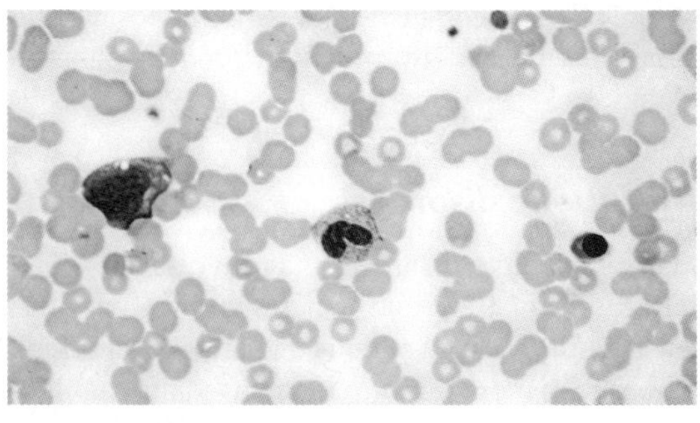

Figure 44.3 Leuco-erythroblastic blood film showing a myelocyte, a metamyelocyte and a nucleated red cell in the peripheral blood

non-specific fibrotic reaction to leukaemic or solid tumour infiltration, and may lead eventually to profound pancytopenia associated with an enlarged liver and spleen which expand in an effort to contribute to haematopoiesis under the erythropoietic drive associated with anaemia. Other more subtle effects may result from release of granulocyte colony-stimulating factors by tumour cells which produce a neutrophil leucocytosis in the absence of direct marrow infiltration. Therefore, any persistent neutrophil leucocytosis or thrombocytosis in the absence of an obvious inflammatory cause is suspicious for possible underlying malignancy.

Rheumatology

The main haematological problems in relation to rheumatological disorders relate to cytopenias, most commonly the anaemia of chronic disease but also neutropenia and thrombocytopenia. The difficulty in relation to these problems is in determining, in each case, whether the problem is part of the autoimmune disorder and related to increased disease activity or whether it is due to either drugs or, more rarely, some other unrelated condition.

Rheumatoid arthritis: anaemia of chronic disease

Rheumatoid arthritis may be associated with anaemia of chronic disease. The haemoglobin in such cases rarely falls much below 80–100 g/L, and the serum ferritin and other haematinic studies are within the normal range. However, anaemia may also occur as a result of iron deficiency associated with the use of non-steroidal anti-inflammatory drugs and chronic gastrointestinal blood loss secondary to gastritis. As with inflammatory bowel disease (see above), the usual values for ferritin may not be appropriate in acute and chronic inflammation. Recent studies suggest that in an elderly population with anaemia for any reason, a cut-off point of 100 μg/L separates those with iron deficiency from those with other disorders. Thus, iron deficiency should be suspected in any patient who has active rheumatoid arthritis with a ferritin level less than 100 μg/L. The variations in associated tests of iron status in various conditions are summarised in Table 44.4.

Autoimmune haemolytic anaemia may also occur as part of the autoimmune disorder. This is diagnosed by finding an increased reticulocyte count, spherocytes on the blood film, a lowered serum haptoglobin and raised LDH levels and bilirubin. Steroids are the usual first-line treatment, but blood transfusion, despite the difficulties encountered in cross-matching, may be necessary if anaemia is progressive and the patient becomes symptomatic. Splenectomy may be appropriate in selected patients.

Neutropenia and/or thrombocytopenia may also be autoimmune or associated with immunosuppressive drugs such as azathioprine. Newer immunomodulatory drugs (e.g. leflunomide) may also cause severe myelosuppression, and blood counts should be monitored regularly. Discontinuing the drug or moderating the dose may be required. Haematological assessment with a bone marrow examination is recommended in severe cases or where there is doubt about the diagnosis. Patients on gold injections are also at risk of severe neutropenia, and in any patient with falling white

Table 44.4 Iron studies in iron deficiency, anaemia of chronic disease and iron overload

Assay	Normal range	Iron deficiency	Chronic disease	Iron overload
Ferritin (μg/L)	10–150	< 10	> 150	> 250
Iron (μmol/L)	8–28	< 8	< 8	> 30
TIBC (μmol/L)	45–72	45–96	< 40	< 45
Transferrin (g/L)[a]	2–3.9	> 4	< 2	< 2
Transferrin saturation (%)	15–48	< 15	< 25	> 60

(a) TIBC (total iron-binding capacity) was used as an estimate of transferrin concentration. However, transferrin is now more commonly measured directly using an immunologic assay.

Note: Anaemia of chronic disease is distinguished by a low serum iron with a raised or high-normal ferritin in association with a low transferrin and transferrin saturation.

cell counts, gold injections should be ceased and haematological review undertaken with bone marrow assessment of cellularity if severe neutropenia ensues. Early use of growth factors such as G-CSF may limit the neutropenia, and in the event of fever, early and aggressive use of intravenous broad-spectrum antibiotics by a physician/haematologist experienced in the care of neutropenic patients is mandatory to avoid disaster.

Felty's syndrome

This is an autoimmune neutropenia and haemolytic anaemia associated with rheumatoid arthritis. There is premature and excessive destruction of cellular elements in the spleen, which is enlarged. Steroids may be successful in maintaining control of the cytopenias, but splenectomy may result in a more definitive response.

Systemic lupus erythematosus (SLE)

This may be associated with any or all of the problems noted above. Autoimmune neutropenia or immune thrombocytopenia may be associated particularly with SLE. Again, steroids and/or splenectomy may be helpful in selected cases.

Drugs

Agranulocytosis

This is one of the most common haematological reactions to drugs. The many different classes of drugs that may be associated with neutropenia and agranulocytosis are listed in Table 44.1.

Thrombocytopenia

Many drugs (over 120) have been implicated with thrombocytopenia, although quinine is one of the few drugs that can be demonstrated *in vitro* to cause a true drug-dependent thrombocytopenia. Another important cause of this phenomenon is heparin-induced thrombocytopenia (HIT).

Heparin-induced thrombocytopenia (HIT)

Heparin may cause a fall in the platelet count by two different mechanisms. The first is benign and may commence almost immediately after heparin has been started. In addition it is usually mild, producing a modest reduction in the platelet count which may or may not become subnormal. The mechanism is due to a non-specific aggregatory affect of heparin on platelets. The second more serious mechanism usually occurs after the fifth day of heparin therapy due to the formation of heparin dependent antibodies against glycoproteins on the platelet surface. The binding of these antibodies to platelet glycoproteins in the presence of heparin causes widespread platelet activation, resulting in microvascular thrombosis and severe thrombocytopenia. Heparin should be stopped immediately (even low-dose heparin employed for flushing intravenous cannulae or central lines), platelet infusions should be avoided, and if anticoagulation must be continued, one of the alternative heparinoids or synthetic alternatives used. Failure to do so can lead to diffuse intravascular coagulopathy with severe thrombocytopenia, major thromboses and bleeding. Severe HIT is most likely to occur with unfractionated heparin, but has also been reported with low molecular weight heparin. Diagnosis has been simplified by newer assays that can detect antibodies in the patient's plasma which are targeted against platelet glycoprotein/heparin conjugates. These are not present in normal patients.

Drug-induced haemolysis

Some drugs, such as α-methyl dopa, may be associated with a positive direct Coomb's test that detects antibody on red cells. Up to 60% of patients may become positive, especially after more than 2 years on the drug, but only 10% of patients will develop a significant degree of haemolysis. Patients on cyclosporin A may also develop a low grade haemolysis with spherocytosis on the blood film.

Oxidative haemolysis may be precipitated by certain oxidant drugs, particularly in patients with glucose-6-phosphate dehydrogenase (G6PD) deficiency, or by the ingestion of fava beans. Haemolysis associated with G6PD deficiency can be idiosyncratic and may rarely occur and present late in life in patients who have never been aware of problems in the past. The blood film may show variable numbers of poikilocytes, red cell fragments and 'bite' cells. These cells are due to degeneration of haemoglobin which produces small clear areas under the red cell membrane and which therefore appear to have a small bite out of their periphery (Figure 44.4).

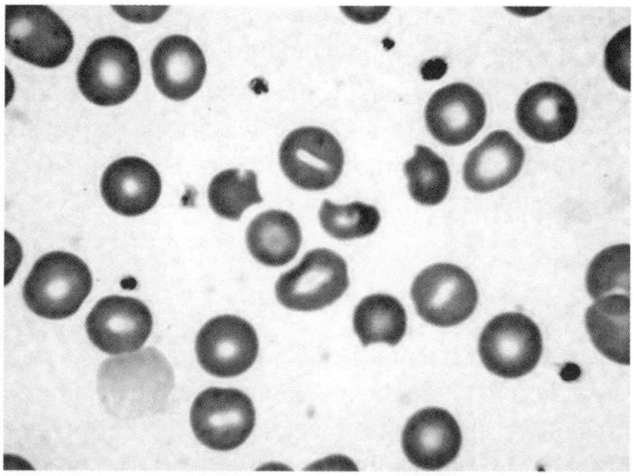

Figure 44.4 Blood film from a patient with severe anaemia (Hb 78 g/L) secondary to oxidative haemolysis showing characteristic 'bite' cells. The patient was found to have G6PD deficiency with a G6PD assay of only 1 U/g Hb whereas the normal range is from 9 to 20 U/g Hb

Poisons

Iron overdose

This presents with epigastric pain, nausea and vomiting with haematemesis. It may proceed to encephalopathy, circulatory collapse, hepatic necrosis and renal failure. Serum iron of greater than 145 μmol/L within 4 hours of ingestion in an adult is indicative of severe poisoning. Treatment is with the administration of desferrioxamine (Desferal) either by intramuscular injection 12 hourly or by continuous intravenous infusion together with gastric lavage and intragastric Desferal solution. The serum iron is monitored and the Desferal continued until levels are within the normal range.

Lead poisoning

Lead poisoning may occur through inhalation, ingestion or absorption (industrial exposure or, rarely, lead-containing cosmetics). It may develop insidiously and present with colicky abdominal pain and a mild normochromic normocytic anaemia. This is due to lead interfering with porphyrin ring metabolism and therefore haemoglobin synthesis. More severe poisoning causes other symptoms such as anorexia, nausea, fatigue, ataxia, paralysis of extensor muscles and encephalopathy. Examination of the blood film suggests the diagnosis if basophilic stippling (due to RNA remnants) is seen in the red cells (Figure 44.5). Diagnosis is confirmed by measurement of blood lead levels (usually greater than 3.9 μmol/L). Treatment involves hydration, analgesia and chelation therapy with D-penicillamine until blood levels return to normal.

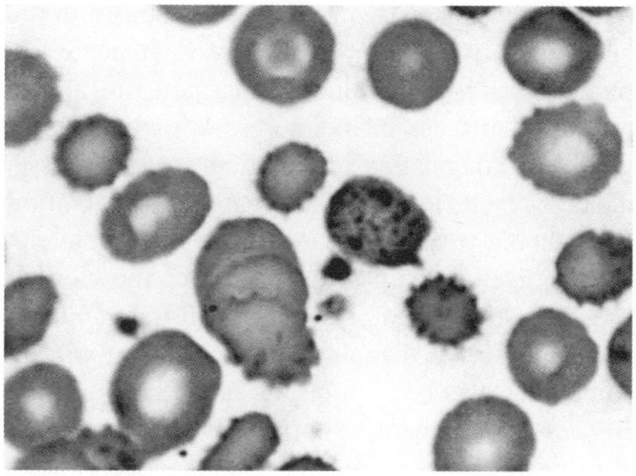

Figure 44.5 This blood film shows some red cell crenation and basophilic stippling associated with lead poisoning. The patient had worked in a small lead foundry in East Asia all his life and had been complaining of vague abdominal pains for several years. He was referred to the haematologists when a normochromic normocytic anaemia (Hb 105 g/L) was discovered on one of his visits to the hospital

Trauma

Severe acute haemorrhage

Trauma can result in vascular damage leading to sudden and dramatic blood loss. The initial response of the body to sudden blood loss is the constriction of both small arterioles and capillaries as well as the larger capacitance vessels to maintain blood pressure. In the otherwise fit young well-hydrated patient, another compensatory mechanism is the shift of extravascular fluid into the blood vessels with the same aim. The older patient's vascular system is not able to perform this fluid shift from the extravascular space with the same rapidity.

Consequently, haemoglobin estimations performed soon after an accident may underestimate seriously the degree of blood loss. A clue to this lies in the assessment of other indicators of volume depletion, such as low blood pressure and tachyarrhythmia. Volume replacement with a plasma volume expander to support the circulation is critical in the emergency situation with replacement of lost red cells as soon as possible.

Fat embolism

Crush injuries release fat globules into the circulation which may cause massive fat embolism in the pulmonary circulation with an associated acute respiratory distress syndrome. Furthermore, the abnormal lipid surfaces in blood vessels of patients in whom the coagulation system is activated by vessel damage results in diffuse intravascular coagulation (DIC) being precipitated. A decline in the platelet count, together with prolongation of the clotting times and the appearance of red cell fragments on the blood film, is diagnostic of DIC. Fat emboli can sometimes also be seen on the blood film in these situations. Treatment is supportive with blood products, including fresh frozen plasma, cryoprecipitate and platelets, in addition to red cells. The use of heparin in these situations to counter the procoagulant stimuli triggering the DIC remains controversial, with strong arguments and opinions voiced by both proponents and opponents.

Infections

Infections may provoke a variety of immune responses beyond the well recognised neutrophil leucocytosis of bacterial sepsis or the production of atypical mononuclear cells and lymphocytes in response to some viral infections. Cold haemagglutinins are associated particularly with mycoplasma infections, and paroxysmal cold haemoglobinuria is most commonly found after childhood viral infections but was described classically in association with syphilis. Severe overwhelming sepsis, particularly in the malnourished individual, may result in myelosuppression with severe leucopenia.

Tuberculosis is one of the most common causes of anaemia in developing countries, especially in its disseminated form. An associated reactive leucocytosis with neutrophilia, monocytosis and reactive thrombocytosis may be present, but cytopenias also occur.

Some, but not all, parasitic infestations—mainly helminths and two enteric protozoans, *Isospora belli* and *Dientamoeba fragilis*—are associated with eosinophilia which should prompt a search in fresh stool specimens for ova, cysts and parasites. The multiplicity of white cell responses in infective and other conditions is detailed in Tables 44.1–44.3.

Haematological system

The common haematological malignancies seen in the elderly include the myeloproliferative disorders, myelodysplasia, acute myeloid leukaemia, myelofibrosis, chronic lymphocytic leukaemia, lymphoma and multiple myeloma. In some cases, hyperleucocytosis can be a major problem, causing cellular sequestration in the microvasculature of vital organs (brain, lungs and kidneys) and requiring urgent treatment with hydration, leucapheresis and the immediate commencement of chemotherapy. In general, however, the main problems associated with these diseases as they progress are cytopenias, infection and haemorrhage. The availability of improved blood products, newer antibiotics and specific remedies for complications, such as hypercalcaemia, has resulted in a great deal of improvement in the quality, if not the extent, of life for these patients over the last 20 years.

Clinical tests

The impact of systemic diseases on the haematological system may be subtle and only apparent on laboratory investigation. However, as well as looking for signs of anaemia, careful examination of the skin, including skin creases, the digits, mucous membranes, optic fundi and bodily orifices is important for detecting a possible skin rash, infection, bruising or petechiae which are important in patients with haematological abnormalities. Particular attention to palpation for enlargement of lymph nodes, liver, spleen or other abdominal or pelvic masses should of course also be part of the routine assessment.

Diagnosis

Any diagnosis will depend on a full assessment of a patient's history, clinical findings and relevant investigations. The importance of taking a full and exhaustive drug history, recording any possible chemical/toxin exposure, details of all employment, and family history cannot be overemphasised in relation to patients with systemic diseases who have co-existent haematological abnormalities.

Treatment

In many cases, reassurance regarding minor abnormalities may be the most important part of a patient's management. For example, many elderly patients are alarmed and embarrassed regarding unsightly bruising associated with fragile capillaries, and benefit from explanation and assurance. In patients with anaemia of chronic disease, exclusion of associated iron deficiency is important and may be worth the inconvenience to the patient of a bone marrow assessment of iron stores, although in most cases this can be avoided. Such iron deficient patients may have a gratifying response to iron supplements, although their haemoglobin may not return completely to normal. Patients with hypersplenism, uncomfortably enlarged spleens, or whose cardiac function is compromised by the increased circulatory load, may benefit from splenectomy. Patients with autoimmune disease and associated cytopenias may also benefit from splenectomy and/or immunosuppression with steroids.

Prognosis

The development of abnormalities in the blood in patients with other systemic disease cannot be easily pigeonholed into correlating with any one particular outcome. Rather, changes in the blood may herald an associated condition or otherwise unexpected complication, the investigation of which may provide valuable information leading to a new diagnosis or the correction of a potentially debilitating complication. The elderly patient, especially one aged over 65 years, has a reduced haemopoietic reserve. The bone marrow consequently acts as a sensitive 'early warning system' which is ignored at the physician's, and more importantly the patient's, peril.

Bibliography and further reading

BKS Iyengar (1976), *Light on Yoga*, 2nd edn, George Allen & Unwin, London.

Hoffbrand, A. V. & Pettit, J. E. (1993), *Essential Haematology*, 3rd edn, Blackwell Scientific, Oxford.

Hoffbrand, A. V., Lewis, S. M. & Tuddenham, E. G. D. (1999), *Postgraduate Haematology*, 4th edn, Butterworth Heinemann International, Oxford.

Hope, R. A., Longmore, J. M., Hodgetts, T. J. & Ramrakha, P. S. (1994), *Oxford Handbook of Clinical Medicine*, 3rd edn, Oxford University Press, Oxford.

Wickham, N. (2000), 'Haematological tests', in Ratnaike, R. (ed.), *Small Bowel Disorders*, Edward Arnold, London.

Chapter 45

Chronic lymphocytic leukaemia

HUSSAIN I. SABA

Introduction

Chronic lymphocytic leukaemia (CLL) is the most common type of leukaemia in the elderly in Western countries and has been reported to account for as much as 31% of all leukaemias. The disease was recognised as early as 1845 and has been described as 'an accumulative disease of immunologically incompetent lymphocytes'. A variable clinical picture with a wide range of prognoses characterises this disease. Elderly patients, with the inherent haematological and physical findings related to age and co-morbid conditions, are at higher risk of a poor CLL prognosis. This chapter provides geriatric physicians with current information about the epidemiology, clinicopathology, diagnosis and treatment of this important and common disease.

CLL is a clonal malignancy, which results from abnormal mature but functionally deficient lymphocyte expansion caused by prolonged cell survival. The affected lymphocytes are normally of the B-cell lineage (85–98% of the reported cases), with T cells being affected in the remaining 2–15% of cases. CLL is the most common leukaemia in the US and Western Europe, and is most common in adults. The incidence of CLL is reported to be 3.5–5.5 per 100 000 population, an increase from the 2.5 per 1000 cases from previously reported series. This increase is most probably due to an increase in the number of cases diagnosed in the early stage.

Epidemiology

While CLL can be found in patients both above and below the age of 50, the vast majority of cases have been found in older patients. The median age at diagnosis has been reported to be 65–70 years, and the disease is rarely observed in patients younger than 35 years. Recently, however, there appears to be a trend towards lower age at diagnosis, particularly in patients at the earlier stages of disease, which is recognised by newly available diagnostic tools. There is a slightly higher incidence of CLL in men, with the male–female ratio being 1.7:1–2.85:1 in patients less than 50 years old, 1.29:1 in patients over 50 and approximately 1:1 in patients of 75 years of age. While it has been reported that race does not appear to play a role in the incidence of CLL in the US, the disease seems to have a higher predilection for Caucasians as compared to Afro-Americans. In the US, it has been estimated that more than 7000 new cases of CLL are reported per year and the frequency is similar to what is seen in other Western countries. The incidence of this leukaemia is much lower in Japan, Korea, China, Latin America and Africa. The cause for these differing frequency rates is unclear and could also be related to the increased longevity of the geriatric population in the Western world.

In general, the aetiology of CLL is unclear, although there are some risk factors that have been associated with the disease. B-lymphocytic CLL (B-CLL) is the only blood malignancy where the incidence does not seem to be increased in atomic bomb survivors. Familial risk appears to be high, with family members of patients with CLL having a twofold to sevenfold higher risk of developing the disease. Family members who do develop the disease usually share the same immunoglobulin rearrangements but not always the same oncogene rearrangements. Familial-association CLL tends to occur at earlier ages in each successive family generation. Attempts have been made to discover if certain HLA patterns are associated with CLL, but no such association has been found. Environmental risks for the development of CLL appear to include chemicals, such as those used in farming. No documented risk has been associated with agents such as radiation, alkylating agents or known leukomogenic chemicals. The development of CLL has been associated with several viruses, including human T-cell lymphotrophic viruses I and II (HTLV-I and HTLV-II) and Epstein-Barr virus (EBV). Although this association has been noted, no evidence that these viruses cause CLL has yet been discovered.

Clinicopathological features

CLL has an insidious onset and approximately 20% of patients are asymptomatic at the time of diagnosis. In these patients, the disease is discovered with routine blood tests. Symptoms, when present, are non-specific and may include fatigue, weakness and malaise. The disease attribute is an immunocompromised state in patients and, therefore, CLL patients have an increased susceptibility to infection. Fever, weight loss and night sweats are not common at the early stages of disease, and therefore are not usually presenting complaints but these symptoms may be present at disease progression. Patients often present with lymphadenopathy. An enlarged spleen may also be present in 30–40% of presenting patients and, less occasionally, hepatomegaly is present in 20% of cases. Massive splenomegaly can be seen in advanced cases, as can other organomegaly, such as of the gastrointestinal tract, prostate, lungs and bones.

B-CLL primarily involves defects in the induction of programmed cell death, with the genetics of the B-CLL cells organised to avoid apoptosis, which is in line with the concept that CLL is a disease of piling up of lymphocytes. Complications in patients with CLL are multiple, including infections, autoimmune cytopenias and pure red blood cell aplasia. It is also known that patients with CLL have a higher frequency of second malignant neoplasms.

Although the disease initially remains indolent, in due time it progresses to the advanced stage. Transformation with time occurs frequently to prolymphocytic leukaemia or Richter's syndrome (i.e. large cell lymphoma). More than 90% of all cases of CLL show a B-cell phenotype. These cells, which have stopped maturation between a pre-B cell and a mature B cell, appear to resemble mature lymphocytes in the peripheral blood.

This is helpful in differentiating CLL from prolymphocytic leukaemia, in which more than 65% of the cells are morphologically less mature prolymphocytes. Flow cytometry is one of the most valuable clinical tools for the diagnosis of CLL. The clonal B lymphocytes express CD19, CD20, CD21 and/or CD24, and co-express CD5, which is more commonly found on T cells. The expression of surface immunoglobulins, such as IgM or IgD, is usually lower than is observed in normal B cells, and with a single light chain only (either κ or λ). Weak expression of interleukin-2 (IL-2) also occurs. Recently, studies on *Bcl-2*, a proto-oncogene and known suppressor of apoptosis, have found it to be over-expressed in cases of B-CLL.

The bone marrow of patients with CLL may be normocellular or hypercellular, but characteristically presents with the presence of at least 30% mature

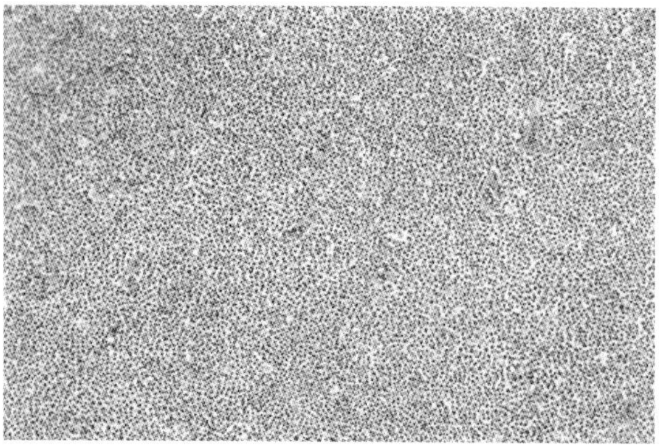

Figure 45.1 Low power view of a lymph node of a patient with CLL showing diffuse effacement of the architecture by small, mature-looking lymphocytes

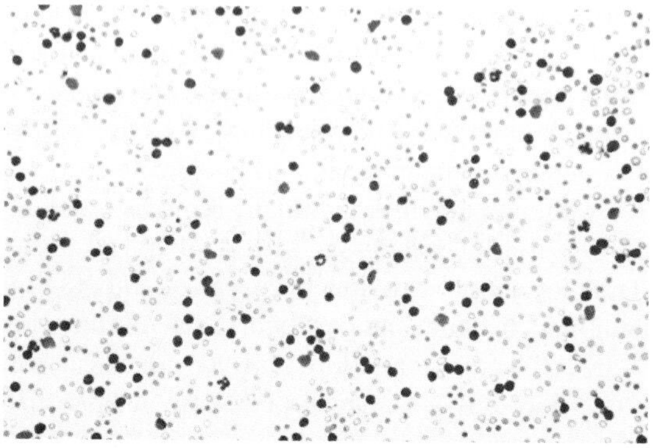

Figure 45.2 Blood film (low power view) of a patient with CLL showing an increased white blood cell count, predominantly composed of small, mature-looking lymphocytes

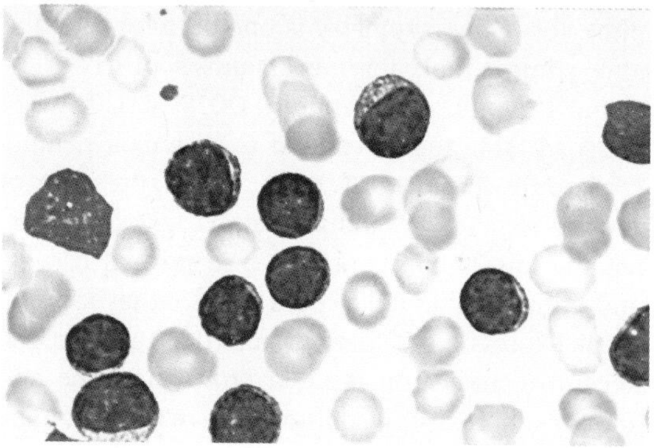

Figure 45.3 Blood film (high power view) of a patient with CLL showing small lymphoid cells with round nuclei, clumped chromatin and scant cytoplasm with an occasional smudge cell present

lymphocytes. This lymphocyte infiltrate may be either interstitial, nodular, mixed interstitial or diffuse.

Other laboratory abnormalities that can be seen include hypogammaglobulinaemia, paraproteinaemia and elevated levels of β_2-microglobulin and/or serum lactate dehydrogenase (LDH). Hypogammaglobulinaemia is the most common of these abnormalities and can be seen in more than 50% of the patients presenting with CLL unless they present with a very early stage of disease, where the levels are usually normal. This hypogammaglobulinaemia most commonly involves lower levels of IgA, followed by IgM and then IgG. A small proportion of these patients (5–10%) may have a small monoclonal peak of gammaglobulin. While elevated LDH levels are only rarely observed in patients at presentation, it is commonly seen at the time of disease transformation and may be used as a marker in transformation.

Cytogenetic abnormalities are also commonly present in approximately 50–65% of patients with CLL. Table 45.1 shows some of the common cytogenetic patterns.

The most common of these abnormalities is trisomy 12, followed by chromosome 13q abnormalities. Structural abnormalities of the long arm of chromosomes 6, 11 and 14 (14q-, t[11;14]) can also

Table 45.1 Common CLL cytogenetic abnormalities and their effects

Cytogenetic abnormality	Effect
Trisomy 12	Activation of dominant proto-oncogene and associated with atypical morphology
13q14 deletions	Inactivation of tumour suppressor gene (*DBM*)
18q21 translocations	Deregulation of the *Bcl-2* gene and overproduction of anti-apoptotic Bcl-2 protein
t(11;14) translocations	Deregulated *Bcl-1* gene activation favouring proliferation
17p alterations	*p53* gene inactivation promoting cell proliferation and survival

be seen, as well as abnormalities of chromosome 17, and numerical abnormalities of chromosomes 3, 8, 18 and 21. More than one cytogenetic abnormality can be seen in 50% of the patients in which one is located.

Although no single gene has been associated with CLL, several genes have been found to be involved in the pathogenesis to differing degrees. Although cytogenetic abnormalities in the long arm of chromosome 13 have been found in patients with CLL, the retinoblastoma 1 gene (*Rb1*) is not usually affected while the telomeric region to *Rb1* (D13S25) is often affected. Few patients have *ras* mutations, even though chromosome 12 is often involved, and the *Bcl-1/PRAD-1* gene is rearranged or amplified in a small number of patients with a t(11;14) mutation. Approximately 40% of patients with CLL overexpress *MDR1* (multi-drug resistance gene).

Diagnosis

CLL is diagnosed by an absolute increase in lymphocytes and/or bone marrow infiltration. Lymphocytosis with small, mature cells ≥ 5000/μL is classically seen. The bone marrow remains involved with 30% or more of these lymphocytes. Clonal expansion of abnormal B lymphocytes, with a low density of surface immunoglobulins (IgM or IgD) with κ or λ light chains, are the hallmark of this clonal expansion. B-cell surface antigens CD19, CD20 and CD23 are strongly positive with flow cytometric studies. CD20 and CD5 are dimly positive. Recently, the US National Cancer Institute and an International Workshop on CLL (IWCLL) have presented precise criteria for the diagnosis of CLL. These are shown in Table 45.2, and include lymphocytosis with a ≥ 5 × 10⁹/L count on peripheral blood. The flow cytometry should show ≥ B-cell markers (CD19, CD20, CD23) plus CD5 positivity. Atypical lymphocytes should be ≤ 55%. Bone marrow lymphocytosis should be ≥ 30%.

With the presence of atypical lymphocytes in the peripheral blood, confusion and concern of the possibility of prolymphocytic leukaemia can exist. This should be ruled out by the difference in their flow cytometry patterns (Table 45.3).

CLL must also be differentiated from hairy cell leukaemia, mantle cell lymphoma, Waldenstrom's macroglobulinaemia and T-cell CLL. While prolymphocytic leukaemia and hairy cell leukaemia can be differentiated on the basis of cell morphology, mantle cell lymphoma is best differentiated on the basis of flow cytometry. Mantle cells typically express FMC-7, in addition to CD5, CD19 and CD20. Waldenstrom's macroglobulinaemia is similar to

Table 45.3 Flow cytometry patterns for different leukaemias

	CLL	PLL[a]	Mantle cell lymphoma
Surface Ig	+	++	++
CD19	++	+	++
CD20	+	++	++
CD35	+	+/–	—
CD5	++	+/–	+

(*a*) PLL = prolymphocytic leukaemia.

Table 45.2 Diagnostic criteria for CLL

	National Cancer Institute	IWCLL
Lymphocytes	≥ 5 × 10⁹/L + ≥ B-cell marker (CD19, CD20, CD23) + CD5	≥ 10 × 10⁹/L and + B-cell phenotype or bone marrow involvement or Lymphocytes < 10 000 and bone marrow involvement and B-cell phenotype
Atypical cells	< 55%	—
Duration of lymphocytosis	≥ 2 months	≥ 1 month
Bone marrow lymphocytes	≥ 30%	≥ 30%

CLL in terms of its natural history and therapeutic options, except for the characteristic hyperviscosity syndrome associated with macroglobulinaemia resulting from an elevated level of IgM.

Patients with T-cell CLL must be differentiated from those with T-prolymphocytic leukaemia or large granular lymphocytic leukaemia. In a 1996 article in which Hoyer described 25 'true T-cell chronic lymphocytic leukaemia' patients, he lists the characteristics of T-cell CLL as median age of 57 years, median presenting lymphocyte count of 36×10^9/L, mild to moderate splenomegaly in 40% of patients and shoddy adenopathy in approximately 50% of patients. The lymphocytes were described as small with a high nuclear:cytoplasmic ratio and round to oval nuclei with absent or small nucleoli. The cytoplasmic granulation was absent, and the cells were of mature T-cell immunophenotype. The most common chromosomal abnormalities were 14q11, 14q32, 7p15 or the long arm of chromosome 8. Immunophenotyping of all CLL patients can be helpful in accurate diagnosis.

Two staging systems have been in use for depicting the prognosis in CLL patients. The Rai staging system (Table 45.4) and the Binet staging system (Table 45.5) are both utilised.

The Binet system integrates the nodal groups involved with the disease with bone marrow failure, acknowledges a predominantly splenic form of the disease, and may be better in terms of depicting prognosis.

The majority of patients with CLL belong to the subset entitled 'smouldering CLL', which is characterised by a haemoglobin level of > 130 g/L, a platelet count of > 150 000/mL, a lymphocyte count of < 30 000/mL and a non-diffuse bone marrow pattern. These patients, in general, have a survival rate that is the same as an age- and sex-matched population. Those patients who have a doubling time of the lymphocyte count of over 1 year may often be observed without treatment.

Treatment

At this stage, no one approach to the treatment of CLL has been proven to be curative. Although CLL normally has a prolonged indolent clinical course,

Table 45.4 The Rai staging system of CLL

	Stage				
	0	**I**	**2**	**3**	**4**
Absolute lymphocytosis (> 15 000/mm^3)	+	+	+	+	+
Lymphadenopathy	–	+	+/–	+/–	+/–
Hepatomegaly and/or splenomegaly	–	–	+	+/–	+/–
Anaemia (< 11 g/dL)	–	–	–	+	+/–
Thrombocytopenia (< 100 000/mm^3)	–	–	–	–	+
Estimated median survival in years	> 10	> 8	6	2	2
Modified stage and risk	Low	Intermediate	Intermediate	High	High

Table 45.5 Binet classification of CLL

		Characteristics			
Binet clinical stage	**Rai stage**	**Anaemia**	**Thrombocytopenia**	**Lymphoid involvement**[(a)]	**Estimated median survival (years)**
A	0, I, II	—	—	< 3 areas	> 10
B	I, II	—	—	≥ 3 areas	6
C	III, IV	One or both		—	2

(*a*) Lymphoid involvement areas: cervical, axillary, inguinal and/or spleen.

disease progression is the norm for almost all patients eventually. In general, early stage disease should not be treated, since patients with early stage CLL have a good long-term prognosis due to the slow progression of the disease in the majority of patients. In general, treatment of early stage disease has not been shown to be effective in terms of long-term survival. The ability to recognise active versus stable disease is of major importance in terms of treatment. The guidelines of the National Cancer Institute's sponsored Working Group define active disease as including a weight loss of more than 10% within 6 months, extreme fatigue, night sweats and a fever of ≥ 100.5°F (38°C) for more than 2 weeks without evidence of infection. Active disease is also defined as including the following criteria:

- anaemia and/or thrombocytopenia indicating bone marrow failure
- autoimmune manifestations
- bulky adenopathy (> 10 cm node clusters or progressive clusters)
- organomegaly (> 6 cm below the costal margin or progressive)
- a > 50% increase in lymphocytes over 2 months or a 6 month doubling time of the lymphocyte count.

Stage-associated treatment options are outlined in Table 45.6.

Conventional chemotherapeutic approaches include both single-agent treatment or combination chemotherapy. Chlorambucil (Leukeran) is the most common single-agent chemotherapeutic drug used in the treatment of CLL. A 1999 meta-analysis of the randomised trials of chemotherapeutic options in CLL by the UK CLL Trialists Collaborative Group concluded that:

- no chemotherapy should be given to most patients with early stage disease
- single-agent chlorambucil should be used as the first line of treatment for most patients with advanced disease
- there is no evidence of benefit from early inclusion of anthracycline.

Chlorambucil is usually given in a daily dose of 0.1 mg/kg or 0.4–1.0 mg/kg every 4 weeks. Higher doses have been associated with a better response rate and longer survival. While the total dose with daily administration is higher, making this a more preferable and possibly more superior treatment regimen, the monthly dosing schedule is still widely used. Chlorambucil has been combined with oral prednisone (30–100 mg/m^2 per day). Although no evidence exists that this is more effective than chlorambucil alone, it can be useful in the treatment of CLL-associated autoimmune cytopenias. Cyclophosphamide has also been used in the treatment of CLL, and is usually given as 1–2 g/m^2 doses every 3–4 weeks in combination with vincristine and steroids (CVP regimen). In 1998, the French Cooperative Group on CLL randomised a total of 1535 patients with previously untreated stage A disease to receive chlorambucil or no treatment. Median follow-up exceeded 11 years for the first trial, and 6 years for the second, and they found no difference between the groups, which is further evidence that observation may be the best treatment approach for early stage patients.

Combination chemotherapy has mainly been utilised in patients with advanced disease, and has overall response rates of 40–85%. The most common combinations used are CVP (cyclophosphamide + vincristine + prednisone) and CHOP (cyclophosphamide, oncovin, prednisone and low dose doxorubicin [25 mg/m^2]). In regimens such as CAP (cyclophosphamide + andriamycin + prednisone) or CHOP, 50 mg/m^2 doxorubicin has been employed. COP (cyclophosphamidet onvocin + prednisone) appears as effective as chlorambucil plus prednisone. CHOP appears to be more effective than COP or chlorambucil plus prednisone in terms of a short-term response, but long-term follow-up has not confirmed this. The French Cooperative Group on CLL randomised 287 stage B-CLL patients between intermittent chlorambucil plus prednisone or CHOP, and 90 stage C patients between CHOP and CHOP plus methotrexate. No difference in survival was seen in the stage B patients, although treatment response in these patients was improved with CHOP. The stage C patients showed no differences in either treatment response or median survival. In general, combination chemotherapy results are similar to those obtained with simple regimens and the current

Table 45.6 CLL treatment

Treatment option	Stage 0	I	II	III	IV
Observation alone	Yes	Yes	Yes, if disease is minimal	—	—
Prophylactic use of hydration and allopurinol	—	Yes, in patients with large lymph masses	Yes, in patients with large lymph masses	Yes, in patients with large lymph masses	Yes, in patients with large lymph masses
Radiation	—	Involved field	Splenic for palliation or hypersplenism	Splenic for hypersplenism, haemolytic anaemia (HA) or idiopathic thrombocytopenic purpura (ITP)[a]	Splenic for hypersplenism, HA or ITP[a]
Chemotherapy with oral alkylating agents such as chlorambucil or cyclophosphamide (prednisone or prednisolone if indicated)	—	Yes	Yes	Yes	Yes
Fludarabine	—	Yes	Yes	Yes	Yes
2-chloro-deoxyadenosine (2-CDA)	—	Yes	Yes	Yes	Yes
Pentostatin	—	Yes	Yes	Yes	Yes
Combination chemotherapy, such as CVP[b] or CHOP[c]	—	—	—	Yes	Yes
Bone marrow transplant	—	Under clinical evaluation	Under clinical evaluation	Under clinical evaluation	Under clinical evaluation
Peripheral stem cell transplantation	—	Under clinical evaluation	Under clinical evaluation	Under clinical evaluation	Under clinical evaluation
Biologic response modifiers	—	—	Under clinical evaluation	Under clinical evaluation	Under clinical evaluation
Clinical trials	—	—	Yes	Yes	Yes

(*a*) Patients failing with alkylating agents and prednisone.

(*b*) CVP: cyclophosphamide + vincristine + prednisone.

(*c*) CHOP: cyclophosphamide + doxorubicin + vincristine + prednisone.

consensus is that early treatment with chlorambucil is not beneficial to patients.

One of the more recent nucleoside analogues, fludarabine (Fludara), has been found to be quite effective. Fludarabine has been studied for its effectiveness as a front-line treatment option. When used alone, it has been shown to have an overall response rate of greater than 50% in patients previously treated with alkylating agents. Patients who are refractory to alkylating agents have overall response rates of 35–40%. When used at a dosage of 25–30 mg/m^2 per day for 5 days every 3–4 weeks in patients who have been previously treated with other agents, responses have been observed in approximately 50% of patients, with 15% of them achieving a complete remission. Previously untreated patients have an approximate response rate of 80%, with 30–65% of the responders having a complete remission, depending upon the study. In a 1996 randomised trial by Rai and his associates, patients receiving fludarabine had a higher response rate (70% versus 43%) and a longer median progression-free survival (27 versus 17 months) than patients treated with chlorambucil. At a median follow-up of 30 months, there was no statistical difference in the overall survival in either group. Follow-up of this study found an increase in the infection-related hospitalisation rate in the fludarabine-treated patients (29% versus 17%, $P > 0.0001$). Fludarabine has been shown to be even more effective when given in combination with cyclophosphamide, with complete remission rates being reported as high as 44% in previously untreated patients and 21% in patients previously treated with alkylating agents. The addition of prednisone to fludarabine therapy, as with other therapeutic combinations, has not improved response rate and may be counterproductive since it has been associated with an increased incidence of opportunistic infections.

Cladribine (2-chlorode-oxyadenosine, 2-CdA [Leustatin]) has also been used in CLL patients. It is most effective in patients with previously untreated CLL, and this has been hypothesised to be due to the poor bone marrow reserve in patients who have received other therapy. It appears effective at doses of either 0.1 mg/kg per day or 4 mg/m^2 per day for 7 days with a minimum of 4 courses, although it is less effective than fludarabine.

Other recent treatment modalities for patients with CLL include bone marrow transplant (BMT), interferon, splenectomy and radiotherapy. Allogeneic BMT is a relatively effective treatment alternative in younger, non-responsive patients suffering from advanced stage CLL.

The European Bone Marrow Transplant Registry and the International Bone Marrow Transplant Registry have shown that patients with allogeneic BMT have a high engraftment rate with a high complete remission rate. Complete remission rates as high as 70% have been reported. If allogeneic BMT is not a possibility due to age, as is the case with the majority of patients with CLL, autologous BMT may be used. Preliminary studies suggest that complete remissions can be obtained in some patients. Investigators from the Dana Farber Cancer Institute in the US have had success with autologous BMT as intensification for patients, achieving a very good remission with front-line induction regimens, while the M. D. Anderson Cancer Center experience in the US has not been as positive. Unfortunately, many studies where BMT has been investigated have had a high rate of treatment-related mortality, including graft versus host disease (GVHD). Although studies on the frequency of GVHD in patients with CLL undergoing BMT have suggested that the use of fludarabine in these patients may lessen the chances of GVHD, specific clinical trials are needed to confirm this. Many questions still must be answered regarding the role of BMT in patients with CLL.

Interferon has been reported to induce some response in patients with early stage CLL. Unfortunately, maintenance regimens with interferon do not appear to prolong remissions after fludarabine treatment. IL-2 has not proven to be effective.

Splenectomy has been shown to be beneficial in treating CLL-associated cytopenias and has been used in palliative therapy when necessary. The procedure has a low perioperative mortality rate that allows benefit to exceed risk in many patients.

Monoclonal antibodies are now being investigated as a potential treatment modality. These include anti-CD52 (Campath-1H) and anti-CD20 (Rituximab). CD52 is a leukocyte antigen expressed on most B- and T-cell lymphocytes. Campath-1H, a humanised monoclonal antibody to CD52, selectively depletes lymphocytes, eventually restoring normal haematopoiesis. Preliminary studies of Campath-1H in patients with CLL resulted in a remarkable decrease in absolute lymphocyte counts and improvement in the haemoglobin levels, neutrophil counts and platelet counts with continued treatment. Side effects of this treatment, while problematic, usually subsided with continued treatment and included shaking chills, fever and transient hypotension. Unfortunately, patients with CLL treated with Campath-1H in this study developed serious opportunistic infections. Further investigation in this therapeutic approach is now under way. This study, entitled CAM-211, has involved intravenous treatment of patients with CLL with a shorter course of Campath-1H in combination with simultaneous prophylaxis against *Pneumocystis carinii* and viral infections. Interim results of this study were published in 1999 and indicate that 20% of the patients with CLL achieved complete remission, 50% have achieved partial remission and 30% of the patients tested had no response in this study. A recent study in Sweden has evaluated the effectiveness of subcutaneous Campath-1H and infection prophylaxis in patients who have never undergone other treatment. Results of this study were also promising. The agent has been approved in the US for refractory CLL patients.

Rituximab (IDEC-C2B8) is approved by the US Food and Drug Administration for the treatment of patients with relapsed or refractory low grade or follicular B-cell non-Hodgkin's lymphoma (NHL). It is reasonably well tolerated, severe adverse effects are rare and it is an effective therapeutic option for these patients. Preliminary results of patients with CLL treated with Rituximab have shown a decrease in the number of peripheral blood lymphocytes. Unfortunately, some patients treated with this anti-CD20 antibody had severe infusion reactions, thrombocytopenia and tumour lysis syndrome.

Conjugation of monoclonal antibodies to toxins or radioactive isotopes has been investigated as a treatment technique to deliver treatment more specifically. This technique has been used in the treatment of other cancers. Anti-B1 is a murine anti-CD20 monoclonal antibody that has been labelled with iodine-131 to enhance the efficacy of therapy for lymphoma. Anti-B1 induces apoptosis and antibody-dependent cytotoxicity, and its radiolabelling allows for specific targeting to CD20-bearing cells. In a 1999 review by Rai, it is theorised that monoclonal antibodies labelled with radioisotopes should have the ability to destroy antigen-positive as well as antigen-negative tumour cells due to the specific characteristics of the radioisotope. Bexxar, an iodine-131 anti-B1 antibody (^{131}I-tositumomab) has initially been studied in patients with NHL, mantle cell lymphoma and follicular lymphoma with promising results. These results suggest that this may be an effective treatment modality for patients with CLL. Lym-1, a monoclonal antibody that preferentially targets malignant lymphocytes, has also been labelled with iodine-131 and tested in patients with NHL and CLL. While preliminary results in this area indicate that this might eventually prove to be effective, further studies are essential in this area.

Several other studies are currently under way in order to investigate new treatment modalities in CLL. The US National Cancer Institute is currently sponsoring a phase II evaluation of bryostatin-1 (a natural product isolated from a marine invertebrate) in patients with relapsed or refractory B-cell CLL. Patients are treated with a 40 μg/m^2 per day continuous infusion for 3 days every 2 weeks as long as there is no disease progression and toxicity is acceptable. A phase II study of antineoplaston A10 and AS2-1 in patients with advanced-stage symptomatic CLL that is refractory to standard chemotherapy is also under way. CI-980, an agent with activity against mitotic spindles, is also being investigated as it is not influenced by the presence of a multi-drug resistance gene. A high-dose deoxycoformycin regimen is being investigated in refractory patients as well. Other investigations involve the study of UCN01, falvorpiridol and depsipeptide since they appear to have cytotoxic activity against CLL cells independent of the *p53* gene.

Unfortunately, infectious complications in patients with advanced CLL play a significant role in survival for such patients. These complications are partially due to hypogammaglobulinaemia and an inability to effectively defend against bacterial or viral agents. These infections, frequently herpes zoster, *Pneumocystis carinii* and *Candida albicans*, should be recognised and treated as early as possible in these patients. Intravenous gammaglobulin (400 mg/kg every 3 weeks for 1 year) has been shown to significantly reduce the number of infections in patients with CLL with hypogammaglobulinaemia, but this did not have a significant effect on survival. The increased expense of this treatment modality has not been shown to be offset by the long-term benefit.

In summary, at this stage there is no curative chemotherapy available for CLL. Chemotherapy should be used with caution and only in advanced and symptomatic patients. Chlorambucil could be a less toxic chemotherapy, but prolonged use should be cautious due to the increased incidence of acute myeloid leukaemia (AML) in this group. Nucleoside analogues and BMT should be considered as second-line therapeutic approaches. Patients with advanced disease (Rai stage II, III or IV) or refractory CLL may be considered to be appropriate candidates for clinical trials.

Prognosis

Patients with CLL succumb to infections and secondary cancers. A 1999 Italian study by Mauro and associates investigated the causes of death in patients with CLL as related to age. This study involved 204 patients 55 years of age or under and 807 patients over 55 years. The results of this study are outlined in Table 45.7.

The most significant age-related differences were found in the deaths related to progressive disease, and no relationship between age and infection-related death was noted.

The small number of patients presenting with each specific feature limits prognosis on the basis of biological parameters. In general, the overall 5-year survival of patients with CLL is approximately 60%, but several factors affect the prognosis of CLL. Generally accepted unfavourable prognostic indicators are summarised in Table 45.8.

Prognostic factors include age, performance status, doubling time of the lymphocytes, bone marrow biopsy pattern and chromogenic abnormalities, among others. Chromosomal abnormalities are generally associated with poor prognosis, and the severity of the prognosis is directly related to the complexity of the karyotype. Therefore,

Table 45.7 Mortality in patients with CLL

	Cause of death			
	Related to CLL (%)			
Age (years)	**Progressive disease**	**Infection**	**Secondary malignancies (i.e. melanoma, soft tissue sarcoma, colorectal and lung)**	**Unrelated to CLL (%)**
≤ 55	85	9	4	2
> 55	49	9	14	28
Statistical significance (*P*)	< 0.0001	Not significant	< 0.05	< 0.0001

Table 45.8 Major unfavourable prognostic indicators in patients with CLL

Clinical	Haematological	Immunological	Other
Older age Hepatomegaly Poor performance	Anaemia Thrombocytopenia Short lymphocyte doubling time Peripheral lymphocytosis Higher bone marrow lymphocyte percentage Diffuse bone marrow pattern Morphological variants	β_2-microglobulin Soluble CD23 Soluble ICAM-1 T-/natural killer-cell number Function Ig gene rearrangements	Cytogenetic abnormalities Molecular abnormalities Multi-drug resistance gene Lymphocyte doubling time CLL with prolymphocytic leukaemia components in the peripheral blood and bone marrow

patients with multiple complex abnormalities have a poorer prognosis than those in which no abnormalities are noted. Particularly, patients with 13q chromosomal abnormalities have prognoses similar to that of patients with normal karyotypes. Recent studies suggest that patients with a single trisomy 12 abnormality may have a poorer prognosis than any other single abnormality, and chromosome 7 abnormalities may be associated with poor prognosis and response to therapy. The abnormalities of 17p and the loss of chromosome 17 seen in some patients may involve the *p53* oncogene and are also associated with a poor prognosis. The presence of multiple chromosomal abnormalities also has a worse prognosis. The TP53 chromosomal mutation, which is seen in approximately 15% of patients, is theorised to be associated with resistance to chemotherapy, and is more common in patients with advanced CLL or CLL in transformation. Patients with CLL who express the T-cell markers CD4 and CD7 and have clonal rearrangements of their T-cell receptor genes have shorter median survival rates (13 months) and poor response to chemotherapy.

The presence of a diffuse lymphocyte infiltration in the bone marrow is also associated with a poor prognosis, as opposed to a nodular or interstitial one. Elevated levels of β_2-microglobulin have also been suggested to be a poor prognostic indicator. In fact, serum β_2-microglobulin levels may be the most important prognostic indicator in patients with CLL in both treated and untreated patients. In a 1999 review by Keating, the β_2-microglobulin level increases as prognosis deteriorates.

Patients who are characterised with extensive bone marrow infiltration and impaired production of red blood cells and platelets leading to thrombocytopenia and/or anaemia (Rai stage III/IV, Binet C) have a poorer prognosis than do patients with immune cytopenias.

Approximately 3–10% of patients with CLL undergo Richter's transformation and progress to large cell lymphoma. This transformation presents with fever of sudden onset, B symptoms (i.e. weight loss, night sweats and fever) and progressive lymphadenopathy, and these patients have a poor prognosis with a median survival rate of less than 1 year. Paraproteinaemia, high LDH levels and extranodal involvement may also occur in these patients. Treatment is often ineffective in these patients at this time, although it has been reported that 20% of these patients may live for more than 5 years after receiving aggressive combination chemotherapy. Studies are currently under way to examine the effect of combination chemotherapy involving nucleoside analogues.

CLL is currently being diagnosed at younger ages due to advances in diagnostic techniques. Therefore, in many cases, observation is no longer an acceptable treatment modality to many. Recent advances in the treatment of CLL, and the investigation of novel therapeutic approaches, may lead to a significant increase in the effective treatment of this disorder.

Acknowledgment

The author would like to acknowledge the efforts of Ms Genevieve A. Morelli in the preparation of this manuscript.

Bibliography and further reading

Bartlett, N. L. & Longo, D. L. (1999), 'T-small lymphocyte disorders', *Seminars in Hematology*, 36(2), pp. 164–70.

Boussiotis, V. A., Freedman, A. S. & Nadler, L. M. (1999), 'Bone marrow transplantation for low-grade lymphoma and chronic lymphocytic leukaemia', *Seminars in Hematology*, 36(2), pp. 209–16.

Caligaris-Cappio, F. & Hamblin, T. J. (1999), 'B-cell chronic lymphocytic leukaemia: a bird of a different feather', *Journal of Clinical Oncology*, 17(1), pp. 399–408.

CLL Trialists Collaborative Group (1999), 'Chemotherapeutic options in chronic lymphocytic leukaemia: a meta-analysis of the randomised trials', *Journal of the National Cancer Institute*, 91(10), pp. 861–8.

Dighireo, G., Maloum, K., Desablens, B., Cazin, B., Navarro, M., Leblay, R., Leporrier, M., Jaubert, J., Lepeu, G., Dreyfus, B., Binet, J. L. & Travade, P. (1998), 'Chloroambucil in indolent chronic lymphocytic leukemia. French Cooperative Group on Chronic Lymphocytic Leukemia', *New England Journal of Medicine*, 339(13), p. 924.

Hoyer, J. D., Ross, C. W., Li, C. Y., Witzig, T. E., Gascoyne, R. D., Dewald, G. W. & Hanson, C. A. (1996), 'True T-cell chronic lymphocytic leukemia: a morphologic and immunophenotypic study of 25 cases', *Blood*, 87(8), pp. 3520–1.

Jurlander, J. (1998), 'The cellular biology of B-cell chronic lymphocytic leukaemia', *Critical Reviews in Oncology Hematology*, 27, pp. 29–52.

Keating, M. J. (1999), 'Chronic lymphocytic leukaemia', *Seminars in Oncology*, 26(5), pp. 107–14.

Mauro, F. R., Foa, R., Giannarelli, D., Cordone, I., Crescenzi, S., Pescarmona, E., Sala, R., Cerretti, R. & Mandelli, F. (1999), 'Clinical characteristics and outcomes of young chronic lymphocyte leukaemia patients: a single institution study of 204 cases', *Blood*, 94(2), pp. 448–54.

Mellstedt, H., Osterborg, A., Lundin, J. et al. (1998), 'Campath-1H therapy of patients with previously untreated chronic lymphocytic leukemia', *Blood*, 92(S1), p. 490a.

Panayiotidis, P. & Kotsi, P. (1999), 'Genetics of small lymphocyte disorders', *Seminars in Hematology*, 36(2), pp. 171–7.

Rai, K. R. (1999), 'New biologic therapies', *Seminars in Hematology*, 36(4), pp. 12–17.

Rai, K. R., Peterson, B., Kolitz, J. et al. (1996), 'A randomized comparison of fludarabine and chloroambucil for patients with previously untreated chronic lymphocytic leukemia. A CALCG, SWOG, CTG/NCI-C and ECOG Inter-Group Study', *Blood*, 88, p. 141.

Reed, J. (1998), 'Molecular biology of chronic lymphocytic leukaemia', *Seminars in Oncology*, 25(1), pp. 11–18.

Zwiebel, J. A. & Cheson, B. D. (1998), 'Chronic lymphocytic leukaemia: staging and prognostic factors', *Seminars in Oncology*, 25(1), pp. 42–59.

Chapter 46
Myelodysplasia

HUSSAIN I. SABA

Introduction

Myelodysplastic syndrome (MDS) is one of the most common haematological malignancies in the aged. It includes a wide spectrum of diverse clonal bone marrow disorders that present with anaemia and other cytopenias. The most serious complication is the transformation of MDS in patients to acute leukaemia. These disorders are characterised by peripheral cytopenias, hypercellular bone marrow and dysplastic changes in all cell lines. MDS may originate due to premalignant or malignant transformation of a pluripotent stem cell and may involve either myeloid or lymphoid cell lines. Alteration of this cell line leads to ineffective haematopoiesis which, in turn, leads to peripheral cytopenias. The disorder runs a chronic indolent course but can terminate in acute leukaemic states with its transformation. Death also occurs due to infection or haemorrhage.

In the earlier literature, the disorder has been referred to with many different terminologies, such as pre-leukaemia, oligoblastic leukaemia, smouldering acute leukaemia, refractory anaemia, refractory anaemia with excess of blasts and sideroblastic anaemia. The term 'myelodysplastic syndrome' was evolved by the efforts of a core group of French, American and British clinicians and haematopathologists (FAB group). The FAB group distinguished acute leukaemia from a group of subacute or chronic disorders that showed some of the characteristics of acute myeloid leukaemia (AML). This group of patients with subacute or chronic disorders was typically comprised of older patients (≥ 60 years) who rarely needed immediate treatment. The FAB group later coined the name 'myelodysplastic syndromes' to describe the disorders. Specific morphologic features and abnormalities in patients with MDS were reviewed by the FAB group in relation to biological behaviour and outcome, and five subgroups of patients with MDS were identified:

1. refractory anaemia (RA)
2. refractory anaemia with ring sideroblasts (RARS)
3. refractory anaemia with excess blasts (RAEB)
4. chronic myelomonocytic leukaemia (CMML)
5. refractory anaemia with excess of blasts in transformation (RAEB-T).

The above FAB subgroups have been further divided into 'low-risk MDS', comprising RA and RARS, and 'high-risk MDS', which includes CMML,

RAEB and RAEB-T. At a recent World Health Organization (WHO) meeting on the classification of haematological malignancies, it was suggested that CMML with high white blood cell counts be removed from the MDS category and placed in the myeloproliferative disorders (MPD) category. It was originally suggested that CMML with lower or normal counts should remain included in the MDS category. The consensus of the meeting participants was that CMML is one disease and should be classified in one category only, and that it be included in a separately established category of disorders with characteristics of both MPD and MDS. The participants at this meeting reached a consensus that RAEB-T be removed from the MDS category and reclassified in the AML group. To discuss this disorder fully, all subtypes originally included will be discussed in this chapter.

Epidemiology

The median age of patients with MDS remains between 60 and 80 years, and the disease has primarily been considered a disease of the aged. However, more recently, MDS is being diagnosed in relatively younger ages in the Third World. In the majority of these patients, the MDS is related to exposure to toxins, chemicals and pollution and is therefore secondary MDS, but this needs to be further defined. In a Belgian study, the relationship of MDS with anaemia has been illuminated. In this report, 24% of a population of 732 elderly patients admitted to geriatric service were found to be anaemic. MDS was found to be the cause of the anaemia observed in 9% of these patients. Myelodysplasia is currently considered to be the most common haematological malignancy in the elderly. It has also been noted that anaemia is the most common presenting factor in patients diagnosed with MDS. The relative frequency reported has varied depending upon the study area and time of study, with the lowest incidence occurring in the population less than 49 years of age (average of 0.5/100 000). The incidence in persons 50–69 years is higher (average of 5.6/100 000), with an increasing frequency in the 60–69 years age group. Most cases of MDS occur in patients 70 years of age or older, with age-related incidences being reported to be an average of 28.9/100 000 in patients 70–79 years of age. The incidence of MDS has been reported to be as high as 89/100 000 for patients older than 80 years.

The incidence of each of the different MDS subtypes also varies with subtype. Table 46.1 shows the average incidence of MDS subgroups as observed in each FAB classification.

Table 46.1 FAB classification and incidence of MDS

Classification	Average incidence (%)
Refractory anaemia (RA)	26
Refractory anaemia with ring sideroblasts (RARS)	19
Chronic myelomonocytic leukaemia (CMML)	14
Refractory anaemia with excess of blasts (RAEB)	23
Refractory anaemia with excess of blasts in transformation (RAEB-T)	11

Clinical manifestations

As many as half of the patients diagnosed with MDS are symptom-free at the time of diagnosis, and are identified only by routine clinical and laboratory tests. The symptomatic patient most commonly presents with anaemia and has many symptoms that may also be attributed to cardiopulmonary disease, such as fatigue and dyspnoea on exertion. One-third of the patients' histories include recurrent infection, which may be due to either neutropenia or neutrophil dysfunction. Bleeding diathesis is less frequently present in patients with MDS. Serious bleeding, including gastrointestinal haemorrhage, haematuria, central nervous system bleeding and retinal haemorrhage, occur in no more than 10% of patients with MDS. Splenomegaly can be seen in 10–20% of patients and hepatomegaly in 5–15% of patients. In cases of CMML, however, the incidences of splenomegaly and hepatomegaly increase to 30–50%, and the spleen may be massively enlarged. In general, lymph node enlargement is seen in not more than 5–15% of these cases.

Clinical tests

The disorder is most frequently diagnosed by routine laboratory tests and bone marrow biopsy. Cytogenetic studies are also used to diagnose MDS and to assess the prognosis of patients with MDS. Flow cytometry with immune markers is also helpful in analysing lymphoid and myeloid cells as it has been utilised in the diagnosis of acute leukaemia.

Table 46.2 summarises the most typical peripheral smear and bone marrow findings in each of the MDS subtypes.

Refractory anaemia

Patients with RA typically have less than 11 g/dL haemoglobin, low neutrophil and platelet counts, and ≤1 % myeloblasts in the peripheral blood. Their bone marrow is usually hypercellular with moderate to marked dyserythropoiesis, dysgranulopoiesis, and megakaryocytopoiesis, but they may present with marrow hypocellularity. Increased bone marrow fibrosis has also been found in a small percentage of these patients.

Refractory anaemia with ring sideroblasts

The characteristic feature of patients in this subgroup is the finding of ring sideroblasts, which are more than 15% of the iron-containing normoblasts in the bone marrow that contain iron granules in a perinuclear distribution. The myeloblast count in the bone marrow is less than 5%. MDS in patients with the RARS subtype has the least likelihood to transform to acute leukaemia.

Chronic myelomonocytic leukaemia

Patients normally have monocyte counts greater than 1×10^9/L, minimal to marked trilineal dyspoiesis and frequent cytogenetic abnormalities. This subgroup also includes patients with chronic monocytic leukaemia (CML). The prognostic correlation between the initial blast count and survival time after diagnosis is unclear, with some studies finding a correlation and others finding little or none. Differentiation between CMML and chronic myeloproliferative disorders is difficult because of the occasional occurrence of hepatosplenomegaly, leucocytosis and myelofibrosis and because some patients with chronic MPD may have monocytosis of greater than 1×10^9/L. According to the WHO classification, CMML with a low proliferative fraction (< 5000 monocytes) is included in MDS and CMML with greater counts is included in the MPD category.

Refractory anaemia with excess of blasts

These patients are characterised by the presence of 5–20% myeloblasts in the bone marrow. The dysgranulopoiesis, dyserythropoiesis and dysmegakaryocytopoiesis are more marked in cases of RAEB than in those of RA, RARS and CMML and there are fewer blasts in circulation than in the bone marrow.

Table 46.2 Peripheral smear and bone marrow findings in patients with MDS

	Peripheral smear	Bone marrow
Low-risk MDS		
RA	Rare monocytes with 1+ dyspoiesis	< 15% ring sideroblasts and < 5% myeloblasts
RARS	Rare monocytes with 1+ dyspoiesis	> 15% ring sideroblasts and < 5% myeloblasts
High-risk MDS		
CMML	Monocytes increased with 2+ dyspoiesis	Ring sideroblasts percentage variable and 1–20% myeloblasts
RAEB	Rare monocytes with 2+ dyspoiesis	Ring sideroblasts percentage variable and 5–20% myeloblasts
RAEB-T	Monocyte number variable with 2+ dyspoiesis	Ring sideroblasts percentage variable and 21–30% myeloblasts

Refractory anaemia with excess blasts in transformation

These patients are characterised by higher bone marrow blast counts and they have a poor median survival time. Younger patients (< 50 years) in this subgroup have been found to respond well to conventional chemotherapy used to treat AML. According to the WHO classification, RAEB-T is no longer considered a subgroup of MDS and is now included in AML.

Diagnosis

Anaemia of unknown origin, leucopenia, and thrombocytopenia generally characterise a diagnosis of MDS. Anaemia of varying level of haemoglobin is the most common finding. Anaemia remains the most common presenting symptom, although isolated thrombocytopenia or, less commonly, isolated leucopenia can also be found at presentation. Therefore, a diagnosis of MDS may be difficult with patients where dysplastic features are obscure. In these cases, the review of an experienced haematopathologist is essential to make the diagnosis. Exposure to cytotoxic agents or heavy metals and deficiencies of vitamin B_{12} and folate should be ruled out during the evaluation of these patients and before a diagnosis of primary MDS is made.

Forty to 70% of patients with MDS are found to have karyotypic anomalies at the time of diagnosis. In secondary MDS, this percentage increases to more than 80% of cases. Chromosomal deletions are more frequent in patients with MDS than in those with AML, and major karyotypic aberrations are more commonly found in more advanced MDS cases. The number of karyotypic abnormalities found varies depending upon MDS subtype, and may relate to prognosis. As many as three or more chromosomal abnormalities are commonly seen in cases of RAEB and RAEB-T, but only rarely is more than one karyotypic anomaly seen in cases of RA. Patients with RARS have the lowest incidence of karyotypic aberration. Chromosomal abnormalities seen in patients with MDS include del(4)(q13q33), del(5)(q13q22q33), monosomy 7, deletion of 7q, del(11)(q14q23) and trisomy 8.

Treatment

Treatment of MDS and its outcome has remained far from spectacular. So far, treatment modalities have included hormonal therapy, the use of differentiating agents, chemotherapy, bone marrow transplant (BMT) and the use of haematopoietic growth factors. Newer strategies have included amifostine, cyclosporin A, anti-thymocyte globulin, and topotecan either alone or in combination with other agents.

Hormonal therapy

Hormonal therapy has been used in patients with MDS in order to improve their haematological parameters. Treatment with androgens and danazol has also been suggested but results have been inconsistent.

Differentiating agents

Differentiating agents have also been used to treat MDS. Many small studies have reported the efficacy of cytarabine in MDS. Careful evaluation of these studies indicates the overall response rate has not been more than 15%, with no significant improvement in survival. In a co-operative, randomised study by the Eastern Cooperative Oncology Group (ECOG) and the Southwest Oncology Group (SWOG) on low-dose cytarabine versus supportive therapy in patients with MDS, the complete response rate for cytarabine therapy was found to be 8% and the overall survival in both groups to be equal.

Other differentiating agents (i.e. interferon-α and interferon-γ) have proved to be disappointing in the treatment of MDS. Methyl transferase inhibitors, 5-aza-2′ deoxycytidine (decitabine) and 5-azacytidine, have also been studied since cytosine can incorporate into the DNA of target cells, thereby inhibiting this enzyme's biochemical activity. Clinical trials of decitabine and 5-azacytidine in patients with leukaemia and MDS suggest that they have anti-leukaemic activity and can induce trilineal differentiation in advanced MDS at a rate superior to that of other differentiating agents in the treatment of MDS. Several multicentre trials using 5-azacytidine and decitabine have reported initial results showing

10–37% complete remission rates and 17–25% partial response rates and relatively low levels of bone marrow hypoplasia or drug-related cytopenia.

Bone marrow transplantation

Bone marrow transplantation (BMT) has been considered a viable treatment alternative for younger patients with MDS. In the past, this treatment modality has been found to have a high mortality and relapse rate in older patients with MDS. A 1998 study by Applebaum et al. investigated the use of allogeneic BMT in 251 patients and found an inverse correlation between age and disease-free survival. Patients who received allogeneic BMT and were less than 20 years of age had a disease-free survival rate of 60% at 6 years. Those patients aged over 60 years had a disease-free survival rate of less than 20% at 6 years. Recently, Deeg et al. investigated BMT in 50 patients with MDS aged 55–66 years and found a relapse-free survival rate of 39% at 3 years follow-up. Recent studies suggest that this may be a viable treatment option in certain patients, but this requires further investigation and follow-up.

Chemotherapy

Chemotherapy regimens have also been utilised to treat patients with MDS and several different regimens have been used with varying degrees of success. Cytosine arabinoside and daunorubicin, alone or in combination with or without 6-thioguanine, have been used to treat patients with MDS during their pre-leukaemic phase. Daunorubicin, cytosine arabinoside and 6-thioguanine (DAT) chemotherapy regimens have been used, and are reported to give complete remission rates of 15–51% with considerable death from toxicity. With high-dose cytosine arabinoside, complete remission rates of 13–53% with death rates from toxicity of greater than 33% have been reported. Although complete remissions can be achieved in patients with MDS with chemotherapy, they are transient and there is a high incidence of toxic deaths. The age of the patients and the biological nature of this disease may be related to the high incidence of toxic death as seen in these patients receiving chemotherapy.

Resistance has been considered to be a determinant for the failure or successful response to chemotherapy in patients with MDS. Over-expression of the multi-drug resistance (*MDR1*) gene product P-glycoprotein (P-gp) has been considered to be one of the causes for chemotherapy resistance. This over-expression has been linked to CD34 expression, cytogenetic pattern and secondary leukaemic processes due to prior cytotoxic therapy. It also leads to cross-resistance to anthracyclines, mitoxantrone and etoposide, drugs commonly used to treat leukaemia. Inhibitors of drug resistance, such as quinine, tamoxifen, cyclosporin A and its stable analogue PSC 833, have been used in an attempt to improve the efficacy of chemotherapeutic agents. A trial of PSC 833 along with standard chemotherapy suggested improved complete response in patients with MDS which transformed to AML. However, in a recent ECOG randomised trial, this improved complete remission rate with PSC 833 was not found. A European trial, however, has indicated that PSC 833 does seem to play an important role in MDS/AML treatment as in patients treated with PSC 833 in this study, once they were in remission, the remission was more durable.

Haematopoietic growth factors

Haematopoietic growth factors, their production and the expression of receptors for these factors on haematopoietic cells are considered to regulate normal haematopoiesis. Haematopoietic growth factors appear to affect different cell progeny at different stages of development. Some (e.g. interleukin-1 (IL-1), interleukin-3 (IL-3) and granulocyte-macrophage colony stimulating factor (GM-CSF), work on earlier progeny leading to proliferation of multipotent haematopoietic cells, while others (e.g. G-CSF, M-CSF) primarily work on more differentiated progenitors.

Most patients with MDS appear to have defective myeloid and erythroid precursor maturation, cytogenetics and enzyme characteristics. The defect in precursor maturation appears to worsen as the patient's condition advances towards acute leukaemic transformation. This defective haematopoietic precursor proliferation may involve the decreased responsiveness or impaired production of haematopoietic growth factors. Therefore, it is possible that growth factors could be beneficial to patients with MDS. These benefits could include stimulation of residual normal bone marrow haematopoietic progenitor cells unable to respond to the physiologically available level of colony stimulating factors and induction of maturation of myelodysplastic cells leading to clonal extinction. They could also act by increasing the sensitivity of these transformed malignant clones to chemotherapy, and increase the rate of bone marrow recovery after treatment.

Recombinant haematopoietic growth factors have been used in the management of patients with MDS to attempt to induce normal differentiation in malignantly transformed cells or to stimulate normal myeloid colonies in the bone marrow. Growth factors can also be used to treat neutropenia and decrease its infection-related morbidity and mortality.

GM-CSF has the ability to stimulate a variety of early progenitor cells. Recombinant GM-CSF has been shown to increase the neutrophil, eosinophil, monocyte and lymphocyte counts in patients with MDS. Response to GM-CSF occurs in a dose-dependent manner, with the most common toxicity reaction observed involving a dose-dependent flu-like syndrome. Fever, bone pain, local erythema, phlebitis with intravenous administration (IV), splenomegaly and adult respiratory distress syndrome (ARDS)-like complications have also been reported.

G-CSF also has the ability to increase the neutrophil count in patients with MDS without affecting the monocyte, eosinophil and lymphocyte numbers. Clinical studies have suggested that G-CSF may not appear as effective as GM-CSF in increasing the cell counts of patients with MDS. G-CSF improves granulocyte function, chemotaxis and phagocytosis in patients with MDS, and can restore the level of the enzyme alkaline phosphatases and the superoxide-generating ability of neutrophils in patients with MDS. Adverse effects with G-CSF are fewer than those observed in patients treated with GM-CSF, and they include bone pain, occasional reports of fluid overload and Sweet's syndrome. Although both GM-CSF and G-CSF have been shown to be effective in decreasing the number of minor life-threatening infections in many patients, they do not appear to affect survival time of patients with MDS or the progression rate to AML.

With anaemia being the most dominant presentation, patients with MDS require significant numbers of red blood cell transfusions. It has been hypothesised that *erythropoietin* (EPO) could be used to overcome the maturation block of red blood cell precursors in the bone marrow of patients with MDS, leading to erythropoiesis, reducing the need for transfusions in these patients, but study results have not been greatly rewarding. A rise of haemoglobin levels has only been observed in 20–30% of patients with MDS.

Recently, there has been an indication that a combination of erythropoietin and G-CSF might be helpful to improve the anaemia observed in some patients where erythropoietin alone has failed. Patients with MDS were treated with G-CSF (starting dose of 1 μg/kg, subcutaneously [SC]), with the dosage adjusted to either normalise or double the neutrophil count (dosage range, 0.2–5.0 μg/kg per day). Erythropoietin (SC, 100 U/kg per day for weeks 1–4, 150 U/kg per day for weeks 5–8, 300 U/kg per day for weeks 8–16) was started once the required absolute neutrophil count (ANC) level was reached, and was given simultaneously with the daily G-CSF dose. All patients showed a myeloid response in the study, with the vast majority showing an increase in their ANC level to over 1800/μL from a baseline of less than 1800/μL. Erythroid responses also occurred in 42% of the patients, with at least an increase in untransfused haemoglobin levels of 1–2g/dL or a 50% decrease in transfusion requirements over the treatment period. Generally, this combined regimen is well tolerated.

Concern has been expressed that haematopoietic growth factors could enhance or induce proliferation of malignant haematopoietic progenitor clones, leading to a treatment-related onset of acute leukaemic transformation. Non-controlled studies have suggested that this may occur in those patients with MDS with greater than 14% blasts in their bone marrow immediately prior to the administration of GM-CSF. Recent and controlled studies have failed to substantiate the concern of enhancing acute leukaemic transformation during usage of GM-CSF and G-CSF in patients with MDS.

In many patients with MDS, there is transformation to frank AML, and palliative treatment with haematopoietic growth factors without chemotherapy may be beneficial in the management of these patients, especially those who are debilitated and significantly older. In our centre, we evaluated the results of 41 patients with MDS/AML who received standard induction chemotherapy, 8 who received chemotherapy and BMT and 11 who were not actively treated. Five of these patients had severe neutropenia and anaemia and received haematopoietic growth factors (G-CSF and/or erythropoietin) without chemotherapy. The average survival time of the patients receiving induction chemotherapy was 8.3 months, as compared to 14.9 months in patients who received only haematopoietic growth factors ($P < 0.007$), and the elderly patients with MDS/AML remained ambulatory and had fewer hospitalisations and a better quality of life. These results suggest that, in some patients with MDS, haematopoietic growth factors alone could be an effective alternative to chemotherapy.

Studies of other haematopoietic growth factors in the treatment of patients with MDS have also been done. These growth factors include IL-1, interleukin-2 (IL-2), interleukin-6 (IL-6), interleukin-8 (IL-8), interleukin-11 (IL-11), interleukin-12 (IL-12) and mast cell growth factor.

The febrile response related to IL-1 treatment has led to the commercial development of interleukin-1α. IL-1α stimulates primitive haematopoietic progenitor cells, as well as accessory cells, such as marrow stromal cells, T cells and macrophages producing endogenous GM-CSF, G-CSF and M-CSF. Treatment with IL-1α in a phase II trial resulted in an initial platelet response of 33–43% in the patients, depending upon dose. The neutrophil response was 40%.

IL-2 studies have shown it can decrease the number of bone marrow blasts, increase the number of colony forming unit granulocyte-macrophages (CFU-GM) and increase the levels of γ-interferon and GM-CSF released by bone marrow mononuclear cells. It does did not induce blast cell proliferation in most patients, but the IL-2 response appears to be heterogeneous in patients with MDS. Patients with low blood-soluble IL-2 receptor levels may respond to IL-2 therapy, and low-risk patients may have a better chance of responding to IL-2 therapy. Although IL-2 does not appear to be promising as a treatment modality for MDS, further investigation is necessary.

In a 1995 study of 22 patients with MDS treated with IL-6, 8 patients (36%) had a significant improvement in their platelet count, and 8 (36%) had a transient rise. IL-6 appeared to enhance the maturation of megakaryocytes without increasing the megakaryocyte number in these patients.

IL-11 is approved for the prevention of severe thrombocytopenia due to chemotherapy, and for the reduction of platelet support in some non-myeloid malignancies. Although this growth factor has been called the 'megakaryocyte growth and development factor' (MGDF) and 'megapoietin' due to its megakaryocytic-specific lineage, studies have shown that it can also enhance erythroid progenitor cell growth and stimulate other progenitors in the presence of other cytokines. The use of this cytokine in patients with MDS has not been established. A recent in-vitro study found that in cases of AML, this cytokine may protect blast cells from programmed cell death.

In-vitro studies of other cytokines in patients with MDS have been done. Neutrophils from 23 patients with MDS were treated with IL-8 in vitro and demonstrated significant functional improvement. The addition of IL-8 did not result in significant stimulation of myeloid growth when IL-8 was added to bone marrow cultures from normal controls and patients with MDS. In an in-vitro study of IL-12, natural killer (NK) cell cytotoxicity of normal controls and some patients with MDS was found to increase in the presence of IL-12, with the addition of IL-2 further enhancing the increase. The effect of mast cell growth factor (MGF, c-kit ligand) on bone marrow progenitor cells has also been studied in vitro. Results suggest that MGF may improve the ability of colony forming units of bone marrow haematopoietic progenitors in patients with MDS. These cytokines require further study before their potential as treatment modalities in cases of MDS can be meaningfully evaluated.

New approaches

Several new therapeutic approaches are under investigation for the treatment of patients with MDS. *Amifostine* (AMF, ethanethiol, 2[(3-aminopropyl)amino] dihydrogen phosphate), a phosphorylated aminothiol, has the ability to stimulate in-vitro growth and survival of haematopoietic stem cells. Studies have indicated that normal marrow mononuclear cells exposed to amifostine show a significant stimulation of Colony forming unit-granulocyte/erythroid/macrophage/megakaryocyte (CFU-GEMM) and burst forming unit-erythroid (BFU-E), as well as stimulation of myeloid progenitors (CFU-GM). Amifostine has also been shown to enhance CFU-GEMM and BFU-E in the bone marrow from patients with MDS. In a phase I/II trial established to study the effects of amifostine on patients with MDS and refractory cytopenias, patients received a 21-day treatment course at different dosages. Fifteen of the 18 patients (83%) in this study had favourable responses, including increases in absolute neutrophil counts, decreases in transfusion requirements, increases in platelet counts and in-vitro progenitor recovery. Most of these patients retained their abnormal clones. Higher amifostine doses produced adverse reactions, while doses less than 200 mg/m^2 were well tolerated. In order to define an optimal route and schedule for long-term amifostine administration, a phase I/II trial of SC amifostine in 20 patients with MDS (RA: 8; RARS: 8; RAEB: 4) was done. These patients received two courses of 200 mg/m^2 amifostine, 5 days per week for 3 consecutive weeks followed by 2 weeks of observation. Forty-five per cent (9 of 20) had single or multiple lineage haematological improvement. Results of this study suggest that, while SC amifostine is well tolerated, IV administration is more haematologically effective. While most studies have illustrated the positive benefits of amifostine as a modality to combat the poor haematopoiesis associated with MDS, a 1998 study showed little response. Further trials on the use of this drug, both alone and in combination with other therapeutic treatments, in patients with MDS are needed to establish its efficacy.

Cyclosporin A (CsA) is a potent immunosuppressive drug and it has been investigated as a possible treatment strategy for patients with MDS. Results of a transfusion-dependent patient with MDS who has been transfusion independent for more than 5 years as a result of cyclosporin A treatment have been noted. In one study, 17 patients with hypoplastic MDS were treated with cyclosporin A. Three patients had serious side effects related to treatment. Eighty-two per cent were reported to have a response, with all transfusion-dependent patients becoming transfusion independent and 23% of the patients having a complete recovery. Two patients with hypoplastic MDS who were treated with cyclosporin A, anti-thymocyte globulin or a combination of both have also been reported. The patients no longer required transfusions, had increased bone marrow cellularity and the disappearance of their dysplastic characteristics.

Anti-thymocyte globulin (ATG) has been studied for its possible efficacy in the treatment of patients with MDS. Eleven of 25 (44%) transfusion-dependent patients with MDS with < 20% blasts treated with ATG in a 1999 study responded and became transfusion-independent: 3 complete responses, 6 partial responses and 2 minimal responses. Sixty-four per cent (9/14) of the responders had RA and 33% (2/6) had RAEB. The side effects of the ATG treatment were mild. It has been theorised that this response of patients with MDS to ATG treatment is related to a loss of lymphocyte-mediated inhibition of CFU-GM and alterations of T-cell-receptor V_β profiles. In another study, 26 'low-risk' patients with MDS were treated with ATG. The regimen was well tolerated with only one patient experiencing acute pulmonary oedema due to fluid overload. Of those patients with adequate follow-up (14), 6 patients had a partial response (43%), 1 had a complete response (7%) and 7 had no response (50%). These results indicate the potential in this treatment modality, and further studies on both cyclosporin A and ATG are warranted.

Other drugs are being investigated for their effectiveness in treating patients with MDS. One study investigated the effectiveness of *topotecan* in combination with ara-C, and found that topotecan added to the effectiveness of ara-C in the treatment of patients with RAEB or RAEB-T, but not to that of those with CMML. High-risk patients with MDS have been treated with a regimen consisting of the addition of topotecan to A-PCD (amifostine + pentoxyfylline + ciprofloxacin + dexamethasone) treatment. A response was noted in 75% of the evaluable patients, and the treatment was well tolerated, suggesting that topotecan in combination with A-PCD treatment may be particularly effective in high-risk patients with MDS. Topotecan has also been tested in combination with fludarabine, ara-C and G-CSF in patients with aggressive MDS. Thirty per cent of the evaluable patients had complete remissions, and 5 had partial remissions at a topotecan dose of 1.5 mg/m^2. Three of the patients with partial remissions were further treated with 2 mg/m^2. All went into complete remission, and 100% of the patients with abnormalities in their chromosomes had cytogenic remissions. Topotecan-based combination chemotherapy in patients with MDS and CMML has been utilised. This treatment appears particularly promising. Thirty-eight patients with advanced MDS and 21 patients with chronic CMML were treated with topotecan and cytarabine. Complete remission occurred in 66% of the patients with MDS, with similar rates in both good-risk and poor-risk patients (79% and 58%, respectively). The complete remission rate in patients with chronic CMML in this study was 48%. Patients with poor prognosis karyotypes and secondary MDS had particularly good complete remission responses to this treatment (63% and 69%, respectively). The median duration of complete remission was 41 weeks in patients with MDS with a median survival of 60 weeks, and the median duration of complete remission in patients with chronic CMML was 33 weeks with a median survival of 41 weeks. This regimen resulted in fever of unknown origin and/or infection in many patients but it was reasonably well tolerated and had a low mortality rate. Topotecan may eventually be important in patients with unfavourable prognoses and warrants further investigation.

Melphalan, *arsenic trioxide* (AS203) and *thalidomide* are also being investigated for their effectiveness in patients with MDS.

Summary on treatment

As this information on treatment illustrates, treatment and management of patients with MDS is difficult and the precise treatment course remains difficult. The only 'cure' for MDS still remains BMT. The National Comprehensive Cancer Network (NCCN) in the US has developed MDS practice guidelines to aid physicians in the diagnosis, evaluation, risk evaluation and treatment of these patients. These guidelines are reviewed and re-evaluated annually. Therapeutic suggestions are recommended on the basis of course type and age. These guidelines include supportive care (i.e. transfusions, cytokine support and/or iron chelation), low-intensity therapy (i.e. low-intensity chemotherapy or biological response modifiers) and high-intensity therapy for high-risk patients (i.e. intensive induction chemotherapy, moderately intense chemotherapy or BMT). It should be recognised that these guidelines are only suggestions and treatment decisions should be based on the characteristics of each individual patient.

Prognosis

The prognosis for different MDS subtypes varies. In general, RA and RARS are considered to have a lower risk associated with them than the CMML, RAEB and RAEB-T subtypes. The reported percentage of AML transformations and the median survival time for each is outlined in Table 46.3.

In general, 10–40% of patients will develop AML and 20–40% will die of infection and/or bleeding. Various attempts have been made to define the prognostic factors to predict the course of patients with MDS. These have included: age, degree of anaemia, neutropenia, thrombocytopenia, bone marrow blast

Table 46.3 The prognosis for different MDS subtypes

MDS subtypes	AML transformation (%)	Median survival (months)
Refractory anaemia (RA)	11–26	17–64
Refractory anaemia with ring sideroblasts (RARS)	5–39	16–52
Chronic myelomonocytic leukaemia (CMML)	15–32	8–22
Refractory anaemia with excess of blasts (RAEB)	27–66	9–17
Refractory anaemia with excess of blasts in transformation (RAEB-T)	50–81	5–10

percentage, extensive dyspoiesis, central clustering of immature precursors and cytogenetic abnormalities. Various scoring systems have been devised to attempt to provide a more objective assessment of the disease, but none of the scoring systems developed have been overly acceptable. Overall, the single most important prognostic parameter appears to be the bone marrow blast count.

Chromosomal abnormalities in patients with MDS may have prognostic significance by directly correlating the number and type with the risk of developing acute leukaemia. In general, aggressive forms of MDS have been found to have more chromosomal aberrations. In a study of de novo patients with MDS, the overall incidence of chromosomal aberration was 69%, with the relative frequency being 100% in patients with RAEB-T, 76% in patients with RAEB, 56% in patients with RA and 42% in patients with CMML. The most common single anomalies were del(5)(q13q22q33), monosomy 7 or deletion of 7q, del(11)(q14q23) and trisomy 8, and complex karyotypic abnormalities were noted. Leukaemic transformation occurred in 66 patients (35%) in this study, although no transformation in this report occurred in patients with a normal karyotype, in those with del(5)(q13q33) or in those with del(11)(q14q23) alone. All of the patients in this study with complex rearrangements, monosomy 7 or del(7q) developed acute leukaemia. The median survival time inversely related to the presence and number of complex abnormalities found. Patients with del(5)(q13q33) had the best survival, and those with monosomy 7 and del(7q) had the worst.

Recently, an International Prognostic Scoring System (IPSS) has been compiled for the more accurate prediction of prognosis. This scoring system generates risk scores for bone marrow blast percentage, karyotype and the number of cytopenias the patient has. The presence of < 5% blasts is scored 0, 5–10% blasts are scored 0.5, 11–20% blasts are scored 1.5, and 21–30% blasts are scored 2.0. Karyotypes are separated by type, such as good (scored 0), intermediate (scored 0.5) and poor (scored 1.0). If the patient has more than one cytopenia, a score of 0.5 is given, and ≤ 1 cytopenia is scored 0. The IPSS system has developed four risk groups based upon the sum of the patient's risk scores for the three major variables. *Low-risk patients* have a total score of 0 and an estimated survival time of 5.7 years. *Intermediate-1 risk patients* score 0.5–1.0 with an estimated survival time of 3.5 years, while *intermediate-2 patients* are considered to be those with a total risk score of 1.5–2.0 and a survival time of 1.2 years. *High-risk patients* have an IPSS score of greater than 2.5 and a projected survival time of 0.4 years. Therefore, according to the IPSS scoring system, a patient with 17% blasts, thrombocytopenia, neutropenia and a good karyotype would receive scores of 1.5, 0.5 and 0 respectively. This patient would receive a total score of 2 and would be ranked in the intermediate-2 IPSS group.

Conclusion

Myelodysplastic syndrome includes a group of heterogeneous clonal bone marrow disorders, characterised by dysplasia and ineffective haematopoiesis. These disorders lead to peripheral cytopenia(s) and hypercellular marrow in the majority of the patients, and further transform into AML in many patients. MDS is primarily a disease of the elderly, with an incidence twice that of acute leukaemia and close to that of chronic lymphocytic leukaemia.

Five subgroups of MDS have been described:

1. RA (refractory anaemia)
2. RARS (refractory anaemia with ring sideroblasts)
3. CMML (chronic myelomonocytic leukaemia)
4. RAEB (refractory anaemia with excess of blasts)
5. RAEB-T (refractory anaemia with excess of blasts in transformation).

Cytogenetic abnormalities occur in at least half the patients with MDS and are helpful in both the diagnosis and the prediction of the clinical course and prognosis.

The current management approaches in the treatment of MDS include the use of differentiating agents, aggressive chemotherapy, BMT and haematopoietic growth factors. Although there has been a great deal of progress in the treatment of this disorder, current treatment strategies are far from optimum. Further studies are needed in this area.

Acknowledgment

The author would like to acknowledge the efforts of Ms Genevieve A. Morelli in the preparation of this manuscript.

Bibliography and further reading

Applebaum, F. R. & Anderson, J. (1998), 'Allogeneic bone marrow transplantation for myelodysplastic syndrome: outcomes analysis according to IPSS score', *Leukemia*, 12(suppl. 1), pp. S25–9.

Bennett, J. M., Catovsky, D., Daniel, M. T., Flandrin, M. T., Galton, D. A., Gralnick, H. R. & Sultan, C. (1982), 'Proposals for the classification of the myelodysplastic syndromes', *British Journal of Haematology*, 51(2), pp. 189–99.

Deeg, H. J., Shulman, H. M., Anderson, J. E., Bryant, E. M., Gooley, T. A., Slattery, J. T., Anasetti, C., Fefer, A., Storb, R. & Applebaum, F. R. (2000), 'Allogeneic and syngenic marrow transplantation for myelodysplastic syndrome in patients 55 to 66 years of age', *Blood*, 95(4), pp. 1188–94.

Fenaux, P. & Preudhomme, C. (1997), 'Molecular abnormalities and clonality in myelodysplastic syndromes', *Pathologie Biologie*, 45(7), pp. 556–60.

Goyal, R., Qawi, H., Ali, I., Dar, S., Mundle, S., Shetty, V., Mativi, Y., Allampallam, K., Lisak, L., Loew, J., Venugopal, P., Gezer, S., Robin, E., Rifkin, S. & Raza, A. (1999), 'Biologic characteristics of patients with hypocellular myelodysplastic syndromes', *Leukemia Research*, 23(4), pp. 357–64.

Greenberg, P., Cox, C., Le Beau, M. M., Fenaux, P., Morel, P., Sanz, G., Sanz, M., Vallespi, T., Hamblin, T., Oscier, D., Ohyashiki, K., Toyama, K., Aul, C., Mufti, G. & Bennett J. (1997), 'International scoring system for evaluating prognosis in myelodysplastic syndrome', *Blood*, 89(6), pp. 2079–88.

Hellstrom-Lindberg, E. (1999), 'Treatment of adult myelodysplastic syndromes', *International Journal of Hematology*, 70(3), pp. 141–54.

Harris, N. L., Jaffe, E. S., Diebold, J., Flandrin, G., Muller-Hermelink, H. K., Vardiman, J., Lister, T. A. & Bloomfield, C. D. (1999), 'World Health Organization classification of neoplastic diseases of the hematopoietic and lymphoid tissues: Report of the Clinical Advisory Committee meeting—Airlie House, Virginia, November, 1997', *Journal of Clinical Oncology*, 17(12), pp. 3835–49.

Kaushansky, K. (2000), 'Use of thrombopoietic growth factors in acute leukemia', *Leukemia*, 14(3), pp. 505–8.

List, A. F., Garewal, H. S. & Sandberg, A. A. (1990), 'The myelodysplastic syndromes: biology and implications for management', *Journal of Clinical Oncology*, 8(8), pp. 1424–41.

Mecucci, C. & Vandèn Berghe, H. (1992), 'Cytogenetics', *Hematology-Oncology Clinics of North America*, 6(3), pp. 523–41.

NCCN (1998), 'NCCN practice guidelines for the myelodysplastic syndromes', *Oncology*, 12(11), pp. 53–80.

Raza, A., Alvi, S., Borok, R. Z., Span, L., Parcharidou, A., Alston, D., Rifkin, S., Robin, E., Shah, R. & Gregory, S. A. (1996), 'Excessive proliferation matched by excess apoptosis in myelodysplastic syndromes: the cause–effect relationship', *Leukemia and Lymphoma*, 27(1–2), pp. 111–8.

Saba, H. I., Ballester, O. F. & Balducci, L. (1992), 'Hemopoietic growth factors in myelodysplasia', *Hematology Reviews*, 37, pp. 207–21.

Sanz, G., Sanz, M. & Greenberg, P. (1998). 'Prognostic factors and scoring systems in myelodysplastic syndromes: recent advances in myelodysplastic syndromes', *Haematologica*, 83, pp. 358–76.

Yoshida, Y. (1996), 'Treatment of the myelodysplastic syndromes: an updated Japanese experience', *Seminars in Hematology*, 33(3), pp. 246–55.

Chapter 47

Malignancy: a pragmatic approach

BRIAN STEIN

Introduction

This chapter provides some background to the issues of cancer in the elderly as well as a pragmatic approach to assessment of the elderly patient with cancer. Although it is written from a specialist point of view, the aim is to provide principles for the generalist. The frequent issues that arise are: firstly, does this patient have cancer?; secondly, what can be done about it?; and thirdly, is this patient a candidate for specific antineoplastic treatment?

My general thesis is that elderly patients should be carefully assessed and the physiologically young should be treated identically to those of a younger chronological age. Thus, there will be significant overlaps with oncology of the younger patient. The two approaches used in this chapter are summarised diagrammatically: the approach to diagnosis (Figure 47.1), and the approach to treatment (Figure 47.2).

Some may consider this an overly aggressive stance. It is if one does not take into account frail older persons, and treat them with due consideration for their age. Furthermore, the approach is reasonable when one considers that in First World countries:

- the average life expectancy for an 80 year old woman is about 9 years
- the average life expectancy for an 80 year old man is about 7 years
- the 5 year survival rate for 90 year old women is about 40%
- the 5 year survival rate for 90 year old men is about 30%.

Treatment of the physiologically old and frail is difficult, with little hard data to guide treatment. There is systematic under-representation of the elderly in clinical trials, and many clinical trials automatically exclude patients on the basis of an arbitrary upper age limit. As the elderly patients included in trials are the most robust people, they cannot serve as a guide for the frail elderly. In the absence of hard data, an approach is to begin by proceeding as outlined in Figure 47.1 and modulated by the approach outlined in Figure 47.2. Be particularly guided by the patient's wishes: in general, the elderly have been shown to have similar preferences for active therapy as younger people. It is also vital to keep a very close eye on the balance between benefit and adverse effects. Hopefully, some sense of this will come through in the various case vignettes.

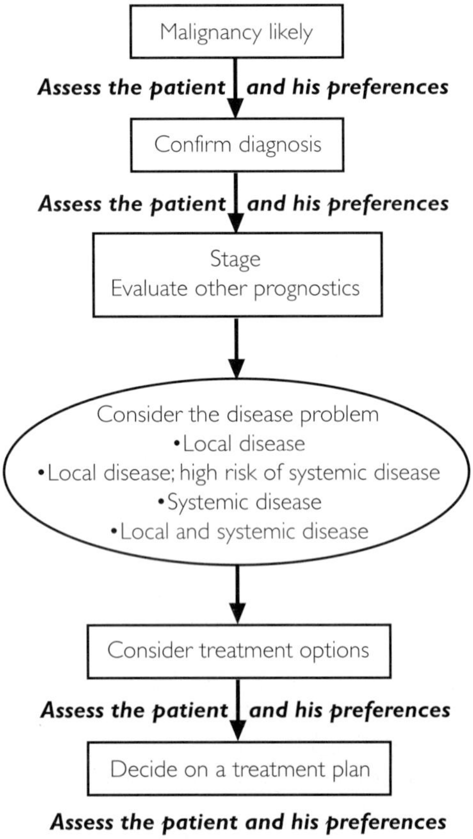

Figure 47.1 An outline of the approach to diagnosis of the elderly patient with suspected malignancy

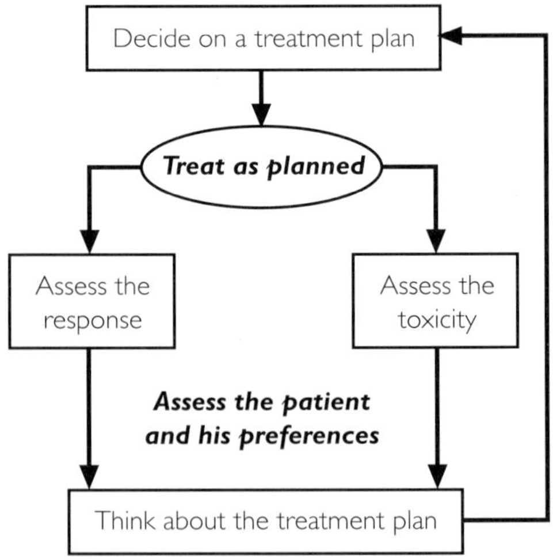

Figure 47.2 An outline of the approach to treating the elderly patient with a malignancy

Table 47.1 The six most commonly diagnosed cancers in South Australia[(a)]

Cancer	Percentage of cases	Peak age of incidence (years)
Colon and rectum	13.9	70–80
Prostate	13.7	70–74
Breast	13.5	50–54
Lung	9.1	70–80
Melanoma	8	no clear peak
Lymphoma	4.4	no clear peak

(a) Data from the South Australian Cancer Registry.

Background

Epidemiology

Cancer is a common disease of the elderly, however one chooses to define that group, but no malignancy is restricted to the elderly. However, the peak incidence of many of the common cancers is found in the later years of life, as shown in Table 47.1.

The total burden of malignant disease in the elderly is also considerable (see Table 47.2).

It is clear that most of those dying from cancer are elderly: about 35% of all deaths from cancer occur in those over the age of 75. Although these figures are taken from South Australia, and thus reflect certain idiosyncrasies of the region (e.g. the high incidence of melanoma), other registries in developed countries show similar patterns of

Table 47.2 Percentage of cancer deaths by age in South Australia[(a)]

Age (years)	Male deaths (%)	Female deaths (%)
< 50	7	10
50–55	5	6
55–59	8	7
60–64	12	10
65–69	16	13
70–74	18	15
75–79	16	15
80–84	11	12
> 85	8	12

(a) Data from South Australian Cancer Registry.

disease. Even though the pattern of malignancy in the developing world is not identical, with some of the more common malignancies (e.g. hepatocellular carcinoma) being more evenly distributed across ages, this does not negate the argument. Even malignancies that do not have their peak incidence in the aged are often a problem in later years. This is illustrated graphically in Figure 47.3. A malignancy such as melanoma is still of importance in the older population, even though it does not show a clear peak of incidence in the elderly, like lung cancer does, with which it is compared.

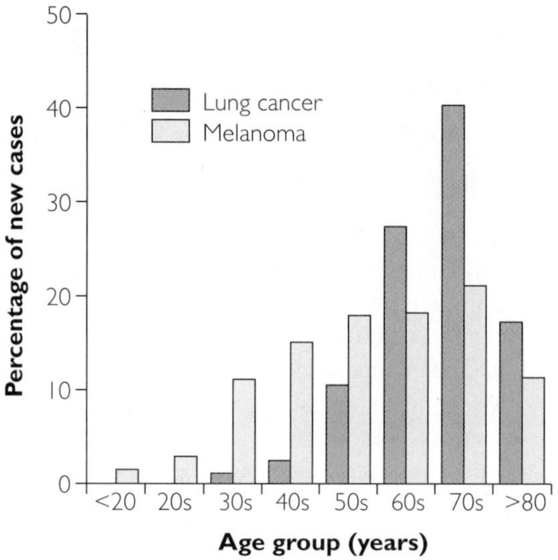

Figure 47.3 Age at diagnosis with melanoma and lung cancer. Data adapted from the South Australian Cancer Registry

Natural history of cancer in the elderly

Geriatric oncology would be of less issue if the natural history of malignant disease were uniformly more slow in the elderly. In some diseases, best exemplified by prostate cancer, this thesis can be argued—up to 70% of 85-year-old males have foci of asymptomatic prostatic carcinoma found at autopsy but the disease does not always have an impact on the patient.

This, however, is not always the norm. Although many have described youth as a poor prognosticator in breast cancer, several workers have found that advanced age is also a predictor for poor outcome. In this case, it is not possible to separate out the potential interaction between age and more aggressive biology from the effects of a more laissez-faire approach to diagnosis and therapy. In patients with non-Hodgkin's lymphoma, however, the case is more clear-cut. When subjected to a uniform policy of staging and treatment, those over 60 have a significantly lower chance of achieving complete remission and cure. This may reflect inability to tolerate the treatment regimen, as seems to be the case in the aggressive regimens used to treat acute myeloid leukaemia; however, with standard lymphoma chemotherapy, the evidence that this is the case is not convincing, as discussed in the next section.

Is treatment of the elderly too toxic?

It is not possible to predict with certainty the toxicity of treatment in any patient. Substantial work has been done in correlating morbidity and mortality with chronological age in relation to both chemotherapy and surgery (see page 685). Elderly patients can tolerate major procedures and aggressive treatment regimens with acceptable levels of complications, but this requires careful selection of patients and closer supervision than in younger patients.

It is also important to consider that under-treatment can have major 'toxicity': failure to control the disease may be even more troublesome than treatment. This is best exemplified in patients with metastatic breast cancer: in a trial, investigators found that stopping chemotherapy after a few cycles led to a worse quality of life than continuing therapy because the 'toxicity' of disease symptoms overrode the toxicity of chemotherapy. Similarly, attempting to design 'gentle' treatments for the elderly may backfire in the longer term by producing poorer outcomes, thus requiring more efforts to try and achieve the original aim. This has been well documented in patients with the aggressive lymphomas: investigators found that 'standard' chemotherapy produced better cure rates than 'gentle' treatment, and thus in the long term was less 'toxic'.

The essential questions of oncology

Conceptually, the approach to any patient with malignancy is not particularly involved. In contrast, the practicalities are often extremely involved and change significantly with time: the aim here is to convey the essence of the approach. This involves setting and answering a series of clinical questions. By necessity these are presented as a sequence; in practice they are often performed concurrently. The approach is summarised in Figures 47.1 and 47.2.

What is the state of the patient?

This is one of the central issues, which must be revisited at each step in the process of evaluating the neoplasm. In some circumstances, the state of the patient (i.e. physical, psychological, social) will prohibit any evaluation, in others it will limit some of the steps in evaluation or treatment, and in others there will be no difference in the approach from the younger patient.

Further discussion of how to assess the state of patients and their likely tolerance of treatment is presented on page 685.

> **Vignette 47.1**
>
> A frail 88-year-old woman was referred with abdominal discomfort, abnormal liver function tests, and para-aortic lymphadenopathy on ultrasound of the abdomen. Physical examination revealed multiple 1–3 cm lymph nodes in the axillae, 1 cm nodes in the neck and groin, but no abdominal mass nor hepatosplenomegaly. A peripheral blood film was normal. A fine-needle aspirate was consistent with a diagnosis of low-grade non-Hodgkin's lymphoma.
>
> After discussion she did not want any invasive procedures, including excision biopsy, nor did she want intensive therapy, but she was prepared to try oral chemotherapy if it had some chance of improving her symptoms. As the fine-needle aspirate suggested a diagnosis of low-grade lymphoma, oral chemotherapy with minimal probability of adverse effects was likely to be effective. A trial of chlorambucil was instituted. She showed significant improvement in her discomfort for 2 months but then developed evidence of progressive disease. After further discussion she declined further active therapy.

Is it a malignant neoplasm?

It is not possible to discuss all the potential presentations of malignancy in the elderly. For the most part, these are similar to those encountered in younger patients. Some non-specific presentations may be more common in the elderly. In particular, systemic symptoms such as weight loss may provoke evaluation for malignant disease, as over 75% of patients with more than 5 kg of weight loss will have serious underlying abnormalities.

Is the diagnosis certain?

The cornerstone of oncology is histopathological or cytological diagnosis. Although imaging techniques have improved enormously in the last 2 decades, they cannot substitute for pathological examination as it has been consistently shown in the literature that serious misdiagnosis remains a problem. Even in the era of computerised tomography (CT) and magnetic resonance imaging (MRI), autopsy studies consistently show clinical diagnosis is seriously in error in at least 10% of cases. Biopsy, therefore, should be the rule not the exception; one advantage of modern imaging is the feasibility of obtaining fine-needle and fine-core biopsies with minimal discomfort to the patient in most circumstances.

Several types of diagnostic errors may be made.

1. Missing a more treatable non-malignant disease.

> **Vignette 47.2**
>
> An 83-year-old man was being investigated for back pain, weight loss and night sweats. A bone scan showed two adjacent abnormal lumbar vertebra and a CT scan suggested either malignancy or possibly an infective process. A needle biopsy was consistent with osteomyelitis, and cultures of biopsy material grew *Staphylococcus aureus*, which was successfully treated with antibiotics.

2. Missing a more treatable malignancy.

Vignette 47.3

A 76-year-old man had undergone a nephrectomy for renal cell carcinoma 4 years previously. He had weight loss, night sweats and vague abdominal pain without any abnormalities on examination. A CT scan of the abdomen showed multiple enlarged para-aortic nodes, which were ascribed to recurrent renal carcinoma, and he was told his condition was incurable and likely to be fatal in the relatively near future. A needle biopsy showed low-grade lymphoma. Although his second neoplasm is also incurable, the prognosis is far better, and he remains in a complete remission some months after completing 6 cycles of chemotherapy.

3. Missing a less treatable malignancy.

Vignette 47.4

A 71-year-old man was referred for treatment of chronic lymphocytic leukaemia, diagnosed on the basis of a peripheral blood count of 210 000 typical lymphocytes/μL. He had also noted a rapidly growing right axillary node that was now about 8 cm in diameter. He had no other lymphadenopathy but did have several 2 cm lung lesions. He was otherwise well, but had had a melanoma excised from the right posterior thorax many years ago. In view of the atypical distribution of disease, the lung lesion was biopsied and this showed melanoma.

What is the oncological problem?

Typically, many texts will proceed on to discuss staging of the neoplasm, and then the results of different treatment modalities. The rationale behind this is not always evident, and presupposes an understanding of the oncological problem faced by the patient and the treating practitioner.

How does one decide what the problem is likely to be? This is determined by the usual natural history of the neoplasm (again the benefit of biopsy!) and the stage of the disease.

The principle oncological problems are:

- predominantly local disease
- predominantly systemic disease
- both local and systemic disease
- local disease is the current problem; systemic disease is a likely issue later.

Which neoplasms cause what oncological problems?

To summarise completely the behaviour of all the common malignancies is impossible, but in Box 47.1 the general behaviour of the common malignancies is presented by grouping them into the oncological problems they most commonly produce. Several malignancies appear in different classifications; this is generally because as the stage advances the behaviour may change.

This classification is of importance in deciding which of the available means of treatment are best suited to dealing with the problem (see page 685).

What else can be determined about the neoplasm?

To determine the oncological problem completely, one must stage the neoplasm. This helps in determining not only the likely oncological problem, but also the prognosis, and the likely success of various therapeutic options. In situations where local disease is evident and occult systemic disease is likely, further information can be of use in judging how likely this is to be a problem.

What stage is the neoplasm?

How does one stage a particular neoplasm? This is done by a combination of history, examination and investigations. These are aimed at determining the stage of the primary lesion and the local nodal systems involved, and examining the likely sites of metastatic involvement (the common sites of spread of some neoplasms are presented in Table 47.3).

Although many manuals have been written discussing the detailed staging of each malignancy, a

Box 47.1 General behaviour of the common malignancies

Local disease is generally the major problem

- Head and neck squamous cell carcinomas[a]
- Non-melanoma skin cancer
- Early stage bladder cancer
- Primary brain neoplasms
- Early stage cervical cancer
- Mesothelioma
- Hepatocellular cancer
- Thyroid cancer

Systemic disease is generally the major problem

- Germ cell neoplasms
- Lymphoma[b]
- Other haematological neoplasms
- Carcinoma of unknown primary

Both local and systemic disease are issues

- Bladder cancer, later stages
- Prostate cancer
- Cervix carcinoma, later stages
- Uterine cancer
- Ovarian cancer
- Colon cancer
- Rectal cancer
- Small-cell lung cancer
- Non-small-cell lung cancer
- Stomach cancer
- Pancreatic cancer
- Sarcomas in the 'axial' region[c]
- Oesophageal cancer
- Breast cancer, more advanced

Local disease is evident; occult systemic disease is likely

- Early breast cancer
- Sarcomas of extremities
- Renal cell cancer
- Melanoma, more advanced stages
- Rectal cancer
- Colon cancer
- Early stage non-small-cell lung cancer

(*a*) Excluding nasopharyngeal cancer.
(*b*) When there are bulky masses, local failure can be a significant problem.
(*c*) Head and neck; retroperitoneum and pelvis; mediastinum and thorax.

Table 47.3 The sites of predilection for metastatic malignancies in order of frequency

Malignancy	Common sites of spread
Thoracic neoplasms	
Non-small-cell lung cancer	Nodes, liver, adrenal glands, bone, brain
Small-cell lung cancer	Nodes, liver, adrenal glands, bone, CNS
Oesophagus	Nodes, lung, liver, adrenal glands
Gastrointestinal neoplasms	
Stomach	Liver, lung, peritoneum
Pancreas	Liver, peritoneum
Colon	Liver, lung, peritoneum
Rectum	Liver, lung, peritoneum, nodes
Genitourinary neoplasms	
Renal	Lung, soft tissue, bone, liver
Bladder	Lung, bone, liver
Prostate	Bone, nodes
Ovary	Peritoneum, nodes, liver, pleura
Uterus	Lung, liver, nodes, peritoneum
Cervix	Nodes, lung
Germ cell tumours	Nodes, lung
Other solid tumours	
Breast	Nodes, liver, lung, bone, CNS
Sarcoma	Lung
Melanoma	Skin, nodes, CNS, lung
Haematological neoplasms	
Lymphoma	Nodes, bone marrow, liver, spleen
Myeloma	Bone marrow
Leukaemias	Bone marrow, nodes, liver, spleen

'rough and ready' outline can be given. This is not a substitute for the official staging systems but is close enough to be of practical use at the bedside, and simple enough in concept to be able to be recalled. Staging varies between neoplasms, but in general the following staging system exists:

- TNM classification—(T)umour, (N)ode and (M)etastasis classification—for malignancies of solid organs and of hollow organs
- lymphomas
- other haematological neoplasms
- specialised staging—gynaecological malignancies, small-cell lung cancer.

The following general principles of TNM staging will generally help give a sensible initial approach.

The tumour (T) stage

Depending on the organ (e.g. hollow viscus, solid), the criteria will vary. The principle issues are:

- size of tumour
- invasion of associated structures (e.g. capsule, serosa)
- invasion into surrounding structures
- fixity.

Table 47.4 shows the typical stages and the characteristics used to determine them.

Example 47.1

A patient was referred for consideration of adjuvant therapy following resection of a rectal cancer. The tumour extended through the serosa but did not involve other organs. It was thus staged as T_3.

Regional lymph node (N) stage

The differentiation of nodes into regional and metastatic disease will depend on the lymphatic anatomy. The principle criteria in determining lymph node stage are:

Table 47.4 Typical tumour stages and their characteristics

Tumour stage	Characteristics
T_0	No evidence of primary tumour[(a)]
T_1	Confined to organ of origin or superficially invasive; ≤ 2 cm; mobile
T_2	Invading associated structures or invading through muscularis mucosae; 2–5 cm; mobile or partially mobile
T_3	Regionally confined but fixed or invading through serosa; > 5 cm but < 10 cm
T_4	Invading into surrounding structures or organs; > 10 cm; invasion of vital structures

(a) This may be associated with the problem of malignancy of unknown primary tumour.

- fixation
- number
- size
- drainage (e.g. unilateral, contralateral)
- nodal station (*Note*: Lymph nodes in the anatomical region of an organ do not consistently receive all the lymph flow from the organ. It is more accurate to think of regular stopping places (stations) in the system of flow. Thus, first nodal stations tend to receive only flow from the organ, second stations receive flow from first station nodes.).

The typical nodal stages and their characteristics are shown in Table 47.5.

Table 47.5 Typical nodal stages and their characteristics

Nodal stage	Characteristics
N_0	No involved lymph nodes
N_1	First echelon nodes; mobile; solitary nodes; ipsilateral to organ; < 2–3 cm
N_2	Multiple nodes; > 3 cm; matted; generally ipsilateral
N_3	Fixed nodes; contralateral or bilateral; second echelon nodes; massive nodes
Metastatic nodes	Nodes distant to the organ are more often metastatic and should be classified as such

Example 47.2

A patient had a painful lesion on the tip of his ear and a 4 cm mobile node in the pre-auricular region. Biopsy confirmed squamous cell carcinoma in both sites, thus the staging was T_1, N_2. Pathological examination showed extensive local invasion, including invasion of the cartilage of the ear: his clinical staging was thus an underestimate, and his pathological tumour stage was T_3.

Example 47.3

A patient with breast cancer was noted to have an ipsilateral supraclavicular node. This has previously been classified as N_3 (second echelon) but is currently staged as metastatic disease.

It is fairly easy to appreciate from the above description that a high T or N stage disease is not generally amenable to resection, although radiotherapy may be an option. Furthermore, it is fairly self-evident that the higher the T or N stage, the grimmer the prognosis, and in most neoplasms the presence of metastatic disease connotes incurability (although not necessarily untreatability).

Metastatic (M) stage

This is a simpler staging: metastases are either detected or not detected, or there is no evaluation. Evaluation is driven by an examination of the likely sites of disease spread (see Table 47.3), which in turn depends on the nature of the neoplasm. Although the routine staging for most diseases does not further subdivide metastases, it is often worth doing so as it is prognostically important (Table 47.6).

Table 47.6 Typical metastatic stages and their characteristics

Metastatic stage	Characteristics
M_0	No evidence of metastases
M_1	Presence of metastases
M_{+1}	Metastases in a single site/organ
M_{+2}	Multiple metastases in a single site or organ
M_{+3}	Multiple organs involved (and it is worth counting the number of organs)
M_x	Inadequate evaluation performed

Example 47.4

An 82-year-old woman was referred for evaluation. She had a mobile 7 × 5 cm breast lump, a 3 cm fixed axillary node, and spinal discomfort with tenderness in several vertebrae and ribs. Thus, in general terms she would be staged as T_3, N_2, M_1 (multiple skeletal lesions) but these should be confirmed by investigation.

Staging of lymphoma

Lymphoma staging is also anatomical in approach (Table 47.7). The issue of note is that early stage disease in low-grade lymphoma may sometimes be cured by radiotherapy alone, and in higher grade lymphoma brief courses of chemotherapy plus irradiation are at least as good as longer treatment. It should be of no surprise that local failure is more frequent with bulky disease; thus, local radiotherapy is often used to combat this.

Staging of other haematological neoplasms

These are essentially all systemic diseases from the outset; staging systems do not reflect anatomical issues and the therapeutic options are determined by their systemic nature.

Under-staging

Under-staging is extremely common in the elderly. As illustrated in Vignettes 47.6 and 47.7, under-staging should be a conscious decision, either because of patient preferences or because management would not be altered. Where it is a reflection of therapeutic ambivalence, difficulties may arise.

Table 47.7 Staging and characteristics of lymphoma

Lymphoma stage	Characteristic
I	One node bearing area involved
II	2 or more node-bearing areas on the same side of the diaphragm involved
III	Node-bearing areas on both sides of the diaphragm involved
IV	Systemic disease, typically bone marrow or liver disease
E disease	Where an extra-nodal site is involved, this suffix is used (e.g. a localised gastric lymphoma is stage I_E)
Bulky disease	Where node masses are > 10 cm or over one-third of the cardiothoracic diameter

Vignette 47.5

A 74-year-old woman noted painless lymphadenopathy in the middle of the anterior triangle. A fine-needle aspirate suggested lymphoma. An excision biopsy confirmed diffuse, large-cell non-Hodgkin's lymphoma (an intermediate grade lymphoma). Staging with physical examination, CT scans of the neck, chest and abdomen, and bone marrow biopsies revealed no other sites of disease. The lymphoma was thus diagnosed as stage I. She was a keen singer and so wished to avoid radiotherapy; a provisional plan was made to give her 6 cycles of chemotherapy to avoid this. Three cycles of standard combination chemotherapy in full doses were given, which resulted in significant fatigue, lethargy and taste changes. She decided that the small risk of vocal toxicity was outweighed by her current experience and local radiation was used, leaving her in complete remission (she has also been able to resume choir singing).

Vignette 47.6

A 68-year-old woman presented with dyspnoea from a large pleural effusion. The effusion was drained and cytology demonstrated a large-cell undifferentiated malignancy. She indicated that she did not wish any further intervention to be made but that only comfort measures were to be employed. No further staging was undertaken. Clinically and biochemically the chest was the only site of disease; a pleurodesis was performed to minimise the chances of local recurrence. At present, she remains well with no evidence of progression.

Vignette 47.7

An 86-year-old woman was referred from a rehabilitation centre. She had become paraplegic over the course of some weeks. Imaging demonstrated a mass adjacent to the L2 vertebra that extended into the spinal canal, causing compression of the cauda equina, and a fine-needle aspirate was consistent with lymphoma. As her sole desire was to walk again, radiotherapy was the most logical treatment. In view of the adequate regional definition of the malignancy, the usual systemic evaluation was dispensed with. Unfortunately, she had little objective return in neurological function after radiotherapy. After some months, her disease progressed systemically and eventually led to her demise.

What other prognostic information is available?

Grade

Good pathology reporting can be invaluable in providing prognostic information. The nuclear grade of solid malignancies clearly has prognostic importance in most situations; the higher the grade, the higher the risk of metastasis, or local failure. In a number of malignancies (e.g. CNS malignancies, sarcomas), histological grade is so important it is a factor explicitly included in the staging system.

Other data

More specialised information can be provided for some neoplasms. In a number of neoplasms, the level of tumour markers is an important prognosticator (e.g. prostate-specific antigen [PSA] in prostatic cancer, β–human chorionic gonadotrophin [β–HCG] in germ cell malignancies). In practice, this information tends to be neoplasm specific.

Generic information

Some pathological information is more generic. The risk of spread or local failure often correlates with the presence of lymphatic, vascular or perineural invasion or infiltration. These factors may be of use in estimating the likelihood of distant spread or in judging the likely behaviour of a neoplasm.

What is the best outcome that can be achieved?

This depends on the answers to the above questions, plus a knowledge of specific outcomes of therapy. In general terms, the nature of the malignancy is the primary determinant, strongly influenced by the stage of the malignancy and the grade. In advanced disease there are important simple clinical indicators: performance status, weight loss > 10% of body weight, and burden or bulk of the disease (measured as either by number of sites involved, involvement of multiple parenchymal organs, or changes in serum markers, such as elevation of lactate dehydrogenase or fall in albumin or haemoglobin levels).

More specifically, malignancies can by broken up by likely outcome, which are outlined below.

1. *Cure is likely*. These include: early stage cancers of the colon, rectum, bladder, kidney, prostate, cervix, uterus, ovary and breast; melanoma and other skin cancers; some head and neck malignancies; some lymphomas and leukaemias; and germ cell tumours.
2. *Cure is possible but less likely*. These include more advanced neoplasms of the above categories, oesophageal cancer, stomach cancer, non-small-cell lung cancer, early stage small-cell lung cancer and sarcomas.
3. *Cure is occasional*. These include locally advanced non-small-cell lung cancer and localised pancreatic cancer.
4. *Cure is impossible but active therapies (arbitrary) are available*. These include: metastatic cancers of the breast, ovary, some thyroid cancers, prostate cancer, and small-cell lung cancer; myeloma, some lymphomas and leukaemias.
5. *Modestly active therapies are available*. These include metastatic cancers of the colon and rectum, metastatic non-small-cell lung cancer, metastatic sarcomas, advanced gynaecological malignancies, advanced head and neck malignancies, and possibly pancreatic cancer.

6. *Few responses are seen with active therapy.* These include metastatic renal malignancies and metastatic melanoma.

Is this elderly patient likely to tolerate treatment?

Unfortunately, there is no treatment recipe that can be followed. The important factors vary somewhat with the proposed modality of therapy. Furthermore, these factors cannot be taken into account without considering the rigour of the proposed therapy: to choose one modality as an example, not all radiation therapy is of equal 'difficulty'. For example, for the patient, the ease of a single fraction of palliative radiotherapy cannot be compared to a radical course of treatment; similarly, the adverse effects from treating a peripheral bone are generally far less than those from treating the abdomen or chest.

Before considering the specifics of each therapeutic modality, some general factors do predict a patient's ability to tolerate treatment. Several of these factors have been derived for predicting toxicity from chemotherapy, but they do seem to 'map' across to the other modalities. Objective global predictors of tolerance include:

1. performance status (see Table 47.8)
2. ability to perform activities of daily living
3. ability to perform instrumental activities of daily living
4. physiological reserve, particularly renal function, but also pulmonary, hepatic, and cardiac function.

Of these, performance status is one of the most important variables. It can be determined quickly, fairly objectively and simply. Patients with a performance status of greater than 2 generally will not tolerate medical therapies well: unless they have particularly treatment-responsive malignancies they are not likely to benefit from chemotherapy. In some situations, for example, in advanced non-small-cell lung cancer, many oncologists will exclude patients with a performance status above 1 unless the decline has been very recent.

Table 47.8 Performance status: Zubrod (or ECOG) scale

Performance status	Description
0	Asymptomatic
1	Symptomatic
2	Symptomatic and in bed or chair less than 50% of the day
3	Symptomatic and in bed or chair more than 50% of the day
4	Completely dependent

More subjective measures of tolerance include:

1. 'Biological age': an assessment of what age the patients look and function at, rather than what chronological age they are.
2. Co-morbidity burden. A count of the number of co-existing medical conditions and the span of organ systems they affect.
3. Co-morbidity severity. The impact of the individual disease processes suffered by the patient.

Co-morbidity burden and severity can both be formally evaluated by a number of scales (see Bibliography and Further Reading for more details). Most of these have reasonable inter-rater reliability and test–retest reliability. Of these, one of the easiest to use is the Charlson score (see Table 47.9). It can predict mortality risk and other outcomes, such as postoperative complications and length of hospital stay. Another brief scoring system is the American Society of Anesthetists' (ASA) score, which is used for the most severe co-morbid conditions. Although less validated outside the operating theatre, it has the great benefit of being almost instantaneously determinable (see Table 47.10).

It is impossible to use these methods as a sieve and leave behind only those patients likely to have few problems from therapy. They are more a starting point before thinking about the specific issues of treatment in the elderly.

Chemotherapy

In several large reviews of treatment experience, many agents appear to have no increase in the rate of adverse effects in the elderly. Indeed, several common and significant adverse effects, such as nausea and vomiting, appear to be less common in the elderly. Where elderly patients do experience an adverse effect, their ability to cope may be lower.

Table 47.9 The Charlson Co-Morbidity Index[(a)]

Co-morbidity	Points
Myocardial infarct	1
Congestive heart failure	1
Peripheral vascular disease	1
Cerebrovascular disease (except hemiplegia)	1
Dementia	1
Chronic pulmonary disease leading to symptomatic dyspnoea	1
Connective tissue disease (excluding mild rheumatoid arthritis)	1
Peptic ulcer disease	1
Chronic hepatitis or cirrhosis without portal hypertension	1
Diabetes—uncomplicated	1
Diabetes with end organ damage	2
Hemiplegia	2
Creatinine clearance > 2× upper normal or dialysis or transplant	2
Second solid tumour (non-metastatic) within 5 years	2
Leukaemia	2
Other haematological malignancy	2
Cirrhosis with portal hypertension or varices	3
Second solid tumour (metastatic)	6
AIDS	6
Total points	
Age (an extension)	**score**
50–59	1
60–69	2
70–79	3
80–89	4
> 90	5
Age points	
Combined total score	

(*a*) The total score is proportional to mortality or can be subdivided into four categories: 0, 1–2, 3–4, > 4. Age can be integrated by adding the score from the age extension.

Table 47.10 American Society of Anesthetists' (ASA) classification of physical status

Class	Description	Estimated anaesthetic related mortality
1	Healthy patient, process requiring operation does not cause significant systemic disturbance	1:25 000
2	Mild/moderate systemic disturbance from the problem or other processes (e.g. treated hypertension without complication)	1:1 000
3	Severe systemic disease that limits activity but is not incapacitating. It may not be possible to define degree of disability with finality (e.g. healed myocardial infarct, diabetes with severe complications)	1:350
4	Incapacitating systemic disease that is a constant threat to life and not always correctable by operation (e.g. cardiac disease with cardiac failure)	1:45
5	Moribund, not expected to survive 24 hours without operation	1:25

Vignette 47.8

A man in his 70s was referred for consideration of therapy for apparently locally advanced non-small-cell lung cancer. He had significant parkinsonism, which was well controlled with levo-dopa; a mitral valve replacement for congestive cardiac failure complicated by atrial fibrillation controlled with digoxin and verapamil; major depression controlled with fluoxetine; and he had had a perioperative stroke after his cardiac surgery 2 years before from which he had little residual disability. His cancer had caused him some chest pain and occasional small haemoptysis, as well as worsening his usual exertional breathlessness. He had lost no weight and was otherwise active (performance status was thus 1). On staging, he had a 1 cm lung lesion, involvement of mediastinal nodes and a supraclavicular node: thus he was staged as T_1, N_2, M_1 (nodal disease).

Excluding his neoplasm, he has significant disease in at least 3 systems; his most severe problem could be graded as ASA class 3. His Charlson score was 2 (+3 for age). He was able to perform all activities of daily living and had a good performance status. After discussion of the pros and cons of active therapy, he elected to try chemotherapy. Single-agent gemcitabine was chosen as this agent has a quality of life benefit over supportive care alone and is generally well tolerated (in particular, having little chance of causing neurological or cardiac toxicity). He had 4 cycles, which caused a minor response (25% reduction in tumour size); treatment was well tolerated, although it was stopped because of increasing depression. He has been treated successfully for this and remains stable off therapy.

Hence, closer observation and a lower threshold for intervention is needed compared with younger patients.

In trying to predict the likelihood of toxicity, the major factor (as discussed above) is performance status. Where the patient has a poor performance status (see Table 47.8), the risk of untoward toxicity increases dramatically. A predictable, and thus avoidable, source of toxicity arises from the characteristic age-associated changes in organ function. These are of most importance in the case of decline of renal function: if the glomerular filtration rate is either calculated (see Chapter 38) or measured and doses adjusted accordingly, chemotherapy can generally be given with no increase in toxicity. Decline in other organ function must usually be of major extent (e.g. hepatic abnormalities resulting in jaundice) before it is necessary to alter the doses of many chemotherapeutic agents.

Vignette 47.9

An 82-year-old man presented with facial oedema, which was found to be secondary to a mass compressing the superior vena cava. He had an implantable defibrillator for symptomatic ventricular tachycardia secondary to ischaemic heart disease. He was otherwise well, and had only recently given up working on his roof at the insistence of his cardiologist. Biopsy confirmed small-cell lung cancer, and staging showed no other sites of disease. He wished to have as active a treatment program as possible. He was given chemotherapy with carboplatin, his dose adjusted to his calculated creatinine clearance of 45 mL/min, and etoposide. He had no significant adverse effects from the first 2 cycles, and re-evaluation showed him to be in complete remission. His treatment was consolidated with 2 further cycles of chemotherapy with concurrent thoracic irradiation. This was complicated by radiation oesophagitis of a mild degree and significant fatigue; at the time of writing he was recovering from these toxicities, but hopes to be out in his garden in a few months.

Surgery

Surgical mortality and complication rates do rise with increasing chronological age. For example, the mortality and complication rates after curative surgery for lung cancer clearly increase with age, as shown in Table 47.11. Against this must be set the general decrease in operative mortality with time: for example, the mortality from gastrectomy declined from about 4% to 1% from the early 1960s to the mid 1980s.

Operative risk can be predicted from a variety of indices. Chief of these is the ASA classification, which is outlined together with the associated mortality from anaesthesia alone in Table 47.10.

A major cause of postoperative complications and deaths are related to cardiac complications. These can be estimated as a means of gaining a better handle on the surgical risk. There are a number of risk indices, which generally involve calculating a number of 'points' and then assigning a patient to a risk class. Two such tables are presented as an appendix (page 692). To try and combine these various indices is difficult but the data in Table 47.12 does do this to some extent, pointing out that far advanced age, poor general state as measured by ASA class, and the nature of the procedure dominate. Most of these factors can be determined at the bedside or in the consulting room.

Table 47.12 Factors influencing early postoperative mortality

Variable	Relative odds of death within 1 week
Patient variables	
Age: > 80 years versus < 60	3.3
ASA 3/4 (see Table 47.10)	10.7
Surgical variables	
Operation: major versus minor	3.8
Emergency versus elective operation	4.4
Procedure of > 2 hours versus less	1.08
Anaesthetic factors	
Technique	Up to 3

Radiotherapy

The data on the effects of age and tolerance to radiation is sparser than that for surgery or chemotherapy. Indeed, one of the standard texts on radiation therapy has no comment on the matter at all. This lack of data must be ameliorated by the observation that where there is a choice between radiotherapy and surgery, it is generally the oldest and most unwell patients who are treated with radiotherapy. The ability to stop treatment during a course of fractionated radiotherapy to allow acute reactions to settle is extremely valuable in this regard.

Table 47.11 Morbidity and mortality of lung resection as a function of age[a]

Age (years)	Mortality (%)	Complications (%)
< 50	1.3	3
50–59	1.3	10.7
60–69	4.1	13
70–79	7	24.5
> 79	8.1	20

(*a*) V. T. DeVita, S. Hellman & S. A. Rosenberg (eds), (1997), *Cancer: Principles and Practice of Oncology*, 5th edn, Lippincott-Raven, Philadelphia.

Radiotherapy can often be recommended in the elderly because it can allow the patient to avoid mutilating surgery, and allow organ preservation. Patients with significant co-morbidity may not be able to cope with a prolonged rehabilitation program after, for example, laryngectomy, and thus radiotherapy adds to its advantages.

What then is the aim of therapy?

The aim of therapy is the end result of working through the above process, and represents integration of the patient's state, the patient's wishes, the best possible outcome that can be achieved, and the ability of the patient to tolerate the treatment used in achieving that outcome. It may be to:

- cure
- attain a prolonged disease-free or stable state
- palliate with antineoplastic therapy with the likelihood of a short stable state
- palliate without specific antineoplastic therapy
- maintain symptom control throughout any or all of the above.

From this the appropriate means to achieve that end can be selected. Typically, treatment options are presented as different modalities, or combinations thereof, as seen in Box 47.2.

Box 47.2 The oncological therapeutic armamentarium

Symptom control without anti-cancer therapy

- Surgery
- Radiation therapy
- Medical therapy
- Chemotherapy
- Endocrine therapy
- Biological agents
- Multimodality therapy
- Simultaneous combinations (usually of chemotherapy and radiation)
- Sequential combinations of any of the above

From a pragmatic viewpoint, it is more useful to organise therapy around the oncological problem as defined on page 685. This is a more stable approach, as the nature of the problem being confronted changes less than changes in available treatment modalities.

1. *Local disease is generally the major problem.* Surgical and/or radiation therapy are generally the mainstay; where radiation therapy alone is inadequate, combinations of medical and radiotherapy (usually simultaneously) may be used to enhance control.

Vignette 47.10

The patient described in Example 47.2 with a painful lesion on the tip of his ear and a 4 cm mobile node in the pre-auricular region from squamous cell carcinoma proved to have a pathological staging of T_3, N_2. In view of the nodal disease, a superficial parotidectomy and limited neck dissection were recommended. Despite his considerable chronic airways disease related to smoking (forced expiratory volume in 1 second, ± 1 L) he was felt to be a reasonable risk for surgery and proved this to be the case. His neck dissection yielded no other pathological nodes. As he was at high risk of having local failure in the neck, radiotherapy was also given.

2. *Systemic disease is generally the major problem.* Medical therapy is the mainstay in this situation.

Vignette 47.11

A 74-year-old woman presented with symptoms from bony and hepatic metastases 5 years after local therapy for breast cancer. A biopsy confirmed recurrent disease. In view of her visceral disease, chemotherapy was felt more appropriate than hormonal manipulation. She was treated with single-agent vinorelbine, an agent well tolerated by the elderly. In view of her bony disease she was enrolled in a clinical trial comparing two bisphosphonates (the established pamidronate, which has been shown to reduce the rates of skeletal morbidity and improve skeletal pain, with a newer agent). She has, thus far, tolerated therapy well, with evidence of improvement in her hepatic lesions.

3. *Both local and systemic disease are issues.* Several options exist: medical therapy with salvage, local therapy, simultaneous medical and radiation therapy, or sequential local and systemic therapy depending on the relative urgency of the situation.

Vignette 47.12

An 81-year-old man with significant mitral valve disease and occasional episodes of congestive cardiac failure was seen with significant lymphoedema and deep venous thrombosis of the left leg. This was secondary to lymphoma in the groin. This had initially been treated only with radiation therapy in view of his general condition, but had rapidly recurred both in and adjacent to the radiation field. He had had fever and had lost approximately 12 kg in weight in recent weeks. A repeat CT scan showed bulky disease in both the iliac and para-aortic regions. As his disease was behaving in an aggressive fashion, it was felt his chances of response to 'mild' chemotherapy were slim; many would treat with a fairly aggressive regimen based on an anthracycline. In view of his cardiac disease this was not an option. A salvage regimen based on etoposide was thus offered to try and palliate his considerable discomfort. He had 5 of a planned 6 cycles of treatment; the only complications experienced were of alopecia, peripheral paraesthesia, and recurrent anaemia requiring transfusion. His nodal disease regressed, and with physical therapy his leg lymphoedema was dramatically reduced. He became pain-free and was able to stop all analgesics after the second cycle of treatment. When he developed new hilar lymphadenopathy and a pulmonary mass lesion, his treatment was stopped. He declined any further therapy, and died about 8 weeks later.

4. *Local disease is evident; occult systemic disease is likely.* Sequential combinations of a local and a systemic modality are generally considered.

Vignette 47.13

A 72-year-old woman noted a breast lump, which was proven to be malignant; after mastectomy and axillary clearance, her pathological stage was T_2 (3 cm tumour), N_1 (4 of 12 nodes positive), and further staging was negative, so she was M_0. Assays showed her tumour expressed both oestrogen and progesterone receptors. As she has about a 40–50% chance of systemic relapse in the next 10 years, and as adjuvant therapy is effective, she was offered tamoxifen, which should improve her chances of staying disease-free to about 65–75%.

Vignette 47.14

A 62-year-old woman presented with dysphagia secondary to a squamous cell carcinoma high in the oesophagus. She did not wish to have an oesophagectomy. A combination of simultaneous chemotherapy with cisplatin and fluoro-uracil plus radical radiotherapy were given as this is superior to radiotherapy alone. She had moderate radiation oesophagitis and moderate nausea but no vomiting. Her major problem was extreme fatigue. Restaging after treatment revealed no evidence of disease. Fourteen months after treatment a pulmonary nodule was noted on follow-up chest X-ray. It was unclear whether this represented a second primary (related to her previous smoking) or metastatic disease. Staging revealed this to be the only lesion and she had a lobectomy, where a 3 cm squamous cell malignancy was removed. She continues disease-free a further year later.

5. *Symptom control alone.* This must be considered at all times for all patients.

Vignette 47.15

An 86-year-old woman was admitted with fever, rigors, bruising and severe dyspnoea secondary to severe anaemia, thrombocytopenia and leucopoenia. She was treated with antibiotics, and was transfused and given diuretics, which improved her dyspnoea. A bone marrow biopsy under neurolept-analgesia confirmed a diagnosis of acute myeloid leukaemia. She felt that symptomatic therapy was the best option, as she did not wish to experience the side effects of chemotherapy. Supportive care was continued as she wished to have a chance to go home but she rapidly deteriorated from uncontrollable sepsis.

Vignette 47.16

A 67-year-old woman was diagnosed with metastatic pancreatic cancer. She decided to try active treatment with gemcitabine; she was also given narcotics for pain as well as a course of dexamethasone to try and improve her sense of wellbeing. Her pain was well controlled. Her disease progressed after 8 weeks with increasing hepatic dysfunction.

Conclusions

It is hoped that some of the thinking employed in oncological practice has been conveyed and thereby provided a practical approach to any patient with a malignant neoplasm. Also, that the vignettes and further discussion have flavoured the bare bones of this approach to provide a more rounded view of the matter. It has not been the intention to be too detailed as the details change and often do so rapidly.

Further general sources of information are provided in the bibliography and further reading, including a discussion of assessment of the elderly and an alternative review. A smattering of original papers cover the potential disadvantages of 'gentle' treatment, patient preferences related to age, and patterns of treatment in the elderly. As the advances in the science of oncology are heavily trial-driven, also included is a 'plug' for some evidence-based medicine resources. There is also some excellent material (and some phenomenal drivel) on the Internet and two of the best sites have been provided as well as a gateway link.

Bibliography and further reading

Association of Cancer Online Resources: http://www.acor.org.

Balducci, L. & Extermann, M. (2000), 'Management of cancer in older patients: a practical approach', *Oncologist*, 5, pp. 224–37.

Cancernet at the National Cancer Institute: http://cancernet.nci.nih.gov.

DeVita, V. T., Hellman, S. & Rosenberg, S. A. (eds), (1997), *Cancer: Principles and Practice of Oncology*, 5th edn, Lippincott-Raven, Philadelphia.

Djulbegovilic, B. & Sullivan, D. M. (eds), (1997), *Decision Making in Oncology: Evidence Based Management*, Churchill-Livingstone, New York.

Extermann, M. (2000), 'Measuring comorbidity in older cancer patients', *European Journal of Cancer*, 36, pp. 453–71.

Extermann, M., Overcash, J., Lyman, G. H., Parr, J. & Balducci, L. (1998), 'Comorbidity and functional status are independent in older cancer patients', *Journal of Clinical Oncology*, 16, pp. 1582–7.

Mandelblatt, J. S., Hadley, J., Kerner, J. F., Schulman, K. A., Gold, K., Dunmore-Griffith, J., Edge, S., Guadagnoli, E., Lynch, J. J., Meropol, N., Weeks, J. C. & Winn, R. (2000), 'Patterns of breast carcinoma treatment in older women: patient preference and clinical and physical influences', *Cancer*, 89, pp. 561–73.

Oncolink at the University of Pennsylvania: http://www.oncolink.com.

Perez, C. A. & Brady, L. W. (eds), (1998), *Principles and Practice of Radiation Oncology*, 3rd edn, Lippincott-Raven, New York.

Sackett, D. L., Richardson, W. S., Rosenberg, W. & Haynes, R. B. (1997), *Evidence-Based Medicine: How to Practice and Teach EBM*, Churchill Livingstone, New York.

Tirelli, U., Errante, D., Van Glabekke, M., Teodorovic, I., Kluin-Nelemans, J., Thomas, J., Bron, D., Rosti, G., Somers, R., Zagonagel, V. & Noordijk, E. (1998), 'Chop is the standard regimen in patients > or = 70 years of age with intermediate grade and high grade Non-Hodgkin's lymphoma: results of a randomized study of the European Organization for Research and Treatment of Cancer Lymphoma Cooperative Study Group', *Journal of Clinical Oncology*, 16, pp. 27–34.

Yellen, S. B., Cella, D. F. & Leslie, W. T. (1994), 'Age and clinical decision making in oncology patients', *Journal of the National Cancer Institute*, 86, pp. 1766–70.

Appendix 47.1: Computation of cardiac risk for surgery

Table 47.13 Computation of cardiac risk index points

Criterion	Points
Patient history	
Age > 70 years	5
Myocardial infarct within 6 months	10
Examination findings	
Clinically significant aortic stenosis	3
Gallop or elevation of venous pressure	11
Electrocardiogram	
Not sinus rhythm	7
More than 5 ventricular premature beats	7
Metabolic indices	
Any of:	
$P_{O_2} < 60$ mmHg or $P_{CO_2} > 50$ mmHg	
$K < 3$ mmol/L or $HCO_3 < 20$ mmol/L	
Urea or creatinine levels > normal	
Abnormal transaminase levels or stigmata of chronic liver disease	
Bedridden	3
Operation	
Emergency surgery	4
Intrathoracic, intra-abdominal or aortic	3

Table 47.14 Cardiac risk index and postoperative life threatening cardiac morbidity and mortality

Class	Points	Complications or deaths
I	0–5	1%
II	6–12	7%
III	13–25	14%
IV	> 26	78%

Part X

Infections

Chapter 48
Common infections

KELLY PAPANAOUM

Introduction

Infectious diseases in the elderly patient pose a number of challenges for the clinician. Individuals at the extremes of age are, in general, more susceptible to the complications and mortality associated with certain infections. The early diagnosis of infections in the elderly often requires attention to symptoms and signs that may be subtle or atypical. The antimicrobial treatment of infections is frequently complicated by the problems of polypharmacy and enhanced toxicity.

This chapter outlines the problems in host defences to infection encountered by the elderly and alterations in their clinical presentation of infection. Important community acquired infections in the older patient are discussed, except for respiratory tract and urinary tract infections, which are covered in Chapters 50 and 51, respectively. The recommended immunisations for older persons are also discussed. Infections associated with hospitalisation or residence in long-term care facilities are discussed in Chapter 49.

Ageing and host defence

Host defence mechanisms against infection, both non-immune and immune, are often impaired in the elderly, particularly in the presence of chronic illness. The biological changes observed with ageing, such as reduced tissue perfusion, decreased chest wall expansion and alveolar elasticity, reduction in skin thickness and reduced gastric acidity (Chapter 34), contribute to the risk of a variety of infections.

More importantly, the frequent presence of chronic illness or disability in elderly individuals predisposes them to infections by a number of mechanisms. For example, the reduced gag and cough reflexes, immobility and incontinence following a stroke may lead to pneumonia, urinary tract infection and infected pressure ulcers. Altered tissue perfusion due to diabetic vasculopathy predisposes to infections in the lower limb. Obstructive abnormalities that may be benign (e.g. prostatic hypertrophy) or malignant (e.g. bronchial carcinoma) lead to stasis and subsequent infection.

Host defences may also be reduced by extrinsic factors. Important examples include medications such as corticosteroids, cytotoxic agents and other immunosuppressive drugs, as well as H-2 receptor blockers and sedatives. Medical devices that breach protective anatomical barriers, such as urinary catheters, intravascular devices and endotracheal tubes, may lead to hospital acquired infections. The elderly are more often exposed to these risk factors given their greater frequency of hospitalisation.

Cell-mediated immune function is reduced in older adults. Decreases in T-cell proliferative response, cytotoxic activity, cytokine production and mononuclear phagocyte function have been demonstrated with ageing. Humoral immunity may also be impaired in the elderly. Serum immunoglobulin responses are normal or tend to increase with ageing. However, there is a blunting of IgG and IgM responses following primary antigenic stimulation or rechallenge. This results in reduced antibody responses following infection or vaccination.

Special issues for infection in the elderly

Alteration in clinical presentation

The diagnosis of infection is more likely to be delayed in the elderly and thus result in more complications and a higher morbidity and mortality. Reasons for this delay include the frequent under-reporting of symptoms, particularly in the setting of dementia or dysphasia. The presence of co-existing illness, such as chronic arthritis or diverticular disease, may serve to confound or obscure the features of infection. Altered host immune responses or immunosuppressive medication may mask or subdue the classic symptoms and signs of infection. An example is intestinal or gall bladder perforation with seemingly minor associated pain and peritonism. As a result, infections in elderly patients often present atypically or non-specifically (e.g. with confusion or collapse).

Fever

The presence of fever in elderly persons is more likely to signify serious bacterial infection compared with younger patients in whom a fever often signifies viral or less serious bacterial infections. Conversely, a blunted or even absent febrile response is much more common in older patients. Approximately a third of bacteraemias occur in the elderly in the absence of fever. A lack of a pyrexial response is also correlated with a poorer survival.

The possible mechanisms for an attenuated febrile reaction include disturbances in thermal homeostasis, altered production and response to pro-inflammatory cytokines such as interleukin-1, and a failure to produce and conserve body heat. A reduced fever may also occur due to a lower basal temperature, which is common in older persons. Thus, patients with a temperature of 37.8°C or greater should be thoroughly investigated to exclude a bacterial infection.

Inflammatory markers

The erythrocyte sedimentation rate (ESR) and C-reactive protein (CRP) level are often used by clinicians as non-specific markers of infections and inflammatory disorders. However, the sensitivity and positive predictive value of these markers are quite low, with neither test convincingly shown to have a particular advantage over the other. If raised, the specificity for infection or inflammation rather than malignancy is generally higher for CRP. However, a normal CRP level does not exclude infection. An elevated CRP level may be monitored (e.g. weekly) to follow the response to therapy in serious infections such as endocarditis and osteomyelitis.

Antibiotic toxicity and drug interactions

Physiological changes with ageing, adverse drug reactions and drug–drug interactions may have a dramatic effect on the safety of certain antibiotics in the elderly. The age-related decline in renal function may be poorly reflected by the serum creatinine level, which does not take lean body weight and age into account. Creatinine clearance should be calculated, especially when using nephrotoxic agents such as aminoglycosides or other parenteral agents that are renally excreted.

Aminoglycosides have excellent bactericidal activity against a variety of aerobic Gram-negative bacilli and are also used with β-lactams for synergy against some Gram-positive infections. Toxicity is more likely to occur in the elderly and is compounded in the presence of dehydration or other nephrotoxic agents. Nephrotoxicity is usually reversible but incurs significant morbidity and costs associated with prolonged hospital stay. Ototoxicity with auditory or vestibular impairment is a less common but dreaded complication as it is often irreversible. Once daily dosing of aminoglycosides improves their bactericidal efficacy and is also associated with lower rates of nephrotoxicity. Regular serum monitoring (i.e. at least 2–3 times a week) is essential for optimising dosing and minimising toxicity. Specific computer programs that aid dosage selection are available. If these are unavailable or impractical, or in the patient with a creatinine clearance rate of < 60–70 mL/minute, aminoglycosides should be avoided. Alternatives include a third generation cephalosporin, ciprofloxacin, carbapenems such as meropenem or imipenem, or the extended-spectrum penicillins, such as piperacillin or ticarcillin. However, an aminoglycoside may still be required for certain multiresistant pathogens, or if synergy is required for serious infections such as enterococcal endocarditis.

Many other antimicrobials have greater toxicity in the elderly. Hepatitis due to amoxycillin-clavulanate and flucloxacillin is more common in the elderly, especially following prolonged courses of therapy. Dicloxacillin appears to have a lower risk of hepatitis than flucloxacillin but is more likely to cause thrombophlebitis when administered intravenously. Benzylpenicillin, imipenem and ciprofloxacin in high dosages intravenously may cause seizures in patients with reduced renal function unless dosage adjustments are made. Ciprofloxacin-induced sedation and confusion is mostly seen in the older patient. *Clostridium difficile* colitis may follow treatment with any antibiotic, but particularly after clindamycin, cephalosporins and amoxycillin-clavulanate. Ototoxicity is also a complication that is usually seen in the elderly following therapy with macrolides such as azithromycin or intravenous erythromycin.

Drug interactions should always be considered before prescribing antibiotics, especially in geriatric practice where patients may be on numerous medications. Examples include an increased effect of warfarin, which is very likely to occur with the co-administration of erythromycin, sulphonamides, ciprofloxacin and metronidazole, requiring frequent monitoring of the prothrombin time. Rifampicin is a potent inducer of hepatic cytochromes and reduces the levels of other drugs metabolised by these pathways, such as warfarin, digoxin and prednisolone. Theophylline levels are increased by ciprofloxacin, erythromycin and clarithromycin. These examples are by no means exhaustive and the product information for the drugs in question should be checked. The elevation of penicillin levels by the drug probenecid may be used therapeutically to boost levels of the penicillins when given orally.

Common infections

Bacteraemia

Aetiology and epidemiology

Bacteraemia is more frequent in the elderly population and is also accompanied by a higher mortality rate. The most frequently occurring organisms isolated in community acquired bacteraemia are *Escherichia coli*, other coliforms (e.g. *Klebsiella* sp. and *Proteus* sp.), *Streptococcus pneumoniae* and *Staphylococcus aureus*. The most common causes of nosocomial bacteraemia are coliforms, *S. aureus* (including methicillin-resistant strains, MRSA) and *Pseudomonas aeruginosa*. Nosocomial bacteraemia is further discussed in Chapter 49.

Community acquired bacteraemia most frequently originates from the urinary tract, followed by intra-abdominal sites and the respiratory tract (Table 48.1). The isolation of a coliform in blood cultures is usually secondary to a urinary, biliary or intestinal source. A community acquired *S. aureus* bacteraemia should prompt a thorough search for endocarditis, osteomyelitis or septic arthritis. *Bacteroides fragilis* is the most common anaerobe causing bacteraemia, indicating an intra-abdominal collection or an infected pressure ulcer. Enterococcal bacteraemia is associated with urinary tract or intra-abdominal sepsis or endocarditis. Pneumonia may cause bacteraemia with *S. pneumoniae*, *H. influenzae* or coliforms.

Clinical features

The clinical presentation of bacteraemia in the elderly is often muted. A high fever with chills and sweats is less common than in younger adults. Hypothermia, which carries a worse prognosis, may

Table 48.1 Infective sources of common organisms causing bacteraemia

	Organisms causing bacteraemia	Clinical source of bacteraemia
Gram-positive	*Staphylococcus aureus*	Endocarditis, osteomyelitis, septic arthritis, cellulitis, abscesses
	Streptococcus pneumoniae	Pneumonia, meningitis, cellulitis
	Enterococcus faecalis	Endocarditis, urinary tract infection, intra-abdominal sepsis
	Streptococci groups A, B, G	Cellulitis, pneumonia
	Viridans streptococci	Endocarditis
Gram-negative	Coliforms	Urinary tract infection, intra-abdominal sepsis
	Haemophilus influenzae	Meningitis, pneumonia, epiglottitis
	Bacteroides fragilis	Intra-abdominal sepsis, infected pressure ulcer

be present. Symptoms and signs of the original site of sepsis, such as abdominal pain with peritonism, cellulitis, or cough with pulmonary crepitations, may or may not be present. Presentation is often atypical with falls, lassitude, confusion or urinary incontinence. There may be a rapid onset to a sepsis syndrome and shock with hypotension, oliguria and increasing confusion. A raised ESR and C-reactive protein level and a leucocytosis with band forms are frequently present but each has a poor specificity for predicting bacteraemia. Blood cultures should be taken prior to commencing antibiotics if patients have a fever or if sepsis is suspected. A 'septic screen', including cultures of urine and chest X-ray, should be performed. Other investigations, such as abdominal ultrasound, lumbar puncture or computerised tomographic (CT) scanning may be required.

Treatment

Treatment should be commenced without delay following initial cultures of blood and other fluids as appropriate. If bacteraemia is confirmed or strongly suspected, antibiotics should be given parenterally until there is clinical improvement. Intensive inpatient monitoring and supportive therapy with intravenous fluids and inotropes may be required if there is a sepsis syndrome. Initial antibiotics should be chosen according to the suspected source of sepsis (Table 48.2). If the source is unknown, antibiotics to cover *S. aureus* and Gram-negative bacilli should be given empirically. Anaerobic cover should be added if an intra-abdominal source or pressure sore is a possibility. Antimicrobial treatment should be reassessed when the antibiotic susceptibility of the organism is reported. Aminoglycosides should be used with caution or avoided in the elderly. They may be used empirically in patients without significant renal impairment (i.e. creatinine clearance >70 mL/minute) or substituted for a less toxic agent after culture results are known.

Prognosis

The mortality rate of bacteraemia in elderly patients is high at a rate of up to 50% in various series. Nosocomial bacteraemia has a worse outcome overall compared with bacteraemia acquired in the community. The best survival rate is from Gram-negative bacteraemia related to a urinary source at approximately 70%. Bacteraemia related to pneumonia has the worst survival rate of 40%. When compared with younger patients, *S. aureus* bacteraemia has twice the mortality in the elderly. The increased mortality is often related to co-existing chronic illness. Early and appropriate antibiotic therapy has been shown to reduce mortality.

Infective endocarditis

Aetiology and epidemiology

Infective endocarditis is now commonly a disease of the aged due to a greater prevalence of degenerative valvular heart disease in the elderly and the increasing use of prosthetic heart valves. The proportion of endocarditis due to rheumatic heart disease in younger patients is also falling. Endocarditis is more likely to be nosocomially acquired in older patients due to their greater frequency of hospitalisation and

Table 48.2 Antibiotic treatment of important community acquired bacterial infections in elderly patients

Infection	Antibiotic(s)	Alternative	Comments
Bacteraemia/ septicaemia			
Unknown source	2 g flucloxacillin[a] IV 6 hourly *plus* 5 mg/kg gentamicin once daily	Penicillin allergy: replace flucloxacillin with 2 g cephazolin[b] IV 8 hourly	Renal impairment: replace gentamicin with ceftriaxone/cefotaxime
Suspected source Urinary tract	1 g ceftriaxone IV daily *or* 1 g cefotaxime IV 8 hourly	2 g amoxycillin IV 6 hourly *plus* 5 mg/kg gentamicin once daily	*E. faecalis* and *P. aeruginosa* not covered by cephalosporin
Pressure ulcer or diabetic foot	2 g flucloxacillin[a] IV 6 hourly *plus* 5 mg/kg gentamicin once daily *plus* 500 mg metronidazole IV 12 hourly	If penicillin allergy: replace penicillin with 1 g cephazolin[b] IV 8 hourly If renal impairment: 3.1 g ticarcillin-clavulanate[c] IV 6 hourly	
Intra-abdominal source	2 g amoxycillin IV 6 hourly *plus* 5 mg/kg gentamicin once daily *plus* 500 mg metronidazole IV 12 hourly	If renal impairment: replace gentamicin with ceftriaxone/cefotaxime	
Lung source	1 g ceftriaxone IV daily *or* 1 g cefotaxime IV 8 hourly *plus* 0.5–1.0 g erythromycin IV 6 hourly		
Urinary tract infection			
Cystitis	300 mg trimethoprim po daily for 3 days *or* 250 mg amoxycillin-clavulanate po 8 hourly for 5 days *or* 500 mg cephalexin po 12 hourly for 5 days	Amoxycillin should be used in preference to amoxycillin-clavulanate if susceptible isolate	Asymptomatic bacteruria usually should not be treated
Pyelonephritis Mild	As for cystitis but continue for 14 days		
Severe	As for bacteraemia, urinary tract source		
Pneumonia — community acquired			
Mild–moderate	500 mg amoxycillin po 8 hourly *or* 1.5 g procaine penicillin IM daily *or* 1.2 g benzylpenicillin IV 6 hourly	500 mg azithromycin × 1 then 250 mg daily *or* 500 mg clarithromycin po 12 hourly *or* 100 mg doxycycline po bd	Duration of 7–14 days
Severe	1 g ceftriaxone IV daily *or* 1 g cefotaxime IV 8 hourly *plus* 0.5–1.0 g erythromycin IV 6 hourly	For aspiration pneumonia, add metronidazole If *S. aureus* suspected, use ticarcillin-clavulanate[c]	Duration of 14–21 days

Table continues

Table 48.2 Antibiotic treatment of important community acquired bacterial infections in elderly patients *(continued)*

Infection	Antibiotic(s)	Alternative	Comments
Meningitis			
Empiric	2 g amoxycillin IV 4 hourly *plus* 2 g ceftriaxone IV 12 hourly *or* 2 g cefotaxime IV 6 hourly	Penicillin allergy: 1.0 g meropenem IV 8 hourly *plus* vancomycin	Amoxycillin added to cover listeriosis
S. pneumoniae			
Penicillin sensitive	2.4 g penicillin IV 4 hourly		Duration of 10–14 days
Penicillin resistant	15 mg/kg vancomycin IV 6 hourly *plus* ceftriaxone/cefotaxime (doses above)		
Cellulitis			
Mild–moderate	500 mg flucloxacillin po 6 hourly[(a)]	Penicillin allergy: 500 mg cephalexin po 6 hourly *or* 500 mg erythromycin po 6 hourly	
Moderate–severe	1–2 g flucloxacillin IV 6 hourly[(a)] Add gentamicin *or* ciproflaxacin if gram negative	1 g cephalothin IV 6 hourly *or* 1 g cefazolin IV 8 hourly	
Diabetic foot infections			
Mild	500 mg cephalexin po 6 hourly 850 mg amoxycillin-clavulanate po bd 150 mg clindamycin po 6 hourly		Duration of 7–14 days
Severe	1 g cephalothin IV 6 hourly *or* 1 g cefazolin IV 8 hourly *plus* 400 mg metronidazole po bd	3.1 g ticarcillin-clavulanate IV 8 hourly[(c)]	Exclude osteomyelitis
Septic arthritis			
Empirical	2 g flucloxacillin[(l)] IV 6 hourly	2 g cefazolin IV 8 hourly[(b)]	Switch to oral after 1–2 weeks to complete 6 weeks. Covers S. aureus
Endocarditis			
Empirical	1.8 g benzylpenicillin IV 4 hourly *plus* 2 g flucloxacillin IV 4 hourly *plus* 1 mg/kg gentamicin IV 8 hourly		Monitor renal function and gentamicin levels closely
Viridans streptococci	1.8 g benzylpenicillin IV 4 hourly If relatively resistant, add 1 mg/kg gentamicin IV 8 hourly		Duration of 4 weeks
Enterococci (e.g. *E. faecalis*)	1.8 g benzylpenicillin IV 4 hourly *plus* 1 mg/kg gentamicin IV 8 hourly	2 g amoxycillin IV 4 hourly *plus* gentamicin	If gentamicin resistant, use penicillin alone

Table 48.2 Antibiotic treatment of important community acquired bacterial infections in elderly patients *(continued)*

Infection	Antibiotic(s)	Alternative	Comments
Penicillin resistant enterococci	1 g vancomycin IV 12 hourly *plus* 1 mg/kg gentamicin IV 8 hourly		
S. aureus	2 g flucloxacillin IV 4 hourly *plus* 1 mg/kg gentamicin IV 8 hourly	If penicillin allergy: 2 g cephazolin IV 8 hourly[(b)] *plus* gentamicin *or* 1 g vancomycin IV 12 hourly *plus* gentamicin	Consider valve replacement surgery early Duration of 6 weeks
Methicillin resistant *S. aureus*	1 g vancomycin IV 12 hourly	800 mg/kg teicoplanin daily	
Prosthetic valve	1 g vancomycin IV 12 hourly *plus* 1 mg/kg gentamicin IV 8 hourly		Consider valve replacement surgery early Duration of 6 weeks

(*a*) Dicloxacillin may be used interchangeably with flucloxacillin and may have a lower risk of hepatotoxicity.

(*b*) 2 g cephalothin IV 6 hourly is an interchangeable first generation cephalosporin.

(*c*) 4.5 g piperacillin-tazobactam IV 8 hourly is an alternative extended spectrum penicillin.

invasive procedures. The most frequent causes of infective endocarditis are viridans streptococci and *S. aureus*. Infection due to *Enterococcus faecalis*, *Streptococcus bovis*, and groups B and G streptococci occurs predominantly in the elderly. Enterococcal endocarditis is more common in men, and is often related to instrumentation of an infected urinary tract. *S. bovis* and group B streptococcal endocarditis are associated with colonic polyps or malignancy. Coagulase-negative staphylococci may cause infection of prosthetic cardiac valves.

Clinical features

Streptococcal and enterococcal endocarditis have a subacute clinical course with non-specific symptoms that are easily misdiagnosed in elderly patients. Fatigue, malaise and weight loss develop over weeks to months. Rheumatologic symptoms of arthralgia, arthritis and myalgias may dominate the clinical picture. *S. aureus* endocarditis presents acutely with fever, confusion, vomiting and frequently embolic disease, especially to the brain. The cardinal signs are fever and heart murmur; however, the heart murmur is often ascribed to calcific aortic lesions, which are very common in the elderly. The development of a fever in a patient with a prosthetic valve should always raise the possibility of endocarditis.

Diagnosis

If endocarditis is suspected or if the source of fever is unknown, blood cultures must be taken prior to antibiotic therapy. Over 90% of cases are positive if three sets of cultures are taken. A normocytic anaemia with a raised ESR and C-reactive protein level are usually present. Microscopic haematuria is also found. Transthoracic echocardiography may show valvular vegetations. However, a trans-oesophageal echocardiogram should be performed if there is a strong suspicion of endocarditis, given its superior sensitivity in detecting vegetations and para-valvular abscesses. The colon should be fully investigated for malignancy if *S. bovis* or group B streptococci endocarditis is diagnosed.

Treatment

Antibiotic therapy for endocarditis should be given empirically if the patient is acutely ill, immediately after 3 sets of blood cultures are drawn. If the onset is over several months and the patient is stable, therapy may await the results of blood cultures.

Once an organism is cultured and sensitivity results are available, therapy may be modified accordingly. Table 48.2 summarises the antimicrobial treatment of endocarditis. Treatment should be given intravenously for 4–6 weeks in most cases. The levels of gentamicin or vancomycin should be regularly monitored to avoid nephrotoxicity. Surgery may be necessary for valve replacement and drainage of abscesses. The indications for surgery include persistent fever or positive blood cultures for more than 1 week despite therapy, recurrent embolism, prosthetic valve endocarditis and fungal endocarditis.

Prognosis

The mortality of infective endocarditis is significantly greater in older than younger patients. This difference may be improved by early investigation with transoesophageal echocardiography and appropriate timely antibiotic therapy.

Prophylaxis

Patients with high risk valvular conditions (e.g. prosthetic valves, previous endocarditis) or with moderate risk conditions (e.g. mitral valve prolapse with regurgitation and congenital, rheumatic and other acquired valve disease) should receive antibiotic prophylaxis prior to certain procedures. These include dental procedures that induce bleeding; surgical procedures breaching respiratory, intestinal or genital mucosa; and urethral catheterisation if urinary tract infection is confirmed or suspected.

Three grams of amoxycillin orally given 1 hour before the procedure is recommended prior to dental and upper respiratory interventions. In patients unable to swallow, 1 g amoxycillin intravenously immediately prior to the procedure and 500 mg intravenously or orally 6 hours later may be given. Six hundred milligrams of clindamycin is an alternative oral agent in cases of penicillin allergy. Patients undergoing genitourinary or gastrointestinal procedures should receive intravenous 2 mg/kg gentamicin and 1 g amoxycillin immediately prior to the procedure and 500 mg amoxycillin 6 hours later. Alternatively, the first doses may be given intramuscularly 30 minutes prior to the procedure. Penicillin-allergic patients may be given 1 g vancomycin plus 2 mg/kg gentamicin prior to the procedure.

Pyrexia of unknown origin

Pyrexia or fever of unknown origin (PUO, FUO) is defined as fever of greater than 38°C occurring for at least 3 weeks. Infections, tumours and multisystem diseases (e.g. temporal arteritis and other vasculitides, rheumatic diseases, connective tissue diseases, sarcoidosis) account for the vast majority of cases of PUO.

Infections and multisystem diseases each account for approximately a third of cases in the elderly. Approximately 20% are due to malignancy. The frequency of malignant disease is greater in older than in younger adults. Less common causes include drug-related fevers and factitious fevers. The frequency of undiagnosed cases is around 10%, which is lower than in younger patients. In the elderly, the most common infections causing PUO are endocarditis, intra-abdominal collections, complicated urinary tract infections and tuberculosis.

A thorough clinical examination combined with targeted investigation is critical for establishing a diagnosis, as more than half the cases are potentially curable. Initial investigations should include a complete blood picture, serum biochemistry, urinalysis and chest X-ray. Cultures of blood, urine and, as appropriate, sputum, faeces, wound swabs, spinal fluid, joint fluid or tissue should be performed. Tuberculosis should be actively excluded by mycobacterial cultures of sputum and urine on 3 consecutive mornings. Abdominal (and pelvic) ultrasound or CT scan are vital for helping to exclude occult abscesses. Echocardiography should be done to assess the presence of valvular disease and vegetations. A transoesophageal echocardiogram has a superior sensitivity and is preferable. Gallium-67 or labelled leucocyte scanning to detect occult abscesses should be considered as the next procedure if the diagnosis remains elusive. Elderly patients without a diagnosis should undergo a temporal artery biopsy to exclude arteritis.

Herpes zoster

Aetiology and epidemiology

Herpes zoster or shingles is a disease that occurs at all ages but most commonly afflicts the elderly. It occurs in individuals who are seropositive for varicella zoster virus (VZV). It may affect up to 25% of elderly persons and its risk increases with age. Individuals with lymphoma or who are taking immunosuppressive therapy are particularly at risk. Post-herpetic neuralgia may occur in as many as 25–50% of patients over the age of 50 years, with a significant proportion having severe pain persistent for more than 1 month. A decline in cell-mediated immunity for VZV is the primary factor responsible for reactivation of latent VZV within the dorsal sensory ganglion.

Clinical features

The onset of the rash is usually heralded by pain within the unilateral dermatome preceding the lesions by 2–3 days. Thoracic and lumbar dermatomes are most commonly involved. The cranial nerves may also be affected, especially the ophthalmic division of the trigeminal nerve (V1). If the nasociliary branch is involved, sight-threatening keratitis or zoster ophthalmicus can occur and ophthalmological review should be obtained. Initially, the rash consists of erythematous macropapular lesions, which rapidly evolve into vesicles. New lesions continue to form over a period of 3–5 days. Crusting of the vesicles follows, with subsequent healing and variable scar formation. Cutaneous dissemination is more likely to occur in the elderly. Occasionally, extracutaneous involvement may occur with the development of meningoencephalitis or myelitis. An occlusive cerebral vasculitis is a rare complication of zoster ophthalmicus.

Diagnosis and treatment

The diagnosis of shingles is usually made on clinical grounds. Confirmation is possible by scraping the base of vesicular lesions and performing viral culture or demonstrating viral antigen by direct immunofluorescence or enzyme immunoassay.

The treatment of herpes zoster consists of ameliorating pain, preventing complications and using specific antiviral therapy. Acyclovir has been shown to accelerate healing of the rash and reduces post-herpetic pain and ocular complications. Treatment with valaciclovir or famciclovir, prodrugs of acyclovir and penciclovir, respectively, is preferred due to their improved oral bioavailability. Both drugs result in faster cutaneous healing and equal or improved pain resolution when compared to acyclovir. The recommended dosages for herpes zoster are 1 g valaciclovir 3 times daily and 500 mg famciclovir 3 times daily for 7–10 days. Treatment should begin within 72 hours of the rash onset. Patients with or at high risk of cutaneous or visceral dissemination should be treated with intravenous 10 mg/kg acyclovir every 8 hours.

Paracetamol with or without codeine should be given initially for control of pain. If this is inadequate, the addition of amitriptyline or an anticonvulsant is often helpful. Other options are transcutaneous nerve stimulation or topical capsaicin.

The use of oral corticosteroid therapy with antiviral therapy is controversial. Previous studies have shown no effect on post-herpetic neuralgia. However, a recent placebo-controlled study showed a beneficial effect of steroids in resolving acute neuritis and reducing analgesic intake. In this study, a tapering dose of prednisolone was used with 60 mg daily, then 30 mg, then 15 mg each for 7 days in combination with acyclovir for 21 days. Patients at risk of steroid-related complications were not included in this study.

Bacterial meningitis

Aetiology and epidemiology

Bacterial meningitis remains an infection with serious immediate and long-term morbidity and mortality. It is more common in elderly individuals than younger adults, and has a higher mortality rate, ranging from 35% to 80% despite antibiotic therapy. The most common organism in the elderly is *Streptococcus pneumoniae*. Meningococcal and *Haemophilus influenzae* meningitis are notably less common in the elderly compared with children and younger adults. Meningitis due to *Listeria monocytogenes* and *Mycobacterium tuberculosis* is more common in older adults, particularly if there is a history of immunocompromise or alcoholism. Both organisms are associated with declining cell-mediated immunity. Gram-negative bacteria, such as *Enterobacter* sp., *E. coli* and *Pseudomonas aeruginosa*, are also more common in the elderly and are often associated with neurosurgical procedures. The recent worldwide increase in infection with antibiotic resistant strains of *S. pneumoniae* continues, with 25% of patients with invasive pneumococcal infection in the US showing penicillin resistance. This has resulted in modified treatment guidelines for suspected pneumococcal meningitis.

Clinical features

The clinical presentation of meningitis in the older patient may be non-specific, with fever and altered conscious state. Meningismus may be absent or difficult to assess in the presence of cervical osteoarthritis. The combination of the classic signs of meningitis with fever, headache and meningismus were noted in less than 20% of elderly patients with bacterial meningitis. Focal neurologic signs were reported in 43% of elderly patients in one series. Papilloedema is unusual. Concurrent infections, including pneumonia or endocarditis, may be present. Infection may also be present in contiguous sites with sinusitis, otitis media or a craniotomy wound infection.

Diagnosis

The diagnosis of bacterial meningitis is based upon examination of the cerebrospinal fluid (CSF), which should be sampled as soon as possible. The CSF white cell count is usually in the range of 1000–5000/mL with a neutrophilic predominance. A lymphocytic predominance is suggestive of listeria, tuberculosis, viral or fungal aetiology. The CSF glucose level is depressed, with a CSF–serum glucose ratio below 0.31. A very low initial CSF glucose level is associated with a poor survival. The CSF Gram stain is positive in 60–90% cases of acute bacterial meningitis, falling to 40–60% if patients have already received antibiotics. CSF cultures are positive in up to 85% of cases. If the CSF protein, glucose and cell count are consistent with acute meningitis but the Gram stain is negative, a latex agglutination test for bacterial antigen may be done to detect *S. pneumoniae*; however, its sensitivity is suboptimal.

A CT scan should be performed prior to lumbar puncture if the patient has papilloedema or focal neurologic signs to rule out an intracranial mass lesion, which carries the risk of cerebral herniation. If this delays treatment, empirical antibiotics should be commenced prior to obtaining the CSF, once blood cultures are taken. In this situation the yield of cultures is only marginally diminished.

Treatment

The empirical antibiotic treatment of purulent meningitis for elderly patients is a third-generation cephalosporin (2 g cefotaxime 6 hourly or 2 g ceftriaxone twice daily) plus 2 g ampicillin (or amoxycillin) 4–6 hourly, the latter to cover listeria infection. If the CSF shows Gram-positive cocci or if pneumococci are grown in culture, 1 g vancomycin twice daily should be added to the cephalosporin until pneumococcal resistance is excluded. Pneumococci that are penicillin susceptible should be treated with 2.4 g benzylpenicillin every 4–6 hours, or a third-generation cephalosporin (see above) for strains of intermediate penicillin sensitivity. Vancomycin must be used for penicillin- and cephalosporin-resistant strains which are emerging in increased frequency. If Gram-negative bacilli are seen, ceftazidime or a carbapenem (e.g. meropenem) should be begun. *Listeria* meningitis should be treated with 3 g amoxycillin 6 hourly plus cotrimoxazole. The duration of therapy for pneumococcal meningitis is 10–14 days or 21 days for *Listeria* or Gram-negative bacilli. Adjunctive dexamethasone treatment remains controversial in adults and is not generally recommended.

Herpes encephalitis

Herpes simplex virus (HSV) is the most common cause of acute viral encephalitis and is mostly due to HSV 1. It has a biphasic age distribution with the second peak in adults over 50 years of age. Most patients have had prior infection with HSV and develop encephalitis following reactivation of latent virus or reinfection with another strain of the virus. The virus causes a necrotising encephalitis with a predilection for the temporal lobes.

The disease usually presents acutely with headache, fever and altered conscious state or personality change. Seizures and focal neurologic signs, especially temporal lobe signs (e.g. aphasia) rapidly ensue.

Diagnosis

CT scans of the brain are often normal at the time of presentation and may need to be repeated after several days to demonstrate changes involving the temporal lobes. Magnetic resonance imaging (MRI) is far more sensitive and is almost always abnormal at presentation. Testing for HSV DNA in the CSF by polymerase chain reaction (PCR) has also obviated the need for a diagnostic brain biopsy. Viral culture of the CSF has a very low yield but should be performed to exclude other viral causes. The CSF also has an elevated mononuclear cell count. A rise in the CSF HSV antibody titre occurs but is not a useful diagnostic tool in practice.

Treatment

Treatment with intravenous 10 mg/kg acyclovir 8 hourly for 14 days is recommended. Given the importance of early therapy to minimise irreversible neurological sequelae, intravenous acyclovir should be given empirically if HSV encephalitis is suspected until HSV is confirmed or an alternative diagnosis is made.

Soft tissue infections

Cellulitis

Aetiology and epidemiology

This infection of the skin and subcutaneous tissues is most commonly caused by group A streptococci (*S. pyogenes*) and *S. aureus*. Groups B, C and G streptococci may also cause cellulitis. It is most common in the elderly due to their reduced skin thickness and elasticity, and it often complicates diabetes and chronic oedema. The causative organism residing on the skin gains access to deeper tissues by a break in the skin, which may not be apparent. Tinea pedis is often overlooked as an entry site. Cellulitis complicating surgical wounds or intravenous catheter sites is usually due to *S. aureus*. Other causes of cellulitis include coliforms and *P. aeruginosa*, which are often seen in neutropenic states. The environmental Gram-negative bacteria, *Vibrio* sp. and *Aeromonas hydrophila*, may cause cellulitis associated with exposure to contaminated salt water or fresh water, respectively.

Clinical features

The diagnosis of cellulitis is usually readily recognised by the presence of rapidly spreading swelling, warmth and redness of the skin. There is associated fever, malaise and chills, which may precede any obvious skin changes. Lymphangitis and proximal lymphadenopathy are common, especially with *S. pyogenes* cellulitis. Recurrent cellulitis can be a troublesome clinical problem in some patients with chronic lymphoedema, such as following surgery or radiation therapy.

Diagnosis

Isolation of the causative organism is difficult to obtain in most cases. Swabs of associated ulcers or abrasions culture a causative organism in about 30% of cases. Blood cultures should be taken if there is a fever or signs of sepsis but are positive in less than a quarter of patients. Aspiration of tissue fluid for culture from the advancing edge of the cellulitis may establish the cause but has a low positive yield.

Treatment

Treatment should be directed towards streptococci as well as *S. aureus* if the latter is thought likely. In mild cases, if *S. pyogenes* is suspected, 500 mg penicillin V 6 hourly may be given alone. A semi-synthetic penicillin, such as flucloxacillin (500 mg–1 g) 6 hourly, covers both streptococci and most strains of *S. aureus*. Patients with a penicillin allergy should receive a first-generation cephalosporin (e.g. cephalexin or cephazolin). If there is serious β-lactam allergy, erythromycin, clindamycin or vancomycin IV are used. Parenteral antibiotics are required for moderate to severe cases or if there is progression while on oral therapy. If MRSA is suspected, 1 g vancomycin IV twice daily may be required. For cellulitis associated with an environmental water source, Gram-negative cover with a quinolone (e.g. 500 mg ciprofloxacin bd, cotrimoxazole or gentamicin IV) should be added.

Patients with recurrent cellulitis should receive good skin hygiene, support stockings to control leg oedema and treatment of any tinea pedis. For recalcitrant cases, long-term prophylaxis with

250–500 mg penicillin twice daily may be required or 250 mg erythromycin twice daily if there is penicillin allergy.

Erysipelas

Erysipelas is a more superficial infection of the skin, due in most cases to *S. pyogenes*. It usually affects older adults, involving the lower limbs or face. It is typically bright red and indurated with a more sharply defined border than cellulitis. Treatment is with 500 mg oral penicillin V 6 hourly, 600 000 units procaine penicillin daily or 1.2–1.8 g IV benzylpenicillin 6 hourly for severe cases. Penicillin-allergic patients should receive oral cephalexin (or intravenous cephalothin/cefazolin) or erythromycin.

Diabetic foot infections

Diabetic foot infections are a common and difficult problem in patients with peripheral neuropathy and/or vascular disease. Cellulitis of varying degree is present, often in association with skin necrosis, ulceration and osteomyelitis. *S. pyogenes* or *S. aureus* is often the initial organism. The infection subsequently involves a mixture of aerobic and anaerobic organisms, especially when it is associated with extensive cellulitis, deep ulceration and limb ischaemia. Organisms frequently isolated include *Bacteroides fragilis*, enterococci, coliforms and *P. aeruginosa*. Cultures of ulcer swabs may not reflect the true infecting pathogens from colonising organisms; therefore a microbial diagnosis from surgically obtained deep tissue or bone cultures is desirable. Osteomyelitis should be excluded by radionuclide scan, MRI or CT scanning. Plain radiographs are usually performed but are insensitive in detecting the early changes of osteomyelitis.

Treatment

Antibiotics should cover streptococci, staphylococci and, in most cases, coliforms and anaerobic bacteria. Oral antibiotic therapy with 500 mg cephalexin 6 hourly plus 200 mg metronidazole po 8 hourly, 875 mg amoxycillin-clavulanate twice daily or 150 mg clindamycin 6 hourly is appropriate for mild to moderate cases. More severe infections should be treated intravenously with 1 g cefazolin 8 hourly (or 1 g cephalothin 6 hourly) plus 500 mg metronidazole twice daily, 3.1 g ticarcillin-clavulanate 6 hourly, 4.5 g piperacillin-tazobactam 8 hourly, 500 mg imipenem 6 hourly or 300 mg ciprofloxacin twice daily plus 500 mg metronidazole twice daily. Necrotic areas should be deroofed and debrided, with deep tissue biopsies sent for culture. Ulcers should be cleaned and dressed regularly with saline-soaked gauze. Control of hyperglycaemia will also assist healing.

Septic arthritis

Aetiology and epidemiology

Septic arthritis is an important infection in elderly patients. Approximately 50% of all cases of non-gonococcal bacterial arthritis in non-prosthetic joints occur in patients over the age of 60 years. The term 'septic arthritis' generally refers to bacterial arthritis. Mycobacterial and fungal agents should also be considered in patients with a chronic monoarticular process. Viral infections such as Ross River virus and rubella usually cause a polyarthritis in association with fevers. Predominant risk factors for acquiring septic arthritis are age ≥ 80 years, diabetes mellitus, rheumatoid arthritis and malignancy.

Infection usually arises in the joint following haematogenous seeding of an organism from a distant site. In prosthetic joint infections the bacteria are acquired directly via the wound at the time of surgery. Postoperatively, haematogenous seeding of organisms from an infected urinary tract or intravascular catheter may also occur. The majority of cases of septic arthritis in non-prosthetic joints are due to *S. aureus* as in younger patients. Streptococcal infection, including groups A, B and G, is also relatively common. Infection due to coliforms and *P. aeruginosa* is also an important cause in elderly patients, particularly those with chronic underlying disease. Prosthetic joint infection is commonly due to *S. aureus* (including MRSA), coagulase-negative staphylococci, coliforms and *P. aeruginosa*.

Clinical features

Septic arthritis usually presents with fever, chills and severe pain and limitation of motion in a single joint. However, in elderly patients these symptoms may be less marked. Fever is commonly absent or low grade, and the white blood cell count is often within the normal range. The knee is the most commonly affected joint, followed by the hip and shoulder. Approximately 10% of patients have multiple joint involvement. This is associated with *S. aureus* endocarditis, rheumatoid arthritis and diabetes.

Diagnosis

Inflammatory markers such as the ESR and C-reactive protein level are almost always elevated. There may be a leucocytosis but the white cell count is often within the normal range. Radionuclide bone scans may be useful. A blood culture should be performed if the patient has a fever or appears toxic. Synovial fluid from the affected joint should be sampled for culture prior to antimicrobial therapy. It usually appears turbid but may be serosanguinous. The synovial fluid leucocyte count is often greater than 50 000/mL with a neutrophil preponderance. However, this finding may also be seen in other inflammatory arthropathies. The Gram stain is only positive in about one-third of patients but cultures are usually positive unless taken after antibiotics are commenced.

Treatment

Early recognition and treatment of septic arthritis is critical for minimising its crippling effects due to the loss of collagen and erosion of the articular surface. Successful treatment of septic arthritis requires timely antimicrobial therapy, drainage of the infected joint and control of associated pain. Initial empirical antibiotic therapy should consist of either 2 g flucloxacillin IV 6 hourly, or in the penicillin-allergic patient, 1 g cephalothin 6 hourly or 1 g cephazolin 8 hourly. If the patient has a severe β-lactam allergy, 600 mg clindamycin IV 8 hourly may be used. Therapy should be re-evaluated as soon as the causative organism is identified by Gram stain or culture. Oral antibiotics (1 g flucloxacillin 6 hourly, 1 g cephalexin 6 hourly or 300 mg clindamycin 6–8 hourly) may be given after 2–4 weeks if there is improvement and should continue for a total of 6 weeks. Early surgical drainage has been shown to improve outcome. If this is not performed, repeated joint aspirations should be performed as needed. Successful treatment of prosthetic joint infection requires removal of the prosthesis and at least 6 weeks of intravenous antibiotics prior to joint revision. In many elderly patients this approach is not feasible and long-term suppression with oral antibiotics is the preferred option.

Prognosis

Despite therapy, elderly patients, especially those with underlying joint disease, tend to do poorly. Many patients have ongoing limitation of movement and persistent pain. Other factors suggesting a poor outcome include infection of the hip or shoulder, duration of symptoms for more than 1 week before treatment, involvement of more than 4 joints and persistently positive cultures despite a week of appropriate antibiotic therapy.

Gastrointestinal infections

Gastroenteritis is a significant cause of morbidity and mortality at the extremes of ages. Achlorhydria, malnutrition, debility due to chronic illness, frequent antibiotic use and residing in nursing homes are some of the factors that make diarrhoeal disease more common and severe in the elderly. Bacterial causes of diarrhoea such as *Salmonella* sp., *Shigella* sp., *Campylobacter jejuni* and *Yersinia enterocolitica* are more likely to cause prolonged diarrhoea and associated bacteraemia in the elderly. Traveller's diarrhoea is also more likely to occur in older adults. Enteropathogenic *E. coli* are particularly common in this setting. Viral agents such as Norwalk virus and rotavirus are common causes of diarrhoea and may cause seasonal outbreaks of diarrhoeal disease in long-term care facilities. Parasitic infection by *Cryptosporidium* sp. has recently also been associated with the elderly, particularly in nursing homes. *Candida albicans* may be found in the stool but even when found in large numbers has not been associated with diarrhoeal disease.

Diagnosis and treatment

Stool samples (up to 3) should be sent for culture, and if there is a history of recent antibiotic use, *C. difficile* toxin testing should be requested. Antimicrobial therapy for bacterial gastroenteritis is recommended in elderly patients with severe or persisting diarrhoea. Acute diarrhoea of unknown cause should be treated empirically with antibiotics if it is severe and there is associated fever, rigors and bloody diarrhoea, suggesting an invasive pathogen. Blood cultures should be drawn prior to therapy. Initial empirical treatment in this setting is with 500 mg oral ciprofloxacin 12 hourly. If oral therapy is not possible, intravenous therapy with 200 mg ciprofloxacin twice daily or ceftriaxone is recommended. Therapy may need to be modified according to culture and sensitivity results. The treatment of choice for severe Campylobacter diarrhoea is 500 mg oral erythromycin 6 hourly. Dysentery due to *Shigella* sp. should be treated in all cases for public health reasons. Treatment options should be guided by susceptibility results and include 400 mg norfloxacin twice daily, 1 g ampicillin 6 hourly or 160/800 mg trimethoprim-sulphamethoxazole twice daily, given orally for 7–10 days. Salmonella gastroenteritis should be treated in severe cases, although therapy carries the risk of prolonged excretion of the organism in the stool. Ciprofloxacin, norfloxacin or cotrimoxazole may be used according to susceptibility, in the doses above. Oral rehydration therapy is vital for preventing dehydration. Diarrhoea due to *C. difficile* is covered in Chapter 34.

Intra-abdominal infection

Intra-abdominal infection usually follows perforation of the gastrointestinal or biliary tract or pancreatitis. It presents as generalised peritonitis or as a localised abscess. It is more common in elderly patients due to their greater risk of developing biliary disease, diverticular disease and colorectal cancer as well as age-related vascular and tissue changes. Older persons are less likely than younger patients to present with the typical features of abdominal pain, fever, nausea, vomiting or diarrhoea. They are also more likely to be given an incorrect extra-abdominal diagnosis at the time that they present, potentially increasing the morbidity and mortality. The finding that elderly patients are more likely to present with gangrenous appendicitis or cholecystitis exemplifies this. Pyogenic liver abscess is also more frequent in the elderly and is often mistaken for metastatic cancer unless an aspirate is performed. Diagnostic investigations for intra-abdominal sepsis include ultrasound, CT scan and radiolabelled white blood cell scans.

Treatment

Optimal management of intra-abdominal infection requires surgical removal of the source of peritoneal contamination and drainage of abscesses. Antibiotics are an adjunct to surgery, to treat the residual contamination of the peritoneum. Percutaneous CT or ultrasound guided drainage may be an alternative in some settings such as pancreatic collections.

Intra-abdominal infection is polymicrobial and reflects bowel flora. Successful therapy requires broad-spectrum cover against streptococci, coliforms and anaerobic Gram-negative bacteria such as *Bacteroides fragilis*. An exception is infection related to cholecystitis or pancreatitis, where anaerobic bacteria are unusual except in complicated cases. Pseudomonas, resistant coliforms, enterococci and yeasts assume a greater role in cases of protracted hospitalisation and prolonged antibiotic therapy.

Triple antibiotic therapy with 2 g amoxycillin 6 hourly, 5 mg/kg gentamicin once daily plus 500 mg metronidazole twice daily intravenously is commonly recommended for community acquired intra-abdominal sepsis. However, the toxicity of aminoglycosides, frequently combined with dehydration and surgery, make alternative options preferable if there is any impairment of the creatinine clearance. Options for community acquired sepsis are 1 g cefotaxime 8 hourly or 1 g ceftriaxone once daily plus metronidazole or cefoxitin alone. Monotherapy with 3.1 g ticarcillin-clavulanate 6 hourly, 4.5 g piperacillin-tazobactam 8 hourly or 500 mg imipenem 6 hourly are more costly alternatives. Imipenem- and ciprofloxacin-containing regimens are best kept in reserve for the therapy of more resistant infections. Antifungal therapy with fluconazole or intravenous amphotericin B may be necessary for the treatment of deep candidal infections. Duration of treatment for 7 days is usually adequate unless surgical drainage is inadequate or if there is prolonged fever.

Prognosis

Increasing age, colonic perforation, malnutrition, post-surgical anastomotic leak and post-operative pneumonia are poor prognostic factors for survival following peritonitis or intra-abdominal abscess. Mortality is up to 60%, depending on the cause of the peritonitis.

Immunisation

Practitioners should endeavour to immunise patients over the age of 65 years with influenza virus vaccine, pneumococcal vaccine and tetanus toxoid in line with current national guidelines. Influenza vaccine has been shown to reduce the rates of influenza-related complications and mortality, and is recommended for all individuals over the age of 65. Annual vaccination prior to the influenza season is required due to the antigenic drift of the virus. Vaccination of staff in hospitals and nursing homes is beneficial in reducing the attack rates in elderly patients. The main contraindications to receiving the vaccine are a history of anaphylactic hypersensitivity to eggs or of Guillain-Barre syndrome. The effectiveness of the vaccine in preventing influenza varies from over 90% for healthy older persons to less than 50% for nursing home residents. However, there is a greater impact on the reduction of influenza-related complications and the vaccine is clearly cost effective.

Pneumococcal vaccine is also recommended for all elderly persons, especially those individuals with chronic illness, such as diabetes mellitus, cardiac disease, chronic lung disease and if immunocompromised. Booster vaccination is recommended every 5 years. The overall efficacy in preventing invasive disease is up to 80%. The increasing problem of penicillin resistance in *S. pneumoniae* underscores the benefit of immunisation as well as the need for more efficacious conjugate pneumococcal vaccines. Influenza and pneumococcal vaccination is also discussed in Chapter 50.

In developed nations, tetanus is more likely to occur in the elderly. This group is at risk due to an absence of prior vaccination or waning vaccine immunity. The case fatality rate is also higher in this age group. Most cases follow either a laceration or puncture wound, although a significant number are cryptogenic. If there is a history of incomplete vaccination, or if vaccination occurred more than 5 years earlier, 250 units tetanus immunoglobulin (TIG) intramuscularly should be administered following a tetanus-prone wound. A schedule of 3 doses of tetanus toxoid should be given to the unvaccinated or to those with an unknown history of vaccination. Thereafter a booster injection every 10 years is recommended. Mild local reactions or a low-grade fever following vaccine administration are common; severe reactions, including hypersensitivity and brachial neuritis, are rare.

Bibliograpy and further reading

Beutner, K. R., et al. (1995), 'Valaciclovir compared with acyclovir for improved therapy for herpes zoster in immunocompetent adults', *Antimicrobial Agents and Chemotherapy*, 39, pp. 1546–53.

Chassagne, P., Perol, M.-B., Doucet, J., et al. (1996), 'Is presentation of bacteraemia in the elderly the same as in younger patients', *American Journal of Medicine*, 100, pp. 65–70.

Cooper, G. S., et al. (1994), 'Intraabdominal infection: Differences in presentation and outcome between younger patients and the elderly', *Clinical Infectious Diseases*, 19, pp. 146–8.

Crossley, K. & Peterson, P. K. (1996), 'Infections in the elderly', *Clinical Infectious Diseases*, 22, pp. 209–15.

Ernst, M. E. & Ernst, E. J. (1999), 'Effectively treating common infections in residents of long term care facilities', *Pharmacotherapy*, 19, pp. 1026–35.

Knockaert, D. C., et al. (1993), 'Fever of unknown origin in elderly patients', *Journal of the American Geriatric Society*, 41, pp. 1187–92.

Kortekangas, P. (1999), 'Bacterial arthritis in the elderly. An overview', *Drugs and Aging*, 14, pp. 165–71.

Norman, D. C. & Toledo, S. D. (1992), 'Infections in the elderly', *Clinics in Geriatric Medicine*, 8, pp. 713–19.

Norman, D. C. & Yoshikawa, T. T. (1996), 'Fever in the elderly', *Infectious Diseases Clinics of North America*, 10, pp. 93–9.

Pioro, M. H. & Mandell, B. F. (1997), 'Septic arthritis', *Rheumatic Disease Clinics of North America*, 23, pp. 239–55.

Selton-Suty, C., Hoen, B., Grentzinger, A., et al. (1997), 'Clinical and bacteriological characteristics of infective endocarditis in the elderly', *Heart*, 77, pp. 260–3.

Therapeutic Guidelines: Antibiotic (1998), 10th edn, Therapeutic Guidelines Limited, Australia.

Tyring, S., et al. (1995), 'Famciclovir for the treatment of acute herpes zoster: Effects on acute disease and post-herpetic neuralgia. A randomized double blind placebo controlled trial', *Annals of Internal Medicine*, 123, pp. 89–96.

Whitley, R. J., et al. (1996), 'Acyclovir with and without prednisone for the treatment of herpes zoster. A randomized placebo-controlled trial', *Annals of Internal Medicine*, 125, pp. 376–83.

Chapter 49

Institutionally acquired infections

KELLY PAPANAOUM

Introduction

Aged individuals suffer a disproportionate burden of nosocomial or hospital acquired infections. The risk of developing a nosocomial infection increases significantly per decade in old age. The morbidity, mortality and excess costs associated with nosocomial infections are likely to increase with the ageing of the population. The incidence of nosocomial infection in the elderly admitted to acute care or the rehabilitation setting has been reported as 10.8–16.9 infections per 1000 patient hospital days. The rate of hospital acquired infection in the elderly increases per day of admission after day 8 and beyond.

Infections in residents of nursing homes are a significant cause of transfer to hospital, or death. Approximately 10–20% of nursing home associated infections occur as part of an outbreak within the institution. In this setting, the incidence of infection ranges from 4–8 infections per 1000 resident days. The prevalence is significantly higher given the chronicity of certain infections, such as catheter-related urinary tract infections and infected pressure ulcers.

Nosocomial pneumonia, urinary tract infection, wound infection and bacteraemia are the major infections seen in hospital. In nursing homes, the spectrum includes urinary tract infections, pressure sores, respiratory infections (often viral) and infective diarrhoea.

Risk factors for developing a nosocomial infection include the following: faecal and urinary incontinence, intravenous lines, urinary catheterisation or instrumentation, recent broad-spectrum antibiotic therapy, steroid therapy, prolonged surgery, continuous ventilator support, chronic airways disease and diabetes mellitus.

This chapter outlines the common infections that are associated with hospitalisation or residence in a long-term care facility. Urinary tract infections are discussed in Chapter 51.

Nosocomial and nursing home acquired infections

Bacteraemia

Epidemiology and aetiology

Bacteraemia acquired during hospitalisation is more likely to occur in older than younger patients and has a higher morbidity and mortality. The most common sources of hospital acquired bacteraemia are intravascular catheters, urinary catheters, surgical wound infections, pneumonia and intra-abdominal sepsis. Additional risk factors for developing nosocomial sepsis are neutropenia, burns, severe underlying disease or immunosuppressive treatment. In nursing homes, the causes of bacteraemia more closely resemble those seen in the community and the most common sources are the urinary tract, skin and soft tissue, lower respiratory tract and intra-abdominal sites.

Staphylococcal bacteraemia, due to *Staphylococcus aureus* and coagulase-negative staphylococci, is the most common cause of nosocomial bacteraemia. It is principally caused by infected intravascular devices, especially central vascular catheters, and to a lesser extent peripheral intravenous lines. Serious complications of nosocomial *S. aureus* bacteraemia include endocarditis, osteomyelitis and septic arthritis. Most cases of hospital acquired endocarditis occur in elderly patients, and are usually acquired from an infected intravascular device. The mortality rate is around 50%.

Other organisms that cause nosocomial bacteraemia from a variety of sources include coliforms (especially *Escherichia coli*, *Proteus* sp., *Enterobacter* sp., *Klebsiella* sp.), enterococci, *Pseudomonas aeruginosa* and *Candida* sp. Increasing numbers of hospital acquired pathogens, such as methicillin-resistant *S. aureus* (MRSA), aminoglycoside- and quinolone-resistant *P. aeruginosa* and vancomycin-resistant enterococci, are multiple-antibiotic resistant.

In long-term care facilities, Gram-negative bacteria such as *E. coli* and *Proteus* sp., usually originating from the urinary tract, are the most common causes of bacteraemia. Gram-positive bacteria causing bloodstream sepsis include *S. pneumoniae*, group A streptococci, enterococci and *S. aureus*.

Diagnosis

The diagnosis of bacteraemia requires the recognition that fever and other sign of sepsis may be attenuated or present atypically (e.g. with confusion) in the aged. A source of sepsis should be sought with particular attention to the skin and respiratory tract. Wounds and intravenous catheter sites must be closely examined. Investigations should include blood cultures, cultures of urine, respiratory secretions, wound or ulcer swabs and a chest X-ray. Intravenous (IV) catheter tips should be removed and sent for culture if IV line infection is suspected.

Treatment

Treatment of suspected septicaemia in the elderly patient in a hospital or long-term care facility should be commenced subsequent to taking at least 2 sets of blood cultures. Parenteral antibiotics should be used initially, especially if there are signs of a sepsis syndrome with hypotension or oliguria. Volume replacement therapy and inotropes may be required. Antibiotic treatment should be directed to the clinical source of sepsis if this is obvious. If the origin is unknown, initial therapy with broad-spectrum cover to include Gram-negative bacteria and *S. aureus* should be commenced until culture results are available. Intravenous flucloxacillin plus gentamicin is recommended unless there is renal impairment. If this is the case, a third-generation cephalosporin such as ceftriaxone should be used, or a carbapenem such as meropenem if resistant Gram-negative bacteria are likely. Vancomycin should be used if there is a high rate of methicillin-resistant *S. aureus* in the institution. Anaerobic cover with metronidazole or other agent should be added if an intra-abdominal cause is likely.

Prevention

Intravascular catheter infection may be minimised by ensuring that the catheter is inserted using a strict aseptic technique. Peripheral catheters should, as a general rule, not be left in situ for more than 48 hours. Central venous catheters impregnated with antibacterial compounds have been shown to reduce the rate of catheter-related bacteraemia but are costly. Other aspects of infection prevention are discussed later in this chapter.

Lower respiratory tract infections

Bacterial pneumonia

Epidemiology

Hospital acquired pneumonia accounts for approximately 20% of nosocomial infections overall, being second in frequency to urinary tract infection. It is the most lethal of all nosocomial infections, and is associated with a mortality rate ranging from 20% to 70%. The highest rates are seen with ventilator-associated Gram-negative pneumonia, especially if complicated by the adult respiratory distress syndrome (ARDS).

Elderly patients are twice as likely to develop nosocomial pneumonia and die than patients under the age of 60 years. Other risk factors for developing pneumonia in addition to age include intubation and ventilation, severity of co-morbid illness, chronic lung disease, neuromuscular disease, thoracic or upper abdominal surgery, prior antibiotic therapy and immunosuppressive treatment. Gram-negative bacteria frequently colonise the upper airway in hospitalised patients, especially after antibiotic therapy. Pneumonia develops after micro-aspiration of contaminated oropharyngeal secretions.

Aetiology

Coliform bacteria (such as *E. coli*, *Klebsiella* sp., *Enterobacter* sp.) and *Pseudomonas aeruginosa* together account for approximately 50% of cases of hospital acquired pneumonia. Other causes include *S. aureus*, *S. pneumoniae*, *Haemophilus influenzae*, anaerobic bacteria (following aspiration) and *Legionella* sp. Viral causes of pneumonia are discussed below. Fungi such as *Cryptococcus neoformans* and *Aspergillus* sp. should be considered in immunosuppressed patients.

In nursing home associated pneumonia, the microbial aetiology is infrequently diagnosed given the difficulty in obtaining good sputum samples. Nevertheless, an attempt to obtain a sample should be made in addition to taking blood cultures. Pneumococcal pneumonia is a common cause of pneumonia in this setting. Other nosocomial pathogens listed above may also occur, in addition to atypical pathogens such as *Mycoplasma pneumoniae* and *Chlamydia pneumoniae*. Aspiration pneumonia is also common in nursing homes.

Diagnosis

The diagnosis of nosocomial pneumonia can be notoriously difficult in the older patient who may have absence of a cough or fever and difficulty in expectorating sputum. Co-existing chronic airways disease, cardiac failure or ARDS may confound the interpretation of clinical and X-ray signs. Investigations that should be performed include a complete blood picture, serum biochemistry, chest X-ray and arterial blood gas. Computerised tomographic (CT) scans may be helpful in defining the pattern of pneumonia or in excluding pulmonary embolism. Blood cultures and, if possible, respiratory secretions (sputum or tracheal aspirate in ventilated patients) for microscopy and culture should be obtained. Positive sputum or tracheal aspirate cultures may reflect organisms colonising the upper airway. A Gram stain is useful for assessing the presence of leucocytes and organisms.

In patients not responding to therapy or in immunosuppressed patients who are susceptible to a wider range of pathogens, a bronchoscopy and bronchoalveolar lavage (BAL) or protected specimen brushing should be considered to obtain an optimal sample for culture.

Treatment

Empirical therapy of nosocomial pneumonia for mild to moderate disease is with oral amoxycillin-clavulanate or a third-generation cephalosporin, such as parenteral ceftriaxone. Severe cases should be treated initially with broader spectrum drugs to cover *P. aeruginosa* and *S. aureus*. Options include piperacillin-tazobactam, imipenem or meropenem. A macrolide such as erythromycin should be added if atypical infection is suspected or if the patient is on high-dose corticosteroids.

Measures to prevent nosocomial pneumonia include elevation of the head of the bed to 30 degrees, avoidance of aspiration, frugal usage of corticosteroids and antibiotics, and avoiding the contamination of respiratory equipment.

Epidemic pneumonia in the nursing home

Outbreaks of viral respiratory infection are common in long-term care facilities and less so in hospitals. Influenza causes significant morbidity and mortality during the winter season. Attack rates in unvaccinated residents are as high as 40% and mortality in up to one-third of patients has been reported. Individuals with suspected influenza should be isolated.

Amantadine prophylaxis may be commenced in other residents. Annual vaccination of all residents and staff is important. Individual cases may be treated within 48 hours of the onset of symptoms, with amantadine or the neuraminidase inhibitor, zanamivir.

Respiratory syncytial virus (RSV) is also a frequent cause of lower respiratory tract infection in the elderly and may cause epidemics in nursing homes in the winter months. The rate of pneumonia and mortality is comparable to influenza. A vaccine is not yet commercially available. Outbreaks of rhinovirus infection are common but usually cause upper respiratory infection.

Tuberculosis can occur from reactivation of latent infection. Epidemics by airborne spread within the nursing home originating from patients with cavitary disease have been reported. Mantoux testing at the time of entry to the nursing home and at regular intervals thereafter is recommended. Residents with a positive Mantoux test but no evidence of active tuberculosis should be carefully followed for the development of fever, cough, weight loss or lymphadenopathy. Isoniazid prophylaxis is required if recent skin test conversion has been shown.

Soft tissue infections and infestations

Pressure ulcers

Epidemiology and aetiology

Pressure or decubitus ulcers frequently develop in elderly patients with reduced mobility and resulting pressure associated soft tissue ischaemia. Most develop in association with an admission to a hospital or nursing home.

The prevalence of skin and soft tissue infections in nursing homes is between 5.6% and 8.4%, the high rate reflecting the chronicity of some problems such as infected pressure ulcers. The incidence of these infections is considerably lower at approximately 1% or less episodes per 1000 patient days. Such surveys are hampered by the clinical problem of differentiating infected ulcers from those colonised with bacteria.

Chronic pressure ulcers are always contaminated by a mixture of bacteria, often reflecting faecal flora, with a mixture of Gram-negative bacilli, anaerobes such as *Bacteroides* sp. and Gram-positive bacteria such as enterococci and staphylococci, as well as yeasts. Thus, cultures of surface swabs are of little value, and taken alone are not an indication for antibiotic therapy. The preferred specimen is a punch biopsy of deep tissue or bone if osteomyelitis is present.

Treatment

The optimal management of pressure ulcers requires attention to several factors. Firstly, the features, location and severity grading of the pressure sore(s) should be assessed (Table 49.1). Reversible systemic factors that may affect tissue healing, such as hypoalbuminaemia, uncontrolled hyperglycaemia, anaemia, incontinence, regional ischaemia and deficiencies in vitamin C, zinc and selenium, should be treated. Reducing the tissue load by regular repositioning and pressure-reducing devices or beds will help minimise further tissue damage and allow healing. Pressure ulcer wound care involves debriding devitalised tissue, cleansing with normal saline and wound dressings. Topical antiseptics, such as povidone iodine, hydrogen peroxide and acetic acid, should be avoided as they may inhibit healing. Dressings should keep the ulcer bed moist but prevent maceration of the surrounding skin. Saline-soaked gauze dressings changed 4 times daily are appropriate. Wound coverings such as hydrogel or hydrocolloid dressings are alternatives that reduce the nursing time required. Surgery may be required for deeper debridement or occasionally for closure of the wound by skin grafting or myocutaneous flaps.

Table 49.1 Grading of pressure ulcers

Grade	Clinical features
I	Non-blanchable erythema
II	Partial thickness skin loss involving epidermis and/or dermis
III	Full thickness skin loss involving necrosis of subcutaneous tissues, not through fascia
IV	Full thickness skin loss with tissue necrosis extending to underlying bone, tendon, joint capsule

Antibiotic therapy should be used if there is associated sepsis, cellulitis or osteomyelitis. Cultures of blood and ulcer tissue (in preference to swabs) must be taken prior to antibiotics. Generalised sepsis with fever, chills and confusion usually signify a bacteraemia. Blood cultures may be positive with a mixture of organisms, usually including *Bacteroides* sp. Underlying osteomyelitis is a common reason for a non-healing ulcer and should be suspected if there is associated fever, or raised C-reactive protein level or erythrocyte sedimentation rate (ESR), although these may be absent. A radionuclide bone scan is useful for confirming the diagnosis of osteomyelitis. In osteomyelitis, a bone biopsy for culture and sensitivity is vital for enabling appropriate antibiotic therapy. Broad-spectrum antibiotics for covering both anaerobes and aerobic Gram-negative bacteria should be started pending culture results if there is generalised sepsis or cellulitis. Suitable choices include amoxycillin-clavulanate, cephazolin plus metronidazole, ticarcillin-clavulanate, piperacillin-tazobactam, or clindamycin plus gentamicin. Treatment should be given parenterally if there is serious sepsis or for proven osteomyelitis. Infection with multiresistant organisms, such as methicillin-resistant *S. aureus* and multiresistant *P. aeruginosa*, is a problem in the hospital and increasingly in the nursing home setting.

Surgical wound infections

Epidemiology

Surgical wound infections account for about a third of hospital acquired infections. Elderly patients are twice as likely as their younger counterparts to develop this complication. Risk factors for developing a wound infection include the type of surgery, duration of surgery and presence of contamination. In the elderly, host risk factors such as poor mobility, malnutrition, diabetes, peripheral vascular disease, cardiopulmonary disease and malignancy are commonly present. Reduction in skin thickness and subcutaneous tissue may also affect wound healing. The increasing trend towards day surgery and shorter postoperative length of stay has meant that many surgical wound infections become apparent after discharge from hospital and often present to the general practitioner.

Diagnosis and treatment

The diagnosis is usually easily recognised by an inflamed wound; a purulent discharge may be present. Any discharge should be swabbed or aspirated for microscopy and culture. Removal of sutures, exploration of the wound and drainage of pus is often required. Such local measures are adequate for minor infections. Antibiotics should be administered, usually intravenously, if there is an associated fever or evidence of sepsis, cellulitis or involvement of deeper structures. Obtaining a microbial aetiology is important given the variety of organisms and increasing frequency of multiresistant organisms. *S. aureus*, including strains resistant to methicillin, are the most common causes of wound infections. Coliforms, enterococci, *P. aeruginosa* and anaerobes may cause wound infections after abdominal, gynaecologic or vascular surgery of the lower limb. Initial therapy with dicloxacillin or flucloxacillin is recommended. If Gram-negative infection is suspected, gentamicin, a third-generation cephalosporin or ciprofloxacin should be added.

Scabies

Outbreaks of scabies are a significant problem in elderly patients and staff in nursing homes and, to a lesser extent, in hospitals. Transmission occurs by skin contact, particularly in debilitated residents who require greater nursing care. Scabies is caused by the mite *Sarcoptes scabiei*, which burrows into the epidermis where it resides and reproduces. The clinical picture of intense itching accompanied by erythematous papules, excoriation marks and linear burrows is extremely variable. Frequently involved sites are the interdigital web spaces, wrists, periumbilical skin, anterior axillary folds and ankles. Norwegian scabies is a severe variant of the disease that can occur in immunosuppressed or very debilitated individuals. It is characterised by widespread hyperkeratotic plaques and nodules and is caused by a very heavy infestation of mites.

Treatment

Permethrin 5% cream is effective against scabies, usually after one application. It should be applied all over the skin from the chin down and washed off after 8–10 hours. Secondary bacterial infection by *S. aureus* may need to be treated. Ivermectin, an oral antiparasitic agent, is also a useful agent, especially in institutional outbreaks. A single dose of 200 μg/kg is adequate in most instances, except for Norwegian scabies where 2–3 treatments (each given 14 days apart) and concomitant topical permethrin twice weekly is recommended. Close contacts should be treated prophylactically.

Staff should wear gloves to handle patients with typical scabies for at least 8 hours after topical treatment. Clothes and linen should be washed and dried in the hot cycle to kill the mites. Patients with Norwegian scabies should be isolated and staff wear disposable gowns and gloves prior to patient contact.

Gastrointestinal infections

Elderly patients are at risk of gastrointestinal infection due to achlorhydria, reduced intestinal motility and frequent antibiotic use. Outbreaks of gastroenteritis are common in geriatric long-term care facilities and to a lesser extent in hospitals. Viruses, especially small, round, structured viruses and rotavirus, cause the majority of these outbreaks. *Clostridium difficile*, *Salmonella* sp., *Shigella* sp. and *Campylobacter* sp. are common bacterial causes of diarrhoea in the nursing home and hospital. Parasitic infections such as cryptosporidiosis, giardiasis and amoebiasis have also caused outbreaks of diarrhoea in long-term care facilities (see also Chapter 34).

Viral gastroenteritis

Small, round, structured viruses (SRSV), such as Norwalk and Norwalk-like viruses, account for the majority of outbreaks of gastroenteritis in the institutional setting. These viruses spread by the faecal–oral route and via aerosols produced by vomiting. Infected food handlers may also play a role in transmission in some cases. Viral spread on the ward is very rapid and extensive, with attack rates of up to 80% in patients and staff reported. The illness is characterised by profuse vomiting and diarrhoea, which typically resolves within 3–4 days.

The organism may be detected in stool samples by electron microscopy or by the polymerase chain reaction. The infection control measures recommended include the use of gloves and gowns for patient care, isolating or cohorting patients and, if necessary, ward closures for at least 48 hours after the last case of diarrhoea. Other viruses that can cause nosocomial diarrhoea include rotavirus, enteric adenoviruses and certain enteroviruses.

Bacterial gastroenteritis

Salmonellosis is a frequent cause of bacterial gastroenteritis in long-term care facilities. If detected, the source of infection is due to an infected resident, contaminated food such as poultry or an infected food handler. Shigellosis is spread only from person to person, while gastroenteritis due to *Campylobacter* sp. and *E. coli* usually originates from a contaminated food source.

Clostridium difficile colitis

Antibiotic-associated diarrhoea due to *C. difficile* is frequently seen in elderly patients who are hospitalised or reside in long-term care facilities. It is rarely fatal but is an important cause of morbidity and prolonged hospital stay. *C. difficile* diarrhoea occurs after virtually any antibiotic but is particularly associated with cephalosporins and clindamycin. The organism may also colonise the bowel asymptomatically in patients. In addition to antibiotic use, the risk factors for *C. difficile* disease are age over 75 years, severe underlying disease, cytotoxic treatment, antacids, nasogastric tubes, intestinal surgery and altered gut motility. Diarrhoea usually occurs within 10 days of commencing antibiotics, but can begin up to 6 weeks after stopping the drug in up to 20% of cases.

Transmission between patients occurs by the faecal–oral route via the hands of health care workers. The patient's environment is also heavily colonised by bacterial spores, thus fomites are also an important means of spread. Infection control precautions are important for preventing spread, particularly when patients are faecally incontinent.

The organism produces two main toxins—toxin A (enterotoxin) and toxin B (cytotoxin)—which are responsible for the colitis. The disease produced ranges from mild diarrhoea to fulminant colitis or toxic megacolon. At sigmoidoscopy, colitis may be present, which in severe cases has the appearance of a pseudomembrane.

The diagnosis of *C. difficile* is obtained by submitting stool for detection of the cytotoxin by cell culture, enzyme immunoassay or polymerase chain reaction. The organism may also be cultured but this is relatively costly and potentially detects non-toxigenic strains.

Treatment should include stopping antibiotic therapy if possible and commencing 200–400 mg metronidazole orally 8 hourly. An alternative is 125 mg vancomycin orally 4 times daily, which should be reserved for relapsing or particularly severe episodes of colitis. Opiates and anti-diarrhoeal agents should be avoided. Relapses or reinfections are common and may require more prolonged treatment.

Prevention of infection is best achieved by limiting the use of broad-spectrum antibiotics, especially cephalosporins and clindamycin. Strict infection control procedures with contact precautions and thorough cleaning of the patient environment are recommended.

Antibiotic-resistant organisms

Important antibiotic-resistant bacteria acquired by the elderly in hospital include methicillin resistant *S. aureus* (MRSA), multiresistant Gram-negative bacteria and enterococci resistant to aminoglycosides and vancomycin. Transfer of patients between nursing homes and hospitals establishes a two-way flow of resistant bacteria between the institutions. The rates of antibiotic-resistant organisms reported in nursing homes varies considerably, with isolation rates varying from < 5% to > 30% of all bacterial isolates.

MRSA is the most common resistant organism identified in hospitals and nursing homes, with colonisation rates of up to 20–30% in some long-term care facilities in the US. MRSA infection, however, is far less common than colonisation, particularly in the non-epidemic or endemic situation usually evident in nursing homes and geriatric wards. Risk factors for being colonised with MRSA include hospital admission or a surgical procedure in the last year, male sex, poor functional status, pressure sores or chronic ulcers, urinary and intravascular catheters, enteric feeding tubes, urinary or faecal incontinence, and recent antibiotic use, especially with cephalosporins. More recently, isolates of *S. aureus* with reduced susceptibility to vancomycin have been reported in hospitals in Asia and the US.

Enterococci resistant to gentamicin and more recently vancomycin are also emerging and may colonise the bowels of elderly patients in hospitals and nursing homes. Avoiding vancomycin usage for *C. difficile* colitis is one factor recommended for helping to minimise the development of vancomycin-resistant enterococci.

Infections due to resistant *P. aeruginosa* and coliforms such as *E. coli*, *Proteus* sp., *Klebsiella* sp., *Enterobacter* sp., *Serratia* sp., *Citrobacter* sp. and *Acinetobacter* sp. are an increasing problem in the elderly in nursing homes. Infection of the urinary tract and respiratory tract, and pressure ulcers are common. Single or multiple resistance to aminoglycosides, quinolones such as norfloxacin, and third-generation cephalosporins make effective therapy difficult, especially with oral antibiotics.

Infection prevention in the hospital and nursing home

The basic principles of infection control include surveillance, hand washing and appropriate isolation and handling of patients colonised with resistant organisms. Standard precautions (previously known as universal precautions) are applicable to all patients and consist of hand washing before and after patient contact, and the use of barrier precautions when handling body fluid. Disinfection and sterilisation of medical equipment should occur in accordance with national published guidelines.

Isolation of patients in hospital is often instituted with the adoption of special precautions such as contact precautions, where staff use of gowns and gloves is required. Respiratory precautions with the use of masks are recommended for infections such as tuberculosis and varicella zoster.

The isolation of elderly patients with resistant organisms such as MRSA can be problematic as it may promote confusion and anxiety and can delay physical therapy and rehabilitation. In the nursing home and geriatric ward setting, MRSA colonisation rarely causes harm, and single room isolation or curtailment of social mixing is not recommended. The exception is for residents with open wounds or urinary or percutaneous catheters, who should not share sleeping areas with individuals colonised with MRSA. MRSA colonisation should also not be a barrier to nursing home admission.

Invasive procedures should be minimised where possible. Intravenous catheters should be inserted using a sterile technique and removed as soon as no longer needed. Peripheral intravenous lines should be re-sited every 48 hours or earlier if phlebitis develops. Urinary catheters should be removed as soon as possible in hospital. Attention should be paid to ensuring adequate nutrition, avoidance of pressure sores and preventing aspiration in patients with neurological disorders. A policy of vaccinating all nursing home residents against influenza and pneumococcus is essential.

Finally, restricting the use of antibiotics is a crucial factor in preventing nosocomial infections. Short courses of antibiotics (e.g. 5–7 days) should be used if symptoms respond quickly. The use of cephalosporins should be minimised with greater use of penicillin, dicloxacillin and trimethoprim as appropriate. Metronidazole should be used instead of vancomycin for the treatment of *C. difficile* colitis. Box 49.1 summarises the factors that reduce the frequency of nosocomial and nursing home associated infections in older patients.

Box 49.1 Measures to reduce institutionally acquired infections in older patients

- Follow standard (universal) precautions
- Limit use of urinary catheters
- Limit use of intravenous catheters
- Minimise hospital stay
- Limit use of corticosteroids
- Limit use of antibiotics, especially those with greatest risk of *C. difficile* superinfection
- Promote mobility
- Prevent pressure sores
- Maintain adequate nutrition and hydration

Bibliography and further reading

AGS Clinical Practice Committee (1996), 'Pressure ulcer in adults: predictions and prevention', *Journal of the American Geriatric Society*, 44, pp. 1118–19.

Allman, R. M. (1989), 'Pressure ulcers among the elderly', *New England Journal of Medicine*, 320, pp. 850–3.

Garibaldi, R. A. (1999), 'Residential care and the elderly: the burden of infection', *Journal of Hospital Infection*, 435, pp. S9–S18.

Gross, P., Levine, J. F., LoPresti, A. & Urdaneta, M. (1997), 'Infections in the elderly', in Wenzel, R. P. (ed.), *Prevention and Control of Nosocomial Infections*, Williams & Wilkins, Baltimore, MD, pp. 1059–97.

Hussain, M., et al. (1996), 'Prospective survey of the incidence, risk factors and outcome of hospital acquired infection in the elderly', *Journal of Hospital Infection*, 32, pp. 117–26.

Lertzman, B. H. & Gaspari, A. A. (1996), 'Drug treatment of skin and soft tissue infections in elderly long term care residents', *Drugs and Aging*, 9, pp. 109–21.

Loeb, M. (1999), 'Risk factors for pneumonia and other lower respiratory tract infections in elderly residents of long term care facilities', *Archives of Internal Medicine*, 159(17), pp. 2058–64.

Smith, P. W. (1989), 'Nosocomial infection in the elderly', *Infectious Diseases Clinics of North America*, 3(4), pp. 763–77.

Stone, S. P. (1999), 'Soil, seed and climate: developing a strategy for preventions and management of infections in UK nursing homes', *Journal of Hospital Infection*, 435, pp. S29–S38.

Strausbaugh, L. J. (2000), 'Nosocomial respiratory infections', in Mandell, G. L., Bennett, J. E. & Dolin, R. (eds), *Principles and Practice of Infectious Diseases*, 5th edn, Churchill Livingstone, Philadelphia, pp. 3020–7.

Therapeutic Guidelines: Antibiotic (1998), 10th edn, Therapeutic Guidelines Limited, Australia.

Thielman, N. M. (2000), 'Antibiotic associated colitis', in Mandell, G. L., Bennett, J. E. & Dolin, R. (eds), *Principles and Practice of Infectious Diseases*, 5th edn, Churchill Livingstone, Philadelphia, pp. 1111–25.

Chapter 50

Infections of the respiratory tract

WAH KIT LAM

The effect of ageing on lung defences against infections

Respiratory diseases, particularly infections, are a major cause of morbidity and mortality in the elderly. Elderly persons are more prone to respiratory tract infections due to multiple factors of alterations of pulmonary host defence and immune status (Table 50.1). Coughing is less effective due to spinal degeneration leading to kyphosis, costochondral joint calcification resulting in a stiff rib cage, increased residual volume, and atrophic, weakened respiratory muscles. Mucociliary clearance is impaired. There is decreased ciliary function and increased frequency of ciliary ultrastructural anomalies with ageing. There is also impaired ability of T-cells to activate and proliferate and to secrete interleukin-2 in response to antigens. B-cell defects cause decreased antibody production (and loss of immune regulation results in increased circulation of autoantibodies in the elderly, e.g. rheumatoid factor).

Neutrophil chemotaxis and phagocytosis are impaired. In addition, elderly people have a number of co-morbidities increasing proneness to respiratory

Table 50.1 Alterations of pulmonary host defence in the elderly

Impaired coughing	Kyphosis Stiff rib cage Increased lung residual volume Weak respiratory muscles
Impaired mucociliary clearance	Impaired coughing Decreased ciliary function Increased ciliary ultrastructural anomalies Increased mucus secretions, especially in chronic smokers and patients with COPD
Impaired T-cell function	Impaired activation and proliferation Impaired interleukin secretions
Impaired B-cell function	Decreased antibody production
Impaired neutrophil function	Impaired chemotaxis Impaired phagocytosis
Co-morbidities	COPD Congestive heart failure Stroke Diabetes mellitus Malnutrition

tract infections. These include chronic obstructive pulmonary disease (COPD), congestive heart failure, stroke (immobility and aspiration), uraemia (impaired macrophage and neutrophil function), diabetes mellitus and malnutrition.

Aetiology and epidemiology

This chapter focuses on three major respiratory tract infections in the elderly: influenza, pneumonia (community acquired and nursing home acquired) and pulmonary tuberculosis.

Influenza

Influenza is the most prevalent cause of acute respiratory illness requiring medical intervention. Worldwide, it is one of the main causes of morbidity, with a large impact on health care services. Most influenza infections are self-limited, but in the elderly it is an important cause of mortality, especially in winter epidemics. These epidemics are characterised by excess mortality occurring rapidly over a short time: for example, 29 000 excess deaths were estimated to have occurred in Britain within 2 months in the influenza epidemic in 1989/90 winter. Most influenza deaths occur in patients aged above 75 years and/or who have chronic medical disorders, and about half of the deaths occur in the elderly in residential nursing homes where an environment of grouping of frail elderly people allows rapid spread of this highly contagious illness in an epidemic.

Influenza viruses possess two surface glycoproteins—haemagglutinin and neuraminidase. Influenza A viruses are subtyped according to the haemagglutinin (H1–H15) and neuraminidase (N1–N9) subtypes. The epidemics and pandemics in humans in the 20th century have been caused by influenza A viruses of the H1/H2/H3 and N1/N2 subtypes, such as the H1N1 flu and the H3N2 flu (e.g. Hong Kong flu and Sydney flu). Influenza A virus is characterised by the periodic antigenic variation of its H and N antigens (antigenic shifts and antigenic drifts). Currently, both the H1N1 and H3N2 subtypes of influenza A viruses, along with influenza B viruses, are circulating.

The last major outbreak of influenza occurred in Europe and North America in the winter of 1999/2000. In Scotland, it was the worst flu outbreak in 6 years with flu rates of up to 800 per 100 000 population. All intensive care unit beds were occupied, and emergency admission to hospital hit record levels, with rates in Edinburgh being 50% higher than normal for this time of the year.

Pneumonia

Pneumonia is common in the elderly, particularly in nursing home residents. Pneumonia is the second most common important infection among nursing home residents after urinary tract infections, accounting for 13–48% of all institutionally acquired infections. Pneumonia in the elderly is also more serious. In a population based study in Rochester in the US, the incidence of pneumonia in patients above the age of 65 years was more than 5400 per 100 000 population, and more than two-thirds of patients were not hospitalised. In a Canadian study, the overall rate of pneumonia requiring hospitalisation was 1 per 1000 total population annually, while the rates for those 75 years of age or older and nursing home residents were 12 and 33, respectively. In the UK, over 90% of patients acutely admitted to hospitals for community acquired pneumonia are aged over 65 years, and the mortality rate is 16–40%, which is 3–6 times that of younger patients. It is the most common cause of death from infections in nursing home residents. In Hong Kong, pneumonia is the third most common cause of death in the elderly (16%) after malignant neoplasms (28%) and cardiovascular diseases (17%).

This chapter will review community acquired pneumonia and nursing home acquired pneumonia managed by general practitioners, but will not include hospital acquired nosocomial pneumonia and pneumonia in the intensive care unit setting.

Risk factors for pneumonia in the elderly include malnutrition (low serum albumin), current smoking, aspiration (due to swallowing disorders, altered consciousness, dementia), immobility, COPD, chronic heart failure, history of myocardial infarction, alcoholism, altered immune status including immunosuppressive therapy, and institutionalisation.

Common pathogens isolated from sputum in elderly patients with pneumonia are *Streptococcus pneumoniae*, *Haemophilus influenzae* and *Staphylococcus aureus*. Gram-negative enteric bacilli are also important in nursing home acquired pneumonia. Anaerobes should be considered in patients with predisposition to aspiration. *Mycoplasma pneumoniae* and *Legionella pneumophila* are important pathogens in some series, and recently *Chlamydia pneumoniae* has been reported to be common in Mediterranean areas.

Tuberculosis

Tuberculosis in elderly people is becoming an important health problem, even in Western countries. The increase in tuberculosis risk in the elderly probably relates to impaired T-cell mediated immunity and to co-morbidities, particularly diabetes mellitus, malignancies, uraemia and use of immunosuppressive drugs. In nursing homes and long-term care facilities, overcrowding with close and prolonged contacts, recirculation of air and few open windows plus lack of isolation facilities are additional risk factors.

In the US, there has been a gradual rise in the average age of patients with tuberculosis, and the case rate of persons older than 65 years is nearly double that of the general population (11.5 versus 6/100 000). In some areas, over 50% of the tuberculosis cases develop in elderly patients. Tuberculosis is the most common notifiable disease among persons older than 65 years of age. In non-Hispanic whites, the peak number of tuberculosis cases occurs at 75 years of age. It is assumed that the majority of these cases are due to reactivation of infection acquired in the 1920s and 1930s before the era of antituberculosis chemotherapy. In Hong Kong, tuberculosis remains a common disease despite an affluent society, and the notification rate remains at the high level of 112/100 000 population in 1999, which is 10 times or more that of most Western countries. There is a marked difference in the rate of tuberculosis between men and women in the elderly population: 75% of the elderly patients are men. Thirty-four per cent of the cases occur in patients over 65 years old, and 76% of deaths occur in this age group. The average age of tuberculosis deaths in Hong Kong has increased from 25 years in 1950 to 57 years in 1970 and 69–70 years in the 1990s.

Elderly residents in nursing homes are at even greater risk. In the US, the case rate for elderly residents in nursing homes is about 4 times that of elderly people living at home and 14 times that of the general population. In Hong Kong, the case rate of tuberculosis among the elderly in nursing homes is an amazing 1200–2600/100 000 population.

Clinical features

Influenza

Typical clinical presentations of influenza include an abrupt onset of fever and chills, malaise and myalgia, sore throat, cough, nasal discharge and headache. Compared to younger subjects, elderly patients tend to have more anorexia, productive cough and dyspnoea, and less sore throat, abdominal pain and diarrhoea. Up to one-third of elderly patients, especially those in nursing homes, have none of the typical signs and symptoms. Instead, they present with non-specific features such as anorexia, confusion or worsening of congestive heart failure or COPD. The elderly patients are also more likely to have post-influenza asthenia with weakness and malaise persisting for weeks after the acute illness.

Major pulmonary complications of influenza include the less common but serious primary viral pneumonia presenting with bloody sputum, tachypnoea and progressive respiratory failure which carries a high mortality rate; the more common but less serious secondary bacterial pneumonia, most commonly due to *S. pneumoniae*, *S. aureus* or *H. influenzae*; and mixed viral and bacterial pneumonia. The clinician must have a high index of suspicion of the complication of pneumonia whenever the patient has a gradual worsening of the acute illness or a recurrence of fever with cough and purulent sputum. Chest radiography is indicated. Non-pulmonary complications include rhabdomyolysis and myoglobinuria and central nervous system complications such as Guillain-Barre syndrome, post-influenza encephalitis and encephalopathy.

Many elderly patients, particularly those with chronic medical diseases, may develop a gradual deterioration of cardiac, pulmonary or renal function after an attack of influenza. Many of these patients ultimately die, and contribute to the remarkable excess mortality with influenza A epidemics in the elderly population.

Pneumonia

The clinical manifestations of pneumonia in the elderly are generally more subtle and non-specific than in younger patients. Up to a third of patients above the age of 65 years with pneumonia show no systemic signs of chest infection. Classical features such as fever, chills, cough with purulent sputum, chest pain and leucocytosis are often lacking. In fact, hypothermia and absence of leucocytosis are not uncommon, and are poor prognostic factors. Generally, patients present with a gradual deterioration in general conditions such as loss of appetite, weakness, dyspnoea, urinary incontinence and change of mental status. Acute confusion is a fairly characteristic presenting feature of pneumonia in the elderly, and may be present in over 50% of nursing home acquired pneumonia. Alternatively, pneumonia may present as a rapid deterioration of the underlying chronic medical condition (e.g. COPD or congestive heart failure).

Physical examination will typically show a dehydrated, confused patient with cyanosis, tachycardia and tachypnoea. An increased respiratory rate has been identified in many studies as a sensitive indicator of the presence of pneumonia. Classical signs of pulmonary consolidation are not commonly present. Auscultation of the chest in elderly patients may be difficult as these patients may be too weak to breathe deeply. Crackles detected may be due to concomitant heart failure or chronic bronchitis.

Complications from pneumonia occur frequently in elderly patients. Complicating pleural effusion or empyema may occur, and bacteraemia leading to acute respiratory distress syndrome is especially common with *S. pneumoniae* and Gram-negative bacilli pneumonia. The clinician should also check for the complications of atrial fibrillation, congestive heart failure, myocardial infarct, deep vein thrombosis and pulmonary embolism.

Tuberculosis

Clinical presentation of tuberculosis in the elderly is often atypical. Cough and sputum are commonly present as in younger patients, but other typical symptoms such as haemoptysis, fever, chills and night sweats are less frequent. Commonly, the primary manifestations are non-specific and may only be anorexia, fatigue, malaise, loss of body weight, shortness of breath, and 'slowly resolving' or 'unresolving' pneumonia. In addition, elderly patients may be unable to give an accurate history, and symptoms are often attributed to other common diseases including heart failure, COPD and malignancy.

Extrapulmonary and miliary tuberculosis are also more common, and similarly may present non-specifically with loss of appetite, weakness and failure to thrive.

As a result of the difficulties in recognising tuberculosis clinically, the diagnosis is frequently delayed or only discovered at post-mortem in the elderly. Ninety per cent of tuberculosis cases not suspected initially were patients older than 65 years old. Health care providers must have a high index of suspicion for tuberculosis in elderly patients who present with non-specific constitutional symptoms, general deterioration in wellbeing, or a chronic wasting or respiratory illness, or whose 'pneumonia' does not respond to the usual antimicrobial agents.

Investigations

Influenza

As a guide to the use of antiviral agents, a definite diagnosis of influenza should be established by laboratory tests. Nasopharyngeal and throat swabs are sampled for virus isolation, viral protein detection and viral RNA detection, and blood may be taken for serological diagnosis.

Virus isolation

Virus isolation (respiratory specimens obtained 1–4 days after illness onset) is the gold standard confirmatory test, and is important also for the purpose of antigenic and genetic characterisation of virus isolates which guides the selection of virus strains for inclusion in vaccine formulations. However, the test results are not rapidly available (usually requiring 48–72 hours) and may not be helpful in early decision making about starting antiviral therapy and infection control measures.

Viral protein detection tests

Viral protein detection tests are rapid and simple to perform, and are available commercially for point-of-case rapid diagnosis (< 1 hour). Thus they are useful for guiding initiation of antiviral therapy, but are less sensitive than culture or viral RNA detection tests (sensitivity 62–96%). The tests detect influenza A, or both types A and B, but do not distinguish between them (e.g. Directigen and Flu A detect influenza A; Biostar and Zstat Flu detect types A and B).

Viral RNA detection

Viral RNA detection by reverse-transcription and polymerase chain reaction (PCR) using gene specific oligonucleotide primers is very sensitive. Specimens must not be contaminated because PCR can actually detect non-viable virus.

Serological diagnosis

Serological diagnosis involves paired serum samples (10–14 days apart) to detect a fourfold or greater rise in specific antibody titres. The test is useful primarily in retrospect.

Chest radiography

Chest radiography in primary viral pneumonia typically shows bilateral interstitial infiltrates. It is also useful for detecting secondary bacterial pneumonia which commonly shows lobar pneumonia.

Pneumonia

Because of the atypical presentation, pneumonia in the elderly is often initially missed and the diagnosis is delayed. Clinicians must have a high index of suspicion. A change in the functional status or mental status or an unexplained rise in respiratory rate may be the only presenting feature of pneumonia and it warrants prompt investigation and treatment.

Chest radiology

A well taken chest radiograph would alert the clinician to the diagnosis of pneumonia in most cases. In the elderly, incomplete consolidation (due to the presence of emphysema) and multilobar involvement occur more commonly than in younger patients, and lower lobe consolidation with associated pleural effusion is also common, particularly with a history of aspiration.

It should be noted that many non-infectious conditions in elderly patients may also have abnormal chest radiological findings, including pulmonary infarct, congestive heart failure, atelectasis and tumours.

Sputum and blood culture

To establish a microbiological diagnosis of pneumonia from sputum studies in the elderly is a challenging task. Firstly, it is difficult to differentiate infection from colonisation of the upper airway. Up to one-third of nursing home residents have colonisation of the oropharynx and tracheobronchial tree by aerobic Gram-negative bacilli. Secondly, the coughing effort in the elderly is often poor or absent. Thirdly, some patients may have polymicrobial infections, and recovery of multiple organisms from sputum culture may mean colonisation or polymicrobial infections. Fourthly, special tests are needed (including blood tests) for some infections (e.g. *Legionella* or *Mycoplasma* infections). Sputum collection with the help of a physiotherapist/respiratory therapist, together with the finding of over 25 neutrophils and less than 10 squamous epithelial cells on low power field under microscope, would indicate a good sample, and a Gram stain to identify the predominant organism may be helpful.

If the patient is febrile and a properly taken blood culture is positive, the microbiological diagnosis is then quite definite.

An aetiological diagnosis is made only in slightly less than half of the patients. The common isolates are *S. pneumoniae*, *H. influenzae*, *S. aureus* and Gram-negative enteric bacilli.

Other tests

Other useful laboratory tests include serology for *Mycoplasma*, *Chlamydia*, *Legionella* infections, white cell counts, serum electrolytes and blood urea/creatinine (to help assess dehydration, detect hyponatraemia, and detect declining renal function in the elderly which may affect choice and dosage of antimicrobials, *vide infra*), blood gases followed by oximetry monitoring, and electrocardiogram.

There is no significant association between the type of isolated microbials and the clinical features and laboratory findings in the elderly.

Tuberculosis

The diagnosis of tuberculosis in the elderly is commonly delayed because of non-specific presenting features, the tendency for the patients to seek medical advice late, and a low index of suspicion of the health care providers. There must be increased awareness of the disease, and the disease should be considered early.

Tuberculosis intradermal skin test (Mantoux test)

Five tuberculin units of stabilised purified protein derivative (PPD) tuberculin are injected intradermally, and the results are read 48–72 hours later by measuring the induration in millimetres (not the area of redness). A 10 mm diameter of induration is taken as the criterion for a positive test. In persons with chest radiographic findings consistent with tuberculosis, a 5 mm diameter of induration is considered positive.

In the interpretation of the Mantoux test, the following should be noted:

1. For tuberculosis, infection should be distinguished from disease. Infection is usually defined by tuberculin skin test reactivity. It indicates the tubercle bacillus is in the body, but there are no clinical features (including radiological evidence) of active tuberculosis, and sputum smear and culture for *M. tuberculosis* are negative. Diagnosis of disease is usually confirmed by microbiologic studies. Only a small minority (less than 15%) of infected persons will ever develop the disease. A positive Mantoux test should therefore be followed by chest radiography and, if indicated, microbiological studies.
2. The Mantoux test is a delayed-type hypersensitivity test, and may be impaired or delayed in the elderly. If the test is negative in the first instance, it should be repeated with the same dose in 1–2 weeks (i.e. '2-step' technique), and it may become positive then (so-called booster phenomenon). The second test should be done early from 1–2 weeks to differentiate a boosted response from a new skin test conversion.

Ten to twenty per cent of elderly patients with tuberculosis disease may have negative reactions, particularly those with miliary disease.

In persons who have previously received BCG vaccinations, and in regions where tuberculosis is endemic, the Mantoux test has limited usefulness as a screening or diagnostic test for active tuberculosis.

A recent conversion (indicated by a 15 mm or more increase in tuberculin test within a 2-year period) even without positive clinical features or microbiological confirmation, is an indication for isoniazid preventive therapy.

Chest radiography

Chest radiography is mandatory in an elderly patient suspected of tuberculosis. Recognition of typical radiographic features, such as cavitary infiltrates in the apical or posterior segment of upper lobes, is relatively simple. However, in at least a third of elderly patients, tuberculosis presents with atypical and non-specific radiological findings such as diffuse mid-zone and lower-zone infiltrates, nodular lesions, peripheral inflammatory lesions and atelectasis (which may be attributed to pneumonia), aspiration, lung malignancy or cardiac failure. The clinician must be cautious of 'slowly resolving or unresolving pneumonia' in the elderly patient. Misinterpretation of radiographic findings is a major reason for delay in the diagnosis of tuberculosis in this group of patients.

It should be noted that chest radiography may be normal in up to a third of patients with miliary tuberculosis.

Sputum for smear and culture

This is the standard method of establishing the diagnosis of pulmonary tuberculosis. Three fresh morning sputum specimens are collected for smears and cultures for *M. tuberculosis*. Sputum for acid-fast bacilli, when available, gives similar positive rates (about 78%) in elderly patients and younger patients, indicating that when the diagnosis is considered, it can often readily be made.

However, because of impaired coughing efforts, elderly patients may not be able to provide a sputum specimen adequate for microbiologic studies. Chest physiotherapy or induction of sputum by inhaled hypertonic saline (beware of patients with asthma or bronchial hyper-reactivity) may be tried. Patients who cannot produce sputum despite these measures may require gastric aspiration or fibreoptic bronchoscopy with washings, bronchoalveolar lavage or transbronchial biopsy when indicated. Post-bronchoscopy sputum may further improve the diagnostic yield.

Rapid BACTEC test

A smear for acid-fast bacilli is fast and simple, but less sensitive and specific compared to cultures. Traditional solid egg-based, medium culture (Lowenstein-Jensen medium), however, takes up to 6–8 weeks for smear negative cases. A recent BACTEC system, which utilises liquid broth media containing ^{14}C-labelled palmitic acid specific for mycobacteria, allows rapid radiometric detection of growth (detection of $^{14}CO_2$ released) in 10–12 days. A further advantage is that the DNA probe identification and antibiotic susceptibility testing can also be performed rapidly.

Treatment

Influenza

Symptomatic and supportive

Patients should be advised to have adequate rest, and hydration should be maintained. Paracetamol is useful for symptomatic control of fever, myalgia and headache.

The possibility of a secondary bacterial pneumonia should always be looked for if chest symptoms persist or recur. The choice of antibiotics is guided by Gram stain or culture of sputum, or empirical antibiotics should be chosen against the most common bacterial pathogens in this situation (*S. pneumoniae*, *S. aureus*, *H. influenzae*) such as amoxycillin-clavulinate or a cephalosporin.

Amantadine and rimantadine

These two antiviral drugs, which act on the M2 protein of influenza A viruses, can reduce the severity and duration of signs and symptoms of influenza A infections when given within 48 hours of the onset of symptoms. Their efficacy is similar, but amantadine gives more side effects (mainly neurological, such as insomnia, anxiety or loss of concentration), particularly in elderly patients with impaired renal function, as the drug is excreted by the kidney. The dose is 100 mg per day (half the usual dose) or less for 3–7 days in the elderly. Emergence of resistant virus strains may be a problem. These drugs are ineffective against influenza B infections.

Neuraminidase inhibitors

Neuraminidase, one of the two surface glycoproteins of influenza viruses, is essential for viral replication and spread as it enables the release of influenza virus from infected cells, prevents the aggregation of the virus, and may also protect the virus from inactivation by respiratory secretions. Neuraminidase inhibitors, both by inhalation and by the oral route, are now available and have been tested in phase III clinical trials. Zanamivir (Relenza, 10 mg bid by inhalation for 5 days) shortens the duration of all major influenza symptoms by one day (4 days versus 5 days) if administered within 48 hours of the onset of an uncomplicated influenza illness. The degree of benefit is greater in patients with a more severe illness (e.g. high fever at onset) and in those treated within 30 hours after the onset of symptoms (3 days shorter duration of major symptoms, 4 days versus 7 days). In high-risk patients who are treated, fewer have complications, and antibiotic use is decreased. Overall, the magnitude of clinical benefit observed (1–2.5 day reductions in time to alleviation of illness) is at least as great as that observed in earlier trials of amantadine and rimantadine for acute febrile influenza A illness in adults. Oseltamivir (Tamiflu, 75 mg bid orally for 5 days) similarly results in statistically significant reductions in the duration and magnitude of viral replication and in the duration (by 1.2–1.4 days, 30%) and severity (30% reduction in scores) of influenza illness when given early. Two additional advantages are that neuraminidase inhibitors are active against both influenza A and B viruses, and appear less likely to induce the development of resistant viruses. Both drugs are well tolerated.

There have been rare reports of patients experiencing bronchospasms or a decline in lung function after using zanamivir inhalation. Such patients should discontinue zanamivir and seek medical advice. Special cautions should be taken when zanamivir is prescribed to patients with chronic lung diseases (especially asthma and COPD) and they should have a fast-acting bronchodilator inhaler available when taking zanamivir. Also, demented, very frail elderly patients may have difficulty using the inhalational device. Transient mild nausea may occur after oseltamivir dosing, but is largely prevented by ingestion with food. The oseltamivir prodrug is metabolised to active oseltamivir carboxylate. In elderly subjects, systemic exposure to oseltamivir carboxylate at steady state is 25% higher than the younger age group, but tolerance is good, and dose reduction is not necessary. It is renally excreted, and dose adjustments are indicated in advanced renal failure.

It should be noted that the efficacy of neuraminidase inhibitors in influenza has only been studied in teenagers aged 12 or more and in healthy, young adults with acute uncomplicated disease. No direct comparison between the two inhibitors has been done. As yet there is no controlled treatment data for elderly subjects. Its efficacy in the elderly and complicated illness remains to be determined.

Pneumonia

Hospitalisation

The first decision is whether to admit the patient to hospital or not. Indications for hospitalisation would include severe vital sign abnormalities (e.g. temperature ≥ 40°C or < 35°C, significant tachypnoea (> 30/min) or tachycardia (> 125/min), and hypotension), significant dehydration or cyanosis, alterations in mental status (e.g. acute confusion), severe laboratory abnormalities (e.g. severe hyponatraemia), chest radiograph showing multilobar consolidation or complicating effusion/empyema, and acute exacerbation of co-morbidities such as COPD or congestive heart failure.

Supportive measures

Hypoxaemia should be corrected by oxygen therapy. If the patient has chronic bronchitis, oxygen therapy should be carefully controlled to ensure that progressive carbon dioxide retention does not occur.

The patient should be adequately rehydrated. This is especially important in the elderly because of alteration in thirst mechanisms and if there are problems with adequate fluid intake due to weakness, anorexia or confusion.

Sputum clearance should be facilitated by physiotherapy and mucolytics. It should be noted that simple rehydration will help sputum expectoration significantly.

Any co-existing medical co-morbidities should be treated appropriately: for example, airflow obstruction by bronchodilators, heart failure or cor pulmonale by diuretics.

Nutritional and vitamin C supplements are additional supportive measures.

Antimicrobial therapy

Appropriate and early antimicrobial therapy is extremely important in the successful treatment of pneumonia in the elderly. Because of the low yield of culture and the delay in microbiological information, empirical antimicrobial treatment is initiated in most cases. The following principles of empirical antimicrobial therapy for pneumonia in the elderly should be noted:

1. Initial empirical antimicrobial therapy should provide broad coverage against the common causative organisms based on the local epidemiological data and information on resistance

patterns. In general, *S. pneumoniae*, *H. influenzae* (30% strains being β-lactamase positive in most countries) and *S. aureus* should be covered. Amoxycillin-clavulinate or second generation cephalosporins are appropriate choices. For nursing home residents, Gram-negative enteric bacilli would be included as the likely causative organisms, and if aspiration is likely, anaerobes should also be covered. Again, amoxycillin-clavulinate would be good therapy. Macrolides, which cover *Mycoplasma*, *Chlamydia* and *Legionella* infections as well, and quinolones, which have antipseudomonal activities, may be considered in the appropriate clinical settings (Table 50.2).

2. Antimicrobial pharmacokinetics in the elderly are altered due to changes in absorption, metabolism and excretion of drugs related to the ageing process. In particular, a gradual decline in renal function in the elderly requires a reduction in dosage of those antimicrobials that are excreted primarily by the kidneys.
3. Aminoglycosides should be given with caution and avoided whenever possible because of their exclusive renal excretion, since elderly persons are very susceptible to renal toxicity and ototoxicity. The ototoxicity of these drugs is increased with the simultaneous use of loop diuretics (e.g. frusemide).
4. Polypharmacy is common in the elderly because of co-morbidities, and all medications must be carefully reviewed for potential drug interactions (Table 50.2).

Approach for a slowly resolving or unresolving pneumonia

Elderly patients commonly recover from pneumonia much more slowly than younger patients. This is due to a combination of factors, including less effective cough, impaired mucociliary clearance of airway secretions, changes in immune function, and associated co-morbidities such as COPD, diabetes mellitus and malnutrition. In addition, treatment is often stalled due to delayed diagnosis because of atypical presentation. Gram-negative bacilli are often the causative organisms that usually resolve more slowly.

We therefore need to know the pattern of resolution of pneumonia in elderly patients so that unnecessary diagnostic procedures can be minimised. In general, clinical improvement precedes radiological improvement. Indeed, some patients may show deterioration in the chest radiograph during the first week of treatment. For bacteraemic pneumococcal pneumonia, radiological clearing may take up to 3 months, and residual radiological abnormalities (atelectasis or pleural based abnormalities) occur in about 30% of cases. Even in non-bacteraemic pneumococcal pneumonia, resolution commonly occurs only after 1 month of starting appropriate antibiotics, and a normal chest radiograph is observed in only a quarter of elderly patients by 1 month. For *S. aureus* and Gram-negative bacilli pneumonia, radiographic resolutions are often delayed beyond 3 months up to 5 months, and residual fibrosis is not uncommon.

When radiographic improvement or resolution of the pneumonia is delayed beyond the expected duration for the presumptive diagnosis, attention should be given to identifying the reason, such as inadequate antimicrobial therapy (compliance, adverse drug interactions), complicating empyema, unexpected organisms such as tuberculosis, and non-infectious causes, such as bronchial carcinoma causing unresolving post-obstructive pneumonia, pulmonary infarction, bronchiolitis obliterans with organising pneumonia (BOOP) or drug-induced (e.g. amiodarone) pulmonary diseases. A drug history should be obtained, sputum should be sent for AFB smear and cytology, and if negative, a fibreoptic bronchoscopy with biopsy and washings would then be appropriate.

Tuberculosis

Recommended treatment of pulmonary tuberculosis is the same in elderly patients as younger patients, with three special points to note:

1. elderly patients are more prone to side effects
2. compliance must be especially monitored because of their impaired vision or memory
3. interactions with other concomitant medications must be carefully screened.

Table 50.2 Commonly used antimicrobials for pneumonia in the elderly in general practice

Antimicrobial	Pharmaco-kinetics	Organisms usually sensitive	Special dose adjustments	Major drug interactions	Other comments
Amoxycillin-clavulinate	Both amoxycillin and clavulinate excreted in urine	P,[a] H,[b] A,[c] G(–),[d] An[e]	Cl cr[f] > 30: no dose change Cl cr 10–30: ↓ dose by 1/3 Cl cr <10: ↓ dose by > ⅔	—	—
Erythromycin	Metabolised in liver Excreted in bile < 5% excreted in urine	P, A, M,[g] C,[h] L[i]	Caution, or avoid in hepatic impairment	Inhibits hepatic cytochrome P450 activity, ↑ serum level of theophylline, digoxin, warfarin, carbamazepine, cyclosporin, phenytoin, disopyramide, valproate, ergots	Hearing loss may occur in elderly, → ↓ dose; concurrent use with cisapride and terfenadine contraindicated
Clarithromycin	Oral absorption not affected by food Metabolised in liver 45% excreted in urine 35% excreted in bile	P, A, H, M, C, L	Hepatic impairment: ↑ urine excretion of parent drug, hence no dose change provided renal function normal Cl cr 30–60: ↓ dose by ½ C cr <30: ↓ dose by ¾	Inhibits hepatic cytochrome P450 activity, drug interactions same as erythromycin	Concurrent use with cisapride and terfenadine contraindicated
Azithromycin	Oral absorption reduced by food and antacids Mainly excreted as unchanged drug in bile	P, A, H, M, C, L	Caution in hepatic impairment	No reports of drug interactions (except digoxin serum level may increase)	Take on an empty stomach; simple daily dose. × 3–5 days regimen Not taken with antacids
Cefaclor	Mainly excreted unchanged in urine	P, H, A, G(–)	Cl cr < 50: ↓ dose by ½	—	False (+)ve urine glucose with Clinitest
Cefuroxime	Mainly excreted unchanged in urine	P, H, A, G(–)	Cl cr 20–60: ↓ dose by ¼ Cl cr < 20: ↓ dose by > ¾	—	False (+)ve urine glucose with Clinitest

Table 50.2 Commonly used antimicrobials for pneumonia in the elderly in general practice (*continued*)

Antimicrobial	Pharmaco-kinetics	Organisms usually sensitive	Special dose adjustments	Major drug interactions	Other comments
Ceftriaxone	50% excreted unchanged in urine 50% excreted unchanged in bile	P, H, A, G(–)	Lone liver or kidney impairment → no dose adjustment needed	—	Convenient daily IM regimen. False (+)ve urine glucose with Clinitest
Ciprofloxacin	Oral absorption ↓↓ (up to 90%) by antacids, iron salts, sucralphate, calcium-containing food 30–50% excreted unchanged in urine 20–40% metabolised in liver and excreted in bile	H, L, G(–), Ps(±)[(j)]	Cl cr 30–50: limit oral dose to < 500 mg 12 hourly Cl cr < 30: limit oral dose to < 500 mg 18 hourly	↑ serum level of theophylline, cyclosporins, (with ↑ serum creatinine), warfarin ↓ serum level of phenytoin	Avoid concomitant ingestion with antacids, iron-salt, sucralphate, calcium-containing food (milk, yogurt). Prone to CNS side-effects in elderly (tremor, restlessness, dizziness, confusion, convulsion)
Levofloxacin	Oral absorption ↓↓ (up to 90%) by antacids, iron salts, calcium-containing food Mainly excreted unchanged in urine	P,[(k)] H, A, M, C, L, G(–), Ps(±)	Cl cr 20–50: ↓ dose by ½ Cl cr < 20: ↓ dose by ¾	↑ serum level of theophylline (one study indicated no effect on theophylline), warfarin, cyclosporin (with ↑ serum creatinine) ↓ serum level of phenytoin	Avoid concomitant ingestion with antacids, iron-salt, calcium-containing food (milk, yogurt); prone to CNS side-effects in elderly (tremor, restlessness, dizziness, confusion, convulsion)

(*a*) P = *S. pneumoniae*.
(*b*) H = *H. influenzae*.
(*c*) A = *S. aureus* (MRSA).
(*d*) G(–) = Gram-negative enteric bacilli (*E. coli, K. pneumoniae, P. mirabilis*).
(*e*) An = anaerobes.
(*f*) Cl cr = creatinine clearance in mL/min.
(*g*) M = *Mycoplasma pneumoniae*.
(*h*) C = *C. pneumoniae*.
(*i*) L = *Legionella pneumophila*.
(*j*) Ps = *Ps. aeruginosa*.
(*k*) Including penicillin-resistant strains.

The recommended drug regimen is shown in Box 50.1. With appropriate and timely treatment, and with full compliance, elderly patients are expected to respond as well as younger patients. In areas with higher prevalence of tuberculosis and in patients with history of previous treatment, particularly when the diagnosis is delayed, the incidence of drug resistance and unfavourable response to antituberculosis therapy would be significantly higher in the older patients.

Box 50.1 Antituberculosis drug regimens for elderly patients with pulmonary tuberculosis

9 month regimen

- H[a] 300 mg + R[a] 450 mg (BW[b] < 50 kg)/ 600 mg (BW > 50 kg) daily × 9 months

or

- H 300 mg + R 450 mg (BW < 50 kg)/600 mg (BW > 50 kg) daily × 2 months

followed by

- H 15 mg/kg (max. 900 mg) + R 10 mg/kg (max. 600 mg) twice weekly (directly supervised) × 7 months

6 month regimen

- H 300 mg + R 600 mg + Z[a] 15–30 mg /kg (max. 2 g/d) × 2 months

followed by

- H 300 mg + R 450 mg (BW < 50 kg)/600 mg (BW > 50 kg) daily × 4 months

or

- H 15 mg/kg (max. 900 mg) + R 10 mg/kg (max. 600 mg) twice weekly (directly supervised) × 4 months

(*a*) H = isoniazid, R = rifampicin, Z = pyrazinamide.
(*b*) BW = body weight.

Notes:

1. If drug resistance is suspected, initial therapy should include ethambutol until results of drug susceptibility testing are available. Dosage of ethambutol is 25 mg/kg, maximum dose 2.5 g × 2 months, then decrease to 15 mg/kg, daily.
2. Streptomycin is avoided in elderly patients if possible for its oto- and nephrotoxicity.

A baseline complete blood count and liver and renal function tests should be obtained before treatment begins. Monitoring of side effects of antituberculosis drugs during therapy is important (Table 50.3). Mildly elevated liver enzymes are common (2–3 times upper limit of normal), and need not cause concern in the absence of symptoms. However, if liver enzymes increase to above 3 times the upper limit, or if nausea and vomiting occurs, isoniazid and rifampicin (and pyrazinamide) should be stopped, and the patient should be referred to a specialist for desensitisation and further management. Elderly patients on ethambutol should have baseline tests of visual acuity and colour discrimination and then be followed up carefully. Baseline visual impairment would be a contraindication for ethambutol.

Prognosis

Only pneumonia will be discussed in this section, but factors such as underlying co-morbidities and low index of suspicion leading to delayed diagnosis also apply to influenza and tuberculosis.

Pneumonia

The mortality rate from hospitalised community acquired pneumonia generally increases with advancing age. In 1995 in England and Wales, 78% and 88% of all deaths in men and women, respectively, due to pneumococcal pneumonia occurred in persons aged 65 years or above. Generally, the mortality rate is high—at 20% for all patients aged 65 years or above, peaking in the age group 81–90 years old (40%). Due to a delay in diagnosis and treatment, the mortality rate of nursing home acquired pneumonia is even higher at 40%, that is, double that of community acquired pneumonia in the same elderly age group.

It is now known that age itself is not a poor prognostic factor for elderly individuals with pneumonia. The important prognostic factors are underlying co-morbidities: COPD, heart failure, stroke, swallowing problems, dementia, diabetes mellitus, immobilisation and malnutrition (hypoalbuminaemia) and decreased body mass index. Other

Table 50.3 Important side effects and drug interactions of the 4 commonly used anti-tuberculosis drugs in the elderly

Drug	Important side effects	Important drug interactions	Other comments
Isoniazid	↑ liver enzymes Hepatitis Peripheral neuropathy Hypersensitivity	↑ Phenytoin serum level	Pyridoxine (25 mg/day) for prevention of peripheral neuropathy Hepatitis risk ↑ with alcohol
Rifampicin	Hepatitis Gastrointestinal upset ↓ platelets Hypersensitivity	↓ serum level of quinidine, digoxin, disopyramide, oral hypoglycaemics, oral anticoagulants, theophylline, protease inhibitor, corticosteroids	Turns body fluids (urine, sweat) orange
Pyrazinamide	Hepatitis Hyperuricaemia Gastrointestinal upset Rash	—	Treat hyperuricaemia only if symptomatic
Ethambutol	Optic neuritis	—	Avoid in patients with pre-existing visual/renal impairment. ↓ dosage after 2 months, and stop drug if visual impairment occurs

poor prognostic factors include absence of fever or hypothermia, tachypnoea (respiratory rate > 30/minute), multilobar consolidation with radiological evidence of deterioration on treatment, hypotension and increasing hypoxaemia. Needless to say, the clinicians' low index of suspicion leading to a delay in diagnosis and late or inadequate antimicrobial treatment also contributes to the high mortality of elderly patients with pneumonia.

Prevention

Elderly individuals are prone to respiratory tract infections because of multiple factors, including co-morbidities and malnutrition. Regular, close medical care of COPD, heart failure, diabetes mellitus, attention to personal hygiene, nutrition and exercise will all be important in reducing respiratory tract infections in elderly patients.

Influenza

Vaccination

Influenza vaccines consist of inactivated influenza virus strains. The recommended composition is updated annually to provide vaccines antigenically matched with influenza virus strains that are circulating and anticipated to cause epidemics. Influenza vaccines licensed in 1999/2000, for instance, are trivalent formulations containing influenza A (H1N1), influenza A (H3N2) (Sydney strain) and influenza B strains. The inactivated vaccine protects 70–90% of healthy young adults, but its efficacy is expected to be lower in elderly subjects with immune senescence and co-morbidities. Overall, influenza vaccination in the elderly can reduce morbidity (hospitalisation) for influenza or co-morbidities (e.g. COPD, heart failure) and mortality by 20–40% and 40–75%, respectively.

Despite the relatively lower efficacy in the elderly, influenza vaccination significantly reduces morbidity and mortality due to the disease, especially in the elderly who are most vulnerable to the infection. Influenza vaccination is highly cost effective in the elderly, both in the community setting and in the nursing home setting, and annual vaccination is now recommended to all people above the age of 65 years before the outbreak season (in autumn). It is in fact also recommended for health care workers and employers of residential nursing homes for the elderly: this is associated with a substantial decrease in mortality among the residents.

Inactivated influenza vaccine is generally well tolerated. A minority of patients will develop a low-grade fever and mild systemic symptoms 8–24 hours after vaccination or mild tenderness at the vaccination site. It is contraindicated in persons with serious egg allergies because the vaccine is grown in eggs.

Other vaccine preparations such as intranasally administered live attenuated vaccines are in use in Russia and are now under development in the US. The easy administration of these vaccines and their ability to produce a mucosal immune response in addition to systemic immune responses makes them an attractive alternative. They enhance local and systemic immune response in elderly subjects when combined with inactivated influenza vaccine. Clinical evidence of efficacy is awaited with great interest.

Amantadine and rimantadine

These antiviral drugs are effective (70%) and licensed for the prevention of influenza A. They are indicated in persons at high risk who have not been vaccinated, especially for nursing home residents to control influenza outbreaks until the effect of the vaccination occurs (which takes 2 weeks), and for persons with severe hypersensitivity to egg proteins who cannot be vaccinated. They are also useful in the special situation when an unexpected change in the circulating virus strain limits the efficacy of the available or administered vaccine preparation.

Neuraminidase inhibitors

Inhaled zanamivir and oral oseltamivir have been shown to be effective in preventing influenza; the US FDA has approved the use oseltamivir in the prevention of influenza in adults and adolescents 13 years and older.

Pneumonia

Pneumococcal vaccine

S. pneumoniae is the most common pathogenic isolate from sputum and blood cultures, and accounts for 30–40% of all community acquired pneumonia in the elderly. It is also very lethal in the aged population, and 78–88% of all deaths due to pneumococcal pneumonia occur in persons 65 years of age or older. Its burden on health care resources is tremendous.

Pneumococcal vaccines currently in use contain 23 different serotypes of *S. pneumoniae*, which cover more than 90% of serotypes most commonly isolated from sputum and blood cultures, including the most prevalent invasive penicillin resistant pneumococcal serotypes. Current evidence indicates that the vaccine can offer about 60–70% protection against pneumococcal pneumonia for low-risk, healthy adults, but its efficacy in the elderly remains unclear. On the other hand, the vaccine has been shown quite clearly to give about 60% protection against invasive pneumococcal disease in subjects above the age of 65 years, including those with chronic medical conditions, such as chronic lung and heart diseases and diabetes mellitus. It probably does not protect those who are immunocompromised.

The analysis of efficacy of pneumococcal vaccine is thus a complex issue. An important consideration is whether it is worthwhile to advocate widespread use of the vaccine in the elderly to prevent invasive pneumococcal disease alone in the absence of good evidence that pneumococcal pneumonia is prevented. The incidence of invasive pneumococcal disease in the elderly is about 2–3 times that of the younger age group, and the high mortality rate of 30% or more is also about double that of the young. Studies in Europe and America have shown that pneumococcal vaccination is cost effective. The Advisory Committee on Immunization Practices of the United States recommends that pneumococcal vaccination is offered to all persons above the age of 65 years, with an additional dose if the patient was immunised at least 5 years previously. Thereafter, the vaccine can be repeated every 6–10 years (more frequently in nursing home residents).

Tuberculosis

The most effective way of preventing spread of tuberculosis in the elderly is an awareness of the disease, avoiding a delay in diagnosis and instituting early and effective treatment to minimise the potential spread of the disease, especially to vulnerable subjects in the community, nursing homes and in hospitals.

The Mantoux skin test is a useful screen for tuberculosis, particularly in nursing homes and in countries of low tuberculosis prevalence in the general population. All elderly persons on admission to nursing homes should be screened for tuberculosis by the two-step Mantoux test (see the 'Investigations' section). If the test is positive, but the chest radiograph is negative, the positive Mantoux test should be kept on file (prominently) to remind health care providers to consider tuberculosis if the resident develops symptoms such as cough, anorexia, weight loss or is just generally unwell.

Preventive therapy in asymptomatic elderly persons (300 mg isoniazid daily for 6–12 months) is indicated in new Mantoux test converters. For other elderly groups, the benefit is less clearly defined, but would be indicated if a positive Mantoux test is associated with loss of body weight of 10% or more, diabetes mellitus, uraemia, recent close contact with an active tuberculosis case, or a chest radiograph consistent with stable old, inactive tuberculosis. Preventive therapy is given to all exposed persons (residents and employees, regardless of age) in the nursing home.

Other preventive measures for nursing homes and long-term care facilities include containment of active cases and active case finding, and education of residents and employees. Improved ventilation and creation of isolation rooms with negative pressure are other measures. If effects directed towards preventing tuberculosis in the elderly population are successful, the incidence of tuberculosis in many countries will decline significantly.

Bibliography and further reading

Cox, N. J. & Subbarao, K. (1999), 'Influenza', *Lancet*, 354, pp. 1277–82.

Gubareva, L. V., Kaiser L. & Hayden F. G. (2000), 'Influenza virus neuraminidase inhibitors', *Lancet*, 355, pp. 827–35.

Gubser, V. L. (1998), 'Tuberculosis and the elderly. A community health perspective', *Journal of Gerontological Nursing*, 24, pp. 36–41.

Marrie, T. J. (1996), 'Pneumonia in the elderly', *Current Opinion in Pulmonary Medicine*, 2, pp. 192–7.

Nguyen-Van-Tam, J. S. & Neal, K. R. (1999), 'Clinical effectiveness, policies and practices for influenza and pneumococcal vaccines', *Seminars in Respiratory Medicine*, 14, pp. 184–95.

Patriarca, P. A. (1999), 'New options for prevention and control of influenza', *Journal of the American Medical Association*, 282, pp. 75–7.

Perez-Guzman, C., Vargas, M. H., Torres-Cruz, A. & Villarreal-Velarde, H. (1999), 'Does aging modify pulmonary tuberculosis? A meta-analytical review', *Chest*, 116, pp. 961–7.

Semla, T. P., Beizer, J. L. & Higbee, M. D. (1998), *Geriatric Dosage Handbook*, 4th edn, Lexi-Comp Inc., American Pharmaceutical Association, Hudson, OH.

Torres, A., El-Ebiary, M., Riquelme, R., Ruiz, M. & Celis, R. (1999), 'Community-acquired pneumonia in the elderly', *Seminars in Respiratory Infections*, 14, pp. 173–83.

Wort, S. J. & Rogers, T. R. (1998), 'Community acquired pneumonia in elderly people', *British Medical Journal*, 316, p. 1690.

Chapter 51
Urinary tract infections

BEN J. BARNETT

Introduction

The commonly used phrase 'urinary tract infection', or UTI, refers to an infection, usually bacterial in aetiology, at any location along the urinary tract from the urethral meatus to the perinephric fascia. Structures in this pathway include the urethra, bladder, ureters, and the renal pelvis and parenchyma. Associated structures that may also become infected and that may serve as foci of recurrent UTI are the prostate, epididymis and perinephric fascia. The term urethritis refers to an infection limited to the urethra. Cystitis is an infection of the urinary bladder. Acute pyelonephritis is a more extensive infection of the renal parenchyma and often presents with systemic signs and symptoms of infection. Chronic pyelonephritis implies renal cortical scarring, which may have active ongoing infection or sterile scarring.

Although these definitions are anatomically descriptive, the terms 'uncomplicated' versus 'complicated' UTI are more useful in a clinical setting. Uncomplicated UTI occurs in patients, usually women, with anatomically normal urinary tracts and resolves with short courses of antibiotics. Although uncomplicated UTI may cause significant morbidity, the long-term effects on renal function are practically nil. This is true both for acute cystitis as well as acute uncomplicated pyelonephritis. Complicated UTI is defined in patients with structurally or functionally abnormal urinary tracts and often is caused by antibiotic-resistant bacteria, and is more common in a geriatric population. This includes intrinsic abnormalities, such as renal calculi or prostatic hypertrophy, as well as the presence of extrinsic devices, such as indwelling urinary catheters. Complicated UTI is often difficult to cure and sometimes necessitates surgery or other resolution of the anatomical abnormality in order to be fully eradicated. The risk of long-term damage to renal function is increased with complicated UTI.

Urine is normally sterile and any bacteria isolated from the urine should be considered abnormal. However, some bacterial isolates may be contaminants from surrounding structures and not the cause of true infection. Furthermore, not all bacteria are equally able to cause infection in the urinary tract. Therefore, to help categorise organisms with differing virulence, a 'uropathogen' is defined as an organism that is likely to be a cause of disease when isolated from urine. Examples of uropathogens are *Escherichia coli* and other Enterobacteriaceae such as *Klebsiella*, *Enterococcus*, *Staphylococcus saprophyticus* and Group B *Streptococcus*. These organisms can possess virulence factors that first allow colonisation and then invasion of the urinary tract epithelium. They then are able to multiply well in urine. Other organisms such as lactobacilli, α-haemolytic streptococci or anaerobes are not uropathogens, and by definition do not grow well in urine. In the absence of evidence of enteric or vaginal fistulae, these are usually considered to be contaminants when isolated in urine.

UTIs are very common in the geriatric population, and as this population expands in number and grows older, will become an increasing problem both in the ambulatory setting and in long-term care facilities. The geriatric population is expected to double over the next 30 years, and an estimated 40% of persons over the age of 65 will require some sort of long-term care in their lifetime. These persons will be susceptible to a variety of infections, with UTI being the most common.

Aetiology

The majority of uncomplicated UTIs are caused by uropathogenic strains of *E. coli*, with as many as 90% of all UTIs caused by this single organism. In the geriatric population, other Enterobacteriaceae, such as *Klebsiella*, *Enterobacter*, *Proteus* and *Providencia*, also are common uropathogens, as is *Pseudomonas*. Gram-positive bacteria, such as *S. saprophyticus* and *Enterococcus*, can produce infection in certain circumstances. Many times, the epidemiological setting of the UTI will give a clue as to the aetiological diagnosis. For example, *S. saprophyticus* causes approximately 10% of UTIs in young adult women, particularly in the late summer and autumn. *Enterococcus* can be a pathogen in uncomplicated UTI but is more likely to be seen in cases of complicated UTI, in patients with indwelling urethral catheters, or in patients receiving broad-spectrum antibiotics for an infection at another site. Often, isolation of *Enterococcus* in the urine is an important signal that a mixed infection or occult urinary tract disease may be present. Sometimes, the urinary tract will become infected as a consequence of a bloodstream infection. In this circumstance, *Staphylococcus aureus* is the most common pathogen, followed by *Candida* and, rarely, *Salmonella* species. Geriatric patients in long-term care facilities are often colonised with and subsequently develop UTIs from antibiotic-resistant organisms, such as methicillin-resistant *S. aureus*, vancomycin-resistant *Enterococcus*, and extended-spectrum β-lactamase-producing and fluoroquinolone-resistant Gram-negative organisms.

UTI in a geriatric population, in both men and women, is also more likely to be complicated UTI. This is due to the increased incidence of anatomical abnormalities, such as prostatic hypertrophy or malignancy, renal calculi, urethral strictures and neurogenic bladder. A large proportion of complicated UTIs result from the use of indwelling urinary catheters. Complicated UTIs of all types are more likely to cause lasting renal damage and are more likely to result in bacteraemia. The bacterial aetiologies of complicated UTI include the same spectrum as for uncomplicated UTI but also include other Gram-negative rods, such as *Acinetobacter*, *Serratia* and *Providencia*, which tend to be more resistant to antimicrobial therapy.

A wide variety of bacteria, mycobacteria, viruses and yeast have been isolated from the urinary tract in patients with complicated UTI and the clinician must be guided by the results of urine culture to make proper treatment decisions. To illustrate the wide variety of organisms that potentially can cause complicated UTI, recent reports have documented *Nocardia asteroides*, *Oligella urethralis*, *Actinomyces bernardiae* and *Mycobacterium terrae* as aetiological agents in patients with structural abnormalities of the urinary tract. A recent case report of UTI caused by a strain of *Enterococcus faecalis* that was dependent on vancomycin for growth emphasises the problems of increasing proliferation of drug-resistant organisms and persistent, complicated UTI caused by indwelling urinary catheters. Recent reports have also emphasised the role of *Aerococcus urinae* as an aetiological agent of UTI in elderly men. This organism is a Gram-positive coccus that produces α-haemolysis on blood agar, and can be misidentified as *Streptococcus*, *Enterococcus* or *Staphylococcus* unless specifically investigated by the microbiology laboratory.

Bacteraemia is a common consequence of UTI, and the microbiological spectrum of bacteraemia originating from a urinary tract source naturally reflects the spectrum of agents that cause primary UTI. Recently published case studies in geriatric populations have documented that 80% of bacteraemic UTIs were with Gram-negative organisms, the majority being caused by *E. coli*. Patients with long-term indwelling urethral catheters have more infections with Gram-positive organisms (32% versus 14% of patients without catheters in one series) and non-*E. coli* Gram-negative infections (35% versus 14% of patients without catheters in the same series).

Geriatric patients also develop non-bacterial UTI, such as with *Candida albicans* and other non-*albicans Candida* species, which can lead to fungaemia. The common risk factors for urinary candidiasis are urinary tract instrumentation, recent antibiotic therapy and advanced age. In one series of patients with *Candida* fungaemia from a urinary tract source, from the Mayo Clinic in 1993, 19% of the patients were infected with *Candida glabrata*, a species sometimes resistant to fluconazole. As the use of fluconazole and other azole compounds continues to increase, resistant *Candida* species are predicted to become increasingly important.

Epidemiology

Infection of the urinary tract is very common, accounting for more than 6 million outpatient physician office visits every year. UTI is the leading cause of nosocomial infection and is the leading cause of Gram-negative sepsis in hospitalised patients. In neonates, UTI is more common in boys, although circumcision significantly reduces the risk. In childhood and into adulthood, girls are at a much higher risk than boys, and the prevalence of bacteriuria in girls rises steadily by approximately 1% per decade of life, reaching 10% in females up to 65 years old. As many as 50% of adult women report having had at least one UTI in their lifetime.

In the elderly population, UTI presents a special problem for both men and women. The incidence of complicated UTI is higher because of a higher prevalence of urinary tract abnormalities. Not surprisingly, UTI is the most common cause of all infections in nursing home residents, with up to one-third of all infections in some series of nursing home resident infections related to UTI. The attack rate in nursing home populations is approximately 15–20% per year. UTI is also the most common source of bacteraemia in the elderly, and up to 50% of all bacteraemias in long-term care residents have a urinary source. As the population ages, the problem of UTI will only continue to grow, as approximately 20–25% of persons aged 85 years or older now reside in nursing homes.

In addition to age, there are several other well-defined risk factors for acquiring infections of the urinary tract. Studies of sexually active young women demonstrate an association between an increased risk of UTI and recent use of a diaphragm with spermicide, spermicide use alone, recent sexual intercourse, maternal history of UTI, and a history of UTI in childhood. The association of UTI with the use of a spermicide has been confirmed in several studies and is most likely caused by a change in the vaginal flora, allowing enhanced vaginal and urethral colonisation by uropathogens. This change in vaginal flora is also likely to be involved in the pathogenesis of UTI in the postmenopausal population.

In postmenopausal women, the lack of oestrogen plays a major role in the epidemiology of UTI. This is due to an alteration of vaginal pH, and colonisation of the periurethral area with uropathogens.

In the geriatric population, a major risk factor for the development of UTI is the presence of indwelling urinary catheters. Bacteriuria develops in approximately 1% of patients after a single catheterisation, while by the thirtieth day of catheterisation there is almost universal bacteriuria, and indwelling catheters greatly increase the risk for development of a symptomatic UTI. The presence of an indwelling urinary catheter is associated with a 39-fold increase in the risk of bacteraemia over a 1 year period in residents of long-term care facilities and has been demonstrated to be an independent risk factor for increased mortality in residents of nursing homes. In hospitals, about 80% of cases of nosocomial UTIs are associated with urethral catheters. Therefore, they should only be used when absolutely necessary and should be promptly removed after their purpose has been served. Other factors in the development of UTI in the elderly are increased rates of incontinence and exposure to antibiotics for other purposes.

Recurrence of UTI is a common problem after a first infection for all populations. This was shown to occur in up to half of women with *E. coli* cystitis in some studies with follow-up to 12 months. In addition, up to one-third of recurrences with *E. coli* are caused by a serologically identical strain. Therefore, although most UTI recurrences are caused by reinfection with a new strain, persistence of the infecting organism after appropriate treatment or reinfection with the same strain occurs in a significant number of patients.

Pathophysiology

The pathophysiology of UTI is a complex interaction between virulence factors of micro-organisms and host defences. Natural host defences against UTI include the pattern of urine flow, which eliminates almost all bacteria attached to the uroepithelium, and the acidic, hypertonic nature of urine itself, which inhibits the growth of most bacteria. Bacterial virulence factors have been characterised best in *E. coli*, but many of the same principles may be applicable to *Klebsiella* and other enteric Gram-negative bacteria.

Most isolates of uropathogenic *E. coli* belong to a specific number of O:K:H serotypes and possess adhesion organelles called fimbriae. Fimbriae protrude from the surface of *E. coli* and mediate attachment to host uroepithelial cells. P-fimbriae bind to P-blood-group receptors, and bacterial strains with P-fimbriae are found most often in patients with acute pyelonephritis (90%) but in relatively few patients with asymptomatic bacteriuria (30%). Also, children with intestinal carriage of P-fimbriated strains of *E. coli* are at a greater risk of developing UTI. Type 1 fimbriae are known to promote bacterial persistence in the bladder as well as in the upper urinary tract, and also enhance the inflammatory response of the host. Type 1 fimbriae probably act in concert with P-fimbriae to cause disease, although the exact mechanism remains to be elucidated.

In addition to fimbriae, the aerobactin-mediated uptake of iron may promote bacterial growth in urinary tissues, but this association with clinical UTI is less clear. Haemolysin also may contribute to host-cell injury by its cytotoxic effect, especially in men with acute pyelonephritis. Many of the bacterial virulence factors, such as P-fimbriae and haemolysin-distinguishing uropathogenic strains of *E. coli*, are found together on 'pathogenicity islands', which are large 35–190 kb segments of DNA that apparently have been acquired by horizontal gene transfer.

The ability to produce ammonia and form struvite stones makes urease-producing bacteria, such as *Proteus*, *Providencia*, *Morganella*, *S. saprophyticus*, and *Corynebacterium urealyticum*, particularly virulent. These bacteria pose a special threat to the geriatric patient because the stones they produce may obstruct urinary catheters or become a persistent nidus of infection that is difficult to eradicate.

Several host factors play a role in the pathogenesis of UTI. In healthy women, behavioural factors, such as sexual activity, spermicide use and voiding practices, can contribute to urethral colonisation with uropathogens and ultimately lead to infection. The role of sexual activity seems to be most important for a subset of young women who are subject to recurrent UTI, but has not been definitively described in older patients. Spermicide use increases the risk of UTI by altering the natural vaginal bacterial flora. A temporal association between UTI and the stage of the menstrual cycle has been observed, most often in the second week of the cycle. It is not clear if this association reflects the variations in sexual activity or the effects of oestrogen. Finally, an increased frequency of blood group non-secretor phenotypes have been observed in women with recurrent UTI. This finding may relate to the differential binding ability of bacteria to uroepithelial cells in these women. Specifically, unique non-secretor-associated glycolipids may serve as binding sites for certain *E. coli* strains and allow better bacterial adherence to uroepithelial cells.

In postmenopausal women, the main host factor that predisposes to UTI is the lack of oestrogen. Oestrogen promotes the normal lactobacilli-dominant vaginal flora, reduces the vaginal pH and decreases *E. coli* colonisation. Other factors involved in this age group are urogenital surgery, stress and urge incontinence, a history of UTI in the premenopausal period, presence of a cystocoele, and post-void residual urine.

In the geriatric population, several host factors are associated with UTI. The use of urethral catheters may counteract natural host defences and predispose patients to UTI. The catheter enhances uropathogenic colonisation and may carry uropathogens up through the urethra and into the bladder. Catheters may also mechanically damage the adjacent epithelium, allow greater numbers of bacteria to adhere to cell surfaces, and inhibit the activity of polymorphonuclear leucocytes. The incidence of bacteriuria is 3–10% per day of indwelling urethral catheterisation, and indwelling catheter use is an independent risk factor for mortality both in acute care hospitals and nursing homes. External, or condom, catheters also are associated with UTI in men, with double the frequency of bacteriuria of non-catheterised men, and overall do not confer much of an advantage over indwelling catheters. This is because of complications such as local skin breakdown and the collection of urine around the condom, which has a very high bacterial colonisation rate. Even in the absence of catheterisation, declining functional status will predispose the geriatric population to UTI. This includes prostatic hypertrophy, concomitant medical illness, neurogenic bladder, urogenital surgery, altered mental status, antimicrobial use for other indications, and importantly, nosocomial acquisition of infection, which may be more difficult to treat given increased antimicrobial resistance.

In all age groups, UTIs are most commonly acquired by bacterial ascension starting at the urethral meatus. The first step is urethral colonisation by enteric organisms that grow well in urine. Women have a shorter urethra than men and are therefore more prone to cystitis. Bacteraemia can result from an infected kidney and produce metastatic abscesses, particularly to the spinal column and psoas muscle. Conversely, the kidney can become infected by haematogenous spread from a distant focus, particularly in the setting of *S. aureus* bacteraemia or candidaemia.

Clinical manifestations

Symptoms of acute cystitis or urethritis most commonly include dysuria and increased frequency of voiding. Fever ($>38.5°C$) is not a common characteristic of uncomplicated acute cystitis. Constitutional symptoms, such as malaise, may also be present but are not prominent. Physical examination may show suprapubic tenderness, but often no revealing physical signs are present. Examination of a voided urine sample often reveals the urine to be cloudy and sometimes it contains frank blood or clots.

Patients with acute pyelonephritis, in contrast, often present with high fever, systemic toxicity and costovertebral pain, without many symptoms directly related to the urinary tract. Gastrointestinal complaints are a common feature and may be misleading. Physical examination may reveal costovertebral angle tenderness and a bulging flank mass can sometimes be palpated in patients with a perinephric abscess. Unexplained Gram-negative bacteraemia should prompt an investigation for pyelonephritis as this is sometimes the only presenting sign. An examination of a voided urine sample is similar to that from the patient with cystitis, but pyelonephritis is accompanied by peripheral blood leucocytosis and sometimes positive blood cultures. Acute renal failure is not a prominent feature unless accompanied by the sepsis syndrome.

As is the case for many infectious syndromes in the geriatric population, the clinician must proceed with caution in evaluating older patients for possible UTI. The ambulatory elderly population often will present with the typical signs and symptoms of UTI that occur in the younger population. However, for many functionally impaired elderly, few, if any, of the classic symptoms and signs of UTI may appear and they are much more likely than younger patients to present with atypical symptoms, such as nausea and vomiting. Older patients may have difficulty in articulating symptoms due to underlying dementia, dysarthria or deafness. Older patients often do not have fever as commonly defined for younger patients, even in the presence of acute pyelonephritis or urosepsis, and the basal body temperature of the frail elderly may be lower than

37°C. For this reason, some authors advocate a definition of fever in the frail elderly to be 1.1°C above the patient's baseline temperature. Many times the only presenting sign of UTI in the elderly patient is altered mental status. Decreased urinary output may be a sign of UTI or of a non-infected but obstructed indwelling urinary catheter. Similarly, bacteraemia in the frail elderly often presents as lethargy, confusion, falling or gastrointestinal symptoms. Any unclear syndrome in an elderly patient should prompt analysis of the urinary tract as a potential source.

After the initiation of appropriate therapy, the signs and symptoms of UTI should resolve within a few days. If fever and flank pain persist after 72 hours in a patient with pyelonephritis, diagnostic imaging should be performed to rule out perinephric abscess. If patients have diabetes mellitus, they are subject to emphysematous pyelonephritis, which can be very destructive and requires surgical evaluation. Vertebral osteomyelitis and abscess can occur as the consequence of pyelonephritis and should also be ruled out in patients who do not respond promptly to antibiotic therapy.

It is important to perform a quantitative bacterial count in the urine for diagnostic and therapeutic purposes. Quantitative colony counts greater than 10^5 colony forming units per millilitre (cfu/mL) traditionally have been used as clinical markers for significant bacteriuria and colony counts less than 10^5 cfu/mL were considered to be contaminants from adjacent structures. This limit has been used in clinical trials and other investigations, but its relevance to the clinician has recently been reassessed. So-called low count bacteriuria, defined as 10^2–10^4 cfu/mL, has been demonstrated to be statistically more frequent in women with urinary complaints than in asymptomatic women. This suggests that, in patients with low bacterial colony counts, infection may not have yet been established in the bladder but rather is in an early phase and some authorities recommend treatment if the patient is symptomatic or if pyuria is present. This would apply to both young patients and the ambulatory elderly.

The clinical manifestation of the 'urethral syndrome' has been used to refer to a syndrome in patients with dysuria and pyuria, and less than 10^5 bacterial cfu/mL of a uropathogen in a urine sample. In addition to early UTI as described above, other causes of acute urethral syndrome are urethritis due to *Chlamydia trachomatis* or *Neisseria gonorrhoea* infection, genital herpes simplex infection, vaginitis, and non-infectious syndromes, such as psychological or allergic illnesses.

Asymptomatic bacteriuria is relatively infrequent (approximately 5% prevalence) in healthy premenopausal women, is often transient, but when present is a strong predictor of the development of subsequent symptomatic UTI when compared to young women without bacteriuria. In contrast, asymptomatic bacteriuria in geriatric patients is quite common and can be the source of many diagnostic and therapeutic dilemmas for the clinician. It is usually accompanied by a host inflammatory response, so it is not strictly speaking 'colonisation' but rather an asymptomatic infection. The prevalence of asymptomatic bacteriuria is 15–50% in non-catheterised residents of long-term care facilities, due in large part to chronic co-morbid conditions with neurogenic bladder and incontinence. For long-term care residents with indwelling urinary catheters, the presence of asymptomatic bacteriuria is almost universal. For geriatric patients who are not in long-term care, approximately 20% of women and 5% of men have asymptomatic bacteriuria.

The diagnosis of asymptomatic bacteriuria requires the isolation of colony counts greater than 10^5 cfu/mL in two consecutive urine specimens, although some authors consider a single culture adequate if there is only one organism isolated in culture. Treatment with antibiotics in these patients has no effect on morbidity or mortality, and prospective studies show that untreated asymptomatic bacteriuria can persist for up to 2 years without any deleterious effect. Furthermore, the progression to symptomatic infection in older patients with asymptomatic bacteriuria has not been demonstrated to be higher than in those without asymptomatic infection. Finally, treatment of asymptomatic patients may lead to future infection with resistant micro-organisms and to side effects caused by antibiotics. An exception to this general rule is the finding of *Proteus* or other urea-splitting bacteria in the asymptomatic patient's urine. Patients with these organisms should be treated with the goal of bacterial eradication because of the organisms' propensity to form urinary stones.

Urinary candidiasis is another common clinical syndrome in the elderly, often presenting the clinician with the problem of deciding which patients would benefit from treatment. It can also be difficult to decide if the infection, when present, is localised to the bladder, has ascended into the upper urinary tract structures, or represents haematogenous spread from underlying candidaemia. Syndromes that may present with candiduria include simple colonisation associated with indwelling urinary catheters, superficial bladder infection, or infection of obstructed ureters as with a fungal ball. More unusually, candiduria can also present as a marker of invasive renal parenchymal disease or acute haematogenous dissemination. Underlying conditions in patients with candiduria are commonly diabetes mellitus, neurogenic bladder, prostatic hypertrophy, malnutrition and neutropenia. Candiduria is very common in patients with indwelling urinary catheters, and often catheter removal alone will result in elimination of the organism. The vast majority of patients with candiduria have received a recent course of antibiotics for a distant infection prior to the onset of candiduria. In most patients, isolation of *Candida* is not accompanied by symptoms of a UTI and is a benign event that simply represents colonisation. Candiduria can, however, lead to ascending infection and systemic candidiasis, especially in patients with obstructive uropathy, and this process should be considered in the persistently febrile patient with candiduria.

Diagnosis

A presumptive diagnosis of UTI can be made based on the presence of typical symptoms and signs, including increased frequency of urination, dysuria, bloody or cloudy urine, suprapubic tenderness, fever or costovertebral pain. A definite diagnosis requires the demonstration of pyuria and bacteriuria. This is accomplished through the urine dipstick test, Gram stain, and in some circumstances, a urine culture.

The urine dipstick test can rapidly check voided urine for pyuria and bacteriuria by detection of leucocyte esterase and nitrite, respectively. The leucocyte esterase test detects pyuria (> 10–20 leucocytes/mL) and indicates inflammation but does not specifically indicate bacterial infection. Generally, it is predictive enough to administer empiric antibiotics to an ambulatory population. For symptomatic patients with a negative leucocyte esterase test result, microscopic evaluation of an unspun urine sample to look for leucocytes is appropriate, and 5 or more leucocytes per high-powered field would indicate pyuria. The urine nitrite dipstick test is highly specific for bacteria but is relatively insensitive. The Gram stain of urine is important for early aetiological assessment. This can be performed on an unspun sample under oil immersion lens, or under the high-dry lens for a centrifuged sample. A finding of more than 20 bacteria per field has a high correlation with the results of urine culture.

In the functionally impaired elderly population and in nursing home residents, special care must be taken in evaluating a urine dipstick test and in the diagnosis of UTI. There is extreme diagnostic uncertainty in impaired elderly patients with regards to UTI, and this uncertainty is responsible for the high rates of often-inappropriate use of antibiotics in this population. In order to prevent clinical dilemmas, urinalysis and culture should not be performed on asymptomatic persons because of the high incidence of asymptomatic bacteriuria. Approximately 30% of elderly nursing home patients have isolated pyuria, and microscopic pyuria or a positive dipstick test result for leucocyte esterase alone are not highly predictive of bacteriuria and true infection. Therefore, pyuria alone is not diagnostic of UTI in this population and cannot be used to differentiate asymptomatic bacteriuria from symptomatic infection since most patients with asymptomatic bacteriuria also have pyuria. However, in conjunction with the acute onset of urinary symptoms, positive results of leucocyte esterase and nitrite tests indicate a high probability for true UTI.

On the other hand, a negative result for pyuria has a high negative predictive value for significant infection, and therefore no urine culture should be requested. The absence of pyuria is useful to exclude a diagnosis of UTI because in patients with symptomatic UTI, the aetiological organism is virtually always accompanied by pyuria. Similarly, a finding of bacteriuria without pyuria should be approached with caution, and if infection of the patient is suspected, this finding should not preclude a search for an alternative source of the infection. Lower UTI alone rarely causes fever, and the positive predictive value of a positive urine culture for patients with fever and no localising symptoms to the urinary tract is low. If urosepsis is suspected, urine and blood cultures should be obtained, and a urine sample should be inspected by Gram stain.

Urine specimens for culture can be collected by a clean-void method in most acutely symptomatic young women and ambulatory elderly. For frail elderly women, who are often unable to provide a midstream urine sample, in-and-out urinary catheterisation may be needed. This method carries a small risk of introducing infection. For elderly men who are functionally well, a midstream urine sample is appropriate and reliable. For functionally impaired men, it is necessary to use a freshly applied clean condom external collection system. If this is done, a quantitative colony count of 10^5 cfu/mL is diagnostic of significant bacteriuria. The use of bedpans for urine collection carries substantial contamination and is not appropriate. For patients with indwelling urinary catheters, the sample should be taken from the catheter port near the entrance to the urethra, not from the collection bag. The value of changing the catheter to obtain a more accurate sample has not been defined and it is not routinely necessary to change the catheter for diagnostic purposes unless obstruction is suspected.

Radiographic tests are generally not indicated for acute uncomplicated UTI. Plain X-rays of the abdomen can demonstrate urinary tract stones, soft tissue masses and gas formations. Ultrasonography can be used to evaluate the urine collecting system and retroperitoneum rapidly, and reliably shows changes consistent with acute pyelonephritis. Computerised tomography is helpful to evaluate the renal parenchyma and surrounding structures for abscesses.

Treatment

Treatment of UTIs has undergone significant changes in recent years and largely depends on the epidemiological setting in which the infection occurs. Treatment recommendations can be divided into five patient groups:

1. women with acute uncomplicated cystitis
2. women with recurrent cystitis
3. women with acute uncomplicated pyelonephritis
4. all adults with complicated UTI
5. all adults with asymptomatic bacteriuria.

Use of empiric antibiotics and duration of therapy depends on the classification of the patient into one of these groups. The ambulatory elderly can be treated under the same guidelines as for younger women. Functionally impaired geriatric patients have a higher incidence of complicated UTI and are often treated for longer periods.

For acutely symptomatic women with cystitis, an abbreviated laboratory analysis, such as simply a dipstick test for pyuria without culture is generally sufficient. It is often prudent also to perform a pretreatment urine culture in ambulatory elderly patients because they often have received courses of antibiotics for other conditions and have a higher likelihood of being infected with a resistant or unusual organism. It is essential to perform pretreatment urine cultures in elderly patients with symptomatic urinary-catheter-related or nosocomial infections. In fully functional patients, treatment can generally be accomplished with a 3-day course of empiric antibiotics, such as with trimethoprim-sulphamethoxazole or a fluoroquinolone, which eradicate *E. coli*, *S. saprophyticus*, *Proteus mirabilis* and *Klebsiella pneumoniae*. Trimethoprim-sulphamethoxazole is given as a double-strength tablet (160/400 mg) every 12 hours. Trimethoprim alone at 200 mg every 12 hours is an equivalent treatment and may have fewer adverse effects than trimethoprim-sulphamethoxazole. Various fluoroquinolones, such as ofloxacin, have been demonstrated to be as effective as trimethoprim-sulphamethoxazole for 3-day courses, as are norfloxacin or ciprofloxacin, but resistance across fluoroquinolone agents is common. Fluoroquinolones are more expensive than trimethoprim-sulphamethoxazole or trimethoprim, and should be reserved for use in patient populations with rates of bacterial resistance greater than 10%. Newer fluoroquinolones with increased activity against respiratory pathogens should not be routinely given for UTI because of the risk of emergence of resistance, which may limit their usefulness for non-urinary infections in the future. Nitrofurantoin sustained-release form (monohydrate macrocrystals) is given at 100 mg every 12 hours but is contraindicated in patients with renal failure. In the US, fosfomycin (a phosphonic acid derivative) given as a single oral dose for uncomplicated cystitis may be useful if resistance to other agents is high. Single-dose therapy with any agent is generally less effective than a 3-day course but can be used early in the disease, and this strategy is known to decrease adverse events. In general, β-lactam agents are less effective for UTI than the agents mentioned above. For patients with diabetes mellitus, a recent history of UTI, or who are older than 65 years (especially men), a 7–10 day course of antibiotics may be more appropriate. Definitive studies of the optimal duration of treatment for uncomplicated cystitis in the ambulatory elderly (>65 years of age) are lacking. For elderly patients in long-term care facilities, a minimum duration of 7 days' treatment is standard.

Treatment recommendations must be interpreted in the light of local patterns of resistance in circulating uropathogens. In some parts of the world, significant levels of resistance to trimethoprim-sulphamethoxazole are emerging, and specific recommendations for antibiotics must depend on local patterns. For example, in Seattle, the prevalence of resistance to trimethoprim-sulphamethoxazole was approximately 20% in 1996 in isolates from women with uncomplicated cystitis. Similarly, resistance to fluoroquinolones has been documented to be increasing and is likely to continue to increase as their use increases. It is important to recognise treatment failure early so urine cultures can be collected and antibiotics changed as necessary.

Antibiotics must be given with care to a geriatric population. Drug–drug interactions are common and must be managed appropriately. For example, the ototoxicity of aminoglycosides is increased in patients taking loop diuretics. Some fluoroquinolones increase theophylline levels, and trimethoprim can increase levels of digoxin. Side effects are also more common in the elderly due to the physiological effects of ageing on the kidney, liver and brain (see Chapter 5).

Recurrences of UTI are fairly common and most represent a reinfection rather than persistence or relapse of the same offending organism. Simple reinfections can be treated with short course therapy as described above. For patients with infrequent recurrences, patient-initiated therapy is an option. For frequently recurrent cystitis (more than 2 UTIs per year) in women, treatment with a continuous or post-coital prophylaxis may be appropriate. This can be accomplished with trimethoprim, trimethoprim-sulphamethoxazole or a fluoroquinolone. Unfortunately, recurrences resume once prophylaxis is stopped. Methenamine or similar urinary antiseptics can be used for prophylaxis but require an acidic urine to be effective. The daily ingestion of cranberry juice has been proposed to decrease bacteriuria in elderly patients (presumably because of the bacteriostatic nature of hippuric acid) but currently there is no clear evidence that this decreases the incidence of symptomatic or asymptomatic infections and cannot be recommended universally. There are also no randomised trials that have evaluated the effectiveness of cranberry juice for the treatment of UTI. In postmenopausal ambulatory women, intravaginal oestrogen has been shown to reduce the incidence of recurrent UTI significantly. This occurs by decreasing the amount of vaginal colonisation by *E. coli*, re-establishing the lactobacillus population, and decreasing the vaginal fluid pH. Topical oestrogens can be a very effective strategy to reduce UTI in the functionally unimpaired geriatric population. The role of intravaginal oestrogen in institutionalised elderly patients is less clear.

For acute uncomplicated pyelonephritis, oral therapy with a fluoroquinolone or trimethoprim-sulphamethoxazole for 7–14 days is recommended. Severe cases should be treated for 14 days, and mild-to-moderate disease can be treated for 7 days. In addition to a urine dipstick test, a urine culture is mandated in all cases of suspected pyelonephritis to document the aetiological agent and antimicrobial sensitivity pattern. Initial treatment with a fluoroquinolone is recommended by most authors, with trimethoprim-sulphamethoxazole reserved for patients infected with an organism known to be susceptible to this agent. It is common practice to initiate treatment with a single dose of intravenous antibiotics (ceftriaxone, gentamicin or a fluoroquinolone) prior to oral therapy, but this strategy has not been studied systematically. If the urine Gram stain indicates possible infection with a Gram-positive organism, amoxicillin or amoxicillin/clavulanic acid is recommended.

Admission to hospital and parenteral antibiotic therapy may be necessary if the patient is nauseated or vomiting and cannot tolerate oral therapy, has otherwise toxic symptoms, or has an underlying illness such as diabetes mellitus. Blood culture should also be obtained in this setting. If the patient requires hospitalisation and the urine Gram stain indicates possible infection with *Enterococcus* or another Gram-positive organism, intravenous ampicillin/sulbactam (a combination of an aminopenicillin and a synthetic penicillamate sulphone with β-lactamase inhibitory activity) with or without an aminoglycoside is recommended as empiric treatment until culture results are returned. If the causative organism is Gram-negative, a fluoroquinolone, an aminoglycoside with or without ampicillin, an extended-spectrum penicillin with a β-lactamase inhibitor, or a third-generation cephalosporin with or without an aminoglycoside is adequate. Once the patient is improved, a prompt change to an oral antibiotic to which the organism is susceptible is indicated to complete the treatment. If fever and flank pain persist for more than 72 hours, evaluation for perinephric abscess is indicated, and if present, may require surgical drainage. Any foreign bodies present in the urinary system usually require removal for successful treatment of pyelonephritis.

For patients with complicated UTI, therapy usually must be guided by the results of urine cultures to obtain the aetiological organism and antibiotic sensitivity because of the wide variety of infecting organisms and variable antimicrobial susceptibilities. In selecting empiric antibiotics, coverage against *Enterococcus* and *Pseudomonas* should be provided while awaiting culture results. Usually a fluoroquinolone such as levofloxacin or ciprofloxacin is recommended for initial empiric therapy, unless prior culture results from a patient indicate possible infection with a fluoroquinolone-resistant organism. In cases of complicated UTI, it is often necessary to correct an anatomical abnormality if possible and certainly remove or at a minimum change an indwelling urinary catheter if present. In general, any obstruction or foreign body must be removed for successful eradication of the aetiological agent. Otherwise, recurrence of the UTI may follow successful initial treatment. For cases of complicated UTI, a treatment course of 10–14 days is the minimum for women, but may require longer treatment, 14–28 days, for men because of the possibility of prostate gland involvement. If the anatomical abnormality (e.g. a stone) cannot be corrected, it is often best not to attempt suppressive therapy as this will inevitably lead to infection with resistant bacteria. In these instances, it is best to treat only when acute symptoms develop.

As stated previously, asymptomatic bacteriuria in a geriatric population is common and does not generally require treatment in the absence of underlying structural or functional abnormalities. The risk for subsequent renal damage is minimal, and the treatment toxicities and costs are substantial. Treatment of asymptomatic bacteriuria does not decrease the frequency of subsequent symptomatic episodes, does not decrease incontinence, and has no demonstrable survival benefit and is therefore not indicated. Only if the patient develops signs and symptoms of active infection should antibiotics be used.

There are a few important exceptions to this general rule. Eradicating asymptomatic bacteriuria in pregnancy will reduce the risk of acute pyelonephritis and prematurity of the newborn. Though no definitive data exist, a 3-day course of oral antibiotics should be sufficient. Patients undergoing urologic surgery or procedures and renal transplant recipients also benefit from eradication of asymptomatic bacteriuria. Finally, treatment may be considered in elderly patients with underlying diseases such as neutropenia, diabetes or structural or functional abnormalities of the urinary tract that would make them more likely to have a complicated UTI should they develop a symptomatic UTI.

Treatment of asymptomatic bacteriuria in these situations must be individualised.

Indwelling catheter-associated bacteriuria is commonly a polymicrobial process, often involving such bacterial organisms as *Providencia*, *Proteus* and *Morganella* in addition to the usual uropathogens. In general, antibiotics should not be used for asymptomatic bacteriuria in the setting of catheterisation because this will simply foster bacterial resistance. However, the same exceptions as discussed above for non-catheterised patients would apply here as well. Antibiotics directed at the organisms isolated in urine or blood culture are indicated in cases of symptomatic UTI in catheterised patients. Clinical and bacteriological outcomes have recently been shown to improve if the catheter is replaced prior to antimicrobial therapy. A treatment duration of 10–14 days is usually enough. Silver alloy catheters can reduce the incidence of UTI by three-fold, and may be cost-effective in short-term catheterisation but their efficacy in long-term catheterisation has been mixed. An alternative for indwelling catheters has been the use of intermittent clean catheterisation, which may decrease febrile episodes and bacteraemia in patients from indwelling catheters.

For asymptomatic candiduria in the non-neutropenic patient with an indwelling urinary catheter, specific antifungal treatment is not indicated and the first step should be to remove or at least change the indwelling catheter. It must be remembered that candiduria rarely may be the only clue to occult disseminated candidiasis, and this can be an important clinical clue in the patient with persistent occult fever. Candiduria should be treated in symptomatic patients especially with positive leucocyte esterase test results, in neutropenic patients, in diabetic patients, or in patients who will soon undergo urologic manipulations. This should be treated as a complicated UTI, and therefore therapy for 7–14 days is recommended. Removal of all urinary instruments is often essential to successful eradication of the organism. Fluconazole (oral or intravenous) at 200 mg per day for 7–14 days is recommended as the initial treatment. For non-*albicans Candida* species, oral flucytosine at a dose of 25 mg per kg 4 times daily may be of benefit, but this must be used with caution in elderly patients due to the difficulty in measuring drug levels and the risk of resulting cytopenias. The use of flucytosine as a single agent is discouraged due to the rapid emergence of resistant organisms. Bladder irrigation with amphotericin B (50–200 μg/mL) is rarely indicated and does not treat infection above the level of the bladder. Relapse of candiduria is very common, especially if an indwelling catheter is maintained. Unnecessary treatment of asymptomatic candiduria may select for resistant organisms and is discouraged.

Unfortunately, modifiable risk factors for UTI in a geriatric population are limited. Intravaginal oestrogen may decrease UTI recurrence in postmenopausal women. Certainly, the use of indwelling catheters must be minimised to those in whom it is absolutely necessary. Understanding of the phenomenon of asymptomatic bacteriuria will limit overuse of antibiotics and possibly decrease the incidence of infection with resistant pathogens. However, much remains to be learned about the pathogenesis, treatment and prevention of UTI.

Bibliography and further reading

Ackermann, R. J. & Monroe, P. W. (1996), 'Bacteremic urinary tract infection in older people', *Journal of the American Geriatrics Society*, 44, pp. 927–33.

Hooton, T. M. (2000), 'Pathogenesis of urinary tract infections: an update', *Journal of Antimicrobial Chemotherapy*, 46(suppl. 1), pp. 1–7.

Kunin, C. M. (1997), *Urinary Tract Infections, Detection, Prevention, and Management*, 5th edn, Williams & Wilkins, Baltimore, MD.

Nicolle, L. E. (1997), 'Asymptomatic bacteriuria in the elderly', *Infectious Disease Clinics of North America*, 11, pp. 647–62.

Nicolle, L. E. (2000), 'Urinary tract infection in long-term care facility residents', *Clinical Infectious Diseases*, 31, pp. 757–61.

Sobel, J. D. (1999), 'Management of asymptomatic candiduria', *International Journal of Antimicrobial Agents*, 11, pp. 285–8.

Sobel, J. D. & Kaye, D. (2000), 'Urinary tract infections', in Mandell, G. L., Bennett, J. E. & Dolin, R. (eds), *Principles and Practice of Infectious Diseases*, 5th edn, Churchill Livingstone, Philadelphia, pp. 773–805.

Warren, J. W. (1997), 'Catheter-associated urinary tract infections', *Infectious Disease Clinics of North America*, 11, pp. 609–22.

Warren, J. W., Abrutyn, E., Hebel, J. R., et al. (1999), 'Guidelines for antimicrobial treatment of uncomplicated acute bacterial cystitis and acute pyelonephritis in women', *Clinical Infectious Diseases*, 29, pp. 745–58.

Wise, G. J. & Silver, D. A. (1993), 'Fungal infections of the genitourinary system', *Journal of Urology*, 149, pp. 1377–88.

Part XI

Musculoskeletal conditions

Chapter 52
The painful shoulder

PETER NASH and KEVIN PILE

Introduction

Soft tissue rheumatism typified by disorders affecting the shoulder has been, in the main, poorly studied in all age groups, particularly the elderly. There has been a paucity of quality randomised trials so that disease definition, clinical 'diagnostic' tests, their interpretation and recommendations for therapy are often based more on dogma than on hard clinical evidence.

Nevertheless, conditions that cause shoulder pain are common, increase in frequency with age and contribute substantially to the musculoskeletal morbidity of the community. Studies of acute admissions of the elderly to an aged care facility not only demonstrated that 1 in 5 had symptomatic shoulder disease but only 1 in 30 had sought medical attention for the problem. Sleep-disturbing night pain was common and chronicity the norm. A community study of the elderly has found that 26% have current shoulder pain, of which three-quarters of patients have rotator cuff disease. Chronicity again was present, with symptom duration from 19 to 50 months, and only one-third had reported their symptoms to their doctor. When these patient populations are followed up to 3 years later:

- three-quarters of the patients had persisting signs
- two-thirds of the patients had not improved or had worsened
- up to one-quarter of patients had impairment of personal care and difficulty with household tasks
- one-third of patients had pain with movement
- the authors concluded that treatment in a community setting had little effect on the long-term prognosis.

The following discussion aims to describe the clinical features of some of the more common problems affecting the shoulder.

Incidence and risk factors

Shoulder pain is an almost unavoidable life experience, with 7% of an adult population aged 25–75 years in one study reporting at least 1 month's shoulder pain over the previous year. The peak annual incidence of shoulder disorders is in the fourth and fifth decades, at a rate of 2.5%. A Dutch study found that 25% of all 85 year olds in Leiden suffered from chronic shoulder pain and restriction.

Community-based surveys concur with this high incidence of soft tissue lesions about the shoulder, with roughly equal sex incidence. Up to 20% of patients with chronic symptoms and 65% of all diagnoses relate to lesions of the rotator cuff. Indeed, post-mortem studies reveal 20% of all shoulders have full thickness rotator cuff rupture. An ultrasound study found rotator cuff tears in 13% of 50–59 year olds, 20% of 60–69 year olds, 31% of 70–79 year olds, and 51% of over 80 year olds even when they were asymptomatic.

Risk factors for shoulder disorders include trauma, surgery, intravenous infusion, impaired consciousness, diabetes mellitus, thyroid diseases, occupation as well as underlying inflammatory rheumatic diseases such as rheumatoid arthritis. Ergonomic factors in acute shoulder complaints include prolonged duration of forward and outward flexion of the arm.

Aetiology

The causes of shoulder pain can be considered in three categories (Table 52.1).

Table 52.1 Causes of shoulder pain

Category	Cause
Extracapsular lesions	Pain arising in the rotator cuff and subacromial bursa (e.g. impingement syndromes, calcific tendinitis, cuff tears, bursitis)
Intracapsular lesions	Pain arising from the glenohumeral joint (e.g. osteoarthritis, sepsis, inflammatory arthritis like rheumatoid arthritis, seronegative spondyloarthritis, gout and pseudogout) or joint capsule (e.g. adhesive capsulitis), and disease of bone (e.g. Paget's disease or metastases)
Referred pain	Pain referred from cervical spine (e.g. facet joint root impingement, tumour), brachial plexus (e.g. brachial amyotrophy), thorax (e.g. Pancoast's tumour), thoracic outlet syndrome, suprascapular nerve entrapment and subdiaphragmatic abnormalities (e.g. abscess, blood, hepatic lesions)

1. Lesions that arise from extracapsular structures (e.g. the rotator cuff and subacromial bursa) are characterised by:
   (a) a painful arc of abduction
   (b) pain on resisted cuff muscle movements with intact passive movements allowing for pain and guarding
   (c) pain produced by impingement tests as the inflamed rotator cuff tendons impinge on the inferior surface of the acromion and coracoacromial arch.
2. Intracapsular lesions produce loss of both active and passive range of movement as well as a reduction in glenohumeral range. Night pain is common and muscle strength, allowing for pain, is intact.
3. Referred pain to the shoulder region (Figure 52.1) is a common clinical problem in the elderly, where cervical abnormalities, in particular, are so common. Suggestive features pointing to referred pain as the problem include:
   (a) arm and hand pain and paraesthesia
   (b) marked muscle wasting and weakness
   (c) neck pain and stiffness
   (d) abdominal pain
   (e) weight loss
   (f) herpes zoster rash
   (g) systemic features.

The localisation of pain may be diagnostically helpful. The pain-sensitive structures of the shoulder are mainly innervated by the fifth cervical (C5) segment, so that pain from these structures is referred to the C5 dermatome, creating the sensation of pain over the anterior arm, especially the deltoid insertion (Figure 52.2). The acromioclavicular joint is innervated by the C4 segment, so that pain arising here is felt at the joint itself and radiates over the top of the shoulder into the trapezius muscle and up the side of the neck (Figure 52.3). Pain at the shoulder tip suggests pain arising from diaphragmatic irritation (Figure 52.4).

Clinical assessment

The history, an examination and simple imaging allow diagnosis in shoulder problems like few other areas of clinical medicine.

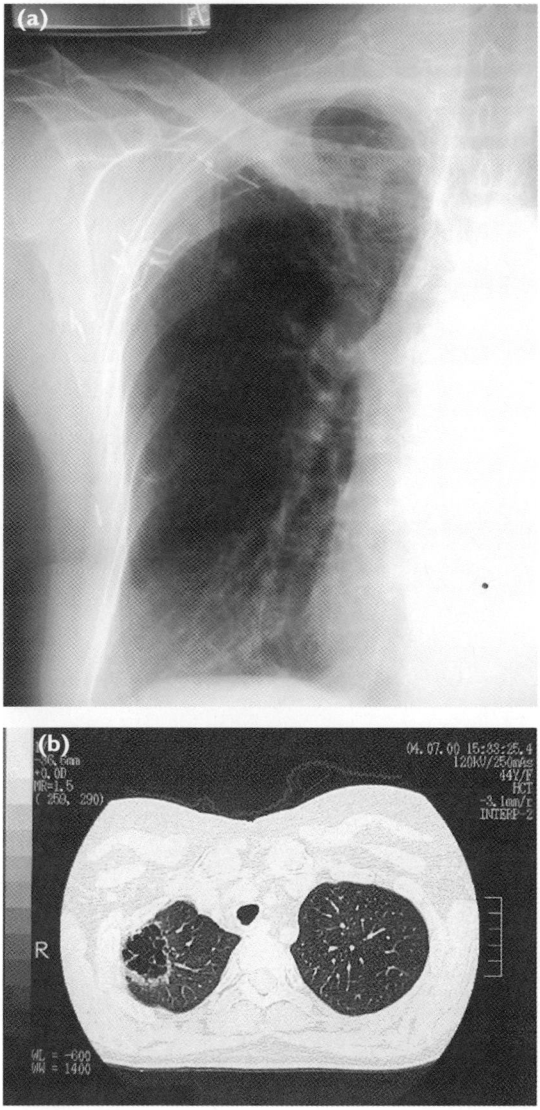

Figure 52.1 Pain referred to the right shoulder from a pulmonary abnormality. **(a)** Chest X-ray shows the right upper lobe infiltrates and clips from axillary surgery. **(b)** Chest CT scan showing cavitating right upper lobe lesion

History

An accurate history is the cornerstone of the clinical assessment and the diagnostic clues to be sought are listed in Box 52.1. In the elderly, a history of trauma, marked night pain and weakness on resisted abduction strongly suggests a rotator cuff tear. The sleeping position that induces night pain is an

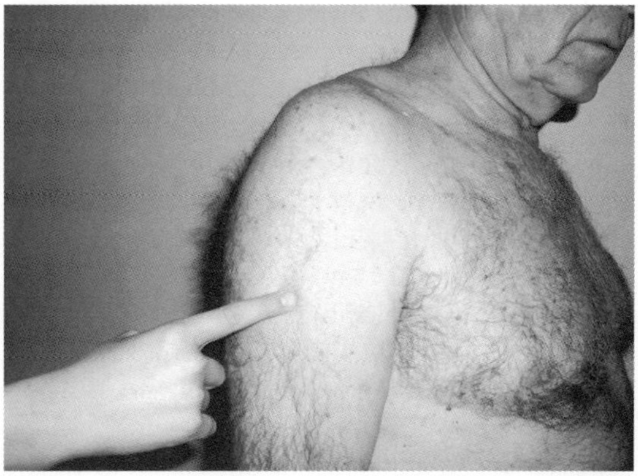

Figure 52.2 Pain is referred to the deltoid insertion from shoulder structures innervated by C5 nerve roots

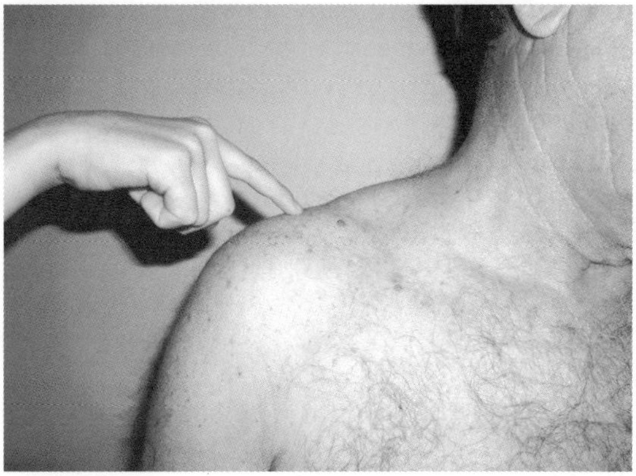

Figure 52.3 Pain referred to the acromioclavicular joint, which is innervated by the C4 segment, is felt over the joint and into the neck

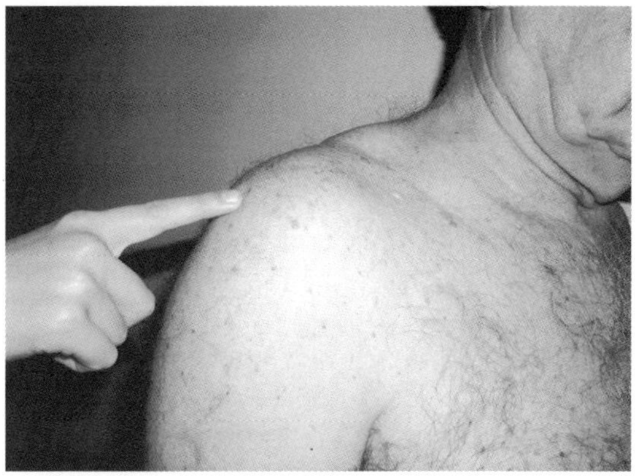

Figure 52.4 Pain referred to the shoulder tip is from a subdiaphragmatic abnormality

important clue in the history. True night pain that results in awakening as a result of a painful shoulder when *not* lying on that shoulder is found in frozen shoulder (adhesive capsulitis) and inflammatory arthritis. Night pain when lying on the affected shoulder is seen in acromioclavicular joint disease and rotator cuff disease. Prior shoulder problems suggest rotator cuff disease with chronic impingement, or calcific tendinitis and recurrent dislocation after trauma. It is a useful rule that frozen shoulder does not recur in the same shoulder. A history of marked shoulder joint swelling suggests an inflammatory arthropathy, with the presence of an anterior bulge in the shoulder, usually secondary to a subacromial bursal effusion. Glenohumeral joint osteoarthritis is characterised by morning stiffness, pain with use and chronicity of symptoms. Osteoarthritis, however, is significantly less common than rotator cuff dysfunction.

Box 52.1 Historical clues in the evaluation of shoulder pain

- History of trauma
- Prior shoulder problems
- Presence of night pain and nocturnal awakening
- Sleep position inducing pain
- Response to corticosteroid injection
- Occupation
- Dead arm of dislocation
- Presence and localisation of shoulder swelling
- Medical history: inflammatory arthritis (e.g. rheumatoid arthritis, Paget's disease (Figure 52.5), metastases)

(a)

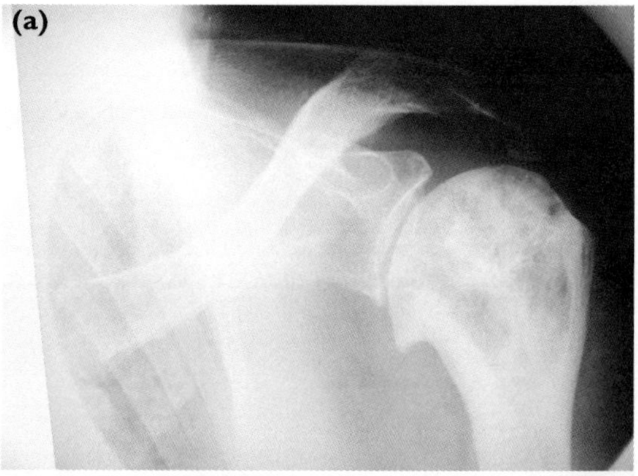

Figure 52.5 (a) Plain X-ray of the left shoulder demonstrating Paget's disease of the humeral head, with enlargement and alteration of the bony texture. **(b)** Bone scan showing widespread Paget's disease, notably in the left humerus, right patella and right tibia

(b)

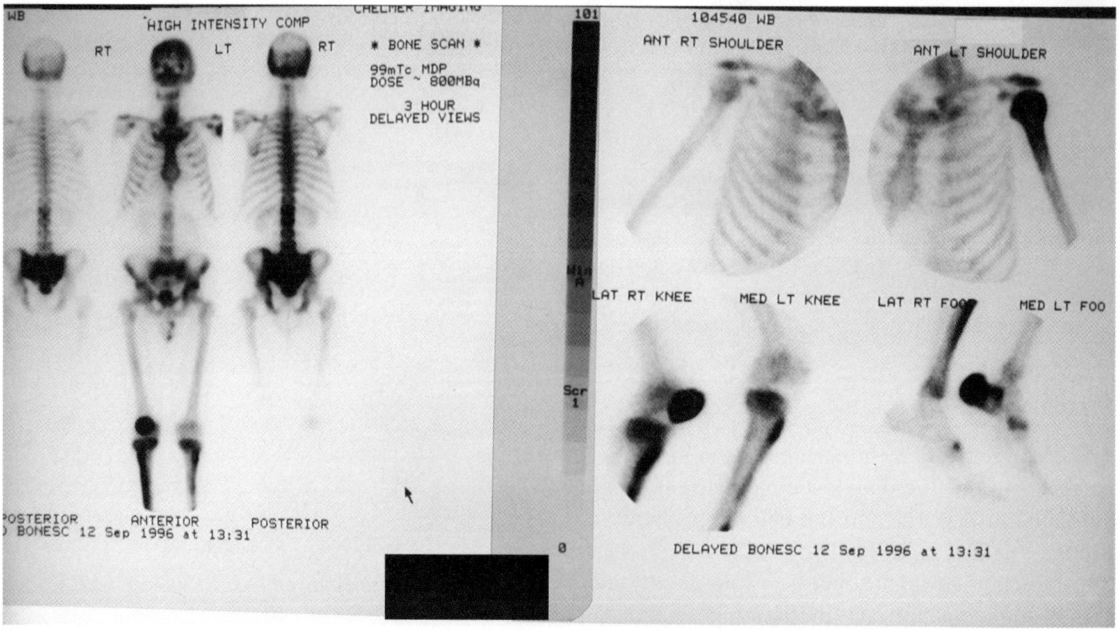

Examination

Examination of the shoulder is best undertaken with males undressed to the waist and women to their bra. The patient may be examined standing or sitting in a chair without arms, which allows full arm movement. The contours of the shoulder should be inspected, noting in women any depression in the trapezius muscles from bra straps. On inspection, look for muscle wasting (Figure 52.6), the result of chronic rotator cuff tear or longstanding glenohumeral joint osteoarthritis. Fasciculations are highly suggestive of cervical disc abnormality, motor neuron disease or brachial amyotrophy (Figure 52.7). Inspect also for rupture of the long head of biceps (Figure 52.8), and the rash of acute herpes zoster infection. After inspection, palpation should proceed from the sternoclavicular joint along the clavicle to the acromioclavicular joint, to the tip of the acromion and the humeral head beneath the acromion. Stressing the acromioclavicular joint can diagnose degenerative problems at this site.

The shoulder range of movement should be examined both passively and actively, with muscle strength and pain on resistance assessed. Active movement should be undertaken first, with the doctor demonstrating the required movements. This allows comparison with your hopefully normal self, and both left and right shoulders in the patient. Complete rotator cuff tears will show no active abduction but near full range when passively moved. During the examination, ask about a painful arc during abduction (Figure 52.9). Abduction of the shoulder includes movement of the glenohumeral joint as well as scapulothoracic movement. The latter can be successfully used in 'trick' movements to overcome significant restriction of the glenohumeral joint. When examining active and passive abduction, you should stand behind the patient and place one hand over the shoulder and scapula. The scapula should not begin to elevate or rotate until at least 90 degrees of abduction has been reached. Early scapulothoracic movement localises the abnormality to the glenohumeral joint or capsule as seen in frozen shoulder (Figure 52.10).

There are essentially three movements to test in the shoulder (Figures 52.11–52.13): abduction due to supraspinatus contraction, external rotation as a

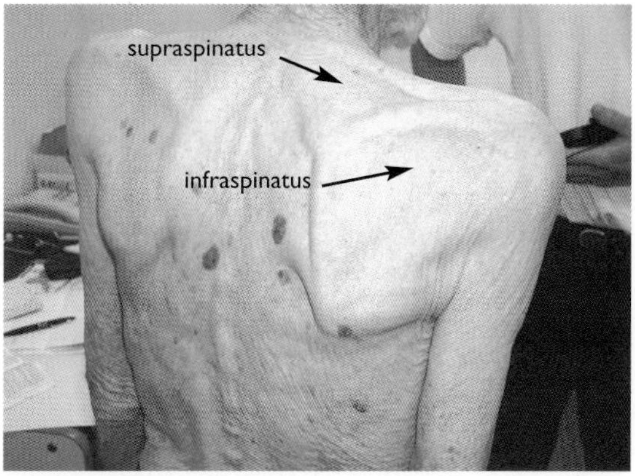

Figure 52.6 Wasting of the supraspinatus and infraspinatus muscles

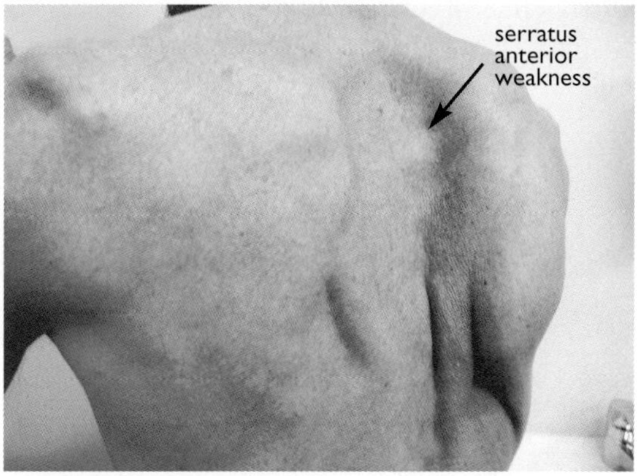

Figure 52.7 Winging of the scapula secondary to weakness of the serratus anterior, due to involvement of the long thoracic nerve

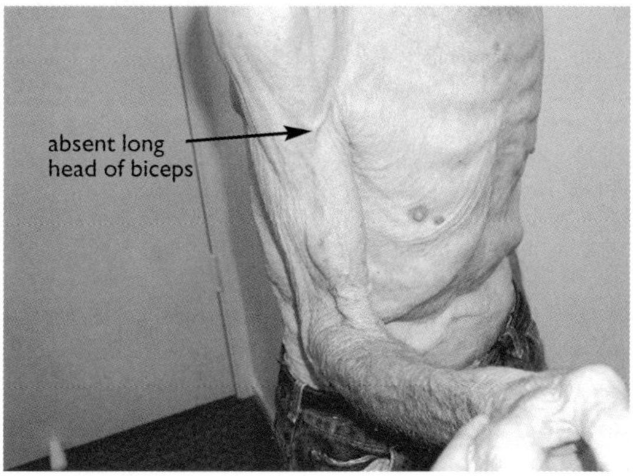

Figure 52. 8 Ruptured long head of biceps

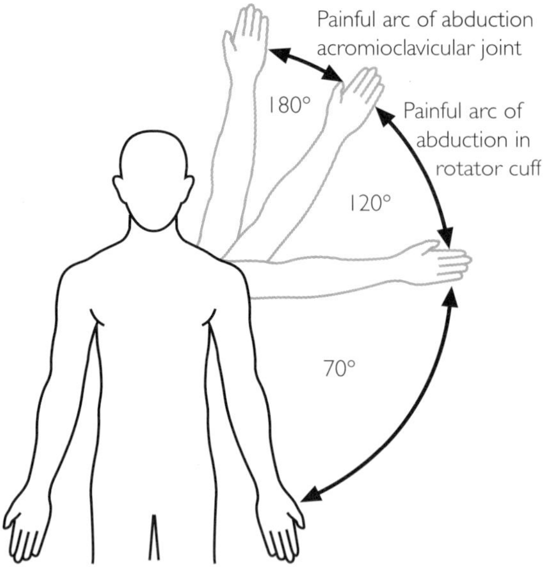

Figure 52.9 Painful arc. The patient slowly abducts the arm as high as possible, describing symptoms as the arm rises

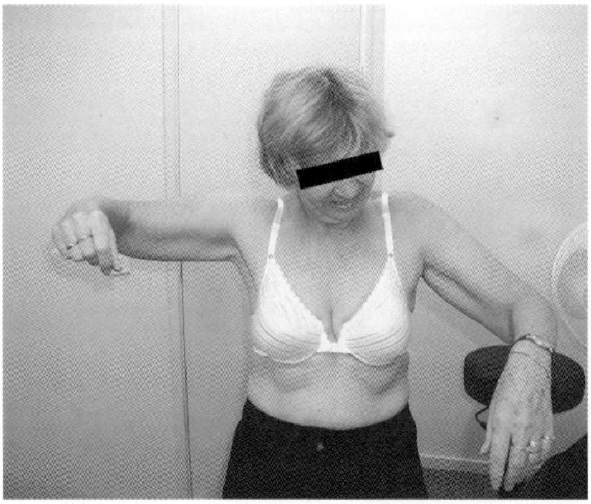

Figure 52.10 Reduced left glenohumeral range, as in frozen shoulder or glenohumeral joint osteoarthritis (ipsilateral girdle lifts when abduction attempted)

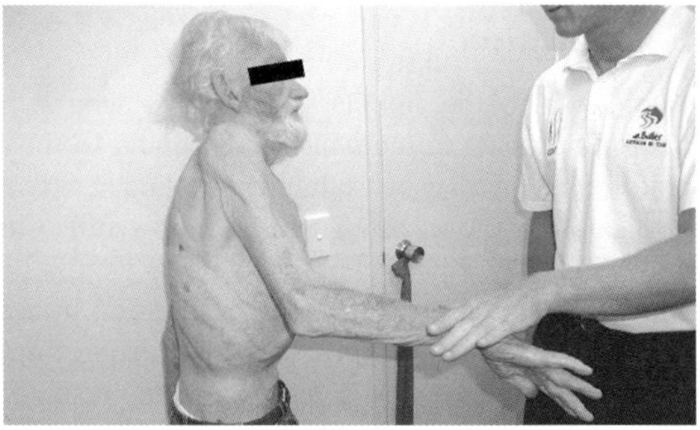

Figure 52.11 Testing supraspinatus strength and pain on resistance. The patient's arm is abducted with the elbow flexed and the patient asked to empty an imaginary can of beer. The examiner attempts to adduct the arm

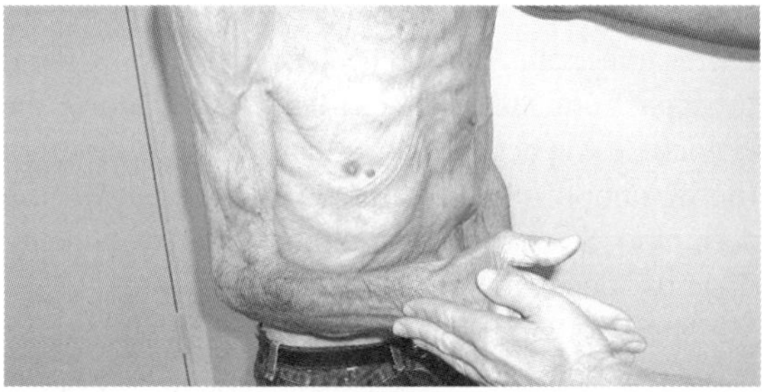

Figure 52.12 Testing infraspinatus strength and pain on resistance. The patient's elbow remains at the side, and the patient attempts to externally rotate the shoulder, which is resisted by the examiner

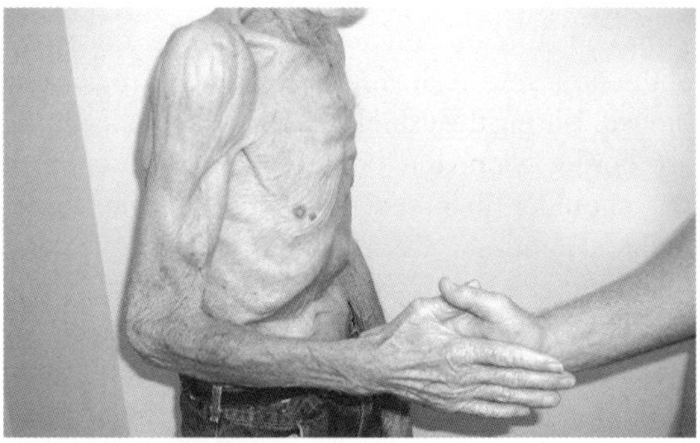

Figure 52.13 Testing subscapularis strength and pain on resistance. The patient's elbow should be at the side, and the patient attempts to internally rotate the shoulder, which is resisted by the examiner

result of infraspinatus and teres minor movement, and internal rotation due to subscapularis movement. Maximal internal rotation is evaluated by having the patient place the hand behind the back, and is notably restricted in glenohumeral joint and capsular abnormalities. You should examine external rotation at 0 degrees abduction, with the elbow beside the chest, and if external rotation is absent, then a frozen shoulder is likely (Figures 52.14). Next re-examine both internal and external rotation at 90 degrees abduction and if both are restricted, a frozen shoulder is again likely. Bicipital tendinitis is examined by testing resisted flexion at 30 degrees external rotation and feeling for tenderness in the bicipital groove.

Shoulder impingement can be reproduced by internally rotating the arm held flexed at 90 degrees and bringing the inflamed rotator cuff against the anterior acromion (Figure 52.15). The 'empty can' test is suggestive of a rotator cuff tear, and shows pain on resisted elevation of the inverted arm held extended at 90 degrees, as if emptying a can of drink (Figure 52.16), while the lift-off test is suggestive of a subscapularis tear, and shows resisted lift of the extended arm off the buttock (Figure 52.17). Apprehension testing in the recurrent dislocator and instability testing in the chronic impinger are more relevant to the young and the athlete. When there is a history of trauma along with painful clunking, lesions of the glenoid labrum need to be considered.

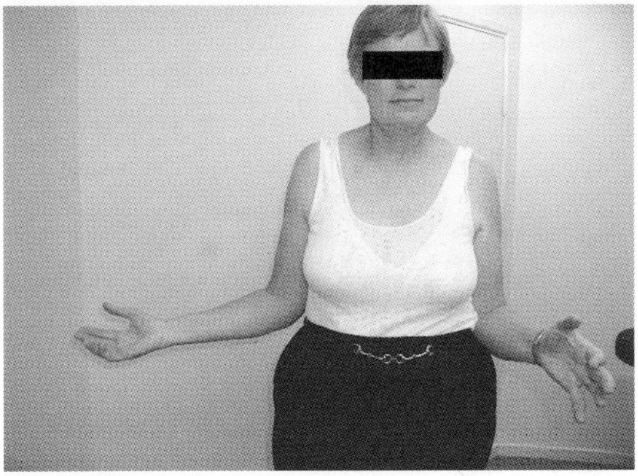

Figure 52.14 Loss of left external rotation at 0 degrees abduction, typical of frozen shoulder or significant glenohumeral osteoarthritis

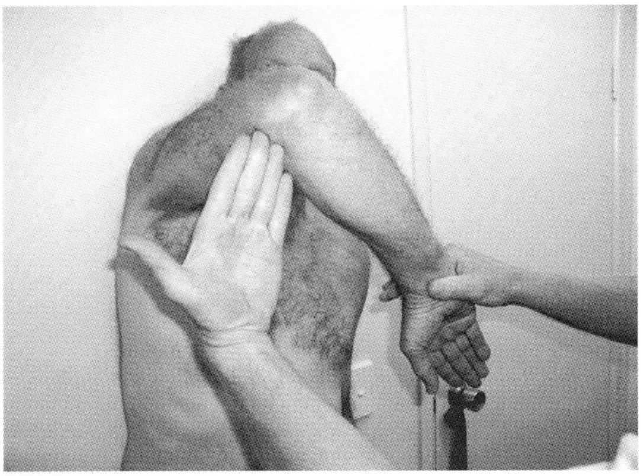

Figure 52.15 Testing for anterior impingement

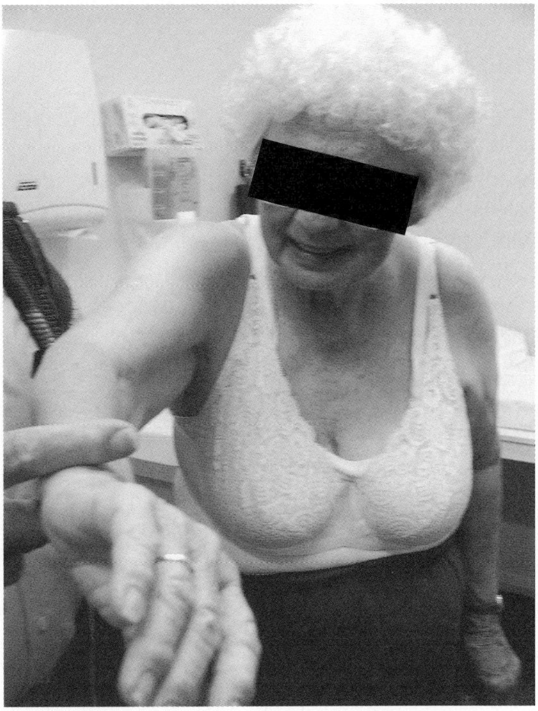

Figure 52.16 The 'empty can' test—rotator cuff tear

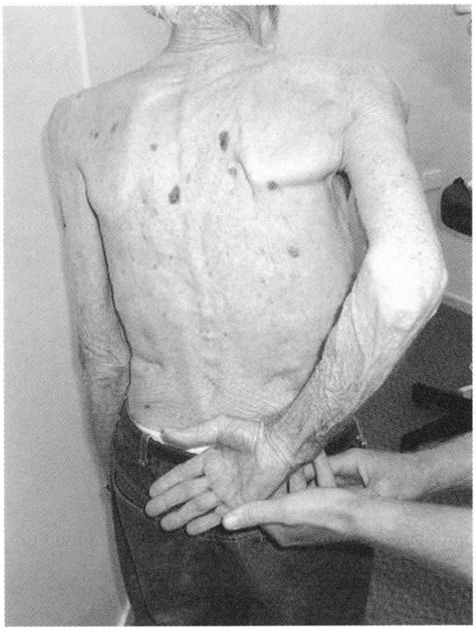

Figure 52.17 The lift-off test—subscapularis tear

Imaging

All imaging modalities have been used to assess shoulder disorders but in the majority of patients, depending upon the clinical features, ultrasound with plain X-ray is all that is generally necessary.

Plain radiography

Plain radiography is simple, quick, cheap and readily available. You can expect plain radiography to demonstrate: fractures, glenohumeral joint osteoarthritis, changes of chronic rotator cuff disease with superior migration of the humeral head, rotator cuff calcification in calcific tendinitis, chondrocalcinosis, joint erosions and effusions, loose bodies, Paget's disease, lytic lesions from infection and both primary and secondary neoplasia. In the setting of recurrent dislocation (Figure 52.18), the presence of a compression fracture of the posterior aspect of the humeral head (Hill-Sach's lesion) is diagnostically helpful. Three varieties of acromial shape are noted on plain X-ray: flat, curved and hooked. The hooked acromion predisposes to rotator cuff impingement and degenerative changes of the acromioclavicular joint, including inferior subacromial spurs.

Ultrasound

Ultrasound (Figures 52.19, 52.20) has evolved as an important diagnostic tool as most clinical problems, especially in the elderly, relate to rotator cuff abnormalities. Ultrasound is cheap, quick and

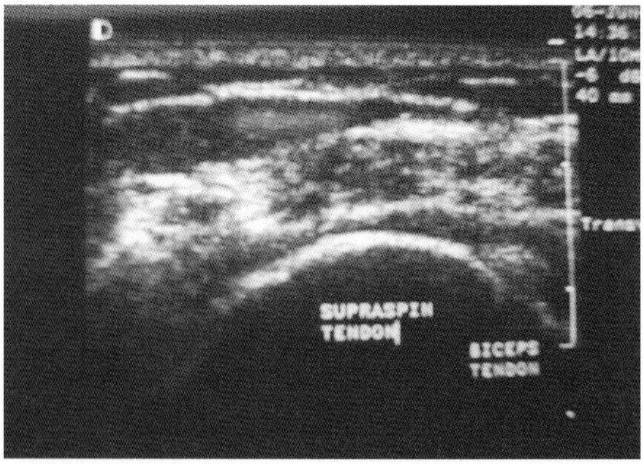

Figure 52.19 Ultrasound showing the supraspinatus tendon and biceps tendon

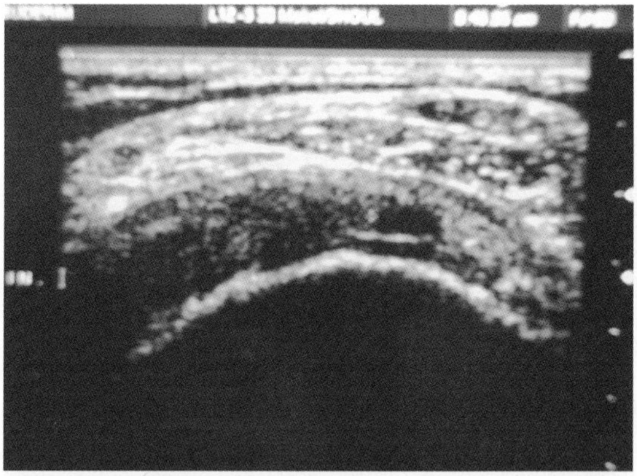

Figure 52.20 Ultrasound showing full thickness supraspinatus tear

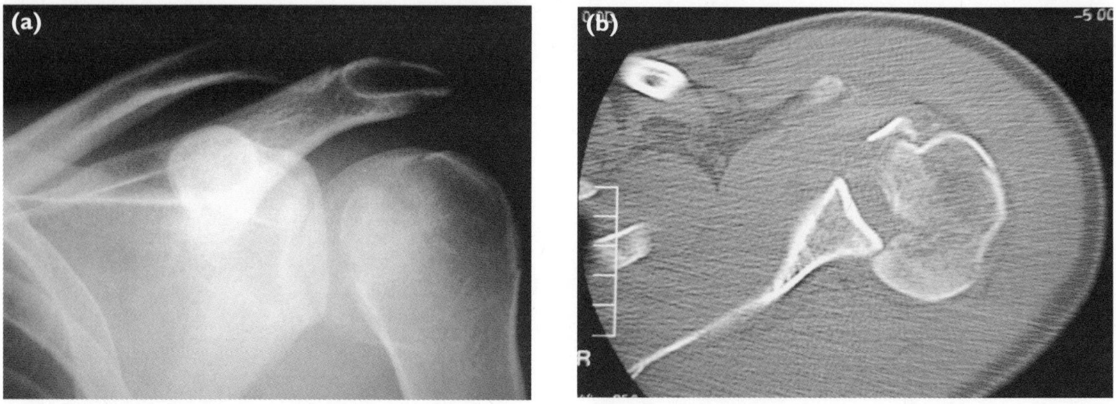

Figure 52.18 (a) Plain X-ray showing posterior dislocation of the shoulder in an epileptic patient. **(b)** CT scan showing posterior dislocation and compression fracture of the humeral head

readily available but is a very operator-dependent examination. If the clinical features strongly suggest rotator cuff tear (i.e. history of trauma, night pain, abduction weakness) but the ultrasound is clear or equivocal, further imaging with either arthrography or magnetic resonance imaging (MRI) with gadolinium may be necessary if this will alter clinical management. As with all investigations, the results must be interpreted in the individual patient. Rotator cuff tears are extremely common in the elderly and the clinical symptoms must match before undue significance is placed on the radiology report. Suprascapular notch cysts are easily demonstrated by ultrasound but the operator needs to be alerted to examine the appropriate area and given a suggestive clinical scenario (i.e. manual worker or sportsperson involved in repetitive above-head loading, posterior shoulder pain, marked infraspinatus weakness and wasting) (Figure 52.21).

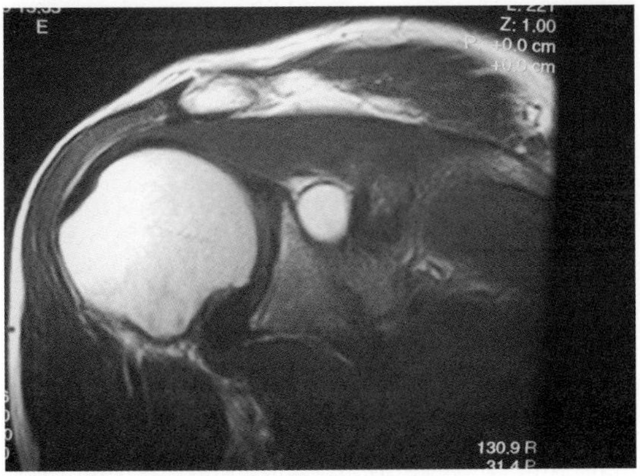

Figure 52.21 Suprascapular notch cyst demonstrated with MRI (although ultrasound is the preferred method)

Arthrography

This investigation remains the gold standard for diagnosis of full thickness rotator cuff tears. However, due to its invasiveness and discomfort, it is likely to be replaced by MRI, with its superior soft tissue imaging of lesions about the cuff as well as being able to demonstrate intra-substance/partial tears. Arthrography will continue to have a role for the very claustrophobic patient where it is important to know if the cuff has a full-thickness tear. It is also helpful diagnostically and occasionally therapeutically in cases of frozen shoulder, where a reduced capsular volume is seen and distension with dye can produce pain relief suggested to be by 'breaking' adhesions. In patients with frozen shoulder, arthrography is painful and is not generally required for a clinical diagnosis, and if required should be performed under mild anaesthesia. Subacromial bursography is rarely required, adding little information to that gained by ultrasound.

MRI and CT imaging

Both MRI and computerised tomography (CT) are relatively expensive and are only indicated if the results will alter management. MRI (often with intra-articular gadolinium) (Figure 52.22) is becoming the investigation of choice in the complicated patient requiring soft tissue imaging, particularly of intra-substance and partial cuff tears. It may also have a role in identifying lesions of the ligamentous/labral complex, bone and joint cysts, as well as assessment of the symptomatic post-surgical patient. CT scanning generally with intra-articular contrast is utilised when MRI is not available.

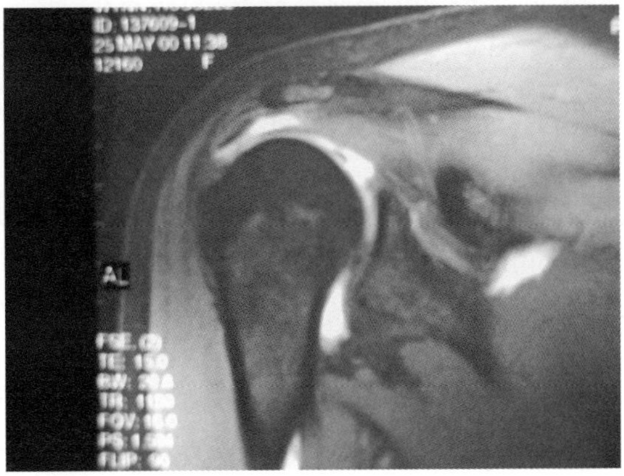

Figure 52.22 MRI with gadolinium showing intra-substance cuff tear

Presentations

Rotator cuff disease

The glenohumeral joint is, by virtue of its anatomical shape, inherently unstable, relying on the joint capsule as well as the rotator cuff muscles (supraspinatus, infraspinatus and subscapularis) for additional stability. Impingement of the rotator cuff occurs when the cuff becomes compressed in the subacromial space as the arm is elevated. As the humeral head rotates, the rotator cuff tendons are compressed between the greater tuberosity of the humerus and the anterior edge of the acromion, the coracoacromial ligament, the under-surface of the acromioclavicular joint and with the reactive inflammatory subacromial bursa. With the arm at the side, the supraspinatus tendon has an avascular area 1 cm proximal to its insertion at the greater tuberosity directly beneath the impingement zone. Chronic irritation in the avascular region produces tendinitis, leading to localised inflammation and further compression. Other causes of tendinitis include trauma, instability and possibly infarction of the cuff in patients with widespread atherosclerosis.

Symptoms vary from pain with activity through to severe night pain, weakness and range restriction. Signs include a painful arc of abduction, pain on resisted cuff muscle movement and wasting, often in the setting of poor scapular control and a round-shouldered posture. With time, wearing and attrition of the cuff leads to poor action of the short rotators stabilising the humeral head into the glenoid so that the deltoid pulls the humerus against the under-surface of the acromion and a vicious impingement cycle is established. The cuff thins, the humeral head migrates superiorly and eventually the cuff tears (Figures 52.23). If the long head of biceps is torn, the associated rotator cuff tear is large.

The history and clinical examination, as detailed above, are the basis of the diagnosis. Plain radiography should precede ultrasound, because if there is marked superior migration of the humeral head, there must be complete rotator cuff disruption. Ultrasound can demonstrate cuff swelling, calcification and partial or full-thickness tears. A sensitive measure of subacromial inflammation is the finding of fluid in the bicipital groove, which is the most dependent part of the subacromial bursa. MRI, with intra-articular gadolinium, is helpful in the diagnosis of intra-substance tears.

Therapy includes patient education as to the cause of the problem and avoidance of repeated abduction, which only worsens the impingement. Advice on moving kitchen items lower, and to brush or wash hair with the elbow against the side of the chest are useful strategies. Simple analgesia or non-steroidal anti-inflammatory drugs (NSAIDs) may relieve symptoms, and physical therapies aimed at distracting rather than compressing the subacromial space may be taught as part of a home exercise program. Interventions such as intra-articular corticosteroid injection are tempting but it has been difficult to prove significant benefit in controlled trials. Arthroscopic decompression acromioplasty has become the treatment of choice for cases of chronic impingement where adequate conservative therapy has failed. Rotator cuff repair is a difficult issue, particularly in the elderly, and is really only viable if the patient presents within a few days of the sudden loss of function, before the tendon ends have retracted. It is unclear which partial tears need repair and whether subacromial injection of corticosteroid is contraindicated in the presence of

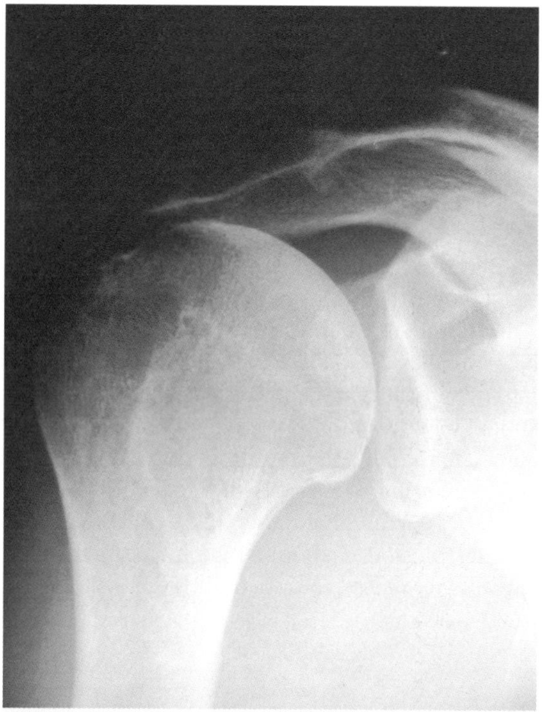

Figure 52.23 Rotator cuff atrophy leading to superior migration of the humeral head

a cuff tear. In the elderly, repair is made more difficult by the poor quality of the avascular tendons, which are difficult to bring together, with an often massive tear size and the patient's poor general medical fitness.

Calcific tendinitis of the shoulder

Calcification of the rotator cuff is seen in 7.5–20% of asymptomatic adults and 7% of those with shoulder pain, making it hard to determine whether it is a symptom-inducing process or a stand-alone condition. It is observed in people in their 50s and 60s, is of unknown causation, not uncommonly bilateral, affecting any cuff tendon, is slightly more common in females and is more likely to be seen in sedentary workers. Hypotheses as to the cause vary from calcification of fibrotic and necrotic degenerative tendon through to theories of self-limiting/self-resorbing calcification of fibrocartilaginous transformed tendon at its 'critical' ischaemic zone. Occasional rupture of calcific material into the subacromial bursa presents with acute pain and restriction due to a crystal-induced synovitis, which has been reported to occasionally progress to secondary adhesive capsulitis. Differing stages have been described (Figure 52.24).

Plain X-ray, often needing anteroposterior views in internal and external rotation, shows dense, well-defined deposits early and ill-defined deposits in resorptive stages. Distinction from dystrophic calcification of cuff rupture, chondrocalcinosis and calcification in bone of glenohumeral joint osteoarthritis is important (Figures 52.25, 52.26). Evidence for currently used therapies is anecdotal and choice tends to be presentation dependent. Subacute presentations are generally treated along the same lines as impingement, with analgesia, NSAIDs, physical therapies and subacromial injections of corticosteroids being used. Subacromial steroid injections seem particularly appropriate in the setting of a crystal-induced reaction. It is possible to use dual-needle washout to aspirate and lavage the intra-tendinous calcium deposits under ultrasound guidance, but whether you are treating the patient or the X-rays remains uncertain. Patients

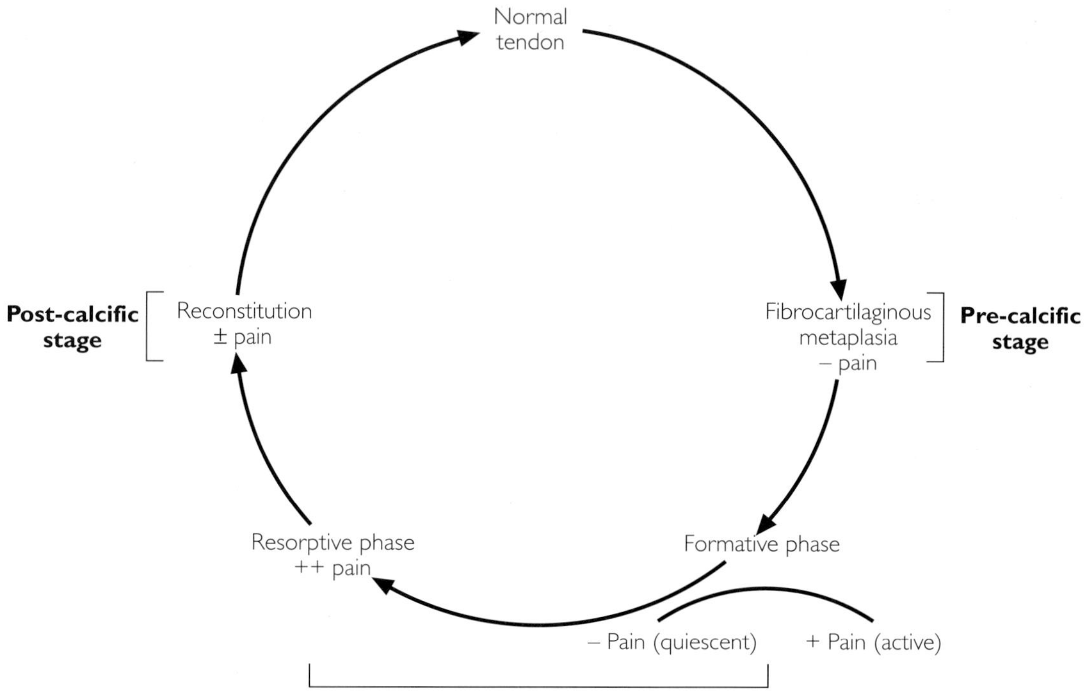

Figure 52.24 Stages of calcific tendinitis

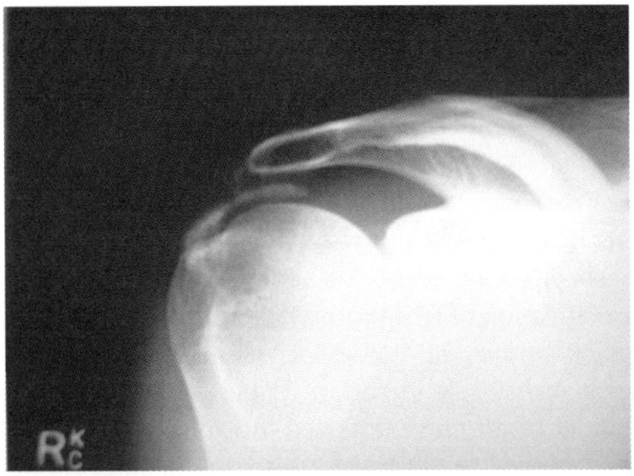

Figure 52.25 Supraspinatus calcification

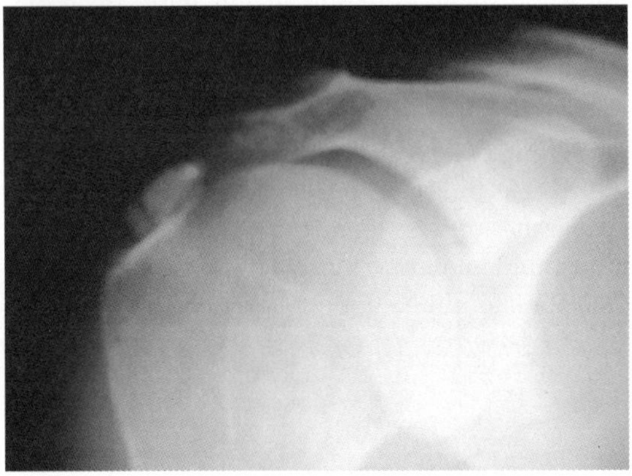

Figure 52.26 Subacromial bursa calcification

with acute presentations have been treated with subacromial injections or oral pulse corticosteroid, suprascapular nerve blockade and extracorporeal shock wave therapy, but all require further study. Pulsed ultrasound has been used in symptomatic patients with demonstrated improvements in pain and quality of life.

Frozen shoulder (adhesive capsulitis)

Initially described in 1872, this enigmatic rheumatological condition remains as 'difficult to treat and difficult to explain from the point of view of pathology' as Codman observed in 1934. This common disorder (2% cumulative risk in an at-risk population annually) is frequently misdiagnosed and is characterised by painful restriction of all shoulder movements, both active and passive, with characteristic restriction in the glenohumeral range (Figure 52.10). There is marked reduction or absence of shoulder external rotation at 0 degrees abduction (Figure 52.14), reduction of both internal and external rotation at 90 degrees abduction, as well as prominent restriction of placing the hand behind the back on internal rotation. Its aetiology is unknown. Box 52.2 lists the diseases associated with frozen shoulder, diabetes being the most significant. Diabetes, particularly longstanding insulin-dependent diabetes, is associated with glycosylation of subcutaneous collagen and the development of soft tissue contraction—so-called limited joint mobility or diabetic cheiroarthropathy. When a diabetic patient presents with adhesive capsulitis, other diabetic complications, especially retinopathy and nephropathy, are seen more frequently and should be searched for.

Box 52.2 Disorders associated with frozen shoulder

- Acute shoulder trauma and shoulder immobilisation
- Diabetes mellitus
- Thyroid disease (both hyper- and hypothyroidism)
- Cardiac disease, particularly after cardiac surgery
- Neurological disease with loss of consciousness or hemiplegia
- Pulmonary disease—tuberculosis and carcinoma
- Reflex sympathetic dystrophy (shoulder–hand syndrome)
- Rotator cuff disease, especially cuff tear
- Acute glenohumeral joint inflammation (e.g. polymyalgia rheumatica, viral polyarthritis)

Three phases of frozen shoulder or adhesive capsulitis are recognised:

1. Painful inflammatory phase. This has an insidious onset, with often only minor injury being recalled (e.g. reaching into the back seat of the car), and pain, especially at night (true nocturnal awakening due to pain). Pain can be constant with the patient unable to lie on the

shoulder. Physiotherapy often aggravates symptoms at this stage and corticosteroid injections are of limited benefit. Studies suggest the painful phase can last 10–36 weeks.

2. Frozen shoulder. With time, night and rest pain eases, but the shoulder remains limited in range. Mean duration 4–12 months.
3. With a mean delay of a further 5–26 months, shoulder limitation slowly recovers in the majority of patients towards normal range. The total duration of symptoms lasts 12–42 months, with a mean disease duration of 30 months.

Imaging is rarely necessary in frozen shoulder as it is a clinical diagnosis. Plain X-ray can be used to exclude significant glenohumeral joint osteoarthritis, as the clinical signs can be similar. Ultrasound establishes the presence or absence of full thickness cuff tear, but remember the high prevalence of this finding in the elderly and rotator cuff tears should not restrict shoulder movement with the arm dependent. It has been demonstrated that 30% of patients with carefully defined frozen shoulder have full thickness rotator cuff tears. Arthrography is technically difficult and painful due to the contracted joint capsule and small intra-articular space. Classic arthrographic features include reduction of joint capacity and a small or non-existent axillary fold. Distending the shoulder joint at arthrography can have therapeutic benefit, with mechanical rupture of the joint capsule occurring with small-volume injections. Arthroscopy shows a spectrum from low-grade synovitis at an early stage through to adhesions in the axillary fold, joint contracture and capsular restriction and thickened fibrotic capsule at later stages. The subacromial bursa is thickened and obliterated by adhesions.

Treatment recommendation is difficult. Analgesia and NSAIDs are of limited benefit. Physiotherapy aggravates symptoms early and helps to recover range later. Corticosteroid injections are of limited benefit. A short course of low-dose oral corticosteroid has been shown to improve symptoms, especially inflammatory night pain, but has little effect on limited range of movement and duration of illness. Double blind placebo-controlled trials assessing the benefit of this therapy are currently in progress. Saline hydrodistension, manipulation under anaesthesia and arthroscopic subcapsular release are employed therapies for frozen shoulder. Saline hydrodistension should be performed with appropriate anaesthesia under X-ray control as the glenohumeral joint is difficult to enter (Figure 52.27). Like all therapies for frozen shoulder, controlled studies are lacking, with a number currently under way. Treatment comparisons are often made on small groups of patients at differing stages of the disease process in poorly blinded and non-controlled studies. Prophylaxis by limiting shoulder immobilisation, with active and passive exercise programs instituted early in high-risk situations (e.g. acute hemiplegia) can be beneficial.

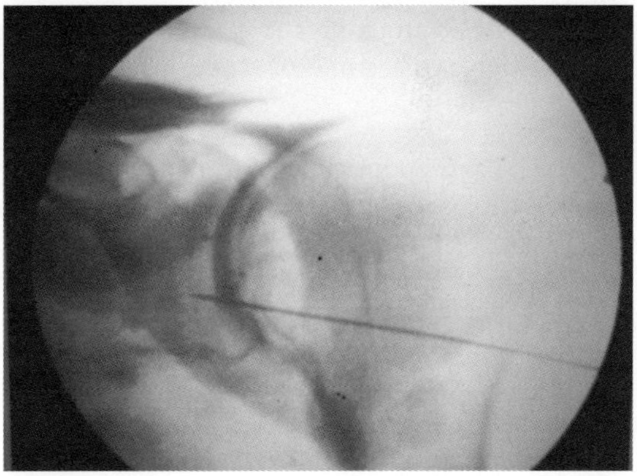

Figure 52.27 Saline distension X-ray control using contrast to localise the glenohumeral joint

Shoulder–hand syndrome

The shoulder joint, when immobilised, such as following a cerebrovascular event or fall, is prone to the development of acute reflex sympathetic dystrophy (also known as the shoulder–hand syndrome). This is manifested by severe pain in the limb, shoulder, arm and hand, which is often constant day and night. Associated features include limb swelling, with cyanosis and changes in temperature control, sweating, and skin hypersensitivity suggestive of sympathetic nerve dysfunction. In a prospective study, a quarter of hemiplegic patients developed this lesion with subluxation, girdle paresis, moderate spasticity and deficits in visual field testing being the major risk factors. In a smaller placebo-controlled trial, low dose oral corticosteroid appeared to improve symptoms significantly, and it was proposed that care with exercises, physiotherapy and limb positioning could prevent its development. There is no specific treatment for shoulder–hand syndrome as demonstrated by the range of options, which include sympathetic blockade, aggressive physiotherapy, analgesia, infusion of bisphosphonates, oral corticosteroids and vasodilators. The aim of therapy is to control any inflammation present, and provide analgesia by any means possible so as to allow preservation of movement and function.

Box 52.4 Causes of glenohumeral osteoarthritis

- Post-traumatic: fracture, recurrent dislocation
- Inflammatory joint disease including rheumatoid arthritis, crystal arthropathies
- Avascular necrosis
- Neuropathic arthropathy
- Rarities: haemophilia, acromegaly, ochronosis, synovial enchondromatosis

Glenohumeral joint arthropathies

A variety of arthropathies can affect the glenohumeral joint as listed in Box 52.3.

Box 52.3 Glenohumeral arthropathies

- Osteoarthritis
- Crystal arthropathies: urate, calcium pyrophosphate, hydroxyapatite
- Inflammatory joint disease: rheumatoid arthritis, psoriatic arthritis, ankylosing spondylitis, systemic lupus erythematosus
- Septic arthritis
- 'Milwaukee shoulder': destructive arthritis of the elderly

Osteoarthritis

Osteoarthritis (OA) of the glenohumeral joint is relatively uncommon and should not be the first diagnostic possibility for a painful shoulder. When OA of the shoulder joint occurs, it is rarely part of the primary nodal osteoarthritic process, and usually an underlying cause is present (Box 52.4). Despite its lower profile clinically, osteoarthritic changes do occur commonly with age, albeit clinically silent. One-quarter of cadaveric humeri showed moderate to severe osteophytes and 14% of a small sample of males over 60 who presented with shoulder pain had moderate to severe osteoarthritis. In life, symptoms of glenohumeral osteoarthritis include pain, particularly with use, morning stiffness, restricted range and loss of function. The global restriction of movement is similar to frozen shoulder, although clinically palpable crepitus or known predisposing factors, as listed in Box 52.4, may provide clues. Plain radiographs provide documentary support if required, with typical OA showing joint space loss, bony sclerosis and osteophyte formation (Figure 52.28). Therapy includes physical therapies, analgesia, NSAIDs, intra-articular corticosteroid injections (hyaluronic acid injections are being analysed) and, when sufficiently symptomatic (disabling pain the primary indication), shoulder joint replacement.

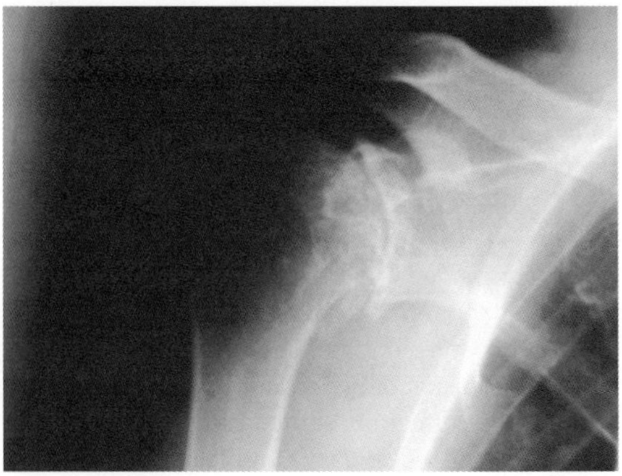

Figure 52.28 Glenohumeral joint osteoarthritis

Crystal arthropathies

Calcium pyrophosphate deposition presents as asymptomatic chondrocalcinosis, attacks of acute pseudogout with acute pain, joint swelling, and crystals in inflammatory joint fluid, or the 'dry' form with destructive joint damage and exuberant osteophyte formation. Treatable causes (e.g. primary hyperparathyroidism, haemochromatosis and hypothyroidism) should be considered.

Hydroxyapatite crystals are found when synovial fluid is specifically examined with alizarin red stain in patients with destructive arthropathies of the shoulder, such as in rheumatoid arthritis, neuropathic arthropathy (Charcot's arthropathy), idiopathic destructive arthropathy of the shoulder and in chronic renal failure.

Inflammatory arthropathies

Rheumatoid arthritis (Figure 52.29) and the seronegative arthropathies (psoriatic, colitic, reactive and ankylosing spondylitis) are characterised by proliferative synovitis, prominent joint effusions, subacromial bursitis, joint erosions, cartilage destruction and attrition, and rupture of the rotator cuff. They never manifest solely as disease of the shoulders, and will always present as part of a more systemic illness. Treatment is aimed at the underlying disease process, with liberal use (any one joint 3 times per annum) of corticosteroid injections to maintain function and quality of life.

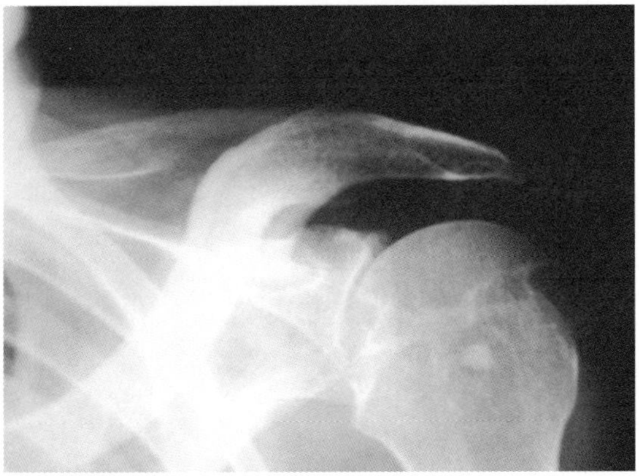

Figure 52.29 Large humeral head erosion in a patient with rheumatoid arthritis

Septic arthritis

Septic arthritis affects the shoulder in isolation rarely, being more common in patients with underlying diseases such as diabetes, alcoholism or immunosuppression. Direct inoculation of the joint can occur post injection but is rare (approximately 1:10 000 injections) and is extremely rare after surgery. Haematogenous spread from sepsis elsewhere or via intravenous drug use needs to be remembered. The expected septic presentation of pain, fevers and rigors may be less dramatic in the elderly and immunosuppressed. The best clue is always marked limitation in movement with a swollen, warm joint. In these circumstances, joint aspiration is mandatory and shows a high neutrophil count (both absolute and percentage) with reduced glucose level and viscosity. Gram stain and culture usually reveal *Staphylococcus aureus*, except in intravenous drug users or the immunosuppressed, in which unusual organisms including fungi can be found. Therapy includes joint drainage, parenteral antibiotics, analgesia and physical therapies to limit joint and cuff damage (Figure 52.30).

Destructive arthritis of the shoulder

This condition is also known as 'Milwaukee shoulder', cuff tear arthropathy and apatite-associated destructive arthritis of the shoulder. The typical patient is an elderly female, with an unstable, painful, markedly swollen joint and full thickness rotator cuff tear. Other joints, including knees, hips and metatarsals, can be affected. Joint aspirate

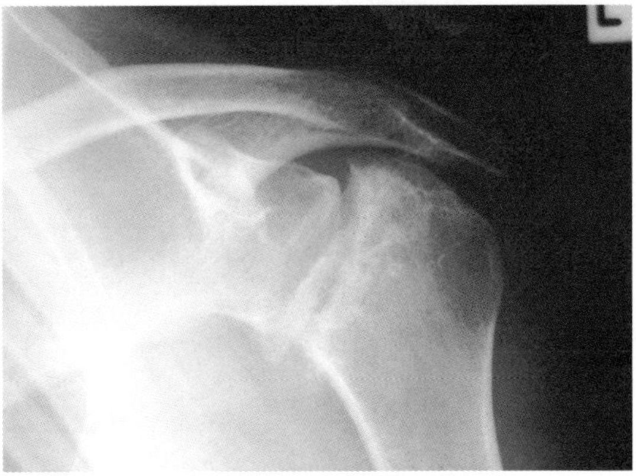

Figure 52.30 Damage resulting from septic arthritis

shows a non-inflammatory, blood-stained fluid with positive alizarin red stain for basic calcium phosphate crystals, typically hydroxyapatite. Severe bone loss of the humeral head and glenoid is also typical. The term 'cuff tear arthropathy' is used to describe glenohumeral osteoarthritis and full thickness rotator cuff tear with superior migration of the humeral head and prominent impingement (Figure 52.31). Codman in 1934 considered that a neglected rotator cuff tear left an exposed humeral head and resulted in chronic synovitis, effusion and destruction of the glenohumeral joint. It has been postulated that glenohumeral osteoarthritis resulted from repetitive trauma as a result of the altered biomechanics associated with the loss of stabilisers of the joint from cuff tear. Cuff tear arthropathy is commonly seen in elderly females with a long duration of shoulder symptoms—joint pain, often at night and worse after activity, restriction in range and recurrent swelling. Bilateral disease is common.

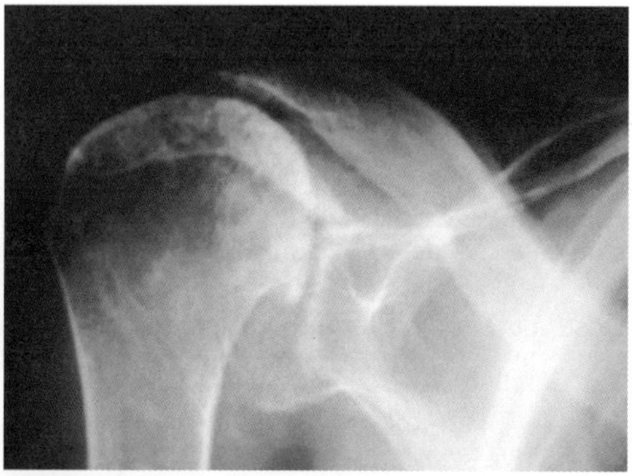

Figure 52.31 Chronic cuff tear with elevated humeral head, false articulation with inferior acromion and secondary degeneration of the glenohumeral joint

It is our opinion that a neglected element in the aetiology of this syndrome is underlying cervical abnormalities. Common bilateral disease points to a central causative factor. These patients commonly have cervical disc abnormality, exit foraminal encroachment, and likely root impingement, particularly at the commonest level of disc abnormality—C5–6—precisely the level that innervates the rotator cuff musculature (Figures 52.32 and 52.33). Root lesions here would result in cuff atrophy, superior humeral head migration and chronic impingement. Chronic impingement, a weak cuff or repeated corticosteroid injection for pain lead to progressive cuff atrophy and rupture. Once initiated, the spiral to glenohumeral joint destruction results. In those individuals whose osteoarthritis process results in a crystal-producing reaction, an apatite-associated disease process results. Some of these patients have features resembling a neuropathic arthropathy—instability, variable pain, hypertrophic osteophyte development and large joint effusions. As cervical disc disease is so common in the elderly, a coincidental occurrence of cervical and shoulder abnormalities is difficult to discount. Electromyographic studies are under way to try to demonstrate more precisely any relationship by trying to document denervation.

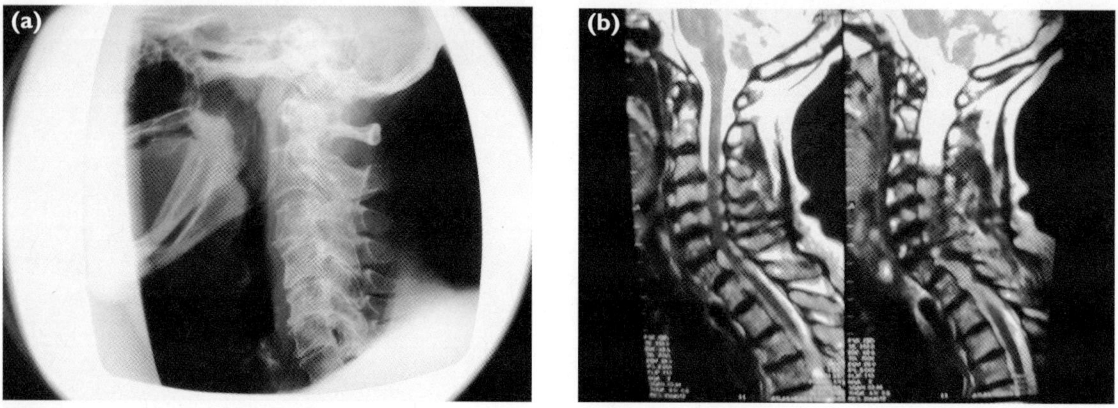

Figure 52.32 Advanced cervical spondylosis shown on **(a)** plain X-ray and **(b)** MRI in a patient with bilateral cuff tear arthropathy

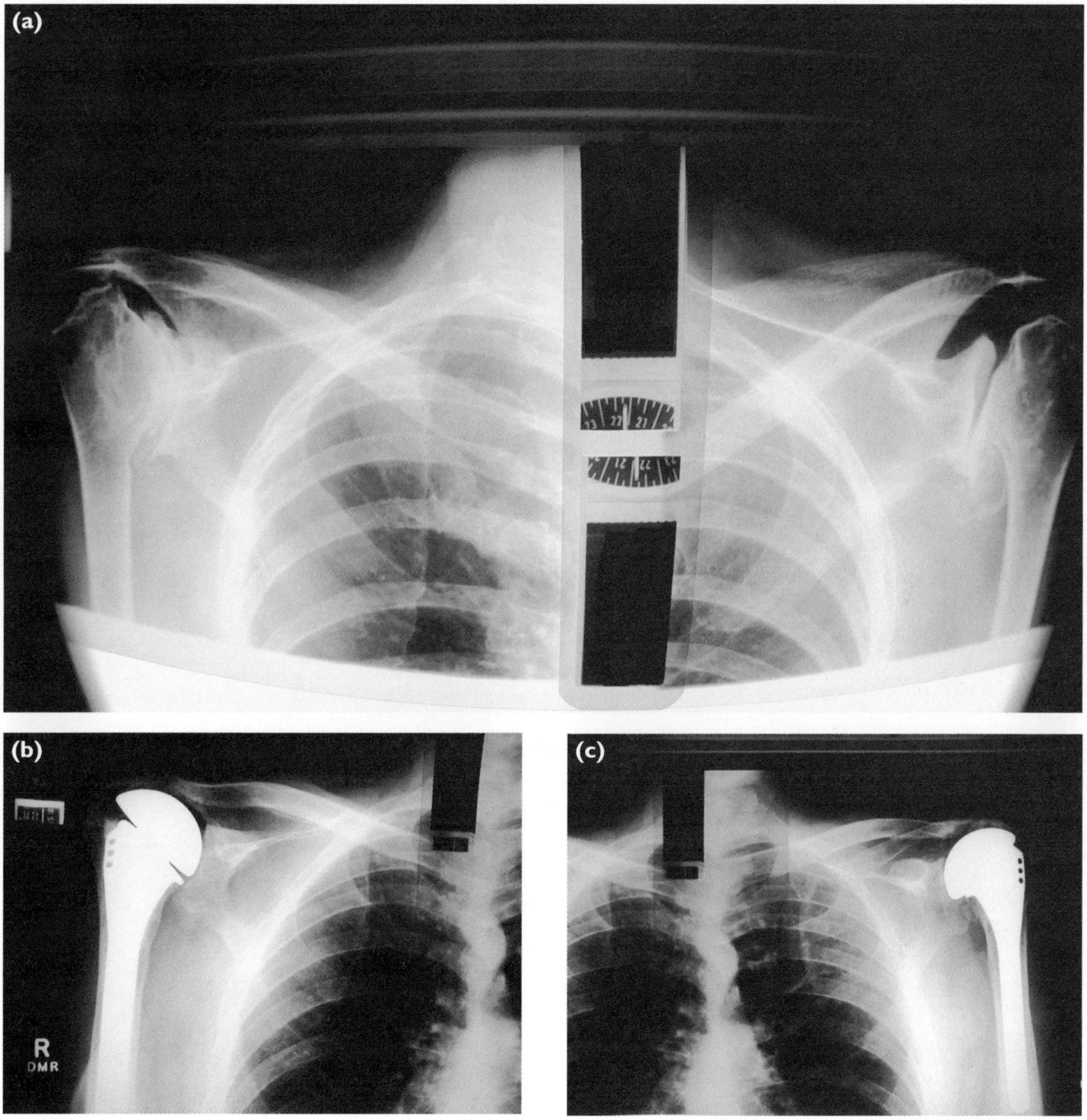

Figure 52.33 **(a)** Chronic bilateral cuff tear arthropathy with **(b, c)** resultant bilateral joint replacement

Conclusion

Problems affecting the shoulder are common and contribute significantly to the community's musculoskeletal morbidity. The challenge for clinicians then, particularly for those who care for the elderly, is to:

- assess by formal study if more accurate and timely diagnosis can improve prognosis
- reappraise 'orthodox' therapeutic approaches in terms of evidence for efficacy
- develop new strategies to improve long-term outcome.

Bibliography and further reading

Green, S., Buchbinder, R., Glazier, R. & Forbes, A. (2000), 'Interventions for shoulder pain', *Cochrane Database of Systematic Reviews*, 2, CD001156.

Nash, P. (1999), 'Shoulder pain', *Current Therapeutics*, 40, pp. 15–23.

Speed, C., Burnet, S. & Hazleman, B. (1999), 'Shoulder pain', *Clinical Evidence, Issue 2*, BMJ Publishing Group, London, pp. 463–75.

Vecchio, P., Kavanagh, R., Hazleman, B. & King, R. (1995), 'Community survey of shoulder disorders in the elderly to assess the natural history and effects of therapy', *Annals of the Rheumatic Diseases*, 54, pp. 152–4.

Watson, E. M. & Sonnabend, D. H. (2000), 'Shoulder problems: a guide to common disorders', *Medicine Today*, 1, pp. 22–30.

Chapter 53
Polyarthritis

KEVIN PILE

Introduction

Arthritis and rheumatism are major physical and psychological burdens in the elderly population. As most forms of arthritis are chronic, the combinations of lifespan, cumulative arthritis incidence, and concomitant disease and treatments create the almost inevitable experience of arthritis. Approximately two-thirds of elderly people experience sufficient symptoms each day to warrant regular use of non-steroidal anti-inflammatory drugs (NSAIDs). This experience of arthritis is sufficient to disrupt the sleep or leisure activities of one-third of the population, with nearly all these people utilising at least one medical, complementary or self-care strategy. In terms of disease burden, arthritis is the most prevalent chronic condition among adults aged over 65 years (48.9 per 100 adults), followed by hypertension (40.3 per 100 adults) and heart disease (28.6 per 100 adults). The psychological burden of arthritis is often underestimated, as people's imaginations conjure images of becoming 'wheelchair bound' or sufficiently restricted so as to be no longer able to look after themselves, with loss of independence.

This chapter reviews the pertinent parts of the history and examination allowing a differential diagnosis for arthritis to be formulated. Only the common forms of polyarthritis in an elderly population are addressed.

History and examination

The purpose of the history and examination has three aims:

1. Production of a differential diagnosis and later a diagnosis.
2. Objective monitoring of the primary outcome of an intervention.
3. Objective monitoring of adverse outcomes of an intervention.

Differential diagnosis

Assuming you have asked whether a diagnosis has previously been made, a careful history and examination is used to determine whether the symptoms are articular or non-articular in nature. Subsequently, the pattern of joint involvement is identified along with 'clues' elicited from the history and examination to distinguish between 'inflammatory' or 'non-inflammatory' arthritis and also to act as a guide within each pattern (Box 53.1).

Non-articular, musculoskeletal soft tissue symptoms are very common, including the local conditions of tendinitis, bursitis, back pain and the more generalised problem of fibromyalgia. Fibromyalgia is one of the most common musculoskeletal problems affecting 5% of women and 3% of men over the age of 50 years. Patients with fibromyalgia report widespread musculoskeletal symptoms that are bilateral, including both upper and lower limbs as well as the axial skeleton. They also experience symptoms involving sleep disturbance, and their gastrointestinal and genitourinary systems. Objectively, the examination is normal, but the patient experiences diffuse sensitivity to pressure applied to their muscles, with more marked tenderness in discrete areas. The overall impression is of abnormal pain perception by the individual to non-noxious external stimuli, and to normal peripheral stimuli created by movement. In contrast, localised soft tissue symptoms are identified by their localisation to a discrete region, with maximum discomfort associated with movement in planes that apply tension on the involved muscles or tendons.

Box 53.1 Patterns of musculoskeletal symptoms

Non-articular

- Localised musculoskeletal symptoms: tendinitis, bursitis, back pain
- Diffuse musculoskeletal symptoms: fibromyalgia

Articular

- Non-inflammatory
  - Symmetrical small joint: nodal osteoarthritis
  - Weight-bearing joints, spine: osteoarthritis
- Inflammatory
- Monoarthritis (1 joint): gout, pseudogout, sepsis, trauma
- Oligoarthritis (2–4 joints): spondyloarthropathies (psoriasis, reactive), crystal arthropathies
- Polyarthritis (> 4 joints): rheumatoid arthritis, psoriatic arthritis, systemic lupus erythematosus, post-viral

Articular symptoms localise to the joint itself, with the number and pattern of joint involvement becoming important. The joint may manifest externally visible changes of swelling, redness, heat and deformity. Pain occurs on movement in the directions allowed by the joint. The distinction between inflammatory and non-inflammatory arthropathies is a useful categorisation, but one that is also misleading, really being inflammatory and relatively non-inflammatory. The commonest 'non-inflammatory' arthritis is osteoarthritis, and compared to gout or septic arthritis it is non-inflammatory, but often inflammation is present clinically and inflammatory cytokines can be identified in the joints involved. Table 53.1 lists the clues that help distinguish inflammatory from non-inflammatory arthritis. These are based on probability and are not absolute! Early morning stiffness is regarded as a key differentiator, although it is a difficult concept for many people to quantify. Less than 10 minutes of early morning stiffness is probably non-inflammatory, and greater than an hour of stiffness probably reflects an inflammatory cause, with the mid range unreliable.

The GALS (gait, arms, legs, spine) rheumatological screen, developed in Nottingham, UK, is an excellent tool for rapidly determining the presence of any relevant musculoskeletal disease. Three questions are asked in the screen:

Table 53.1 Features suggestive of inflammatory and non-inflammatory arthropathies

Inflammatory	Non-inflammatory
Systemic illness Joint erythema Joint heat Diurnal variation Symptoms reduced with activity Prolonged early morning stiffness Joints stiffen after inactivity	Symptoms worsen with activity Brief early morning stiffness

1. Have you had any pain or stiffness in your muscles, joints or back?
2. Can you dress yourself completely without any difficulty?
3. Can you walk up and down stairs without any difficulty?

Positive responses are followed with relevant questions, which include: 'Where is the pain (localised or widespread)?', 'How severe is the pain, stiffness or swelling?', 'When is the discomfort most difficult (early morning, after activities, late in the day)?', 'How did the pain, stiffness or swelling begin (acute or chronic)?'.

There are other points to note within the history additional to those directly related to the polyarthritis:

- Recent infectious exposure—viral infections, vaccinations, mosquito or tick bites, gastrointestinal or genitourinary infections. In humans, various viruses are known to cause arthritis. Rubella virus can lead to a rheumatoid arthritis-like syndrome after either wild-type rubella infection or vaccination with attenuated virus. In some cases, the virus can be cultured from within the joint and as such is a form of septic arthritis.
- Past and current medications resulting in hyperuricaemia—diuretics, low-dose aspirin, cyclosporin.
- Personal or family history of psoriasis, inflammatory bowel disease, arthritis.

Next, the patient's gait, arms, legs and spine are systematically inspected. The patient is first examined standing still, and then responding to instructions (Table 53.2). Any abnormalities on screening are followed by a more detailed regional examination. A brief physical examination can identify most problems of the musculoskeletal system. Examination of affected areas should involve palpation for tenderness and swelling and a check of range of movement. Arthritis is suggested by pain in all motions of a joint. Tendinitis or bursitis are suggested by point tenderness and pain in only one plane of motion. Fibromyalgia is suggested by diffuse muscle spasm and tender points. A brief, gentle 'squeeze' of each proximal interphalangeal (PIP) joint and metacarpophalangeal (MCP) joint requires no more than 30 seconds and can detect subtle inflammation, as seen in early rheumatoid arthritis.

The patient can be asked to squeeze the finger of the examiner to assess hand strength and then move his arms above the head, behind the back, and in a wing span test for shoulder flexion, abduction, and internal and external rotation.

Clinicians should make a point of observing their patients walking towards the consultation room and their mobility in the room, particularly undressing or mounting an examination couch. A patient who cannot arise from a chair without holding on to a support has an abnormality, which may exist in the joints, muscles or nerves—your task is to characterise the problem.

Investigations

Unfortunately, blood tests in patients with rheumatic diseases are often imprecise and non-specific in guiding the clinician to a diagnosis. Tests will alter the diagnostic probabilities in some circumstances if the clinician is able to calculate the effect a particular test result will have, considering the diagnostic certainty before the test and the sensitivity and specificity of the test.

Markers of inflammation, such as erythrocyte sedimentation rate (ESR) and C-reactive protein (CRP), are non-specific indicators of systemic inflammation, with the ESR increasing physiologically with age (male normal is age halved, female normal is age plus 10, halved) and being affected by red cell morphology and serum protein alterations. Rheumatoid factor (RF) is, by quality control definition, positive in 5% of the overall population, but closer to 10% in the elderly. At least 25% of patients with proven rheumatoid arthritis (RA) are consistently RF negative, and half of the patients with RA are RF negative in the first 6 months. Similar problems exist for anti-nuclear antibody (ANA) tests and hyperuricaemia, where a positive test result does not make a specific diagnosis, and many patients with positive test results never develop any identifiable disease process.

Abnormal radiographs are also to be expected in an elderly population. Seventy per cent of 70 year olds will manifest radiographic evidence of osteoarthritis in X-rays of the hand, hips or knees,

Table 53.2 The GALS examination guide

Position/activity	Observation
Gait	Symmetry, smoothness of movement (legs, arm swing, pelvic tilting) Normal stride length Normal heel strike, stance, toe-off, swing through Ability to turn quickly
Inspection from behind	Straight spine (no scoliosis) Normal, symmetrical paraspinal muscles Normal shoulder and gluteal muscle bulk/symmetry Level iliac crests No popliteal swelling No hindfoot swelling/deformity Inspection from the side
'Touch toes'	Normal cervical and lumbar lordosis Normal (mild) thoracic kyphosis Normal lumbar spine (and hip) flexion
Inspection from in front	
Spine	
'Head on shoulders'	Normal cervical lateral flexion
Arms	
'Arms behind head'	Normal glenohumeral, sternoclavicular, and acromioclavicular joint movement
'Arms straight'	Full elbow extension
'Hands in front'	No wrist/finger swelling or deformity Ability to fully extend fingers
'Turn hands over'	Normal supination/pronation (superior and inferior radio ulnar joints) Normal palms (no swelling, muscle wasting, erythema)
'Make a fist'	Normal power grip
'Fingers on thumb'	Normal fine precision pinch/dexterity
Legs	Normal quadriceps bulk/symmetry No knee swelling or deformity (varus/valgus) No forefoot/midfoot deformity Normal arches

and when this is combined with intervertebral disc narrowing or bulging and degenerative changes in the spinal facet joints it is universal. The identification of an abnormality with the use of higher definition imaging techniques is only clinically relevant if it relates to your clinical assessment.

Monitoring of treatment outcome

In short, the aims of almost all treatments are to improve or maintain a person's quality of life, both in the short and longer terms. Doctors routinely evaluate this at each consultation with general questions such as 'How are you doing today?' or 'What are your joints like?'. This can be better quantified in a reproducible way utilising visual analogue scores of pain or function, and short questionnaires for quality of life. In patients with inflammatory arthritis, the number of tender and swollen joints can be counted and/or marked on a mannequin to objectively follow treatment. Rheumatologists are increasingly using the number of swollen and tender joints as an objective marker of outcome, counting bilaterally the PIP joints, MCP joints, wrists, elbows, shoulders and knees to give an objective tender and swollen joint count out of a maximum of 28.

Similarly, objective markers of inflammation such as ESR or CRP can be followed. Radiographs can be utilised at baseline to help establish the diagnosis and to monitor progression of radiological damage. The dilemma here is that while intuitively it is easy to accept that prevention or retardation of damage shown on X-ray will lead to improved quality of life in the future, this link has not been proven. All clinicians will have noted marked discrepancies between a person's symptoms and function and what is shown on their actual X-ray.

Osteoarthritis

Epidemiology

Osteoarthritis (OA) is the commonest condition to affect synovial joints and the single most important cause of locomotor disability. Although not an inevitable consequence of ageing, OA is strongly related to age, which may represent cumulative insult to the joint, possibly aggravated by decline in neuromuscular function or senescence of homeostatic repair mechanisms.

In general, OA is uncommon and multiple joint OA is rare in persons aged less than 45 years. The prevalence of OA does vary in different populations, but on average affects 60–70% of people aged over 45 years. The prevalence of radiographic OA exceeds that of clinical OA, and is almost universal in the elderly population if distal interphalangeal (DIP) joints and knees are examined. The prevalence of symptomatic OA also increases with age, with, for example, 15% of those aged over 55 years having symptomatic knee OA.

There is a pronounced female preponderance after the age of 55 years for severe radiographic grades of OA, notably in the hand and knee, as well as symptomatic OA. This has suggested that oestrogen deficiency may play a role in aetiology. Occupation predisposes to OA of specific joints (e.g. hip OA in farmers, shoulder OA in baseball pitchers). The best characterised OA risk factor is obesity, with OA in the knee and to a lesser extent in the hip correlating with higher body weights.

Pathophysiology

There is no generally accepted definition of OA, but pathologically it is a condition of synovial joints characterised by focal cartilage loss and an accompanying reparative bone response. The final common pathway of OA is cartilage degradation. Composed of water, collagen, proteoglycans and chondrocytes, the individual cartilage components can be studied to derive both OA aetiology and potential therapy (see Figure 53.1).

Type II collagen fibres create the structural integrity of cartilage, with fibrous arcs forming a mesh. Held within this 'string bag' are the large, heavily charged proteoglycans and the water that they attract in the form of a gel. The basic building blocks of the proteoglycans are glycosaminoglycans (GAGs), such as chondroitin sulphate and keratan sulphate; up to 100 GAG chains asymmetrically attach to a core protein, forming a bottlebrush-like molecule called aggrecan. In turn, 200 or more of the aggrecan molecules join to the chain-like molecule hyaluronan to create an enormous structure with tremendous water-attracting potential. Hyaluronan itself is a repeating disaccharide found in cartilage complexed with aggrecan and also in synovial fluid where it is responsible for the viscoelastic and lubricant properties of synovial fluid. The source of both collagen and the proteoglycans are the chondrocytes. Notable absences from cartilage are blood vessels and nerves, with nutrition deriving from movement-enhanced diffusion from synovial fluid. Stretching of the joint capsule and ligaments, trabecular microfractures and periosteal irritation are all postulated as sources of OA joint pain.

The role of inflammation in OA pathogenesis is a source of contention. At one extreme in arthropathies, such as RA, potent cytokines stimulate the production of matrix metalloproteinase enzymes such as collagenases and aggrecanase, with resultant cartilage degradation. To a lesser extent, the same inflammatory processes are present in OA as a result of cartilage wear particles and hypoxia-reperfusion injury.

Biomechanical factors also contribute to OA, with the rate and area of loading probably more important than total load. Additional to physical disruption, mechanical loading also decreases proteoglycan synthesis and increases proteinase production. The activities of the neuromuscular system also influence cartilage loading and are a focus of research, due to the observation of reduced proprioception and muscle strength as risk factors for OA. Age increases the risk of OA secondary to cumulative

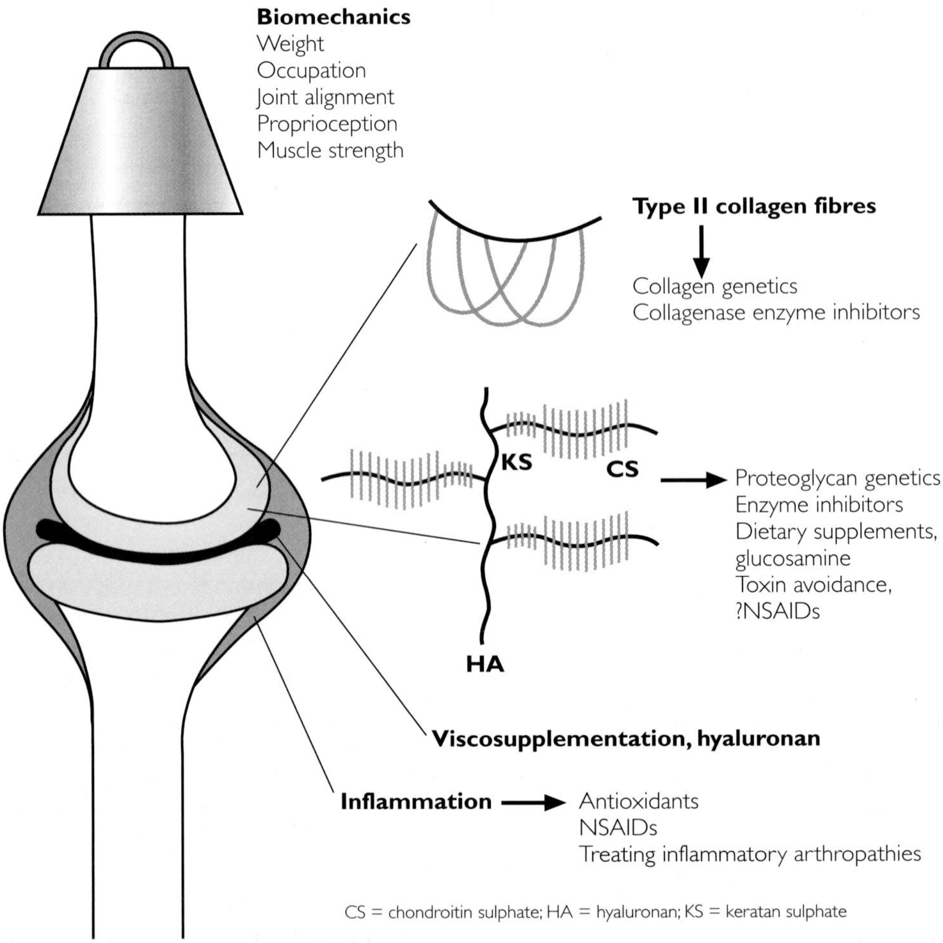

Figure 53.1 Pathophysiology of osteoarthritis

trauma combined with age-related loss of muscle strength, proprioception and chondrocyte function.

Diagnosis

Diagnosis is based on the identification of a 'relatively' non-inflammatory arthropathy that is frequently polyarticular, involving the DIP joints of the hand, the base of the thumb at the first carpometacarpal (CMC) joint, and the hips, knees, cervical and lumbar spines. The primary reason for consultation may be localised inflammation of individual joints, but it is the overall pattern that provides the diagnosis. Clinical examination identifies restriction of joint movement, with palpable and audible crepitus due to the underlying focal cartilage loss, and palpable osteophytes (notably Heberden's and Bouchard's nodes of DIP and PIP joints respectively).

The typical patient with OA is late middle aged to elderly with pain and stiffness in and around a joint accompanied by limitation of function. The pain is gradual or insidious in onset, usually mild in intensity, and worsens with activity and improves with rest.

Clinical tests

The diagnosis of OA can almost always be made by history and physical examination. Routine testing adds little to diagnostic certainty. If a superimposed crystal arthropathy (gout or pseudogout) is suspected, then synovial fluid aspiration and microscopy is required. Radiographs will reinforce the results of clinical examination but rarely change the diagnosis. Radiographs will document the pattern of joint involvement, as well as irregular joint space narrowing, subchondral bone sclerosis and osteophytic bony proliferation at the joint margins.

Treatment

Non-pharmacological treatment strategies

Correction of biomechanical factors is a mainstay of OA treatment and prevention. Obesity is a documented risk factor for knee and hip OA, as are occupational factors such as farming for hip OA. Weight loss of only 5 kg is associated with a 50% reduction in the odds of developing knee OA, and in symptomatic subjects will reduce the severity of knee pain. Strategies aimed at correcting malalignment of joints, stabilisation of subluxing joints or load redistribution can be achieved via diet, orthoses, shock-absorbing footwear or surgical means. New treatment strategies involve muscle strengthening and proprioception training in the elderly. Such physical measures may have a favourable effect on the pathology and symptoms of osteoarthritis, and could enhance the efficacy of disease-modifying drugs (see below). Physical therapies consisting of weight training and aerobic walking can also improve balance and reduce swaying movement in the elderly, thereby reducing the risk of falls. A combination of manual physical therapy and supervised exercise yields functional benefits for patients with osteoarthritis of the knee and may delay or prevent the need for surgical intervention.

Inflammation in OA: the anti-inflammatory or analgesia debate

Current published guidelines from both the US and UK recommend paracetamol as the first-line treatment for OA on a risk–benefit analysis; yet NSAIDs remain preferred agents for pharmacological treatment of patients with OA. Two systematic reviews examined randomised controlled trials of pharmacological therapy in OA of the hip and knee. Comparison between NSAIDs and placebo showed NSAIDs to be superior for pain relief. Surveys of consumers with OA, RA or fibromyalgia also confirm the superior efficacy of NSAIDs. Only one-third of people report moderate to good pain relief from paracetamol alone, and when compared to NSAIDs only one-quarter reported a better result from paracetamol. Nevertheless, a risk minimisation strategy supports a trial of paracetamol with prompt initiation of NSAIDs in those without significant improvement in symptoms. The reticence to recommend NSAIDs as first-line therapy relates to their significant potential toxicity, particularly in the elderly population. As well as their documented gastrointestinal toxicity, NSAIDs have been implicated as having a deleterious effect on proteoglycan synthesis. Shortly after the introduction of indomethacin in 1965, its use was associated with a rapidly developing hip arthropathy. Subsequent studies did not support analgesia-related increased activity as the cause but that the reduction of vasodilating prostaglandins resulted in reduced joint perfusion. In a comparison of the potent prostaglandin inhibitor, indomethacin, with a weak inhibitor, azapropazone, those patients on indomethacin reached the arthroplasty endpoint faster. In a study of the catabolic effects of NSAIDs on in-vitro cartilage cultures, three categories were identified: stimulants of proteoglycan synthesis, such as tolmetin, aceclofenac, tenidap; neutral effects on proteoglycan synthesis, such as diclofenac, piroxicam, tiaprofenic acid, aspirin; and significant inhibitors of proteoglycan synthesis, such as naproxen, ibuprofen, indomethacin. While there are a number of considerations before extrapolating these results to clinical use, they should be considered when planning long-term therapy.

If inflammation plays any role in OA, is there a role for intra-articular steroid injection? Unfortunately, randomised controlled trials show only a 1–2 week benefit from intra-articular steroid injections in the management of knee OA. Even then, not all short-term studies have shown a benefit and this may be due to the strong beneficial response to placebo injections.

In summary, no individual NSAID has been shown to be unequivocally superior when prescribed in appropriate doses. The trend is for

NSAIDs to be more efficacious than paracetamol, but due to NSAID toxicity, paracetamol is the first-choice agent on a risk–benefit ratio. The recent development of the specific cyclo-oxygenase-2 (COX2) inhibitors, celecoxib and rofecoxib, may significantly alter the treatment algorithm, as they appear to have efficacies the same as existing NSAIDs and an ulceration or bleed risk the same as placebo. It is important to remember that the 'coxib' medications do less than existing NSAIDs when considering anti-platelet action and they do not replace aspirin's role. Whenever commencing or changing to a coxib, a separate evaluation of the need for an anti-platelet agent needs to be made.

Current therapies, however, are only symptomatic and it is novel and potential OA-modifying therapies that are of real interest.

Enzyme inhibitors

Aggrecan and collagen are the major molecular constituents of articular cartilage conferring stiffness on compression and tensile strength. Evidence of an increased turnover rate of these molecules in cases of OA led investigators to search for degradative enzymes, so that inhibitors might be developed to prevent or slow the progression of osteoarthritis. Doxycycline is a non-specific inhibitor of matrix metalloproteinases by chelating zinc at the catalytic site, and also reduces total enzyme load within cartilage. Animal models confirm the efficacy of doxycycline in reducing the severity of OA, with human studies showing beneficial biochemical changes in cartilage, but none have documented clinical or radiographic benefits. Specific inhibitors of both collagenase and its activator, stromelysin, have been developed and long-term efficacy and safety data are awaited.

Viscosupplementation

Hyaluronic acid (HA) in articular tissue and synovial fluid plays a critical role in joint homeostasis and normal function. In patients with OA, the concentration and molecular weight of synovial fluid HA is diminished secondary to dilution, enzymatic degradation and reduced production by synoviocytes. Identification of these deficits led to the concept of viscosupplementation by intra-articular injection of HA-based products, and was first used in race horses and humans in the early 1970s. There are currently two types of HA-based products: a relatively low molecular weight product (0.5–1.2 million MW) and a high molecular weight cross-linked HA product (hylan, 6 million MW). The intra-articular residence time of the injected HA is related to molecular weight, ranging from hours to several days. After injection, high concentrations of HA may transiently improve the rheological properties of lubrication and shock absorption. This, however, would not explain a benefit greater than 1 week post-injection, yet most studies to date have shown benefits persisting for months. Accumulating evidence supports anti-inflammatory and anti-nociceptive effects of HA, as well as helping to normalise in-vivo HA synthesis.

Studies of viscosupplementation with either HA or hylan have shown them to be better than placebo and as effective as NSAIDs, being effective in about 70% of those treated for varying periods of time. Randomised control trials highlight the dramatic placebo effect of intra-articular injection, and while a statistical significance may be noted in an appropriately powered study, the clinical significance is less impressive. Mild and self-limited local flare reactions and bruising are very common and may relate to injection technique. A clinical benefit is most likely in those with lesser radiographic evidence of damage but an individual cost–benefit analysis is mandatory.

Nutritional supplements

The production of reactive oxygen species (ROS) is a physiological event, which has been implicated in the pathophysiology of OA. Chondrocytes and synovium are both capable of producing ROS, with macro- and microinflammation-enhancing production of ROS, as does hypoxia-reperfusion injury. Both lipid-soluble vitamin E and water-soluble vitamin C are effective antioxidants, particularly in the extracellular space, and it has been postulated that they may have an anti-ageing effect. In the Framingham knee OA study, over an 8-year period those in the highest tertile of vitamin C intake (mean = 465 mg) were significantly less likely to show progressive X-ray changes or develop knee pain (both odds ratio = 0.3). However, the development of radiographic change in those starting with normal X-rays was not reduced. Similar results were noted with vitamin D, with subjects with the lowest dietary vitamin D intake and those in the lowest tertile of serum 25-hydroxy-vitamin D having 3–4 times the risk of radiologic progression, but again there was no influence on the development of new OA changes. The authors postulated that the mechanism of action was protection in situations with ROS production, but not the initial steps of OA development.

A major growth area in the self-management of OA is the use of dietary supplements containing glucosamine and chondroitin sulphate, both of which are extolled in *The Arthritis Cure Handbook*. Glucosamine is one of the sugars forming the disaccharide pair in HA and several other GAGs.

In-vitro glucosamine stimulates cartilage cells to synthesise GAGs and proteoglycans. Bioavailability is 26% following first-pass metabolism, with tropism for cartilage in humans. A randomised controlled trial comparison of 1500 mg/day of glucosamine to placebo showed significant improvement in joint tenderness, swelling and restriction of active movement beginning at day 14 and continuing throughout the 30-day trial. Comparison of glucosamine 1500 mg/day with low-dose ibuprofen (1200 mg/day) showed a faster analgesic benefit from ibuprofen, which quickly plateaued and was stable over the 8-week trial. At 2 weeks, the group taking glucosamine had fewer symptoms than at baseline, with a continual improvement to become significantly better than those taking ibuprofen at between 4 and 8 weeks. Several glucosamine preparations also contain chondroitin sulphate, which has a high molecular weight and is unlikely to be absorbed intact from the gastrointestinal tract. Recent meta-analyses provide the best summary, noting that many of the studies have low numbers but concluding that both glucosamine and chondroitin sulphate were superior to placebo and at least similar in efficacy to ibuprofen for the treatment of symptomatic OA. The enzyme aggrecanase is partially inhibited by glucosamine, so in theory supplementation could both enhance proteoglycan production and inhibit aggrecanase-mediated proteoglycan degradation. Long-term comparative observational studies utilising accurate radiological measures of joint space and cartilage volume will be necessary to determine if this translates into a clinical impact on disease progression.

When to refer

Due to the almost ubiquitous nature of OA, general practitioners are the primary practitioner for diagnosis, education and management. A referral to allied health professionals will often be made to assist in biomechanical correction using orthoses. A rheumatological referral is not required but may aid in the diagnosis and management of superimposed crystal arthropathies and management of functional loss.

Urgent referral to an orthopaedic or rheumatological colleague is required for sudden pain and loss of function in a patient with knee or hip OA when infection or avascular necrosis is suspected.

A frequent clinical dilemma is when to refer for consideration of joint replacement. The primary reason for joint replacement is pain relief, and pain experienced at night and with activity is the basis on which to determine referral to an orthopaedic surgeon. The primary practitioner will also need to take account of the co-morbidities in the individual, which may influence anaesthetic risk and postoperative rehabilitation.

Rheumatoid arthritis

Epidemiology

Rheumatoid arthritis (RA) is one of the commonest forms of polyarthritis, with a worldwide prevalence of approximately 1%, and occurs 3 times more commonly in women. While the disease can begin at any stage of life, it becomes noticeable in the third decade in women, and has its greatest onset in the fifth to sixth decades. Genetic factors make a substantial contribution to RA in the population, accounting for approximately 60% of the variation in liability to disease.

The strongest genetic association in RA is that with the major histocompatibility complex HLA-DR genes, and they seem to associate with disease severity. HLA-DR1 and specific subtypes of HLA-DR4 (Dw4, Dw14, Dw15) have been consistently reported, with combinations of the susceptibility genes leading to greater risk. The HLA types associating with RA susceptibility or severity have a marked similarity within amino acids 70–74 forming the β-protein of the HLA class II molecule. The shared sequence, coded QKRAA, is strategically located near the antigen-binding site, and may affect the ability of the HLA molecule to present certain antigens. The key function of the HLA-DR molecule is to present antigens to CD4-positive T lymphocytes (T-helper cells). The inherited motif QKRAA may selectively present arthritis-causing peptides or result in a defect in the immune system by failing to present an immunogenic peptide and hence allow an arthritis-inducing pathogen to proliferate and disseminate due to the absence of an appropriate T-cell response.

Aetiology

The concept of a genetic predisposition and an environmental trigger has been applied to nearly all autoimmune diseases, including RA. Despite an intensive search for transmissible agents that might cause RA, an infectious source has yet to be proven. The worldwide distribution of RA has been interpreted as meaning the environmental trigger is ubiquitous, or that multiple triggers are involved. A common environmental trigger will be almost impossible to identify if both RA and non-RA subjects are universally exposed. Due to its universality, Epstein-Barr virus (EBV) has been implicated in RA. Patients with RA have higher serum antibody levels for EBV proteins, and their peripheral blood lymphocytes show a specific defect in the immune response to EBV. One of the EBV coat proteins contains the QKRAA amino acid sequence that is found in HLA-DR4, suggesting that mimicry or cross-reaction between the two similar proteins may be important.

Pathophysiology

The pathogenesis of RA is that of synovial inflammation or synovitis. The normal synovium is a thin and delicate layer that reflects off the cartilage periosteal border on to the underlying fibrous joint capsule. Synovium is composed of cells of both fibroblast and macrophage origin, and it has two major functions: the provision of oxygen and nutrients to cartilage via the synovial fluid, and to produce lubricant factors, notably HA, that allow the articular surfaces to glide smoothly across one another.

In patients with RA, the synovium is transformed into a chronically inflamed tissue. The thin synovial layer thickens dramatically due to cell proliferation and accumulation, and the subsynovial layer becomes oedematous, hypervascular and hypercellular. Mononuclear cells accumulate, particularly T cells, B cells and macrophages. While neutrophils are abundant in the rheumatoid synovial fluid, they are sparse within the synovium. The cell-to-cell interaction results in proliferation of T and B cells, and production of inflammatory and chemotactic cytokines, RF autoantibodies, prostaglandins and matrix metalloproteinases. The net result is both local amplification of the inflammatory cascade, systemic recruitment of cells to the joint and systemic disease.

A current model of RA pathogenesis is shown in Figure 53.2, with an initiation phase resulting from antigen presentation via HLA molecules leading to an antigen-specific T-cell response and an inflammatory cascade. The perpetuation of this process is more complex and might involve T-cell independent processes.

Diagnosis and clinical tests

The diagnosis is based on suspicion in the presence of an insidious-onset inflammatory polyarthropathy symmetrically affecting the peripheral small joints (PIP, MCP, metatarsophalangeal [MTP]). This picture is by no means absolute, and monoarthritis or oligoarthritis may wax and wane for several months before a definitive pattern is established. Duration of disease and persistence of clinical and laboratory markers of inflammation are key features in distinguishing RA from a self-limited arthropathy. Persistence of synovitis for more than 8–10 weeks significantly reduces the likelihood of a reactive or viral arthropathy. Psoriatic arthritis is a great mimic, always necessitating a review of a personal and family history for psoriasis, as well as directed clinical examination. The small joints of the hand (PIP, MCP) need to be

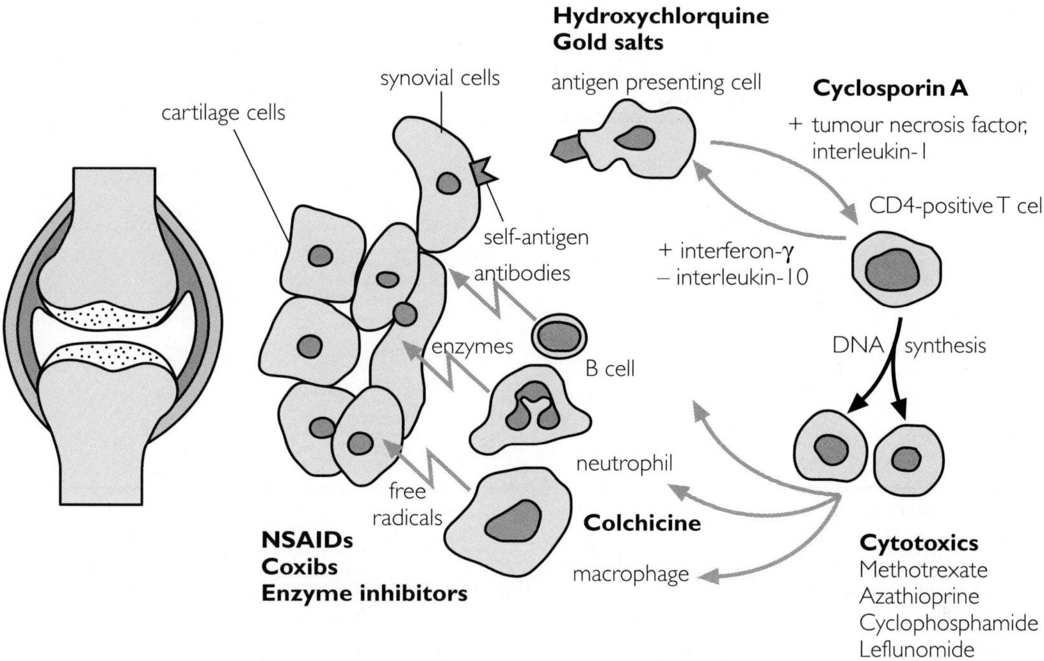

Figure 53.2 Current model of RA pathogenesis indicating site of action of therapeutic drugs

carefully examined for tenderness, swelling and synovial hypertrophy. The presence of prominent inflammatory changes in the DIP joints indicates psoriatic arthritis as the likely diagnosis. The presence of rheumatoid nodules or the classic swan-neck or boutonniere deformities make the diagnosis easy. Despite the common patient focus on hand symptoms, the small joints of the feet must always be examined. Identification of unreported synovitis at the MTP joints supports the diagnosis, while toe interphalangeal synovitis supports psoriatic arthritis.

As noted above, there are no specific tests for RA. RF positivity supports the diagnosis in the appropriate clinical setting. Other laboratory tests will non-specifically identify an inflammatory process and can be used to support other diagnoses, such as polyarticular gout, polyarticular sepsis or viral arthritis. If symptoms have been present for some months, plain radiographs of the hands and feet may identify inflammation-induced periarticular osteopenia or erosions. The pattern of joints affected by erosions can provide major support for the diagnosis.

Rheumatoid arthritis in the elderly

The onset of RA is often abrupt in elderly patients, and although the classic peripheral symmetrical small joint polyarthritis develops, shoulder symptoms may predominate initially and prominent hand oedema may obscure the diagnosis. Conditions that may mimic each other are late-onset RA, remitting seronegative symmetric synovitis with pitting oedema (so-called RS3PE) and polymyalgia rheumatica (PMR). Table 53.3 compares these entities. Both gout and calcium pyrophosphate pseudogout may have a rheumatoid-like presentation in the elderly, making joint aspiration an important diagnostic procedure whenever possible. Paraneoplastic polyarthritis due to lung cancer or colon cancer necessitates review of these possibilities in the history and examination.

Treatment

The aim of treatment is to improve the patient's quality of life both in the short and long term. This begins with patient education and active involvement of individuals with their own self-management

Table 53.3 Differences and similarities between late-onset RA, PMR, and remitting seronegative symmetrical synovitis with pitting oedema

	Late onset RA	PMR	RS3PE
Age of onset	Over 60 years	Over 50 years	Over 60 years
Sex ratio (F:M)	1:1	2.5:1	1:4
Mode of onset	Acute or subtle	Acute	Acute
Predominant joint pattern	Peripheral joints in upper limbs and shoulders	Shoulders, lower back, hips, knees	Hands, wrists, shoulders, knees
Distal oedema	May be present	May be present	Present
RF positivity	In 50%	Negative	Negative
HLA association	DR4	?	? B7
Course	Severe in RF+ Mild in RF–	Self-limited 1–3 years. Giant cell arteritis in 15–20%	Self-limited 1–2 years
Response to low-dose corticosteroids	Poor in RF+ Good in RF–	Good	Good

Source: J. J. Canoso, (1997), *Rheumatology in Primary Care*, W. B. Saunders Co., Philadelphia.

and in the decision-making process with the doctor. Sources of patient information are the Arthritis Foundations, Arthritis Care, and the worldwide web. Allied health professionals play a critical role in the provision of education on joint protection and of orthoses to improve and maintain hand and foot function. Rehabilitation measures should be applied early to attain the goal of maintaining independence.

Pain relief is important at all stages of the disease, and while this is intimately related to suppression of overall inflammatory activity, it needs addressing in its own right. Treatment also needs to take into account age-related factors and co-morbidities. To obtain adequate analgesia with paracetamol requires ongoing dialogue to achieve the required frequency of tablet taking. Most patients assume that 8 tablets (4 g) per day is too many, or are concerned about addiction or side effects. NSAIDs are an important symptomatic treatment, primarily relegated to second position in the elderly due to gastrointestinal and renal toxicity, which are both poorly tolerated in this age group. Of the standard NSAIDs, the shorter-acting medications of ibuprofen and diclofenac are recommended. However, with the development of cyclo-oxygenase-2 (COX2) selective medications, such as celecoxib and rofecoxib, there are now options that are equally efficacious and significantly less likely to induce frank peptic ulceration. It is crucial to note that these medications appear to impair renal function in the elderly similar to existing therapies, do not replace the cardioprotective or CNS protective effect of low-dose aspirin, and do not prevent gastrointestinal toxicity which is not related to COX1 inhibition.

The overriding goal is to suppress the inflammatory process as much as possible within the practical considerations of medication compliance and toxicity. Figure 53.2 details a model of disease pathogenesis, and included are the probable major sites of action of those anti-rheumatic medications in which a method of action has been proposed.

In prescribing treatment for RA, it is useful to imagine 3 heaps of medications. The first contains simple analgesics, such as paracetamol, while the second contains NSAIDs or coxibs. Neither medication alters the underlying disease process and they provide symptomatic relief only. Medications from these groups may be combined together, and with the third heap. Patients can also start and stop and adjust the dose within prescribed limits according to symptoms. The third heap is the slow-acting medications intended to alter the disease process, and which must be taken regularly without patient-initiated dose alteration. For seronegative RA patients with minor evidence of inflammation, the anti-malarial hydroxychloroquine could be considered. In the presence of significant inflammation, there are three first line agents: sulphasalazine, methotrexate and leflunomide. Their efficacy is similar in terms of reduction in swollen and tender joints and slowing of radiographic progression. The actual order of treatment will often be decided on 'toxicity' factors such as alcohol use, sulphur sensitivity, family planning and cost. Initiation of these agents should ideally be undertaken in liaison with a specialist rheumatologist who can advise both yourself and your patient on expected outcomes, adverse effects and requirement for monitoring. Using the analogy of anti-cancer therapy, in which multiple processes are targeted simultaneously to achieve greater tumour reduction and reduced likelihood of disease resistance, combination therapies are increasingly used for the treatment of RA.

Prognosis

Once established, about 70% of patients have a chronic remitting disease, while 10–20% have a very aggressive and destructive form of disease with few clinical remissions. A minority of patients have spontaneous long-lived remissions after the initial diagnosis and this occurs primarily to those who experience an abrupt onset.

The morbidity from RA continues to be significant despite treatment advances. Approximately one-third of patients have to retire from paid employment within 5 years of diagnosis, increasing to half at 10 years. Persons primarily utilising heavy manual skills are disproportionately made unemployable. Morbidity is greatest in those who are RF positive, and positive for one or more of the HLA susceptibility genes.

The overall mortality rate of patients is modestly higher than that of the normal population and is proportional to the disease activity. Patients with a very large proportion of their joints actively inflamed have a mortality similar to patients with stage IV Hodgkin's disease.

When to refer

RA is a potentially disabling condition that markedly reduces life expectancy. All patients with suspected RA require ongoing combined care for monitoring of joint function, disease complications and toxicity of therapy. An inflammatory symmetrical small joint arthritis affecting MTP and MCP joints is highly suspicious of rheumatoid arthritis and early rheumatologic evaluation is important for retardation of joint damage. Physiotherapy and occupational therapy referral should occur when diagnosis is confirmed.

Additional reasons for referral include:

- systemic manifestations: scleritis and episcleritis, pulmonary disease or any forms of vasculitis
- medication toxicity identified clinically or via laboratory tests that persist upon testing at 1 week interval
- when considering corticosteroids, urgent referral is warranted
- other systemic manifestations: anaemia, muscle atrophy and weight loss
- persistent carpal tunnel syndrome failing conservative treatment for 2 weeks
- loss of disease control identified clinically or via laboratory tests for 2 weeks
- patient education on disease process, prognosis and self-management.

Gout

Epidemiology

Gout is one of the common forms of arthritis occurring in the elderly and is often inaccurately used as a blanket explanation for any inflammatory arthritis for which the diagnosis is uncertain. It is the most common inflammatory arthropathy of males over the age of 40 years, and the ratio of male to female (5:1) is reducing. It is rare in children and premenopausal women, and uncommon in males under 30. The prevalence of gout in both sexes mirrors the serum urate level, which begins to climb in males from the early 20s but does not begin to climb in females until the menopause, when the reduction in oestrogen reduces renal excretion of uric acid. The peak ages for gout in males is 40–50 years and 2 decades later for females. Because of increased longevity and the frequent long-term use of thiazide diuretics, the prevalence of gout is rising among elderly women in Western countries.

The overall prevalence of gout is 10–20 per 1000 males, and 2–5 per 1000 females. Racial differences in the rates of hyperuricaemia due to both genetic and environmental factors influence the subsequent prevalence of gout.

Aetiology

Gout is the clinical condition that results when the serum uric acid levels chronically exceed the local tissue saturation, resulting in crystal precipitation. These crystals are then available for phagocytosis by polymorphonuclear (PMN) leucocytes, a step that is enhanced by coating the crystals with protein, particularly IgG. Enzymatic reactions within the PMN phagolysosome and mechanical disruption due to the sharp-pointed crystals lead to cell lysis and release of potent chemoattractant and inflammatory mediators. Some of these stimulate the influx of further PMN leucocytes and prostaglandin production.

Pathophysiology

The serum uric acid level is dynamically balanced between production and excretion. Box 53.2 lists the factors that are important in the overproduction and underexcretion of uric acid, highlighting those that are important in the elderly. While hyperuricaemia is the major risk factor for gout, by itself it does not equate with a diagnosis of gout. Approximately 10% of elderly are hyperuricaemic, with the majority never developing gout.

Box 53.2 Risk factors for gout in the elderly

Uric acid overproduction (10% of primary gout)

- Overweight
- Diet rich in purines
- Alcohol
- Proliferative lesions (psoriasis, haemolysis, myeloproliferative disease, lymphoma)

Decreased excretion (90% of primary gout)

- Overweight
- Renal insufficiency: renal disease, pre-renal volume insufficiency, low urine volume
- Drug induced: alcohol, diuretics (thiazide, frusemide), low-dose aspirin, cyclosporin, nicotinic acid
- Hypothyroidism
- Acidosis: respiratory or metabolic (lactate, acetoacetate, β-hydroxybutyrate)

Uric acid is itself a weak acid which is ionised at normal body pH and can form salts with various cations, with 98% in the form of monosodium urate. The balance of urate to uric acid is pH dependent, with the solubility of uric acid in urine rising exponentially as the pH increases above 4. However, in body fluids such as serum, synovial fluid and tissues, the variation in pH has little effect on solubility. The key factors in determining crystal formation are the local concentration of urate, the local temperature and local factors such as proteoglycans, which appear to increase urate solubility, and the presence of cations such as sodium and calcium, which facilitate crystal seeding.

Uric acid production results from purine nucleotide metabolism, producing hypoxanthine which forms xanthine, which in turn forms uric acid. These last steps are catalysed by the enzyme xanthine oxidase. Purines can be derived directly from the diet (uric acid is not a normal component of food and is poorly absorbed) or by synthesis from small molecular precursors. Purine bases derived from tissue turnover may be reutilised, with these amounts greatly increased in proliferative lesions (skin or haematologic). Inherited disorders of purine metabolism which shunt to the production of uric acid are fascinating, particularly with their link to the self-mutilating Lesch-Nyhan syndrome, but overall are extremely rare.

In order to maintain uric acid balance, urate must be excreted as there is no metabolism of urate in human tissues. Underexcretion is the major factor in the development of hyperuricaemia and gout. Two-thirds of urate is eliminated via the kidneys, the other third passively excreted via the gastrointestinal tract and degraded by colonic bacteria. Plasma urate is essentially completely filtered by the glomerulus and completely reabsorbed in the proximal tubule, with the maintenance of urate excretion depending on active tubular secretion of urate. The exact site of or means of secretion is uncertain, as is the subsequent reabsorption of the tubular secreted urate. The net result is that approximately 10% of the filtered urate is ultimately excreted in the urine.

Alcohol results in hyperuricaemia by shifting the pyruvate–lactate balance towards lactate, which reduces the renal excretion of urate. It also increases urate production by increasing the degradation of adenine nucleotides. In addition, beers contain significant amounts of the purine guanosine, which acts as a purine load. Obesity is linked to hyperuricaemia from excessive dietary purines and alcohol, but obesity per se is also associated with a decreased renal excretion of urate.

Diagnosis

Acute gout

The clinical features of acute gout are very well known and the classic description by Sydenham is available in many texts. In over half the initial attacks, the first joint involved is the MTP in the great toe, with an abrupt red swelling associated with intense pain developing over a few hours, often preceded by a slight niggle in the joint. Subsequently, the swelling may spread to the forefoot, with desquamation of the skin overlying the MTP. Nearly all patients with gout will experience MTP involvement at some time. The cooler, more peripheral lower limb joints are predominantly affected, but soft tissues of the olecranon bursa and Achilles tendon may also be involved. Several factors are recognised as precipitants of acute gout and include acute illness, trauma, surgery, dehydration, alcohol and drugs that either increase or decrease the plasma urate concentration leading to alterations in the solute–solvent balance. The gold standard for the diagnosis of gout is the aspiration of synovial fluid, with microscopy demonstrating the presence of intracellular, negatively birefringent, needle-shaped uric acid crystals. The added trauma of aspiration of an acutely involved joint is only required when the diagnosis of septic arthritis really needs exclusion (noting that sepsis of the first MTP is rare). Large joints can be aspirated relatively atraumatically, with the aspiration alone leading to significant temporary relief.

In the elderly, gout is often more indolent and may be mistaken for osteoarthritis, resulting in a delay in accurate diagnosis and treatment. This is complicated by the high prevalence of OA in the elderly. Where monoarticular initial attacks are the norm in the younger population, attacks in two or more joints are the norm in the elderly. Polyarticular onset is more common in women, although this reflects the initial onset in women usually being over the age of 60. In addition, it appears that tophi and concurrent diuretic use is more common in females than males. Fever and leucocytosis relate to the number of involved joints.

Chronic gout

Chronic gout develops as a consequence of prolonged hyperuricaemia. Tophi usually develop after 8–10 years of gout, with the exception of massive urate production as a result of myeloproliferative disorders on a background of renal impairment. Tophi may occur at any site but are most common in the digits of the hands and feet. When close to the surface they appear yellowish, and may invoke periodic local skin inflammation or discharge a white chalky material.

Clinical tests

Laboratory measurement of urate has little role in the diagnosis of gout as the majority of hyperuricaemic patients will not develop gout, and one-third of patients with acute gout have normal uric acid levels at the time of the attack. Its utility is in the management of chronic gout and in the dissolution of tophi. Baseline investigations should also include renal function, blood sugar and fasting lipid levels and urinalysis.

Microscopic analysis of joint fluid or tophi aspirates can be used to confirm the presence of urate crystals and identify whether they are intra- or extracellular. While the purist will require intracellular crystal identification for the diagnosis of gout, the presence of synovial fluid crystals within the appropriate clinical setting will pass for most clinicians. The skill and diligence of the laboratory technician in searching for crystals and examining spun synovial fluid significantly affects the yield.

Synovial fluid analysis also allows for cell counts, cell differentials, Gram stains and culture.

Radiology is usually not required for the diagnosis of gout. The joint distribution and soft tissue changes mirror the clinical examination. In contrast to RA, the joint space is well preserved and there is no juxta-articular osteopenia. The erosions seen with gout are characteristically described as 'punched out' with sclerotic margins and overhanging edges, and are larger than with RA.

Treatment

The management of gout can be strategically divided into the treatment of acute gout, which does not attempt to modify plasma urate concentrations, and management of recurrent gout, which requires a protracted multidimensional approach.

Acute gout

The management of the acute attack is aimed at a reduction of pain and inflammation and is the same regardless of the cause of the gout. Systemic treatments comprise NSAIDs that block prostaglandin production, and colchicine, which inhibits the PMN cytoskeletal system and reduces migration to the joint and phagocytosis of crystals. NSAIDs are superior to colchicine in speed of action, with the latter invariably causing diarrhoea if a fast onset of action is attempted by frequent dosing. Colchicine has been recommended in elderly patients at risk of gastrointestinal ulceration, although the selective COX2 inhibitors are likely to be used in that setting now. Indomethacin is still widely regarded as the NSAID of choice in treating acute gout, with a dose of 50 mg qid at onset and reduced according to response. The choice, however, is wide, and nearly any NSAID can be used with a starting dose at the upper limit of recommended or just above, and reducing when the attack becomes under control.

If the joint can be successfully injected, then the administration of corticosteroids is a particularly effective means of treatment. Injection of steroids at the time of joint aspiration places you at risk of eventually injecting a septic joint, and it is wiser to await the Gram stain result or overnight culture result before injecting. An alternative to direct injection, particularly if there are multiple joints involved, or the injection is beyond the technical skills of the patient and practitioner, is an intramuscular injection of a depot steroid. A key aspect of the management of the acute attack of gout is *not* to commence a urate-lowering agent while any joint is inflamed, or to discontinue or alter a urate-lowering agent that has been previously commenced. Both increases and decreases in plasma urate concentration may precipitate or prolong an attack of gout.

Chronic gout

The dilemma in gout management is to know when to consider a chronic management plan, which in essence is aimed at reducing the plasma urate concentration. Factors to consider in this decision are the frequency of attacks, the severity and impact on the individual's lifestyle these attacks have and the ease with which the chronic management plan could be introduced in that individual. In many cases, it may be easier to manage the acute attacks as they occur.

Once the decision has been made for chronic management, the first step is combining patient education on the production and excretion of uric acid with a review of the relevant causative factors in that individual (see Box 53.2) and the role of medications in each part of the strategy.

A concept that many patients are not exposed to is that of the urate load. It has invariably taken many years of hyperuricaemia before an acute attack of gout occurs or a tophi develops. The chronic management strategies will shift the balance of production and excretion in favour of excretion, but this in itself will not instantly deplete the urate load that was present before initiating treatment. Thus, acute attacks of gout will not immediately be abolished, but their frequency will progressively decline to zero.

Medication risk factors should be reviewed and where possible alternative medications found, although on occasion the decision analysis favours persisting with a medication in spite of hyperuricaemia. Dietary factors (see Box 53.3) and alcohol use should be addressed with tact, and advice given

Box 53.3 Low purine diet guide

Eat as much as you need
- Milk
- Egg
- Cereal (except whole wheat)
- Most vegetables
- Fruit
- Enriched bread
- Butter or margarine

Restrict your intake of
- Asparagus
- Mushrooms
- Cauliflower
- Oatmeal
- Lentils
- Whole wheat cereal
- Beans
- Meat (1 serving per day)
- Spinach
- Fish and seafood (1 serving per day)
- Beer and distilled liquors

Avoid
- Sweetbreads
- Liver
- Sardines
- Brain
- Anchovies
- Meat extracts
- Kidney
- Gravies

aimed at increasing the urine volume towards 2000 mL per day. The relative purine content of foods needs to be balanced against the absolute amount consumed. Many practitioners remember that anchovies are bad for gout but do not consider that the few grams consumed is an insignificant purine load compared to the kilograms of peas, beans or lentils that may be consumed per week.

The choice of long-term management is between allopurinol, a xanthine oxidase inhibitor, which reduces new production of uric acid, and the uricosuric agents probenecid and sulphinpyrazone, which competitively inhibit renal tubular urate reabsorption. Uricosurics are, in theory, the treatment of choice for hyperuricaemia of under-excretion, which is the majority of cases, yet it is the lesser-used approach for gout. The reason for this is that to work, uricosurics require near normal renal function, a sufficient urine volume and a pH to prevent uric acid renal stone formation and are contraindicated in anyone with renal stones of any type. Therefore, investigations to identify renal calculi, and measurement of urine volume, urine pH and renal function should be undertaken prior to their use. Uricosurics will not work with concomitant salicylates, and the twice-daily regimen reduces compliance. Therefore, allopurinol is usually the drug of choice, although requiring dose reduction if significant renal impairment exists, as its active metabolite oxypurinol accumulates. Maculopapular rashes develop commonly with allopurinol and 1 in 1000 patients may develop an exfoliative dermatitis. Azathioprine is metabolised by xanthine oxidase and the dose must be reduced by 80% if allopurinol is commenced.

My treatment strategy for chronic gout is to treat the acute attack and when that has settled to commence prophylactic treatment with either a low-dose NSAID (e.g. indomethacin 25 mg bd or diclofenac 25 mg bd) or colchicine 0.5 mg bd. This is continued throughout the introduction and adjustment of allopurinol and for 3 months after the final adjustment. After 1 month of prophylaxis and quiet joints, allopurinol 100 mg per day is commenced in addition to the colchicine/NSAID. At 1 month the urate level is measured, and if greater than 0.4 mmol/L, the dose of allopurinol is increased to 200 mg/day while continuing the NSAID/colchicine. This continues monthly until the urate level is below 0.4 mmol/L or 400 mg/day of allopurinol is reached. Three months after the allopurinol dose is stabilised, the prophylaxis is withdrawn. Patients are strongly advised that in the event of an acute attack of gout, they must not discontinue or alter their allopurinol dose but rather reinstitute their acute management plan with either a NSAID or colchicine and arrange urgent review by yourself. If you are aiming for tophi dissolution, then the plasma urate level needs to be lowered towards the lower limit of normal. The current recommendation is for lifelong therapy, which makes the initial decision to commence therapy all the more onerous.

Prognosis

The critical role of patient education cannot be overstated if you wish to obtain a good prognosis. Incomplete knowledge of the precipitating factors, the expected effect of agents such as allopurinol on future attacks and what to do during an acute attack often leaves the person bewildered and frustrated, leading to abandonment of the treatment strategy. If dietary and lifestyle modifications can be made, and the patient adequately informed about the use of his medications, then the prognosis for most patients with gout is excellent symptom relief.

When to refer

In most circumstances, gout is best treated by the patient's general practitioner providing the necessary patient education and consistency of management. Urgent referral is required to aspirate joints (if they are technically outside your area of expertise) to document crystals so as to confirm the diagnosis but more importantly to exclude infection. Other reasons to refer include:

- guidance and education reinforcement in cases of recurrent gout or polyarticular gout
- therapeutic guidance in patients with organ failure or multiple concomitant medications
- patient education on underlying processes and medication strategies
- accurate diagnosis, with appropriate prognostic information and a treatment plan covering common eventualities.

Bibliography and further reading

Brook, P. (ed.) (1997), *MJA Practice Essential: Rheumatology*, Sydney: Australasian Medical Publishing Group.

Doherty, M., Dacre, J., Dieppe, P. & Snaith, M. (1992), 'The "GALS" locomotor screen', *Annals of the Rheumatic Diseases*, 51, pp. 1165–9.

Pile, K. D. (2000), 'Osteoarthritis: analgesics, lubricants and vitamins', *Current Therapeutics*, 41, pp. 34–9.

Snaith, M. (ed.) (1996), *ABC of Rheumatology*, London: BMJ Publishing Group.

Chapter 54

Polymyalgia rheumatica and giant cell arteritis

SIMON BURNET and BRIAN HAZLEMAN

Introduction

The earliest description of giant cell arteritis may have been in the 10th century in the *Tadkwat* of Ali Iba Isu, where removal of the temporal artery was recommended as treatment. Jan Van Eyck's work depicting the *Holy Virgin with Canon Van der Paele* (1436) (Figure 54.1) and Pieri di Cosimo's portrait of *Fracesco Gamberti* (1505) (Figure 54.2) both show signs of prominent temporal arteries. Contemporary accounts document rheumatic pains and difficulty attending morning service with possible stiffness and general ill health.

No further evidence for the existence of either polymyalgia rheumatica or giant cell arteritis exists until the late 19th century, when recognisable descriptions of each were documented in opposite ends of the British Isles. In 1888 Bruce described five cases of 'severe rheumatic gout'. Patients were aged from 60 to 70 years and suffered from widespread muscular and joint pains. Jonathan Hutchinson in 1890 described 'a peculiar form of thrombotic arteritis of the aged, which is sometimes productive of gangrene'.

For 40 years there seem to be no published reports until Horton and colleagues (1932) described the typical histologic appearances at temporal artery biopsy. In the early 1950s several authors used a variety of names to describe a similar condition, adding constitutional symptoms and an elevated erythrocyte sedimentation rate (ESR) to the symptom complex, but it was Barber (1957) who suggested the present name. It was not until 1963 that any cases of polymyalgia rheumatica were reported in the US under its new name.

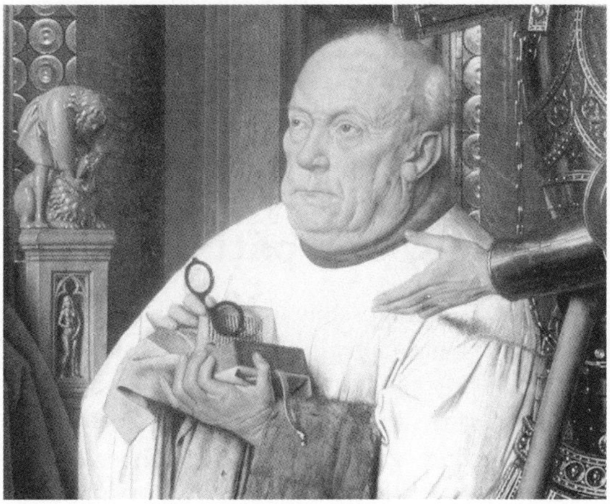

Figure 54.1 Jan Van Eyck's *Holy Virgin with Canon Van der Paele* (1436)

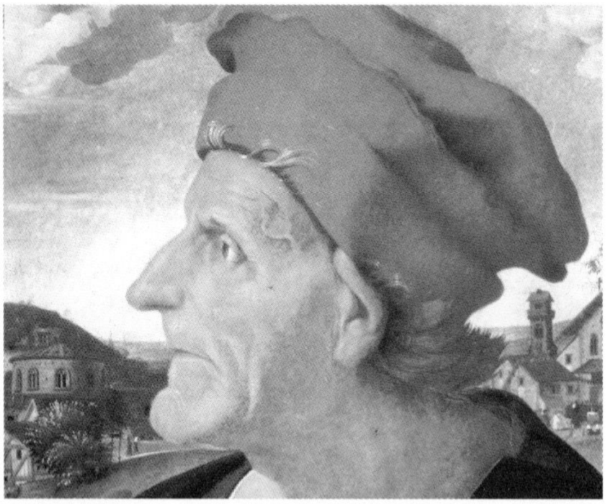

Figure 54.2 Pieri di Cosimo's *Fracesco Gamberti* (1505)

Several authors mentioned myalgic symptoms in early reports of temporal arteritis but Porsman (1951) first pointed out the similarity between temporal arteritis and 'arthritis of the aged'. In 1960 a report on 67 patients emphasised the occurrence of 'anarthritic rheumatism' in giant cell arteritis, providing more solid clinical evidence for the relationship between polymyalgia rheumatica and giant cell arteritis. Histologic support confirmed the coexistence of the two conditions.

Aetiology and pathogenesis

At present it is impossible to define the underlying pathologic abnormality in polymyalgia and, indeed, it may well be that there are several different mechanisms responsible for a largely similar pattern of pain. Large geographical differences in the frequency of positive temporal artery biopsy in polymyalgia rheumatica (PMR) suggest that the clinical syndrome of PMR may comprise a heterogeneous group of conditions, not all of which are associated with giant cell arteritis (GCA). The relative homogeneity of groups of patients, and the apparent rapid clinical response to corticosteroids, does not exclude this possibility. Although the increasing incidence of GCA and PMR after the age of 50 implies a relationship with ageing, the significance of this observation is not understood.

A distinct prodromal event resembling influenza or viral pneumonia is often noted by patients. However, viral studies have produced negative results. The known association of hepatitis B with polyarteritis nodosa led investigators to seek a similar association in polymyalgia. Inconsistent results were the outcome. It has been suggested that contact with pet birds, especially parakeets, might be a factor in aetiology, representing some immunological reaction to psittacosis or constituent of their food. Others have been unable to support this suggestion. Reports of case clustering are few, and seasonal variation in disease onset has not been confirmed in most larger studies.

Both the humoral and cellular immune systems have been implicated in pathogenesis. The latter seems the most important. GCA is limited to vessels with an internal elastic lamina, and electron microscopy shows fragmentation of this with mononuclear cell accumulation compatible with cell mediated injury. Fragments of elastic tissue can be demonstrated within giant cells.

Increased numbers of circulating lymphoblasts are seen in patients with active PMR and immunoglobulins are also elevated. These observations have led to the suggestion that these diseases may have an immunologic basis, perhaps an age-related autoimmune process directed against arterial wall constituents. There is no difference in *in vitro* lymphocytotoxicity to arterial smooth muscle between the cells from patients with active untreated GCA/PMR and normal controls. The lymphocytes in the arteritic lesions express the T-cell phenotype and only a few B-cells are found.

Ageing of the immune and neuroendocrine systems may be important factors in the late onset of GCA. Breakdown in tolerance, increased susceptibility to infectious triggers or perpetuation of

Box 54.1 Essential points

- There is often a distinct prodromal event resembling influenza, but results of viral studies are negative.
- Lymphocytes in arteritic lesions express the T-cell phenotype and the CD4 subset predominates.
- Frequency of HLA-DR4 is increased.

inflammation as a result of relative cortisol deficiency are possible mechanisms. Basal cortisol levels are increased in the elderly but the release of cortisol in response to stress is attenuated. The balance of pro- and anti-inflammatory mediators can determine the development of disease in animal models of inflammation and autoimmunity. The increased prevalence of cases of PMR and GCA in individuals of European background compared to other populations, and reports of multiple family cases, has suggested a genetic relationship, possibly linked to the immune system. In cases of PMR, most studies of HLA typing have used serological methods. Class I antigens have shown variable results, which suggests that a significant relationship is unlikely. It has been found that HLA-B8 was significantly more common in cases of PMR (59%) and GCA (50%) than in arthritis (27%).

Several workers have found the frequency of the class II antigen HLA-DR4 in cases of PMR and GCA to be about twice that in normal controls. In some reports, HLA-DR4 has been increased in patients with PMR and not in those with GCA. Patients rarely suffer from both GCA and rheumatoid arthritis, and this is consistent with the view that different and distinct domains of the HLA-DR molecule are important in determining susceptibility to the two diseases.

Box 54.2 Essential points

- Peak incidence at ages 60–75 years.
- Sex distribution of 3 women to 1 man.
- Annual incidence and prevalence of biopsy proven GCA is 17 and 223/100 000.
- Mainly affects white people, but can occur worldwide.
- Familial aggregation has been reported, suggesting a genetic association.

Epidemiology

GCA affects the white population almost exclusively. Most reports originate from northern Europe and parts of the northern US; however, the diseases are recognisable worldwide. Both PMR and GCA affect elderly people and are seldom diagnosed below the age of 50 years. A study of biopsy proven GCA diagnosed from 1950 through to 1985 in Olmsted County, Minnesota, demonstrated an average annual incidence and prevalence of 17 and 223, respectively, per 100 000 inhabitants aged 50 years or more. The age-adjusted incidence rates were approximately 3 times higher in women than in men. In addition, the incidence increased with higher age in both sexes. The incidence also increased significantly during the period 1950–85 for females but decreased for males over the same period. The incidence rates reported from Olmsted County are similar to those in Göteborg, Sweden. Between 1970 and 1975, the incidence rate was 16.8 per 100 000 inhabitants in Sweden versus 18.3 per 100 000 in Minnesota.

The temporal arteries and aorta of all adults who died in Malmö throughout 1 year were examined, and although active GCA was not found, evidence of previous arteritis was found in 1.7% of the 889 cases. It was found that in 75% of these subjects there had been either biopsy evidence or a clinical history suggestive of GCA. This study certainly suggests that GCA may be underdiagnosed, but further studies are required.

The variety of symptoms and lack of specificity of signs and symptoms contribute to make such studies difficult, and indeed the epidemiology of PMR has been less well defined. One group, using a questionnaire in 656 patients over 65 years, found a prevalence of arteritis/polymyalgia of 3300/100 000. PMR has been found to account for 1.3–4.5% of the patients attending rheumatic disease clinics, but clearly these figures are influenced by the type of clinical load.

Familial aggregation of cases of PMR and GCA has been reported by several workers. Clustering of cases in time and space suggests that, in addition to a genetic predisposition, environmental factors may be important. One author noted that 9 of 11 cases seen over 6 years in a practice of 3000 lived in one small part of the same village, and of these, 2 lived in the same house, 2 were neighbours and 2 others close friends.

Pathophysiology

Box 54.3 Essential points

- Histologically, there is a panarteritis with giant cell granuloma.
- The involvement is patchy and 'skip lesions' are often found.
- Clinically, the artery is enlarged and nodular with a reduced or absent lumen.
- The aorta and other arteries are involved.

The histologic appearance of GCA is one of the most distinctive of vascular disorders. The dense granulomatous inflammatory infiltrates that characterise the acute stages of the disease resemble those of Takayasu's arteritis, but the clinicopathologic features in patients with positive temporal artery biopsies are diagnostic. The arteritis is histologically a panarteritis with giant cell granuloma formation, often in close proximity to a disrupted internal elastic lamina. Large and medium sized arteries are affected, the involvement is patchy and 'skip lesions' are often found. More patients with 'skip lesions' have normal arteries to palpation but do not have a more benign disease.

The gross features are not characteristic. The vessels are enlarged and nodular and have little or no lumen. Thrombosis often develops at sites of active inflammation. Later, these areas may recanalise. The lumen is narrowed by intimal proliferation (Figure 54.3). This is a common finding in arteries and may result from advancing age, nearby chronic inflammation or low blood flow. The adventitia is usually invaded by mononuclear and occasionally polymorphonuclear inflammatory cells, often cuffing the vasa vasorum; here fibrous proliferation is frequent. The changes in the media are dominated by the giant cells, which vary from small cells with 2–3 nuclei up to masses of 100 nm containing many nuclei. Here there is invasion by mononuclear cells resembling histiocytes. Fibrinoid necrosis is infrequent. Giant cells are not seen in all sections and therefore are not required for the diagnosis if other features are compatible. The more sections that are examined in the area of arteritis, the more likely it is that giant cells will be found. Fragments of elastic tissue can be demonstrated within giant cells which are surrounded with plasma cell and lymphocytic infiltration (Figure 54.4).

Corticosteroids reduce the inflammatory cell infiltrate so temporal artery biopsy should, if possible, be carried out before treatment is started. Therapy should not be delayed until a biopsy has been performed.

Involvement of the aorta and its branches, the abdominal vessels and the coronary arteries have all been described. GCA as a cause of aortic dissection has been recorded rarely at autopsy, and most exceptionally during life. This probably reflects the relatively low incidence of aortic involvement in GCA. It is of note that most patients have a history of hypertension in life or features of hypertensive disease at autopsy. None appear to have had hypertension

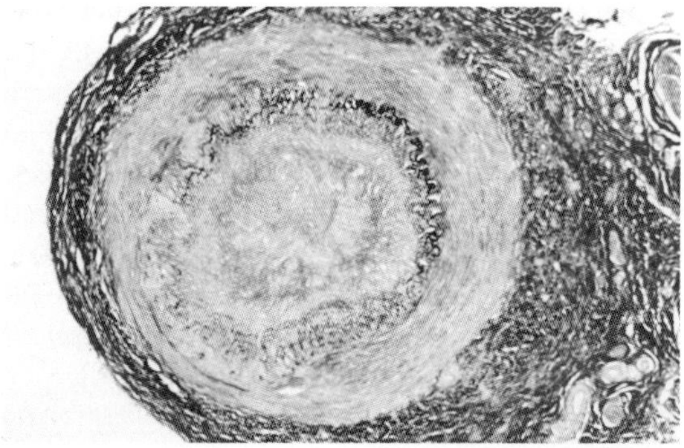

Figure 54.3 Low-powered view of the arterial wall in giant cell arteritis showing narrowing of the lumen

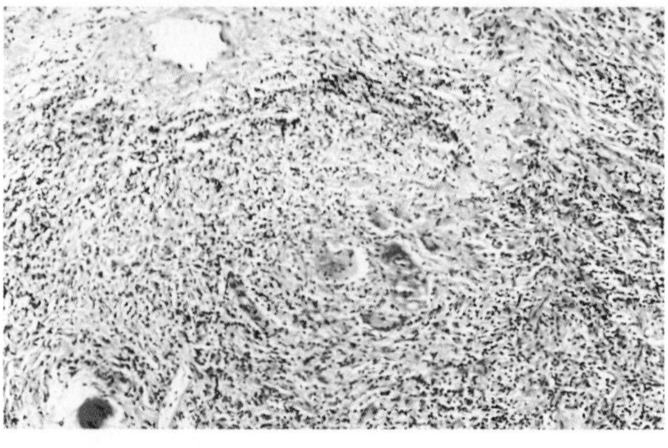

Figure 54.4 High-powered view of the arterial wall in giant cell arteritis showing giant cells in close relationship to elastic lamina

secondary to steroid treatment for GCA. In addition, 14 of the 18 patients described in the literature are women: this is a higher proportion of females than is found for GCA. This suggests that clinicians should be aware of potential life-threatening large vessel disease in cases of GCA, particularly in female patients with hypertension.

There has been little to support a concept of primary muscle disease in PMR. Serum aldolase and creatine phosphokinase levels are normal and there is no abnormality on electromyography. Muscle biopsy has shown type II atrophy alone and there is no evidence of inflammatory changes. Recently there have been reports of focal changes in muscle ultrastructure and abnormalities of mitochondrial form and function, similar to those associated with inherited mitochondrial myopathies (MM). These abnormalities are not due to gene deletions or mutations associated with MM and persist even after successful treatment. The significance of these changes is unclear. Arteritis in skeletal muscle appears to be uncommon.

Liver biopsy can show non-specific inflammatory changes or focal liver cell necrosis. There are occasional reports of granulomata and hepatic arteritis. Synovial biopsy has shown non-specific inflammatory changes with lymphocytic infiltration of knees, sternoclavicular joints and shoulders.

Clinical tests

Essential tests

The following are baseline clinical investigations, used to help make the diagnosis and exclude other conditions:

- full blood count
- biochemical profile
- protein electrophoretic strip
- urinary Bence Jones protein
- thyroid function test
- rheumatoid factor
- chest radiograph
- ESR measurement
- acute phase protein (e.g. C-reactive protein) measurement
- muscle enzymes (if indicated)
- specific investigations
- temporal artery biopsy: for suspected GCA, not for PMR.

The ESR is usually greatly elevated and provides a useful means of monitoring treatment, although it must be appreciated that some elevation of the ESR may occur in otherwise healthy elderly people. A normal ESR is occasionally found in patients with active biopsy proven disease. Repeated measurements may show raised ESRs after an initial normal value.

Anaemia, usually of a mild hypochromic type, is common and resolves without specific treatment, but a more marked normochromic anaemia occasionally occurs and may be a presenting symptom. Leucocyte and differential counts are generally normal; platelet counts are also usually normal but may be increased. Protein electrophoresis may show a non-specific rise in α-2-globulin with less frequent elevation of α-1-globulin and γ-globulin. Quantification of acute phase proteins and α-1-antitrypsin, orosomucoid, haptoglobin and C-reactive protein (CRP) are no more helpful than the ESR in the assessment of disease activity.

Abnormalities of thyroid and liver function have also been well described. In a retrospective survey of 59 cases of GCA, 5 patients with hyperthyroidism were identified. The arteritis followed the thyrotoxicosis by intervals of 4–15 years in 3 cases, and in 2 occurred simultaneously. In 250 patients with autoimmune thyroid disease, 7 cases of PMR or GCA were identified. All cases occurred in women over 60, giving a prevalence of 9.3% in this age group.

Raised serum values for alkaline phosphatase were found in up to 70% of patients with PMR, and transaminases may be mildly elevated. Liver biopsies have shown portal and intralobular inflammation with focal liver cell necrosis and small epithelioid cell granuloma. The pathologic significance of these abnormalities is unclear.

The choice of patients for biopsy depends on local circumstances, but a pragmatic policy would be to select only patients with suspected GCA (not those with obvious clinical features). Patients with PMR alone would need to be monitored carefully for development of clinical GCA, but not have a biopsy.

Box 54.4 Essential points for biopsy in GCA

- Perform biopsy if diagnosis is in doubt, particularly if systemic symptoms predominate.
- Biopsy is most useful within 24 hours of starting treatment, but do not delay treatment for sake of biopsy.
- A negative biopsy result does not exclude GCA.
- A positive result helps to prevent later doubts about diagnosis, particularly if treatment causes complications.

Box 54.5 Essential points in PMR

- The musculoskeletal symptoms are usually bilateral and symmetrical.
- Stiffness is usually the predominant feature; it is particularly severe after rest and may prevent the patient getting out of bed in the morning.
- Muscle strength is unimpaired although the pain makes interpretation of muscle testing difficult.
- Systemic features include low-grade fever, fatigue, weight loss and an elevated ESR.

A third of patients with signs and symptoms of cranial arteritis may have negative temporal artery biopsies, which may be due to the localised involvement of arteries in the head and neck. Temporal artery biopsy may show arteritis even after 14 days of corticosteroid treatment, so biopsy may be worthwhile for up to 2 weeks of treatment. However, the biopsy should be obtained as soon as possible and treatment for suspected GCA should not be delayed simply to allow a biopsy to be carried out.

Clinicians vary greatly in their approach to temporal artery biopsy. Some consider it emphasises the value of a positive histological diagnosis, especially months or years later when side effects of the steroid treatment have developed. Others feel that a high false-negative rate diminishes the value of the procedure. In most instances, the high false-negative rate can be attributed to the focal nature of involvement of the superficial temporal artery by the inflammatory process.

Box 54.6 Essential points in GCA

- There are a wide range of symptoms, but most patients have clinical findings related to involved arteries.
- Frequent features include fatigue, headaches, jaw claudication, loss of vision, scalp tenderness, PMR and aortic arch syndrome (decrease or absence of peripheral pulses, discrepancies of blood pressure, arterial bruits).
- Unlike other forms of vasculitis, GCA rarely involves the skin, kidneys and lungs.
- The ESR is usually highly elevated but may infrequently be normal.

Diagnosis

Age, sex and onset

The mean age at onset of GCA and PMR is approximately 70 years, with a range of about 50 to more than 90 years of age. Younger patients have been reported but these are atypical. Women are affected about twice as often as men. The onset of the disease can be dramatic and some patients can give the date and hour of their first symptom. Equally, the onset can be insidious. In most instances the symptoms have been present for weeks or months before the diagnosis is established, a mean of 6.2 months in one series.

Constitutional symptoms, including fever, fatigue, anorexia and weight loss and depression, are present in the majority of patients and may be an early or even an initial finding and can lead to delay in diagnosis. They may be striking and suggest many different conditions. These patients may be labelled pyrexia of unknown origin (PUO) and subjected to many investigations. GCA was found in 15% of patients over 65 presenting with PUO. A hidden malignancy can mimic the symptoms of PMR but these patients do not usually respond to corticosteroids. Although at present there is no evidence to suggest that malignancy is more common in patients with PMR than in other people, deterioration in health or a poor initial response to corticosteroids must always be taken seriously and a search for an occult neoplasm made.

Polymyalgia rheumatica

Patients usually locate the source of their pain and stiffness to the muscles. The onset is most common in the shoulder region and neck, with eventual involvement of the shoulder and pelvic girdles and the corresponding proximal muscle groups. Involvement of distal limb muscles is unusual. The symptoms are usually bilateral and symmetrical. Stiffness is usually the predominant feature, is particularly severe after rest, and may prevent the patient getting out of bed in the morning. The muscular pain is often diffuse and movement accentuates the pain; pain at night is common. Muscle strength is usually unimpaired, although the pain makes interpretation of muscle testing difficult. There is tenderness of involved structures, including periarticular structures such as bursae, tendons and joint capsules, although the muscle tenderness is generally not as severe as that in myositis. In late stages muscle atrophy may develop, with restriction of shoulder movement. An improvement of shoulder range is rapid with corticosteroid therapy, unlike that seen in frozen shoulder. Occasionally the painful arc sign of subacromial bursitis is present; this is important to recognise, as a local injection of corticosteroid will give relief and save the patient from an increase in systemic corticosteroid dosage.

PMR has traditionally been viewed as a condition affecting muscles and many reports have emphasised the rarity of joint involvement. Recent emphasis has been given to a possible association between synovitis and the muscle symptoms in PMR. It has also been suggested that both axial and peripheral synovitis often occur.

Inflammatory synovitis and effusions have been noted by several authors, the reported incidence varying from 0% to 100% in various series. Synovitis of the knees, wrists and sternoclavicular joints is most common, but involvement is transient and mild. Erosive changes in joints and/or sclerosis of the sacroiliac joints have been reported, although they are difficult to demonstrate in the sternoclavicular joints except by tomography. Abnormal technetium pertechnetate scintigrams have shown widespread uptake over several joints, particularly shoulders, knees, wrists and hands. Abnormalities persisted after treatment, suggesting they are due to concurrent osteoarthritis.

Giant cell arteritis

This condition causes a wide range of symptoms, but most patients have clinical features related to affected arteries. Common features include fatigue, headache and tenderness of the scalp, particularly around the temporal and occipital arteries.

Headache is the most common symptom and is present in two-thirds or more of patients. It usually begins early in the course of the disease and may be the presenting symptom. The pain is severe and localised to the temple. However, it may be occipital or be less defined and precipitated by brushing the hair. It can be severe even when the arteries are clinically normal and, conversely, may subside even though the disease remains active. The nature of the pain varies; some patients describe it as shooting and others as a more steady ache. Scalp tenderness is common, particularly around the temporal and occipital arteries, and may disturb sleep. Tender spots or nodules or even small skin infarcts may be present for several days. The vessels are thickened, tender and nodular with absent or reduced pulsation (Figure 54.5). Occasionally they are red and clearly visible.

Visual disturbances have been described in 25–50% of cases, although the incidence of visual loss is now regarded as much lower, about 6–10% in most series. This is probably because of earlier recognition and treatment.

Visual symptoms are an ophthalmic emergency; if they are identified and treated urgently, blindness is almost entirely preventable. The variety of ocular lesions is essentially due to occlusion of the various orbital or ocular arteries. Blindness is the most serious and irreversible feature. The visual loss is

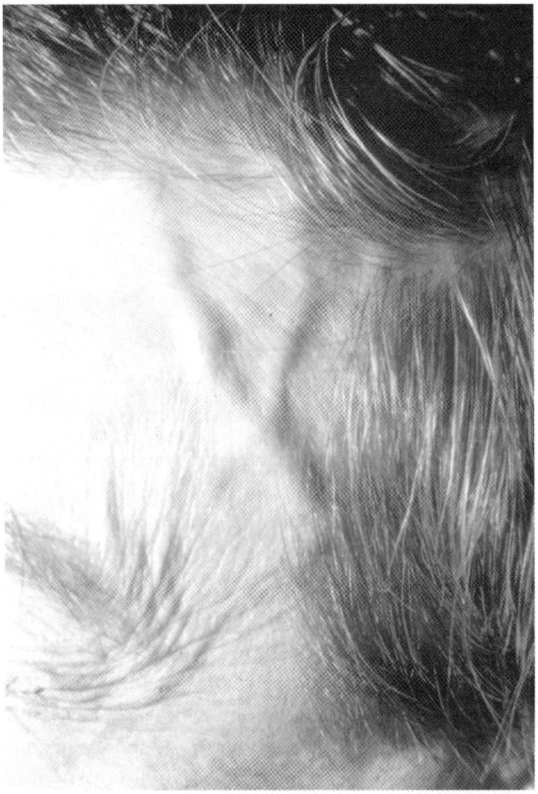

Figure 54.5 Photograph of dilated temporal arteries in a patient with giant cell arteritis

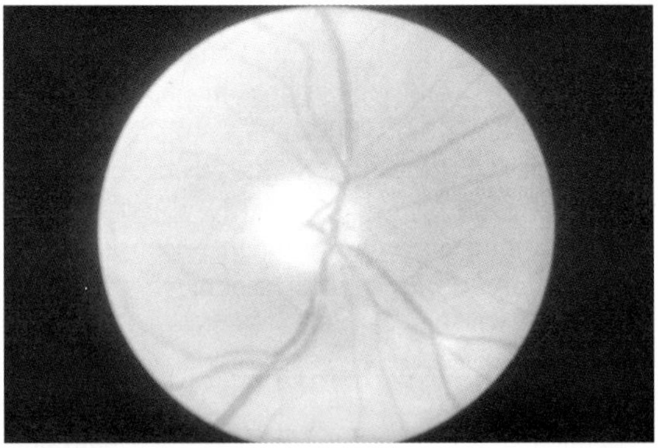

Figure 54.6 A fundus photograph showing optic atrophy secondary to giant cell arteritis

usually sudden, painless and permanent; it may vary from mistiness of vision, or involvement of a part of the visual field, to complete blindness. There is a risk of the second eye being involved if the patient is not treated aggressively. Involvement of the second eye can occur within 24 hours. Blindness may be the initial presentation in cases of GCA but tends to follow other symptoms by several weeks or months (Figure 54.6).

The incidence of various ocular manifestations given in the literature varies widely because the incidence depends on a number of factors, the most important of which is how early the diagnosis of GCA is established and the treatment started. It also depends upon the rigour with which cases are diagnosed. The most common are optic nerve ischaemic lesions. These are usually anterior and are associated with partial or more frequently complete visual loss. They can occasionally be posterior which can lead to partial or complete loss. Extraocular mobility disorders are usually transient and not associated with visual loss. Papillary abnormalities can be seen secondary to visual loss. Cerebral ischaemic lesions producing visual loss are rare, as are anterior segment ischaemic lesions and choroidal infarcts. Retinal ischaemic lesions can affect the central retinal artery, and this is associated with severe visual loss. The cilioretinal artery can be occluded but is invariably associated with anterior ischaemic optic neuropathy (AION).

Pain on chewing, due to claudication of the jaw muscles, occurs in up to two-thirds of patients. Tingling in the tongue, loss of taste, and pain in the mouth and throat can also occur, presumably due to vascular insufficiency.

The widespread nature of the vasculitis has been previously mentioned. Clinical evidence of large artery involvement is present in 10–15% of cases (Figure 54.7), and in some instances aortic dissection and rupture occur.

Less common features of GCA include hemiparesis, peripheral neuropathy, deafness, depression and confusion. Involvement of the coronary arteries may lead to myocardial infarction. Aortic regurgitation and congestive cardiac failure may also occur. Abnormalities of thyroid and liver function are well described. An association between carpal tunnel syndrome and PMR has been noted by several authors. Local corticosteroid injection and/or surgical decompression are sometimes necessary.

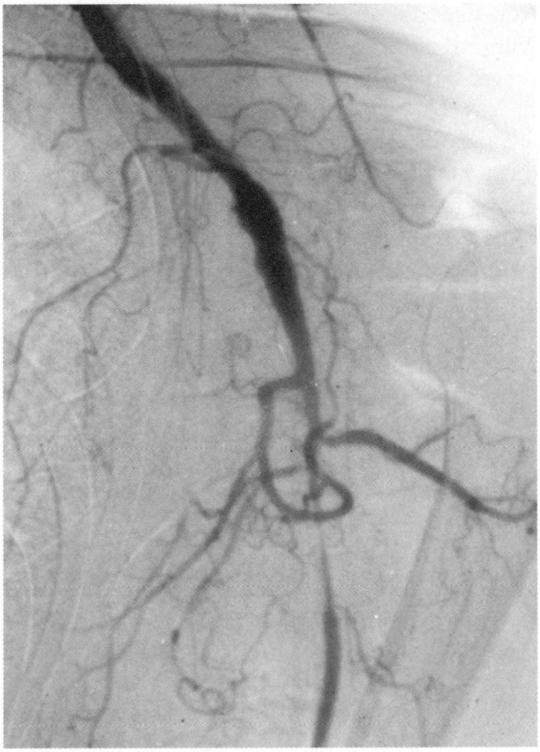

Figure 54.7 Arteriogram showing narrowing of axillary artery in giant cell arteritis

Relationship between PMR and GCA

In recent years, GCA and PMR have increasingly been considered as closely related conditions. The two syndromes form a spectrum of diseases and affect the same types of patient. The conditions may occur independently or may occur in the same patient, either together or separated by time.

In patients with PMR who have no symptoms or signs of GCA, positive temporal biopsies are found in 10–15%. Those wishing to preserve the identity of the two diseases base their argument on the latter figure and on the failure to find evidence of arteritis in many patients with polymyalgia followed for many years. Conversely, there are many similarities between the two conditions. The age and sex distribution is similar, the biopsy findings show an identical pattern and the laboratory features are similar, even though many are non-specific inflammatory changes. In addition, there is similarity in the myalgia, the associated systemic features, and in the response to corticosteroid therapy.

The onset of myalgic symptoms may precede, coincide with, or follow that of the arteritic symptoms. No difference has been found between the characteristics of those myalgic patients with a positive biopsy and those with no histologic evidence of arteritis. Mild aching and stiffness may persist for months after other features of giant cell arteritis have remitted. There is little evidence to suggest that the musculoskeletal symptoms are related to vasculitis. Many patients with giant cell arteritis do not have PMR, even when large vessels are involved. In addition, the finding of joint swelling in some patients and the production of pain by the injection of 5% saline solution into the acromioclavicular, sternoclavicular and manubriosternal joints suggests that PMR in some patients may be a particular form of proximal synovitis.

Differential diagnosis

The diagnosis of PMR is initially one of exclusion. The differential diagnosis (Box 54.7) in an elderly patient with muscle pain, stiffness and a raised ESR

Box 54.7 Differential diagnosis of polymyalgia rheumatica

- Neoplastic disease
- Muscle disease
- Joint disease
- Polymyositis
- Osteoarthritis, particularly cervical spine
- Myopathy
- Rheumatoid arthritis
- Infections (e.g. bacterial endocarditis)
- Connective tissue disease
- Bone disease, particularly osteomyelitis
- Multiple myeloma
- Hypothyroidism
- Leukaemia
- Parkinsonism
- Lymphoma
- Functional

is wide because the prodromal phases of several serious conditions can mimic it. In practice, non-specific clinical features and the frequent absence of physical signs make diagnosis difficult.

Despite a typical pattern of musculoskeletal symptoms and the presence in many of significant systemic features, there is often a considerable delay of several months before diagnosis. Patients and physicians also tend to ascribe the symptoms to degenerative joint disease expected in an older population, or even to psychological illness. In others, the systemic features of the disease and the laboratory abnormalities can lead to diagnostic confusion and often extensive investigation.

Treatment

Corticosteroids are mandatory in the treatment of GCA; they reduce the incidence of complications, such as blindness, and rapidly relieve symptoms. Non-steroidal anti-inflammatory drugs (NSAIDs) will lessen the painful symptoms, but they do not prevent arteritic complications. The response to corticosteroids is usually dramatic and occurs within days. Corticosteroid treatment has improved the quality of life for patients, although there is no evidence that therapy reduces the duration of the disease. A fear of vascular complications in those patients with a positive biopsy often leads to the use of high doses of corticosteroids. Recent studies have emphasised the importance of adopting a cautious and individual treatment schedule, and have highlighted the efficacy of lower doses of prednisolone.

Initially, the corticosteroids should be given in a sufficient dosage to control the disease and then maintained at the lowest dose that will control the symptoms and lower the ESR. In patients with GCA, corticosteroids should preferably be given after the diagnosis has been confirmed histologically. However, where GCA is strongly suspected, there should be no delay in starting therapy as the artery

Box 54.8 Treatment of PMR and GCA

Polymyalgia rheumatica

Initial dose	Prednisolone 10–20 mg daily for 1 month
Reduce dose	By 2.5 mg every 2–4 weeks until dose is 10 mg, then by 1 mg every 4–6 weeks (or until symptoms return)
Maintenance dose	About 10 mg by 6 months after start of treatment and 5–7.5 mg by 1 year. Most patients require treatment for 3–4 years, but withdrawal after 2 years is worth attempting.
Special points	In patients who cannot reduce prednisolone dosage because of recurring symptoms or who develop serious steroid related side effects, azathioprine has been shown to have a modest steroid-sparing effect, and methotrexate may be more effective.
Main side effects	Weight gain, skin atrophy, oedema, increased intraocular pressure, cataracts, gastrointestinal disturbances, diabetes, osteoporosis
Risk of side effects	Increased risk with high initial doses (> 30 mg) of prednisolone, maintenance doses of 10 mg, and high cumulative doses. Maintenance doses of 5 mg are relatively safe.

Giant cell arteritis

Initial dose	Prednisolone 20–40 mg daily for 8 weeks. Patients with ocular symptoms may need up to 50 mg daily.
Reduce dose	By 5 mg every 3–4 weeks until dose is 10 mg daily; then as for PMR.
Maintenance dose	About 3 mg daily may be required.

Note: Recurrence of symptoms requires an increase in the prescribed dose.

biopsy will still show inflammatory changes for several days after corticosteroids have been started and the result is unlikely to alter therapeutic decisions. If the temporal (or other) artery biopsy shows no arteritis, but the suspicion of disease is strong, corticosteroid treatment should be started. The great danger is delaying therapy as blindness may occur at any time.

There are few clinical trials to help decide on the correct initial dose. Most clinicians have strong views on the dose required but some are based on tradition and anecdote. The recommended initial dose for PMR/GCA varies from 10 mg to 100 mg prednisolone daily. Intravenous corticosteroids are occasionally used if there are visual complications. In practice, most studies report using 10–20 mg prednisolone daily to treat PMR and 40–60 mg for GCA because of the higher risk of arteritic complications in cases of GCA. Some ophthalmologists suggest an initial dose of at least 60 mg as they have seen blindness occur at a lower dose. However, this has to be balanced against the potential complication of high dosage in this older age group. Patients should be advised that while they are taking a maintenance dose of steroids, any sudden exacerbation of symptoms, particularly sudden visual deterioration, requires an immediate increase in dose.

Prognosis

Rapid reduction or withdrawal of corticosteroids has been reported to contribute to deaths in patients with GCA. Thirteen of 17 deaths were felt to be due to using an inadequate dose of corticosteroids or reducing the dose too rapidly. Fortunately, complications are rare and the activity of the disease seems to decline steadily. Relapses are more likely during the initial 18 months of treatment and within 1 year of withdrawal of corticosteroids. There is no reliable method of predicting those most at risk, but arteritic relapses in patients who presented with pure PMR are unusual. Temporal artery biopsy does not seem helpful in predicting outcome.

Controversy exists over the expected duration of the disease. Most European studies within the last 20 years report that between one-third and one-half of the patients are able to discontinue corticosteroids after 2 years of treatment. Studies from the Mayo Clinic in the US have reported a shorter duration of disease for both PMR (11 months was the median duration of treatment and three-quarters of patients had stopped taking corticosteroids by 2 years) and GCA (most patients had stopped taking corticosteroids within 2 years). The consensus view seems to be that stopping treatment is feasible from 2 years onwards.

Patients who are unable to reduce the dosage of prednisolone because of recurring symptoms, or who develop serious corticosteroid-related side effects, pose particular problems. Azathioprine and methotrexate have been shown to exert a corticosteroid-sparing effect in 'corticosteroid resistant' cases of PMR/GCA.

Between one-fifth and one-half of patients may experience serious treatment-related side effects. A recent study suggested that if the initial dose of prednisolone is 10 mg or less, and maintenance doses of less than 7.5 mg are used, patients were virtually free of side effects. Serious side effects are significantly related to high initial doses, maintenance doses, cumulative doses and increased duration of treatment. Side effects can be minimised by using low doses of prednisolone whenever possible and giving corticosteroid-sparing drugs such as azathioprine and methotrexate when necessary.

In elderly people corticosteroid treatment carries the risk of increasing osteoporosis. Glucocorticoids have more effect on the spine than on the femur. Bisphosphonates such as etidronate and alendronate have been shown to be useful in retarding bone loss in the setting of prolonged corticosteroid use.

Summary

In summary, patients should be warned to expect treatment for at least 2 years, and most should be able to stop taking corticosteroids after 4–5 years. Monitoring for relapse should continue for 6 months to 1 year after stopping corticosteroids; thereafter patients should be asked to report back urgently if arteritic symptoms occur. The risk of this happening is small and unpredictable. A few patients may need low-dose treatment indefinitely.

PMR and GCA are among the more satisfying diseases for clinicians to diagnose and treat because the unpleasant effects and serious consequences of these conditions can be almost entirely prevented by corticosteroid therapy. Unfortunately, there is no objective means of determining the prognosis in the individual and decisions concerning duration of treatment remain empirical.

Bibliography and further reading

Achkar, A., Lie, J., Hunder, G. et al. (1994), 'How does previous corticosteroid treatment affect the biopsy findings in giant cell (temporal) arteritis?', *Annals of Internal Medicine*, 120, pp. 987–92.

Bahlas, S., Ramos-Remus, C. & Davis, P. (1997), 'Clinical outcome of 149 patients with polymyalgia and giant cell arteritis', *The Journal of Rheumatology*, 25, pp. 99–104.

Barber, H. S. (1957), 'Myalgic syndrome with constitutional effects. Polymyalgia rheumatica', *Annals of Rheumatic Disease*, 16, pp. 230–7.

Buchbinder, R. & Detsky, A. (1992), 'Management of suspected giant cell arteritis: a decision analysis', *The Journal of Rheumatology*, 19, pp. 1220–8.

Homik, J., Cranney, A. & Shea, B. et al. (1999), 'A metaanalysis on the use of bisphosphonates in corticosteroid induced osteoporosis', *The Journal of Rheumatology*, 26, pp. 1148–57.

Horton, B. T., Magath, T. B. & Brown, G. E. (1932), 'An undescribed form of arteritis of the temporal vessels', *Mayo Clinic Proceedings*, 7, pp. 700–1.

Kyle, V., Cawston, T. E. & Hazleman, B. L. (1989), 'ESR and C-reactive protein in the assessment of polymyalgia rheumatica/giant cell arteritis on presentation and during follow up', *Annals of the Rheumatic Diseases*, 48, pp. 408–9.

Kyle, V. & Hazleman, B. L. (1989a), 'Treatment of polymyalgia rheumatica and giant cell arteritis. I. Steroid regimes in the first 2 months', *Annals of the Rheumatic Diseases*, 48, pp. 658–61.

Kyle, V. & Hazleman, B. L. (1989b), 'Treatment of polymyalgia rheumatica and giant cell arteritis. II. The relationship between steroid dose and steroid associated side effects', *Annals of the Rheumatic Diseases*, 48, pp. 662–6.

Kyle, V., Silverman, B., Silman, A. et al. (1985), 'Polymyalgia rheumatica/giant cell arteritis in general practice', *British Medical Journal*, 13, pp. 385–8.

Machedo, E. B., Michet, C. J., Ballard, D. J. et al. (1988), 'Trends in incidence and clinical presentation of temporal arteritis in Olmsted County, Minnesota 1950–1985', *Arthritis and Rheumatism*, 31, pp. 745–9.

Paulley, J. W. & Hughes, J. P. (1960), 'Giant cell arteritis, or arteritis of the aged', *British Medical Journal*, 2, pp. 1562–5.

Porsman, V. A. (1951), 'Arthritis in old age', 2nd European Congress of Rheumatology, Barcelona, Editorial Scientia, col. 1, p. 479.

Chapter 55

Osteoporosis

PENELOPE COATES and GARY WITTERT

Introduction

Osteoporosis is a systemic skeletal condition characterised by low bone mass and microarchitectural deterioration of bone tissue, with increased bone fragility and risk of fracture. The alternative clinical definition of osteoporosis adopted by the World Health Organization is a bone mineral density (BMD) that is more than 2.5 standard deviations (SDs) below the young adult mean. A second category, osteopenia, is defined as a BMD between 1 and 2.5 SDs below the mean for young adults. This 'operational' definition allows patients at risk of fracture to be identified, and also provides a means of monitoring both the natural history and treatment of this condition. Non-traumatic fracture is sometimes used as an additional marker of severity of disease. A fall from standing height, however, generates enough force to cause fracture even where bone density is normal, if the body's normal protective responses are inadequate—for example, because of muscle weakness. There is a need for a defined treatment threshold age and other non-BMD related fracture risk factors to be taken into account.

Epidemiology of osteoporosis and fracture

Osteoporosis is the most common metabolic disease in the developed world. More than half the female and more than a third of the male population are likely to sustain a fracture due to osteoporosis. The total number of fractures is even higher, as many people will experience more than one. The incidence and prevalence of non-traumatic (or minimally traumatic) fracture increases with age, with a doubling of fracture risk every 5–10 years. The magnitude of the problem will increase with the progressive ageing of the population unless efforts in prevention and treatment are successful.

By definition, only 0.6% of young people have osteoporosis as defined by a bone density of greater than 2.5 standard deviations below the young adult mean. Approximately 30% of 60–70-year-old women in the US have osteoporosis and that figure increases to 70% by the age of 80. Similarly, Australian data obtained in 1997 estimated that 15% of women and 1.6% of men between 60 and 64 years have osteoporosis, increasing to 71% of women and 19% of men over 80 years. There is still no universally accepted definition of osteoporosis or osteopenia in men. The lower prevalence in men is consistent with their lower rate of hip fracture and also reflects greater bone density at the hip in men. In nursing home residents, the prevalence of osteoporosis is even higher, with an increase from 63.5% in women between 65 and 74 years to 85.8% in women over 85 years.

The risk of hip fracture is the same for men and women for a given bone density, controlled for age. In the US the rate increases from 2 per 1000 patient years at age 65 to 30 per 1000 patient years after age 85. More than 50% of 50-year-old women will live another 30 years and a significant number will reach the age of 90 or more. Thus, in the US, 55% of all hip fractures occur in people over 80, and 33% in people over 85 years. A similar percentage of hip fracture occurs in institutionalised patients of both sexes. Hip fracture accounts for more than 20% of orthopaedic hospital admissions, and hospital bed occupancy is higher than for many other common disorders, such as myocardial infarction, diabetes or breast cancer. In a large prospective study in Edinburgh over a 2 year period, 15 000 patients of both sexes sustained a fracture, with a female to male ratio of 2.3:1. In 1990 approximately 1.7 million hip fractures occurred worldwide, 30% in men. Osteoporosis contributes to 90% of hip fractures in women and 80% in men. Approximately 1.2 million hip fractures are predicted to occur in men and 2.8 million in women in 2025. Even allowing for the increasing age of the population, the age and sex specific incidence of hip fracture continues to increase more in men than in women. Possible reasons include reduced activity levels, increases in height and possibly in hip axis length, and other environmental and locomotor factors. Men and women with hip fracture tend to be frail, with a higher rate of co-existent medical problems than an age matched population. Compared with women, elderly men with hip fracture have a higher mortality.

The spine is the most common site of osteoporotic fracture, but numbers are clinically underestimated, as only half of all people with radiological vertebral deformity can recall any back pain or injury. A 20–25% decrease in vertebral body height or a greater than 3 or 4 SDs from population values for anterior, posterior or mid-vertebral height are both accepted definitions for vertebral deformity. The difference in fracture rates between men and women is less marked for vertebral deformity than for other types of osteoporotic fracture. Based on the less stringent of these criteria, 30–50% of women and 20–30% of men will experience a vertebral fracture in their lifetime. Using a stricter radiological definition of fracture, the investigators in the Dubbo study in Australia demonstrated an increase in the prevalence of fracture rates from 8% in men aged 60–64, to 22% in men over 80, with similar rates in women. About a third of vertebral fractures are diagnosed clinically, 8% require hospitalisation and 2% require long-term nursing care. At age 65 or over, 14.5 per 10 000 people were hospitalised for vertebral fractures in the US in 1997. Half of all patients with vertebral fractures have 2 or more deformities.

The incidence of wrist fractures increases sharply at the time of the menopause, but reaches a plateau after the age of 60. The reason for this may be that women soon after the menopause are more mobile and are thus more likely to fall on an outstretched hand than the very elderly.

Morbidity, mortality and cost of osteoporotic fracture

Among elderly Australian women, 80% stated that they would rather be dead than experience loss of independence and quality of life due to a 'bad' hip fracture. Death rate (all cause mortality) increases by two- to fivefold in the first year after hip fracture compared to an age and sex matched population. The risk of dying from hip fracture was similar to the death rate from breast cancer in one survey. In another study involving 131 men after hip fracture, hospital mortality was 11.5% and 30 day mortality 16%, with 79% of survivors still in nursing homes 1 year later. The 1 year survival was 58%, compared with 94% for matched controls. The risk of death was increased with co-existing illness and low activity levels at the time of fracture. Prospective studies have also reported increased all cause mortality in both sexes associated with low BMD. These patients seemed to be generally frailer and osteoporosis was not cited as the main cause of death. Low BMD was associated with a 1.39-fold increase in mortality for each SD reduction in bone density in a Swedish prospective population based study; low BMD was a stronger predictor of death than either blood pressure or cholesterol and may therefore be a marker of general frailty.

Morbidity from osteoporotic fractures is also significant. Hospitalisation, rehabilitation or nursing home treatment, pain, disability and loss of independence are of major concern. The costs have been most accurately estimated in hip fracture because virtually all patients are treated in hospital. The average hospital stay in Australia is 13 days, with 20–26% of patients remaining in nursing homes for the rest of their lives. More than a third of patients are readmitted to hospital within a year of hip fracture, for reasons unrelated to their fracture in about half the cases. Even if a patient survives a hip fracture, the long-term prospects are poor. For example, in one prospective study, half the patients did not regain their ability to walk independently and 87% were unable to climb stairs, 1 year after hip fracture. Predictors of recovery include pre-fracture cognitive function, the existence of social networks, and mood. There is a higher rate of mortality and institutionalisation after hip fracture in men than women.

Projected frequency of osteoporosis and fracture

Several studies in the US, Europe and Australia have estimated future rates of osteoporosis and fracture based on existing rates and census population data. In an Australian study the number of fractures was projected to increase by 25% from 1996 to 2006, assuming current age specific fracture rates persist. The rate of hip fracture is expected to double by 2026 and increase fourfold by 2051. Other Australian and US studies showed a similar doubling of risk by 2026.

The aetiology of osteoporosis and approach to patient evaluation

A number of lifestyle, hormonal and biochemical factors are known to affect bone metabolism. Reduced physical activity, reduced total and muscle mass, and an increase in other illnesses with age contribute not only to changes in bone metabolism but also to an increased risk of falls.

The risk of hip fractures in men is increased more than twofold by the presence of a metabolic disorder associated with abnormal bone mineral density, and by nearly sevenfold by a movement or balance disorder. The age related increase in risk of falling is of major importance in the exponential increase in hip fracture rates with age. Approximately 20% of women between the ages of 60 and 64 fall each year; this rises to more than 30% over age 80. In nursing home residents, the rate of falling may be more than 60%.

Falling is a less significant factor in vertebral fracture than hip fracture, accounting for about a quarter of clinically detected cases. Increasing age is the predominant risk factor for vertebral fracture. After adjusting for age, independent predictors of vertebral fracture include weight, height, history of other osteoporotic fractures, or use of anticoagulants. Metabolic factors account for only a 1.2-fold age adjusted increased risk of spinal fracture.

Body composition

Low body weight and tall stature are both associated with increased fracture risk. Falls are more likely to result in fracture in taller persons because of the greater impact. It has been suggested that 1 in 4 low-energy fractures in women are attributable to gains in height this century. Similarly, in the Study of Osteoporotic Fractures, which followed 8011 elderly women prospectively for a mean of 5.2 years, those in the lowest quartile of weight had a relative fracture risk of 1.93 compared to women in the highest quartile. This difference is almost entirely due to lower BMD in the thinner subjects; there was no change after adjustment for height, smoking or physical activity.

Gonadal steroids

A sharp drop in oestrogen levels at the menopause is a major treatable cause of bone loss in women. Similarly, early menopause and late menarche are associated with a higher risk of osteoporosis. In women, in the first few years after the menopause, rapid loss of bone of about 2–4% per year is superimposed on the gradual age related loss of BMD of 1–2% per year. Free and, to a lesser extent, total testosterone levels decline with age. A threshold for testosterone below which there is an increased risk of osteoporosis and fracture has not been defined, as not all investigators have been able to find a correlation between testosterone and bone mineral density. Up to 50% of men with hip fracture and 20% with vertebral fracture are hypogonadal. Oestrogen is also important for the maintenance of BMD in men.

Growth hormone and IGF-1

Plasma levels of growth hormone (GH) and IGF-1 decline with age. Growth hormone activates osteoblasts to increase local production of IGF-1, which acts to enhance bone matrix formation. Thus GH deficiency in the elderly may be of significance in the development of osteoporosis. There is no direct evidence that decreased GH activity alters bone remodelling.

Calciotrophic hormones

Parathyroid hormone (PTH) has been shown to increase with age, at least in part due to a decrease in 25-hydroxy vitamin D. Vitamin D facilitates intestinal calcium as well as new bone formation. Vitamin D insufficiency is a particular problem in the institutionalised elderly population, because of reduced sun exposure and reduced skin thickness (and therefore reduced capacity for vitamin D synthesis). Primary hyperparathyroidism is associated with reduced (predominantly cortical) BMD and this is exacerbated by concomitant vitamin D deficiency.

Dietary factors

A low dietary calcium intake is associated with an increased fracture risk. Requirements for calcium increase with increasing age, possibly because of a gradual reduction in calcium-absorbing capacity. The recommended daily calcium allowance for people aged 65 and over determined by the National Institutes of Health Consensus Conference in 1994 is 1500 mg, similar to the requirement in adolescence. High sodium and animal protein intakes increase urinary calcium loss. Protein-calorie malnutrition is a significant factor in osteoporotic fracture, even in developed countries and particularly in the elderly. Malnourished patients are more likely to fall, and if they do fall, they have less soft tissue padding over bony prominences and are more disposed to fracture. A low serum albumin level confers a lower survival after hip fracture.

Caffeine intake was associated with low BMD and increased fracture risk in the Framingham study, possibly mediated through increased calcium loss in the urine.

Exercise

Immobility causes a rapid loss of bone. At the opposite extreme, elite athletes involved in strength training have a high bone mass. There is some correlation between the extent of walking or weight-bearing exercise and BMD.

Smoking and alcohol consumption

Cigarette smoking has been repeatedly shown to be associated with an increased rate of bone loss and a low BMD, independent of body weight or other lifestyle factors. One consequence of smoking is to reduce calcium absorption. In men, past smokers had a BMD similar to smokers at the lumbar spine, and intermediate between current smokers and those who never smoked at the femoral neck, whereas women who had stopped smoking had a BMD indistinguishable from those who had never smoked.

Heavy alcohol intake is a strong risk factor for osteoporosis in both sexes due to its direct effects on bone formation and calcium absorption, and indirectly through reduced testosterone levels in men, deterioration in liver function, and co-existent protein-calorie malnutrition. The threshold for adverse effects is lower in women than men. The risk of falling is also significantly higher in heavy drinkers. Moderate alcohol intake has been paradoxically associated with increased BMD. One possible explanation for this effect is increased endogenous oestrogen production in moderate drinkers.

Medications

Long-term use of glucocorticoids predominantly decreases trabecular, rather than cortical, bone. In patients taking high doses of steroids for longer than 6 months, subsequent fracture incidence may be between 30% and 50%. Although there is substantial individual variation, approximately 7.5 mg prednisolone (or its equivalent) daily will cause significant bone loss in most people. Patients on corticosteroids for more than 2 months should be considered at risk. Corticosteroids have multiple effects on bone metabolism, including inhibition of osteoblast function and therefore new bone formation, stimulation of bone resorption, impaired active calcium absorption by the gut, and increased renal calcium loss.

Anticonvulsants increase metabolism of 25-hydroxy vitamin D, with secondary hyperparathyroidism in several patients. Commonly used medications implicated in bone loss are listed in Table 55.1.

Biomechanical factors

Various structural and qualitative abnormalities contribute to the loss of bone strength in osteoporosis. These include unremodelled fatigue damage, loss of trabeculae and reduced trabecular thickness, which reduce the strength and load-bearing capacity of bone. The geometry of bone is also a factor. For example, there is a positive relationship between hip axis length (the distance between the trochanter and the pelvis) and fracture risk in women. This amounts to a doubling of fracture risk for each SD increase in hip axis length, independent of BMD. The force experienced by the bone depends on the direction of the fall. In hip fracture, it has been calculated that a fall from standing height directly on to the hip generates sufficient force to fracture even the hip of a young adult. Preventing frailty and decreasing falls is therefore of paramount importance.

Previous history of fracture

A previous fracture with absent or minimal trauma is a strong predictor of future fractures. This may reflect individual bone structure and geometry, increased risk of falling, or both. The risk of future fractures increases about two- to threefold for each prevalent fracture, independent of BMD. The high prevalence of vertebral fracture in the elderly, combined with the fact that only a third of these fractures cause symptoms, argues for the use of spinal radiographs or morphometric analysis of spinal BMD in risk assessment.

Genetic factors

Inherited factors play a role in determining peak bone mass, although the mechanism of such an effect is unclear. A history of osteoporotic fracture in close family members almost doubles the risk of fracture in an individual of either sex.

Table 55.1 Commonly used medications implicated in osteoporotic fracture

Medication	Comments
Corticosteroids	Inhibit calcium absorption, increase excretion Inhibition of new bone formation Reduced gonadal steroids
Heparin	Enhancement of bone resorption with prolonged use Low molecular weight heparin appears to cause less bone loss
Anticonvulsants (phenytoin, carbamazepine)	Increased vitamin D clearance
Exchange resins (cholestyramine)	Reduced vitamin D absorption
Warfarin	Independent predictor of vertebral and rib fracture ? Reduced bone formation
Cyclosporin	
Methotrexate	
Thyroid hormone in excess (suppressed TSH)	
Long-acting benzodiazepines	Increased risk of falling

Cognitive factors

In one study, osteoporotic women had poorer results on formal cognitive testing after adjustment for age and other factors compared to age matched controls, and a greater risk for cognitive deterioration over time. The risk of fracture is likely to be further increased because of an increased risk of falling and poorer balance in this population. An increased frequency of the apolipoprotein E4 allele, previously associated with an increased frequency of Alzheimer's disease, occurs in women who sustained a fracture independent of falls, cognitive function and age. The women with this allele were also more likely to report a maternal history of fracture.

Metabolic disease

Primary hyperparathyroidism (elevated plasma calcium and an inappropriate PTH) is a relatively common condition with a prevalence of 1 to 2 per 1000. Cortical bone is resorbed more than trabecular bone. Primary hyperparathyroidism is usually asymptomatic, but is readily screened for by measuring plasma calcium. Osteoporosis as a bony manifestation of the disease is more common than the previously described erosions and subperiosteal resorption. Secondary hyperparathyroidism (low plasma, or low-normal plasma calcium and an elevated PTH) has a similar effect on the skeleton. Secondary hyperparathyroidism may result from calcium malabsorption consequent to small bowel pathology or vitamin D deficiency, renal failure or a calcium malabsorption syndrome unique to the elderly.

Hyperthyroidism increases both bone resorption and bone formation rates. However, as the latter process takes longer to complete, there is net loss of bone. Women, especially older women, are more severely affected than men. There is debate about the effects of excessive thyroid replacement. In a meta-analysis of patients who received thyroxine in doses that suppressed thyroid stimulating hormone (TSH), there was a 1% annual increase in bone loss in postmenopausal women but not in other groups.

Approach to the evaluation of patients for osteoporosis

BMD measurement and assessment of fracture risk

Plain X-rays predict osteoporosis accurately only 30–50% of the time. A variety of accurate, non-invasive techniques are available for measurement of bone mass and bone density. No technique gives an accurate measurement of true bone density. Dual X-ray absorptiometry (DXA) is the most commonly used modality at present. Radiation exposure is less than 10% that of a standard chest X-ray. DXA measures bone mineral content from a single projection and BMD is then estimated using this and the cross-sectional area to give an apparent areal density (g/cm^2). Using this technique, differences in bone size can lead to underestimation of bone density.

Based on densitometric measurements, several different approaches to diagnosis can be employed. One is to compare patients to young or age adjusted reference ranges; another is to define a 'fracture threshold' based on bone density measurements in patients with fracture, and a third is to estimate a lifetime fracture risk for a patient. Some standardisation has been attempted using standard deviation (SD) units. However, individuals will still be classified differently depending on the site measured, technique, instrument and calibration used and the reference population. It is common for individuals to be diagnosed as osteoporotic at one skeletal site but not at another, for example. Systematic errors occur in some clinical situations. Major sources of error include osteoarthrosis, scoliosis, vascular calcification, overlying contrast material and altered soft tissue distribution. Bone mineral content is underestimated in obese subjects unless the amount of fat is corrected for.

Bone mineral density has a continuous Gaussian distribution. There is an overlap between BMD of populations with and without fracture. Thus, although risk can be estimated, there is no absolute BMD cut-off which will determine if an individual will sustain a fracture. There is no agreed cut-off in men. For any given BMD, fracture risk is higher in elderly than in younger individuals.

Using both single and dual X-ray absorptiometry, the fracture risk increases from 1.5- to threefold for each SD fall in BMD. BMD has high specificity (there is a high lifetime fracture rate in women below arbitrarily determined cut-offs), but low sensitivity (a high proportion of fractures occur in women designated 'low risk' by this technique alone). Thus BMD has not been recommended for universal population screening.

Quantitative calcaneal (heel) ultrasound offers the advantages of no ionising radiation to the patient, portability and low cost. Prospective studies in elderly women in the US and Europe showed an increase in fracture risk (similar to DXA) for each SD change. The predictive value of heel ultrasound in younger patients, particularly women soon after the menopause, is less clear and therefore this technique has not been adopted as a universal clinical practice.

Biochemical markers of bone resorption

Bone is a metabolically active organ that is continuously remodelled. Increased bone resorption magnifies the small negative balance in bone turnover and can cause a net loss of bone. Treatments effective in preventing fracture result in a far greater reduction in fracture risk than can be accounted for by changes in bone density alone. This implies that antiresorptive therapy may correct microarchitectural abnormalities in osteoporotic bone that are at least partly due to the bone turnover rate.

The biochemical markers are usually products of mature bone collagen, released into the bloodstream after bone resorption by the osteoclast, and measured in urine and more recently in blood (Box 55.1). High levels of bone resorption markers are related to high rates of bone loss and fracture, and this relationship may become stronger with advancing age. In one cross-sectional study, biochemical markers of bone turnover accounted for only 10% of the variance in BMD in premenopausal women, but this increased to 52% in women 30 years after the menopause. There is still considerable debate about the applicability of bone resorption markers to risk assessment in individual patients. Part of the difficulty in interpreting the results of these investigations lies in the considerable diurnal and day-to-day variability of many of the markers of bone resorption. However, a clearly elevated level of one of the resorption markers (Box 55.1) may be used as additional supporting evidence of risk and may be useful in monitoring response to therapy. These markers all have roughly equivalent utility and the one most readily available in the local laboratory is the best to use.

Box 55.1 Biochemical markers of bone resorption

Urine (specimen collected fasting, 2 hours after first morning void)

- Pyridinium cross-links (total or free)
  - Pyridinoline
  - Deoxypyridinoline
- Peptide fragments
  - N-telopeptide to helix (NTx, Osteomark®)
  - C-telopeptide (CrossLaps®)
- Hydroxyproline
- Galactosyl-hydroxylysine

Serum

- C-telopeptide to helix (ICTP)
- Tartrate resistant acid phosphatase
- N-telopeptide to helix
- C-telopeptide

Prevention and management of osteoporosis in the elderly

Exercise

Exercise is important for both the prevention and treatment of osteoporosis. Twenty to 30 minutes of walking, jumping, step or low-impact aerobics 2 or 3 times a week helps improve muscular strength and balance—changes which, in turn, reduce the chances of fall and fracture. Whether BMD can substantially increase with a continuous exercise regimen alone (without medical therapy) is still somewhat uncertain; some exercise studies indicate an increase in bone density, others do not. Weight-bearing exercise—with whatever degree of impact is possible, such as that from walking, jumping or jogging, according to fitness and ability—appears to be the most effective type of exercise for osteoporosis.

Diet, calcium and vitamin D

Premenopausal women, postmenopausal women taking oestrogen and all men need at least 1000–1200 mg of calcium daily. Retrospective, cross-sectional and prospective studies suggest that increasing calcium intake during the premenopausal period ensures that women enter menopause with greater bone density. Postmenopausal women who are not taking oestrogen should receive 1500–2000 mg of calcium daily, although a recent study has shown that supplementation of 800 mg of calcium daily may prevent bone loss in postmenopausal women. Furthermore, the results of clinical trials also suggest that such supplementation may prevent hip and vertebral fractures in the elderly. The benefits of calcium on bone mass are also supported by epidemiological data, which suggest that a lifetime of adequate calcium intake decreases fracture risk. The more soluble calcium salts appear to be the most effective. In early postmenopause (< 4 years since the menopause), calcium alone is ineffective, but it reduces bone loss by 25–30% in the late menopause. A National Institute of Health Consensus Statement recommends 800 mg of elemental calcium per day for premenopausal women and 1500 mg per day for postmenopausal women. Most, if not all, postmenopausal women should take calcium supplements to achieve this intake.

Patients at risk for osteoporosis should also receive 400–800 units of vitamin D daily, particularly during winter, and higher doses may be needed when there is vitamin D deficiency.

Although the combination of calcium (1.2 g/day) with vitamin D_3 (800 IU/day) has been reported to prevent fractures in elderly women, a recent meta-analysis concluded that uncertainty remains about the efficacy of regimens that include vitamin D or its analogues in fracture prevention. Particularly if co-supplementation of calcium is required, significant cost differences are likely to exist between regimens. Further randomised trials with economic evaluation are desirable.

In the case of steroid induced osteoporosis, studies have clearly demonstrated a clinically and statistically significant prevention of bone loss at the lumbar spine and forearm with vitamin D and calcium. Because of low toxicity and cost, all patients being started on corticosteroids should receive prophylactic therapy with calcium and vitamin D.

Calcium absorption is optimal when no more than 600 mg of calcium is taken at once; one dose before breakfast and another at bedtime is optimal. Habitual dietary intake improves the efficacy of supplementation.

Drug therapy

Prevention of osteoporosis

Apart from the role of vitamin D and calcium, a number of medical therapies have now been approved (by the FDA) for the prevention of osteoporosis. These agents all reduce bone resorption, and include oestrogen replacement therapy (ERT) (orally or by patch) with or without a progestin, alendronate (Fosamax, a bisphosphonate), 5 mg orally in the morning, and raloxifene (Evista, a selective oestrogen receptor modulator, or SERM), 60 mg orally daily.

Treatment of established osteoporosis

In a recent analysis of more than 35 randomised trials for different therapies, only alendronate and vitamin D plus calcium have clearly demonstrated an overall fracture benefit, with alendronate providing the greatest relative risk reduction. Quality clinical trial fracture data for calcitonin, etidronate, hormone replacement therapy, parathyroid hormone, calcitriol (and other vitamin D preparations), vitamin D and calcium monotherapy, and selective oestrogen receptor modulators are either lacking, inconclusive or published only as abstracts. Two very recently completed European studies have demonstrated reductions in forearm, vertebral and overall fracture risk in women treated with hormone replacement therapy (HRT). HRT is considered the most cost effective treatment. Medical practitioners should inform people that exercise, in addition to its other benefits, would help prevent osteoporosis. Smokers should be helped to quit.

Calcitriol

Calcitriol, or 1,25-$(OH)_2$-vitamin D_3, is the active metabolite of vitamin D. Calcitriol increases intestinal calcium absorption and decreases bone resorption secondary to an increase in calcium absorption. Calcitriol improves and may normalise impaired calcitonin secretion in mildly vitamin D deficient elderly subjects. Calcitriol may be an indirect stimulator of bone resorption via receptor mediated activity on osteoblasts, and enhances the differentiation of preosteoclasts to osteoclasts. If calcium nutrition is inadequate, the net effect of calcitriol will be to mobilise calcium from bone, and therefore calcitriol should be prescribed in a small dose, for example 0.25 µg daily, together with supplemental calcium.

Calcitriol appears to prevent vertebral fractures in patients with osteoporosis. More information is needed on its mechanism of action and efficacy in preventing hip fractures. Recent data show that a combination of cyclical therapy with the bisphosphonate etidronate and calcitriol is better than cyclical etidronate alone in terms of changes in BMD at both spine and femoral neck sites. Further data are needed on fracture efficacy. There is some data to support the concept that low calcium absorption is a cause of negative calcium balance in postmenopausal osteoporosis and that the effectiveness of calcitriol therapy is inversely related to the initial rate of calcium absorption, suggesting that therapy may be specifically tailored for subgroups of women. At present this approach is limited to a few research clinics.

In patients commencing long-term treatment with glucocorticoids, calcitriol 0.5 µg/day plus calcium 1000 mg/day prevents steroid induced bone loss. At recommended dosages hypercalcaemia is infrequent and mild, generally responding to reductions in calcium intake and/or calcitriol dosage. Periodic monitoring of serum calcium and creatinine levels is indicated.

Oestrogen

Hormone replacement therapy (oestrogen (ERT) alone or a combination of oestrogen and progestin (HRT)) reduces bone loss and increases BMD by 2–6% in postmenopausal women. The positive skeletal effects of oestrogen replacement in women have not been supported by large, prospective clinical trials. Past studies indicating an enhanced skeletal effect of oestrogens were mainly observational. Previous efforts have also been criticised because of the small number of women enrolled, the nonrandomisation of study participants, and the use of retrospective analyses. Two recent, relatively small, European studies demonstrated reductions in forearm, vertebral and overall fracture risk in women treated with HRT. The Women's Health Initiative (WHI), a large, multicentre, prospective trial of HRT, is expected to provide definitive data for addressing the uncertainty surrounding the skeletal benefits associated with oestrogen replacement.

There is observational evidence that HRT decreases cardiovascular disease, but not in women with established coronary artery disease. Oestrogen increases the risks of thromboembolic disease and breast cancer.

Selective oestrogen receptor modulators

Oestrogen receptors are ubiquitous. However, some oestrogenic effects are undesirable in certain disease states and after the menopause. For example, the addition of oestrogen should be avoided in women with disorders such as leiomyomata and endometriosis. In postmenopausal women, oestrogenic stimulation of the breast and uterus increases the risk for breast and uterine cancers. Compounds (selective oestrogen response modifiers, or SERMS) have been designed to have selective agonist or antagonist effects at the oestrogen receptor in different organs.

Raloxifene

The effect of raloxifene on preventing bone loss and reducing fracture risk is superior to placebo but inferior to premarin. The effects of raloxifene (60 mg/day) are approximately 50–60% those of conjugated equine oestrogens (0.625 mg/day) on the basis of BMD measurements. However, raloxifene has been shown to significantly reduce vertebral fractures. Raloxifene lowers total cholesterol, low-density lipoprotein-C (LDL-C), and triglycerides, but it does not increase high-density lipoprotein-C (HDL-C). Raloxifene does not stimulate endometrial proliferation, and it reduced the risk of breast cancer by approximately 80% in a 5 year trial, but is not beneficial for hot flushes (and may induce these symptoms), nor is it beneficial for vaginal atrophy. Raloxifene may also induce leg cramps, although one study showed that this effect did not cause participants to discontinue taking the drug. It is not known whether there are cognitive beneficial effects, such as have been associated with oestrogen use. Raloxifene does not appear to impair cognition or affect mood in postmenopausal women. There is a small increase in the risk for venous thrombosis with raloxifene. Raloxifene is therefore an option for some women, particularly those who are at high risk for osteoporosis or breast cancer or who have had breast cancer in the past and are not bothered by hot flushes.

Phyto-oestrogens

Although human data are limited, certain phyto-oestrogens, particularly isoflavones, might also be considered selective oestrogen response modifiers. Isoflavones may have some positive effects on the brain, bone and the cardiovascular system, but have no appreciable stimulatory effects on the breast or uterus. Soy-based phyto-oestrogens have also been shown to be beneficial for hot flushes, although there is a strong dose effect, with higher doses being required to achieve a statistically significant beneficial effect.

Progesterone

Progesterone receptors are present in osteoblasts and there is evidence that progesterone may stimulate new bone formation. Some women have side effects, mainly mood change, irritability and depression. A reduction in the dose and/or change in the type of progestogen, for example, from medroxyprogesterone acetate to norethindrone, norethisterone or natural progesterone, may ameliorate the side effects.

Bisphosphonates

Bisphosphonates are pyrophosphate analogues in which a carbon has replaced the oxygen in P-O-P, resulting in a P-C-P structure. They are characterised by a strong antiosteoclastic activity. Etidronate (intermittently) and alendronate (continuously) are extensively used for the prevention and treatment of osteoporosis. The aminobisphosphonate, risedronate (5 mg) also prevents postmenopausal bone loss. Similar effects have been observed with an intermittent dosage regimen of oral risedronate 30 mg/day for 2 out of 12 weeks, which corresponds to 5 mg/day in terms of cumulative dose. With lower doses (5 mg daily on alternate fortnights) the prevention of bone loss was half that observed with continuous 5 mg/day therapy.

Etidronate and alendronate increase spinal BMD in postmenopausal women with osteoporosis. In one study, etidronate decreased the number of women sustaining new radiographic vertebral fractures over 2 years, but this effect was lost after 3 years of treatment. Alendronate reduces the number of radiographic vertebral fractures in postmenopausal women with a low bone mass. In women with pre-existing fractures, alendronate decreases the number of patients with radiographic vertebral fractures, clinical (i.e. symptomatic vertebral and non-vertebral) fractures, and hip fractures. A significant reduction in the overall number of non-vertebral fractures has not been demonstrated in clinical trials evaluating either alendronate or etidronate. The efficacies of alendronate and etidronate have not been directly compared, and long-term data comparable with that available for HRT have not been published. Based on the results obtained in clinical trials using fracture as an end point, alendronate appears to be the bisphosphonate of choice. Safety profiles and cost should also be considered in the choice of etidronate or alendronate for the treatment of postmenopausal osteoporosis. Etidronate is free of significant side effects. Adverse events with alendronate tend to be transient and usually associated with the upper gastrointestinal tract, most commonly dyspepsia. Of potential concern are a small number of reports of patients developing oesophageal ulceration.

Other treatments and new developments

Calcitonin

Nasal spray calcitonin (NS-CT) is marketed in a few countries, including the US, for the treatment of postmenopausal osteoporosis. The recommended dosage is 200 IU/day. At this dosage, NS-CT has been shown to lower vertebral fracture by 36%, despite a modest 1.2% increase in spine BMD and no effect on femoral neck, over 5 years. The value of NS-CT for the treatment of osteoporosis has not been adequately studied. NS-CT is effective at reducing the pain of osteoporotic vertebral fracture.

Tibolone

Tibolone is a steroidal synthetic compound exerting an oestrogenic, progestogenic or androgenic effect, depending on the tissue. Tibolone therapy also has been evaluated for prevention and treatment of postmenopausal osteoporosis, with results on BMD comparable to those obtained with the traditional oestrogen/progesterone combinations or oestrogen alone. Tibolone has no effect on LDL cholesterol, and it significantly decreases both lipoprotein (a) and HDL cholesterol. Tibolone is effective in treating symptoms of the menopause. Its use is not associated with periodic bleeding, although moderate spotting is observed within the first months of treatment. Tibolone has minimal effect on the breast.

Osteoprotogerin (OPG)

OPG is a naturally occurring protein synthesised by osteoblasts but expressed also by a wide variety of tissue cells. It strongly inhibits osteoclast recruitment, formation and activity. OPG may have a potential role in the treatment of osteoporosis. In a preliminary study of 52 postmenopausal women, up to 3 mg/kg OPG given in a single infusion reduced levels of a marker of bone resorption (urinary N-telopeptide/creatinine) by 80% within 5 days. This marker remained significantly suppressed for approximately 1 month. The infusions were well tolerated, and no appreciable immunologic changes were observed.

Statins

In vitro and *in vivo* statins appear to stimulate bone formation and inhibit bone resorption. Patients taking statin therapy have a reduced risk of hip fracture (*post hoc* analysis).

Strontium

Strontium ranelate concentrates at the mineral phase of bone tissue, substituting for calcium in hydroxyapatite crystals. It inhibits osteoclastic bone resorption without affecting bone formation. The changes in BMD as measured by DXA in preliminary studies have been also attributed to the greater atomic weight of strontium as compared with calcium. For this reason, the value of strontium in the treatment of osteoporosis can be assessed only by fracture trials. Two of such trials are ongoing and will be completed in a couple of years.

Non-steroidal anti-inflammatory drugs (NSAIDs)

There is some indirect evidence that NSAIDs may decrease bone turnover and be associated with greater BMD values. This effect seems to be related to inhibition of cyclo-oxygenase-2 activity (COX2) activity. The availability of better tolerated COX2-specific inhibitors may open a new area of investigation for the treatment of osteoporosis.

Parathyroid hormone (PTH) and analogues

A series of experiments from different centres have demonstrated an anabolic action of PTH on bone when given alone or in combination with oestrogens, vitamin D or calcitonin. Intermittent injection of PTH appears to be a critical factor in the process of stimulating bone formation.

The results of a large, multicentre trial using recombinant human PTH have demonstrated a 65% reduction in vertebral fractures and a 54% reduction in non-vertebral fractures within 1–2 years of PTH therapy.

Bibliography and further reading

Bauer, D. C., Mundy, G. R., Jamal, S. A. et al. (1999), 'Statin use, bone mass and fracture: an analysis of two prospective studies', *Journal of Bone and Mineral Research*, 14(suppl. 1), p. S179.

Bekker, P. J., Holloway, D., Nalanishi, A., Arrighi, H. M. & Dunstan, C. R. (1999), 'Osteoprotegerin (OPG) has potent and sustained anti-resorptive activity in postmenopausal women', *Journal of Bone and Mineral Research*, 14, p. S180.

Bjarnason, N. H., Bjarnason, K., Haarbo, J., Rosenquist, C. & Christiansen, C. (1996), 'Tibolone: prevention of bone loss in late postmenopausal women', *The Journal of Clinical Endocrinology and Metabolism*, 81, pp. 2419–22.

Bouillon, R. A., Auwerx, J. H., Lissens, W. D. & Pelemans, W. K. (1987), 'Vitamin status in the elderly: seasonal substrate deficiency causes 1,25-dihydroxycholecalciferol deficiency', *The American Journal of Clinical Nutrition*, 45, pp. 755–63.

Center, J. R., Nguyen, T. V., Sambrook, P. N. & Eisman, J. A. (1999), 'Hormonal and biochemical parameters in the determination of osteoporosis in elderly men', *The Journal of Clinical Endocrinology and Metabolism*, 84(10), pp. 3626–35.

Center, J. R., Nguyen, T. V., Schneider, D., Sambrook, P. N. & Eisman, J. A. (1999), 'Mortality after all major types of osteoporotic fracture: An observational study', *Lancet*, 353, pp. 878–82.

Cummings, S. R., Browner, W. S., Bauer, D., Stone, K., Ensrud, K., Jamal, S. et al. (1998), 'Endogenous hormones and the risk of hip and vertebral fractures among older women', *The New England Journal of Medicine*, 339(11), pp. 733–8.

Cummings, S. R., Eckert, S., Krueger, K. A. et al. (1999), 'The effect of raloxifene on risk of breast cancer in postmenopausal women. Results from the MORE randomized trial. Multiple Outcomes of Raloxifene Evaluation', *Journal of the American Medical Association*, 281, pp. 2187–97.

Cummings, S. R., Nevitt, M. C., Browner, W. S. et al. (1995), 'Risk factors for hip fracture in white women', *The New England Journal of Medicine*, 332, pp. 767–73.

Dawson-Hughes, B., Harris, S. S., Krall, E. A. & Dallal, G. E. (1997), 'Effect of Ca and vitamin D supplementation on bone density in men and women 65 years of age or older', *The New England Journal of Medicine*, 337, pp. 670–6.

Eastell, R., Reid, D. M., Compston, J. et al. (1998), 'A UK Consensus Group on management of glucocorticoid-induced osteoporosis: An update', *Journal of Internal Medicine*, 244, pp. 271–9.

Ensrud, K. E., Lipschutz, R. C., Cauley, J. A., Seeley, D., Nevitt, M. C., Scott, J. et al. (1997), 'Body size and hip fracture risk in older women: A prospective study', *The American Journal of Medicine*, 103(4), pp. 274–80.

Ettinger, B., Black, D. M., Knickerbocker, R. K. et al. (1999), 'Reduction of vertebral fracture risk in postmenopausal women with osteoporosis treated with raloxifene. Results from a 3-year randomised clinical trial', *Journal of the American Medical Association*, 282, pp. 637–45.

Faber, J. & Galloe, A. M. (1994), 'Changes in bone mass during prolonged sub-clinical hyperthyroidism due to L-thyroxine treatment: A meta-analysis', *European Journal of Endocrinology*, 130, pp. 350–6.

Garnero, P., Hausherr, E., Chapuy, M.-C. et al. (1996), 'Markers of bone turnover predict hip fracture in elderly women: the EPIDOS prospective study', *Journal of Bone and Mineral Research*, 11, pp. 1531–8.

Harris, S. T., Watts, N. B., Jackson, R. D. et al. (1993), 'Four-year study of intermittent cyclic etidronate treatment of postmenopausal osteoporosis: three years of blinded therapy followed by one year of open therapy', *The American Journal of Medicine*, 95, pp. 557–67.

Holbrook, T. L., Barrett-Connor, E. & Wingard, D. L. (1988), 'Dietary calcium and risk of hip fracture: 14-year prospective population study', *Lancet*, 2, pp. 1046–9.

Hulley, S., Grady, D., Bush, T. et al. (1998), 'Randomized trial of estrogen plus progestin for secondary prevention of coronary heart disease in postmenopausal women', *Journal of the American Medical Association*, 208, pp. 605–13.

Lips, P., Graafmans, W. C., Ooms, M. E., Bezemer, D. & Bouter, L. M. (1996), 'Vitamin D supplementation and fracture incidence in elderly persons. A randomized, placebo-controlled clinical trial', *Annals of Internal Medicine*, 124, pp. 400–6.

Looker, A. C., Orwoll, E. S., Johnston Jnr, C. C., Lindsay, R. L., Wahner, H. W., Dunn, W. L. et al. (1997), 'Prevalence of low femoral neck bone density in older US adults from NHANES III', *Journal of Bone and Mineral Research*, 12, pp. 1761–8.

Melton III, L. J., Khosla, S., Atkinson, E. J., O'Fallon, W. M., Riggs, B. L. (1997), 'Relationship of bone turnover to bone density and fractures', *Journal of Bone and Mineral Research*, 12, pp. 1083–91.

Minne, H. W., Pfeifer, M., Begerow, B., Nachtigall, D. & Hansen, C. (2000), 'Vitamin D and calcium supplementation reduces falls in elderly women via improvement of body sway and normalisation of blood pressure: a prospective, randomized and double-blind study', *Osteoporosis International*, 11(suppl. 2), p. S115.

National Institutes of Health Consensus Development Conference Statement, 'Osteoporosis Prevention, Diagosis and Therapy', 27–29 March 2000, 17(1).

Available at: http://odp.od.nih.gov/consensus/cons/111/111_intro.htm (accessed 12 July 2000).

Pols, H. A. P., Felsenberg, D., Hanley, D. A., Step, N. J., Munoz-Torres, M., Wilkin, T. J., Qin-sheng, G., Galich, A. M., Vandormael, K., Yates, A. J. & Stych, B. (1999), 'Multinational, placebo-controlled, randomized trial of the effects of alendronate on bone density and fracture risk in postmenopausal women with low bone mass: results of the FOSIT study', *Osteoporosis International*, 9, pp. 461–8.

Poor, G., Atkinson, E. J., O'Fallon, W. M. & Melton III, L. J. (1995), 'Predictors of hip fractures in elderly men', *Journal of Bone and Mineral Research*, 10, pp. 1900–7.

Sanders, K. M., Nicholson, G. C., Ugoni, A. M., Pasco, J. A., Seeman, E. & Kotowicz, M. A. (2000), 'Health burden of hip and other fractures in Australia beyond 2000', *The Medical Journal of Australia*, 170, pp. 467–70.

Silverman, S. L., Chesnut, C., Andriano, K. et al. (1998), 'Salmon calcitonin nasal spray reduces risk of vertebral fracture(s) in established osteoporosis and has continuous efficacy with prolonged treatment: accrued 5 year world wide data of the PROOF study', *Bone*, 23(Suppl. 5), p. S174.

Yaffe, K., Browner, W., Cauley, J., Launer, L. & Harris, T. (1999), 'Association between bone mineral density and cognitive decline in older women', *The Journal of the American Geriatrics Society*, 47(10), pp. 1176–82.

Chapter 56
Neck and back pain

MICHAEL AHERN and FIONA GOLDBLATT

Introduction

Neck pain and low back pain are common in the elderly and are usually caused by localised musculoskeletal problems. However, they may also be due to a variety of systemic illnesses. This can present a difficult diagnostic challenge for the physician, to avoid missing serious causes, while also avoiding over-investigation of the patient with a self-limited musculoskeletal problem. This chapter aims to define the major aetiologies of neck and back pain in the elderly population and to outline therapeutic managements.

Neck pain

Mechanical disorders of the cervical spine are frequent in the ageing population. The causes are multiple and include osteoarthritis, myelopathy and disc herniation. There are few studies of the natural history of cervical pain, particularly in the elderly. In patients without neurological deficits and where the pain is not due to malignancy or rheumatoid arthritis, neck pain is relatively benign, with 43% of patients recovering fully within 10 years, 25% continuing to have moderate symptoms, 7% remaining or becoming severely disabled and 25% continuing to have mild symptoms.

Mechanical disorders of the cervical spine

Cervical pain of unknown origin ('neck strain')

Neck strain is a non-specific term for soft tissue pain in the middle or lower part of the posterior aspect of the neck, which may be uni- or bilateral. Pain may also radiate to the head and shoulders, tending to spare the arms. Symptoms are often triggered by sleeping in an awkward position or turning the head rapidly.

Physical examination reveals local tenderness in the para-cervical muscles, decreased range of motion and loss of cervical lordosis. There is no neurological abnormality and laboratory tests and radiology investigations are normal.

Treatment

Cervical spine manipulation and mobilisation provide a short-term benefit for some patients with neck pain. Physical therapies, such as electromagnetic therapy, laser therapy, transcutaneous nerve stimulation and ultrasound, have no proof of reversing lesions of the vertebral column. At best they constitute forms of analgesia. There is also no evidence to support the use of traction, magnetic necklaces or collars. Simple analgesics or non-steroidal anti-inflammatory drugs (NSAIDs), used with caution in the elderly, provide analgesia while patients undergo natural improvement. There is no evidence to support the use of major tranquillisers or tricyclic antidepressants, so they should therefore be avoided.

Prolapsed intervertebral disc

Intervertebral cervical disc herniation causes severe radicular pain that radiates from the shoulder to the forearm and hand. Generally, neck pain is minimal or absent. It is precipitated by sudden exertion, such as heavy lifting.

Physical examination reveals increased radicular pain with any movement that places tension on the affected nerve. Neurological examination is variable but may reveal a sensory deficit, reflex asymmetry or motor weakness (Table 56.1). Magnetic resonance imaging (MRI) is the best technique to identify the location of disc herniation and nerve root impingement.

Treatment

Natural history

Few studies have been conducted into the natural history of prolapsed intervertebral discs. Forty-five per cent of patients obtained satisfactory pain relief after 5 years, while 55% continued to have pain and loss of function and 25% were unable to return to work. Cervical disc protrusions do diminish in size with time.

Conservative therapy

Conservative treatment refers to the use of NSAIDs, analgesics, physical therapy, traction, bed rest and transcutaneous nerve stimulation. However, no systematic reviews have been conducted and it is difficult to distinguish between treatment effect and natural history. There is no evidence of superiority of one form of therapy over another. However, patients with acute cervical radicular pain should be offered the above conservative therapy. No data is available to support the use of oral prednisolone. Some patients respond to cervical epidural steroid injections—the best results have been obtained in those with radicular pain—while the evidence of efficacy is stronger with peri-radicular steroids (fluoroscopic-guided injections of steroids into the intervertebral foramen of the affected nerve).

Table 56.1 Radicular symptoms and signs

Vertebra	Pain distribution	Sensory loss	Motor loss	Reflex loss
C2	Occipital pain			
C5	Neck to outer shoulder, arm	Shoulder	Deltoid	Biceps, supinator
C6	Outer arm to thumb, index finger	Thumb, index finger	Biceps, wrist extensors	Triceps
C7	Outer arm to middle finger	Index, middle fingers	Triceps	Triceps
C8	Inner arm to ring, little fingers	Ring, little fingers	Hand muscles	None
L2–4	Anterior thigh–medial leg	Medial leg–medial malleolus	Hip flexion, knee extension (anterior tibialis)	Patellar (knee jerk)
L5	Lateral leg to dorsal foot and great toe	Lateral leg to dorsal foot	Dorsiflexion (extensor hallucis longus)	None
S1	Lateral foot	Lateral foot/sole	Plantar flexion (peroneus longus and brevis)	Achilles (ankle jerk)

Surgical therapy

The indications for surgical therapy are:

- failed conservative therapy
- arm pain or radicular pain with paraesthesia or neurological signs
- radicular or neurological signs matched by corresponding lesion on computerised tomography (CT) or MRI (e.g. cervical disc herniation).

Surgery offers rapid relief of cervical radicular pain and improvement can be expected in 60–80% of cases. Surgery is not usually indicated for acute cervical radicular pain unless the pain is refractory to conservative measures. Surgery, however, does not alter the long-term prognosis.

Cervical spondylosis

Cervical spondylosis is a degenerative condition of the synovial intervertebral joints and ligaments, resulting in the narrowing of the disc space and the formation of osteophytes, which can pressure nerve roots and the cord itself. Factors associated with the development of cervical spondylosis include heavy labour, posture and genetic predisposition.

Symptoms

The symptoms of cervical spondylosis are often chronic, developing insidiously over years, and are characterised by neck stiffness and upper shoulder and arm pain. Pain occasionally radiates to the interscapular muscles, anterior chest or the occiput. Less commonly associated features may include vertebral ischaemia and brachial neuralgia. Patients may also have features of osteoarthritis (pain and stiffness) elsewhere, in particular in the lumbar spine.

The prognosis of cervical spondylosis suggests that 28% of patients will have troublesome symptoms or moderate disability for 2–19 years after the onset of symptoms.

Clinical examination

On clinical examination, there is often little to find except midline tenderness and limitation of neck movements, including flexion/extension/rotation/lateral flexion (ear to shoulder). The C5–6 and C6–7 levels are most commonly affected. Nerve root signs may be present, including pain in the arms and fingers, reduced reflexes and dermatomal sensory loss (Table 56.1).

Investigations

Lateral cervical X-ray demonstrates intervertebral narrowing and facet joint sclerosis. Oblique plain X-ray views are useful if nerve root encroachment is suspected. MRI is not warranted in the absence of nerve root signs and may result in overdiagnosis.

Studies demonstrate that the majority of people over 50 years have radiological evidence of osteoarthritis of the cervical spine, with osteophyte formation and disc narrowing (especially at C5–6). In individuals over 40 there is a greater than 50% chance of degenerative cervical discs showing on MRI. Therefore, it is important to correlate clinical features and radiological changes in the cervical spine. Differential diagnosis of cervical spondylosis can include polymyalgia rheumatica (PMR) and septic discitis.

Cervical myelopathy

Cervical myelopathy is a common cause of disability in older persons, and although the exact prevalence is unknown, it is thought to be the most common cause of spinal cord dysfunction in individuals over 55 years.

Cervical myelopathy is a sequela of cervical spondylosis and results from spinal cord compression by osteophytes, ligamentum flavum or intervertebral discs. With ageing, disc degeneration results in a loss of disc height. Subsequently, osteophytes develop posteriorly and project into the spinal canal, compressing the spinal cord and its vascular supply. There are three important pathophysiological factors in the development of cervical myelopathy:

1. static mechanical factors (e.g. size of the spinal canal)
2. dynamic mechanical factors—related to the effect of normal cervical motion (flexion and extension) on the already compromised spinal cord
3. spinal cord ischaemia.

Symptoms

The symptoms are believed to develop when the spinal cord has been reduced by at least 30% or to an anteroposterior diameter of 10 mm or less. Neck pain/stiffness (from cervical spondylosis) is mentioned in only about one-third of patients with myelopathy. A history of peculiar sensations in the arms and hands associated with weakness and inco-ordination may also be described. Patients may develop leg stiffness, spasticity, gait disturbances and spontaneous leg movements. Loss of sphincter control is rare.

Clinical examination

Flexion of the neck may result in a generalised 'electric shock' sensation down the centre of the back (Lhermitte's sign). Leg and arm weakness, a stiff spastic gait and long tract signs (i.e. spasticity, clonus and upgoing plantar reflexes) indicate compression of the spinal cord. A characteristic sign is of hyper-reflexia. For example, a C5–6 level spondylosis and cord compression results in absent biceps and supinator reflexes (C5–6) with a brisk triceps reflex (C7). An underlying peripheral neuropathy, such as in a diabetic patient, may mask hyper-reflexia. Sensory abnormalities are variable with deficits, including decreased dermatomal sensation and loss of proprioception (Table 56.1).

Investigations

Plain radiographs demonstrate the advanced degenerative disease of cervical spondylosis with narrowed disc spaces, osteophytes, facet joint sclerosis and cervical instability. MRI is the investigation of choice, and can detect the degree of spinal cord compression and the effects on the integrity of the cord (Figure 56.1). It can exclude other causes of myelopathy, such as metastatic tumours, syringomyelia and spinal cord infarction.

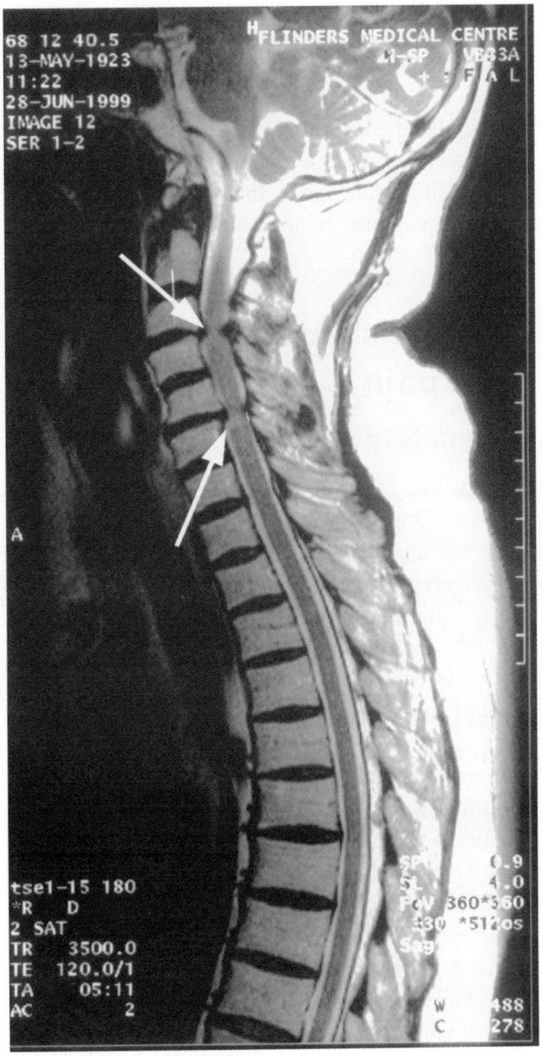

Figure 56.1 T2-weighted sagittal midline MRI of the cervicothoracic spine. Arrows indicate spinal canal stenosis with increased signal intensity within the cord (C5–6 level) consistent with cervical myelopathy

Treatment of cervical myelopathy due to spondylosis

Natural history

Eighteen per cent of patients with cervical myelopathy improve spontaneously, while 40% of patients remain stable and 42% progress.

Conservative therapy

Conservative therapy includes cervical traction, immobilisation (collar or neck brace), skull traction and physical therapy. However, no randomised studies have been conducted and it is difficult to distinguish between treatment effects and natural history.

Surgical therapy

The aim of surgical treatment is to decompress the spinal cord, however, only 50% of patients have successful outcomes. Prognostic factors for a poor postoperative outcome include severe neurological deficits, abnormal signal changes in the spinal cord and/or spinal cord atrophy on MRI.

Other disorders causing neck pain

Rheumatoid arthritis

Cervical involvement with rheumatoid arthritis is common. The symptoms of early disease are mainly neck stiffness in all directions of movement. Tenosynovitis of the transverse ligament of C1, which stabilises the odontoid process of C2, may produce significant C1–2 instability (atlanto-axial subluxation). Cervical myelopathy also may develop as a result of erosion of the odontoid process, ligament laxity or ligament rupture. Neck pain without neurological involvement tends to be self-limiting.

Subluxation is best detected with the neck in flexion, when the lateral view will demonstrate a separation of the odontoid process from the arch of the atlas greater than 3 mm.

All patients with rheumatoid arthritis requiring a general anaesthetic should have a preoperative cervical spine X-ray in flexion and the anaesthetist informed if cervical involvement is present.

Polymyalgia rheumatica

Polymyalgia rheumatica (PMR) is a clinical syndrome characterised by symmetrical pain and stiffness in the muscles of the pelvis and shoulder girdles without evidence of a primary muscle disorder. Its incidence increases with age, being rarely diagnosed in people under 50 years.

There are no specific clinical signs or laboratory findings in cases of PMR. The diagnosis is based on the typical history of an elderly person who has acute pain and stiffness of the neck, with symmetrical shoulder and hip girdle involvement. Symptoms are significantly worse in the morning and there are variable systemic manifestations of fever, fatigue, depression and malaise. Laboratory markers include a high erythrocyte sedimentation rate (ESR) and high C-reactive protein (CRP) levels. Most important is the association with giant cell arteritis and the associated risk of blindness.

A good response to 15 mg prednisolone within 24–48 hours is typical. Treatment should continue for 12–24 months and the patient weaned according to symptoms and the CRP level or ESR. Higher dose steroids (prednisolone 50–60 mg/day) are required if the patient also has giant cell arteritis or develops it subsequently.

Back pain

Back pain is a common complaint among the elderly, affecting up to 70% of the population. The duration of symptoms is variable, with recovery from non-specific low back pain generally the rule, with an estimated 70% recovering within several weeks, although recurrence is common (40% within 6 months). The National Health Survey, however, reported that 11% of the elderly population had back pain that persisted or was expected to persist for a period of 6 months or more. There are numerous causes of back pain (Box 56.1). Mechanical disorders are the commonest cause of low back pain in the elderly and include disc degeneration, osteoarthritis and spinal stenosis. Malignancy is the most common systemic disease affecting the spine, and although it accounts for less than 1% of episodes of low back pain, 80% of cases are in patients over the age of 50 years.

The history and physical examination are important influences on diagnostic imaging, laboratory testing, therapeutic choices and specialist referral. Key questions when taking the history include:

1. Was the onset sudden (e.g. trauma) or gradual?
2. What is the character of the pain?
3. Is the pain localised, symmetrical, asymmetrical, radicular?
4. Is the pain worsened or relieved by activity?
5. What time of day is the pain at its worst—morning stiffness, rest pain, night pain?

Box 56.1 Back pain in the elderly

Degenerative
- Disc degeneration
- Prolapsed intervertebral disc
- Facet joint osteoarthritis
- Spinal stenosis
- Spondylolisthesis

Metabolic
- Osteoporosis
- Osteomalacia
- Paget's disease

Neoplastic
- Metastasis
- Myeloma
- Pancreatic carcinoma
- Retroperitoneal tumours

Infective
- Septic discitis
- Osteomyelitis
- Epidural or paraspinal abscesses

Referred pain
- Abdominal pathology
  - Gastric or duodenal ulcers
  - Pancreatitis
  - Cholecystitis
  - Aortic aneurysm
- Retroperitoneal
  - Sarcoma
  - Fibrosis
- Pelvic
  - Infection
  - Malignancy

6. Are motor or sensory symptoms present or not?
7. Is claudication present or not?
8. Are the bowel or bladder affected?

Other important questions relate to identifying an underlying systemic disease include questions on weight loss, fever, chills, night sweats and pain elsewhere.

The specific history and examination details that can aid the doctor to identify a subgroup of patients with an increased probability of having a serious underlying cause of back pain are referred to as 'red flags'. Presence of one or more 'red flags' corresponds to a pre-test probability of serious systemic disease of up to 10% (Box 56.2).

Box 56.2 Indicators of high risk: red flags

- Age > 50 years
- A past/current history of cancer
- Unexplained weight loss
- Duration of pain more than 1 month
- Absence of response to treatment/unresponsive to narcotics
- Pain worse at rest or unrelieved by bed rest
- History of intravenous drug use
- Presence of urinary tract or other infection
- Nocturnal pain
- Elevated ESR

The majority of elderly people will have radiographic evidence of degenerative spine disease (e.g. facet joint osteoarthritis or disc space narrowing) and the anatomical abnormalities need to be correlated with the patient's clinical presentation in order to avoid incorrect diagnosis or over-interpretation.

There is consensus that plain X-ray is not necessary for every patient with acute low back pain, as it has a low yield of useful findings and frequent potentially misleading results. In patients presenting over 50 years of age or with neurological deficits, fever, trauma or signs of neoplasm, early imaging is advised. Failure to improve in 6 weeks should also be an indication to proceed to imaging.

CT and MRI are more sensitive to detect spinal infections and cancer, spinal stenosis and herniated discs.

Degenerative disorders of the lumbosacral spine

Facet joint osteoarthritis, disc degeneration and spinal stenosis are the most common degenerative disorders of the lumbosacral spine to affect the elderly.

Lumbosacral spondylosis

Arthritis in the facet joints is common in the elderly and symptoms may vary from mild low back pain to nerve root compression to spinal claudication. The most commonly involved level is L4–5.

Symptoms

Patients describe recurrent or chronic low back pain often referred to the gluteal region or into the posterior thigh (although usually not below the knee). Pain increases towards the end of the day and on prolonged standing or sitting.

Clinical examination

Examination typically reveals reduced lumbar extension and exacerbation of pain on lumbar extension and ipsilateral bending to one side with the osteoarthritic joints (facet joint disease) (Table 56.2). Neurological examination is normal.

Investigations

Plain X-rays invariably show spondylosis in patients aged over 40 years. These show one or more areas of disc space narrowing, osteophyte formation and degenerative changes in posterior joints. It is therefore difficult to use radiology for diagnosis, with the association between symptoms and imaging being weak.

Table 56.2 Examination of the (lumbar) spine

Examination	Procedure
Inspection	Examine the spine when patient is erect looking for lumbar lordosis, kyphosis and scoliosis
Palpation	Palpate spinous processes and paraspinal muscle for tenderness and spasm, for scoliosis and local bone pain (due to e.g. osteoporosis, fracture, neoplasia)
Mobilise	Reduced lumbar extension suggests facet joint degeneration Straight leg raise (SLR): lift leg with the knee fully extended while patient is supine—normal is 90 degrees
Neurological examination	Nerve root impingement is suggested by dermatomal sensory loss, asymmetrical reduction in reflexes and myotomal weakness
Systemic review	Full general physical (multisystem) examination

Treatment

Treatment is generally with regular use of NSAIDs or paracetamol. Beware of potential side effects of NSAIDs, particularly aggravation of pre-existing renal disease, hypertension, cardiac failure, fluid retention and gastrointestinal side effects, including perforation and haemorrhage. Other side effects of NSAIDs in the elderly involve the central nervous system, such as headaches and confusion. Beware of the potential interaction of NSAIDs with diuretics and antihypertensive medications. Some patients respond to muscle relaxants but these are best avoided in the elderly because of falls and sedation. Spinal manipulation may benefit some patients but beware of the patient with osteoporosis. It is recommended that patients return to all normal activities, avoid bed rest and avoid exercise in the acute phase. Conventional traction, facet joint injections and transcutaneous nerve stimulation are ineffective or minimally effective.

Prolapsed intervertebral discs

Intervertebral disc herniation can result in nerve root irritation and impingement resulting in radicular pain. Prolapsed intervertebral discs can occur at any level, but are most common in the neck and low back. The majority of clinically important lumbar disc herniations are at the L4–5 or L5–S1 level and result in sciatica (a sharp or burning pain radiating down the posterior or lateral aspect of the leg, usually to the foot or ankle). Sciatica is often more prominent than the back pain. The natural history of prolapsed intervertebral discs is generally favourable and improvement is usual. Sequential MRI studies have revealed that the herniated portion of the disc tends to regress with time, with partial or complete resolution in two-thirds of people after 6 months.

Clinical examination

On straight leg raising (SLR) pain is a result of the disc tethering the nerve root and a typically positive SLR sign is one that reproduces the patient's pain at 30–60 degrees elevation. The lower the angle, the more specific the test becomes. The femoral nerve stretch test (flexing the knee with the patient face down) is performed to test for irritation of the higher lumbar roots L2 and L3. Neurological examination is performed to identify nerve root impingement (Table 56.1).

Treatment

Natural history

Ten per cent of patients have continuing pain after 6 months. MRI studies show partial or complete resolution in two-thirds of patients after 6 months.

Therapy

Therapy involves non-surgical treatment initially for 6 weeks. Early treatment is as above for non-specific back pain, but safety and efficacy of spinal manipulation is not established in prolapsed intervertebral discs. If progressive neurological deficit occurs or cauda equina syndrome, the patients should be referred for consideration for surgery, after CT or MRI examination. Narcotic analgesics may be necessary but for limited periods only. Epidural corticosteroids help some patients. Discectomy provides pain relief for up to 4 years but has questionable benefits after 10 years.

Spinal canal stenosis

Spinal canal stenosis is common in the elderly, although the exact prevalence is unknown. It is usually degenerative with growth of osteophytes, redundancy of the ligamentum flavum and posterior bulging of the intervertebral discs resulting in symptoms. With central disc protrusion lesions are usually multiple, although they can occur at a single level.

Symptoms

The pattern of the radicular pain depends on the location of nerve compression. With central canal stenosis, pain in one or both legs occurs with walking (pseudoclaudication). Lateral stenosis causes unilateral leg pain with standing while stenosis of the intervertebral foramen causes leg pain that is persistent regardless of the patient's position. Unlike vascular claudication, the pain appears after walking variable distances and can occur on standing alone (without ambulation). To relieve pain, the patient tends to need to flex forward or sit down, which increases the room in the spinal canal and restores blood flow to the spinal nerve roots, decreasing pain. Symptoms are characteristically not present when the hips are flexed. In the elderly, the differences in symptoms with vascular claudication, however, are not always so clear-cut because the two conditions may co-exist.

Clinical examination

The diagnosis of spinal canal stenosis tends to be based on symptoms, as clinical findings are few or absent. Few data are available on the accuracy of physical examination, as the condition has only been widely recognised in the past 10 years. Physical examination may be unremarkable unless the patient exercises to the point of developing symptoms. There is often evidence of lumbar degenerative disease and the SLR is usually negative. While symptoms are present, motor weakness (in up to one-third of patients) and reflex abnormalities (in half of patients) can be demonstrated, which resolve when the episode of pain resolves. It is important to examine the peripheral pulses.

Investigations

Plain X-rays may demonstrate degenerative disc disease with facet joint narrowing (Figure 56.2a). CT scans demonstrate facet joint disease and reduced dimensions of the spinal canal (Figure 56.2b) and MRI can show neural compression.

Abnormal findings of spinal canal stenosis are very common on spinal imaging, even in those who are asymptomatic, and again the physician needs to correlate symptoms and radiological findings. Radiographic alterations of canal stenosis are only significant if the patient has corresponding symptoms.

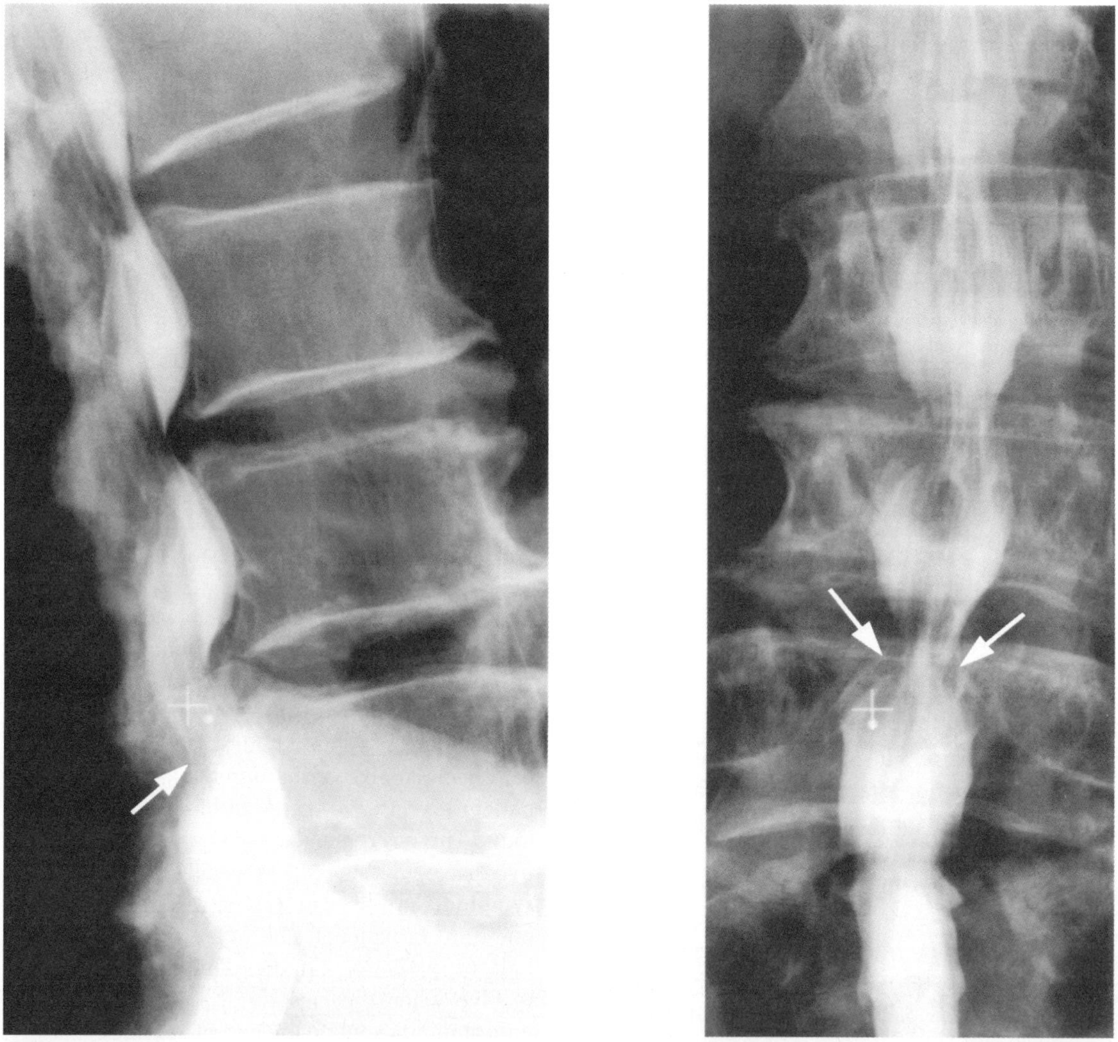

Figure 56.2 (a) Lateral and AP views of a lumbar myelogram. There is multilevel waisting of the thecal sac most prominent at the L4–5 disc level consistent with moderate to severe canal stenosis

Treatment

Natural history

The patient's condition is usually stable or gradually worsens—over 4 years 15% improve, 70% are stable and 15% get worse.

Therapy

Therapy includes simple analgesics (e.g. paracetamol), NSAIDs, epidural steroids. Back and leg strengthening exercises help to maintain mobility and prevent falls. In cases of persistent severe pain, the patients should be referred for consideration of laminectomy. If degenerative spondylolisthesis is present, spinal fusion and decompression should be considered. Symptoms often recur after several years even when surgery is initially beneficial.

Spondylolisthesis/spondylolysis

Spondylolisthesis is the displacement of a vertebral body in relation to the underlying vertebra. It is

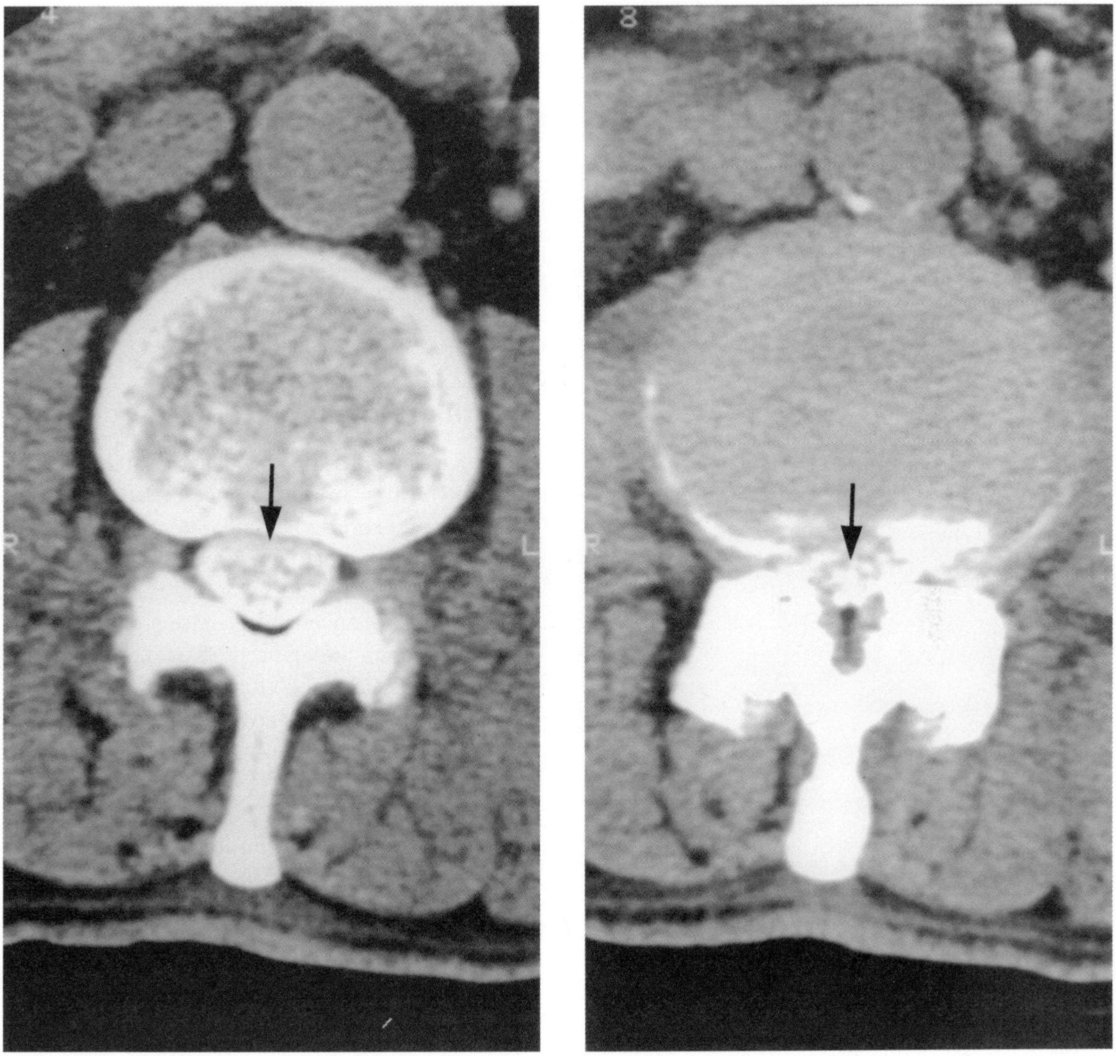

Figure 56.2 (b) Lumbar CT scan with intrathecal contrast. In the left image, the L2 body and thecal sac are within normal limits. At the L2–3 disc level, severe canal stenosis is evident due to short pedicles and hypertrophy of the facet joints and ligamentum flava

usually secondary to degeneration of intervertebral discs and deterioration of the plane of motion of the facet joints. It may also occur as a developmental abnormality in association with spondylolysis, a separation of the pars interarticularis. A stress fracture may also occur in the pars interarticularis.

Symptoms

Patients describe low back pain in both conditions exacerbated by standing and relieved with rest. With severe subluxation patients can also have leg pain. From the history it is not possible to differentiate between a pars fracture and other causes of mechanical back pain.

Clinical examination

Increased lordosis with a 'step up' may be evident in patients with spondylolisthesis. Pars fractures cannot be detected clinically (Figure 56.3). There are usually no neurological abnormalities in either condition.

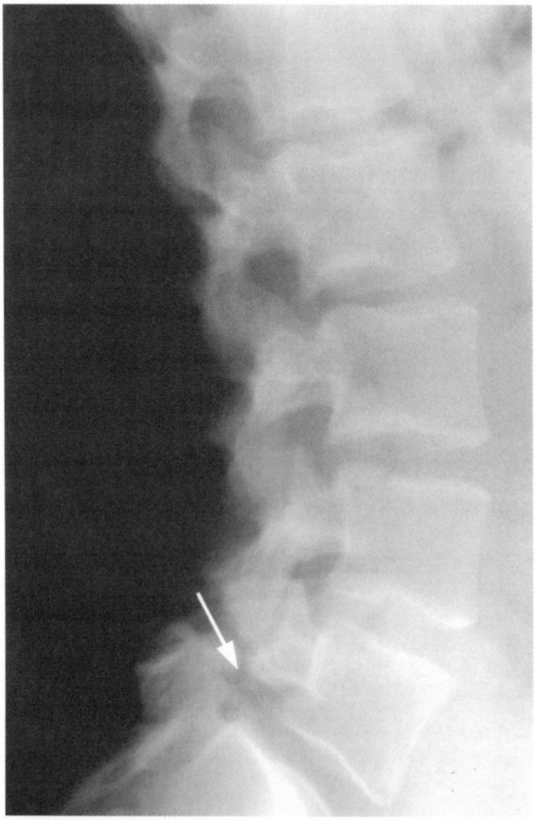

Figure 56.3 Lateral X-ray of the lumbar spine. The arrow indicates a grade I spondylolisthesis with bilateral pars interarticularis defects of L5

Investigations

Plain X-rays are adequate to demonstrate the defect in the pars interarticularis (collar on the Scottie dog), and lateral views demonstrate the degree of subluxation (Figure 56.3). Bone scan is required to detect recent fractures. MRI can detect entrapment and direct impingement of spinal nerve roots associated with the spondylolisthesis.

Treatment

See treatment under the sections on lumbosacral spondylosis (above) and chronic low back pain (below).

Scoliosis

A scoliosis is defined as a lateral curvature of the spine in excess of 10 degrees and most commonly begins to develop in adolescence. In the elderly, patients describe symptoms of osteoarthritis and subsequent back pain related to the longstanding scoliosis. The symptoms are increasing back pain relieved by bed rest. Nerve compression can occur in more seriously affected individuals, with demonstration of appropriate neurological findings.

Plain X-ray allows evaluation of the degree of scoliosis. In patients with less than 40 degrees of scoliosis, exercises and NSAIDs may be effective in reducing pain and maintaining function.

Treatment of chronic low back pain

Treatment includes simple analgesics and, if unsuccessful, NSAIDs. In the absence of radiculopathy, conditioning exercise has the potential benefits of weight loss, reducing pain, improving functioning, increasing mobility and avoiding a sick role, but long-term compliance with exercise programs is difficult. Narcotics and muscle relaxants should be avoided in the elderly. Multidisciplinary pain clinics and back schools are effective and helpful (e.g. cognitive behavioural therapy, patient education, supervised exercise and selective nerve blocks).

Indications for surgery in low back pain

The indications for surgery include:

- cauda equina syndrome (surgical emergency)
- progressive or severe neurological deficit
- failed conservative treatment after 6 weeks with persistent neuromotor deficit
- progressive or severe neurological deficit associated with spinal stenosis, spondylolisthesis or herniated discs.

Metabolic disorders of the spine

Osteoporotic vertebral compression fractures

Osteoporosis (reduced bone mass per unit volume, with normal mineralisation) is the most common metabolic bone disease seen in the elderly, affecting about 15% of postmenopausal white women. A common clinical manifestation of osteoporosis is a vertebral crush fracture that occurs in about 20% of affected postmenopausal women. Osteoporosis causing vertebral crush fractures may be primary (e.g. age, postmenopausal) or secondary (e.g. long-term corticosteroids use, endocrine disorders). Such fractures often occur without a history of identifiable trauma.

Symptoms

The symptoms relate to the bone collapse and subsequent vertebral fracture. Symptoms of a crush fracture may range from none to an acute severe pain in the area of the affected vertebrae. Pain is typically worse on movement, is decreased on lying flat and may be accompanied by symptoms of nerve root compression.

Clinical examination

Examination may reveal tenderness over affected vertebrae and a progressive thoracic kyphosis.

Investigations

Bone mineral density is used to assess osteoporosis and is used as a guide for risk of fracture. The differential diagnosis includes pathological fractures due to malignancy.

Treatment

Management of osteoporosis is discussed in Chapter 55. Back pain due to osteoporotic fracture may be severe and require narcotic analgesics and bed rest in the short term. Prolonged bed rest is discouraged.

Paget's disease

Paget's disease is a focal disorder of bone remodelling that typically begins with excessive bone resorption followed by excessive bone formation. The primary disturbance is an exaggeration of osteoclastic bone resorption, initially producing a localised bone loss. The condition is often first noticed when bone formation is pronounced, resulting in enlarged and deformed bones. The disease prevalence increases with age, occurring in over 10% of those over 80 years.

Symptoms

The disease is typically asymptomatic, with only 5–10% developing symptoms. It is often detected on an X-ray performed for another cause or with an elevated serum alkaline phosphatase level detected on routine biochemical testing. Clinical symptoms depend on the bone involved and include pain, deformity, nerve root compression, spinal cord compression (rarely) and osteoarthritis. It may be monostotic, affecting only a single bone, or polyostotic, involving two or more bones. The most common sites of involvement include the pelvis, femur, spine, skull and tibia.

Investigations

Screening demonstrates an increased blood alkaline phosphatase level, normal calcium and phosphate levels and an increased urinary hydroxyproline level. Plain X-ray initially shows radiolucency followed by increased density and coarsened trabeculae. A bone scan can be useful in demonstrating the extent of disease.

Treatment

Specific anti-pagetic therapy consists of agents that suppress the activity of pagetic osteoclasts. These treatments include salmon and human calcitonin and bisphosphonate compounds: oral etidronate, alendronate, risedronate and intravenously administered pamidronate. These drugs ameliorate bone pain, low back pain secondary to pagetic vertebral changes and some syndromes of neural compression (e.g. radiculopathy).

Other symptomatic treatments for Paget's disease include analgesics, NSAIDs and surgery.

Osteomalacia

Osteomalacia describes a condition of qualitatively abnormal bone with inadequate mineralisation of osteoid due to vitamin D deficiency. This can be due to many causes, such as decreased production due to inadequate sunlight or reduced vitamin D dietary intake. The rheumatic manifestations include bone pain and muscle weakness (myopathy). X-rays demonstrate osteoporosis (later) and pseudofractures (Looser zones).

Neoplastic disorders

Metastases

Breast, lung or prostate carcinomas most commonly metastasise to bone. The history is generally more useful than examination for detecting underlying cancer, except in later stages. It is important to obtain a detailed past medical history in addition to the high-risk features listed in Box 56.2.

Myeloma

Multiple myeloma, the commonest primary tumour of bone, is a plasma cell dyscrasia that has frequent bony involvement in the form of lytic lesions, osteoporosis and pathological fractures. Bone pain (particularly back or chest wall) is present in up to 60% of patients. Up to one-third of patients have generalised bone loss secondary to cytokines (osteoclastic activating factors, e.g. interleukin-1, tumour necrosis factor, lymphotoxin).

Investigations

If multiple myeloma is suspected, serum and urinary electrophoresis and screening for urinary Bence-Jones protein should be performed. Further investigations would include a bone marrow biopsy. Plain X-rays are more useful for the skeletal survey than radioisotope bone scans, which are generally negative, as myeloma lesions are lytic rather than blastic.

Infective disorders

Septic discitis and osteomyelitis

Spinal infections (discitis or osteomyelitis) are a rare cause of back pain ($< 0.01\%$ in the primary care setting), however, physicians need to consider infection in older patients as they often do not demonstrate the typical features of infection, such as fever or elevated white cell count. The infective source is usually blood-borne from other sites, such as urinary tract infections, indwelling catheter infections and skin infections. The organisms involved are mostly Gram-negative bacilli or *Staphylococcus aureus*.

Epidural or paraspinal abscesses

Spinal osteomyelitis can be the precipitant for the formation of an abscess that may enlarge to compress the spinal cord. Initial symptoms include mild backache and unexplained fever followed by radicular pain. Treatment includes decompression by laminectomy, drainage and appropriate antibiotics.

Miscellaneous

Diffuse idiopathic skeletal hyperostosis

Diffuse idiopathic skeletal hyperostosis (DISH) is a disease of the later middle aged and elderly. Affected individuals may experience stiffness and restricted range of movement and there may also be extra-spinal involvement, such as tendinitis or enthesitis. A characteristic radiological finding is of flowing calcification and ossification of the anterior and lateral ligaments involving four contiguous vertebrae ('dripping candle wax'), preservation of disc height and absence of sacroiliac joint ankylosis.

Bibliography and further reading

Ahern, M. J. & Rischmueller, M. (1992), 'Problems of age in rheumatology', *Modern Medicine of Australia*, July, pp. 94–101.

Borenstein, D. G. (1997), 'Disorders of the low back and neck', in Klippel, J. (ed.), *Primer on the Rheumatic Diseases*, 11th edn, Arthritis Foundation, Atlanta, pp. 130–6.

Deyo, R. A., Rainville, J. & Kent, D. L. (1992), 'What can the history and physical examination tell us about low back pain?', *Journal of the American Medical Association*, 268(6), pp. 760–5.

Deyo, R. A. & Weinstein, J. N. (2001), 'Low back pain', *New England Journal of Medicine*, 344(5), pp. 363–70.

Edmonds, J. & Hughes, G. (1985), 'Neck and back pain', in *Lecture Notes on Rheumatology*, Blackwell Scientific Publications, Oxford, pp. 233–41.

Lane, M. J., Werntz, J. R., Healey, J. H. & Vigorita, V. J. (1986), 'Metabolic bone disease and Paget's disease in the elderly', *Clinics in Rheumatological Diseases*, 12, pp. 49–96.

Lurie, J. D., Gerber, P. D. & Sox, H. C. (2000), 'A pain in the back', *New England Journal of Medicine*, 343(10), pp. 723–6.

Olhagen, B. (1986), 'Polymyalgia rheumatica', *Clinics in Rheumatological Diseases*, 12, pp. 33–47.

Young, W. F. (2000), 'Cervical spondylotic myelopathy: a common cause of spinal cord dysfunction in older persons', *American Family Physician*, 62(5), pp. 1064–70.

Wipf, J. E. & Deyo, R. A. (1995), 'Low back pain', *Medical Clinics of North America*, 79, pp. 231–46.

Part XII

Other issues

Chapter 57
Ethical dilemmas

LESLEY BOWKER, CLAIRE PRICE, KEVIN STEWART AND GURCHARAN S. RAI

Introduction

This chapter deals with ethical dilemmas that may arise in dealing with elderly patients. We hope to take a pragmatic, patient centred approach to common ethical dilemmas by focusing the discussion on case histories. By the nature of the subject there is often not one clear answer to each problem. In addition, this chapter gives a brief overview of background ethical principles and relevant differences in law in different jurisdictions, although readers looking for more in-depth coverage of these subjects should consult specialist texts.

General ethical principles

The moral or ethical duties of doctors were first defined by Hippocrates (c. 460–c. 377 BC). There are four moral values that are particularly pertinent to medicine (see Box 57.1), and in clinical practice the extent to which each principle applies varies, depending on the situation.

Box 57.1 The four basic principles

1. Respect for patient autonomy
2. Beneficence
3. Non-maleficence
4. Justice

Patient autonomy refers to the right of individuals to dictate what happens to them and, in the context of medicine, what treatment they do and do not have. Hence, fully informed, competent patients are entitled to be asked to consent to medical examination and treatment. Treatment cannot usually be given without such consent. They are also entitled to refuse treatment, even though doing so may lead to deterioration in their condition, or even their death. Although it is an important principle, respect for autonomy is not absolute. For example, patients cannot demand treatment that is not clinically indicated. They are also unable to demand treatment which is illegal (e.g. euthanasia) or to refuse measures as in the case of controlling an infectious disease that may harm others.

Beneficence and non-maleficence refer to the need for treatment to do good and not to do harm, or at least be likely to do more good than harm. Traditionally, medicine has been practised with reference to these principles, perhaps at the expense of respect for autonomy.

The principle of justice refers to the need to consider not just the individual patient but also the health of the community as a whole; this is especially relevant where 'socialised' medicine exists, as in the UK. For example, allocating scarce resources to a very expensive treatment for one individual may deprive many others of less expensive treatment.

Ethical choices necessarily involve value judgments rather than scientific fact. Since society consists of individuals who differ in their personal views of right and wrong, conflict of opinion is inevitable.

Although many of the principles of medical ethics are ancient, views and practices have changed substantially over the centuries. The trend in recent years for more openness among the medical profession marks a move away from unilateral 'paternalistic' decisions based on beneficence/non-maleficence towards a greater emphasis on patient autonomy.

Medical ethics has particular relevance to geriatric medicine because of:

1. the frequency of end-of-life decisions in an older population
2. the frequency of making decisions for temporarily or permanently incompetent patients
3. the challenge of ensuring that discrimination (ageism) is not being practised.

Case 1: Exercising autonomy

Mr CR is a fit, active 89-year-old retired engineer who has had a myocardial infarction. On admission to hospital he tells the coronary care unit (CCU) staff that he will have thrombolytic treatment but does not want cardiopulmonary resuscitation (CPR) should he have a cardiac arrest. He seems to be mentally lucid and know all about myocardial infarction and its treatment, which he learnt about from the Internet after his brother died a few years earlier from a heart attack. He is adamant that he doesn't want to be resuscitated since he thinks that he doesn't really want to live into his 90s. Staff are unsure what to do; the attending doctor says that it is illogical for him to refuse CPR but want thrombolysis, since having this will also reduce his risk of dying. Mr CR listens to this argument and seems to understand, but maintains his position.

Comment

The patient seems mentally competent and well informed about the treatment on offer as well as the consequences of having or not having treatment. He is exercising his autonomy, which overrules the doctor's beneficence in trying to offer him the best available treatment. He is entitled to withhold consent for whatever treatment he decides (in this instance CPR), even if the staff feel it is illogical or against his own best interest.

A do not resuscitate (DNR) order should have been written. The patient should have received all other usual treatment as requested. Staff should have ensured that their discussions with him were clearly documented. They could have asked him to put his wishes in writing and also explain them to family members and others if necessary.

Case 2: Competent adult refusing treatment

Mr JS is 70 and lives alone. He develops increasing shortness of breath and his general practitioner (GP) diagnoses pneumonia and says he requires admission to hospital, but the patient wants to remain at home. The GP explains that without intravenous antibiotics he may deteriorate and could even die. Mr JS says he would rather take his chances at home with any treatment he could have there. He understands that he might die but he just does not want to go in to the hospital. He is not confused, and he is adamant that he will not go to hospital. He gives no reason for his refusal.

Comment

Mr JS appears to be competent to refuse admission to hospital. He understands the nature of his problem, the advised treatment and the consequences of not having the treatment. He is therefore refusing consent to be admitted. His GP should ensure that Mr JS knows that he is also able to change his mind and consent to admission at a later stage should he wish to do so. The GP should carefully document the decision and the discussions, and he should consider asking Mr JS to inform family members of his decision, or ask permission to inform them himself.

The principles of consent

Fully informed, competent patients are entitled to be asked to consent to medical examination and treatment. Treatment cannot usually be given without such consent. Patients are entitled to refuse treatment against the advice of a doctor, even though doing so may lead to deterioration in their condition, or even their death. Although it is an important principle, respect for autonomy is not absolute; patients cannot demand treatment that is not clinically indicated or is illegal. Nor does patient autonomy equate to patients refusing treatment that may result in their condition harming others, as in the case of a contagious disease. In many instances consent is implied rather than explicit: for example, by attending the doctor's consulting rooms or undressing and lying on the examination couch, the patient implies that he consents to examination. Explicit written consent is commonly sought for certain higher-risk procedures, such as surgical operations. Consent is not required for emergency treatment in which case doctors are covered by common law, providing they act with good intent. Patients may withhold consent to specific examinations or treatments and there is no obligation for them to either accept or refuse the whole 'package of treatment' (i.e. either take all the usual treatment for the condition, or none of it). For consent to be valid, patients must be mentally competent (see below) and fully informed. 'Fully informed' implies that they have been made aware of the proposed treatment and likely outcome in straightforward language, and that they are also aware of the potential adverse effects and complications. Patients may give or withhold consent contemporaneously or in advance (an advance directive).

Case 3: Competence/proxy decisions

Mrs AT is an 85-year-old woman who lives alone; she has no close family. She has had increasing problems with her memory over the last 3 years and this has been getting worse. She often wanders and her neighbours are worried about her safety. She falls at home and is admitted with a fractured neck of femur. On arrival in hospital she is drowsy and very confused. The orthopaedic surgeon wishes to operate the following day but asks the geriatrician to review the patient as he's unsure about how to obtain consent for surgery.

Comment

The patient probably has progressive dementia. Since she is now even more confused than normal, she is certainly incompetent to give consent. It would appear that surgery is probably in the patient's best interest given that mortality is very high if these patients are not operated on and that she is likely to be in considerable pain. She is not in a position to exercise autonomy, so the surgeon should balance the beneficence/non-maleficence principles. The surgeon should document the situation carefully, then operate without consent 'in the best interest' of the patient. Although in this case no proxy decision maker is available, others may sometimes decide on behalf of incompetent patients, depending on the jurisdiction (see below). In addition an advance directive might have been useful here if one had been available.

Case 4: Competency assessment

Mrs LT is 85 and lives in a hostel (residential home). She is mildly confused but functions independently. Her general practitioner finds her to have a severe microcytic anaemia after she complains of breathlessness. She agrees to a blood transfusion. Underlying malignancy is suspected but a gastroscopy is normal; colonoscopy is felt to be indicated. The registrar explains this to Mrs LT and she seems to understand. She says several times that she definitely does not want any more tests and that she would not want to go through an operation, even if a very serious condition was detected. She knows her memory is deteriorating and will probably get worse. Mrs LT's daughter is upset that her mother is not having any further tests; she says that her mother is confused and couldn't possibly take responsibility for this decision.

Comment

The issue here is competence. Although the patient is mildly confused, she appears to understand the proposed treatment options and the consequences of not having an operation. She is therefore probably competent to refuse treatment. She may have made this decision because she is aware that she probably has dementia and does not want to survive with severe confusion.

To help clarify the situation, the doctors might consider seeing her on several occasions in relaxed or familiar circumstances to discuss the decision. They should assess her understanding of the situation and the options available to her. They should explore the reasoning behind her decision, which needs to be valid but not necessarily the same as anyone else's. They should ensure that she understands the outcome of her decision and that she shows consistency. All these aspects of the assessment should be recorded. It might be helpful to ask for a second opinion from an independent doctor, such as a psychiatrist, on the patient's competence to make this specific decision.

Having the family member present would be useful for trying to improve their understanding of the process, although the doctor would have to ensure that the daughter didn't exert undue duress on her mother.

Competence

Competence may be defined as an ability to understand the proposed treatment, its consequences and complications, and an ability to use that understanding to make and communicate a decision. The decision of a competent patient must be stable over time. Competence is decision specific, that is, patients may be competent to decide on some issues and incompetent on others. The assumption is in favour of competence if there is doubt, although the degree of certainty required varies, depending on the gravity of the decision; a greater degree of certainty about competence would be required, for example, if the decision involved refusing cancer surgery rather than refusing varicose vein stripping.

Case 5: Proxy decision making or 'in the best interest'

Mr AS has Parkinson's disease and chronic bronchitis. He develops a chest infection and becomes very confused. On hospital admission, pneumonia and toxic confusional state (delirium) is diagnosed. His condition continues to deteriorate despite IV antibiotics, and 24 hours later, he goes into respiratory failure. His doctors feel that if he's going to survive he'll need artificial ventilation in the intensive care unit. The only two family members who are available are the daughter from his first marriage and a son from his second one; they have a very poor relationship and disagree strongly about what is best for him now.

Comment

The patient is clearly incompetent. Presumably his doctors feel that ventilation has at least some chance of helping him survive. The decision whether to proceed seems to be based on whether he would want life-prolonging treatment given his severe medical problems and whether he would consider his quality of life to warrant the treatment at this stage. He is incapable of exercising autonomy and there is no advance directive to use as a guide. In these circumstances family members seem unlikely to be a useful source of information about what he would have wanted.

Depending on the jurisdiction, the role of family members may be to act as proxy decision makers; alternatively, it may be to inform medical staff about the patient's wishes so they can then decide 'in the patient's best interest'.

Proxy decision making

The role of proxy decision makers varies, depending on the jurisdiction. In England and Wales the decision rests with the treating doctor who acts 'in the best interest' of the patient. To ascertain the patient's best interest, the doctor will usually consult family members about the patient's previously stated views, although it is recognised that there are circumstances when consensus is unlikely to be achieved.

In some states of Australia and in most states in the US, the next of kin may legally make proxy decisions for incompetent patients. The 'person responsible' who is empowered to give or withhold consent for incompetent patients is identified from a hierarchy of relatives/carers. In the above case, the doctor may have to act in the best interest of the patient.

In many jurisdictions it is possible for patients to nominate proxy decision makers in an enduring medical power of attorney or in some advance directives.

Advance directives

Advance directives (sometimes called living wills) are a way for patients to continue to exercise their autonomy in decision making, even after they have become incompetent to do so contemporaneously. Patients may nominate a proxy decision maker or stipulate which treatment they accept/refuse, or both. Advance directives cannot override contemporaneous decisions. They usually contain a statement about the circumstances in which they would not want them to come into force, for example, in the case of incompetence and irreversible dementia or terminal malignancy. Most advance directives contain refusal of treatment statements, but there is no reason why a patient may not request continuation of treatment within the bounds of normal clinical practice.

In the UK certain types of advance directive (advance refusals of treatment) carry weight under common law. In some states in Australia there is legislation for advance directives, but there is little uniformity between states. This has proved to be an area of rapidly changing legislation and doctors should obtain up-to-date local information when assessing the legality of living wills.

Directives need to have been made when the patient was competent and not acting under duress (e.g. from family members). For an advance directive to be acted upon, the circumstances which have arisen need to be as envisaged by the patient when the directive was drafted. If, for example, a new treatment has been introduced since the drafting of the directive, then this may invalidate it. Advance directives cannot request treatment that is illegal, unethical or not clinically indicated.

Case 6: Advance directive

Mrs AR is 73 and was still working as a psychotherapist until she had a severe stroke; this caused a dense right hemiparesis and severe mixed expressive and receptive dysphasia; she also has dysphagia and is now tube fed. On her second day in hospital she went into cardiac failure that was eventually controlled with digoxin and diuretics. On the seventh day she had a pulmonary embolism for which she was anticoagulated. Venography showed extensive thrombosis in proximal veins in both legs.

Despite 2 months' rehabilitation in the stroke unit, she made little progress; when she was discharged to a nursing home she remained unable to use her arm or leg at all, required tube feeds and had severe expressive and receptive dysphasia.

At the nursing home her husband asked to see the medical officer; he produced an advance directive, which his wife had completed some years before, stating that she would not want life-prolonging treatment if she became severely dependent with little chance of recovery to independent living. He said that this was now the case and that all treatment, the drugs and the tube feed, should be withdrawn in accordance with her wishes.

Comment

Even though she is incompetent, the patient is expressing her autonomous opinion through the advance directive. Medical staff should ensure the validity of the directive and question any witnesses. They might also want to speak with other family members or her regular family doctor to determine her previously held views and the likelihood that she would complete such a directive. It seems strange that her husband did not produce the directive until after her acute treatment was over, and he should be asked about this.

If the document's validity is established, then it seems reasonable to at least withdraw anticoagulation, which is given specifically to prevent further pulmonary embolism. Withdrawal of heart failure drugs may not be sensible; they do not prolong life and further episodes of acute pulmonary oedema could make the patient severely distressed and breathless. The diuretics might almost be regarded as having a palliative role here. Likewise, tube feeding is regarded as a medical treatment in most jurisdictions, but withdrawal may lead to severe distress in a fully conscious patient. This should all be carefully documented, along with decisions about other potentially life-prolonging treatment (e.g. antibiotics).

Case 7: Advance directive/demand for treatment not clinically indicated

Mrs KS is 81 and has been a member of the Voluntary Euthanasia Society for the past 25 years. She completed an advance directive 5 years ago at the onset of her Alzheimer's disease. She is now very severely affected and is admitted to hospital when she develops pneumonia. Her son immediately produces her advance directive and, since it appears to be valid and in keeping with previously documented wishes, no active treatment is given. She deteriorates, but appears to staff to be comfortable. Her son insists that she is in pain and asks that she be given high-dose opiate analgesia. The staff are of the view that his intent is to hasten her death (i.e. active euthanasia). The doctors or nurses should explain their position to the son compassionately but frankly, and reassure him that all attempts will be made to ensure his mother will not be in pain, and that she will die with dignity.

Comment

Mrs KS is clearly exercising her autonomy through her advance directive and medical staff are obliged to follow her wishes by not giving active treatment for the pneumonia. However, there does not appear to be any rationale for opiate analgesia, other than to end her life. This is clearly something that she believes in. However, she cannot, either contemporaneously or in advance, insist on treatment which is illegal or involves doctors in doing something that is unethical.

Rationing health care by age

In the face of a limited health budget, it is essential to ensure that money is spent according to the principle of 'justice'. This means that it is necessary to ration some treatments for everyone (such as cosmetic surgery) or select which individuals would most benefit from other treatments. The decision about which individuals should benefit should be made on physiological/clinical grounds. It may be reasonable, for example, to withhold intensive treatment from an elderly patient with multiple organ failure on the basis that the treatment is medically futile. Older people are more likely to have multiple pathology and smaller physiological reserves, and will therefore more commonly be excluded from such treatment. However, people age at different rates, and using age as a surrogate marker for physiological frailty is little different to using hair colour or sex as a marker of educational achievement. Because elderly patients have a higher risk of illness, some treatments (e.g. for hypertension or atrial fibrillation) are actually of more benefit than the same treatment in a younger patient. In other areas (e.g. lowering cholesterol) there is little or no information on whether older patients benefit as much as a younger group since they are/have been excluded from clinical trials. Rationing should be explicit and defensible on the basis of medical facts; where it appears to be based on prejudice, ignorance or because it is an easy way of cost cutting, the physician should stand against it.

Case 8: Ageism

Mr K is a 74-year-old retired schoolteacher who is enjoying a physically and intellectually active retirement. He collapses with chest pain at a football match and is assessed in the casualty department. He is diagnosed as having an anterior myocardial infarction, and thrombolytic therapy is planned. When the treating doctor tries to obtain a bed for him in the CCU, she is told by the ward sister that the ward is full and that the protocol would not allow her to move a younger, day 3 post-infarction patient off the ward to make room for a 74-year-old.

Comment

The withholding of a beneficial treatment purely on the basis of age is unacceptable discrimination. The doctor should point out that the patient has as much to gain from the best level of care as a younger patient. She should explain that the younger day 3 patient is at significantly lower risk of complications and therefore has less to gain by staying in CCU. The doctor should insist that someone else be moved out of CCU to create room for her patient, and she should examine the admission protocol and ensure it is revised if there is a purely age based exclusion policy. (In the UK it is common in CCUs to move patients with an uncomplicated myocardial infarction to an 'ordinary' medical ward following the first 24–48 hours after thrombolysis when the risk of arrythmia is much lower.)

Case 9: Withdrawal of artificial nutrition

Mrs HC suffered a very disabling stroke during surgery for bowel obstruction due to adhesions. She was noticed to have a dense right hemiparesis and was unresponsive after the operation. A CT scan shows a large left middle cerebral artery infarct. After 10 days she is able to open her eyes but does not obey commands or interact with her visitors. She is unable to speak and cannot swallow. The surgical team is happy that her bowels are working normally and ask you if they should commence nasogastric feeding. The patient's husband is very upset and concerned that his wife doesn't 'end up as a vegetable'.

Comment

Artificial nutrition is regarded as a medical treatment rather than 'basic care' (which includes oral food and drink, hygiene, shelter and symptom control) and as such can theoretically be withheld or withdrawn in the same way as other treatment. However, feeding is a very emotive area and the legal position is not as clear as for most other medical treatment. Treatment should not be withheld, because it is easier to withhold than to withdraw it once it has been initiated. A trial of feeding over a pre-defined period of time will allow an assessment of what recovery, if any, is going to occur after the combined insult of stroke and the operation. Continual assessment of the relative risks and benefits of the artificial feeding should be made and the decision regularly reviewed. If the patient were to deteriorate and death was considered to be imminent, then artificial feeding would cease to benefit the patient and it could be withdrawn as part of palliative care. On the other hand, the patient may improve, in which case the benefit of feeding becomes obvious.

If the husband's worst fear is realised and the patient lives on with very poor conscious level and function, then a very difficult decision has to be made. This is an area of enormous ethical and legal uncertainty, but there is a responsible body of medical opinion that would support withdrawal of artificial nutrition from incompetent patients under certain circumstances. In the UK the courts have ruled that withdrawal of artificial nutrition from patients in a persistent vegetative state requires a court ruling but this is not the case for other, much more common, forms of severe brain damage, such as stroke or dementia. The doctor needs to consider if there is a net benefit for the patient, taking into account the burdens of treatment and the possibility of future improvement. The doctor will need to talk with the family and the nurses, and should determine if there is any evidence of what the patient's choice would have been. It would be wise to seek a second opinion from a senior colleague and document the discussions and decisions carefully. If there is conflict of opinion, treatment should be continued and legal advice sought.

Current legal situation in the UK and Australia

The United Kingdom

Contemporaneous decisions

The right of a competent adult to accept or refuse treatment has been established by case law. A patient who refuses treatment need not justify his choice; his decision doesn't have to be rational.

Advance decision making

An advance decision has the same legal weight as a contemporaneous one, providing the patient:

- is adult and mentally competent at the time the advance refusal was made
- knows the nature and consequences of the refusal
- intended the refusal to apply in the circumstances that subsequently arise
- has not revoked the advance refusal
- is now incompetent to make a decision.

The legality of advance decision making is through case law. So far the UK government has avoided legislating for advance decision making, although it proposes to legislate for a form of proxy decision making.

Decisions for incompetent patients

In England and Wales no one can legally make a decision about medical treatment for another adult, even when the patient is judged incompetent to make his own decisions. Relatives and even guardians appointed by the Guardianship Board have no right to make proxy decisions regarding medical matters. In these cases doctors are expected to make decisions in the 'best interest' of their incompetent patients. A new continuing power of attorney to cover medical and lifestyle decisions, as well as financial ones, has been proposed. In parallel with this, a court appointed manager could make welfare and healthcare decisions for an incompetent patient where one had not been previously nominated by a patient. This policy has not yet been heard in parliament.

In Scotland the law is slightly different and a tutor dative can be theoretically appointed by the Court of Session to make decisions for an incompetent person, although this has never been tested in court.

Euthanasia

Advance directives can be used to promote a form of passive euthanasia (not providing treatment that would prolong life and therefore allowing death to occur 'naturally'), which is legal. Active euthanasia (in which a person is assisted to commit suicide) is illegal, and doctors are liable to manslaughter charges in such cases.

Australia

Contemporaneous decisions

As in the UK, common law dictates that mentally competent adults have the right to consent to or refuse medical treatment throughout the continent. In three states (Victoria, South Australia and the Australian Capital Territory) there is also legislation to support contemporaneous medical decisions.

Decisions for incompetent patients/advance decision making

The law regarding advance decision making and decision making for incompetent patients varies between the five states and two territories of Australia (see Table 57.1). Western Australia is similar to the UK in having very little legislation, while many of the other states have legislation for some kind of written directive or appointment of a proxy decision maker. This is a rapidly changing area and many of these laws were passed in the last 5 years, with further changes planned in many states.

Euthanasia

In May 1995 the Northern Territory passed the *Rights of the Terminally Ill Act*, which allowed doctors to assist a terminally ill person to terminate his own life (voluntary active euthanasia). There was massive public outcry and, in March 1997, a private member's Bill in the Senate overturned the Northern Territory ruling and there is now no provision for legal assisted suicide anywhere in Australia.

Table 57.1 Summary of legislation regarding medical decision making for incompetent adults in the United Kingdom and Australia

Country/state		Written instructional directive about future medical treatment	Appointment of proxy decision maker	Provision for next of kin to make decisions when no official guardian available	State appointed guardian
UK	England	No legislation (valid under common law)	No	No	No
	Scotland	No	No	No	Yes, possibly a tutor dative. Not tested
Australia	New South Wales	No	Yes, 'enduring guardian'	Yes, 'responsible person'	Yes
	Western Australia	No	No	No	Yes
	South Australia	Yes but only for palliative care and persistent vegetative state	Yes, enduring guardian or medical power of attorney	No	Yes
	Tasmania	No but can make conditions on an enduring guardian	Yes, 'enduring guardian'	Yes 'person responsible'	Yes
	Australian Capital Territory	Yes but only for current medical condition. Oral statements also valid	Yes, enduring power of attorney	No	Yes
	Northern Territories	Yes but only for terminal illness	No	No	Yes
	Victoria	No. Refusal of treatment certificate for treatment of current condition only	Yes, enduring power of attorney for medical treatment	Yes 'person responsible'	Yes
	Queensland	Yes but only if patient terminally ill or unconscious. Standard form	Yes, enduring power of attorney for personal/health matters	Yes 'statutory health attorney'	Yes—from July 2000

Bibliography and further reading

(1999), 'Making decisions', The government's proposals for making decisions on behalf of mentally incapacitated adults, October, Cm 4465, http://www.open.gov.uk/lcd/family/mdecisions/indexfr.htm.

Benevolent Society of NSW and the Centre for Education and Research on Ageing (1999), *Taking Charge: Making Decisions for Later Life*, NSW Committee on Ageing, Sydney.

Biegler, P., Stewart, C., Savulescu, J. & Skene, L. (2000), 'Determining the validity of advance directives', *Medical Journal of Australia*, 172, pp. 545–8.

British Medical Association (1995a), *Advance Statements About Medical Treatment*, British Medical Journal Publishing Group, London.

British Medical Association (1995b), *Medical Ethics Today: Its Practice and Philosophy*, British Medical Journal Publishing Group, London.

British Medical Association (1999), *Withholding and Withdrawing Life-Prolonging Medical Treatment (Guidance for Decision Making)*, British Medical Journal Publishing Group, London.

Evans, J. G. (1997), 'The rationing debate; Rationing health care by age: the case against', *British Medical Journal*, 314, p. 822.

Gillon, R. (1995), *Philosophical Medical Ethics*, Whiley Medical Publication, London.

Molloy, D. W., Darzins, P. & Strang, D. (1999), *Capacity to Decide*, New Grange Press, Troy, Ontario.

Rai, G. S. (ed.) (1999), *Medical Ethics and the Elderly*, Harwood Academic Publishers, London.

The Royal Australasian College of Physicians (1992), *Ethics: A Manual for Consultant Physicians*, The Royal Australasian College of Physicians, Sydney

Chapter 58
Rehabilitation

PHILIP J. HENSCHKE and PAUL FINUCANE

Introduction

Definitions of the term rehabilitation abound. Dictionaries describe rehabilitation as 'acts by which a person is restored to a previous standing'. An examination of the derivation of the word provides associations with the reclothing of the penitent heretic or the reissue of uniforms to the disgraced soldier. For disabled people, their return to personally satisfying, normal or near normal living is the aim. To this end, an interdisciplinary approach is typically needed due to the multiple interventions required.

The World Health Organization (WHO) definition of rehabilitation is most often used:

> *As applied to disability, rehabilitation is the combined and coordinated use of medical, social, educational and vocational measures for the training and retraining of the individual to the highest possible level of functional ability.*

The WHO also refers to the concepts of impairment, disability and handicap. *Impairment* refers to the pathological defect in an organ or tissue. *Disability* arises when an impairment is sufficiently strategic and severe to affect a person's functional status. *Handicap* refers to the restriction of social role as a consequence of the disability. As a practical example, a person with rheumatoid arthritis (an impairment) may have major problems in coping with the activities of daily living (i.e. be disabled) and may therefore be unable to continue to pursue former activities and interests (i.e. be handicapped). Societal arrangements restricting access to resources and venues handicap individuals.

The relationship between impairment, disability and handicap is often complex. For example, some people may have several impairments without any residual disability or handicap. Similarly, disability and handicap can result from the sum effect of several different impairments. Thus, immobility (motor disability) may be due to a combination of osteoarthritis of the hips, Parkinson's disease and permanent neurological deficit following a stroke.

The philosophy and approach to rehabilitation in elderly people

The main stimuli to the development of rehabilitation medicine in Europe and in other countries were

World Wars I and II, which resulted in the return home of vast numbers of mutilated soldiers with ongoing disabilities. Early rehabilitation services were therefore developed to meet the needs of previously fit young men, whose care needs were principally met by therapists. Rehabilitation subsequently evolved to meet the changing population needs. In developed societies, disabling diseases are concentrated in the elderly population and typically in older women. Contemporary geriatric rehabilitation must confront the reality of dealing with disability in the context of multiple diseases in people with decreased physiological reserve and with social supports that are often tenuous. Health care systems are sometimes poorly adapted to meet the needs of such people. For example, hospitals are increasingly funded on their output, which creates an incentive to discharge older patients to the community before they have attained optimal levels of function. In other instances, premature and inappropriate referral for long-term residential care may be made as an expedient solution and to avoid a prolonged hospital stay. The economic and personal costs of overlooking opportunities for rehabilitation are high. The intern or geriatrician must often act as a patient advocate in such situations. The relevant points to consider are as follows:

- The number of disabling disorders affecting an individual tends to increase with age. For this and other reasons, acute illness in the older person is often associated with delayed recovery. Health care in this context requires a consideration of all co-existing disabling conditions and the need for rehabilitation before a successful return to previous accommodation can be anticipated.
- For elderly people, there is an increased likelihood of living alone, with limited support and in accommodation unsuited to their disabilities. The rehabilitation team must take account of these realities. A patient's performance in the security of the hospital ward may not be replicated at home. The ultimate outcome of rehabilitation is measured in terms of what the patient does and continues to do at home, and not what he does in hospital.
- Attitudes exist among health care workers that potentially threaten the independence of the older patient. The acute hospital, with its emphasis on bed-centred care, is often unsuited to the optimal recovery of the older patient. Ward policies and practices often encourage people to assume the role of an invalid. Bed-centred care, if prolonged, places the older person at risk of 'deconditioning', a term used to describe a loss of cardiorespiratory and/or neuromuscular fitness. Restorative care of the older patient has been termed 'the informed withdrawal of support'. This means that whenever possible, and as part of the rehabilitation process, people should be encouraged to undertake tasks themselves rather than to rely on others. Each self-care activity should, therefore, be viewed as a therapeutic opportunity.
- Attitudes exist among some older patients that may threaten their independence. Faced with the burden of illness and the losses that often accompany ageing, the enthusiasm of the older person to retrain and regain physical capacity is easily lost. Depression is common and needs to be countered by a realistic optimism in others.
- There needs to be a realisation that the human and economic cost of avoidable dependency in elderly people is high. This cost is also borne by the family and friends of people with disability and by society in general. In all countries and cultures, families and friends provide most aged care, and formal rehabilitation and support services primarily exist to sustain this commitment. In addition to providing community-based services, most societies have developed institutional or residential care to provide care and shelter for those with severe and continuing disability and without adequate family support.
- Those providing rehabilitation programs are sustained by the reality that strategies to reduce disability and handicap in older people are generally successful. Even a small change in performance often produces a significant reduction in handicap with attendant improvement in quality of life.

Steps in the rehabilitation process

The principles of rehabilitation and the steps in the process are broadly similar, irrespective of the specific rehabilitation problem with which one is dealing. The essential steps are listed in Box 58.1 and are described further. Although these steps are discussed in isolation and in sequence, in reality many of the steps overlap and need to be dealt with concurrently.

Box 58.1 Steps in the rehabilitation process

1. Stabilise the primary disorder.
2. Minimise the impact of co-morbidities.
3. Prevent disabling secondary events.
4. Treat the functional deficits.
5. Promote adaptation of the person to the disability.
6. Help adapt the environment.
7. Help carers adapt to the disabled person.

Stabilise the primary disorder

The first consideration should be to ensure that, whenever possible, the main impairment does not progress further. Thus, for the person who has had a stroke, strategies should be put in place to minimise the risk of extension of or another stroke. This should involve an accurate assessment of the impairment (e.g. nature and site of a stroke) as well as the identification and management of underlying risk factors.

Minimise the impact of co-morbidities

Co-morbid conditions can further contribute to the disability and handicap resulting from an impairment. For example, conditions that impair mobility, such as Parkinson's disease or osteoarthritis, can increase the immobility in a person who has had a stroke. Co-morbid conditions should be identified from the outset and appropriately managed. In this regard, it is crucially important to review the medications being prescribed and to ensure that these are not contributing to the impairment or disability.

Prevent disabling secondary events

The onset of impairment sometimes triggers a series of events that produce further disability and handicap. As an example, shoulder subluxation is a common complication of stroke, particularly when there is significant associated sensory inattention. A secondary event may cause more disability and handicap than the original impairment and is sometimes fatal (e.g. a pulmonary embolus in an immobile person following a stroke). There should be careful consideration of likely secondary events and implementation of strategies to prevent them.

Treat the functional deficits

This is perhaps the principal and best understood component of rehabilitation. It involves the assessment of mobility deficits, functional deficits in activities of daily living, speech and swallowing deficits, and psychological deficits. These tend to be addressed by physiotherapists, occupational therapists, speech pathologists and clinical psychologists respectively. A detailed description of their roles is beyond the scope of this chapter.

Promote adaptation of the person to the disability

For people whose disability and handicap cannot be fully reversed, the rehabilitation process needs to focus on helping them adapt to their disability. One strategy is the prescription of personal aids, such as mobility aids and aids that promote independence with activities of daily living. Care must be taken to ensure that such aids are prescribed appropriately as their inappropriate use can reinforce disability rather than reduce it. The promotion of psychological adaptation should not be forgotten.

Help adapt the environment

Environmental modifications might also be required. In the person's home, the provision of ramps can facilitate wheelchair access and rails can make walking easier and safer. Bathroom and kitchen aids promote independence with personal care. In many societies, much has been done in recent years to make the wider environment more accessible to people with mobility and other disabilities. However, in this regard much more needs to be done.

Help carers adapt to the disabled person

It is often as difficult for spouses, family and other carers to come to terms with the onset of disability and handicap. In attempting to adjust, a bereavement-type reaction is often observed with recognisable elements of denial, anger and depression before acceptance is finally reached. As part of a rehabilitation strategy, support and counselling should be offered to those in need.

Measuring function

As part of a consistent trend towards greater accountability in health care, the providers of rehabilitation are increasingly expected to measure what they are doing and thereby prove their effectiveness and efficiency. This has stimulated attempts to develop objective markers of disability and handicap, so that the literature on rehabilitation is now plagued by an oversupply of assessment scales. Among the scales in common use are:

- The Katz Activities of Daily Living (ADL) scale. This was first described in 1963 and was one of the first assessment scales. Its simplicity has ensured its survival and popularity. It rates six activities of daily living: bathing, dressing, toileting, transfers, continence and feeding. Functional status is graded from A (totally independent) to G (totally dependent). The scale has practical utility but is mainly a descriptive and not a quantitative instrument.
- The Barthel Index. This was first described in 1965 and is one of the best known and frequently used functional assessment scales. It rates 10 aspects of function, using different weights for each variable, with possible scores ranging from 0 (totally dependent) to 100 (totally independent). The original Barthel Index, as well as a number of subsequent modified versions, have been extensively studied, show high degrees of validity and reliability, are sensitive to changes in function over time, and are useful across a variety of diagnostic groups.
- The Functional Improvement Measure (FIM). This was developed by the American Association of Physical Medicine and Rehabilitation. The scale consists of 18 categories of function grouped under self-care, sphincter control, mobility, locomotion, communication and social cognition. Each item is scored on a scale ranging from 1 (dependent) to 7 (independent). The FIM incorporates components of the Barthel Index but is more sensitive and inclusive. However, it is more time-consuming to administer and this has limited its application in settings where patient throughput is high. It has become particularly popular in specialised rehabilitation settings (e.g. head injury and spinal injury rehabilitation units).
- Instrumental activities of daily living (IADL). These were described by Lawton and Brody in 1969 when they recognised the need for a secondary scale that included more complex activities which allowed people to live independently in the community. Such skills included shopping, cooking and competence with finances. IADL scales have emerged as more sensitive in detecting disability in older persons than simple self-care scales. The functions measured in IADL scales tend to be lost first and with milder levels of disability. A limitation of IADL scales is their influence by gender, cultural and environmental factors. A wide range of scales has been developed for particular groups and situations.

Use of outcome measures to fund rehabilitation programs

In recent years, attempts have been made in Australia and in other countries to fund clinical activity according to clinical output measures. The 'casemix' formula classifies patients into groups based on the principal medical disorder that requires treatment (so-called diagnosis-related groups, DRGs) and to fund health service providers according to the number of people treated in each DRG. A similar formula has been applied to residential care, using resource-utilisation groups (RUGs). However, such formulae do not accurately predict resource utilisation or cost in the inpatient rehabilitation setting. A formula that relies on functional status rather than on the nature of the impairment has been found to be a better predictor of length of hospital stay and resource utilisation in the context of rehabilitation. A new case-mix measure, unique to inpatient rehabilitation, is being developed that incorporates FIM data into function-related groups (FIM-FRGs). In the future, FIM-FRGs may provide a basis for prospective payment for inpatient rehabilitation, and facilitate inter-hospital comparisons of resource utilisation and patient outcomes.

Common disabling conditions in the older person

Hip fracture rehabilitation

The risk of hip fracture rises with age. Every year, 2–3 men per 1000 and 3–6 women per 1000 aged 65–74 years will fracture a hip. For those aged 85 and over the rates are notably higher, with 15–20 fractures per 1000 males and 25–40 per 1000 females per year.

Early initiatives in the rehabilitation of patients with hip fracture are summarised in Box 58.2. Physiotherapy should start on the first postoperative day with a careful assessment of hip movement. An active range of movement of the unaffected leg, of both ankles and of the upper limbs can begin, together with isometric exercises of the quadriceps and gluteal muscles of the affected leg. On day 2 post surgery, transfers and bed mobility are taught and assisted standing can occur subject to the approval of the orthopaedic surgical team. On day 3 after surgery, the patient starts to walk short distances with a frame, observing partial weight-bearing. Mobilisation should start with a standard walking frame (i.e. one without wheels).

Box 58.2 Early initiatives in hip fracture rehabilitation

- Prophylaxis to limit deep vein thromboses.
- Avoidance of pressure areas.
- Avoidance of constipation.
- Chest physiotherapy to decrease atelectasis and pneumonia.
- Removal of indwelling catheters within 48 hours.

During week 2 when the patient is near full weight-bearing, the use of a wheeled walker allows faster walking and an improved gait pattern. Later, a stick can be used, which should be held in the hand opposite to the fractured hip.

Weight-bearing

Surgical decisions in this matter are not standardised, being dependent on the type of fixation, bone quality, fracture location and the patient's cognitive and physical ability to comply with graded degrees of weight-bearing. The provision of adequate analgesia is an important consideration. Weight-bearing 'as tolerated' with a walking frame is the aim within the first week after effective fracture reduction and fixation. Where fixation is less secure or where severe osteoporosis exists, more gradual progression to full weight-bearing should occur over a more gradual period (e.g. 2 weeks).

Early precautions following hip fracture surgery

Femoral head replacement demands precautions if the risk of posterior hip dislocation is to be minimised. The key principles are as follows:

- Avoid hip flexion of more than 90 degrees (e.g. when performing chest examination). Reaching forward should be avoided when the person is transferring from a chair or bed edge. Toilet seats should be raised and low chairs should be avoided. Long-handled devices such as shoehorns, stocking aids for donning socks and long-handled washers for the feet should be provided when necessary. Prolonged sitting should be avoided.

- Patients should avoid leg adduction past the midline. To ensure this, a triangular pillow should be placed between the knees for the first 5 days. Rolling to the affected side should not exceed 45 degrees. Patients should not roll fully to the unaffected side, as the affected side will then be adducted by gravity.
- Combined movements such as flexion and internal rotation should also be avoided.

These precautions are usually continued for at least 6 weeks and for up to 3 months.

Later precautions following hip fracture surgery

The prevention of further falls is a crucial issue and many clinical services now operate Falls and Balance Clinics that specifically target people who have sustained a fracture. Exercise programs improve balance and co-ordination. They are effective in reducing falls, particularly when coupled with other falls reduction strategies that focus on both the fallers and on their environment. Those with a fractured hip have a substantially increased risk of a further lower limb fracture. In such people in particular, the use of psychotropic medications (e.g. sedatives, major tranquillisers, antidepressants) should be avoided whenever possible. Postural hypotension and falls are not closely linked but, where relevant, the need for the continued use of antihypertensive drugs should be reviewed. Additional preventative steps include strategies to improve vision, correct the use of inappropriate footwear and remove hazards from the home environment. Hip protectors have not been shown to reduce the risk of hip fracture among people living at home and in those who have already had one hip fracture.

Effective therapies now exist for osteoporosis and their use can reduce the risk of fractures. Such risk reductions vary from 5% over 3 years for calcium and vitamin D supplementation to 40% for more potent agents such as bisphosphonates. Where life expectancy exceeds 2–3 years, the use of such therapies should be considered. Unless contraindicated by the presence of co-morbid conditions (e.g. advanced dementia), all elderly patients with fractures other than those caused by major trauma should be screened for osteoporosis.

Stroke rehabilitation

Stroke is primarily a disease of old people and its incidence rises exponentially with age. Trends towards increased stroke incidence appear to have stabilised since the early 1990s, perhaps due to improved attention to risk factors. Ischaemia accounts for 70–80% of all strokes and most ischaemic strokes are caused by embolisation from atherosclerotic extracranial and intracranial arteries to distal cerebral vessels. In other cases, lacunar infarcts occur due to disease of small penetrating arteries in the brain, commonly in patients who smoke, or with hypertension or diabetes. Approximately 30% of ischaemic strokes occur as a result of cardiac emboli, particularly in association with atrial fibrillation, mitral valve disease, cardiomyopathy or endocarditis.

Although the efficacy of stroke rehabilitation has not been proven unequivocally, there is a strong and prevailing belief that rehabilitation improves functional ability and reduces the need for long-term residential care. Studies of stroke illness reveal a hospital mortality rate of about 15%, and of those who survive, some 50% are discharged home with the remainder requiring some form of supportive accommodation. Evidence is emerging that for people with lower levels of disability, home-based stroke rehabilitation can be delivered with reduced costs and improved patient satisfaction.

A major regional hospital with some 500 beds serving some 150 000 people can expect to treat about 300 stroke patients each year. Some 100 people are likely to require a formal rehabilitation program. On average, such patients will need 3–4 weeks of intensive inpatient rehabilitation before being able to return home. A 10-bed rehabilitation ward would be required for such stroke care.

Stroke rehabilitation should be regarded as part of a continuum of care rather than as a separate phase in the illness. Specific rehabilitation measures are required in the early phase of care and these will now be described.

Early stroke rehabilitation strategies

- If the conscious state permits, the risk of swallowing should be evaluated. A sip of water from a cup or spoon with the patient sitting upright and with the neck partially flexed (to protect the airway) is a safe and appropriate step before allowing the unsupervised intake of food and fluids. The outcome of such an assessment should be documented in the case notes.
- Aphasic patients are a particular rehabilitation challenge and the extent of the receptive ability in particular needs to be defined early.
- Condom or catheter drainage of urine should be instituted when incontinence persists for more than 48 hours or when there is immediate concern about skin integrity.
- Measures to avoid constipation should be instituted. These include promoting a good fluid intake, minimising the use of constipating agents and perhaps using an aperient.
- Prophylaxis against venous thromboembolism is advised when cerebral bleeding has been excluded through brain imaging.
- Correct positioning of a flaccid or weakened upper limb is important, particularly to protect the shoulder. If the muscles of the rotator cuff, which elevates the shoulder and holds the head of the humerus in the glenoid fossa, are paralysed and flaccid, the humerus will subluxate downwards, causing distension of the joint capsule and painful traumatic synovitis. When sitting, the arm needs to be supported on pillows, and when the patient is upright, treating staff should support the limb and shoulder. Traction on the shoulder joint must be avoided. Shoulder pain can occur despite proper handling and can affect patients such that their rehabilitation is compromised. Treatment methods are controversial and include slings, anti-inflammatory medication or intra-articular steroid injection.
- Correct posturing of a paralysed limb so as to promote 'antispastic' positions appears to limit the emergence of post-stroke spasticity (Figure 58.1). Over time, a spastic upper limb will tend to be flexed and adducted at the shoulder joint, and flexed at the elbow, wrist and hand. Supporting the outstretched upper limb on a pillow promotes abduction at the shoulder and extension at the other joints, which inhibits spasticity. A spastic lower limb tends to develop extension in the hip, knee and ankle. Having the person sitting 'normally' in a chair, the height of which is adjusted so that the foot is in contact with the floor, will keep the ankle, knee and hip in flexion and thus inhibit spasticity. A long mirror placed in front may help the patient correct his own position.

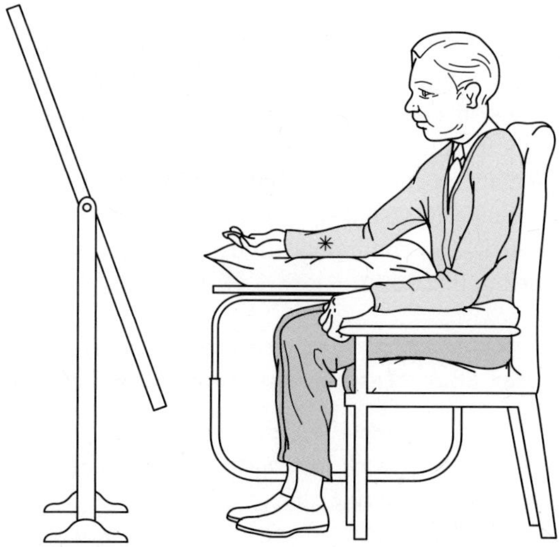

Figure 58.1 Correct posturing of a paretic upper limb assists in reducing spasticity

Assessment for rehabilitation

Rehabilitation requires interdisciplinary care and is therefore costly. Like intensive care and other highly specialised and costly treatment programs, the selection of people for rehabilitation needs to balance costs with the potential benefits. In estimating cost, non-monetary factors, such as the physical and emotional cost to the patient, should be considered. It is unfair to all concerned, and particularly to the patient, to admit a person to a rehabilitation program from which he cannot benefit. Of those appropriately admitted to a rehabilitation program, some 80% can expect to achieve independence in walking and 65–70% will become independent in activities of daily living. It is usually argued that appropriate patient selection for a designated stroke rehabilitation unit should aim to achieve a result wherein 85–90% of those selected for such inpatient rehabilitation return to their former accommodation.

As in other situations, assessment of stroke patients should consider the patient's physical, mental, functional and social status. Assessment for possible visual–spatial deficits is often overlooked. The commonly used techniques are outlined in Box 58.3.

Box 58.3 Tests of visual–spatial deficits

- Copy a simple stylised house.
- Draw a clock face and apply the hands to show a specific time (e.g. 3.40).
- Draw a face.
- Ask the patient to bisect a line drawn across the page.
- The examiner draws a series of 1 cm short lines randomly over an A4 page (20–30 lines). The patient is shown how to draw a similar line to bisect one of the examiner's strokes, thereby creating a cross. Ask the patient to cross off all the lines.

Factors predicting the prognosis following stroke

The prognosis concerning functional improvement is difficult to predict, especially in the first week or two following a stroke. However, older age, a history of prior stroke, urinary and faecal incontinence and visual–spatial deficits are recognised adverse prognostic factors. The impact of the severity of paralysis on the ultimate outcome is uncertain. However, severe dysphasia and reduced cardiorespiratory capacity can interfere with the ability to participate in and benefit from an intensive rehabilitation program, as can reduced mental capacity from dementia or psychiatric illness. Furthermore, the capacity for a highly motivated person to overcome even very major impairment should not be underestimated.

The final outcome in terms of returning home or moving to residential care is strongly influenced by psychosocial variables. The best predictors of nursing home placement or hospital readmission after stroke are the number of co-morbid chronic conditions, poor mental status and psychiatric co-morbidity. Although these observations are useful, ultimately the clinician is left with the difficult task of judging rehabilitation potential. Funding bodies increasingly require objective evidence of functional gain from rehabilitation. Those with uncertain rehabilitation potential should at least be offered a time-limited trial of rehabilitation.

Emotional problems after stroke

Emotional lability is common after stroke, particularly in those with bilateral vascular lesions. In many cases this is seen in the early weeks and lessens over time. In persistent cases, the use of selective serotonin reuptake inhibitors appears useful even in the absence of depressive features. Depression is commonly reported in stroke and is an expected reaction to such an illness. In this context, its prevalence has been consistently estimated at about 30%, a rate similar to that observed in other illnesses with comparable levels of disability. The decision to add antidepressant medication to supportive therapy should be based on the intensity and duration of the mood disorder and its negative impact on the patient's rehabilitation effort.

Poor impulse control and impatience are particularly seen in patients with frontal lobe involvement. In others, more subtle personality changes occur. The ability to interpret and appropriately respond to non-verbal facial communication can be lost and carers can interpret this as indifference. Sexual concerns do not often surface in the hectic atmosphere of a rehabilitation unit but should be raised for possible discussion at later reviews. The severity of the motor paralysis does not correlate well with alterations in sexual activity. It seems that stroke illness does reduce sexual activity, partly through changes in touch sensation but probably also through its effects on the respective roles of the partners. If the victim is perceived as a 'child-like' and dependent person, sexual activity may no longer be deemed appropriate. Inappropriate fears of possible stroke recurrence during sexual activity should be discussed.

Rheumatological rehabilitation

Surveys from the UK reveal that half of all adults aged 75 years or over have disability due to locomotor system disease. Osteoarthrosis (OA) is the most common arthritic joint disease and OA of the knees often causes considerable pain, loss of mobility and function. In this situation, rehabilitation aims to decrease pain, increase function, and reduce handicap and potential social isolation. Pain relief with simple analgesics ahead of scheduled activity is recommended and this should be interspersed with periods of rest. Physiotherapy of the affected knee consists principally of quadriceps strengthening exercises, performed at least daily to ensure that both strength and endurance are improved. For those who fail to respond to such conservative management, age alone should be no barrier to surgery. Prosthetic joints usually relieve pain dramatically and reduce dependency. With elective joint replacement, 'rehabilitation' begins in the presurgical period, with exercise programs that increase muscle strength and improve cardiorespiratory fitness.

In patients with rheumatoid arthritis (RA), specific therapeutic measures include initial rest, particularly for the inflamed joint. The use of exercise in inactive joint disease is increasingly emphasised. Some 30% of muscle bulk is lost in a week and muscle strength is lost at the rate of 5% per day when patients are subjected to strict bed rest. Exercise programs seek to increase joint stability and biomechanical function as well as promote physical endurance and overall functional ability.

Hydrotherapy is particularly useful in rheumatological rehabilitation. Water buoyancy reduces the effect of gravity and reduces joint compression and pain. Evidence exists that hydrotherapy improves patients' sense of self-efficacy or sense of mastery over their disease, as opposed to the concept of having the disease control or dominate them. Local heat application is also often recommended. While there is no evidence that this produces any long-term benefit, in the short term patients report reduced pain and improved range of motion. Recreational exercise should build on the benefits of physiotherapy. Patients without inflamed joints should be encouraged to walk and to participate in low-impact sports, such as swimming and dancing.

Amputee rehabilitation

People undergoing lower limb amputation have an average age of 70 years and some 25% are aged over 80. The vast majority have peripheral vascular disease and many will have associated cerebrovascular and cardiovascular disease. Some 30–50% have diabetes mellitus and many will have smoking-induced lung disease. While the loss of a limb is a major psychological blow at any age, for the elderly person it seriously threatens independent living. Successful rehabilitation outcomes are most likely to emerge when a single person, either a rehabilitation consultant, a geriatrician or a vascular surgeon, co-ordinate and assume responsibility for the program. This includes preoperative limb assessment, the postoperative period and the continuing care over the prosthetic phase.

Preoperative care

Referral should be made to physiotherapy, ideally some weeks in advance, to improve strength in the other limbs and to optimise mobility and functional status. Additionally, the physiotherapist can inform the patient and carers of the probable rehabilitation program and expected outcome. For example, the presence of joint contractures or arthritic changes may preclude prosthetic fitting. Nutritional supplements may be indicated in some cases.

Postoperative care

Following limb amputation, it is important that early physical therapy be directed at stabilising residual limb volume by decreasing oedema and thus promoting healing. This is achieved with rigid or soft dressings such as 'shrinkers' (i.e. fitted elasticised stump socks) together with elastic figure of 8 bandaging. The use of early walking aids (EWAs) greatly improves the rate of functional recovery. A typical program is shown below:

- Days 1–3: Bed exercises while sitting and lying aim to strengthen the arms, abdominal muscles, lower back and the remaining leg.

Balance training begins in the sitting position. Maintenance of joint mobility and the avoidance of contractures is promoted by a full range of knee and hip extension. The patient should avoid long periods of inert sitting. Prone lying for 20–30 minutes twice per day promotes optimum knee and hip extension.

- Days 4–6. Training in transfers from bed to chair is initiated. The patient is also trained in wheelchair mobility with a stump board or with an attachment to support the amputee stump. Balance and walking training with a walking frame is begun.
- Days 7–10. An EWA is introduced. The most commonly used device is a pneumatic post-amputation walking aid (Figure 58.2). The EWA is used initially twice daily for 10 minutes, increasing to 1 hour twice per day over the next 1–2 weeks. The stump is checked after each effort to detect any pressure problems or healing delay. Most patients who demonstrate walking capacity with an EWA quickly adapt to walking with a prosthesis.

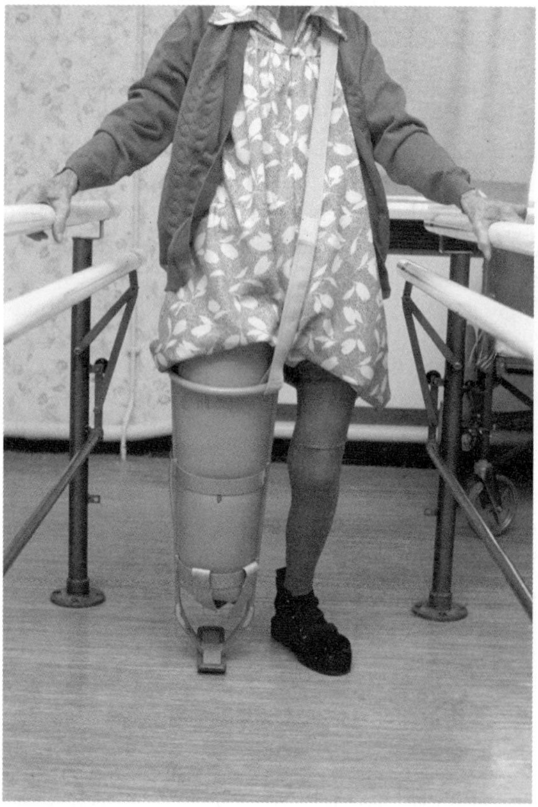

Figure 58.2 A pneumatic post-amputation walking aid

Prosthetic program

Fitting a prosthesis is almost always indicated, even in the presence of other limiting medical problems, as it facilitates transfers and standing and has added cosmetic value. It is sometimes argued that an older amputee should be able to walk with crutches before a prosthesis is offered. However, as walking with crutches involves far higher energy expenditure than walking on a below-knee prosthesis, this criterion is neither rational nor fair to the individual. Some older patients decline the offer of a prosthetic program and opt for wheelchair mobility, while others, given a prosthesis, fail to use it, particularly in the home setting. As always, any medical intervention should only be prescribed following consideration of the unique needs and wishes of each patient.

Limb-fitting typically begins about 3 weeks postoperatively for trans-tibial (i.e. below-knee) amputees. In some cases where healing is delayed and the stump shape is uncertain, a temporary limb pylon is employed. Prosthetic training focuses on stump care and bandaging, transferring, and if feasible, hopping with the use of an aid (i.e. crutches or a frame). The ability to hop is a useful skill when the patient needs to get up at night to toilet or while the prosthesis is being repaired. Walking on slopes and over rough ground and improving general balance and fitness complete the scope of prosthetic training.

Common postoperative and rehabilitation problems

- *Stump pain*. This is pain felt in the residual limb and may be due to ischaemia, infection, a neuroma or to a poorly fitting prosthesis. The underlying cause needs to be identified and managed.
- *Phantom sensations*. These occur in about 70% of amputees. Initially, they can be so deceptive that the patient may inadvertently attempt to walk or reach to scratch the missing limb. They often become more proximal (telescope) when people start to walk and may eventually disappear. Conventional management involves

explanation, desensitising the stump with massage, vibration, percussion and transcutaneous electrical nerve stimulation (TENS).

- *Phantom pain*. Pain felt in the missing limb is reported by 60–70% of amputees in the year after amputation and then diminishes with time. It may be continuous or intermittent. It can usually be differentiated from stump pain as it is localised in the amputated limb and is variously described as burning, crushing or lancinating. The limb may be perceived as twisted or deformed. The pathophysiology is unclear but current treatment approaches assume that it results from functional or structural changes in the central nervous system in response to noxious somatosensory input. Although early regional treatments (e.g. epidurals and nerve blocks) are widely believed to reduce the incidence of long-term phantom pain, this has not been conclusively demonstrated. Debilitating phantom pain persists in less than 1% of amputees. Sometimes a neuroma can be identified and removed surgically. Reliable and effective treatment is lacking for patients with phantom pain, particularly when pain persists beyond 6 months. Physical treatments such as desensitising massage and the use of TENS should be taught. Walking on a temporary prosthesis often reduces pain and psychological interventions (e.g. relaxation therapy, biofeedback) sometimes help. Drugs with membrane-stabilising properties drawn from anticonvulsant or tricyclic antidepressant categories (e.g. carbamazepine, amitryptyline) are sometimes effective to a variable degree. Such therapy is thought to operate by modifying pain transmission in the central nervous system. In resistant cases, psychiatric treatment incorporating techniques of self-hypnosis, distraction, conditioning and psychotherapy may be helpful. Many neurosurgical procedures have been advocated but none consistently give relief.
- *Other vascular problems*. Elderly amputees with peripheral vascular disease are a high-risk group, with some 50% dying within 3 years, generally as a result of vascular disease. The remaining limb is often critically ischaemic, such that 25% of non-diabetic amputees and over 50% of diabetic amputees require a second lower limb amputation within 5 years. The viability of the remaining leg can often be enhanced by surgery and by minimising risk factors for vascular disease (e.g. poor diabetic control, cigarette smoking, etc.). It is important that amputees receive advice on foot care and appropriate footwear to further reduce risks to the remaining limb.

Outcome of amputee rehabilitation

The functional outcome depends on the level of amputation, the pre-morbid health (particularly cardiovascular status), co-morbidities, psychosocial factors and the patient's motivation. The energy expenditure required for mobilising with an above-knee amputation is such as to place mobilisation beyond the capacity of most elderly patients, particularly if they are compromised by cardiorespiratory disease or advanced age. With appropriate rehabilitation and social support on discharge, the majority of elderly amputees return home to lead functionally useful lives. However, elderly amputees are a high risk group: 50% die within 3 years of amputation often due to ischaemic heart disease, cerebrovascular disease or malignancy. Of the survivors, 25% of non-diabetic amputees and over 50% of diabetic amputees will need another amputation within 5 years.

Rehabilitation in idiopathic Parkinson's disease

The judicious use of an expanding array of medication remains the cornerstone of management in Parkinson's disease. However, as the disease progresses, medication tends to have reducing efficacy. Timely referral to remedial therapy can do much to reduce attendant disability and prevent secondary morbidity.

Regrettably, many patients with the disease are not introduced to the skills available through outpatient rehabilitation departments. The physiotherapist can provide an exercise program that aims to increase strength, flexibility and endurance, and this should become part of a daily routine. The patient can be taught to consciously correct head and trunk flexion. Gait and balance training helps to prevent falls, as does advice on the best form of walking aid. Occupational therapists can inform patients about a range of assistive devices and adapted clothing. Speech therapy can help to improve speech volume and clarity.

Cardiac rehabilitation

As evidence for its efficacy, an overview of 22 randomised trials of exercise-based rehabilitation after myocardial infarction found a 20% reduction in overall mortality at 3 years. Elderly people were once excluded from cardiac rehabilitation on the false assumption that the associated risks were high and that the potential benefits were low. Such attitudes are now changing, due at least in part to the recognition that both in-hospital mortality and later death from myocardial infarction is twice as high in older people than in the young. Submaximal exercise testing before hospital discharge is now more freely available and can reassure older patients of their ability to exercise safely. Function, related to symptom severity in heart failure, is typically classified by means of the New York Heart Association system. In this system, class 1 patients become dyspnoeic with heavy exertion, those in class 2 develop symptoms with above average or moderate effort, those in class 3 have symptoms on mild exertion, and those in class 4 are limited by symptoms at rest. Evidence has emerged that patients with stable class 2 and 3 heart failure can safely improve exercise tolerance, attenuate an overactive sympathetic nervous system, partially reverse skeletal muscle abnormalities and enhance health-related quality of life. The principles of cardiac rehabilitation are the same for all age groups:

- Early mobilisation.
- Participation in exercise programs. Most elderly patients can benefit from relatively informal exercise programs. Beneficial outcomes are seen with moderate doses of physical activity, such as 30–60 minutes of walking or cycling on 3–5 days per week at an intensity of 60–70% of peak oxygen consumption. Patients with unstable angina, valvular stenosis or with a history of cardiac arrhythmia are most at risk of adverse exercise-induced cardiac events. A cardiological opinion and regular review is indicated for such patients.
- Psychological support.
- Education, including secondary prevention. Most of the success in preventing recurrent cardiac illness in elderly patients resides in investing time and energy in ensuring that they or their carers understand the medication, its rationale and dosing. In all but rare instances, medication can be simplified to a once-daily regimen. Written instructions on matters such as diet, activities and follow-up arrangements are markers of quality care. Monitoring of weight in the patient with congestive heart failure is a further preventative measure. In the latter setting, when patients are discharged from hospital they should be told to weigh themselves daily on their usual scales. They should be given limits to weight gain and loss. When they exceed these limits, advice on increasing or decreasing diuretic doses can be followed. Failure to maintain weight within the agreed limits is an indication for medical review.

Respiratory rehabilitation

Chronic obstructive pulmonary disease (COPD) leads to increased dyspnoea, reduced activity, secondary deconditioning and social isolation. Respiratory rehabilitation can interrupt a vicious cycle of further inactivity and deconditioning. An interdisciplinary team approach to respiratory rehabilitation has been shown to be beneficial in improving both health-related quality of life and exercise capacity. Evidence of feasibility in older persons, even in cases of severe COPD, has emerged. Anxiety, depression and feelings of alienation, rather than symptoms of dyspnoea and fatigue, emerged as important reasons for withdrawal from such programs.

Meta-analysis strongly supports the view that respiratory rehabilitation (with at least 4 weeks of exercise training) is capable of producing greater improvements in health-related quality of life and functional exercise capacity than other important components of care, such as bronchodilator therapy. The elements of pulmonary rehabilitation can be classified as 'initial', 'interventional' or 'follow-up' as indicated in Table 58.1.

Table 58.1 Elements of respiratory rehabilitation

Initial measures	Interventional measures	Follow-up measures
Assessment of the nature and severity of lung disease, co-morbidities, nutritional and immunisation status (i.e. against pneumococcus and influenza)	Optimise medical management	Identify benefits achieved through the program
Assessment of lifestyle factors contributing to disability and handicap	Exercise program	Establish possible need for a repeat program
Exercise testing with blood gas analysis/ oximetry and ECG monitoring	Breathing exercises	Patient education Lifestyle and dietary advice Psychosocial support

Community-based care rehabilitation alternatives

The last decade has seen a trend towards providing community-based alternatives to inpatient rehabilitation. Such initiatives appear largely driven by economic pressures and rehabilitation programs involving relatively long lengths of hospital stay (e.g. following stroke and fractured neck of femur) have been particular targets for trials of home-based rehabilitation. Attempts to transfer rehabilitation from the hospital to the community have theoretical advantages. Hospitals are potentially dangerous places, particularly for surgical patients exposed to antibiotic-resistant pathogens. Furthermore, elderly people are more prone to falls and confusion when placed in unfamiliar surroundings. To date, there is no clear proof that community-based rehabilitation services are cost-effective. Savings in hospital accommodation costs need to be considered alongside reduced contact time with key health professionals and an increased burden on carers. In time, it may emerge that selected patients recovering from a stroke or a lower limb fracture can be efficiently rehabilitated at home provided that their social supports are adequate.

In this setting, it will be important to develop strategies to address quality assurance and professional liability issues. Much remains to be done in educating and otherwise supporting family physicians and other community-based professionals in dealing with disabled elderly people at home. While aids and appliances are increasingly available, significant numbers of elderly persons, even in affluent societies, lack basic and low-cost items, such as safety railing in bathing areas and chair raises (including raised toilet seating).

The field of rehabilitation medicine continues to evolve in response to new challenges, new technologies and new therapeutic strategies. While some of today's dogma will undoubtedly be challenged and superseded at some future time, the successful implementation of the principles described in this chapter will undoubtedly free many impaired elderly people from unnecessary disability and handicap.

Bibliography and further reading

Afzal, A., Brawner, C. A. & Keteyian, S. J. (1998), 'Exercise training in heart failure', *Progress in Cardiovascular Diseases*, 41, pp. 175–90.

Barer, D. (1993), 'Assessment in rehabilitation', *Reviews in Clinical Gerontology*, 3, pp. 169–86.

Brandstater, M. E. (1990), 'An overview of stroke rehabilitation', *Stroke*, 21(suppl. II), pp. 40–2.

Ethans, K. & Powell, C. (1996), 'Rehabilitation of patients with hip fracture', *Reviews in Clinical Gerontology*, 6, pp. 371–88.

Jongbloed, L. (1986), 'Prediction of function after stroke: a critical review', *Stroke*, 17, pp. 765–6.

Lacasse, Y., Goldstein, R. S. & Guyatt, G. H. (1997), 'Respiratory rehabilitation in chronic obstructive pulmonary disease: summary of a systematic overview of the literature', *Reviews in Clinical Gerontology*, 7, pp. 327–47.

Lafferty, G. (1996), 'Community-based alternatives to hospital rehabilitation services: a review of the evidence and suggestions for approaching future evaluations', *Reviews in Clinical Gerontology*, 6, pp. 183–94.

Mulley, G. P. (ed.) (1986), 'Provision of aids', in *Everyday Aids and Appliances*, British Medical Journal Publications, London.

O'Connor, G. T., Buring, J. E., Yusuf, S., et al. (1989), 'An overview of randomized trials of rehabilitation with exercise after myocardial infarction', *Circulation*, 880, pp. 234–44.

Parker, M. J. (2000), 'Managing an elderly patient with a fractured femur', *British Medical Journal*, 320, pp. 102–3.

Roy, C. W. (1988), 'Shoulder pain in hemiplegia: a literature review', *Clinical Rehabilitation*, 2, pp. 35–44.

Stewart, C. P. U. & Condie, M. E. (1996), 'Amputee rehabilitation', *Reviews in Clinical Gerontology*, 6, pp. 273–83.

Wade, D. T. (1998), 'A framework for considering rehabilitation interventions', *Clinical Rehabilitation*, 12, pp. 368–86.

Ward, G., Jagger, C. & Harper, W. (1998), 'A review of instrumental ADL assessments for use with elderly people', *Reviews in Clinical Gerontology*, 8, pp. 65–71.

Wasti, S. A. & Chamberlain, M. A. (1996), 'Rheumatological rehabilitation of older adults', *Reviews in Clinical Gerontology*, 6, pp. 255–71.

World Health Organization (1980), *International Classification of Impairment, Disability and Handicap*, WHO, Geneva.

Chapter 59

Abuse and neglect: Identification, screening and intervention

DAPHNE M. NAHMIASH IN COLLABORATION with SUSAN KURRLE

Introduction

This chapter addresses the phenomenon of violence against dependent older adults who live in the community and are being cared for by a family member, friend or neighbour. It is hard for us to imagine that such violence exists and, in fact, has always existed. As a society, we are becoming more and more aware of domestic violence, and violence against older adults is yet another manifestation of this. It is particularly important for doctors and other health care professionals to be aware of the signs and symptoms of such violence. They are the best placed professionals to detect the presence of such a problem and thus enable patients to get the help they need. Even though some cases of abuse and neglect are perpetrated by paid caregivers in institutional milieux, most older adults are abused by an unpaid caregiver living in the community. Therefore this chapter focuses only on community based abuse.

We begin by explaining the prevalence of the problem. Next, we address definitions and the difficulties in arriving at a common terminology. A brief discussion on the probable causes follows. We then present the main risk factors that have been identified in the research. Some discussion of tools for identifying suspected victims and suspected abusers is presented, along with an example of one screening tool. A discussion of how to approach persons who are identified and screened follows, and the barriers to reporting abuse and neglect are listed. Finally, an approach to empowering abused or neglected victims is outlined, with examples of interventions.

Prevalence

Why are we talking about violence towards older adults right now? Is the phenomenon more prevalent than it was? It is important to note that violence against older adults is not a new phenomenon. In fact, a recent study from Greece notes that 'ancient Greek history reveals clear cases of selfish carelessness or coarse insolence toward the old and offers instances of children taking over their parents' property...without proof of incapacity in the elders'.

In spite of that, abuse and neglect of older adults has only come to the attention of researchers and practitioners in the past 3 decades. Estimates in

Canada note that approximately 1 in 25 older persons (over the age of 65) are victims of abuse and neglect. Similar estimates have been made for the US. In the past few years, more and more countries have been identifying the problem and finding ways to bring it to public attention. A British study observed that work on abuse of older adults has been reported in 22 European countries, even though much of the work is still in the formative stages. Compiled research from 10 countries in different parts of the world from international and cross-cultural perspectives concludes that the problem will probably augment as a major world social problem as populations age and the number and proportion of older adults increase, especially the oldest of the old.

However, few studies have actually measured the incidence or prevalence of the phenomenon. Of those studies that have attempted to measure the problem, the descriptions vary according to the methodology used. For example, it is difficult to distinguish in the studies between the incidence of cases and the prevalence. North American studies, however, do seem to agree that between 3% and 5% of persons over the age of 65 years are victims of abuse and/or neglect. In the US alone, this represents over 1 million persons. Thus, abuse of older adults is a serious social problem and practitioners should be aware of its existence in order to identify, treat and prevent it. Authors have also noted in all studies that the phenomenon of abuse and neglect is extremely taboo among the older population and rarely reported. Furthermore, since most cases are hidden and difficult to find, the reported estimates of 3–5% are probably underestimates. For this reason it is extremely important that doctors and health care professionals become familiar with the signs and symptoms of suspected abuse.

Definitions of abuse and neglect

Definitions of abuse and neglect are problematic. There are no agreed upon intrinsic or extrinsic definitions, or standardised conceptualisations of the phenomenon as yet, although several authors have attempted this. Definitions are nevertheless important for giving a clear understanding of the problem in question and differentiating that area of concern from others. One of the main reasons why definitions differ is that their meanings are interpreted differently by each researcher; definitions also depend upon the purpose of the study. Some people use the word 'mistreatment' and others use the term 'abuse and neglect'. Stones (1991) offers the following general definition of abuse: 'a misdemeanor against acknowledged standards by someone a senior has reason to trust'. The most systematically developed Canadian framework for abuse and neglect consists of the definitions in the EAST tool, which contains 71 items grouped into the following 9 categories: physical assault, excessive restraint, putting health at risk, failure to give care by someone acting as a paid or unpaid caretaker under pressure, undue pressure, humiliating behaviour, abuse in an institution, material exploitation and verbal humiliation. Stones found high agreement among seniors and professionals on items that indicate greater or lesser abuse, and the items rated as most abusive were mainly examples of physical abuse. However, most researchers have opted to use the following definitions to operationalise the types of abuse and neglect encountered.

- *Physical abuse* includes hitting, burning, assault, rough handling, etc.
- *Sexual abuse* includes any form of assault of the person in a sexual way or forcing him to perform or engage in any sexual activity against his wishes. Sexual abuse is often part of physical abuse. However, practitioners frequently do not identify it as a form of abuse and therefore it should be kept as a separate category.
- *Psychological abuse* is where the older person is subject to repeated or chronic verbal assault which insults, threatens, humiliates or excludes. Lack of affection, betrayal, social isolation or denying the person the chance to make or participate in decisions which are in his own interests are included.
- *Material/financial abuse* involves misuse of the person's money, possessions or property. It includes fraud or using the older adult's funds for purposes contrary to his needs and interests.

This type of abuse has been noted as the most common among older adults.

- *Passive or active neglect* involves the withholding of items or care necessary for daily living and can be intentional (active or physical) or non-intentional (passive).
- *Self-neglect* has also been identified as a form of abuse. It is where a person fails to provide adequate care for himself. This form of abuse is different from the others in that there is no abuser involved. However, relatives or others may be aware of the problem and fail to help.
- *Violation of a person's rights* has also been recognised as a form of abuse. This consists of forcing a person to do something against his wishes or preventing him from making his own decisions, such as forcing him to go to a nursing home. Other authors include this in the psychological abuse category.
- *Social, systemic or collective abuse* has been identified as a societal form of abuse. It includes ageism and other ways of treating elderly persons that affect their personal dignity and identity. This type of abuse was highlighted in a British study, which pointed out that abuse and neglect are socially structured through a range of policies and professional ideologies relating to dependency in old age. Some authors include this type of abuse and neglect in a category termed 'psychosocial abuse'.
- *Carer abuse* is abuse which is perpetrated by the care receiver towards the caregiver. It is usually reported to be among caregivers who are taking care of a person suffering from dementia and was reported by one study to represent about 3% of the overall abuse.

Finally, it is important to note that few studies have observed how multicultural or Aboriginal groups define abuse and neglect. Most studies ignore the cultural aspects and seem to assume that all older adults are similar in their attitudes and perceptions. Thus work in this area should pay attention to these aspects as each society and group has different standards and norms as to what constitutes abusive and neglectful behaviour. Some standards and norms are laid down in the criminal code or the charter of rights, others are laid down by organisations and in professional codes of ethics, but those presenting most difficulty are usually defined by common consensus of the society or group. Psychological abuse and some types of neglect or self-neglect tend to fall mainly into this latter category. For this reason it is a good idea to discuss the definitions with other multidisciplinary team members to try to arrive at common meanings for the definitions used. It is important to note that often several types of abuse and/or neglect are present and there is sometimes more than one abuser. Occasionally, abuse is mutually perpetrated by the older adults and the caregivers, especially in cases in which there is mental illness or dementia.

Identification of abuse and neglect in older adults

A brief screening tool named the CASE (Caregiver Abuse Screen) was created in Project CARE to identify suspected abusive caregivers. It was found to discriminate them from non-abusive caregivers more effectively than a screening tool used to discriminate abused older adults from non-abused older adults. The tool can be administered in 2–3 minutes and merely consists of asking all caregivers 8 questions at the end of the assessment interview (see Box 59.1).

The CASE can also be used over the telephone when the caregiver is not available for an interview. To score the CASE the responses are tallied: the more 'Yes' responses, the more likely the presence of abuse and/or neglect. The mean 'Yes' score for a group of abuser caregivers in Project CARE was 3.3, and the median score was 4. Each 'Yes' response should be probed for clinical information. The physician should ask the caregiver to explain her answer and try to assess the specific situation.

The screen contains items relating to the main categories of abuse and neglect, and it also correlates with other abuse scales. No specific question refers to financial abuse in the CASE, as the question originally included was not found to be significant. However, financial dependency is an indicator in the Indicator of Abuse (IOA) tool

Box 59.1 The Caregiver Abuse Screen (CASE)

Please answer the following questions as a helper or caregiver:

	Yes	No
1. Do you sometimes have trouble making (______) control his/her temper or aggression?	☐	☐
2. Do you often feel you are being forced to act out of character or do things you feel bad about?	☐	☐
3. Do you find it difficult to manage (______'s) behaviour?	☐	☐
4. Do you sometimes feel that you are forced to be rough with (______)?	☐	☐
5. Do you sometimes feel you can't do what is really necessary or what should be done for (______)?	☐	☐
6. Do you often feel you have to reject or ignore (______)?	☐	☐
7. Do you often feel so tired and exhausted that you cannot meet (______'s) needs?	☐	☐
8. Do you often feel you have to yell at (______)?	☐	☐

presented subsequently in this chapter, both for the caregiver and the care receiver.

Even when abuse and neglect are discovered, the older adult and/or the caregiver are usually reluctant to acknowledge the mistreatment, and the situation has to be handled very delicately. This is even more pertinent in the case of an adult who is deemed competent to make his own decisions. Sometimes the suspicion of abuse may only emerge over time. The physician must also try to gather as much information as possible from the older adult, family members, friends and others to confirm the evidence of mistreatment. All evidence must be carefully documented and accumulated. Other service providers, if available, should also be consulted. The older adult may be afraid to acknowledge the abuse through fear of retaliation by the abuser or through fear of losing the relationship with the caregiver abuser. Parent/child relationships which are abusive are particularly difficult for the parent to acknowledge on account of feelings of guilt, such as: 'I was a bad mother', 'It's my fault', 'I don't want my son to go to prison', 'I'd like to give him one last chance', etc. However, the doctor–patient relationship is the ideal setting in which to encourage the patient and/or caregiver to break the silence and acknowledge the abusive behaviour.

In cases where the abused older adult is found not to be competent because of dementia or another mental health condition and the family caregiver is suspected to be the abuser, the situation is particularly difficult to deal with. It is important to attempt to find another family member, neighbour, friend or other person who may have witnessed the abusive behaviour and who can help in the intervention plan. However, in Project CARE we were surprised to find the caregiver abuser was often willing to admit the abusive behaviour with all kinds of justifications, such as: 'I did it because I was at the end of my rope' or 'because of her behaviour' or 'I did it because she wouldn't eat' (as in the case of a husband who forced a spoon into his wife's mouth).

Causes of abuse and neglect of older adults

Several causes have been attributed to abuse and neglect of older adults. The explanations are complex and vary according to the theoretical perspective of the researchers or professionals. The major causes are reported to fall into the following broad categories:

- *The situational model* suggests that mistreatment is an irrational response to environmental conditions and situational life crises. The model is said to have its roots in the child abuse and intrafamily violence literature. The situational variables include caregiver related factors, elder related factors and sociostructural factors. Caregiver related factors may stem from transgenerational or learnt violence, personality traits, web of dependencies, filial crises and internal stress. Elder related factors tend to stem primarily from a web of dependencies, although they may also result from transgenerational violence or internal stress. Sociostructural factors may include external stressors and societal attitudes towards the elderly. This model is the most widely used perspective by professionals and researchers. It emphasises present social conditions rather than past problems. However, the model does not account for the fact that individuals experience similar situations and similar environmental crises but respond differently. In addition, it has been observed that environmental factors alone cannot explain elder abuse although they may contribute to it.
- *Social exchange theory* posits that as older people age they have less access to power, fewer resources and are progressively less able to perform instrumental tasks. As ageing progresses, the imbalance grows and the elderly generally become more powerless, dependent and vulnerable than their caregivers. However, research has observed that dependency sometimes operates in the other direction in abuse cases and abusive caregivers are often dependent on the abused older adult: for example, a son who is a substance abuser may depend upon his mother for financial assistance.
- *Symbolic interaction* is a little used theory that describes a process between at least two individuals who are in constant interaction with one another. The relationship occurs over time and there are identifiable phases that recur and interrelate and require constant negotiation and renegotiation. In this model, mistreatment is seen as a recurring phenomenon in a family and is related to the family's history of violent relationships. This theory has been challenged, as not all types of abuse and neglect fit with the model.
- *An empowerment perspective* based on systems theory has also been used to explain how abuse and neglect occurs. This seems to be the approach favoured by most practitioners since it relates to intervention in addition to explaining what factors contribute to the violent situation. Empowerment is described as an outcome and a process. According to this perspective, an abused person and the abusive caregiver are described as being in a process of powerlessness defined as 'a continuous interaction between the abused person, the abuser caregiver and their environment and results in an inability to act or move out of the situation and an inability to manage emotions, skills, knowledge and/or material resources'. The powerlessness is caused by a number of interacting indicators related to the abused person, the abuser and the cultural, economic and social context. These indicators will be identified in the next section. Not all the indicators interact in every situation, but in each situation of abuse and neglect we can identify some interacting indicators which are present and contribute to the abuse.

Empowerment is described as the process that 'helps people assure or claim control over their destinies, which entails maximising their confidence, skills and abilities and making informed decisions that are in their best interests, having access to choices and available, accessible resources and options...for the attainment of both personal and collective goals'. Abused persons move out of the process of powerlessness to empowerment with the assistance of a facilitator (health professional).

As we have already mentioned, few studies have validated these approaches to explain the causes of abuse and neglect. The choice for this chapter is the empowerment perspective. It was used in two studies, Project CARE and Powerlessness and Abuse, because of its relevance to all types of abuse and neglect of older adults, and also its relevance to intervention.

Indicators of abuse and neglect

Indicators are important for predicting which older adults are likely to be abused and which caregivers are likely to become abusive. This section will mainly alert doctors and health professionals to the main indicators which have been found to be present in the abused older adult, the abuser and the context. We will subsequently suggest a tool which may be useful for doctors and health professionals for screening clinically those who are suspected victims of abuse, and for screening out the caregivers likely to be abusers. The role of the family physician in the identification and management of elder abuse has been recognised as an important one. The following indicators will help the physician know who is at risk of abuse or behaving abusively.

The abused

Ten indicators have been identified as being present in abused older adults:

1. gender (most are women, although some studies have found more men)
2. marital status (most are widows or spouses)
3. poor health (physical or mental)
4. advanced age
5. substance abuse
6. living arrangements (the abuser often lives with or close to the older adult)
7. psychological factors (depression or resignation)
8. presence of problem behaviour
9. dependence (e.g. regarding activities of daily living)
10. social isolation.

The abuser

Ten indicators have been identified as being present in abusers of older adults. These are:

1. substance abuse (mainly alcohol)
2. emotional illness (depression especially has been found to be present in caregiver abusers)
3. caregiving inexperience
4. caregiving reluctance
5. history of abuse
6. dependency (often financial) on the care recipient
7. confusion and dementia
8. burden and stress of caregiving
9. personality traits (related to control, depression, blame, being overly critical and unsympathetic)
10. lack of social support.

The social context

Six indicators have been observed to be related to the social context of the care situation:

1. financial problems (from unemployment)
2. family violence (especially related to physical and psychological abuse)
3. lack of social support
4. family disharmony
5. living arrangements (lack of privacy, overcrowding, substandard housing conditions)
6. intergenerational transmission of violence.

The cultural context of care

Attitudes, beliefs and values can also influence individuals to engage in, or deter them from engaging in, the abuse and neglect of older adults. Six such indicators have been identified in the literature:

1. ageism
2. sexism
3. cultural beliefs and attitudes about violence (abuse is often perceived as 'a family affair')
4. reactions towards abuse (personal beliefs due to religious convictions, family or cultural backgrounds may influence help-seeking patterns)
5. negative attitudes towards the disabled and imperatives for family caregiving (expectations about obligations to give care).

The economic context of care

Four indicators that influence the abuse situation have been observed:

1. poverty
2. limited finances

3. lack of informal resources (other family members who could help)
4. a lack of formal resources.

Having noted these indicators, we have also observed that 6 indicators have occurred more frequently in the overall abuse studies:

1. dependency of care recipient and caregiver (often in a co-dependent relationship)
2. gender (often female victims and male or female abusers)
3. social isolation/lack of family support (of the care recipient and the caregiver)
4. substance abuse of the caregiver
5. depression of the caregiver
6. living arrangements that are shared between caregiver and care recipient or in close proximity to one another.

Figure 59.1 presents all the indicators listed above; those in bold note the 6 most frequent ones associated with abuse of older adults.

The studies also note that chronic verbal aggression is more common among spouses, both male and female, and that physical abuse, although affecting more males than females, is more violent towards females.

Also according to the studies, in older adults with Alzheimer's disease the risk for abuse increased with caregiver depression, poor self-esteem, shared living arrangements and presence of spousal violence.

Tools for identifying abused older adults and their abusers

The paucity of case controlled studies has limited the development of effective screening tools for abused older adults, as it is not clear which markers must be screened. In a systematic overview of assessment and screening tools for elder abuse, only 6 tools demonstrated evidence of reliability and/or validity. Project CARE, a large study done in Montreal, Canada, is one of the 6 studies that validated

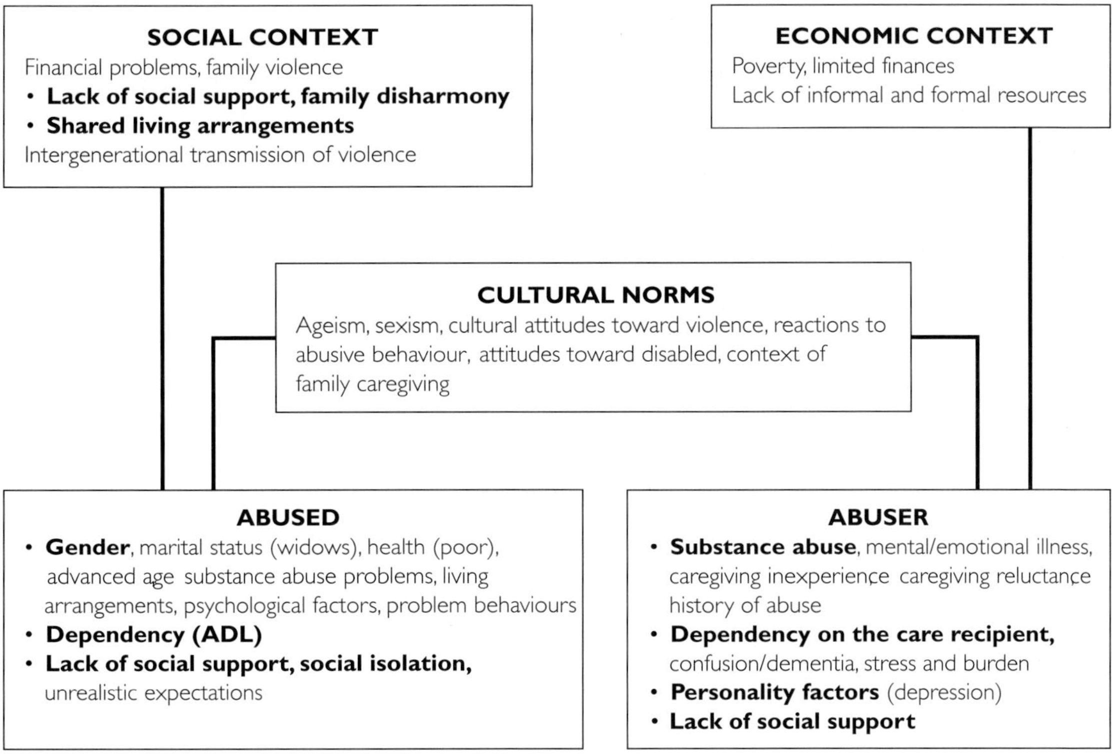

Figure 59.1 Interacting indicators present in abused, abusers and the context

the checklist of indicators, based on the list above, found in the research. Subsequently, the study developed a clinical tool named the IOA (Indicators of Abuse) (Box 59.2), based on those indicators which were found to be most significant in identifying abused older adults and their caregiver abusers, in order to signal mistreatment of seniors as well as suspected caregiver abusers.

It is not difficult to use the IOA screen and it only takes a few minutes to complete. The physician or practitioner, as part of her regular assessment with the older adult and the caregiver, rates each of the 27 indicators on a scale of 0–4 (as described on the tool) according to her current opinion. In the Project CARE study, caregiver items were found to be more important than care receiver items. The total overall score is a maximum of 88 points, and for caregivers and care receivers in Project CARE, a mean score of 16 or over denoted abuse situations, whereas a score of 4 or less denoted non-abuse situations. Although problems could be present, each of the indicators denotes a specific problem and those that are rated as moderate or severe should be followed up with appropriate referrals or interventions. For example, substance abuse is one of the most important indicators of abuse and neglect of older adults, and if this is noted to be a problem, the caregiver would be referred to Alcoholics

Box 59.2 The Indicators of Abuse (IOA) screen

Indicators of abuse are listed below, numbered in order of importance.[a] After a 2–3 hour home assessment (or other intensive assessment), please rate each of the following items on a scale of 0 to 4. Do not omit any items. Rate according to your *current opinion*.

Scale: Estimated extent of problem:

0 = non-existent
1 = slight
2 = moderate
3 = probably/severe
4 = yes/severe

00 = not-applicable
000 = don't know

Caregiver age: ______ years
Caregiver and care receiver kinship: ______ non-spouse
______ spouse

Caregiver

______ 1. Has behaviour problems
______ 2. Is financially dependent
______ 3. Has mental/emotional difficulties
______ 6. Has alcohol/medication problem
______ 7. Has unrealistic expectations
______ 9. Lacks understanding of medical condition
______ 10. Caregiving reluctancy
______ 12. Has marital/family conflict
______ 13. Has poor current relationship
______ 14. Caregiving inexperience
______ 17. Is a blamer
______ 24. Had poor past relationship

Care receiver

______ 4. Has been abused in the past
______ 5. Has marital/family conflict
______ 8. Lacks understanding of medical condition
______ 11. Is socially isolated
______ 15. Lacks social support
______ 16. Has behaviour problems
______ 18. Is financially dependent
______ 19. Has unrealistic expectations
______ 20. Has alcohol/medication problem
______ 21. Has poor current relationship
______ 22. Has suspicious falls/injuries
______ 23. Has mental/emotional difficulties
______ 25. Is a blamer
______ 26. Is emotionally dependent
______ 27. Has no regular doctor

(*a*) The majority of the most important indicators are the caregiver ones.

Anonymous or an appropriate treatment centre or program. An example of caregiver problem behaviour could be a spouse who does not understand why his wife, who is diagnosed with Alzheimer's disease, is refusing to eat, so he forces a spoon into her mouth, causing her to have ulcers. The treatment for such behaviour could be to educate the abusive spouse regarding her medical condition and teach him other ways of enticing her to eat. In addition, he could be referred to a support group for caregivers for ongoing support and follow-up. He could also be referred to the local Alzheimer's Society. In this way, each indicator designates an area to be followed up by an intervention plan.

Symptoms and signs of abuse

One of the major problems in dealing with abuse is the difficulty in recognising it. It is necessary to be on the alert because symptoms and signs of abuse are often subtle, and are attributed to the ageing process because the person is old and frail. Older people may be reluctant to admit that they are being abused by a family member or caregiver on whom they rely for their basic needs.

Physical and sexual abuse

This type of abuse includes punching, kicking, beating, biting, burning, pushing, dragging, scratching, shaking, arm twisting, sexual assault and any other physical harm to an older person. It also includes physical restraint, such as being tied to a bed or chair, or being locked in a room.

- Look for a history of unexplained accidents or injuries. Has the older person been to several different doctors or hospitals? It is important to check on conflicting stories from the older person and caregiver, and on discrepancies between the injury and the history. There may have been a long delay between the injury occurring and reporting for treatment.
- Any story of an elderly person being accident prone should be viewed with suspicion, as should multiple injuries, especially at different stages of healing, and untreated old injuries.
- Medical and nursing staff should undertake a good physical examination where possible. However, in the absence of a formal physical examination, other practitioners can note the presence of bruising and abrasions on exposed areas, such as the face, neck, forearms and lower legs.
- On the head, look for bald patches, and signs of bruising on the scalp. This may be indicative of hair pulling.
- Watch for black eyes and bleeding in the white part of the eye. Look at the nose and lips for swelling, bruising, lacerations and missing teeth. Fractures of the skull, nose and facial bones should always alert one to the possibility of abuse.
- On the arms look for bruising, especially bruises of an unusual shape. Consider belt buckles, walking sticks, hair brushes or ropes as instruments of injury. Look for pinch marks and grip marks on the upper arms. Victims of abuse are sometimes shaken. Look for bite marks or scratches.
- Look for burns from cigarettes, or chemical burns from caustic substances. Glove or stocking distributions of burns suggest immersion in hot or boiling water.
- Look for rope or chain burns, or other signs of physical restraint, especially on the wrists or around the waist. Older people may be tied to a bed, to a chair, even to a toilet.
- On the trunk look for bruises, abrasions, cigarette burns. Ribs may be fractured if the victim is pushed or shoved against an object or piece of furniture.
- Medical or nursing staff should examine the genital area for bruising, bleeding and painful areas. Check for torn, stained or blood-stained underwear. Look for evidence of sexually transmitted disease. Watch for difficulty with walking or sitting. Any of these signs may be indicative of sexual abuse.
- On the lower limbs look for bruising, rope burns, abrasions, lacerations or evidence of past or present fractures.

Psychological abuse

This is said to have occurred when an older person suffers mental anguish as a result of being shouted at, threatened, humiliated, emotionally isolated by withdrawal of affection, or emotionally blackmailed. Psychological abuse is usually characterised by a pattern of behaviour repeated over time and intended to maintain a hold of fear over the older person.

- The older person may be huddled when sitting, and nervous with the family member or caregiver nearby.
- Insomnia, sleep deprivation and loss of interest in self or environment may occur.
- Look for fearfulness, helplessness, hopelessness, passivity, apathy, resignation, withdrawal. Look for paranoid behaviour or confusion. Look for anger, agitation or anxiety. Many of these signs may be attributed to psychiatric disorders.
- Watch how the older person behaves when the caregiver enters or leaves the room. There may be ambivalence towards a family member or caregiver. Often there is reluctance to talk openly, and the older person avoids facial or eye contact with both practitioner and caregiver.

Material/financial abuse

This is the improper use of an older person's money, property, or assets by someone else. This may be more easily detected when older people are visited in their own homes.

- There may be loss of money, ranging from removal of cash from a wallet to the cashing of cheques for large amounts of money.
- Sudden or unexplained withdrawal of money from a bank account may occur.
- There may be a sudden inability to pay bills or buy food.
- Bank books, credit cards and cheque books may be 'lost'.
- There may be a loss of jewellery, silverware, paintings, even furniture.
- An unprecedented transfer of money or property to another person may have occurred.
- A new will may have been made in favour of a new friend or another family member. Power of attorney may be obtained improperly from an older person who is not mentally competent.

Active or passive neglect

This is where an older person is deprived by the caregiver of the necessities of life.

- If food or drinks are being withheld there is malnourishment, weight loss, wasting and dehydration, all without an illness related cause. The older person may have constipation or faecal impaction.
- There may be evidence of inadequate or inappropriate use of medication: for instance, the older person may be oversedated in the middle of the day.
- There may be evidence of unmet physical needs, such as decaying teeth or overgrown nails.
- The older person may be lacking necessary aids such as spectacles, dentures, hearing aids or walking frame.
- There may be poor hygiene or inadequate skin care. The older person may be very dirty or smell strongly of urine or be infested with lice. There may be a urine rash with excoriation and chafing.
- Clothing may be dirty and in poor repair; it may be inappropriate for the weather or for the person's gender.
- In some cases where the older person is immobile, he may develop pressure areas over the sacrum, hips, heels or elbows. Sometimes medical care and attention are withheld until the older person is almost moribund.

It is important to remember that the presence of one or more of the signs listed above does not necessarily establish that abuse is occurring, as many of these are seen in frail older people with chronic disease. Ageing skin may bruise more readily, bones may fracture more easily due to osteoporosis, and falls may occur more often due to degenerative changes or disease in the central nervous system. It should also be noted that the severity of abuse can vary substantially. In some cases one incident may constitute abuse (e.g. theft or physical assault); in other cases one incident may not be abusive (e.g. the case of a stressed carer shouting once at a relative with dementia). However, the presence of any of the signs listed above should alert one to the possibility of abuse.

Interventions and referral

In another study entitled Powerlessness and Abuse, we interviewed abused older adults and some abuser caregivers, referred by community agencies, to identify which intervention strategies were perceived to be successful in helping them out of their abusive situations and which were not. We discovered several simple steps for the physician to follow which may make intervention or referral easier. These are described in 7 steps, shown in Box 59.3.

Naming abuse and moving out

1. The older adult comes to see the doctor: Identification of the abuse

We found in our study that doctors and nurses are very helpful in being able to identify and screen for signs of abuse and neglect. They are most able to check for physical signs of abuse, such as bruises, cuts or burns on the body, etc. during the physical examination. Other types of abuse can be detected through the trusting relationship between doctor and patient. Usually the patient does not report the abuse but it is discovered when the patient comes for other health problems. If the doctor discovers bruises or cuts or unusual marks on the body, the person may explain this by saying the marks are the result of a fall, since this seems to be a more acceptable answer to them. The doctor should investigate further the exact circumstances of the fall through questions, such as: 'Where did you fall?', 'In what room did you fall?', 'Who was present when the fall occurred?', 'What was happening just before you fell?', 'Where was your daughter/spouse at the time?' Without this investigation the doctor may not uncover the abuse incident. The patient may say he cannot explain the physical signs of abuse, but if the doctor asks many questions about the circumstances of the fall, she may find out the older person was pushed by a drunk caregiver. Doctors should be especially vigilant when the patient has several unexplained falls or events occurring during several months or a year. Using the IOA tool and the CASE helps pinpoint and confirm the suspected abusive behaviour so that an appropriate intervention plan can be administered for the abused older adult and the abusive caregiver. If the patient is found to be incompetent through the administration of a mental health test, such as the Folstein Mini-Mental State Examination, the doctor needs to interview the caregiver to assess for possible abuse or neglect.

2. Verbalisation: Helping the older person tell her story

The most important step in helping the older adult acknowledge his abusive situation is to take the time to let the person talk freely about his life situation and about his relationship with the caregiver. This should be done in the absence of the caregiver. The caregiver will be asked to wait and be given time later to talk to the doctor. Since the doctor usually does not have a great deal of time to spend talking with patients, these interviews may have to be specially arranged. Telling the story may take a long time, since it is important to go into many aspects of the situation. The doctor explores the past history of the relationship between the caregiver and the older person. Questions such as 'How did you get along with your husband before you became sick?', or 'Have things changed between you and your husband/daughter since he/she is taking care of you?', or 'How do you feel about being cared for by your son/wife when you used to be the one who took care of everyone in the family?' are important questions in helping the older person talk about the abusive relationship with the caregiver. The older person may have always experienced a violent or conflicted relationship with his spouse or daughter, but the situation may have escalated due to the fact that the dependencies between the pair have become more pronounced since the older person became frail or sick. Therefore the doctor must be on the lookout for any significant events that may have recently occurred, affecting the relationship between the care receiver and caregiver. For example, the relationship may have recently become abusive since they started to share living arrangements. In the study Powerlessness and Abuse, a mother and daughter's relationship became violent when they both bought a duplex and moved in together. Their relationship had always been difficult on account of the daughter's drug dependency,

Box 59.3 Steps to move to empowerment

1. Abused older adult visits health professional
- interaction with facilitator (doctor, social worker or community worker)
- transmission of information and knowledge using humour
- identification of abuse and neglect

2. Verbalisation
- facilitator encourages verbalisation (telling the story) by asking critical questions, measuring the situation
- understanding of historical oppression, learnt violence, gender roles and cultural attitudes to violence, health, ageing, etc.
- disclosing family secrets
- family history
- exploring drinking patterns and depression in the family

3. Preparing to acknowledge and name the abuse: Transformed energy
- insight into situation of abuse and neglect
- critical awareness of one's realities and environment (getting rid of the past garbage)
- reliving past feelings and letting them go
- naming abuse
- knowing one's limits
- reversal of self-blame

4. Taking action
- make complaint about abuse/neglect
- knowledge of law and rights
- knowledge and use of criminal justice system
- breaking isolation: joining Golden Age club or social activities
- self-help strategies (joining support group)
- self-education (attending school or getting a job)
- knowledge about and referral to abuse-trained workers

5. Documentation of problems and the problem-solving process
- documentation in medical file
- letter writing
- picture taking of crimes
- concrete actions (e.g. changing the locks, direct bank deposits, court order to remove the abuser, etc.)
- consultation with experts (lawyers, etc.)
- accompaniment through process of problem solving when necessary

6. Offering resources and referral to other services
- respite services
- divorce, separation services
- advocacy groups and lobbying for improved services
- joining elder abuse committee to prevent abuse/neglect of others
- giving information about abuse/neglect of others

7. Self-control
- new or repaired identity (liberation)
- free time for her/himself
- taking care of one's own needs

but after living together they became co-dependent on one another, each invading the other's privacy, which gradually evolved into the daughter's violent behaviour towards her mother.

It is also important to explore the cultural aspects of the relationship between the caregiver and the care receiver to find out how the older person's beliefs and values may be keeping him in an abusive situation. For example, we found in the same study that some older adults, who had survived the Holocaust, believed their reasons for surviving were to care for their family. Thus, even though their relationships with their children, who were now in their 40s, were abusive, they felt they could not leave the relationship and that they must sacrifice themselves for the good of the children. Similarly, spouses who believed that marriage is 'for better and for worse' and that 'divorce is wrong' stayed in violent relationships rather than move out because of their religious beliefs. Other cultural beliefs also played a role in relationships: for example, an older gentleman from Asia, who had attended British schools when he was young, had been caned and received harsh punishments at school. These past events influenced his belief about not punishing children, despite his being the victim of an abusive situation between him and his North American born spouse and her children from a previous marriage. His own philosophy of the need to be 'resigned to one's situation' made him reluctant to move out of the house.

During the process of 'telling their story', the older adults are encouraged to express their feelings about their situation through simple questions, such as: 'How did that make you feel?' It is the process of being able to name the feeling or situation or past events leading up to the abuse which helps the person to understand what is happening to him, what led up to the present and to acknowledge that he is not to blame for what has happened. The doctor assures them that whatever the circumstances, no one deserves to be abused. Thus, the physician must have a non-judgmental attitude and listen with empathy to what the person is saying, asking occasional important questions to guide the story telling. Humour is a great 'shock absorber', and it can sometimes be appropriate for diffusing a tense situation that may arise during the verbalisation of painful experiences.

It is essential to look into the drinking patterns of the family members, as alcohol has been said to be the single most important risk factor associated with abusive behaviour. Similarly, if one of the family members has a gambling habit or a problem with drugs, the impact of these lifestyle habits must be explored closely to identify any financial or other types of abuse related to the patterns of behaviour. In our study the profiles of abusive gamblers, drug takers and problem drinkers showed similar characteristics. An example of abuse associated with drinking is a mother who called the health care professionals to say her daughter had got drunk the night before, had trashed her mother's house, hit her head against the wall and left. The next day the daughter called to apologise to her mother and asked to come back. The mother felt badly and invited her daughter back home. For a while all went well, until the daughter went on a drinking binge again and the abusive behaviour was repeated. It was also noted that the mother was giving money to her daughter to buy beer. Very often the abusive behaviour is kept a family secret and the older adult is encouraged by the abuser to keep the abuse and neglect hidden, even from other family members who may not be aware of what is going on. Violence and neglect usually occur in isolation and the abuser often even isolates the victim from the supports he may have.

The process of verbalisation is the most important step in discovering abusive behaviour, and it may take several weeks to allow the patient to trust the doctor enough to confide in her. The same interview process is also used with the caregiver. The doctor tries to find out how the caregiver sees her situation. For example, to guide her in telling her story, ask questions like these:

- Is the caregiving difficult for the daughter/spouse?
- Does it impede on other areas of her life?
- What other areas of her life does caregiving impede upon?
- How much does she understand about the care receiver's condition?
- What impact does her demented mother's behaviour have on her and how is she dealing with it?
- How is the relationship between mother and daughter?

- Has it changed since the mother became more dependent on the daughter?

Towards the end of the conversation, the doctor also asks the questions on the CASE tool to explore the areas of abusive behaviour.

It is important for the doctor to allow enough time for both the care receiver and/or caregiver to express their feelings, to talk about the relationship between caregiver and care receiver, and to discuss the broader context within which she is giving care.

3. Preparing the person to acknowledge and name the abuse

Sharing feelings and facts about the abuse situation helps to free the care receiver/caregiver of guilty feelings. It also enables him to release blocked emotions and negative experiences and energy from the past, so that he is able to think about doing something with regards to the abusive situation. The person is able to gain some insight into what led him and his family members into the difficulties and he begins to have some positive energy which can help him make a decision about how to change the situation. Sometimes the care receiver and the caregiver are able to name the abuse specifically, even though they previously denied it. It is important that the doctor reassures the care receiver that he is not to blame for the abuse and that no matter what he did, no one deserves to be abused. Often a mother will have difficulty taking action against one of her children and may believe she has to sacrifice herself to help the son. One mother in our study stated: 'I am not strong when it comes to a son. I spoiled him all my life, my mother spoiled me too. I've given my life for him.' When the person is able to stop blaming herself and realise she does not deserve to be beaten by her son, she is able to move to the next step, which is to act.

4. Taking action

When the abused person is ready to act, he is ready to begin looking at ways of changing the situation. If he is able to make a rational decision, he will begin to discuss with the doctor what possible actions can be taken. In cases of severe physical or financial abuse or neglect, it is important to act quickly and to ensure the person is not in any immediate danger. The first action should be to call the police to the scene of the crime while evidence is still clearly visible. The doctor must be careful to not remove any important evidence that could be necessary for the prosecution of the abuser. The abused person may also need to be admitted to hospital on account of serious injuries.

In all cases of abuse and neglect, the doctor should refer the case to an appropriate social worker or a professional trained in abuse as soon as possible for further investigation. In most US states and some Canadian provinces (in the Maritimes), there are adult protection workers. These are specially trained workers legislated by the government to act in cases of abuse and neglect of older adults, including cases of self-neglect. In such areas the doctor should immediately inform the workers. It is important for doctors to know what the adult protection laws are in their state or province and what they are required by law to do, as each legislative body is different and has different requirements. Some have mandatory reporting procedures while others do not. The workers will accompany the senior through the process of resolving her problem, whether it is a crime or a case of mild neglect in which the caregiver may change his behaviour fairly quickly through education or being referred to a family support group. In areas where there are no adult protection teams, contact community based abuse teams or a social worker to refer cases. Trained volunteers may also be available to help the person reduce his isolation and help him through the problem-solving process.

5. Documentation of problems and the problem-solving process

It is essential that the doctor document her findings on physical examination and also during the interview with the patient and caregiver. This information will be needed to resolve the case. It is also important to ask the abused person to document everything that has happened to him while it is still fresh in his mind. In addition, he should collect any proof that will help him give evidence about his case. Photographs or videos are effective for producing hard evidence. Some simple strategies can also be suggested by the doctor or other health professional: for example, he may need to change the locks of his doors to prevent the abusive caregiver from returning to the house. He might want to make immediate arrangements for his pension cheques to be deposited directly into his bank account to prevent an abusive nephew from stealing them. He may need to take out a court order to remove an abusive relative from the home. These concrete actions can be suggested by the doctor or by a social worker in the case. The person may need a volunteer to accompany him through the steps he has to take and to offer support and encouragement that he is doing the right thing. The person may be referred to other specialists, such as lawyers, psychiatrists or financial experts, to assist him. The doctor's role is to encourage this.

In less serious cases, the doctor should also refer the older adult to the appropriate person or social worker to help him through the conflicts in his relationship with the caregiver, and to figure out the best way of resolving her problems. Very often the older adult refuses to separate from the abusive caregiver even if the person does not have the best interests of the person at heart. The decision of the older person must be affirmed unless the person is in danger or unable to make a decision. The role of the doctor is to offer choices to the person and help him to understand the implications and possible consequences of whatever choices he makes.

6. *Offering resources and referral to other services*

The abused older adult or the caregiver may need a variety of public or private services to support him during this time. For example, a range of home care and respite services were used in our former study for both abused older adults and their caregivers. Some older adults used lawyers to obtain separations or divorces from their abusive spouses. Some caregivers joined support groups to learn how to modify their frustrated feelings and behaviour. Abused older adults joined 'empowerment' groups where they met with other older adults who had similar experiences and learnt self-help strategies. Sometimes when they had solved their own problems they found it to be therapeutic to help others by joining community committees to fight against abuse and neglect.

Caregivers who had alcohol or drug or gambling addictions were referred to suitable treatment programs. Day centres and activities for older adults will prevent the person from becoming isolated and possibly abused again. The doctor needs to keep a handy list of all such referral centres and programs in her office. Giving the correct information in a timely way to older adults and their caregivers not only helps when abuse is present but may even prevent it. Group support for caregivers may be a way of preventing abusive behaviour, as well as preventing the isolation of caregivers. It may be a way of helping those caregivers who do not wish to continue giving care but are doing so out of feelings of guilt, duty or obligation, to acknowledge their limits and make other arrangements for the person to receive care.

7. *Self-control*

In this final step, the older person and/or the caregiver has solved his problem and is once again in control of his own life. This step may entail finding time for oneself—as one caregiver stated: 'I didn't think nothing for myself, I only think about someone else'. Another expressed his joy at finally being able to have lunch once a week with his friends. A third talked about planting a small garden and the pleasure he gained from tending the flowers. These examples are all very simple ways of enjoying oneself as an individual and not being dependent on another person for one's pleasure. It means thinking of and satisfying one's own needs and not only those of others. The doctor should encourage older adults and caregivers to find some such pleasurable activities for themselves and to sometimes find ways to separate themselves from the other person, even though it may be difficult.

Conclusion

In this chapter we discussed the prevalence of abuse and neglect of older adults living in the community by a person in a position of trust, defined as a caregiver. We noted that the present estimates of abuse may be just the tip of the iceberg and that the percentage of abuse in the population of older adults is higher among those who are frail and cannot defend themselves. Next we defined the different manifestations of mistreatment of older adults and noted that often more than one type of abuse and neglect is perpetrated against older adults, and also that there may be more than one perpetrator.

We discussed the possible causes of abuse and neglect, and that there is no single explanation for all the types of mistreatment. We described over 40 different indicators that have been associated with the phenomenon and observed that 6 of these indicators appear most frequently in the studies and often interact with one another. These are dependence, sex, depression (of the caregiver), alcohol/drug addiction, gambling (caregiver), shared living arrangements and social isolation/lack of support. We offered 2 screening tools (CASE and IOA) to screen abusive from non-abusive caregivers so those patients who have abusive caregivers can be targeted for assistance. Finally, we offered some suggestions in a 7 step model to help physicians assist abused older adults and their abusive caregivers. We particularly emphasised the importance of enabling older adults to 'tell their stories'. This model is only in the developmental stages but we hope it may be helpful to physicians and other health professionals in preventing, identifying and treating this outrageous social phenomenon.

Acknowledgment

This text includes work submitted in fulfilment of the degree of Doctor of Philosophy at Laval University, Quebec: 'Powerlessness and Abuse: A Descriptive Qualitative Study Which Explores Abuse and Neglect of Older Adults in the Community in Relation to the Social Context' by D. Nahmiash (1997).

Bibliography and further reading

Council of Europe (1992), *Violence Against Elderly People*, Council of Europe, Brussels.

Health Canada (1993), *Older Canadians and The Abuse of Seniors: A Continuum from Participation to Empowerment*, Family Violence Prevention Division, Ottawa.

Hudson, M. & Johnson, T. F. (1986), 'Elder abuse and neglect: a review of the literature', *Annual Review of Gerontology and Geriatrics*, 6(1), pp. 55–83.

Kosberg, J. I. & Garcia, J. L. (eds) (1995), *Elder Abuse: International and Crosscultural Perspectives*, The Haworth Press, New York.

Kosberg, J. I. & Nahmiash, D. (1996), 'Characteristics of victims and perpetrators', in Baumhover, L. A. & Beal, S. C. (eds), *Assessing Elder Abuse in Health Care Settings*, Health Professions Press, Baltimore, MD, pp. 31–50.

McDonald, P. L., Hornick, J. P., Robertson, G. B. & Wallace, J. E. (1991), *Elder Abuse and Neglect in Canada*, Butterworths Canada Ltd, Toronto.

Nahmiash, D. (1997), 'Powerlessness and Abuse: a descriptive qualitative study which explores abuse and neglect of older adults in the community in relation to the social context', doctoral dissertation, Laval University, Quebec.

Paveza, G. D., Cohen, D., Eisdorfer, C., Freels, S., Semla, T., Ashford, W. J., Gorelick, P., Hirschman, R., Luchins, D. & Levy, P. (1992), 'Severe family violence and Alzheimer's disease: prevalence and risk factors', *The Gerontologist*, 32(4), pp. 493–7.

Pillemer, K. A. (1986), 'Risk factors in elder abuse: results from a case-control study', in Pillemer, K. A. & Wolf, R. S. (eds), *Elder Abuse: Conflict in the Family*, Auburn House Publishing Co, Dover, MA.

Pillemer, K. A. & Wolf, R. S. (1986), 'Major findings from three model projects on elderly abuse', in Pillemer, K. A. & Wolf, R. S. (eds), op. cit., pp. 197–217.

Pitsiou, V., Darrough, E. N. & Spinellis, C. D. (1995), 'Mistreatment of the elderly in Greece', in Kosberg, J. I. & Garcia, J. L. (eds), op. cit., pp. 45–64.

Podnieks, E., Pillemer, K. A., Nicholson, J., Shillington, T. & Frizzell, A. F. (1989), *National Survey on Abuse of the Elderly in Canada*, Office of Research and Innovation, Ryerson Polytechnical Institute, Toronto.

Reis, M. & Nahmiash, D. (1995), *When Seniors are Abused*, Captus Press, Toronto.

Select Committee on Aging (1981), *Elder Abuse: An Examination of a Hidden Problem*, US Government Printing Office, Washington, DC, pp. 99–502.

Solomon, B. B. (1976), *Black Empowerment: Social Work in Oppressed Communities*, Columbia University Press, New York.

Sonkin, D. J., Martin, P. & Walker, E. A. (1985), *The Male Batterer*, Springer, New York.

Stones, M. (1991), *A Lexicon for Elder Mistreatment*, written for St. John's provincial work committee, Newfoundland

Chapter 60
Palliative care

JOSE PEREIRA

Defining palliative care

Palliative care is the care of patients for whom cure is not possible and the disease is progressive. The World Health Organization defines palliative care as: 'The active total care of patients whose disease is not responsive to curative treatment. Control of pain, of other symptoms and of psychological, social and spiritual problems is paramount. The goal of palliative care is the achievement of the best quality of life for patients and their families.'

The palliative approach is relevant to all patients with incurable conditions. It emphasises the importance of considering the physical, psychological, social and spiritual aspects of the patient's illness experience and is best delivered within an interdisciplinary team approach. Palliative care affirms life and regards dying as a normal process. It offers a support system to help patients live as actively as possible until death. It neither intentionally hastens nor unnecessarily prolongs life. It includes consideration of family and carers. The principles of palliative care are the same whether the patient is in a hospice, palliative care unit, hospital or at home. Palliative care should be available to patients at all stages of disease, and not just in the terminal phases. It should become activated at the point that the illness is deemed incurable. Most primary care practitioners will look after patients with life-threatening disease and a palliative approach should be a core skill of every clinician.

Although modern palliative care has its roots in oncology, there is increasing recognition that patients with other incurable illnesses also deserve good end-of-life care. While this chapter will focus on palliative care within the oncological setting, readers are reminded that many of the principles are applicable to patients with other incurable illnesses, including those with various advanced, end-stage neuromuscular, cardiac, pulmonary and renal diseases. A key difference between cancer related palliative care and non-cancer palliative care relates to the illness trajectory. Whereas the former is generally more predictable (predictable steady decline with a relatively short 'terminal phase'), the latter is generally, with some exceptions, a slow decline punctuated by periodic crises.

Palliative care is active care and even when 'active' anticancer treatment is no longer being given, palliative care remains medical active therapy requiring regular assessments and ongoing care. Active interventions such as palliative radiotherapy, treatment of delirium, surgery for pathological fractures and infusions of packed red cells may be offered to selected patients under certain circumstances.

Tasks in palliative care

Communication and disclosure

Effective communication skills are core to the delivery of good palliative care. Palliative care begins the moment a patient is found to have incurable cancer, and breaking the news of the diagnosis to a patient and family is one of the first tasks in the care process. A step-by-step approach adopted from Buckman (1994) is given in Box 60.1.

Modern medical ethics emphasises the patient's right to be fully informed of her own medical condition. The rationale for this is that it protects the autonomy of the patient, allows her to play a greater role in making decisions related to her illness and care, and respects her personal wishes and goals. Truth telling, once regarded as the source of distress, is now thought by many to be morally obligatory. However, one must recognise that people handle information differently. While some prefer all the information, including the prognosis, up front, others may be distressed and overwhelmed by this approach. Providing all the raw details may be inappropriate. Cultural influences need to be recognised. Clinicians should therefore first identify what, how and at what pace the patient wants the information shared.

Clinicians should create opportunities for patients to express their concerns, fears and expectations. Skills that promote disclosure by patients of psychological distress include the use of open questions, questions with a psychological focus, clarification of psychological comments, the use of educated guesses, and empathy. On the other hand, techniques that inhibit disclosure and should therefore not be used include the use of closed questions, leading questions, questioning with physical focus only, selective attention to only physical aspects, premature advice and unreasonable reassurances. Listening and silence can be effective strategies at times.

Box 60.1 Key steps in breaking bad news

- Create an environment conducive to effective communication.
- Ensure that the right people are present (e.g. supportive family members or friends).
- Find out what the patient suspects or knows.
- Find out how much the patient wants to know.
- Find out how and at what pace and detail the patient wants to find out.
- Share the information in a sensitive but honest way.
- Respond to the patient's and family's feelings. Be empathetic and validate their concerns and feelings.
- Communicate prognosis, treatment options. Emphasise ongoing supportive treatment.
- Establish a management plan.
- Allow patients and families to ask questions.
- At all times ensure they understand what is being said.
- Plan follow-up.

Note: This approach needs to be individualised to the patient and circumstances.

Source: R. Buckman (1994), 'Communication in palliative care: A practical guide', in Doyle, D., Hanks, G. & Macdonald, N. (eds), *Oxford Textbook of Palliative Medicine*, 1st edn, Oxford University Press, Oxford, pp. 47–61.

'How long do I have to live?' is a common question from patients and families. In responding to this, it must be noted that accurate assessments of life expectancy are not possible. Generalisations, such as days to weeks, or weeks to months, or many months, are more appropriate.

Multidimensional assessment

Palliative care focuses on the alleviation of suffering. Suffering can be conceptualised as having physical, social, spiritual and psychological components. Consequently, assessment must include all these aspects. Untreated or unresolved problems in one domain will affect the others. Ignoring this interdependence results in inadequate care and unrealistic care goals. Psychological or spiritual distress can alter the pain experience and aggravate the expression of pain and its intensity while uncontrolled pain, on the other hand, may affect the patient's psychological wellbeing. Assessments should include a review of the frequency, intensity and character of the various physical and psychological symptoms, as well as other areas such as coping resources, cognition, spiritual concerns, preferred setting of care and general quality of life, among others.

The key areas of assessment are shown in Box 60.2. A prior history of alcohol or drug abuse, for example, may alert the clinician to maladaptive coping mechanisms when confronted with life stressors. Cognitive impairment, whether it is due to delirium or dementia, alters a patient's expression of symptoms. The agitation and grimacing that is sometimes associated with delirium may easily be misinterpreted as uncontrolled pain. On the other hand, cognitively impaired individuals may have difficulties reporting their symptoms. Cognitive impairment limits the opportunity for counselling. Clinicians should therefore routinely screen for delirium and cognitive impairment in palliative patients, particularly given the high prevalence of delirium in these patients.

Box 60.2 Key assessment areas

Disease history
Physical symptoms
Physical functioning
Psychological symptoms
Psychological functioning
Social circumstances
Financial issues
Past physical and psychiatric history
Personality, life views, goals
Family structure and functioning
Support and coping resources
Decision-making capacity
Information sharing
Preferred setting of care
Identifying local resources
Quality of life

Self-reporting by cognitively intact patients should be encouraged. It has been shown that health care professionals tend to underestimate symptom intensity while family members tend to overestimate it. The use of simple visual analogue scales (VAS), numerical rating scales (NRS) and verbal descriptor scales have proven to be effective and reproducible means of measuring pain and other symptoms. One such system that allows for regular evaluation is the Edmonton Symptom Assessment Scale. This system consists of 9 numerical rating scales that assess 9 frequently occurring symptoms and problems (see Figure 60.1). Patients are encouraged to complete these regularly.

Interdisciplinary care

An interdisciplinary approach that values the input from a variety of disciplines, including nursing, social work, pastoral care, psychology, volunteers, nutritional services, occupational therapy and physiotherapy, is very valuable. In the community, primary physicians can play an important role in identifying the resources available and co-ordinating them so as to ensure comprehensive care.

Advanced planning

The process of planning for future medical care is an integral aspect of palliative care. The topic should be introduced in a sensitive manner and should be followed by discussions covering potential scenarios and treatment issues. Patients should identify a proxy to make decisions on their behalf should they become cognitively incapacitated. Patient and proxy education is paramount and involves defining key medical terms, discussing possible scenarios and treatments, and explaining the benefits and burdens of these treatments. One important area to cover is that of cardiopulmonary resuscitation in the event of cardiopulmonary arrest. The futility of resuscitation attempts in palliative patients, particularly those with advanced disease, should be borne in mind. A 'do not resuscitate' (DNR) preference is optimal in these patients, but other palliative goals and therapies

Please circle the number that best describes the severity of the various symptoms for you.

No pain	1	2	3	4	5	6	7	8	9	10	Worst possible pain
Not tired	1	2	3	4	5	6	7	8	9	10	Worst possible tiredness
Not nauseated	1	2	3	4	5	6	7	8	9	10	Worst possible nausea
Not depressed	1	2	3	4	5	6	7	8	9	10	Worst possible depression
Not anxious	1	2	3	4	5	6	7	8	9	10	Worst possible anxiety
Not drowsy	1	2	3	4	5	6	7	8	9	10	Worst possible drowsiness
Best appetite	1	2	3	4	5	6	7	8	9	10	Worst possible appetite
Best feeling of wellbeing	1	2	3	4	5	6	7	8	9	10	Worst possible feeling of wellbeing
No shortness of breath	1	2	3	4	5	6	7	8	9	10	Worst possible shortness of breath
Other problem	1	2	3	4	5	6	7	8	9	10	Other problem

Figure 60.1 Edmonton Symptom Assessment Scale

should be stressed. These preferences should be documented. The goals of care should be reviewed at regular intervals.

Advanced planning also includes practical issues such as getting financial and legal affairs in order and planning funeral arrangements. Choices regarding care settings, the resources to support these and the burdens and benefits should be discussed. Family and other caregivers should be informed about what to expect, particularly in the last hours of life.

Decision making

Palliative care and the transition into palliative care require an ongoing sequence of decisions, many of which are difficult and some of which result in ethical dilemmas. Consider, for example, the following scenarios: a terminally ill patient who is symptomatic from pneumonia; a patient who requests a full code status despite advanced incurable disease; a patient with intractable symptoms where active sedation is being considered; a cachectic patient with incurable illness who requests artificial nutrition intravenously; or a patient or family member requesting euthanasia. One should avoid overly aggressive treatment (such as aggressive chemotherapy in an elderly, frail patient with an advanced cancer that is resistant to chemotherapy) and under-treatment (and miss the opportunity to improve quality of life). The potential benefits and risks of treatments should be considered in individual cases. It must be noted that adequate symptom management can be achieved without causing death.

A working framework has been proposed in the form of a grid that attempts to identify and recognise medical problems, patient preferences and expectations, quality of life and other contextual considerations for ethical decision making (see Box 60.3). This framework allows for individualisation of decisions and care. The wishes of the patient (as long as they are competent) have a greater weight in the process than the wishes of others. Decision making is largely consensual and most patients and families appear to favour a shared decision-making model with their healthcare providers.

Some of the more frequently encountered issues include those related to life-sustaining treatments, such as cardiopulmonary resuscitation (CPR), mechanical ventilation, dialysis, artificial feeding and hydration. Very few patients with advanced cancer survive CPR and those who do are often subject to impaired quality of life related to advancing disease. In the case of artificial nutrition, irreversible metabolic changes induced by advanced cancer generally make artificial nutrition by enteral or parenteral feeding redundant. There is much debate regarding the appropriateness of artificial hydration by the intravenous or subcutaneous (hypodermoclysis) routes in the palliative setting. While indiscriminate artificial hydration of all terminally ill patients is discouraged, some terminally ill patients may benefit from hydration, particularly those with opioid related neurotoxicity or those with delirium resulting from, or aggravated by, dehydration.

Bereavement care

Bereavement care is an integral part of palliative care. It is discussed in detail in Chapter 11 of this book. Readers are reminded to monitor family members for anticipatory grief.

Box 60.3 An ethical grid for decision making

Decisions should be made within the ethical frameworks of beneficence ('do good'), non-maleficence ('do no harm'), equality (equal access to care and treatments) and autonomy (respecting patient's wishes).

Medical indications

What are the facts of the medical history and the condition, including the prognosis?
What is the overall disease and symptom burden?
Are the symptoms or complications reversible?
What treatment is being proposed?
What are the risks and benefits related to treatment versus non-treatment?
What is the functional level?

Patient (and family) factors and preferences

Is the patient competent? Does he/they comprehend the situation?
What is his understanding of his illness?
What are his expectations?
Does he have an advanced directive?

Quality of life

What does quality of life mean for the patient (and family)?
What are the physical, psychological, social and spiritual statuses?
What is realistic or achievable with regard to the patient's preferences and expectations?

Contextual features

Has an incurable illness been confirmed?
Whose interests are affected?
What are the thoughts of the caregivers on the issues/problems?
What does the law state?
What are the societal norms and expectations?

Source: Adopted from the work of Jonsen, Siegler and Winslade; and adopted from D. R. Kuhl & P. Wilensky (1999), 'Decision making at the end of life: A model using an ethical grid and principles of group process', Journal of Palliative Medicine, 2, pp. 75–86.

Cancer pain

Pain occurs in about 80% of patients with advanced cancer. A quarter to a third of these patients experience severe pain. Adequate pain relief is possible in approximately 80–85% of these patients by adhering to well-established management guidelines. Unfortunately, insufficient training and lack of skills on the part of health care professionals continues to present a barrier to adequate pain control. Patients' and families' fears about opioid treatment often present additional barriers. Some patients, for example, may be reluctant to take morphine for fear of becoming addicted. Others perceive morphine use as a sign that death is close or that morphine will hasten death. The appropriate use of an opioid neither causes addiction nor does it hasten death. The optimal management of cancer pain requires a thorough assessment, the establishment and implementation of an individualised management plan that relies on some basic principles, reassessment and ongoing modification to meet changing needs.

Assessment of cancer pain

The management of cancer pain depends on a comprehensive multidimensional assessment that characterises the symptom and assesses the relation between the pain, the disease, other symptoms and the psychological, social and spiritual status of the patient.

The initial step of assessing pain requires characterisation of the pain/s. Basic features such as location, onset, duration (constant or episodic), quality (e.g. burning, stabbing, dull), ameliorating factors (e.g. response to analgesics), factors that exacerbate it (e.g. weight bearing, coughing, supine position, etc.) and radiation should be documented, as should its intensity. Because pain is inherently subjective, a patient's self-report is the gold standard for assessment. In the presence of significant cognitive impairment, self-reporting becomes problematic. Intensity can be assessed using various scales. Visual or numerical rating scales (see 'Multidimensional assessment') are often used and should be plotted on a regular basis in patients' charts. The intensity of the pain, at its best and at its worst, as well as the level to which a patient can tolerate it, and its effect on functioning, need to be noted. Investigations such as plain X-rays or more specialised investigations, such as computerised tomography and magnetic resonance imaging scans, are sometimes helpful in determining the underlying cause of the pain. The characteristics, combined with information from the physical examination and review of laboratory and imaging studies, usually define a discrete pain syndrome, clarify the extent of disease and the relation between the pain and specific lesions, and allow inferences about pain pathophysiology.

Classifying pain according to the inferred underlying mechanism (see Table 60.1) is helpful in guiding treatment. Adjuvant analgesics, for example, can be selected according to the type of pain. Most patients will experience a combination of the different pain syndromes outlined in Table 60.1.

Understanding the underlying cause is also helpful. Pain is caused by direct tumour involvement of various structures in approximately 75% of patients, and by treatment of the cancer in approximately 20% (e.g. radiation therapy induced neuritis or surgical transection of a nerve). In a small group of patients pain may be unrelated to the cancer (e.g. pre-existing arthritis, chronic pain syndromes or post-herpetic neuralgia). Most patients with advanced cancer often have multiple causes and sites of pain.

It is important to recognise that pain and other symptoms are a multidimensional construct. Pain is only one of a range of issues that contribute to suffering of the patient and family, and impairments or problems in multiple domains, including the physical, psychological, social and spiritual, need to be identified. Psychological distress, for example, including fear and anxiety, can exacerbate pain or other symptoms and vice versa. An approach that assumes all the pain a patient expresses reflects tissue injury fails to recognise the impact of other factors such as fear and anxiety on the pain experience and expression. Differentiating between the various underlying influences on the expression of pain can be challenging. It is in the 10–30% of cases that show limited response to well established regimens that the concern arises about the presence of psychosocial components to

Table 60.1 The classification of pain according to the inferred underlying mechanism[(a)]

Type of pain	Mechanism	Subtype	Characteristics	Example
Nociceptive	Activation of nociceptive receptors	Somatic	Constant or intermittent, often gnawing or aching. Well localised	Bone metastases, muscle/ soft tissue infiltration
		Visceral	Constant or cramping, occasionally aching or squeezing. Often poorly localised, may be referred	Liver metastases, bowel obstruction, pancreatic cancer
Neuropathic	Destruction/ infiltration/ compression of nerve	Dysaesthetic/ deafferentation	Constant burning ± hyperalgesia or allodynia, occasionally radiating	
		Lancinating	Episodic lancinating pain Shock-like paroxysms, often on a background of burning pain	

(*a*) Patients commonly present with more than one type of pain concurrently.

the pain and the presence of other poor prognostic factors. These prognostic factors include the presence of a neuropathic component to the pain, incident pain (pain induced by a specific action such as the movement of coughing), cognitive dysfunction, psychological distress and a history of drug or alcohol abuse. A history of alcohol or other drug abuse may indicate poor coping styles when faced with stressors. Routine assessment of cognitive functioning and screening for cognitive dysfunction is paramount, since this will alter the pain expression and experience. An individual's coping style needs to be assessed. Knowledge of renal function may help guide opioid therapy since renal impairment is a risk factor for opioid-induced neurotoxicity.

Selecting an analgesic regimen

To assist in selecting an appropriate drug, the World Health Organization has defined a therapeutic ladder. It involves a stepped approach based on the severity of the pain (see Figure 60.2). The experience with the application of this ladder has shown that the simple principles of escalating from non-opioid to strong opioid analgesics and titrating the doses to achieve pain control is safe and effective in approximately 75–90% of cases.

If the pain is mild (e.g. < 4/10 on a numerical scale), one may begin by prescribing a step 1 analgesic such as aspirin, acetaminophen (paracetamol) or non-steroidal anti-inflammatory drug (NSAID). Potential adverse effects need to be noted, particularly the renal and gastrointestinal adverse effects of the NSAIDs. Patients with advanced cancer appear to be at increased risk of developing these. If pain persists or worsens despite appropriate dose increases, consider changing to a step 2 analgesic such as codeine. The utility of step 1 agents is generally limited by ceiling doses, and the majority of patients with cancer pain will require a step 2 or 3 analgesic (weak or strong opioid). In those patients presenting initially with moderate to severe pain, step 1 can be skipped in favour of steps 2 or 3. Patients receiving step 2 analgesics (weak opioids) can be switched to a step 3 analgesic (strong opioid) if pain persists or worsens despite appropriate dose titration. At each step, an adjuvant drug or modality such as radiation therapy may be considered in selected patients to enhance analgesia (see section on 'Adjuvant analgesics and therapies').

Opioid analgesics remain the mainstay of treatment and, given their effectiveness and safety, opioids should be administered routinely to patients with moderate to severe cancer pain. The principles of cancer pain management and opioid use are listed in Box 60.4. Morphine is generally recommended as the strong opioid of choice. This is based

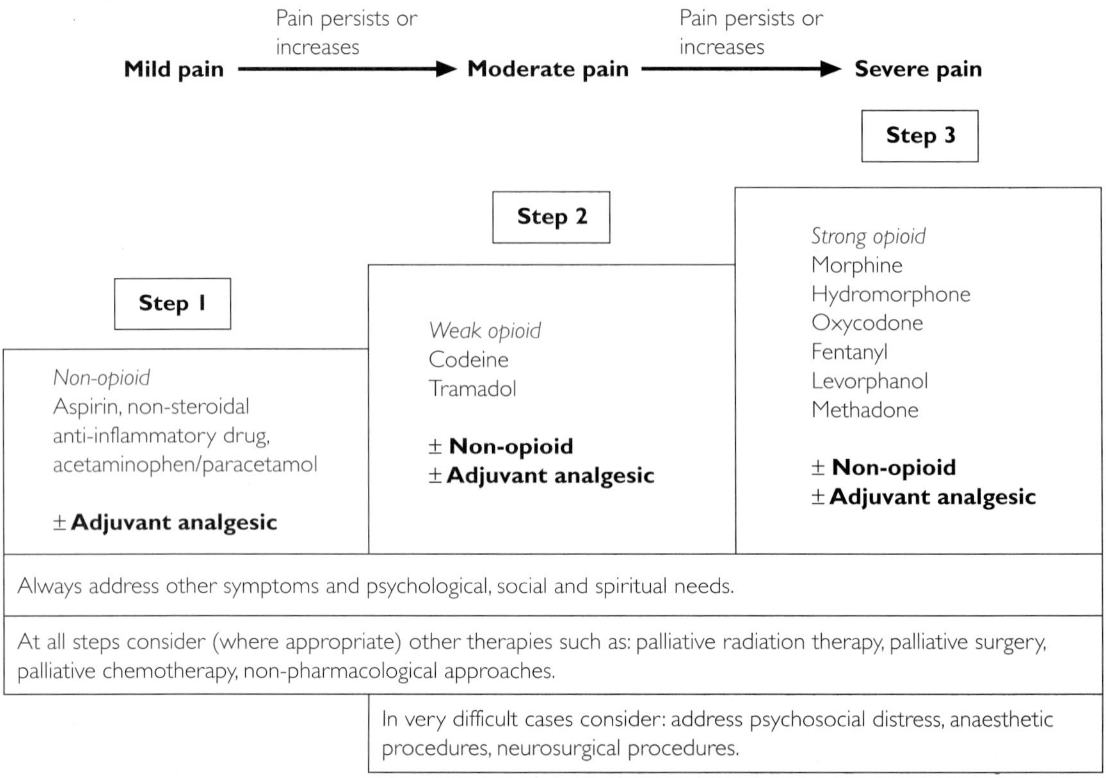

Figure 60.2 WHO analgesic ladder (modified)

on its availability and physicians' familiarity with it. However, other opioids such as hydromorphone, oxycodone and fentanyl are equally effective and have similar efficacy and adverse effect profiles to morphine. A typical starting dose of morphine is 5 mg or 10 mg orally every 4 hours and 2.5 mg or 5 mg every hour as needed for breakthrough pain (see 'Opioid administration, titration and maintenance'). In the case of oxycodone and hydromorphone, an appropriate starting dose would be 2.5 mg or 5 mg and 1 mg, respectively, every 4 hours orally. Equianalgesic doses of other opioids relative to morphine are to be found in Table 60.2.

The dosing intervals depend on the pharmacokinetics of the opioid selected. Generally, immediate release formulations of morphine, oxycodone, hydromorphone and codeine need to be administered every 4 hours. Fentanyl cannot be ingested orally and is available either as a transdermal (patch) formulation or parenteral formulation. The transdermal formulation needs to be changed only every 3 days while the parenteral formulation, because of its rapid onset of action and short half-life, requires a continuous infusion (subcutaneously or intravenously). A transmucosal buccal formulation (in the form of a lozenge) is becoming available for the management of breakthrough pain. Methadone is a very useful and potent opioid that is gaining much interest. However, its unpredictable and long half-life makes it more difficult to use, especially when initiating treatment. It is much more potent than morphine and its equianalgesic dose ratio relative to other opioids changes, depending on the dose of the previous opioid. It should be used under the guidance of a clinician experienced in its use. Oxycodone is sometimes available in combination with aspirin or acetaminophen. This limits the ability to titrate oxycodone doses up. Oxycodone is approximately 1.5–2 times more potent than morphine and therefore belongs in the

Box 60.4 Principles for opioid treatment in cancer pain

- Avoid delay in treatment.
- Administer the opioid regularly around the clock.
- Schedule the appropriate dosing interval according to the formulation.
- The oral route is preferred where possible.
- Start with a low dose and increase until adequate analgesia occurs or dose-limiting side effects occur.
- Titrate the dose individually.
- Allow for extra rescue (breakthrough) doses for rescue analgesia.
- Anticipate and prevent common side effects. Prevent nausea and constipation.
- Educate patients regarding addiction, the possible need for future dose increases and side effects.
- Consider opioids as only one part of the total pain management plan.
- Consider the addition of adjuvant analgesics in selected patients.
- Monitor treatment efficacy and pain status over time and consider modifications if necessary.

Table 60.2 Equianalgesic doses of opioids

Drug	Oral dose	Subcutaneous dose	Half-life (hrs)	Duration of action (hrs)
Morphine	10 mg	5 mg	2–3	3–4
Codeine	200 mg	100 mg	2–3	3–4
Hydromorphone	2 mg	1 mg	2–3	3–4
Oxycodone	5–7.5 mg	2.5 mg	2–3	3–4
Fentanyl (parenteral)		± 50–75 μg	± 1–2	± 1–3
Fentanyl (transdermal)	See manufacturer's tables	See manufacturer's tables ± 50–75 μg		48–72
Methadone	±1 mg	N/A	15–120	6–8

Notes:

1. There is a wide variation in different individuals' responses to different opioids. Close monitoring during switching from one opioid to another is therefore important.
2. A further 25–50% decrease in opioid dose from the equianalgesic dose is required when switching from one opioid to another.

third step of the WHO Ladder. Codeine is often available in combination with acetaminophen (paracetamol). These tend to limit the upward titration of this drug. An appropriate starting dose of codeine is approximately 8 mg or 15 mg orally every 4 hours. There appears to be a diminishing return of benefits when increasing codeine doses beyond 60 mg orally per dose. When using codeine and oxycodone, it must be noted that certain individuals (± 10% Caucasians) have a genetic deficiency of the enzyme CYP2D6. This enzyme is required to metabolise codeine to its active forms (including morphine) and oxycodone to its analgesic metabolite (oxymorphone). Drugs such as selective serotonin reuptake inhibitor antidepressant agents (SSRIs) and cimetidine may inhibit this enzyme, thereby diminishing the effectiveness of these opioids.

Opioids that are not recommended for use in the control of cancer pain include pethidine (meperidine), the partial agonist opioids such as buprenorphine, and the mixed agonist-antagonist opioids such as pentazocine, butarphanol and nalbuphine. They have low maximal efficacy and exhibit a ceiling effect. Mixed agonist-antagonists have the potential to reverse analgesia and precipitate withdrawal reactions in patients taking opioid agonists. They are also associated with a high degree of dose dependent neurotoxic adverse effects. Long-term administration of meperidine (pethidine) is associated with a high incidence of neurotoxicity, as is propoxyphene. This is due to their nor-metabolites. Propoxyphene is not preferred. It is approximately half as potent as codeine.

Controlled or slow release formulations of opioids are generally taken every 12 hours but there are some formulations of morphine that can be taken once a day. Their less frequent dosing is convenient and may improve compliance. However, it is generally suggested that these formulations be used only when the pain is relatively stable (e.g. good pain control and the absence of a delirium or significant renal impairment). Unlike immediate release formulations, their longer half-lives make rapid dose titrations more precarious.

Route of opioid administration

The oral route for opioid delivery is effective and acceptable to most patients and is generally preferred for chronic opioid therapy. However, other routes may be required in selected patients, particularly those who are unable to swallow.

The subcutaneous route is as safe and effective as the intravenous route and arguably more convenient. When administered subcutaneously, opioids can be given either intermittently or continuously with preprogrammed pumps or syringe drivers. To facilitate the subcutaneous administration of opioids, a butterfly needle can be inserted subcutaneously and this single site can be used for several days. The bioavailability of parenterally administered opioids (morphine, hydromorphone, oxycodone, codeine) are generally 2–3 times that of the oral route and when switching from the oral route to the subcutaneous route, the dose needs to be halved or decreased to a third (Table 60.2). Intramuscular administration of opioids is not recommended.

Fentanyl is a highly potent semisynthetic opioid. It is administered via the transdermal or parenteral routes. Transderm fentanyl can control pain for up to 72 hours. This delivery method is particularly useful in patients with stable pain. Transdermal fentanyl is generally not appropriate for patients being initiated on opioid therapy or patients with very unstable pain syndromes. This is due to the considerable delay in reaching steady-state plasma levels when administered transdermally, making rapid dose titrations not possible. Once a dose of 600 μg per hour is reached, patch application becomes impractical. When switching to transdermal fentanyl patch from an immediate release formulation of another opioid, the previous opioid and the patch should overlap for up to 12 hours. Conversely, when switching from transdermal fentanyl to another opioid, a period of up to 12 hours may be required from the time the patch is removed to when the new opioid is started. In the interim, pain should be managed with breakthrough doses.

The rectal route can be useful for selected patients when the medication is administered as suppositories or liquid solutions. One of the major limitations of this route is the inconvenience and discomfort to some patients, especially when it is needed on a regular 4 hourly basis. There is currently a lack of adequate evidence to support opioid administration by inhalation. This route of delivery has poor bioavailability and is unreliable. The absorption of morphine and, to a lesser extent, hydromorphone and oxycodone is poor via the sublingual or buccal routes and therefore not recommended. Fentanyl appears to be an exception. Its high liphophilicity makes it a potentially useful opioid to be administered sublingually or buccally. While the lozenge form is available in some countries, the parenteral formulation can be used sublingually. The maximum volume that can be taken sublingually without spilling into the oral cavity appears to be 1 mL. Doses of 25 μg, titrated up to 50 μg, can be tried for incident pain: for example, prior to a procedure that elicits pain for a patient, such as turning in bed.

A very small, select group of patients may benefit from opioids administered epidurally or intrathecally. It has been reported that approximately 3–10% of patients' cancer pain will require opioids via these two routes, particularly those patients who are responsive to opioids but develop excessive side effects to oral or parenteral administration. However, prospective studies have not shown a clear advantage of the intraspinal or epidural routes over the more conventional parenteral or oral ones and opioid toxicity can often be managed by less invasive methods, such as switching opioids. The more generalised use of the epidural and intraspinal routes is limited by various factors. These include high costs, the risk of introducing infections into the spinal cord, the potential for catheter blockage, and the invasiveness of the procedure. Furthermore, specialised services that will insert and maintain the epidural and spinal catheters are seldom available outside large centres.

Opioid administration, titration and maintenance

Most patients with cancer pain require fixed scheduled dosing to manage the constant pain and prevent the pain from worsening. An as-needed rescue dose (breakthrough dose) should be combined with the regular fixed schedule opioid to control the episodic exacerbation of pain, often referred to as breakthrough pain. When this pain is elicited by an action such as weight-bearing, breathing or defecation, it is termed 'incident' pain. Rescue or breakthrough doses can be on an hourly as-needed basis. The breakthrough dose is generally calculated to be 10% or 1/6 of the total dose of the breakthrough.

There is no maximum dose or ceiling dose for the strong opioid agonists. Dose titration should continue until good pain relief is achieved or intolerable side effects intervene. The goal is to achieve a favourable balance between analgesia and side effects through gradual adjustments of the dose.

The appropriate dosing interval is determined by the opioid used and its formulation. The analgesic effects of short-acting oral opioids such as morphine, hydromorphone, codeine and oxycodone begin within a half-hour after administration and usually last for approximately 4 hours. The dosing interval of these drugs is therefore usually 4 hours. In patients given controlled release formulations of morphine, hydromorphone, codeine or oxycodone, relief should begin in 1 hour, peak in 2–3 hours and last for 12 hours. They are therefore usually prescribed in 12 hourly intervals. However, there is a small group of patients (10–20% of those on 12 hourly controlled release formulations) who may require administration every 8 hours. A new formulation of morphine is now available that allows for once daily administration. The analgesic effect of transdermal fentanyl begins approximately 12 hours after the application of the patch, peaks in 24–48 hours, and lasts for about 72 hours. Patches are therefore changed every 72 hours.

The severity of the pain and the opioid formulation chosen determines the rate of titration. The dose of immediate release formulations can be increased on a daily basis if necessary until pain relief is adequate. Patients with moderate uncontrolled pain require daily increases of between 25% and 50% to their previous dose while patients with severe uncontrolled pain may require a higher increase. This refers to lower doses. At higher opioid doses, increases of 25–30% are prudent. Occasionally doses may need to be reduced or withheld. Indications for dose reductions include renal failure, significant pain relief following a procedure such as irradiation, and significant opioid related sedation that is accompanied by good pain control.

Opioid adverse effects

The most common side effects of opioids include constipation, nausea and somnolence. There are numerous strategies for preventing or managing these. Constipation is probably the most common adverse effect and very little, if any at all, tolerance develops to it. Therefore, patients on long-term opioid therapy require an ongoing regular bowel care regimen, including laxatives. Bowel care should include a stimulant (e.g. sennoside) as well as a stool softener (e.g. docusate). Bulk-forming agents such as fibre require a large fluid intake and are not well tolerated by patients with advanced cancer. The doses of the laxatives need to be adjusted in order to provide a bowel movement at least every 3 days. If no bowel movement has occurred after 3 days, a fleet-enema or bisacodyl suppository may be required. Sedation and nausea are frequent adverse effects during initial exposure to opioid analgesics or on increasing opioid doses. However, tolerance to these effects develops rapidly and they both tend to resolve spontaneously within a few days. Patients should be warned not to drive for the first few weeks following initiation of opioid therapy or increases in opioid dose. Antiemetics may be prescribed on an as-needed basis or a regular basis for the first few days. Antiemetic agents that have antidopamine properties (to counteract the opioid's stimulation of the chemoreceptor trigger zone) and pro-motility action on the gut are recommended. Examples of these are metoclopramide and domperidone. The former may cause some extrapyramidal adverse effects, yet these are not seen frequently in palliative patients.

In the process of titrating an opioid, some patients may develop intolerable adverse effects. These may be in the form of opioid-related neurotoxicity. They manifest clinically as myoclonus, hallucinations, cognitive impairment, agitated behaviour, hyperalgesia and/or allodynia. They have been described in patients taking a variety of opioids, including morphine, hydromorphone, oxycodone and fentanyl. Patients with renal impairment are at a higher risk of developing these, as are those on higher doses. Myoclonus presents as muscle jerks. The clinical implications of these toxicities are significant. Apart from their inherent morbidity, hyperalgesia or allodynia can erroneously be interpreted as uncontrolled pain, as can delirious agitation and grimacing. It is suspected that active opioid metabolites, and to a lesser degree the opioids themselves, are responsible for these toxicities.

Several strategies are suggested for managing the neurotoxicities. Switching from the offending opioid (e.g. morphine) to an alternative opioid (e.g. hydromorphone or oxycodone) is gaining acceptance as one such strategy, particularly when the toxicity is severe or pain is poorly controlled. When switching from one opioid to another, equianalgesic dose tables are used to calculate the dose of the new opioid. A further 25–50% dose decrease is suggested. For example, a patient who is on 100 mg of oral morphine per day may be switched to 2 mg hydromorphone orally every 4 hours (a total of 12 mg/day). Hydromorphone is 5 times more potent than morphine. (In this example, the equivalent dose of hydromorphone is 20 mg orally per day. A further 40% decrease brings the new dose to 12 mg per day, which when divided into 4-hourly doses, gives 2 mg of hydromorphone every 4 hours.) When switching, clinicians should note that the tables serve as guidelines and patients should therefore be seen more regularly during the switching process. An alternative option, particularly if the toxicity is not severe and pain is well controlled, is to reduce the opioid dose. Adequate hydration is helpful in facilitating the renal elimination of the opioid metabolites. Hydration may be done by hypodermoclysis. This technique requires the placement of a subcutaneous needle and the administration of fluid subcutaneously at volumes of up to 80–100 mL per hour or 2 or 3 daily doses of 500 mL. Some patients prefer that the fluid is administered overnight only. This technique is convenient and effective for patients where intravenous lines are not easily accessible (e.g. in the home or hospice settings). The use of benzodiazepines and other agents such as baclofen to manage opioid induced myoclonus or delirium is not recommended, neither is the use of opioid-antagonists such as naloxone. It must be stressed that opioids remain effective and safe agents, and the management of these adverse effects when they do occur is straightforward and effective.

Adjuvant analgesics and therapies

In patients with cancer pain, these drugs tend to be administered in combination with a primary analgesic, usually an opioid. They include medications from diverse classes of drugs. Adjuvant analgesics are generally less reliable than the opioids and should be considered after treatment with an opioid has been initiated. The decreased reliability of the adjuvants is reflected by a smaller proportion of treated patients who respond adequately, and slower onset of action. There exists large inter- and intraindividual variability in the response to the various adjuvant analgesics, sometimes requiring sequential therapeutic trials to identify the most useful one. Few studies have compared one with the other in the various syndromes and, despite their popularity, they have been subjected to limited clinical trials in the setting of cancer pain. The choice of a first-line adjuvant analgesic is therefore largely based on safety, potential interactions with other agents, and the experience and familiarity of the clinician with cancer pain management.

Numerous adjuvant analgesics are suggested for the management of neuropathic pain. Traditionally, the antidepressants (particularly amitriptyline and imipramine) have been used first line for the management of dysaesthetic pain. It is not clear whether newer antidepressant agents such as the SSRIs are as effective. It is generally suggested that the antidepressants be started at low doses and, particularly in the elderly, titrated slowly up. Analgesic effects usually manifest at doses lower than those used for the management of depression. Second-line agents would include the anticonvulsants and corticosteroids. Palliative radiation therapy can be useful where tumours are affecting large neurological structures (e.g. brachial plexopathy). The anti-convulsants, particularly gabapentin and carbamazepine, are suggested as first-line adjuvant agents for the lancinating type of neuropathic pain. Gabapentin starting doses of 100 mg orally 3 times a day are suggested, followed by dose titration up to 1800–2400 mg per day. Corticosteroids may also be helpful in select patients. Dexamethasone is usually used. The optimal dose is unknown but starting doses of between 4 mg and 8 mg twice to three times a day are acceptable, followed by a tapering regimen.

In recent years, N-methyl-D-aspartic acid (NMDA) receptor antagonists have received much attention and show great promise in the setting of neuropathic pain. Currently available NMDA antagonist agents, with the exception of methadone that has both opioid receptor agonist and NMDA antagonist properties, cause too many central nervous system side effects. Other second line adjuvant agents for neuropathic pain are oral local anaesthetics such as mexiletine and α-2 adrenergic agents such as clonidine.

The optimal time to add an adjuvant analgesic to an opioid regimen, particularly in neuropathic pain, is not clear. One school of thought suggests that an adjuvant analgesic be added as soon as neuropathic pain is diagnosed, while another suggests that (given that approximately two-thirds of patients with neuropathic pain respond to opioids alone, albeit at higher doses) the opioid should first be titrated up before an adjuvant analgesic is considered.

Localised metastatic bone pain is best treated with external palliative radiation therapy. Up to 85% of patients receiving this therapy will experience a response with as many as 30% of patients experiencing complete resolution of pain. Adverse effects, unlike in the setting of radical radiation therapy, are minimal. Single fractions to the affected long bones appear as effective and more convenient than multiple fractions. NSAIDs have traditionally been used as adjuvant analgesics for bone pain. However, their use is limited by side effects and concerns about gastrointestinal and renal toxicity, particularly in vulnerable elderly patients with advanced cancer. The use of these drugs is likely to improve with the advent of cyclogenase-2 selective inhibitors, which lack significant gastrointestinal effects but do not entirely protect the kidneys. Generalised bone pain from extensive bone metastases deserves the consideration of a bisphosphonate such as clodronate or pamidronate. These agents have been shown to decrease the risk of skeletal events such as pathological fractures, hypercalcaemia and pain when administered regularly, every 2–3 weeks in the case of clodronate and every 4–6 weeks in the case of pamidronate. Clodronate, unlike pamidronate that requires intravenous administration, can be administered subcutaneously. Calcitonin is frequently touted for malignant bone pain but the little evidence that exists in the setting of cancer pain is contradictory. Once again, corticosteroids can be useful as well. Radioactive nuclides, such as strontium, are systematic treatments that can be useful when there is extensive bone involvement. However, they are expensive and may cause bone suppression in patients with very advanced cancer.

Colicky pain associated with complete, irreversible malignant bowel obstruction may require an antispasmodic, such as hyoscine butylbromide.

An approach to optimising the adjuvant analgesics is as follows:

- Optimise opioids as first-line agents before considering an adjuvant analgesic.
- One adjuvant should be added at a time to avoid drug interactions and polypharmacy.
- Side effects should be monitored for and the drug discontinued if intolerable adverse effects occur.

Other non-pharmacological methods apart from radiation therapy include anaesthetic procedures, neurosurgical procedures, occupational/physiotherapy modalities (such as relaxation therapy) and transcutaneous electrical nerve stimulation. Coeliac plexus blocks can be useful for patients with pancreatic cancer, while local anaesthetics administered intraspinally may help refractory cases of incident pain, particularly if the pain originates in the pelvis.

Cordotomies may be performed for patients with severe unilateral pain, especially pain in the pelvis or lower limbs. These options are third-line strategies and are to be considered only in patients with refractory symptoms. Local blocks such as intercostal blocks, brachial plexus blocks and femoral blocks have limited value in these patients.

In some cases, particularly those involving pathological fractures of the hips and lower extremities, surgery offers definitive therapy for controlling pain and providing mobility. An expected survival of only weeks to months is not necessarily a contraindication to surgery. As with any treatment modality, the potential benefits to be gained with surgery need to be weighed against the potential risks and drawbacks.

Difficult pain problems and spinal cord compression

Incident pain has been defined as pain that occurs following certain activities, such as moving, weight-bearing, swallowing or defecation. Opioid doses often need to be increased to control these episodes of pain. The frequency of these episodes can range from a few times a day to many times a day, incapacitating patients. The use of short-acting, potent opioids such as fentanyl administered sublingually or parenterally may be useful for a select group of patients. Neuropathic pain often results in the use of higher opioid doses and the addition of adjuvant analgesics.

Any cancer patient who presents with back pain or limb weakness needs to be assessed for the presence of spinal cord compression. If the clinical signs are suggestive of a spinal cord compression (motor and sensory deficits, loss of bladder/bowel control, tenderness of vertebral column), the patient should be started on a relatively high dose of corticosteroids (e.g. 10 mg dexamethasone 4 times a day orally or subcutaneously) and be transferred immediately for further investigations (MRI) at the closest oncology referral centre. The degree to which neurological status will improve is directly dependent on the promptness of diagnosis and definitive management, which in most cases consists of decompression by irradiation.

Pain management and opioid use in the elderly

Two issues related specifically to the assessment and management of elderly palliative patients with opioids need to be highlighted. The first one is the challenge of assessing pain in cognitively impaired patients and the second one is the increased sensitivity of elderly patients to the effects of opioids and their increased vulnerability to drug interactions between opioids and other drugs.

The inability of cognitively impaired patients to communicate and report pain is a substantial barrier to pain assessment and leads to suboptimal therapy. A major difficulty in assessing and managing pain in the presence of cognitive impairment is the inability of these patients to self-report their experience of pain. Nevertheless, studies suggest that cognitive impairment, including that related to dementia, does not alter the fundamental experience of pain and pain perception does not change with advancing age. Patients with dementia are often unable to express pain adequately, recall painful episodes and request analgesics. Although some investigators have attempted to assess pain in these patients with mixed results, the tools and scales rely upon caregivers or health care professionals who are quite familiar with the patient. They can note and respond to subtle changes in a patient's affect and behaviour. In the absence of a reliable measurement, clinicians should be vigilant about the needs of these patients and be proactive in their care.

It has been suggested by some that opioid requirements decrease with advancing age. Rather, it appears the elderly experience similar pain intensity to their younger counterparts, but may require a smaller amount of opioid analgesia. Pharmacokinetic (e.g. changes in body composition and/or in function of drug-eliminating organs) or pharmacodynamic (e.g. increased sensitivity of the central nervous system to opioids and their metabolites) factors could be responsible, at least in part.

The elderly are more likely to be affected by the acute and chronic toxicities of opioids. The elderly generally show decreased opioid clearance with a trend to a smaller volume of distribution. Given doses of an opioid may be clinically effective for longer periods. This is compatible with decreased first-pass metabolism and clearance in the elderly.

Other symptoms in advanced cancer

Delirium

Delirium is one of the most common neuropsychiatric complications of advanced cancer and occurs in up to 85% of patients in their last weeks of life. It frequently goes unrecognised and imposes an additional burden of distress on the patient, family and staff. Awareness and attention deficits impede communication with families and caregivers, and hinder participation in symptom assessment, treatment decisions and counselling.

The clinical features of delirium are numerous and are discussed in Chapter 16 of this book. Three clinical presentations of delirium are recognised: a hyperactive form, a hypoactive form and a mixed form with alternating agitation and hypoactivity. The latter is the most common in palliative care. The hyperactive form and its accompanying restlessness, agitation and groaning may be misdiagnosed as uncontrolled pain, while the hypoactive form may be misinterpreted as depression with withdrawal. The need for maintaining a high vigilance needs to be emphasised. Early recognition requires regular screening and monitoring.

The approach to managing delirium in patients with advanced disease includes a search for underlying causes, correction of those factors (if appropriate) and the management of symptoms such as hallucinations, paranoia, agitation and confusion. The desired outcome is a patient who is able to communicate coherently, is alert, free of psychotic features and comfortable, or, at the very least, a patient who is not agitated. Family members need to be educated about the problem and kept up to date with the process.

The most common aetiologies in the palliative care setting include drugs, infections, organ failure (e.g. hepatic and uraemic encephalopathy), electrolyte imbalances (e.g. severe hyponatraemia and hypercalcaemia), dehydration, hypoxia and central nervous system involvement (e.g. brain metastases). The aetiology is usually multifactorial. The drugs that are most commonly implicated are the opioids, antidepressants, benzodiazepines and anticonvulsants. When opioid induced toxicity is deemed to be an underlying cause, switching from one opioid agonist to another has been demonstrated to be helpful.

A combination of hydration and the administration of a bisphosphonate such as clodronate or pamidronate is used to treat hypercalcaemia. Clodronate, unlike pamidronate, can be administered subcutaneously. The patient's medications should be reviewed and drugs such as antidepressants and benzodiazepines be discontinued where possible. Investigations that may assist in identifying the underlying causes can be useful. These include the blood levels of electrolytes, calcium, albumin and indicators of renal functioning such as urea and creatinine. Imaging studies of the brain may be required where metastatic brain involvement is suspected. It must be noted that in the setting of advanced cancer, the underlying aetiologies of delirium may not be easily identifiable.

In a patient who does not have incurable disease, it is clear that attempts should be made to seek and reverse underlying causes. However, this decision can be challenging in a patient deemed to be in the terminal stages of cancer. On the one hand, delirium is viewed by some to be a natural part of the dying process that should not be altered, while on the other hand it is recognised that delirium is a very distressing problem and that a significant number of episodes are reversible with interventions of relatively low invasiveness. In those cases that are deemed irreversible, the goal is to minimise agitation, hallucinations and overall discomfort.

In addition to addressing the underlying causes of delirium, symptomatic and supportive therapies are required. Symptomatic treatment with neuroleptic drugs is generally required. Neuroleptics such as haloperidol and loxapine can be useful. These should be considered temporary measures while the strategies described above are being implemented. Benzodiazepines, with the exception of midazolam (see below), should be avoided.

Palliative sedation has been defined as the intention to induce sleep in a patient with refractory symptoms who is perceived to be close to death. All attempts should be made to reverse or control the delirium prior to considering this form of sedation, and palliative sedation should be viewed as a last resort in patients close to death. The more common reasons for initiating palliative sedation are severe, intractable agitated delirium and shortness of breath. The role of palliative sedation for profound spiritual or existential anguish that is not amenable to spiritual or psychological counselling is unclear and requires further ethical considerations. Midazolam can be titrated rapidly to achieve the goal of inducing rest without respiratory depression. It can be administered subcutaneously. Starting doses of 1–4 mg per hour are generally adequate. Sometimes, sedation could be a short-term measure while underlying causes are being addressed. The decision to use this approach should be undertaken with the patient's and/or family's consent (if the patient cannot make the decision). Patients and their families should be informed that palliative sedation is not intended to shorten a person's life and generally does not have that effect. The clinician needs to clearly document the indications, the attempts at using other management means and the intent of the sedation treatment.

Dyspnoea and coughing

Dyspnoea (see Chapter 27) is defined as an uncomfortable awareness of breathing. Dyspnoea, therefore, like pain, is a subjective experience. Patients with comparable degrees of functional lung impairment and disease burden may express varying intensities of dyspnoea. Dyspnoea is a common symptom, especially in advanced cancer patients, occurring in approximately 28–70% of these patients. About two-thirds of these patients rate the intensity of that symptom as moderate to severe. Dyspnoea can seriously affect the quality of life of these patients and a fear of suffocation is a frequent concern.

Assessment of this symptom is complicated by several factors. Objective signs such as tachypnoea or the use of accessory breathing muscles may not match the patient's perception of dyspnoea and the degree of functional impairment it causes. The multidimensional nature of this symptom must be noted. Numerous factors, including psychosocial ones, may impact upon the patient's expression of this symptom. Pulmonary function tests, with a few exceptions, generally play a limited role in the assessment of this syndrome. The temporal onset, the qualities of the symptom, associated symptoms, precipitating and relieving events or activities and responses to medications should be reviewed. Sudden onset may indicate a pulmonary embolism or infection, while gradual onset may suggest the development of a pleural effusion. A history of obstructive airways or cardiac disease can shed some light on possible underlying causes. Investigations, such as measuring oxygen saturation, can be useful in determining whether a patient is hypoxic or not. In the setting of advanced, incurable cancer, arterial blood gases play a limited role.

An attempt should be made to identify the underlying causes. A helpful approach is to divide them into 4 groups:

1. dyspnoea resulting from direct tumour effects, such as intrinsic or extrinsic airway obstruction, pleural involvement, parenchymal involvement either by primary or metastatic disease, and superior vena cava syndrome
2. dyspnoea caused by indirect tumour effects such as pneumonia or a pulmonary embolus
3. treatment related causes such as pulmonary fibrosis secondary to radiation therapy or chemotherapy or chemotherapy induced cardiomyopathy
4. causes unrelated to the cancer. These include chronic obstructive airway disease and congestive heart failure.

Another approach is to consider the causes of dyspnoea as originating either from the lung, systemically from factors, such as a severe anaemia, or from extrapulmonary causes, such as cardiac failure, pericardial tamponade, severe ascites (that restricts the diaphragm) or severe cachexia.

Diagnostic tests that may be helpful in determining the aetiology of dyspnoea include chest imaging by radiography, computerised tomography, complete blood counts, oxygen saturation at rest and with exercise, and to a much lesser extent, pulmonary function tests. Maximal inspiratory pressure (MIP) is sometimes severely impaired in cancer patients with cachexia.

Management should include interventions that are directed at both the underlying causes and the symptom. Specific treatments for the underlying causes should be considered and these are described in detail elsewhere. They include thoracenteses and pleurodeses for exudative pleural effusions; optimal management of chronic obstructive airway disease with bronchodilators and corticosteroids; antibiotic treatment of pneumonia; paracentesis for severe ascites; and the management of superior vena cava syndromes. Corticosteroids may be useful for managing dyspnoea related to lymphangitic carcinomatosis. However, their role here has not been well studied.

Symptomatic management of dyspnoea relies on oxygen therapy, opioid therapy, the correction of aggravating factors such as anaemia, and general, non-pharmacological modalities. A number of randomised controlled trials have provided compelling evidence to support the use of oxygen for the symptomatic treatment of hypoxia. The role of oxygen in the treatment of non-hypoxia related dyspnoea in cancer patients is less clear. Several randomised controlled trials have demonstrated the benefit of systemic opioids for patients with cancer related dyspnoea. Initiation and maintenance of opioid therapy for this indication is done similarly to, and is often concurrent with, the use of opioids for pain control. Nebulised opioids have not been shown to be more effective than systematically administered opioids in palliative patients. Chlorpromazine and promethazine have been shown to decrease dyspnoea without affecting ventilation in non-cancer patients, but their role in cancer related dyspnoea is unclear. The role of benzodiazepines appears to be limited to where dyspnoea is considered a somatic manifestation of a panic disorder or when a patient has concurrent severe anxiety.

In addition to adequate pharmacological therapies, a number of non-pharmacological measures are suggested. These include pursed lip breathing, diaphragmatic and muscle training, cold air directed across the cheek, meditation, relaxation training, biofeedback techniques and psychotherapy. The effectiveness of these in relieving breathlessness appears to be variable.

In some patients, chronic coughing may be the source of major suffering. It can cause pain, interfere with sleep, aggravate dyspnoea and worsen fatigue. The causes of cough can be classified much the same way as the causes of dyspnoea and the optimal therapy, as for dyspnoea, is the treatment of the underlying disorder. Cough-suppressing agents such as opioids are commonly utilised. Anecdotal evidence suggests a role for inhaled local anaesthetics. However, these should be utilised judiciously and sparingly: they are unpleasant to the taste, anaphylactic reactions to preservatives in these solutions have been documented and they obtund the gag reflex. Recently, inhaled sodium cromoglycate has shown promise as a safe method of controlling chronic coughing related to lung cancer.

Nausea, vomiting and bowel obstruction

Nausea and vomiting is a common symptom in patients with advanced cancer. The prevalence varies from 21% to 68% in these patients and the underlying pathophysiological processes often differ from those of nausea related to chemotherapy or radiation therapy.

Chronic nausea in the setting of advanced cancer is a multicausal condition and attempts should be made to identify and manage underlying factors. In the setting of advanced cancer nausea it is often associated with the anorexia-cachexia syndrome, the clinical manifestations of which include nausea, anorexia, asthenia and autonomic failure. Autonomic dysfunction gives rise to decreased gastrointestinal motility and this may manifest as chronic nausea, constipation and early satiety. Concurrent treatments such as opioid therapy further compromise gastrointestinal motility. Apart from decreasing gastrointestinal motility, opioids cause nausea by direct stimulation of the chemoreceptor trigger zone (CTZ) and, to a much lesser degree, the vestibular apparatus. Nausea may follow the initiation of opioid therapy or increases in opioid doses, but this is generally short-lived. Other causes of chronic nausea in these patients include other metabolic abnormalities, such as hypercalcaemia and uraemia, increased intracranial pressure and gastroduodenal ulcers. The accumulation of active opioid metabolites, such as morphine-6-glucuronide, may cause nausea.

In cases where chronic nausea appears refractory, continuous subcutaneous infusion of metoclopramide, at doses of 60–120 mg per day, may be helpful. The judicious concomitant use of corticosteroids in selected patients can augment the above regimen. The exact mechanism of action and the optimal dose of corticosteroids for this indication has not been elucidated. Although 5-hydroxytryptamine ($5HT_3$) antagonists such as ondansetron have proven to be very useful for the management of chemo- and radiation-induced nausea, their role in treating chronic nausea in advanced cancer has not been well established.

A basic working knowledge of the emetic pathways and identification of possible underlying causes should guide antiemetic selection. For example, since opioids induce nausea mostly via the CTZ, an antiemetic that has antidopamine properties, such as metoclopramide or domperidone, should be the first-line treatment of opioid induced nausea. A further advantage of these drugs is that they have gastrointestinal prokinetic properties.

A comprehensive history that includes determining the frequency and effectiveness of bowel movements and laxative therapy is essential. Examination should, among others, attempt to exclude bowel obstruction, faecal impaction, dehydration and raised intracranial pressure. Examination should include a digital rectal examination. Concurrent medications should be reviewed for drugs such as NSAIDs and SSRIs. History taking and physical examination are poor at determining the extent to which constipation may be an underlying problem. A simple flat-plate X-ray of the abdomen has been demonstrated to be a useful tool in assessing faecal load. Surgical views of the abdomen may be helpful if a bowel obstruction is suspected. Investigations to determine blood levels of calcium, urea and renal parameters may be helpful.

On occasion, patients may present with refractory narcotic bowel syndromes that do not appear to improve, even with optimal combinations of prokinetic agents and laxative regimens. It appears that fentanyl may be associated with less constipation than other opioids. Oral administration of an opioid antagonist, specifically naloxone, may be able to ameliorate opioid induced constipation. However, there exists a risk of precipitating systemic opioid withdrawal.

The initial approach to assessing and managing malignant bowel obstruction in advanced cancer involves determining whether the obstruction is reversible or not, and whether the obstruction is partial or complete. In determining the potential for reversibility, suitability for surgery such as resection or intestinal bypassing should be assessed. Several medical options are available for improving the comfort of patients with inoperable bowel obstructions. Less aggressive palliative surgical procedures, such as the insertion of a venting gastrostomy tube, can provide considerable relief. Nasogastric tubes may be used temporarily until the obstruction resolves or a gastrostomy tube is inserted. Antiemetic agents with prokinetic properties are contraindicated in the presence of a complete obstruction, and alternative agents such as an antihistamine or haloperidol are required. A prokinetic agent, with close monitoring, may be useful if the obstruction is not complete. Corticosteroids (e.g. dexamethasone at starting dose of 6–10 mg subcutaneously 3–4 times a day) may be useful. The optimal dose and duration of treatment has not been clarified. Hydration and other drugs, such as opioids and antiemetics, should be administered via routes other than the oral one. The subcutaneous route can be very convenient and effective for both hydration and opioid administration. This route is as effective as the intravenous one, is less invasive and requires less maintenance than the intravenous one. Octreotide, a somatostatin analogue, can be useful at doses of 100–200 μg subcutaneously 3 times a day for refractory obstruction. If the obstruction causes severe colic, hyoscine butylbromide should be considered.

Asthenia

Asthenia is a broad symptom that appears to possess both physical and mental dimensions. It is characterised by:

1. fatigue or lassitude, which is defined as easy tiring occurring after usual or minimal effort and decreased capacity to maintain adequate performance accompanied by

2. generalised weakness, which is defined as the anticipatory sensation of difficulty in initiating activity and
3. mental fatigue, defined as the presence of impaired concentration, loss of memory and emotional lability. This can be confused with lethargy, which is defined as the difficulty in maintaining arousal.

Asthenia is one of the most common symptoms occurring in advanced malignancy. It is reported to occur in 40–70% of cancer patients who are not receiving antineoplastic therapy. The pathophysiology of asthenia is complex and appears to be mediated by a combination of direct tumour effects, tumour induced host responses, and other cancer related factors. Asthenia and cachexia, although distinct symptoms, share aetiological mechanisms. Tumour derived products and host derived cytokines appear to play a central role. Most patients with advanced cancer experience symptoms of both asthenia and cachexia simultaneously, but some patients, such as those with breast cancer, may experience asthenia but no cachexia.

Asthenia is elusive and difficult to assess. Fatigue is often found as a single item or scale in self-report measures of symptoms, mood and functional status, reflecting the effect of fatigue and the interaction of fatigue with other symptoms or concepts related to quality of life. An important aspect to the assessment is identifying possible underlying causes or factors aggravating it. These include anaemia, infection, hypoxia, autonomic dysfunction, overexertion, psychological distress, and electrolyte disorders such as hyponatraemia.

The therapeutic approach to managing asthenia involves identifying and treating, where possible, specific underlying causes, as well as treating specific symptoms by pharmacological and non-pharmacological means. The goal is to decrease the intensity of asthenia and improve functioning. Appropriate, realistic goals of intervention need to be established. Corticosteroids may be of benefit, albeit temporarily. Psychostimulants may also help improve activity. At the forefront of the management are non-pharmacological measures and communication. These consist of keeping the patient informed about her condition and allowing the patient to develop realistic expectations. Adapting the activities of daily living and occupational therapy are suggested.

Cachexia, anorexia and artificial nutrition

Over 80% of patients with advanced cancer develop cachexia, and anorexia has been reported in up to 85% of these patients. In general, the frequency of anorexia/cachexia is higher in solid tumours compared with haematological malignancies. Apart from weight loss, cachexia is associated with fatigue, anorexia and chronic nausea, and is a source of psychological distress for patients and families because of the associated symptoms and altered body image. A common fear on the part of patients and families is that they will 'starve to death'. This fear may prompt aggressive nutritional supplementation in patients with advanced cancer.

Cachexia was previously thought to result primarily from direct tumour effects, such as consumption of calories and production of substances capable of disturbing metabolism and appetite. Based upon this assumption, aggressive nutrition was encouraged in an attempt to restore the energy balance—even for patients with advanced cancer. It is now recognised that the pathophysiology of cachexia is far more complex. It appears that metabolic abnormalities and central effects due to the production of cytokines (e.g. tumour necrosis factor, interleukin-1, interleukin-2 and interferon-γ) and tumour products (e.g. lipid-mobilising factor and protein-mobilising factor) play a central role. The result is catabolism of adipose tissue and skeletal muscle. In most patients, anorexia is more likely the result of the catabolic process than the cause of the cachexia. In most, anorexia is a symptom of cachexia. Aggressive nutritional support with the intent of increasing caloric intake has generally failed to improve survival, reduce treatment related toxicity and morbidity, and reverse cachexia in patients with advanced cancer. It is unclear if intensive artificial nutrition confers any symptomatic benefits. In the past the outcome measures were increased survival, tumour response, treatment toxicity and nutritional status. Improvements in anorexia along with improvements in other symptoms and functional status are now the main outcomes measured in patients with advanced cancer.

Although aggressive nutrition is generally not recommended in patients with end-stage cancer, a very select group of patients may benefit from this intervention: for example, patients with head and neck tumours that advance locally but metastasise slowly; patients recovering from surgery; and patients awaiting active oncological treatment. In patients deemed unsuitable for aggressive nutritional support, symptomatic treatment and supportive counselling of both patients and families is required. Several therapeutic options have been shown to improve the symptoms related to cachexia.

Objective tests are not routinely required in patients with advanced cancer. Symptom intensity can often be the most useful measurement in patients with advanced cancer. Visual analogue scales and numerical rating scales can be applied.

In the absence of evidence that aggressive nutritional support improves advanced cancer patients' outcomes, the goal of nutritional management should be to alleviate any hunger, to reduce anxiety about starvation, and to preserve the social aspects of mealtime. There are no benefits to forcing intake of meals or high-calorie oral preparations in these patients. Enteral nutrition may be useful in patients who have mechanical swallowing difficulties, but who retain good appetite and performance status, such as with head and neck cancer. A gastrostomy tube may be placed. Two main complications of this technique are aspiration and diarrhoea. These may be managed respectively by monitoring gastric residual and diluting hypertonic nutrient solutions. It is suggested that supplementation of water soluble vitamins such as B and C, as well as fat soluble vitamins such as E and K in severely cachectic patients, may be worth considering. It is proposed that the depletion of these vitamins contributes to the increased morbidity of these patients.

Several randomised placebo controlled trials have demonstrated the effects of different types of corticosteroids on cachexia-anorexia. Although appetite improvement was the most significant effect in these studies, none of the studies demonstrated weight gain. Numerous randomised controlled trials have demonstrated the benefits of progestational agents in terms of improved appetite, caloric intake and weight gain in cachectic patients. The nutritional effects of megestrol acetate are dose related and improvements have been noted with doses of 480 mg/day. Adverse effects include thromboembolism and peripheral oedema. Their high costs are problematic.

Depression

Some degree of emotional distress is a normal response to a cancer diagnosis, particularly if the cancer is deemed to be incurable. For most, the distress is transient and resolves with time and with general supportive care. The challenge is differentiating between the expected emotional distress associated with a cancer diagnosis (such as shock, sadness, grief, bereavement and anger) and a major depression. Research suggests that approximately half the patients diagnosed with cancer or with recurrence of cancer will adjust adequately without symptoms beyond those regarded as normal. The symptoms abate as the crisis resolves. In approximately 15–20% of palliative patients, depression becomes a major symptom. The incidence may be higher in patients with very advanced disease or with pancreatic cancer.

The exact frequency of depression in patients with advanced cancer is not well known. Research in the area has been hampered by the lack of standardised methodology and diagnostic criteria, as well as significant differences in the nature of patient populations studied. The belief that 'all patients with advanced cancer are depressed' grossly overestimates the prevalence of major depression in patients with advanced cancer. However, it is also recognised that depression as a major symptom is often poorly managed in patients with advanced cancer.

The largest challenge in assessing for depression in patients with cancer, particularly advanced cancer, is how best to interpret the physical (somatic) symptoms of depression. Commonly utilised criteria for diagnosing major depression include both somatic (physical) and psychological criteria. However, it is argued that in the context of advanced cancer, somatic symptoms such as anorexia, weight loss, psychomotor retardation, insomnia and fatigue are highly prevalent and therefore lose their reliability and specificity for identifying a major depression in these patients. Utilising both the psychological and somatic criteria would increase the sensitivity but result in overdiagnosis. The question then is what should a clinician use. Some suggest focusing on the psychological symptoms of persistent dysphoria, feelings of helplessness and/or hopelessness, loss of self-esteem, feelings of worthlessness, and wishes to die as reliable diagnostic indicators. When these symptoms overwhelm the patient or interfere with functioning, treatment is indicated.

The issue of symptom severity threshold is relevant. For example, hopelessness that is pervasive and profound is suggestive of a major depressive disorder. A major depression should also be considered if a patient is incapacitated by recurrent feelings of hopelessness, guilt, worthlessness and a wish to die. Suicidal ideation, even when mild, is likely to be associated with significant degrees of depression in patients with advanced cancer. Anhedonia appears to be another salient factor in identifying depression in these patients. A past history of a major depressive disorder is perhaps one of the most important factors associated with increased vulnerability to developing depression during the course of a cancer illness.

Chochinov and colleagues have suggested that a single item—namely the question 'Are you depressed?'—correlates well with various tools when screening for depression in terminally ill patients. The authors emphasise that this approach cannot be used for diagnosis.

Assessment of suicide risk, followed by prompt management, is critical. Suicidal ideation, when it occurs, is frightening for the patient, family and for the caregivers. Uncontrolled pain and symptoms for prolonged periods of time in cancer patients is an important risk factor for suicide, as are loss of control, profound feelings of hopelessness, helplessness, pre-existing psychopathology, family history of suicide, previous attempts, inadequate social supports and delirium. The role depression plays in cancer suicide is significant and all patients should be asked for the presence of profound psychological symptoms, including hopelessness, guilt, worthlessness, death wish and suicidal ideation.

Depression in cancer patients is optimally managed through a combination of supportive psychotherapy and pharmacological interventions. Numerous factors are involved in selecting the type of antidepressant for a particular patient. Various classes of antidepressants have been utilised, including conventional agents such as the tricyclic antidepressants (TCAs) and the SSRIs. The lower frequency of sedative and autonomic effects as compared with tricyclics make SSRIs particularly interesting for use in patients with advanced cancer. Unfortunately, there is limited experience with this group of drugs in patients with advanced cancer. Nausea and increasing anxiety may occur, however. Fluvoxamine has been reported to cause more nausea than the others. Fluoxetine generally has a stimulating effect while sertraline, fluvoxamine and fluoxetine are more sedating. Interindividual variation with respect to the emergence of various adverse effects and antidepressant response has been noted. Fluoxetine has a long half-life and its use in these patients is discouraged. The advantages of paroxetine relative to other SSRIs are its short half-life and lack of active metabolites. One should note that withdrawal symptoms consisting of abdominal cramps and flu-like symptoms have been described following abrupt discontinuation of SSRIs. It should also be noted that SSRIs (particularly paroxetine and fluoxetine) are active inhibitors of the enzyme responsible for metabolising oxycodone and codeine to active analgesic forms. It is recommended that, to decrease the risk of untoward effects, the SSRIs and TCA be started at the lowest possible doses and then be titrated gradually upwards. Unfortunately, there is a paucity of data with respect to the use of SSRIs in cancer patients. Tricyclic antidepressants have been better studied in patients with advanced cancer. Although nearly 70% of patients treated with a TCA improved, these drugs have side effect profiles that limit their usefulness in advanced cancer patients. The main side effects relate to the central and peripheral anticholinergic side effects, capable of causing or aggravating delirium, constipation, dry mouth, urinary retention and postural hypotension. In cancer patients, the usual recommendation, as with most other patient groups, is to 'start low and go slow'.

Psychostimulants as a class offer an alternative pharmacological approach to the treatment of depression in the terminally ill, particularly those with limited life expectancy. The most commonly utilised psychostimulants are methylphenidate and dextroamphetamine. These agents are particularly useful in cancer patients who are suffering from depressed mood accompanied by significant psychomotor retardation, decreased energy and poor concentration. The psychostimulants exert an effect within a few hours to 2–3 days—far more rapidly than the 4–6 week latency period of the more conventional antidepressants. Methylphenidate is generally started at a dose of 5 mg at 8 am and 5 mg at noon. This is preceded by a test dose of 2.5–5 mg and the course is continued if no intolerable adverse effects such as severe anxiety, tremors or psychoses occur. Contraindications include the presence of an agitated delirium. The dose may need to be titrated with time and seldom needs to exceed 30 mg per day.

Conclusion

Terminally ill patients may experience multiple physical and psychological symptoms, functional decline, spiritual or existential distress, family disruption, financial concerns, spiritual distress and many other issues and problems that may affect the quality of their lives and those of their families. Optimum care should be viewed from the broad perspective of palliative care that aims to maintain quality of life throughout the course of the disease. All clinicians who treat patients with cancer and other incurable illnesses must acknowledge the importance of palliative care as part of good medical practice and focus appropriately on the knowledge and practical skills needed to address concerns about quality of life.

Assessing and managing difficult symptoms in patients with cancer, particularly in the setting of advanced disease, depends on a systematic approach. This approach should include regular monitoring and documentation of symptom intensity, effect on functioning and other parameters such as cognitive functioning. This allows for prompt response to the appearance of symptoms and problems and the ability to monitor responses to therapeutic interventions. Most of the symptoms experienced in advanced cancer have multiple causes, and the assessment and management revolves around identifying underlying causes and addressing these while providing symptomatic relief. The multidimensional nature of most of the symptoms must be appreciated, as well as their impact on other symptoms and other dimensions, such as psychological status. It is also recognised that psychological concerns can also impact dramatically on the expression of symptoms.

Bibliography and further reading

Bozzetti, F., Amadori, D., Bruera, E. et al. (1996), 'Guidelines on artificial nutrition versus hydration in terminal cancer patients', *Nutrition*, 12, pp. 163–7.

Breitbart, W., Bruera, E., Chochinov, H. & Lynch, M. (1995), 'Neuropsychiatric syndromes and psychological symptoms in patients with advanced cancer', *Journal of Pain and Symptom Management*, 10, pp. 131–41.

Breitbart, W. & Sparrow, B. (1998), 'Management of delirium in the terminally ill', *Progress in Palliative Care*, 6, pp. 107–13.

Bruera, E. (1997), 'ABC of palliative care: anorexia, cachexia and nutrition', *British Medical Journal*, 315, pp. 1219–22.

Bruera, E. & Higginson, E. (eds) (1996), *Cachexia-Anorexia in Cancer Patients*, Oxford University Press, Oxford, pp. 128–40.

Bruera, E., Kuehn, N., Miller, M. J., Selmser, P. & Macmillan, K. (1991), 'The Edmonton Symptom Assessment System (ESAS): a simple method for the assessment of palliative care patients', *Journal of Palliative Care*, 7, pp. 6–9.

Bruera, E. & Pereira, J. (1998), 'Recent developments in palliative cancer care', *Acta Oncologica*, 37, pp. 749–57.

Buckman, R. (1994), 'Communication in palliative care: a practical guide', in Doyle, D., Hanks, G. & Macdonald, N. (eds), *Oxford Textbook of Palliative Medicine*, 1st edn, Oxford University Press, Oxford, pp. 47–61.

Cherny, N., Arbit, E. & Jain, S. (1996), 'Invasive techniques in the management of cancer pain', in Cherny, N. & Foley, K. M. (eds), *Hematology/Oncology Clinics of North America — Pain and Palliative Care*, Vol. 10, W. B. Saunders, Philadelphia, pp. 121–37.

Cherny, N. & Foley, K. M. (eds) (1996), *Hematology/Oncology Clinics of North America—Pain and Palliative*

Care, Vol. 10, W. B. Saunders, Philadelphia, pp. 158–71.

Cherny, N. & Portenoy, R. K. (1994), 'Sedation in the management of refractory symptoms: Guidelines for evaluation and treatment', *Journal of Palliative Care*, 10, pp. 31–9.

Chochinov, H. M., Wilson, K. G., Enns, M. et al. (1994), 'Prevalence of depression in the terminally ill: Effects of diagnostic criteria and symptom threshold judgements', *American Journal of Psychiatry*, 151, pp. 537–40.

Derby, S. & Portenoy, R. K. (1997), 'Assessment and management of opioid-induced constipation', in Portenoy, R. K. & Bruera, E. (eds), *Topics in Palliative Care*, Vol. 1, Oxford University Press, New York, pp. 95–112.

Dudgeon, D. J. & Lertzman, N. (1998), 'Dyspnoea in the advanced cancer patient', *Journal of Pain and Symptom Management*, 16, pp. 212–19.

Fainsinger, R. L. (1996), 'Pharmacological approach to cancer anorexia and cachexia', in Bruera, E. & Higginson, E. (eds), *Cachexia-Anorexia in Cancer Patients*, Oxford University Press, Oxford, pp. 128–40.

Fainsinger, R. L. & Bruera, E. (1997), 'When to treat dehydration in a terminally ill patient?', *Supportive Care in Cancer*, 5, pp. 205–11.

Fainsinger, R. L., Schoeller, T. & Bruera, E. (1993), 'Methadone in the management of cancer pain: A review', *Pain*, 52, pp. 137–47.

Kuhl, D. R. & Wilensky, P. (1999), 'Decision making at the end of life: a model using an ethical grid and principles of group process', *Journal of Palliative Medicine*, 2, pp. 75–86.

MacDonald, N. (1998), 'Ethical issues in hydration and nutrition', in Portenoy, R. K. & Bruera, E. (eds), *Topics in Palliative Care*, Vol. 2, Oxford University Press, New York, pp. 153–63.

Maguire, P. (1985), 'Barriers to psychological care of the dying', *British Medical Journal*, 291, pp. 1711–13.

Maguire, P., Faulkner, A., Booth, K. et al. (1996), 'Helping cancer patients disclose their concerns', *European Journal of Cancer*, 32A, pp. 78–81.

Neuenschwander, H. & Bruera, E. (1998), 'Asthenia', in Doyle, D., Hanks, G. W. C. & Macdonald, N. (eds), *Oxford Textbook of Palliative Medicine*, Oxford University Press, Oxford, pp. 573–81.

Pereira, J. (1998), 'The management of cancer bone pain', in Portenoy, R. K. & Bruera, E. (eds), *Topics in Palliative Care*, Vol. 3, Oxford University Press, New York, pp. 213–27.

Pereira, J. & Bruera, E. (1996), 'Chronic nausea', in Bruera, E. & Higginson, E. (eds), *Cachexia-Anorexia in Cancer Patients*, Oxford University Press, Oxford, pp. 23–37.

Pereira, J. & Bruera, E. (1997), 'Emerging neuropsychiatric toxicities of opioids', *Journal of Pharmaceutical Care in Pain and Symptom Control*, 5, pp. 3–29.

Portenoy, R. (1996), 'Adjuvant analgesic agents', in Cherny, N. & Foley, K. (eds), *Hematology/Oncology Clinics of North America: Pain and Palliative Care*, Vol. 10, No. 1, W. B. Saunders Company, Philadelphia, pp. 103–20.

Portenoy, R. K., Thaler, H. T., Kornblith, A. B. et al. (1994), 'Symptom prevalence, characteristics and distress in a cancer population', *Quality of Life Research*, 3, pp. 183–9.

Watanabe, S. (1997), 'Intraindividual variability in opioid response: A role for sequential opioid trials in patient care', in Portenoy, R. & Bruera, E. (eds), *Topics in Palliative Care*, Vol. 1, Oxford University Press, New York, pp. 195–212.

Watanabe, S. & Bruera, E. (1996), 'Anorexia and cachexia, asthenia, and lethargy', in Cherny, N. & Foley, K. (eds), *Hematology/Oncology Clinics of North America: Pain and Palliative Care*, W. B. Saunders, Philadelphia, 10, pp. 189–206.

World Health Organization (1996), *Cancer Pain Relief*, 2nd edn, World Health Organization, Geneva.

Chapter 61

Euthanasia and physician assisted suicide: psychiatric conditions

LEONARD SCHWARTZ and HARVEY MAX CHOCHINOV

Box 61.1 Case presentation

An elderly widower with a complex medical history and a previous diagnosis of depression was referred for psychiatric consultation. He lived alone in an apartment, and while his family was out of town, he took a mixed overdose of various medications. He was discovered the next day on the floor of his apartment by the cleaning staff, who became suspicious when he did not answer his door.

The patient was taken to the emergency room where he was treated with gastric lavage, as well as respiratory and fluid support. He was admitted first to a medical ward, and was then transferred to a psychiatry ward.

Introduction

Euthanasia is defined as a positive act of commission, such as a lethal injection, which is undertaken deliberately by a physician to end the life of a patient who has asked to die. Physician assisted suicide (PAS) is the provision of advice or the means for an individual to take his own life. The essential distinction between euthanasia and PAS is that, in the former, the physician undertakes the final act that causes the patient's death, whereas in the latter case, the patient must take that final step. The conceptual distinction between these two acts is important; supporters of PAS argue that compared to euthanasia, PAS reduces the power imbalance between the physician and patient, limits the risk of undue coercion because of social or financial pressures, and offers greater protection to physicians in the event of legal action against them.

There are compelling reasons both for and against the provision of euthanasia and PAS, which reflect the deep divisions between proponents on either side of this debate. Supporters of voluntary euthanasia argue that it is a beneficent and compassionate act, which respects autonomy by preserving the patient's control over the manner, method and timing of his death. Furthermore, it takes the matter outside the reach of 'medical power' and prevents the injustice that allows some patients to choose death by refusing life support measures, while denying others the right to do so.

However, the opponents of voluntary euthanasia argue that it undermines the value of, and respect for, human life. There is a concern that allowing such practices will lead to a 'slippery slope', which could result in involuntary euthanasia and the selective elimination of society's most vulnerable citizens. The practice of euthanasia requires the definition and clarification of the patient's underlying medical diagnosis and prognosis, demonstration of intolerable suffering and freedom to give his informed consent. Furthermore, the wish for euthanasia based on concerns regarding pain and fear of overly aggressive treatment could be addressed by better palliative care, analgesia and living wills. The opponents further argue that euthanasia undermines the physician–patient relationship, and defends socially sanctioned killing. Finally, many opponents base their arguments on the religious belief that human life is the gift of the Creator, and the decision to end life is not ours to make.

Attitudes towards euthanasia

The general public

It is now clear that the majority of the general public favour the decriminalising of euthanasia and PAS. In 1950, only about 30% of the American public favoured the legalisation of euthanasia for people with advanced terminal illness. By 1973, this number had risen to 53%, and had further risen to 63% by 1991. Recent Canadian data showed public support for legalisation is at least comparable to that in the US, with 65–79% of respondents in various parts of the country reporting that they would support the overall principle of voluntary euthanasia for the terminally ill. A recent survey of 100 American patients with amyotrophic lateral sclerosis (ALS) showed that 56% stated that they would consider assisted suicide, and 44% agreed with the statement: 'if physician assisted suicide were legal, I would request a lethal prescription from a physician' (although not necessarily for imminent use). Patients in favour of PAS were more likely to be male, have a higher level of education, and be less religious than those who were opposed to this practice.

Religious involvement appears to be the most consistent factor predicting one's stance on the legalisation of euthanasia and PAS. According to US opinion polls, highly educated, liberal respondents who were less religious were most likely to accept the notion of euthanasia or suicide of a terminally ill person. Age appears to be another relevant factor, with younger respondents expressing stronger endorsement of euthanasia than older adults. It is important to note that the response to the issue of euthanasia in public surveys differs markedly, depending on the hypothetical circumstances to which the decision is being applied. The most supportive opinions are expressed regarding scenarios involving patients with a terminal illness and unbearable pain. However, in situations involving non-terminal illness or physical disability and psychiatric disorders, opposition to euthanasia remains high.

Medical practitioners

A number of surveys of physician attitudes towards euthanasia and PAS have also been conducted. In general, the results show that physicians as a group are less favourably disposed towards these practices than is the public at large, but the profession remains evenly split over this issue. The level of support in studies that have asked physicians whether euthanasia or PAS would be acceptable in any circumstance has ranged from 44–60%. If it is legalised, 22–50% of physicians have reported they would be willing to practise either euthanasia or PAS. In one Canadian study of almost 1400 physicians, 51% stated that the law in Canada should be changed to permit patients to receive euthanasia, although only 28% of physicians reported they would be willing to personally participate in such practices.

In the American state of Oregon, residents who are adults can request assistance for suicide if they expect to die within 6 months, are capable of making and communicating to physicians decisions about their health care, and are able to take an oral dose of medication. In a survey of all 418 Oregon psychiatrists carried out prior to the legalisation of PAS, two-thirds of respondents agreed that PAS should be available, but one-third thought that it should never be allowed. Several large-scale American surveys have also been carried out. One recent survey showed that under current American law, 11% of doctors would be willing to hasten death by prescribing medication, while 7% would be willing to do so by lethal injection. These numbers rose to 36% and 24%, respectively, if this practice were to become legal. Almost 20% of the doctors who responded to the survey had received requests for PAS, and 11% had received requests for euthanasia. About 6% of the respondents acknowledged having either prescribed the medication for hastened death or administered a lethal injection to a terminally ill patient.

The rate of participation by doctors who practise euthanasia and PAS is much higher in some studies than in others. For example, over 50% of physicians working with AIDS patients in San Francisco have assisted in at least one suicide. These findings indicate that relatively large numbers of physicians have been in the position of having to respond in some way to a request for euthanasia or PAS, and some have taken part in these practices.

Patients with terminal illness

Only a handful of studies to date have been conducted with patients who actually have cancer or other potentially fatal illnesses. The majority of the participants in those studies consider it acceptable, at least in some circumstances, for physicians to provide terminally ill patients with euthanasia or PAS. Rates of approval ranged from 63% to 80%. These numbers are roughly equivalent to the responses found in surveys of the general public. The results also indicate that 32–56% of patients with life-threatening conditions would seriously consider asking for euthanasia or PAS at some future point in time, should such practices become legally available.

As noted earlier, persons with strong religious convictions are less likely to consider euthanasia or PAS than those who are not as religious. Pain intensity and other physical symptoms do not necessarily increase the patient's desire for euthanasia or PAS, although correlations between pain severity and a desire to die have been reported.

The survey of patients with ALS described above reported that the majority of respondents with this disorder would approve of assisted suicide in some circumstances. Patients in favour of PAS had higher levels of hopelessness and rated their quality of life as lower, compared with patients who were opposed to this practice. However, there was no difference found in the prevalence of depression. Other studies of terminally ill patients and ambulatory AIDS patients have demonstrated that depression and psychological distress was the most significant predictor of support for PAS. Patients request euthanasia and PAS for a variety of reasons. In a majority of cases, these reasons appear not to be related solely to physical suffering, although they do occur in the context of increasing frailty. Instead, patients' reasons are often related to existential concerns and psychosocial issues, such as loss of dignity or becoming a burden to their family—issues that are often, but not always, accompanied by depression.

Legal perspectives

Canada

In Canada, the Criminal Code regards euthanasia as an act of murder, subject to a mandatory life sentence. Assisted suicide is covered under Section 241 of the Criminal Code and is punishable by up to 14 years of imprisonment. In 1993, the Supreme Court of Canada upheld the legality of this provision, in response to an application by a 43-year-old woman named Sue Rodriguez, who at the time was suffering from ALS. The patient asked that a qualified physician set up the technological means by which she might, by her own hand, end her life at a time of her choosing. In their decision, a majority of the Supreme Court held that the provision against assisted suicide does not contravene the Canadian Charter of Rights and Freedoms.

United States

Approximately 30 of the 50 states have statutes that specifically prohibit suicide. States that do not proscribe assisted suicide by statute treat this conduct as murder or manslaughter under the general criminal law statutes. All forms of euthanasia are classified as murder in every state, even when performed at the victim's request and with his consent. American courts have considered petitions from patients seeking assisted suicide. The results are mixed: some courts allowed this practice, while others held that there was no constitutional right to PAS.

As noted earlier, only the state of Oregon allows physician assisted suicide. Oregon's *Death With Dignity Act* allows residents of the state who are 18 years of age or older to request PAS, provided certain requirements are met. Patients must be able to take an oral dose of medication, and they must voluntarily express the wish to die (with 2 oral requests that are at least 15 days apart), as well as one witnessed, and a written request for the attending physician to prescribe a lethal medication. A consulting physician must confirm the diagnosis, prognosis and capacity to make an informed choice. The attending doctor is required to review alternatives such as hospice and pain control, as well as outline the risks and results of a lethal dose with the patient. Referral to a mental health professional is mandatory if either the attending or consulting doctor is concerned that the patient's judgment may be impaired by a mental disorder.

A recent review was carried out on the cases of 33 patients who had received prescriptions for lethal medications after the law came into effect. The most frequent illnesses were cancer, ALS and chronic obstructive pulmonary disease. According to physicians and family members, patients requested PAS for several reasons, including loss of autonomy, loss of control of bodily functions and inability to participate in enjoyable activities, and the determination to control the manner of their death. A survey of over 4000 Oregon physicians found that 144 doctors had received 221 requests for lethal medications since the law came into effect. Eighteen per cent of the patients who requested lethal prescriptions received them. None of the patients who received a lethal prescription had symptoms of depression, but 20% of the patients who requested the medication did have such symptoms. The most important symptoms in the patients' decision to request a lethal prescription were pain, fatigue and shortness of breath. The most common conditions and values that were important to the patients' decision were loss of independence, poor quality of life, readiness to die, and the desire to control the manner of death. It is important to note that 46% of the patients for whom substantive palliative intervention (e.g. pain and symptom control) were made changed their minds about assisted suicide, compared with 15% of those for whom no substantive interventions were made.

Australia: The Northern Territory legislation

In Australia, the administration of the criminal justice system is a matter of individual state and territorial responsibility. In 1995, the State Legislature of the Northern Territory of Australia approved a Bill containing most of the same procedural safeguards as Oregon's *Death With Dignity Act*, but also providing for direct physician participation in euthanasia. The legislation gave a terminally ill person the right to voluntarily request assistance from a medically qualified person to terminate his life. The patient had to be at least 18 years of age, and the medical practitioner had to be satisfied that the patient suffered from a terminal illness, that there was no medical measure acceptable to the patient which could be reasonably undertaken in the hope of effecting a cure, and that any available treatment was purely for relief of pain, suffering and/or distress. Further investigation and examination by a second medical practitioner who confirmed the first doctor's diagnosis and prognosis was mandatory. Furthermore, the patient had to be of sound mind as attested to by a medical practitioner. For a 9 month period in 1996–97, the Northern Territory permitted lawful access to both euthanasia and PAS. During this time, 7 patients made application for physician hastened death under the *Rights of the Terminally Ill Act* and 4 of these patients died as a result. A study of the Australian experience noted that there could be wide differences of opinion among physicians about basic considerations as to whether an illness is terminal, and the extent of the individual patient's life expectancy. Secondly, mental health considerations represented significant concern in cases of euthanasia requests, as reflected in the fact that 4 of the 7 applicants had significant symptoms of depression. Finally, pain was not reported as a prominent clinical issue for these patients. Rather fatigue, frailty and other symptoms contributed more to their sense of suffering.

The Netherlands

In the Netherlands, euthanasia and PAS remain technically illegal, but are not prosecuted, provided extensive guidelines have been followed. These guidelines include that the patient is competent, freely initiates the request, that the request is persistent over time, and that the physical or mental suffering of the patient is unbearable. Furthermore, all alternatives must have been exhausted or refused and a second consulting physician must concur with the decision to perform euthanasia. The circumstances of the patient's death must be carefully documented. However, the Dutch law does not require that euthanasia be restricted only to patients who are terminally ill. The issue is framed more in terms of quality of life rather than medical prognosis.

Studies of the Dutch experience estimate that about 2.8% of all deaths in the Netherlands now occur from euthanasia, and these numbers are increasing over time. A further 0.3% of deaths occur as a result of PAS. In addition, another 0.7% of all deaths can be characterised as life-terminating acts, without the explicit request of the patients. A majority of these cases involve patients who are within days or hours of death and who are too ill to make their wishes known. The Dutch studies found that 68% of euthanasia or PAS deaths involved patients with the medical diagnosis of cancer. It would appear that 6–8% of all deaths among Dutch patients with advanced cancer can be attributed to euthanasia and related medical decisions. Surveys of Dutch medical practitioners have shown that between 48% and 63% of respondents have acknowledged participating in at least one act of euthanasia or PAS. Patients request these practices not so much because of physical suffering, but for reasons that include loss of dignity, 'unworthy dying', being dependent on others, and feeling 'tired of life'.

Pain and symptom management

Proponents of palliative care point out that only a small number of patients who are suffering from a terminal illness receive comprehensive palliative care. They argue that 'until all dying patients and their families have ready access to the full continuum of skilled and effective palliative services', the euthanasia and PAS debate is premature and cannot be addressed appropriately.

The argument is that terminally ill patients rarely request euthanasia when comprehensive palliative care is provided. Such care should include optimal symptom management, and an attentive, involved health care team in an appropriate setting. Some studies have shown that uncontrolled symptoms, especially uncontrolled pain, are major risk factors for suicide among advanced cancer patients. It is estimated that 60–90% of patients with advanced malignant disease will have pain of moderate or greater severity, and that 25% of patients will die without adequate pain relief. Lack of adequate knowledge and experience among physicians regarding pain management, combined with an unreasonable fear concerning opioid addiction (among patients and physicians) are thought to be common barriers to good pain control.

It is also important to consider uncontrolled symptoms besides pain that may influence the patient's request for PAS, or desire for death. In our case presentation (see Box 61.1), the patient was suffering not from uncontrolled pain, but from daily gastrointestinal difficulties stemming from his surgery for cancer. His physical wellbeing impacted significantly on his psychological wellbeing. In this context, it is interesting to note that many patients in the Netherlands withdraw their request for euthanasia after receiving better symptom control. Improved access to comprehensive terminal care might result in fewer patients requesting a hastening of their death.

Uncontrolled pain can cause patients to feel desperate, pushing them to desire death. Thus, palliative care management must address not only the actual physical pain, but also respond to the fear of having intractable pain. One-third of cancer patients in active therapy, and two-thirds of cancer patients with far advanced disease, have significant pain. Pain in AIDS patients is highly prevalent, affecting 40–60% of patients. Pain in AIDS is also dramatically undertreated: a recent study indicated that 40% of AIDS patients who were experiencing moderate to severe pain were not receiving any analgesics.

It has been demonstrated that over 90% of cancer pain can be managed with uncomplicated drug therapies. Yet there still remains an unacceptable level of undertreatment. Barriers include a lack of knowledge and training among health care professionals in the use of pain medications, and fear of addiction by physicians and patients. Unnecessary fear of opioid addiction has prevented many patients from receiving adequate treatment. Patients need to be educated about the differences between physical dependence, psychological dependence and tolerance. Clinicians who are familiar and comfortable with the use of opioids and adjuvant analgesics can help assure their patients that pain and comfort needs will be met, without fear of addiction. Availability of palliative care interventions should also be explained. It is helpful for the clinician to introduce the topic, taking an active role early on in treatment in order to identify patient concerns, and to make a commitment to patients that their pain and other distressing symptoms will be properly treated. Patients will then feel more supported and gain more confidence in their treatment.

Finally, physicians need to be able to distinguish—for both the patient and themselves—between pain control and euthanasia. Pain control serves the function of relieving pain and suffering; the administration of opioids and other adjuvant medication is often necessary for providing comfort. Treatment of pain is never a form of euthanasia; aggressive and appropriate treatment will be curtailed if physicians do not accept this differentiation. When discussing issues of pain and symptoms management with the patient, physicians should explore the patient's feelings about his level of alertness in the event that induced drowsiness or sedation are required for the relief of pain. Limitations in providing appropriate pain management can leave a patient susceptible to suffering, and exacerbate thoughts of suicide and requests for euthanasia.

Depression and other psychiatric symptoms

Appropriate screening for depression

Patients with cancer or other terminal illness are at increased risk of suicide compared with the general population. Suicide risk factors include pain, depression, delirium and deficit symptoms. In one study of psychiatric disorders among suicidal cancer patients, 39% were found to have a major depression, 54% were diagnosed with adjustment disorder with anxious and/or depressed features, and 20% were delirious. While a severe confusional state may render some patients unable to carry out self-destructive acts, mild delirium can place patients at higher risk due to its disinhibiting effect.

Depression plays a significant role in cancer suicide. It is thought that these patients are at up to 25 times greater risk of completed suicide than the general population. Depressive symptoms occur in approximately 25% of patients with advanced cancer, with 6–10% of patients meeting diagnostic criteria for major depression. Apart from an increased risk for suicide in some patients, depression also appears to be important in terms of the patient's choices for treatment. Among elderly depressed patients, an increase in desire for life-sustaining medical therapy followed appropriate treatment of depression in those patients who had initially been more severely depressed, or hopeless, and more likely to overestimate the risks and underestimate the benefits of treatment. Although patients with mild to moderate depression may be less likely to alter their decisions regarding life-sustaining treatment, severely depressed patients (especially those whose situations are hopeless) should be encouraged to defer making advance treatment directives. In these patients, decisions about life-sustaining treatment should be discouraged until the depression has been treated.

Given the importance of detecting depression in patients with terminal illness, how should the clinician go about making the diagnosis? In one recent study, 4 brief screening measures for depression in terminally ill patients were compared.

These measures were a single item interview, a 2-item interview, the Beck Depression Inventory (BDI)—Short Form (score greater than 7) and a Visual Analogue Scale Score (score less than 56). The equivalent of the single item interview was a question which, in essence, asked if patients were feeling depressed most of the time. These measures were administered to 197 patients receiving palliative care for advanced cancer; patients were also assessed using a diagnostic interview that contained items pertaining to the diagnoses of major and minor depression. The results from the screening measures were then compared to the results of the structured diagnostic interviews. The researchers found that the best way to identify depression was the single item interview, which correctly identified the eventual diagnostic outcome of every patient. Inclusion of questions concerning loss of interest or pleasure in activities did not improve diagnostic accuracy, but might be appropriate in a brief screening interview. Inclusion of those questions provides for complete coverage of core depressive symptoms, and decreases the possibility of missing the diagnosis in patients suffering from depression.

Fluctuation of the will to live

The 'will to live' of a dying patient is not a static construct, and may fluctuate according to the patient's clinical progress and subjective experience of his symptoms. One recent study of will to live among the terminally ill used a series of visual analogue scales to assess pain, anxiety, depression, wellbeing, dyspnoea, nausea, activity, drowsiness, appetite and their will to live. The study found that will to live in patients nearing death fluctuated substantially. The predictor variables of the will to live scores also fluctuated significantly over time. The main variables that were associated with fluctuation in will to live included depression, anxiety and dyspnoea, and sense of wellbeing. Initially, anxiety was the most significant predictor of fluctuation in will to live, but later depression, and finally dyspnoea were the most important determinants of the patients' endorsement of their will to live. This finding has important ramifications for the clinician. If the patient's will to live is dependent upon his symptoms, it may well be that appropriate symptom management, together with reassurance and fostering of a good patient–physician relationship, may impact significantly on a patient's will to live or corresponding desire for death.

Hopelessness as a predictor of suicidal intent

The elderly male patient described in the case presentation (Box 61.1) experienced almost daily passive suicidal ideation, which at times became active. Even while in hospital, he expressed strong suicidal ideation. However, at the same time, he was willing to contract for safety during the course of his hospital admission. He described a life that was lonely, restricted and a significant deterioration from his previous life. Yet, while the possibility of amelioration of his physical symptoms existed, there remained within him a glimmer of hope.

In a recent study of almost 200 patients with advanced terminal cancer, each patient underwent an interview to assess hopelessness and suicidal ideation, and also completed the BDI (Beck Depression Inventory)—Short Form. A correlation was found between measures of suicidal ideation and depression. However, the correlation between suicidal ideation and hopelessness was even stronger. The study hypothesis, that suicidal ideation would correlate more highly with hopelessness than with depression, was confirmed in subsequent analysis. This finding has important implications for the evaluation of suicidality in patients with advanced disease. The simple existence of a depression, either major or minor, may not be as significant as the existence of hopelessness in attempting to predict suicidal ideation and intent in severely ill patients.

This being said, depression remains an important factor in understanding and predicting a patient's desire for death. Significant numbers of terminally ill patients in palliative care facilities experience or express at least a fleeting or occasional desire to die. In most cases, these episodes are brief and do not reflect a sustained or committed desire. However, almost 10% of patients in one study reported an unequivocal desire for death to come soon, and indicated that this desire was consistent over time. A strong association was found between desire-for-death ratings and clinical depression, based on interviews from the Schedule of Affective Disorders and Schizophrenia (SADS). About 60% of patients who had a genuine desire for death met criteria for clinical depression. However, among patients who did not endorse a genuine, consistent desire for early death, the prevalence of clinical depression was about 7%. Depression was a more important factor than either pain or low family support in estimating the desire for death. It is possible that prolonged pain may increase the risk for depression, while family support may offer protection against it. However, once depression has developed, the emergence of a desire for death may be a more direct step.

Assessing suicidal intent in a palliative care setting

Evaluating suicidal ideation in a palliative care setting requires the consideration of several issues. Numerous risk factors for suicide have been identified among patients with advanced disease. These include physical problems, such as pain, delirium and fatigue; social factors, such as the extent of emotional or family support; and prior psychopathology and psychiatric history. However, depression is the one factor that has the most empirical support. Studies of oncology outpatients have found that depression, not pain, was related to hoarding drugs in preparation for a possible future suicide attempt. Indeed, the patient discussed in our case presentation (Box 61.1) clearly met the criteria for the diagnosis of major depression, and hoarded drugs in preparation for a future suicide attempt.

It is also important for the physician to consider asking the patient directly about suicidal thoughts or the desire to die. There is no empirical evidence to support the notion, held by some clinicians, that simply asking about suicidal thoughts will somehow implant the idea of committing suicide or self-harm. In fact, such inquiry will be likely to decrease the patient's sense of psychological isolation, and will demonstrate his care provider's willingness to engage in a frank discussion of even the most difficult of issues.

As noted, hopelessness is a good clinical marker for suicidal ideation. When hopelessness becomes the focus of one's psychological response to issues of death and dying then, in some cases, suicide may be seen by the patient as a rational and appropriate alternative, compared with the decline towards a natural death. Thus, the assessment of hopelessness is an important tool in understanding suicidal intent in the terminally ill. The meaning of hope, and its preservation even in the face of impending death, are important issues to be addressed in the care of the dying.

Dependency and other losses

The fear of becoming a burden on family members can be very distressing for terminally ill patients. Surveys of non-cancer patients (i.e. patients with ischaemic heart disease, strokes, respiratory diseases and Alzheimer's disease) found that the desire for earlier death, as well as requests for euthanasia, related predominantly to issues of dependency. Information regarding persons who received prescriptions for lethal medication under Oregon's *Death With Dignity Act* noted that, according to physicians and family members, patients requested PAS for several reasons, including loss of autonomy, loss of control of bodily functions, an inability to participate in enjoyable activities, and a determination to control the manner of death. Indeed, the patient referred to in the case presentation (Box 61.1) also stated a desire not to become a burden to his family as one of the reasons for his suicide attempt.

A patient's relationship with family and others close to him may become strained during the latter course of the illness. Family members must deal with their own feelings of anger, confusion, grief and hopelessness, while also trying to assist their ill loved one. The patient may sense these feelings, and become concerned that he is the unwitting cause and source of this distress. A request for euthanasia or PAS may be seen as the patient's attempt to protect his family against the despair, financial expense and any further sacrifice that continued care might inflict.

When there is concern about the burden of care, this issue should be fully discussed with the patient and his family. Additional resources, such as home health aides and visiting nurses, may be offered. Moving the patient from home to hospital and providing respite care are further possibilities. It is also appropriate to reassure family members and other caregivers that stress and disappointment are natural reactions, and that availing themselves of support may allow them to stay the course for the benefit of their dying loved one.

Loss of autonomy and loss of dignity are often cited by advocates for euthanasia and PAS as reasons for supporting these practices. Patients are required to make accommodations for the health care system, including having to relinquish their privacy, and conform to hospital routines. Loss of bodily functions, and the inability to engage in activities that were previously enjoyable can also contribute to the patient's sense of lost autonomy and diminished significance. It is important to discuss these issues with both patients and caregivers, and to anticipate the feelings of dependency and loss that may accompany terminal illness. To bolster his sense of autonomy, it is important to identify and support those facets of care, decision making and personal routine that are still within the patient's grasp.

Isolation and abandonment

Seriously ill patients have a tremendous fear of being abandoned, left to face their illness alone. Feelings of isolation and abandonment may lead to the development of hopelessness, which can be a harbinger of suicidal intent. Caring for those who are dying can be taxing for family members and health care providers alike. A terminal course can be accompanied by many advances and setbacks. Both family members and health care providers may feel anticipatory grief, apprehension and guilt brought on by a belief that 'something more could have been done'. Response to these feelings may lead to a premature withdrawal from the patient, causing him to experience additional suffering and despair. The physician must make a commitment to the patient and his family to provide continuous, ongoing care. Unwavering commitment to continuing care is a vital foundation of comprehensive end-of-life care. Support of this kind ensures that the patient will be provided with any necessary comfort measures, offers him an opportunity to express his feelings and emotions, and tangibly demonstrates that his life continues to be valuable and thus worthy of receiving care.

Existential suffering

Patients may feel that due to the illness, their lives are rendered without meaning. In this context, a request for euthanasia or PAS may reflect a deeper question or anxiety, namely 'Does my life still have value?'. An agreement by a physician, nurse or other party to provide euthanasia or PAS may validate the patient's fear that his life is meaningless. The patient may then question whether to continue treatment as opposed to seeking a hastened death option. To relieve existential suffering, it is important to explore the patient's sense of meaning or purpose in life. Cognitive therapies may help some patients strengthen their coping abilities, while cognitive restructuring can help others to approach potentially stressful events with the belief that they are able to endure. For example, patients who fear loss of control and dependency might learn to appreciate that by receiving help, they are allowing others to express feelings of love for them. It is important to encourage patients to identify realistic short-term objectives. These might include goals of increasing mobility, or resuming some responsibility for personal care needs, or resolving a family issue or conflict. Engaging in life review, completing important life projects, or simply taking the time to say or document particularly cherished words or feelings, may enhance the patient's sense of meaning and purpose, even as his life approaches its end.

Summary

Right to die versus the right to quality palliative care

We have already discussed the issue of appropriate comprehensive terminal care as a means of alleviating a desire for death in a seriously ill patient. The goal for health care providers faced with death-hastening requests is to identify, understand and, when possible, treat the root cause of the request. Care is based on two principles: the patient should be free of unwanted intervention, and the physician is obligated to provide a suffering patient with comfort care. It has been argued that care based on these principles does not include PAS, because this practice is not justified by the principle of non-intrusion, or by the obligation to relieve suffering. Patients may refuse oral intake in specific situations, especially when they have lost hunger and thirst as a result of their advancing illness. According to some commentators, the right to refuse oral intake should only be available for persons with a non-curable illness, and a life expectancy of 6 months or less.

Perhaps the most critical task facing health care providers attending to patients making a death-hastening request is that of establishing a good physician–patient relationship. This allows the patient to openly express his concerns and anxieties. A patient needs to have confidence in his caregivers, and he needs to feel he will not be abandoned as his disease progresses. It is also important to fully explore end-of-life issues with the patient early in treatment. This should include discussions with the patient about what he can expect as the disease progresses, and options for his care and treatment such as hospitalisation or hospice care. If euthanasia or PAS is requested, it is important to do a comprehensive evaluation, including screening for depression, hopelessness, and suicidal ideation and generalised symptom distress. Obtaining a consultation from palliative care or psychiatry is advisable. Finally, the primary care physician must identify and (where possible) treat the underlying causes of the desire to die.

Underlying or reversible causes of the desire to die

Organic mental disorders

Organic mental disorders are highly prevalent in those with advanced disease. The presence of these syndromes in a patient who is requesting death via assisted suicide or euthanasia calls into question the patient's capacity to make such a request. The most common organic mental syndromes in patients with advanced disease include delirium, dementia, and organic mood and anxiety disorders. However, the diagnosis of an organic mental syndrome may be overlooked because symptoms of dementia are often mistaken for a functional psychiatric disturbance. Feelings of disbelief, denial, numbness, irritability, hopelessness and suicidal ideation may occur in patients who are reacting to the diagnosis of a terminal illness. These symptoms are also common in major depression, anxiety disorders and adjustment disorders (Chapter 10). However, as dementia progresses, the organic nature of psychiatric symptoms becomes more obvious. Formal neuropsychological testing may be helpful in documenting and distinguishing dementia from a depression or adjustment disorder.

An organic mental syndrome interferes with the assessment of a desire for death in patients with terminal illness. It may be difficult to assess whether the mental syndrome is transient or static, whether it affects competence, and whether the wishes expressed by the patient are similar to those that were held prior to the development of the cognitive problem. Collateral from family and friends can be of importance in helping to determine these issues. It is incumbent upon a physician, when faced with a request for euthanasia or PAS, to do a thorough assessment, specifically looking for the presence of dementia or delirium (Chapter 10 and Chapters 15, 16 and 17). When one considers that approximately 25% of hospitalised medical and surgical patients suffer from dementia, and that the prevalence of delirium in dying patients approaches 80%, it is easy to appreciate the significance of this problem.

Depression

See also Chapter 10.

We have already examined the association between depression and terminal illness, and the extent to which it can predict suicidal ideation. Brief screening measures for the assessment of depression have already been discussed. It is important to recognise that a patient who is requesting assistance for a hastened death may be suffering from depression. In these instances, clinical evaluation is of obvious importance. A survey of Oregon psychiatrists, prior to the passage of the *Death With*

Dignity Act, found that only 6% of respondents believed that a single evaluation would be adequate for assessing whether a psychiatric disorder was impairing a patient's judgment. Interestingly, those who felt that such an evaluation could be accomplished in a single session were far more likely to be supportive of the Act itself. However, only 3% of respondents believed that a request for PAS was prima facie evidence of a mental disorder.

The message for the clinician is clear: if there is any concern as to whether the patient is suffering from a clinical depression, a psychiatric consultation should be initiated. Research has shown that treatment of a diagnosed clinical depression can relieve or reverse the desire for death. It is thus incumbent upon the physician to make sure that appropriate measures have been taken to rule out the presence of a clinical depression.

Effective relief of physical suffering

We have already discussed that appropriate comprehensive terminal care may alleviate or reverse a desire for death. The physician must consider whether she is adequately attending to pain relief for the patient, and whether a referral to either a pain specialist or a hospice setting is warranted. Consultation with colleagues who are skilled in comprehensive symptom management is recommended when treating a terminally ill patient who is expressing a desire to die (addressing the spiritual concerns and needs of these patients is also clearly important, and lies beyond the scope of this review). Pain may not be the only symptom that is causing distress; in our case presentation (Box 61.1), chronic abdominal discomfort, combined with a loss of the ability to engage in everyday activities, were important contributing factors to the patient's wish for death.

The physician's own feelings

The physician must recognise that his own feelings play an important role in responding to a patient with a terminal illness who voices a desire to die. Physicians are often uncomfortable with the notion of death, and see it as a personal defeat or failure. This can in turn alter one's clinical decisions and affect the relationship with patients who are obviously close to death.

There are at least two possibilities that may confound the treatment of a patient with a terminal illness. Firstly, the physician may aggressively attempt to stave off an outcome that cannot be prevented. Such a stance, and the physician's own discomfort with the patient's condition, will have an adverse effect on the patient–physician relationship. While it is important to aggressively treat pain and relieve other physical and psychological symptoms, it is also important to consult the patient's own feelings with respect to any life-prolonging measures, and the manner in which the patient wishes to live out his final days.

Conversely, some physicians may withdraw from the patient who is nearing the end of his life, because of feelings of inadequacy or personal discomfort. Because death cannot be prevented, the physician may well feel a sense of failure, and unconsciously avoid dealing with the patient's need for an open and honest discussion of the feasible treatment alternatives, including the full spectrum of palliative care alternatives. Failure to engage and accompany the patient through these difficult discussions can further contribute to his sense of isolation and feelings of abandonment. It is important to be aware of the conflicting feelings and impulses—both conscious and unconscious—that can arise in the course of treating a patient whose death is imminent. Physicians who acknowledge these feelings and pay close attention to their potential effect on the physician–patient relationship will be better able to significantly ease the patient's suffering through his final stage of life.

Bibliography and further reading

Alvin, S. A. D., et al. (2000), 'Legalized physician-assisted suicide in Oregon — The second year', *New England Journal of Medicine*, 342, pp. 598–604.

Breitbart, W. (1987), 'Suicide in cancer patients', *Oncology*, 1, pp. 49–53.

Breitbart, W., et al. (1994), 'Undertreatment of pain in AIDS', American Pain Society, 13th Annual Meeting, 1–13 November, Miami, FL, Abstract.

Breitbart, W., et al. (1996), 'Interest in physician-assisted suicide among ambulatory HIV infected patients', *American Journal of Psychiatry*, 153, pp. 238–42.

Chochinov, H. M., et al. (1997), '"Are you depressed?": screening for depression in the terminally ill', *American Journal of Psychiatry*, 154, pp. 674–6.

Chochinov, H. M., et al. (1998), 'Depression, hopelessness, and suicidal ideation in the terminally ill', *Psychomatics*, 39, pp. 366–70.

Chochinov, H. M., et al. (1999), 'Will to live in the terminally ill', *Lancet*, 354, pp. 816–19.

Chochinov, H. M., Wilson, K. G., et al. (1995), 'Desire for death in the terminally ill', *American Journal of Psychiatry*, 152, pp. 1185–91.

Derogatis, L. R., et al. (1983), 'The prevalence of psychiatric disorders among cancer patients', *Journal of the American Medical Association*, 249, pp. 751–7.

Emanuel, L. L. (1998), 'Facing requests for physician-assisted suicide: toward a practical and principled clinical skill set', *Journal of the American Medical Association*, 280, pp. 643–7.

Foley, K. M. (1985), 'The treatment of cancer pain', *New England Journal of Medicine*, 313, pp. 84–9.

Ganzini L., et al. (1996), 'Attitudes of Oregon psychiatrists towards physician-assisted suicide', *American Journal of Psychiatry*, 153, pp. 1469–75.

Ganzini, L., et al. (1998), 'Attitudes of patients with ALS and their care givers towards assisted suicide', *New England Journal of Medicine*, 339, pp. 963–73.

Ganzini, L., et al. (2000), 'Physicians' experiences with the Oregon *Death with Dignity Act*', *New England Journal of Medicine*, 342, pp. 557–63.

Ganzini, L., Lee, M. A., Heintz, R. T., et al. (1994), 'The effects of depression treatment on elderly patients' preferences for life-sustaining medical therapy', *American Journal of Psychiatry*, 151, pp. 1631–6.

Grond, S., Zech, V., Schug, S. A., et al. (1991), 'Validation of World Health Organization's guidelines for cancer pain relief during the last days of life', *Journal of Pain and Symptom Management*, 6, pp. 411–42.

Helig, S. (1988), 'The San Francisco Medical Society Euthanasia Survey: results and analysis', *San Francisco Medicine*, 61, pp. 24–34.

Kinsella, T. D. & Verhoef, M. J. (1993), 'Alberta Euthanasia Survey: 1. Physicians' opinions about the morality and legalization of Act Euthanasia', *Canadian Medical Journal*, 148, pp. 1921–6.

Latimer, E. J. & McGregor, J. (1994), 'Euthanasia, physician-assisted suicide and the ethical care of dying patients', *Canadian Medical Journal*, 151, p. 1134.

Marks, R. M. & Sacher, E. S. (1973), 'Undertreatment of inpatients with analgesics', *Annals of Internal Medicine*, 78, pp. 173–81.

McDonald, M. V., Passik, S. D. & Coyle, N. (2000), 'Addressing the needs of the patient who requests physician-assisted suicide or euthanasia', in Chochinov, H. M. & Breitbart, W. (eds), *Handbook of Psychiatry in Palliative Medicine*, Oxford University Press, New York.

Meier, D. E., et al. (1998), 'A national survey of physician-assisted suicide and euthanasia in the U.S.', *The New England Journal of Medicine*, 338, pp. 1193–206.

Oregon *Death With Dignity Act*, Oregon Revised Statutes, 127.800–127.995.

Pellegrino, E. D. (1991), 'Ethics', *Journal of the American Medical Association*, 265, pp. 3118–19.

Pijenborg, L., et al. (1993), 'Life-terminating acts without explicit request of patient', *Lancet*, 341, pp. 1196–9.

Van der Maas, P. J., et al. (1991), 'Euthanasia and other medical decisions concerning the end of life', *Lancet*, 338, pp. 669–74.

Index

Page numbers in **bold** print refer to main entries. Page numbers in *italics* refer to tables, figures and boxes

T

V